# Skin Immune System

## Cutaneous Immunology and Clinical Immunodermatology

*Third Edition*

**Edited by**

**Jan D. Bos**

University of Amsterdam
Academic Medical Center
Amsterdam, Netherlands

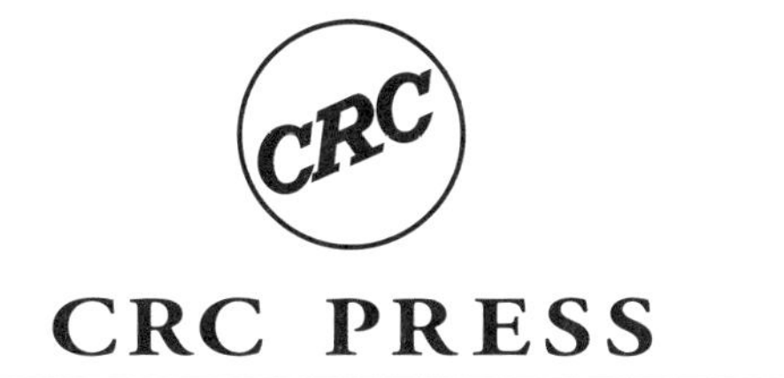


CRC PRESS

Boca Raton London New York Washington, D.C.

**Library of Congress Cataloging-in-Publication Data**

Skin immune system (SIS) : cutaneous immunology and clinical immunodermatology / editor, Jan D. Bos. — 3rd ed.

p. ; cm.

Includes bibliographical references and index.

ISBN 0-8493-1959-5 (alk. paper)

1. Skin—Diseases—Immunological aspects. 2. Skin—Immunology.

[DNLM: 1. Skin Diseases—immunology. 2. Skin—immunology. 3. Skin—physiopathology. 4. Skin Diseases—physiopathology. WR 140 S62785 2004] I. Box, Jan D. II. Title.

RL97 .S65 2004

616.5'079—dc22 2004051938



Direct all inquiries to CRC Press LLC, 2000 N.W. Corporate Blvd., Boca Raton, Florida 33431.



**Visit the CRC Press Web site at www.crcpress.com**



International Standard Book Number 0-8493-1959-5

Library of Congress Card Number 2004051938

Printed in the United States of America 1 2 3 4 5 6 7 8 9 0

Printed on acid-free paper

# Preface to the Third Edition

Since the publication of the first (1990) and second (1997) editions of *Skin Immune System*, significant new knowledge has become available in almost all fields of cutaneous immunology and clinical immunodermatology. Therefore, all authors of the second edition were asked to update their chapters and I am grateful that most accepted the invitation. In addition, and reflecting the progress in this discipline, there are a number of entirely new chapters.

In this third edition, the subdivision into six sections or parts has been maintained. The book starts with Part I (Introduction), with chapters on the definition of the "Skin Immune System (SIS)," a short "History of Immunodermatology," and "Comparative Immunology of the Integument" with fascinating data from cutaneous immunology in other species. Part I now has a new chapter entitled "Immunogenetics of Inflammatory Skin Disease," which reflects the recent and tremendous progress in the area of human genomics. In Part II, the cellular elements of SIS are covered in individual chapters. New cells have not been discovered, so there are no new chapters in this section, but newly defined functional subclasses of cells are included. In Part III, the humoral elements of SIS are described. Captivating recent developments in the area of humoral immunology are represented in two new chapters, "Defensins and Cathelicidins" and "Chemokines of Human Skin."

Part IV contains various concepts of how these cellular and humoral elements of SIS interact under different circumstances. New here is a chapter entitled "Signal Transduction Pathways in Cutaneous Immunology." In Part V, dermatological diseases with a significant immunological background are covered in individual chapters. The selection is a personal one. A new chapter entitled "Immunology of Cutaneous Drug Eruptions" is included, on one of the most difficult and clinically relevant immunodermatological issues. Finally, in Part VI, immunotherapy in dermatology is the theme, with a new chapter reflecting the recent wave of products from biotechnology, "Biologicals for the Treatment of Immune Mediated Skin Diseases."

In this Internet age, one might wonder whether there is a need for a complex book such as this. It is my view that the Internet makes it easy to find specific bits and bytes of information. But this book contains the result of reading all that information by individual experts and teams, who have personally processed it, enabling them to put all the knowledge into perspective. Without a vision, there is no progress in our understanding, as imagination is essential for finding new ways in science, also thus in cutaneous immunology and clinical immunodermatology.

I am indebted to all authors for their efforts; they have made it possible to come with this update. The editorial staff of CRC Press, especially Erika Dery, Stephen Zollo, and Barbara Norwitz are acknowledged for their help in the production process. My gratitude extends to the staff and secretariat of the Department of Dermatology, Academic Medical Center, University of Amsterdam, who together form the stimulating environment I work in. I wish to mention the names of Marja Veltkamp, Mariska Schaap, and Robert Rodenburg, who were always ready to help me with logistical matters in the challenging process of editing this book now in your hands.

**Jan D. Bos**

# The Editor

**Jan D. Bos, M.D., Ph.D., F.R.C.P.,** has been Professor and Chairman of the Department of Dermatology, Academic Medical Center, University of Amsterdam, since 1990. He is a member of several medical societies, including the Netherlands Association of Dermatology and Venereology, the European Academy of Dermatology and Venereology, the European Immunodermatology Society (which he founded), and the European Society for Dermatological Research.

Professor Bos has been the recipient of numerous awards and honors. To name a few, he is a fellow of two Royal Colleges of Physicians (Edinburgh, London), is an honorary member of the Polish, Hungarian, and German Dermatological Societies, and has been awarded with the degree of doctor honoris causa by the University of Szeged, Hungary. Among his other responsibilities, Professor Bos serves on the editorial board of several journals, including the *Archives of Dermatological Research, Experimental Dermatology,* and *Skin Therapy Letter.* Principal areas of his research include the definition and immunology of atopic dermatitis, immunopathogenesis of psoriasis, human photoimmunology, and developments in immunotherapy.

Over the years, he has authored or co-authored more than 300 original articles and book chapters and has spoken at numerous international conferences, many of which were co-organized by him.

# Contributors

**Cristina Albanesi**
Laboratory of Immunology
Istituto Dermopatico dell'Immacolata
Rome, Italy

**Syed Shafi Asghar**
Department of Dermatology
Academic Medical Center
University of Amsterdam
Amsterdam, The Netherlands

**James N. Baraniuk**
Division of Rheumatology, Immunology, and Allergy
Georgetown University
Washington, D.C., U.S.A.

**Jonathan N.W.N. Barker**
St John's Institute of Dermatology
St Thomas Hospital
London, United Kingdom

**Stephan Beissert**
Department of Dermatology
University of Münster
Münster, Germany

**Frédéric Berard**
Clinical Immunology and Allergy Unit
Centre Hospitalier Lyon Sud
Lyon, France

**Jan D. Bos**
Department of Dermatology
Academic Medical Center
University of Amsterdam
Amsterdam, The Netherlands

**Anne C. Bowcock**
Department of Genetics, Pediatrics and Medicine
Washington University School of Medicine
St. Louis, Missouri, U.S.A.

**Raúl M. Cabrera**
Department of Dermatology
Clinica Alemana de Santiago
Universidad del Desarrollo
Santiago, Chile

**Emanuela Camera**
San Gallicano Dermatological Institute
Rome, Italy

**Andrés Castell**
Departemento de Biología Celular y Tisular
Facultad de Medicina
Universidad Nacional Autónoma de México
México, D.F., México

**Andrea Cavani**
Laboratory of Immunology
Istituto Dermopatico dell'Immacolata
Rome, Italy

**George W. Cherry**
Department of Dermatology
Oxford Wound Healing Institute
The Churchill
Oxford, United Kingdom

**Anthony C. Chu**
Unit of Dermatology
Imperial College of Science, Technology and Medicine
Hammersmith Hospital
London, United Kingdom

**William O.C.M. Cookson**
Wellcome Trust Centre for Human Genetics
University of Oxford
Oxford, United Kingdom

**Edwin L. Cooper**
Department of Neurobiology
Laboratory of Comparative Immunology
UCLA Medical Center
Los Angeles, California, U.S.A.

**Kevin D. Cooper**
Department of Dermatology
Case Western Reserve University
University Hospitals of Cleveland
Cleveland, Ohio, U.S.A.

**Guiseppe De Panfilis**
Department of Dermatology
University of Parma
Parma, Italy

**Maria Lucia Dell'Anna**
San Gallicano Dermatological Institute
Rome, Italy

**Sergio Di Nuzzo**
Department of Dermatology
University of Parma
Parma, Italy

**Bertrand Dubois**
Bioscience Lyon-Gerland
Lyon, France

**Stefan Eichmüller**
Skin Cancer Unit
German Cancer Research Center (DKFZ)
Mannheim, Germany

**Lionel Fry**
Consultant Dermatology
Harley Street
London, United Kingdom

**Anita C. Gilliam**
Department of Dermatology
Case Western Reserve University
University Hospitals of Cleveland
Cleveland, Ohio, U.S.A.

**Giampiero Girolomoni**
Laboratory of Immunology
Istituto Dermopatico dell'Immacolata
Rome, Italy

**Sergio B. González**
Department of Dermatopathology
Pontificia Universidad Catolica de Chile
Santiago, Chile

**Kenneth B. Gordon**
Department of Pathology
Loyola University of Chicago
Medical Center
Maywood, Illinois, U.S.A.

**Richard D. Granstein**
Department of Dermatology
Joan and Sanford I. Weill Medical College
Cornell University
New York, New York, U.S.A.

**Rubén T. Guarda**
Department of Dermatology
Clinica Alemana de Santiago
Universidad del Desarrollo
Santiago, Chile

**Ewa Guigné**
Service de Dermatologie
Hôpital Henri Mondor
Créteil, France

**Norbert Haas**
Department of Dermatology
University Hospital Charité
University Medicine of Berlin
Berlin, Germany

**Gary M. Halliday**
Department of Dermatology
University of Sydney
Royal Prince Alfred Hospital
Sydney, Australia

**John I. Harper**
Great Ormond Street Hospital and the Institute for Child Health
London, United Kingdom

**Roderick J. Hay**
Faculty of Medicine and Health Sciences
Queens University Belfast
Belfast, Northern Ireland, United Kingdom

**Maurice W. van der Heijden**
Department of Pharmacology and Pathophysiology
Utrecht Institute for Pharmaceutical Sciences
Utrecht University
Utrecht, The Netherlands

**Beate M. Henz**
Department of Dermatology
University Hospital Charité
University Medicine of Berlin
Berlin, Germany

**Rick Hoekzema**
Department of Dermatology
Academic Medical Center
University of Amsterdam
Amsterdam, The Netherlands

**Lars Iversen**
Department of Dermatology
University of Aarhus
Aarhus, Denmark

**Barbara A. Jakobczak**
Department of Chemistry
University of Michigan
Ann Arbor, Michigan, U.S.A.

**Dominique Kaiserlian**
Bioscience Lyon-Gerland
Lyon, France

**Kefei Kang**
Department of Dermatology
Case Western Reserve University
University Hospitals of Cleveland
Cleveland, Ohio, U.S.A.

**Kevin O. Kisich**
Department of Pediatrics
The National Jewish Medical and Research Center
Denver, Colorado, U.S.A.

**Hanneke P.M. van der Kleij**
Department of Pharmacology and Pathophysiology
Utrecht Institute for Pharmaceutical Sciences
Utrecht University
Utrecht, The Netherlands

**Edward F. Knol**
Department of Dermatology and Allergy
University Medical Center
Utrecht, The Netherlands

**Sreedevi Kodali**
Department of Dermatology
Joan and Sanford I. Weill Medical College
Cornell University
New York, New York, U.S.A.

**Gerhard Kolde**
Department of Dermatology and Allergy
Charité University of Medicine
Berlin, Germany

**Knud Kragballe**
Department of Dermatology
Marselisborg Hospital
University of Aarhus
Aarhus, Denmark

**Maya Krasteva**
Clinical Immunology and Allergy Unit
Centre Hospitalier Lyon Sud
Lyon, France

**Taco W. Kuijpers**
Emma Children's Hospital
Academic Medical Center
University of Amsterdam
Amsterdam, The Netherlands

**Donald Y.M. Leung**
Department of Pediatrics
The National Jewish Medical and Research Center
Denver, Colorado, U.S.A.

**Kurt Q. Lu**
Department of Dermatology
Case Western Reserve University
University Hospitals of Cleveland
Cleveland, Ohio, U.S.A.

**Thomas A. Luger**
Department of Dermatology
Ludwig Boltzmann Institute of Cell Biology and Immunobiology of the Skin
University of Münster
Münster, Germany

**Thomas S. McCormick**
Department of Dermatology
Case Western Reserve University
University Hospitals of Cleveland
Cleveland, Ohio, U.S.A.

**Miriam F. Moffatt**
Wellcome Trust Centre for Human Genetics
University of Oxford
Oxford, United Kingdom

**Jenny F. Morris**
Unit of Dermatology
Imperial College of Science, Technology and Medicine
Hammersmith Hospital
London, United Kingdom

**H. Konrad Muller**
Discipline of Pathology
University of Tasmania
Hobart, Tasmania, Australia

**Brian J. Nickoloff**
Department of Pathology
Loyola University of Chicago
Medical Center
Maywood, Illinois, U.S.A.

**Jean-François Nicolas**
Clinical Immunology and Allergy Unit
Centre Hospitalier Lyon Sud
Lyon, France

**Mary Norval**
Department of Medical Microbiology
University of Edinburgh Medical School
Edinburgh, Scotland
United Kingdom

**Graham S. Ogg**
Weatherall Institute of Molecular Medicine
Oxford, United Kingdom

**Francis E. Palisson**
Department of Dermatology
Clínica Alemana de Santiago
Universidad del Desarrollo
Santiago, Chile

**Marcel Christian Pasch**
Department of Dermatology
University Medical Center, University of Nijmegen
Nijmegen, The Netherlands

**Annette Paschen**
Skin Cancer Unit
German Cancer Research Center (DKFZ)
Mannheim, Germany

**Saveria Pastore**
Laboratory of Immunology
Istituto Dermopatico dell'Immacolata
Rome, Italy

**Krystyna A. Pasyk**
Institute of Gerontology
University of Michigan
Ann Arbor, Michigan, U.S.A.

**Armando Pérez**
Departemento de Biología Celular y Tisular
Facultad de Medicina
Universidad Nacional Autónoma de México
México, D.F., México

**Mauro Picardo**
San Gallicano Dermatological Institute
Rome, Italy

**Jörg Christoph Prinz**
Department of Dermatology and Allergy
Ludwig Maximilian University
Munich, Germany

**Frank A. Redegeld**
Department of Pharmacology and Pathophysiology
Utrecht Institute for Pharmaceutical Sciences
Utrecht University
Utrecht, The Netherlands

**Jean Revuz**
Service de Dermatologie
Hôpital Henri Mondor
Créteil, France

**Menno A. de Rie**
Department of Dermatology
Academic Medical Center
University of Amsterdam
Amsterdam, The Netherlands

**Martin Röcken**
Department of Dermatology
Eberhard Karls University
Tübingen, Germany

**Dirk Roos**
Sanquin Research at CLB Landsteiner Laboratory
Academic Medical Center
University of Amsterdam
Amsterdam, The Netherlands

**Jean-Claude Roujeau**
Service de Dermatologie
Hôpital Henri Mondor
Créteil, France

**Pierre Saint-Mezard**
Clinical Immunology and Allergy Unit
Centre Hospitalier Lyon Sud
Lyon, France

**Dirk Schadendorf**
Skin Cancer Unit
German Cancer Research Center (DKFZ)
Mannheim, Germany

**J. Henk Sillevis Smitt**
Department of Dermatology
Academic Medical Center
University of Amsterdam
Amsterdam, The Netherlands

**Martin Steinhoff**
Department of Dermatology
Ludwig Boltzmann Institute of Cell Biology and Immunobiology of the Skin
University of Münster
Münster, Germany

**Cord Sunderkötter**
Department of Dermatology and Allergology
University of Ulm
Ulm, Germany

**Bhupendra Tank**
Department of Dermatology
Erasmus University Medical Center
Rotterdam, The Netherlands

**Marcel B.M. Teunissen**
Department of Dermatology
Academic Medical Center
University of Amsterdam
Amsterdam, The Netherlands

**Kristian Thestrup-Pedersen**
University of Aarhus
Aarhus, Denmark
and King Faisal Specialist Hospital and Research Centre
Riyadh, Saudi Arabia

**Krisztina Klára Timár**
Academic Medical Center
University of Amsterdam
Amsterdam, The Netherlands

**Henry J.C. de Vries**
Department of Dermatology
Academic Medical Center
University of Amsterdam
Amsterdam, The Netherlands

**Sarah Wakelin**
Dermatology Department
The Oxford Radcliffe Hospital
The Churchill
Oxford, United Kingdom

**Rein Willemze**
Department of Dermatology
Leiden University Medical Center
Leiden, The Netherlands

**Samantha Winsey**
Dermatology Department
The Oxford Radcliffe Hospital
The Churchill
Oxford, United Kingdom

**Fenella Wojnarowska**
Dermatology Department
The Oxford Radcliffe Hospital
The Churchill
Oxford, United Kingdom

**Gregory M. Woods**
Discipline of Pathology
University of Tasmania
Hobart, Tasmania, Australia

**Torsten Zuberbier**
Department of Dermatology and Allergy
Charité Universitätsdiedizin Berlin
Berlin, Germany

# Contents

## PART I Introduction



## PART II Cellular Constituents of the Skin Immune System

## *PART III Humoral Constituents of the Skin Immune System*



## *PART IV Response Patterns of the Skin Immune System*

## *PART V Immunodermatological Diseases*

## *PART VI Immunotherapy in Dermatology*

# *Part I*

## *Introduction*

# 1 Skin Immune System (SIS)

*Jan D. Bos*

## CONTENTS



## I. THE SKIN AS AN ORGAN OF DEFENSE

The skin is the largest organ of the human body and its principal physical function is that of a barrier. This principal function is most prominent in the skin's relative impermeability for water and water-soluble compounds as well as in its structural integrity despite frequent mechanical trauma. Its surface is relatively hostile to potentially pathogenic microorganisms. Its optic properties make it relatively insensitive to the potential damage of sun exposure.

Its resistance to exogenous harmful influences is mainly due to the physicochemical properties of its outermost layer, the corneal layer of the epidermis (stratum corneum). In addition to its function as a barrier against potentially harmful exogenous effects, the skin also serves in maintaining the homeostasis of the *milieu intérieure* by preventing desiccation. Its physical strength depends largely on the vivid and dynamic connective tissue called the dermis, which is mainly composed of highly intertwining collagen and elastin fibers.

The prevention of undesirable water vapor loss and the formation of a true obstacle to the penetration of exogenous water and soluble compounds are indeed localized in superficial extremity. This barrier function is ascribed to the production of ceramide-containing sphingolipid sheets that are continuously packed between the corneocytes of the stratum corneum during keratinization of the epidermis. It is assumed that compounds larger than 500 Da cannot easily penetrate normal stratum corneum. In addition, the lower the lipophilicity, the more difficult it will be for a compound to enter the human skin.

Sunlight, especially its shortwave ultraviolet (UV) part, induces the formation of damaging free radicals, but a variety of defense mechanisms have evolved including free radical–trapping molecules, thiols, melanin, and enzyme systems that can almost perfectly absorb and eliminate these DNA-damaging, potentially carcinogenous elements.

Major physiological functions include maintenance of body temperature, regulation of stable circulation, production of endocrine mediators, and the bearing of peripheral neural receptors and nerve endings. The skin thus serves as the central nervous system's largest outpost and is a major sensory organ. Psychological and social functions are so evident that they do not need, in the context of this introduction, further explanation.

0-8493-1959-5/05/$0.00+$1.50

In addition, and perhaps most importantly, the skin has a complicated defense function, which is best denominated as "immunological." Its capacity to discern self from nonself is indeed challenging to the imagination when one considers the rich variety of exogenous substances to which it is continuously exposed.

The immunological function of the integument, related to both physiology and pathology, is the subject of the present volume. The intimate relationship during evolution between the general defense function and the more specifically acting immune system of the integument is almost unknown territory. A primer of this important aspect of immunodermatology is given in the introductory chapter, which describes comparative immunology of the skin by Cooper et al. (Chapter 3).

## II. CONCEPTS OF THE SKIN AS AN IMMUNOLOGICAL ORGAN

Although some of the history of immunodermatology is covered in Chapter 2, the development of concepts of the skin as an organ of immunity needs special consideration. According to Silverstein (1989), Alexandre Besredka was perhaps the first to realize the existence of organ-specific immunity, early in this century. While working in the Institut Pasteur with the cellular immunologist Ilya Metchnikoff, Besredka wrote at least two books on the subject, but the skin apparently escaped to his attention.

In 1970, Fichtelius and co-workers published a classic article in which they suggested that the skin is to be considered as a *first-level lymphoid organ*, comparable to the primary lymphoid tissue thymus. They referred to lymphoepithelial microorgans in the skin of newborns and human fetuses, which were detected at orifices of the body such as under the nails, in the preputial fornix, in the fornix vaginae, at the conjunctival fold, around the glandular tissue of the external ear canal, around the pilosebaceous units of the lower ear lobes as well as scrotal skin, and around the primitive mammary gland tissue. These collections of lymphocytes were suggested to reflect educational lymphoid environments in which systemic immunity to exogenous agents was formed and in which cells were educated to discern self from nonself antigens. Their localization near the openings of the body suggests that these sites are particularly vulnerable. Development of specific immunity at these sites might need less time when compared to other localizations within the skin.

In adults, these lymphoid accumulations may recur and are then diagnosed as benign lymphoproliferative skin tumors (lymphadenosis cutis benigna). For dermatologists, this still forms a most attractive hypothesis as to the origin of certain benign cutaneous lymphomas. The concept of the skin as a first-level lymphoid organ, however, has yet to be further substantiated.

Can the skin then be a *second-level lymphoid organ*? It has been suggested that in the classical type IV hapten-induced hypersensitivity reaction, sensitization may take place entirely within the skin, without the need for the involvement of regional skin draining lymph nodes. However, such a phenomenon of "peripheral" sensitization has yet to be definitively proved to be a common event *in vivo*. Confirmation of this concept would categorize the skin as a secondary lymphoid organ such as lymph node tissue and spleen.

At the present time, there is no definite evidence for the skin to be either a primary or secondary lymphoid organ. The observations by Fichtelius and his co-workers do not exclude a primary lymphoid role during embryogenesis or later in fetal life.

If, then, the integument is not part of the central organs of the immune system, many features of it have led to the development of concepts that try to give the skin its deserved and distinct place in immunology. A variety of models have been proposed to catch that special place. These are, in order of their appearance in the literature: SALT, SIS, DMU, and DIS. In the remaining part of this chapter, these concepts are discussed. Streilein, in 1978, coined the term *skin associated lymphoid tissues* (SALT) to include keratinocytes, the intraepidermal Langerhans cells (LCs) as antigen-presenting cells (APCs), the skin-seeking T lymphocytes suspected to exist since the first observations on cutaneous T-cell malignancies, the endothelial cells of the skin directing these skin-

**TABLE 1.1**
**Normal Human Skin: Overview of Cell Types Present and Differentiation between Immune Response–Associated and Not Immune Response–Associated Cells**

| Immune Response Associated | Not Immune Response Associated |
|---|---|
| Keratinocytes | Merkel cells |
| Immature dendritic cells (LCs) | Melanocytes |
| T lymphocytes | Fibroblasts/fibrocytes/myofibroblasts |
| Vascular/lymphatic endothelial cells | Pericytes |
| Granulocytes | Eccrine glandular cells |
| Tissue macrophages | Apocrine glandular cells |
| Monocytes | Sebocytes |
| Mature tissue dendritic cells | Schwann cells |
| Mast cells | Smooth muscle cells |

seeking cells into the dermis, and the skin-draining lymph nodes, as the specific localization of induction of immunity by antigens that have been processed and transported by LCs. Later, Streilein extended his concept of SALT by defining two subsystems entitled endoSALT and exoSALT (1990). In this subdivision, dendritic epidermal T-cell receptor (TCR) γ-expressing T cells are crucial. These dendritic TCR γ cells are very common in the epidermis of mice and might serve a function in primary immune defense. However, their human equivalent does not seem to exist, indicating that such a subdivision is less attractive for the envisioning of the role of human skin in immunological defense.

In 1986, we proposed *skin immune system* (SIS) as the denomination of the complexity of immune response–associated cells present in normal human skin. By making a qualitative inventory of cell types present in normal human skin, it became evident that approximately half of them have immune functions and thus are part of the immune system (Table 1.1). Such a simple observation underlines the importance of the role of the integument in immunology. The concept of SIS was later strengthened by adding its humoral constituents. Table 1.2 summarizes both the cellular and humoral constituents of SIS as we at present know them.

Since the introduction of the SALT concept, several authors have entirely focused on the epidermis and suggested it to be an immunological organ with its combination of keratinocytes, dendritic cells, and T lymphocytes. Obviously, concepts focusing solely on the epidermis are incomplete as they exclude the major site of immunological action in skin. The preferential

**TABLE 1.2**
**Cellular and Humoral Constituents of the Skin Immune System**

| Cellular Constituents | Humoral Constituents |
|---|---|
| Keratinocytes | Defensins, cathelicidins |
| Immature dendritic cells (LCs) | Complement and complement regulatory proteins |
| Mature tissue dendritic cells | Mannose binding lectins |
| Monocytes/macrophages | Immunoglobulins |
| Granulocytes | Cytokines, chemokines |
| Mast cells | Neuropeptides |
| Vascular/lymphatic endothelial cells | Eicosanoids and prostaglandins |
| T lymphocytes | Free radicals |

**TABLE 1.3**
**A Comparison of the Proposed Constituents of the Skin-Associated Lymphoid Tissues (SALT), the Dermal Microvascular Unit (DMU), the Dermal Immune System (DIS), and Skin Immune System (SIS)**

| | SALT | DMU | DIS | SIS |
|---|---|---|---|---|
| Keratinocytes | + | – | – | + |
| Langerhans cells | + | – | – | + |
| Epidermal T lymphocytes | + | – | – | + |
| Dermal T lymphocytes | – | + | + | + |
| Mast cells | – | + | + | + |
| Vascular endothelial cells | + | + | + | + |
| Lymphatic endothelial cells | + | – | – | + |
| Tissue dendritic cells | – | + | + | + |
| Monocytes/macrophages | – | + | + | + |
| Fibroblasts | – | – | + | – |
| Granulocytes | – | – | – | + |
| Free radicals | – | – | – | + |
| Secretory immunoglobulins | – | – | – | + |
| Complement factors | – | – | – | + |
| Eicosanoids | – | – | – | + |
| Cytokine network | – | – | + | + |
| Coagulation/fibrinolysis system | – | – | – | + |
| Neuropeptides | – | – | + | + |
| Skin draining lymph nodes | + | – | – | – |

*Source:* Modified from Bos, J.D. The skin immune system: lupus erythematosus as a paradigm, *Arch. Dermatol. Res.*, 287: 23–27, 1994.

distribution of T cells, monocytes, and most other cellular constituents of the skin immune system can be found in the dermis, especially in its papillary part. Thus, Sontheimer in 1989 gave his definition of the *dermal microvascular unit* (DMU), which was to point to the very center of immunological reactivity in most immunodermatoses. Directly around the postcapillary venules, we find accumulations of T cells, monocytes and tissue macrophages, mast cells, and dendritic cells. All elements of immune reactivity are present and it is no surprise that most inflammatory skin diseases show expansion of the cellular elements of the DMU. Thus, DMU might be considered a subsystem of SIS.

Nickoloff (1993) proposed the term *dermal immune system* (DIS) to be the cellular and humoral counterpart of SALT. It included fibroblasts, mainly because they are intrinsically related to homeostasis of other skin components such as epidermis. With the exception of the SALT lymph nodes and the DIS fibroblasts, these two concepts might also be considered functional subsystems of SIS. The conceptual differences in terms of components between SALT, DMU, DIS, and SIS are given in Table 1.3.

## III. THE SKIN IMMUNE SYSTEM

### A. Resident, Recruited, and Recirculating Cells

The concept of SIS might be regarded as a rather static one. Of course, there is intense and vivid activity in it, which can best be illustrated by looking at its cellular constituents. Some of them are

**TABLE 1.4**
**Innate and Adaptive Cells of the Skin Immune System, Divided into Resident, Recruited, and Recirculating Populations**

| | Resident | Recruited | Recirculating |
|---|---|---|---|
| Innate | Keratinocytes | Monocytes | Natural killer cells |
| | Endothelial cells | Granulocytes | Dendritic cells |
| | Vascular | Basophilic | |
| | Lymphatic | Eosinophilic | |
| | | Neutrophilic | |
| | Mast cells | Mast cells | ?Promonocytes |
| | Tissue macrophages | Epitheloid cells | |
| Adaptive | T lymphocytes | T lymphocytes | T lymphocytes |
| | Dendritic cells | B lymphocytes | |

resident, others can be recruited, and one might also delineate a category of recirculating cells. Despite some overlap between these categories, it is helpful to make this subdivision because it is a reflection of essential steps in the development of inflammatory and immune events.

Immunocompetent cells of the skin may also be divided in cells of the innate skin immune system as well as cells of the adaptive skin immune system, each having recirculating, recruitable, and resident subpopulations (Table 1.4). Eosinophilic granulocytes, for example, are a recruited cellular subpopulation, being present within the skin in certain pathological states only. Tissue macrophages (histiocytes) are generally believed to be resident, although they are derived from bone marrow. T lymphocytes are the best example of a cellular constituent of SIS that is thought to be recirculating, especially between the skin and the secondary immune organs, the skin-draining lymph nodes.

In addition to the cellular constituents of the skin immune system, a wide variety of inflammatory and immune mediators are present within the normal integument. A part of them reaches the skin by the circulatory route, while many are constitutively produced within the organ itself. Humoral constituents of SIS may also be looked upon as those mediators present in the normal physiological state ("resident"), while others reach the skin from originating elsewhere (recruited and/or recirculating).

### B. Innate and Adaptive Subcompartments

An objective approach to the description of the cellular and humoral elements of the skin immune system would then be to divide them into innate and adaptive subsystems, as described above. Innate immunity of the integument is represented by a number of biochemical and physical factors, some of them secreted by the sebaceous and sweat glands, orchestrating with cellular constituents such as phagocytes and killer cells in eliminating the invading, potentially harmful compounds and microorganisms. The adaptive subsystem would then include those elements that are essential in the preservation of a natural homeostasis, limiting sensitization to autoantigens as well as alloantigens.

## IV. THE DISTINCTION BETWEEN CUTANEOUS AND SYSTEMIC IMMUNITY

One might argue that the simple presence of T lymphocytes, dendritic cells, mast cells, and monocytes in the environment of vascular endothelial cells is not skin specific. In other words, these are normal elements of connective tissues and there is no difference between the dermis and the supporting connective tissue of other organs.

However, there are a few distinctions that can be made. First of all, the skin shares only with the eyes its almost continuous exposure to light and UV irradiation. During evolution, this has led to adaptation as exemplified by the presence of melanocytes. Another presumably adaptive evolutionary development is reflected in the relative insensitivity of keratinocytes to the DNA-damaging effects of UV exposure. Especially their capacity to recover from damage by UV is high as compared to other immune response–associated cells. The study of UV effects on cutaneous immune function is the major focus of interest in photoimmunology. It is generally believed that UV has an "immunosuppressive" effect on cutaneous immune responses, but there are immunostimulatory effects as well. The precise pathways by which these effects occur are partly characterized.

A second major distinction is that the skin is continuously exposed to an infinite variety of antigens, either in the form of infections or from the environment such as from plants or chemicals. Although the skin shares this characteristic with the pulmonary and gastrointestinal tracts, there is clearly a distinction in the way the skin has developed its immune responses to these antigens. In pulmonary and gastrointestinal immunology, the term *mucosal immune systems* (MIS) has developed. A major characteristic is the directly submucosal localization of lymphoid accumulations. These extranodal lymphoid tissue accumulations are thought to play a major role in the production of secretory IgA, independent of systemic immunity. However, although secretory IgA has been detected in human cutaneous excretions, the quantity is uncomparable and subepidermal extranodular lymphoid tissues are not part of normal human skin. Thus, the innate and adaptive subsystems of SIS are highly distinct from those of MIS.

A third major characteristic of SIS, which sets it apart, is the presence of Langerhans cells. These cells are immature dendritic cells, which in themselves are a subset of APCs, nowadays often referred to as professional APCs. Dendritic cells have the unique capacity to induce primary immune responses, and they are divided into those homing the connective tissues (tissue dendritic cells), the lymphoid organs (lymphoid dendritic cells), and those homing in epithelia (epithelial dendritic cells: Langerhans cells). Although we are not entirely certain why the epidermis would need such a dense infiltration of these dendritic cells, it is evident that these cells play a major role in inducing primary immune responses. There is now evidence that these cells are themselves making a distinction regarding which antigens are to be recognized and which ones can be discarded. Such a function is discordant with present paradigms of immunity, which give T cells the role of being the cells making such an important distinction.

In addition to these three major points of difference between cutaneous and systemic immunity, one might point to the existence of organ-specific T lymphocytes. These are recirculating between the lymphoid organs and their natural home base. These skin-seeking T cells, so long suspected to be there because of the existence of cutaneous T-cell lymphomas, have now been further defined with their skin-specific homing addressins.

## V. SKIN-SPECIFIC RECIRCULATING T CELLS

T cells are present in very small numbers in normal human epidermis. They are also regularly present in normal human dermis, where small clusters of T cells can be detected around the postcapillary venules. It has been known for more than 10 years now that T cells as they occur in the peripheral circulation have a subset (estimated as 16%) that undergo skin tissue-specific lymphocyte recirculation. The recognition of cutaneous lymphocyte antigen (CLA) on a subset of circulating T cells and the expression of its ligand E-selectin on endothelial cells of the dermis gave rise to a series of studies that have further elucidated this phenomenon.

The very existence of tissue-specific recirculating T cells is thought to serve different purposes: increase the effectiveness of regional immune responses; decrease the possibility of tissue antigen cross-reactivity; and allow functional immune specialization of particular tissues, i.e., the skin. The precise mechanisms of cutaneous T-cell homing have been described and the different adhesion molecules and chemokines involved have now been partly characterized.

T-cell homing is generally described in different stages. Endothelial cells express different adhesion molecules that have roles in the different stages of T-cell adherence and transendothelial migration into the dermis. Tethering occurs when CLA expressed on microvilli of fast-moving T cells binds to E-selectin present on the luminal surface of endothelial cells. Subsequent rolling, arrest, and transendothelial migration occur through binding of various adhesion molecules on endothelial cells and their counterstructures on T cells ($\alpha 4\beta 7$/VCAM-1, LFA-1/ICAM, PECAM/PECAM). Migration of T cells through the connective tissue of the dermis is in part dependent on binding of T cells to counterstructures on matrix proteins.

Chemokines and their receptors have subsequently been identified as key elements of this process, adding tissue specificity to the migration of T-cell subpopulations. $CLA^+$ T cells have preferential expression of chemokine receptors CCR4, CXCR3, and CCR10. In human skin, especially in inflammatory states, there is preferential expression of the chemokines specific for these skin T-cell chemokine receptors. Recognition of the endothelial cell expressed chemokine TARC (CCL17) by T-cell receptor CCR4 forms an integral part of the rolling and migration process. After arrival in the dermis, monocyte-derived chemokine MDC (CCL22) activates the migration of T cells by binding to CCR4. Finally, subsequent intraepidermal immigration is stimulated by keratinocyte-derived chemokine CTACK (CCL27) that binds to $CLA^+$ T-cell chemokine receptors CXCR3 and CCR10.

Skin T-cell homing is thought to be particularly necessary for immunosurveillance, serving effective acquired responses to microbial infestation and preventing the development of different cutaneous, particularly keratinocyte malignancies. To the contrary, T-cell homing is seen as disadvantageous in T-cell-mediated skin diseases, of which there are many.

Knowledge of the molecular processes involved in T-cell homing may be of use in different situations. Detection of circulating adhesion molecules has been found to be correlated with disease activity in a variety of skin diseases, notably atopic dermatitis. Upregulation of adhesion molecules in disease states can be used for advanced diagnostic imaging. Understanding of chemokine and adhesion molecule genetic polymorphisms might contribute to our understanding of the variability that skin diseases have in different individuals affected. And finally, adhesion molecules and chemokines might form targets of therapy. The new insights into the mechanisms of cutaneous T-cell homing thus have resulted in the development of innovative therapeutic approaches aimed at preventing skin T-cell immigration. Highly prevalent T-cell-mediated diseases such as psoriasis and atopic dermatitis have been selected for the development of such anti-T-cell immigration therapies.

## VI. CONCLUSION

In conclusion, we believe it is essential for our understanding of cutaneous immunology to keep in mind what distinguishes the skin from other organs. From such a platform of specific immunophysiology of the skin, we might try to understand its dysregulations as we know them in the form of a surprisingly large number of inflammatory and immunodermatological diseases. The science of cutaneous immunophysiopathology can best be further developed by taking into consideration the complete picture of cutaneous immunity, as reflected in its large variety of cellular and humoral factors, that are summarized under the heading "SIS."

## BIBLIOGRAPHY

Besredka, A., *Immunisation Locale; Pensements Specifiques,* Masson, Paris, 1925.
Besredka, A., *Les Immunités Locales*, Masson, Paris, 1937.
Beutner, E.H., Ed., *Autoimmunity in Psoriasis*, CRC Press, Boca Raton, FL, 1982, 313 pp.

Beutner, E.H., Chorzelski, T.P., and Kumar, V., Eds., *Immunopathology of the Skin*, 3rd ed., John Wiley & Sons, New York, 1987, 769 pp.

Bieber, Th. and Leung, D.Y.M., Eds., *Atopic Dermatitis*, Marcel Dekker, New York, 2002, 633 pp.

Bos, J.D., Ed., *Skin Immune System (SIS),* CRC Press, Boca Raton, FL, 1990, 501 pp.

Bos, J.D., Ed., *Skin Immune System (SIS): Cutaneous Immunology and Clinical Immunodermatology*, CRC Press, Boca Raton, FL, 1997, 719 pp.

Bos, J.D., Système immunitaire cutané (SIC), in *Immunologie Cutanée,* Thivolet, J. and Nicolas, J.-F., Eds., John Libbey Eurotext, Paris, 2002, 6–11.

Bos, J.D. and Kapsenberg, M.L., The skin immune system (SIS): its cellular constituents and their interactions. *Immunol. Today*, 7, 235, 1986.

Bos, J.D. and Kapsenberg, M.L., The skin immune system: progress in cutaneous biology, *Immunol. Today*, 14, 75, 1993.

Bos, J.D. and Meinardi, M.M.H.M., The 500 Dalton rule for the skin penetration of chemical compounds and drugs, *Exp. Dermatol.,* 9, 224–228, 2000.

Bruijnzeel-Koomen, C.A.F.M. and Knol, E.F., Eds., *Immunology and Drug Therapy of Allergic Skin Diseases,* Birkhaüser Verlag, Basel, 2000, 204 pp.

Burg, G. and Dummer, R.G., Eds., *Strategies for Immunointerventions in Dermatology,* Springer, Berlin, 1997, 418 pp.

Caputo, R., Ed., *Immunodermatology*, CIC Edizioni Internazionali, Rome, 1987, 286 pp.

Charlesworth, E.N., Ed., *Cutaneous Allergy*, Blackwell, Cambridge, U.K., 1996, 363 pp.

Clements, Ph.J. and Furst, D.E., Eds., *Systemic Sclerosis*, Williams & Wilkins, Baltimore, 1996, 657 pp.

Cormane, R.H. and Asghar, S.S., *Immunology and Skin Diseases*, Edward Arnold, London, 1981, 230 pp.

Crissey, J.T. and Parish, L.C., *The Dermatology and Syphilology of the Nineteenth Century*, Praeger, New York, 1981, 439 pp.

Czernielewski, J.M., Ed., *Immunological and Pharmacological Aspects of Atopic and Contact Eczema*, Karger, Basel, 1991, 253 pp.

Dahl, M.V., *Clinical Immunodermatology*, 2nd ed., Year Book Medical Publishers, Chicago, 1988, 422 pp.

Edelson, R.L. and Fink, J.M., The immunological function of skin, *Sci. Am.*, 34, 1985.

Euvrard, S., Kanitakis, J., and Claudy, A., Eds., *Skin Diseases after Organ Transplantation,* John Libbey, London, 1998, 231 pp.

Fellner, M.J., *Immunology of Skin Diseases,* Elsevier, New York, 1980, 317 pp.

Fichtelius, K.E., Groth, O., and Liden, S., The skin, a first level lymphoid organ? *Int. Arch. Allergy*, 37, 607, 1970.

Fry, L. and Seah, P.P., Eds., *Immunological Aspects of Skin Diseases*, MTP, London, 1974, 289 pp.

Gigli, I.N., Miescher, P.A., and Muller-Eberhard, H.J., Eds., *Immunodermatology*, Springer, Berlin, 1983, 183 pp.

Grabbe, S. and Luger, Th.A., The skin as an immunological organ as well as a target for immune responses, in *Multi-Systemic Auto-Immune Diseases: An Integrated Approach*, Kater, L. and Baart de la Faille, H., Eds., Elsevier, Amsterdam, 1995, chap. 2.

Jordon, R.E., *Immunologic Diseases of the Skin*. Appleton & Lange, Norwalk, CT, 1991, 646 pp.

Katz, S.I., The skin as an immunological organ: a tribute to Marion B. Sulzberger. *J. Am. Acad. Dermatol.,* 13, 530, 1985.

Krutmann, J. and Elmets, C.A., Eds., *Photoimmunology*, Blackwell, Oxford, 1995, 303 pp.

Leung, D.Y.M., Ed., *Atopic Dermatitis: From Pathogenesis to Treatment,* Springer-Verlag, Heidelberg, 1996.

Luger, Th.A. and Schwarz, Th., Eds., *Epidermal Growth Factors and Cytokines,* Marcel Dekker, New York, 1994, 486 pp.

MacDonald, D.M., Ed., *Immunodermatology*, Butterworths, London, 1984, 291 pp.

MacKie, R.M., Ed., *Current Perspectives in Immunodermatology*, Churchill Livingstone, Edinburgh, 1984, 289 pp.

Montagna, W. and Billingham, R.E., Eds., *Immunology and the Skin. Advances in Biology of Skin*, Vol. XI, Plenum Press, New York, 1971, 296 pp.

Nickoloff, B.J., Ed., *Dermal Immune System*. CRC Press, Boca Raton, FL, 1993, 340 pp.

Norris, D.A., Ed., *Immune Mechanisms in Cutaneous Disease*, Marcel Dekker, New York, 1989, 680 pp.

Parrish, J.A., Ed., *The Effect of Ultraviolet Radiation on the Immune System,* Johnson & Johnson Co., Skillman, NJ, 1983, 423 pp.

Ray, M.C., Ed., *Applied Immunodermatology*, Igaku-Shoin, New York, 1992, 215 pp.
Roenigk, H.H., Jr., and Maibach, H.I., *Psoriasis*, Marcel Dekker, New York 1998, 851 pp.
Rowden, G., The Langerhans cell, *CRC Crit. Rev. Immunol.*, 3, 95, 1981.
Safai, B. and Good, R.A., Eds., *Immunodermatology*, Plenum Press, New York, 1981, 717 pp.
Schuler, G., Ed., *Epidermal Langerhans Cells,* CRC Press, Boca Raton, FL, 1991, 336 pp.
Shimada, S. and Katz, S.I., The skin as an immunologic organ, *Arch. Pathol. Lab. Med.*, 112, 231, 1988.
Silverstein, A.M., *A History of Immunology*, Academic Press, San Diego, 1989.
Sontheimer, R.D., Perivascular dendritic macrophages as immunobiological constituents of the human dermal perivascular unit, *J. Invest. Dermatol.*, 93, 96S, 1989.
Stone, J. Ed., *Dermatologic Immunology and Allergy*, C.V. Mosby, St. Louis, MO, 1985, 996 pp.
Streilein, J.W., Lymphocyte traffic, T cell malignancies and the skin, *J. Invest. Dermatol.*, 71, 167, 1978.
Streilein, J.W., Skin-associated lymphoid tissues (SALT): the next generation, in *Skin Immune System (SIS)*, Bos, J.D., Ed., CRC Press, Boca Raton, FL, 1990.
Sulzberger, M.B., *Dermatologic Allergy*, Charles C Thomas, Springfield, IL, 1940, 540 pp.
Sutton, R.L., Jr., *Sixteenth Century Physician and His Methods. Mercurialis on Diseases of the Skin,* Lowell Press, Kansas City, MO, 1986, 226 pp.
Thivolet, J. and Schmitt, D., Eds., *Langerhans Cells*, John Libbey, London, 1988, 512 pp.
Valenzuela, R. et al., Eds., *Interpretation of Immunofluorescent Patterns in Skin Diseases,* American Society of Clinical Pathology, Chicago, 1984, 176 pp.
Van de Kerkhof, P.C.M., Ed., *Textbook of Psoriasis*, Blackwell, Oxford, 1999, 292 pp.
Van Joost, Th., Bos, J.D., and Starink, Th.M., *T-Cell Mediated Dermatoses*, Bohn Stafleu van Loghem, Houten, 1993, 110 pp.
Wallace, D.J. and Hannahs Hahn, B., Eds., *Dubois' Lupus Erythematosus*, Williams & Wilkins, Baltimore, 1997, 1289 pp.
Williams, H.C., Ed., *Atopic Dermatitis*, Cambridge University Press, Cambridge, U.K., 2000, 271 pp.
Wojnarowska, F. and Briggaman, R.A., Eds., *Management of Blistering Diseases*, Chapman & Hall, London, 1990, 308 pp.
Wolff, K., Immunorgan epidermis, *Der Hautartz*, 39, 534, 1988.
Wuepper, K., Gilliam, J.N., Rittenberg, M.B., and Katz, S.I., Eds., Cutaneous Immunobiology, *J. Invest. Dermatol.,* 85(Suppl.), 1–182, 1985.

# 2 A History of Immunodermatology

*Jan D. Bos*

## CONTENTS



## I. INTRODUCTION

The history of medicine is complex. It begins with the earliest written texts that have remained. These include ancient Egyptian, Mesopotamian, Indian, Chinese, biblical, Greek, Roman, and Arabic sources.[1] Although there is regular mention of skin disease, the field of immunodermatology as such, of course, cannot be found in these original sources of medical history. Such is the logical result of dermatology's relatively recent introduction as a clinical and investigative field in medicine and medical biology, the word *dermology* not being found before 1764.[2] Immunology appeared even much later, in the second half of the 19th century.

The immunology of today was established originally as a branch of microbiology.[3] Late in the 19th century, scientists started to identify large numbers of different microbes. Cultures of these microorganisms made them accessible for vaccination and *in vitro* studies. The role of white blood cells in their destruction was soon recognized. Serum factors that were capable of enhancing leukocytes' capacity to ingest and destroy these microbes were subsequently detected, and their study soon became the major focus of interest.

Thus, already by the end of the 19th century, the distinction between cellular and humoral defense mechanisms was made. Scientists, especially in the first half of the 20th century, focused on humoral immunity, describing the various subsets of antibodies in terms of their *in vitro* or experimental *in vivo* function. Opsonizing, reaginic, precipitating, and other classes were to precede the present categorization, in humans, into immunoglobulin classes G, A, M, D, and E.

Although the interest in the cellular elements of immunity continued, it lasted until the second half of the 20th century before progress in distinguishing important subsets of these immune response-related cells gathered momentum. The distinction between T (thymus-dependent) and B (bursa-dependent) lymphocytes, the recognition of dendritic antigen-presenting cells including epidermal Langerhans cells (LCs) as the inducers of primary immune responses, and the molecular characterization of T-cell receptors, all occurred after 1950.

The skin, so visible as it is, was not so much an object of studies in these early immunology years. Although cutaneous anaphylaxis, hapten sensitization, leprosy, and delayed type skin testing

0-8493-1959-5/05/$0.00+$1.50

all were regularly the focus of investigations, dermatologically specific immunology developed relatively late. Nevertheless, dermatology was one of the first specialties in which immunology became clinically incorporated.

It is difficult to set a date for the birth of modern immunodermatology. The recognition, in 1963, of autoantibody deposition in skin of lupus erythematosus[4,5] and of bullous dermatoses such as pemphigus[6] and pemphigoid,[7] with their recognition as presumably autoimmune skin diseases, might be taken as the beginning of modern immunodermatology. From that time on, the development of cutaneous immunology as a distinct area of interest within immunology exploded in terms of numbers of scientists involved and published studies available.

In this chapter, modern immunodermatology as it developed after 1963 is not described in historical detail. This field is so relatively new that describing its history would be like writing a biography of a newborn.

## II. MAJOR SHIFTS IN MEDICAL PARADIGMS

The role of skin in general defense mechanisms was, naturally, recognized in ancient times. Its structure was found to be responsible for general protection against harmful events and influences from outside. The only other physiological function that was ascribed to the integument was, wrongfully, the assumption that it forms a net, a covering structure that holds all body parts together. Without the skin, it was believed that the intestines and other internal organs would fall out, as well as that the limbs and head would be separated from the trunk. Such a fisherman's net function of skin is, of course, no longer seen as realistic, but according to Mercurialis (1530–1606) in his treatise *De Morbis Cutaneis* (1572), such a view had been common since the days of Hippocrates (460–377 B.C.).[8] Plato (428–348 B.C.) and Galen (A.D. 130–?200) both believed that skin not only had a physical protective function, but also provided the binding for the otherwise individual body parts.

This old misunderstanding of the basic function of the integument was complicated by another now-discarded paradigm.[9] Diseases were seen as dyscrasias, improper mixtures of the four juices of life: blood, mucus, yellow and black gall. Skin disorders were thus interpreted as the consequence of an improper mixing of the life juices. Such a dyscrasia would then logically seek its way out of the body through the skin. This antique view of disease, known as classical humoral pathology, was also represented in the four major temperaments: sanguine, phlegmatic, choleric, and melancholic. The paradigm was already evident in Hippocrates's days, and influenced Western medicine through the work of Galenus of Pergamum until well into the 19th century.[10] Even today, many of our patients wonder whether their skin disease is the result of something wrong inside, e.g., certain foods seeking their way out.

It is understandable that two such fundamental misunderstandings regarding the function of skin and the pathomechanisms of disease thwarted progress in what we now see as modern scientific medical thinking. A major development was the recognition of diseases as distinct entities and their description in an orderly and logical form. Such a categorization of disease, better known as "nosology," probably started with Paracelsus (1493–1541).[11] Every disease could be seen as a plant, with its own cause (seed), its specific symptomatology (flower and fruit), and its own course (lifespan). Nosological thinking slowly replaced ancient humoral pathology, and gave rise to etiological thinking and studies of physiology and pathology.

It flourished, concurrent with Linnaeus's binominal description of plant and animal life, in the 18th century, and nosological thinking was first applied in general medicine by F. Boissier de Sauvages.[12] Following these lines, the binominal classification of skin diseases gradually became established. A quartet of protodermatologists served as the founding fathers of the specialty to be: Daniel Turner (1667–1740), Jean Astruc (1684–1766), Anne-Charles Lorry (1726–1783), and Joseph Plenck (1735–1807).[13] By introducing a system of primary and secondary efflorescences, a binominal system of dermatological disease classification became available through the pioneering work of J.J. Plenck in Vienna (1776),[14] perfected by Willan in London (1798 onwards).[15,16]

The nosological basis of disease, established in the 18th century, formed the groundwork for physiopathological developments in the subsequent century. Individual disease categories can thus be followed throughout history, and a beautiful example is Karl Holubar's description of the historical development of the concept of blistering diseases, with emphasis on the autoimmune bullous dermatoses.[17]

In the 19th century, cellular pathology, microbiology, and chemical pathology became major investigative fields, in which the different disease entities could be related to different etiological categories. And, early in the 20th century, disease description and etiological thinking were established far enough to enable the development of a new discipline in medicine, that of immunology.

## III. EARLY DAYS OF IMMUNOLOGY

The Latin words *immunitas* and *immunis* originally had the meaning of exemption, as from military services or from taxes, otherwise obligatory for certain categories of people. The word may first have been used in the context of disease in the 14th century, when a plague epidemic was described and survivors were described as being immunis.[18]

Thus, long before the dawn of immunology, one of the basic functions of the immune system had already been recognized. Mention of individuals escaping from serious epidemics while being extensively exposed to what we now know have been microbial agents may be regularly traced in the historical literature. In fact, this knowledge gave impetus to Jenner's experiments with vaccination against smallpox at the end of the 18th century, when the existence of viruses was not known, and contagious diseases were seen as the result of bad air (miasma).[19] As a consequence of his pioneering work, Jenner is now regarded as one of the forefathers of immunology.

As described above, immunology started as a branch of microbiology and, right from the beginning of modern immunology, the science was divided into two different schools. The major issue was how to explain the molecular basis of immunological specificity. On the one hand, there was the immunochemical school, of which Paul Ehrlich (1854–1915) was the most prominent representative. On the other hand, there was Ilya Metchnikoff (1845–1916) who is seen as the major representative of the cellular immunology school.[20,21] It was Metchnikoff who discovered, on a Saturday afternoon in December 1882 the principle of cellular phagocytosis.

Somehow, the cellular and humoral schools entered into a rivalry situation and the immunochemical school prevailed, leaving attention to the cellular elements of the immune system to a modest number of investigators until well into the 20th century. Immunochemical studies were directed to antibody definition and explanation of their diversity and presence in body fluids. Antibodies, of course, were recognized as part of acquired (vs. innate) immunity. Cellular immunology made little progress.

## IV. APPLICATION OF IMMUNOLOGICAL PRINCIPLES TO DERMATOLOGY

It is possible to make a distinction between cutaneous immunology and immunodermatology. In cutaneous immunology, emphasis is on immunophysiology, as in the definition of the skin immune system, where the elements of immune activity, operating in skin, are encompassed in a larger concept. In immunodermatology, application of knowledge derived from immunophysiology to immune-mediated skin disease and immuno-intervention are the focus of interest. Historically, development of knowledge in these areas is not simultaneous. Cutaneous immunology generally follows, and sometimes leads, developments in general immunology, with some exemptions. Immunodermatology in general follows, and sometimes leads, developments in clinical immunology, but as such is always new because it develops knowledge of particular skin diseases not available before.

Humoral immunology as applied to the skin became especially important with the recognition of autoantibody deposits in the skin lesions of a variety of diseases from the 1960s onward. This has grown into an area where present molecular biological tools enable the identification of the target molecules with which these autoantibodies react. As such, new disease entities have originated, such as certain variants of autoimmune bullous dermatoses.

Cellular immunology, as applied to dermatology, followed the developments in general immunology and thus lagged behind. The delay in cellular immunology is well illustrated with the developments in our thinking of the role of LCs. These cells were first recognized in 1868 by Paul Langerhans, who used gold chloride staining techniques, which were originally developed for neural tissue identification.[22] They were thought to have a relation to neural tissues, and were also seen as cells with a possible function in maintaining epidermal tissue homeostasis. When it was found that these cells contain specific granules when studied at the ultrastructural level, these Birbeck granules became the major feature for recognizing these cells.[23]

Silberberg and co-workers[24] were the first to point to a possible immunological role for Langerhans cells. Their studies at the ultrastructural level identified intimate contact between LCs and lymphocytes during elicitation of contact allergic reactions. Subsequently, Stingl et al.[25] identified receptors for IgG and C3 on LCs, placing them in the category of antigen-presenting cells (APCs). We now know, after a wealth of studies that have followed these early steps in the recognition of LCs as immunocompetent cells, that they form part of the class of professional APCs, distinguishing them from other APCs because they are capable of priming virgin T cells, naive T cells that have not earlier seen the antigen for which they have specific T-cell receptors.

## V. MODERN IMMUNODERMATOLOGY

From the above, it is evident that immunodermatology follows developments in immunology, with some exceptions. The history of the development of knowledge in this field cannot be dissociated from its origin in 1963. From that point in time, immunodermatology emerged as a new area of interest with, since then, an ever-increasing number of scientists involved as well as increasing numbers of disease entities under study.

It is impossible to review a rapidly evolving and relatively new field such as immunodermatology as from these early days. Weekly, we encounter new findings within the field as well as in areas of investigation related to it. A history of modern immunodermatology may probably be only written later in this 21st century.

## ACKNOWLEDGMENTS

Professor Karl Holubar (Vienna) is gratefully acknowledged for his comments after critical reading of the manuscript. I would also like to memorialize the late B. Mesander (1926–2000) for the many stimulating discussions on the history of medicine and dermatology.

## REFERENCES

1. Sierra Valenti, X., *Historia de la Dermatologia,* MRA, Spain, 1994.
2. Schmidt, C. and Holubar, K., Dermatology — the name of the game. *J. Invest. Dermatol.*, 98, 403, 1992.
3. Bos, J.D., *Huid en Afweer/Skin and Defence*, Bohn, Stafleu, van Loghum, Antwerp, 1991.
4. Burnham, T.K., Neblett, T.R., and Fine, G., Application of fluorescent antibody technique to the investigation of lupus erythematosus and various dermatoses, *J. Invest. Dermatol.*, 41, 451, 1963.

5. Cormane, R.H., "Bound" globulin in the skin of patients with chronic discoid lupus erythematosus and systemic lupus erythematosus, *Lancet*, 1, 534, 1964.
6. Beutner, E.H. and Jordon, R.E., Demonstration of skin antibodies in sera of pemphigus vulgaris patients by indirect immunofluorescent staining. *Proc. Soc. Exp. Biol. Med.*, 117, 505, 1964.
7. Jordon, R.E., Beutner, E.H., Witebsky, E. et al., Basement zone antibodies in bullous pemphigoid, *J. Am. Med. Assoc.*, 200, 751, 1967.
8. Sutton, R.L., *Sixteenth Century Physician and His Methods: Mercurialis on Diseases of the Skin*, Lowell Press, Kansas City, MO, 1986.
9. Kuhn, T., *The Structure of Scientific Revolutions*, University of Chicago Press, Chicago, 1970.
10. Crissey, J.T. and Parrish, L.C., *The Dermatology and Syphilology of the Nineteenth Century*, Praeger, New York, 1981.
11. Pagel, W., *Paracelsus: An Introduction to Philosophical Medicine in the Era of the Renaissance*, Karger, Basel, 1958.
12. Sauvages, F.B. de, *Nosologia Methodica Sistens Morborum Classes,* Amstelodami, 1768.
13. Holubar, K., An imperial and royal prelude, in *Challenge Dermatology,* Holubar, K., Schmidt, C., and Wolff, K., Eds., Austrian Academy of Sciences, Vienna, 15, 1993.
14. Plenck, J.J., *Doctrina de morbis cutaneis qua hi morbi in suas classes, genera et species rediguntur*, R. Graeffer, Vienna, 1776.
15. Willan, R., *Cutaneous Diseases,* Vol. 1, J. Johnson, London, 1808.
16. Tilles, G., *La naissance de la dermatologie (1776–1880),* Editions Dacosta, Paris, 1990.
17. Holubar, K., Historical background, in *Management of Blistering Diseases*, Wojnarowska, F. and Briggaman, R.A., Eds., Chapman & Hall, London, 1990, 1.
18. Stettler, A., The history of concepts of infections and defense, *Gesnerus,* 29, 255, 1972.
19. Jenner, E., *An Inquiry into the Causes and Effects of the Variolae Vaccinae, a Disease Discovered in Some of the Western Countries of England, Particularly Gloucestershire, and Known by the Name of Cow Pox*, Samson Law, London, 1798.
20. Silverstein, A. M.,. *A History of Immunology*, Academic Press, San Diego, CA, 1989.
21. Mazumdar, P.M.H., Ed., *Immunology 1930–1980*, Wall & Thomson, Toronto, 1989.
22. Langerhans, P., Über die Nerven des menschlichen Haut, *Virchows Arch. (Pathol. Anat.)*, 44, 325, 1868.
23. Birbeck, M.S., Breathnach, A.S., Everall, J.D., An electron microscopic study of basal melanocytes and high level clear cells (Langerhans cells) in vitiligo, *J. Invest. Dermatol.*, 37, 51, 1961.
24. Silberberg, L., Baer, R.L., and Rosenthal, S.A., The role of Langerhans cells in allergic contact hypersensitivity. A review of findings in man and guinea pigs, *J. Invest. Dermatol.*, 66, 210, 1976.
25. Stingl, G., Wolff-Schreiner, E.Ch., Pichler, W.J., Gschnait, F., Knapp, W., and Wolff, K., Epidermal Langerhans cells bear Fc and C3 receptors, *Nature*, 268, 245, 1977.

# 3 Comparative Immunology of the Integument

*Edwin L. Cooper, Armando Pérez, and Andrés Castell*

## CONTENTS



0-8493-1959-5/05/$0.00+$1.50

## I. INTRODUCTION

The skin is the largest organ of the human body and functions as a general defense system. Components of the immune system have evolved as a complementary line of defense.[1] Fichtelius and co-workers[2] suggested that the skin was a first-level lymphoid organ. They hypothesized that those lymphocytes that reach the epidermis may to a large extent be noncompetent lymphoid cells. Later, they become competent during or shortly after a stay in the epidermis or in the corium close to it. The skin also contains other cells of the immune system including endothelial cells, mast cells, tissue macrophages, and granulocytes. Excluding afferent and efferent lymphatic vessels associated with the ubiquitous lymph nodes, these several cell types form an intricate and complex system called the "skin immune system" (SIS). Skin-associated lymphoid tissue (SALT) consists of (epidermal) lymphocytes, Langerhans cells (LC), keratinocytes, and the skin-draining regional lymph nodes.

Invertebrates and other animals that live in the water or in moist environments have, in general, a soft outer layer, whereas those that live on dry land have a hard outer covering. In this respect, for example, the dry land mammals and birds are comparable to dry land insects, while fishes and amphibians are more comparable to many of the lower invertebrates such as the primitive flatworms and earthworms. The beginnings of skin in vertebrates must be looked for in those animals that are related to our remote ancestors, namely, the lower chordates, which will be presented in the following discussion. Thus, the skin, along with the nervous and endocrine systems, forms a continuous network of immunodefense.[3,4] Now that SALT is established, it is highly appropriate to trace its evolutionary origin by comparing its structure and function in representative animal groups. A generalized view of the integument is presented first, followed by examples of how it is involved in various immune responses, particularly transplantation immunity. What should emerge based on the limited evidence is the concept that SALT as we know it in mammals underwent evolutionary changes comparable to other organ systems of vertebrates.

## II. PHYLOGENETIC DEVELOPMENT OF THE SKIN

### A. Protochordates

The skin of amphioxus consists of an epidermis, which is simple columnar epithelium, and a dermis of fibrous connective tissue. The skin of the enteropneusta (*Balanoglossus*, *Saccoglossus*, *Ptychodora*) also has a simple columnar epithelium, but cilia are present over the entire body and numerous gland cells occur, which contain a copious, slimy secretion with an unpleasant odor. Surely this secretion functions in defense, but its relationship to immunity is obscure. Since these are burrowing animals, this type of skin is well suited for their activities.

In tunicates, or urochordates, the entire body is surrounded by a gelatinous casing or tunic. The material that comprises most of it is a carbohydrate called tunicin, which is closely related to cellulose. Tunicin forms about 50% of the tunic; the rest is composed of nitrogen-containing substances. Tunicin is secreted by mesenchyme-like cells, which give rise to most of the immune system[4] in vertebrates. However, some authors insist that these are epithelial cells, which have migrated inward. Although the epidermis of lower chordates differs considerably from that of even the lowest vertebrates, the dermis does not show such a marked difference. Just beneath the epidermis of amphioxus is a thin layer (2 to 4 mm) of fine connective tissue fibers, generally without cells, which run in an interlacing fashion usually at an angle of about 45° with the body's long axis; the fibers are not arrayed in bundles. Beneath this fibrous layer, or "cutis," is a gelatinous layer, rich in mucoid material, which varies, according to the region of the body, from about the same thickness as that of the cutis to 25 times as great. This layer often appears homogeneous, probably because of the abundant matrix. In many places, small groups of cells are arranged about canal-like structures in the matrix, which probably contain lymph. Deep to the gelatinous layer is another narrow layer of fiber bundles and beneath that a single layer of cells. The subcutaneous layer of dermis beneath the thin subepidermal fibrous layer, from the comparative standpoint, apparently does not correspond with the subcutaneous tissue of vertebrates, which first appears in the cyclostomes.

### B. Cyclostome Fishes

The cyclostome fishes have a slimy and scaleless skin. Beginning with these primitive fishes the epidermis in all of the vertebrates is a stratified covering but with many variations within the different classes. Among the fishes from primitive to advanced, the two outstanding features of the stratified epidermis are (1) the small amount or even lack of cornification of the more superficial layers and (2) the presence of a variety of cell types, including gland cells such as mucous cells, whose function we can recognize readily, and many others, whose exact role is still obscure.

### C. The Elasmobranchs

The elasmobranchs, like all higher fishes, have hard protective structures, the scales in skin. The structure of the elasmobranch scale reveals its dual origin from mesoderm and ectoderm. So striking is the resemblance of these scales to the teeth that the same terms are used in describing the adult conditions and the embryonic cell layers from which they are derived. In elasmobranchs it is only in embryonic development that the epidermis shows a striated cuticular border or the presence of cilia. The epidermis of elasmobranchs is usually thin as compared to that of many cyclostomes, often only four to six cells thick. In some species, however, it is many cells thick, and they are joined together by intercellular bridges. Between the epidermal cells are found leukocytes, including many eosinophils whose precise function is unknown, but it is assumed that in this group as in other vertebrates eosinophils are a part of the immune system.[4]

## D. The Bony Fishes

In teleosts the epidermis varies greatly in thickness in different species. The immense range can be observed when we consider *Hippocampus*, the sea horse, where the thickness is 20 μm, and *Acipenser* in the barbed lip region, where the thickness may be 3 mm. The epidermis contains ordinary epidermal cells, gland cells, and sensory cells. The basal layers are multipotent, able to give rise to different cell types in the higher layers. A genuine cuticular layer, reminiscent of the invertebrates, does exist on the superficial cells in some teleosts, as shown conclusively by the presence of actual cuticular spines. In most species, such a layer cannot be demonstrated; however, the cuticle of *Lepadogaster* is limited to the copulatory apparatus, but offers a striking example of many potencies of fish epidermis. While the cells in the upper layers in many teleosteans are greatly flattened, the presence of superficial layers of definitely dead, keratinized cells seems to be a rare occurrence and has been described only for certain parts of the body, such as lips. Nuclei are generally visible in even the most superficial layers of fish epidermis.

## E. Amphibians

One can hardly imagine a more drastic change for the skin of an animal than the emergence from a watery environment to a dry one on land. In vertebrates this occurs in the Amphibia. Not only did it happen many million years ago, but also it still continues during the life history of many species in this class. The amphibians, then, are terrestrial pioneers, albeit cautious ones. They generally do not go far from the water, and the hopping frog is a figurative as well as an actual sign of the readiness to dive back into the old aquatic medium. The skin of adult amphibians differs from that of fishes in two important respects: the superficial layer is cornified, usually a single layer of cells undergoing this change prior to being "shed." Also, secretory function is taken over in many species by special globular glands permitting the epidermal cells to assume the rather uniform character and appearance that are found in the epidermis of higher vertebrates.

The epidermis of urodelan larvae (tailed amphibians) differs from that of the larvae of anurans (frogs and toads) in its generally greater thickness, which may be four or five cells, and in the presence of the specialized Leydig cells. In the stratum germinativum, ordinary epidermal cells possess intercellular bridges and a change from columnar to polyhedral to flattened forms as one proceeds from the basement membrane. Leukocytes, especially lymphocytes, are observed commonly among cells of the basal layer and presumably enter it by ameboid motion. Several cell types are found in the loose layer. Fibroblasts form a network composed of finer processes that make contact with their neighboring cells, and melanophores form a second, independent network. Leukocytes of various kinds including wandering macrophages are also present. Elastic fibers constitute a network, and beneath the epidermis they form rich anastomoses. The subcutaneous layer contains melanophores, lipophores, guanophores, mast cells, and networks of blood vessels and nerves. Of particular importance are large lymph spaces found in the subcutaneous layer, where there are also lymph sacs. The immune system of amphibians including transplantation immunology is reviewed by Cooper.[5,6]

## F. Reptiles

Although reptiles and birds are alike in many ways and are grouped together as the *Sauropsida*, similarities between the integument of the two classes are few. One important feature in which the skin of birds and of reptiles is similar is the almost complete lack of glands, and this feature distinguishes their skin from that of the other vertebrate classes. The epidermis of reptiles is characterized by an especially high degree of cornification. There are commonly three layers: a stratum germinativum where division of cells occurs; a stratum granulosum where basophilic granules of keratohyalin are found; and a stratum corneum of hard and keratinized dead cells. In the Squamata and in the Rhynchocephalia represented by *Sphenodon*, the entire horny layer is shed at given intervals. Cast skins show a perfect continuity of the body surface including even that of the eye. This molting process reminds us of the similar process in arthropods when they too shed the tough outer cuticle. In crocodiles and turtles, desquamation is usually a slow and inconspicuous process. In reptiles, in contrast to amphibians, horny scales are found throughout the integument. Once again, the integument has been considered in great detail when describing the immune system and transplantation reactions in reptiles.[7]

### G. Birds

Members of the great class Aves, while apparently descended from reptilian ancestors, have developed the splendid property of flight, which has been aided greatly by modifications of their integument. In birds only two layers can be distinguished in the epidermis as a rule, namely, the stratum germinativum and stratum corneum. Pigment cells are usually numerous and tend to accompany blood vessels. Birds have no sweat glands and no sebaceous glands. The dermis frequently shows solitary lymph follicles and masses of diffuse lymphoid tissue, both on feathered and naked parts of the body. Obviously, this arrangement of central elements of the immune system reveals the potential of avian skin.

## III. AMPHIBIAN SKIN

### A. General Considerations Concerning the Presence of Langerhans Cells

For a long time the skin was considered as a relatively inert organ, only having a mechanical function in protecting the body. However, investigations of skin immunobiology have revealed that this organ constitutes a very complex system, which plays an extremely important role in the development of immunologic responses to different antigens. LC have been the axis for the establishment of two concepts: SALT[8] and SIS.[1,9]

Mammalian LC carries out an immunosurveillance function in the skin and in other epithelia. These bone marrow–derived cells constitute 2 to 4% of all the epidermal cells, play an essential role in antigen presentation to lymphocytes, and are critical for the induction and elicitation of contact hypersensitivity (reviewed in Reference 10). LC possess a characteristic morphology that includes a dendritic profile, with numerous and thin cytoplasmic projections; intense enzymatic activities located in the plasma membrane for both formalin-resistant $Ca^{2+}/Mg^{2+}$-dependent adenosine triphosphatase[11,12] and for nonspecific esterase.[13] They also constitutively express class II molecules of the major histocompatibility complex, and other immunologically important molecules such as CD1a, langerin, and DEC-205 (reviewed in Reference 14). At the ultrastructural level, LC possess a clear cytoplasm, a convoluted nucleus, absence of desmosomes and tonofilaments, but presence of a characteristic organelle called Birbeck granule.[15]

Despite increasing knowledge about mammalian LC, only a few studies have examined the possible presence of Langerhans cells or their equivalents in lower vertebrates. In particular in amphibians, LC were probably observed first by Farqhuar and Palade.[16] They examined the location of ATPase activity at the ultrastructural level in skin of different anurans and they found it in the plasma membrane of keratinocytes. Nonetheless, they observed a more intense reaction in cells with dendritic projections located between the germinative and spinosum strata. These cells were characterized by the absence of desmosomes and by a poorly preserved cytoplasm. Unfortunately, because they considered these cells unimportant, no detailed descriptions were made.

Later, Banerjee and Hoshino[17] looked intentionally for the presence of LC in the epidermis of the frog *Rana catesbeiana* using three different techniques: impregnation with zinc-iodine-osmium (ZIO), ATPase enzyme histochemistry, and electron microscopy. They detected no cells similar to LC and only occasionally observed migratory cells comparable to lymphocytes between epidermal cells. They concluded that there were no cells that resembled mammalian LC in the skin of *R.*

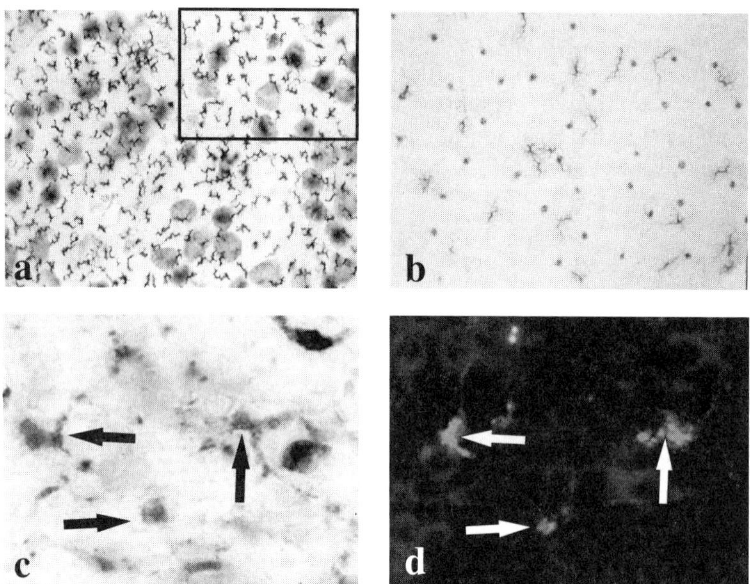


**FIGURE 3.1** Epidermal sheets of *Rana pipiens* separated by incubation in EDTA. (a) ATPase enzymatic histochemistry technique showed cells with dendritic profile scattered between the keratinocytes. In the magnification of these cells the clear appearance and their long cytoplasmic projections are noted. (b) Epidermal sheet processed to demonstrate class II molecules of the MHC of *Rana pipiens* (with the monoclonal antibody AM20). (Courtesy of Martin F. Flajnik, Maryland University.) Note that the long dendritic processes of the cells extend between the epithelial sheets. In a and in b the gland secretion channels are positive for both ATPase and class II molecules. (c and d) Epidermal sheets processed for double class II-FITC/ATPase stain. Positive cells for both markers are shown (arrows); nonetheless, not all ATPase$^+$ cells have mark to class II molecules. (Original magnification: a = 100×; b = 100×; c and d = 1000×.)

*catesbeiana*. Thus, the emergence of these cells was linked to SALT development, assuming it to appear first in birds.

## B. Characteristics of Langerhans-Like Cells of Amphibians

The first formal demonstration of Langerhans-like cells in amphibians was made in *R. catesbeiana* skin using epidermal sheets obtained by EDTA separation.[18,19] These samples were processed to demonstrate the activity of ATPase. When the sheets were examined, the presence of ATPase$^+$ dendritic cells was observed homogeneously scattered between keratinocytes and clearly different from melanocytes (Figure 3.1a). This difference was evident in their size and form as well as in their localization since melanocytes were always located in the basal region. Furthermore, when enzymatic histochemistry for ATPase was applied to ultrathin sections, electron microscopic analysis showed a very specific localization of the enzymatic activity in the plasma membrane of dendritic cells with clear cytoplasm, lacking desmosomes or tonofilaments, and with an indented nucleus (Figure 3.2a). These cells possessed no Birbeck granules; however, they did have all other features of mammalian LC.

## C. Co-Expression of MHC Class II Molecules and ATPase in Relation to Putative Langerhans Cells

Later, Du Pasquier and Flajnik,[20] examining the ontogeny of the class II molecules of the major histocompatibility complex (MHC) with the monoclonal antibody AM-20, demonstrated the presence of class II$^+$ cells in the epidermis of *Xenopus laevis*. They considered that they were probably

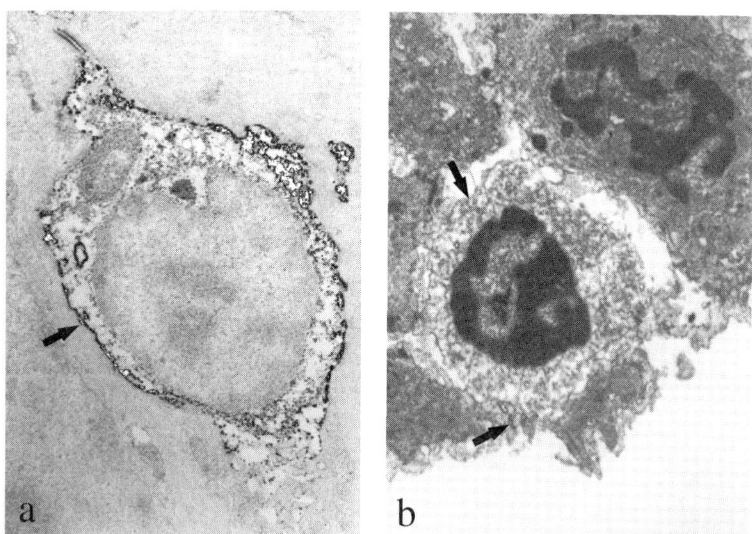


**FIGURE 3.2** Electron micrographs of *Rana pipiens* Langerhans-like cells. (a) ATPase$^+$ cell with the electron-dense reaction product (arrow) delineating the free-desmosomes plasmatic membrane. The cytoplasm of the cell has no tonofilaments. (b) Epidermal sheet processed for demonstrate class II molecules. The mark is weak (arrows) but the cells have similar features to the cell showed in a. (Original magnification: a = 12,500×; b = 10,000×.)

the homologue of the mammalian LC. Recently, we demonstrated in juvenile *R. pipiens,* the expression of class II molecules of MHC as well as ATPase activity in epidermal dendritic cells[21] (Figure 3.1b). When we counted dendritic cells, we found interesting differences. Numbers of class II$^+$ dendritic cells were 119 ± 45/mm$^2$ and numbers of ATPase$^+$ cells were 646 ± 186/mm$^2$. These results suggest that there were probably two different cellular types; however, when both techniques were made in the same epithelial sheet, all class II$^+$ dendritic cells were also positive for ATPase activity (Figures 3.1c,d). Obviously, not all ATPase$^+$ cells were class II$^+$. Other epidermal sheets, after ATPase histochemistry and class II immunohistochemistry, were processed to obtain paraffin sections. We observed that ATPase$^+$ dendritic cells were located in basal and suprabasal regions while class II$^+$ dendritic cells were only located basally (Figures 3.3a,b). With electron microscopy, morphologic features of dendritic cells positive for both markers were similar: a desmosome-free plasma membrane, with an indent nucleus and a clear cytoplasm without tonofilaments (Figure 3.2b). No Birbeck granules were observed. In this sense, the coexistence of ATPase$^+$/class II$^+$ dendritic cells with ATPase$^+$/class II$^-$ with the same morphology, strongly suggests the existence of LC subsets in amphibian skin. There is evidence that in mammals LC cannot form an entirely homogeneous population. For example, different glycoconjugates have been characterized in the plasma membrane of LC of the guinea pigs using different lectins, providing evidence that they could represent different LC subsets.[22]

## D. Are There LC Subsets Based on Class II Differences?

Evidence for the existence of LC subsets in humans and mice is derived from ultrastructural, immunofluorescence and flow cytometry analyses for class II molecules of the MHC. It is evident that there exists a subset that is strongly positive for class II molecules of the MHC[23] and another that is weakly positive. The weakly positive population is more abundant and suprabasally located in the epidermis. On the other hand, the ranges reported for the strongly class II$^+$ subset vary from 5%[23] up to the 25%[24] of all the LC. These LC that are strongly positive for class II molecules differ from the rest of the epidermal LC in four aspects: (1) they are located in a more basal position; (2) as much in humans as in mice, they contain few granules of LC; (3) by their phenotype

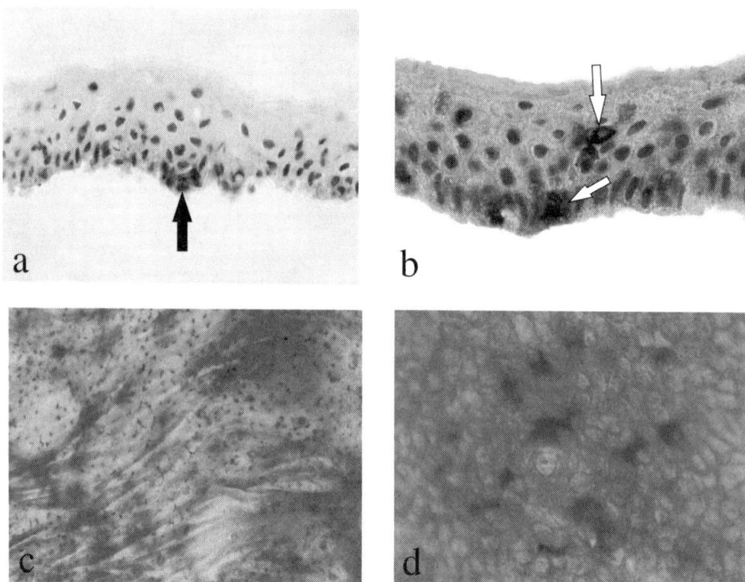


**FIGURE 3.3** (a). Section of *Rana pipiens* epidermal sheet showing basal and suprabasal ATPase$^+$ cells (arrows). (b) Section of epidermal sheet processed for class II immunohistochemistry. Positive cells are located in the basal layer of epidermis. (c) Nonspecific esterase-positive dendritic cells are scattered between keratinocytes and sometimes form clusters. Melanocytes and Langerhans cells are clearly different by the color. (d) A cluster of nonspecific esterase-positive dendritic cells. (Original magnification: a = 400×; b = 400×; c = 40×; d = 1000×.)

these cells resemble both LC that have been in culture several days and lymphoid dendritic cells; and (4) there are studies that suggest that they are very potent in the stimulation of the mixed lymphocyte reaction.[25]

## E. Is the Mammalian Model for LC Emigration Relevant?

The morphological and functional relevance of these LC subsets in mice and humans is still not established; however, it has been suggested that LC strongly positive for class II molecules could be cells that recently have arrived into the epidermis or, more likely, they could be cells that have captured antigens and are migrating from the epidermis via the lymphatic afferent vessels, toward the regional lymph nodes where they will present antigens to lymphocytes in paracortical areas.[26] This could be the case of the dendritic cell subsets observed in *R. pipiens*, where the ATPase$^+$/class II$^-$ cells, located suprabasally, may endocytose antigens, while ATPase$^+$/class II$^+$ cells, located basally, may migrate and present antigens to T lymphocytes. However, this assumption may not be clear in the strictest sense since amphibians lack lymph nodes and presumably all the other necessary anatomical features, i.e., afferent and efferent lymphatic vessels (Reviewed in Reference 36).

## F. An Experimental Model for Demonstrating Putative LC Subsets in Frog Skin

We searched for modifications of epidermal Langerhans-like cells subsets of *R. pipiens*. Frogs were painted with the hapten dinitrofluorobenzene (DNFB) and epidermal sheets obtained at 0.5, 1, 1.5, and 2 h.[27] Epidermal sheets were treated to demonstrate ATPase and class II molecules. We observed a diminution of ATPase$^+$ cells and an increase in class II$^+$ cells. We also observed an increased number of class II$^+$ dendritic cells in the underlying connective tissue. These results suggest that ATPase$^+$ dendritic cells diminished as a consequence of depleting the enzyme caused by the continuous endocytic process, whereas class II+ dendritic cells increased by the amplified synthesis and membrane expression of class II molecules for antigen presentation. It has been suggested that the function of the enzyme ATPase in the plasmatic membrane of mammalian LC is related to the capture of antigenic material carried out by receptor-mediated endocytosis.[28] Also, in mammals a decrease in ATPase activity occurs after the epicutaneous application of an antigen.[29] In mammals, after antigen endocytosis, LC become more positive for class II molecules,[30] and shortly after the application of DNFB there is an increase in dendritic cell numbers in the upper dermis.[31,32] In our study we observed the same phenomenon. In this sense, two possibilities exist: either that class II+ dendritic cells are leaving the epidermis with the captured antigen or that new cells are arriving into it. There are studies that support both possibilities;[33,34] however, it is necessary to question, in the case of amphibians, if the cells are leaving the epidermis, where are they migrating to? In mammals this migration is carried out toward the lymph nodes, but there are strong results that regional lymph nodes do not exist in amphibians (see above). However, anurans possess lymphmyeloid neck organs and the spleen with T and B zones.[35,36] A possible explanation suggests that dendritic cell migration is carried out via blood vessels, toward some lymphmyeloid organs of the neck or to the spleen. This seems highly plausible because the lymphmyeloid organs and spleen are blood-filtering organs, and presumably the bone marrow at least in ranids functions similarly. On the other hand, another possibility should be considered, that the presentation of antigens to lymphocytes is effected in the skin. In this sense, it would be interesting to analyze the amphibians' skin T-cell phenotypes as well as the number of them and their relationship with dendritic cells.

### G. What Is the Situation of the Characteristic Birbeck Granules?

It is of interest that when frog's skin was observed at the ultrastructural level, no organelles similar to the Birbeck granule were observed. However, when examining a sample of the skin of a tadpole we found a structure in a dendritic cell that vaguely resembles a Birbeck granule.[37] This organelle was tennis racket shaped and possessed a hairy cover inside the vesicular portion. These characteristics are similar to those of the mammalian LC. If this organelle is a counterpart of a Birbeck granule, then this is the first formal communication of this organelle in amphibian LC. On the other hand, should we recognize that this discovery was fortuitous, it is necessary to wonder why similar organelles were not observed in dendritic cells of mature frogs in which serial sections were made. It is not easy to offer explanations. This could be due to lack of observing a sufficient number of serial sections, or that the number of these granules is so low that they pass unnoticed. It is not strange that in different mammalian species the number of Birbeck granules varies. There are reports that in humans the number of Birbeck granules may vary significantly, or even be lacking,[38] There is also evidence that the density of these organelles in some mammals can be extremely low,[39–41] that could be the case of amphibian's dendritic cells. We can conclude that the absence of this organelle is not a definitive probe to consider that a cell that has the other characteristics of a LC is not truly an LC.

### H. Ontogeny of Dendritic Cells

To analyze the ontogeny of frog skin dendritic cells, we sacrificed *R. pipiens* at different larval stages.[37] Dendritic cells were observed from early stages of the larval development. Positive cells, both for ATPase and class II molecules, were observed from stage 26 of premetamorphosis; later, in the prometamorphosis, these cells increased until climax of metamorphosis when they diminished drastically. Last, in postmetamorphosis, these cells increased in number again. In mammals and particularly in humans, LC appears from the 14th week of gestation;[42] however, these cells increase gradually until the moment of birth when the number of LC is practically equal to that of adults. In *R. pipiens*, a dramatic fall in the number of LC is observed in the climax of metamorphosis. How can we explain this? It is important to point out that amphibian larvae are free-living animals immersed in a potentially antigenic environment for which it is very important to have cells specialized in antigen capture and processing, precisely in those areas exposed to antigens.[20,29] However, when arriving to the climax of metamorphosis, there is a decrease in hematopoietic activity and an atrophy of lymphoid organs.[43] These changes in lymphoid organs during climax of metamorphosis could explain the decrease of LC number. But it is necessary to keep in mind another possibility: the antigen rearrangement.[44] At climax, some larval antigens are disappearing while others are appearing. In this sense, it is possible that amphibian skin dendritic cell number diminishes in order to inhibit the recognition and presentation of new antigens and with this to avoid immune responses. Once antigens have been suppressed and other new ones have appeared at the end of the metamorphosis, antigen-presenting dendritic cells increase in number again, as was demonstrated in our data. If the above-mentioned model is correct, then these vertebrates could be used in these stages, mainly during the climax of metamorphosis, as excellent analytic models for scrutinizing the phenomenon of tolerance and of antigen presentation.[45]

## I. Expression of Nonspecific Esterase in Langerhans Cells

Recently, we demonstrated that ATPase$^+$ and class II$^+$ dendritic cells express nonspecific esterase activity[46] (Figure 3.3c,d). Besides the epidermis, these cells were also located in other squamous stratified epithelia such as the cornea and the nictitating membrane.[21,46] Interestingly enough, two aspects regarding the activity of this enzyme should be emphasized between the mammalian LC and Langerhans-like cells of *R. pipiens*: the substrate of the enzyme and the ultrastructural localization. The enzyme nonspecific esterase on mammalian LC uses α-naphthyl acetate as substrate, and the inhibitor NaF blocks this reaction.[47] On the other hand, this enzyme has been located, ultrastructurally, in the plasma membrane of mammalian LC and very little in some cytoplasmic vesicles, but not in lysosomes.[13] The activity of the enzyme nonspecific esterase on Langerhans-like cells of *R. pipiens* had the same pattern because it was inhibited by the same inhibitor and was located in the plasma membrane and in certain cytoplasmic vesicles. Interestingly, the enzymatic activities of the ATPase and of the nonspecific esterase, as well as the expression of class II molecules are present in cells that have the same morphological characteristics of mammalian LC, indicating a phylogenetic conservation and suggesting that the function of these cells possibly emerged earlier in vertebrates as components of the immune system.

## J. Functional Development of LC

In mammals clearly there is a family of antigen-presenting cells that originate from a bone marrow precursor. It is generally accepted that this precursor enters tissues in a relatively immature state. These cells basically are located in three corporal compartments: (1) nonlymphoid tissues: as LC in the epidermis and interstitial dendritic cells of lung[48,49] and heart;[50,51] (2) the circulation: as blood dendritic cells[52] and veiled cells of the afferent lymphatic vessels;[53,54] and (3) lymphoid organs: as interdigitating cells of T-dependent areas of lymph nodes, spleen, and thymic cortico-medullary border.[55–57] These cells are defined by their similar morphological characteristics and for their pattern of surface markers and function, so they form a system that connects one another by their mobility. Information about this cellular group in ectothermic vertebrates is scarce. However, the fact that they are present not only in the epidermis, but also in other stratified epithelia as the cornea and the nictitating membrane suggests the establishment of this cellular system in the amphibians. On the other hand, dendritic cells have been described, in amphibians, only at the ultrastructural level, but not using surface markers. Interdigitating cells in the thymus[58–61] and spleen[62] of amphibians have been described, but we have information that these dendritic cells in lymphoid organs coexpress class II molecules and S-100 protein.[63] Taking into account all these results we suggest the existence of a dendritic cellular system that presents antigens in amphibians, similar to that of mammals.

The extraordinarily important physiological role of LC, profusely documented in mammals, strongly suggests that their existence and complex organization may be a homeostatic trait largely preserved along evolution. Therefore, their characterization in species phylogenetically separated from mammals represents an important cornerstone in the comprehension of LC, in the immune system as a whole and, particularly, in the evolution of the skin immune system.

### K. How Do We Resolve Unanswered Questions Concerning LC in Amphibians?

1. There is a need for more-detailed ultrastructural studies, using serial sections with different doses of DNFB applied epicutaneously to amphibian skin, to verify if antigens induce formation of Birbeck granules. Demonstration of more granules will complete the morphological study of these cells in amphibians.
2. It is very important to demonstrate if Langerhans-like cells of amphibians are capable of inducing immune responses against antigens in a similar manner as mammals. It would be interesting to verify the presence of other molecules necessary for antigen presentation on these cells.
3. With the purpose of settling down, in a definitive way, if in the amphibians exist a dendritic cellular system, it would be very interesting to verify if the interdigitating cells of the thymus and of cervical lymphoid organs possess markers of dendritic cells. In spleen of *R. pipiens*, we have verified it previously.
4. The study of behavior of dendritic epidermal cells at the climax of the metamorphosis would help us to understand the establishment of a very important phenomenon as immunological tolerance and histocompatibility.

### L. Cytoplasmic Lectins

As lectins have been used as probes to analyze the function of lymphocytes, it is appropriate to mention the possible role of lectins in the epidermis of selected animal groups. Soluble lectins are widely distributed in vertebrates.[64] Immunohistochemical studies of their distribution generally demonstrate both intracellular and extracellular lectin in a given tissue.[64] As skin is a major secretory organ in *Xenopus*,[65] this provided a potential opportunity to study lectin secretion. Bols et al.[66] described purification and immunohistochemical localization of a β-galactoside-binding lectin from *Xenopus* skin. The lectin is highly concentrated in the cytoplasm of the granular gland, from which it is secreted upon systematic injection with epinephrine.

The skin of *X. laevis* contains a soluble β-galactoside-binding lectin with a 16,000 mol wt subunit. It resembles similar lectins purified from a variety of other vertebrate tissues and differs from two other soluble *X. laevis* lectins from oocytes and serum that bind α-galactosides. The skin lectin is concentrated in the cytoplasm of granular gland and mucous gland cells, as demonstrated by immunohistochemistry with the electron microscope. Upon injection with epinephrine, there is massive secretion of cytoplasmic lectin from granular gland cells. The results provide a dramatic example of secretion of a cytoplasmic lectin without packaging in vesicles.

The function of lectin secreted by granular glands is unknown. Indeed, we cannot rule out the possibility that the function is in the cytoplasm, and that it just happens to be released along with other cellular contents. The secretion is rich in a variety of biologically active peptides and amines,[65,67,68] many of which are also found in mammalian gastrointestinal tract and brain,[67] and which can act as toxins. Massive release of these compounds is believed to act as a defense against predators,[67] which frequently drop frogs that have secreted their cutaneous toxins and learn to avoid them. This raises the possibility that lectin in *Xenopus* skin itself may have a toxic effect like that found in snake venoms.[69,70] The lectin could also serve to organize glycoconjugates in cutaneous mucins, providing a meshwork to hold toxin granules on the skin. Another possibility is that lectin acts like the carbohydrate-binding subunits of the plant lectins ricin and abrin, which combine with toxins. Association of the carbohydrate-binding sites of these lectins with glycoconjugates on the surface of cells serves to deliver the toxins to their targets. In the case of the plant lectins, toxin association is via disulfide bonds. These results and interpretations are a major departure from the work using *Xenopus* as a model for explaining immunity in amphibians and ectotherms.[71]

## IV. LANGERHANS CELLS IN REPTILIAN EPIDERMIS

Based on histochemical and ultrastructural features considered unique to mammalian LC, the epidermis of terrestrial turtles, *Kinosternum integrum*, has been used to search for the presence of LC.[72] ATPase histochemistry has been employed extensively as a reliable assay to identify LC in mammals,[73] especially when epidermal sheets are used.[11] Ultrastructural features of LC include a lobulated nucleus, lysosomes, and mitochondria. According to one proposal, however, LCG (Birbeck granules) are the most characteristic features of LC at the electron microscopy level.[15] These granules are rod-shaped organelles with a central zipper-like striation, which occasionally have a vesicular dilatation at one end which gives them a racket-like appearance.[74] LCG are derived from the invagination of LC cytomembranes,[75–77] maintaining a temporal continuity with the extracellular compartment and then transporting captured external material to the endosomal system.[78] LCG formation also seems to be the morphological aspect of a specialized form of receptor-mediated endocytosis.[79–81] Nevertheless, the significance of LCG is still enigmatic. Furthermore, some mammalian LC have few or none of these granules,[40,41,82–84] so they may not be a prerequisite for the identification of LC.[85–87]

Uniformly distributed ATPase$^+$ dendritic cells have been observed in the epidermis of the turtle with cytoplasmic processes interdigitating with keratinocytes (Figure 3.4). Thus, histochemically and morphologically, these cells are similar to LC. Electron microscopy has shown that ATPase$^+$ dendritic cells exhibited enough ultrastructural criteria to be considered equivalents of LC, including LCG-like organelles, although these structures were less frequently observed in ATPase$^-$ cells or in LC of control samples (Figure 3.5). We are unable to explain this observation, although the disappearance of the ATPase activity associated with increased numbers of LCG and other endocytic organelles in LC after epicutaneous application of a hapten[28] suggests that it might be related to the endocytic activity of the cells.

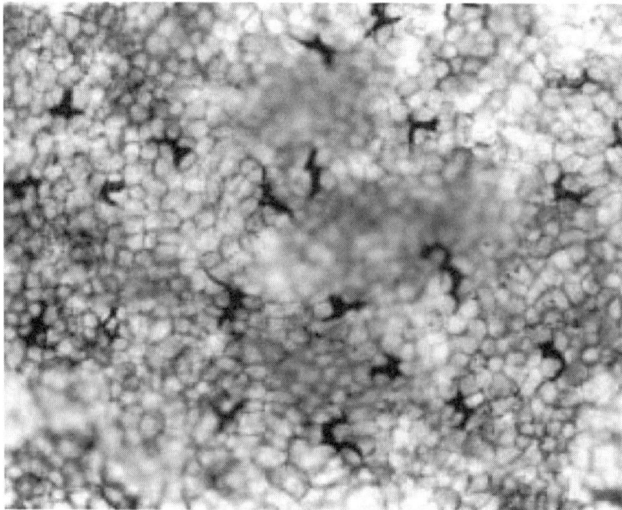

**FIGURE 3.4** ATPase$^+$ dendritic LC in an epidermal sheet of the turtle *Kinosternum integrum*. The background is formed by keratinocytes. (Original magnification: 320×.) (From Pérez-Torres, A. et al., *Dev. Comp. Immunol.,* 19, 225, 1995. With permission.)

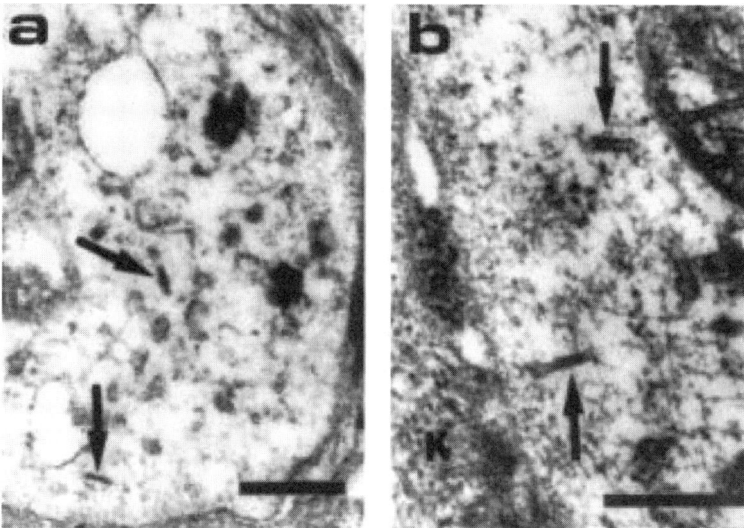


**FIGURE 3.5** Transmission electron micrograph of a dendritic process (a) and the cell body (b) of LC of the turtle *Kinosternum integrum,* containing rod-shaped organelles (arrows) similar to the Birbeck or LC granules. K, keratinocyte. Bar: 500 nm. (From Pérez-Torres, A. et al., *Dev. Comp. Immunol.,* 19, 225, 1995. With permission.)

Surprisingly, seasonal changes were observed to affect the number of LC and intensities of ATPase reactions of epidermal dendritic cells. Cells were numerous and strongly positive in May and November and scarce and weakly stained during the summer and winter. However, electron microscopy suggested that this depletion of dendritic cells in the turtle epidermis was more apparent than real, as we could easily identify LC with a trace of electron-dense precipitate localized in the plasma membrane (Figure 3.6).

In mammals, topical and systemic administration of corticosteroids[88,89] and testosterone propionate[90] reduces the number and changes the morphology of LC, probably by a selective impairment in enzyme expression and immunologically important LC markers. Increasing information suggests a relationship between environmental factors (mainly photoperiod and temperature) and variations in the immune system of lower vertebrates, which is probably mediated by circulating testosterone or corticosteroid levels during critical periods (reviewed in References 91 and 92). Perhaps a possible high level of these steroid hormones in turtles is responsible for a decrease in ATPase activity in LC, and is therefore "absent" during the summer and winter months. Certain circumstantial findings, i.e., seasonal-dependent numerical and enzymatic modifications in epidermal LC of the turtle, should be evaluated strictly with respect to seasonal changes that influence lymphoid organs (and nonlymphoid components) and the immune response of reptiles (reviewed in Reference 91). These results are the first formal evidence of the presence of LC in turtle skin. Once the functional properties of these cells are determined, this might represent an excellent *in vivo* natural model to study the neuroendocrine modulation of antigen presentation in ectothermic vertebrates.

## V. INTEGUMENTARY REACTIVITY IN SELECTED INVERTEBRATES AND VERTEBRATES

### A. Rejection of Allografts and Xenografts in Invertebrates

Although a number of invertebrates have been used to study graft rejection, controversy has surrounded the results in certain insects. Several investigators have utilized integumental transplan-

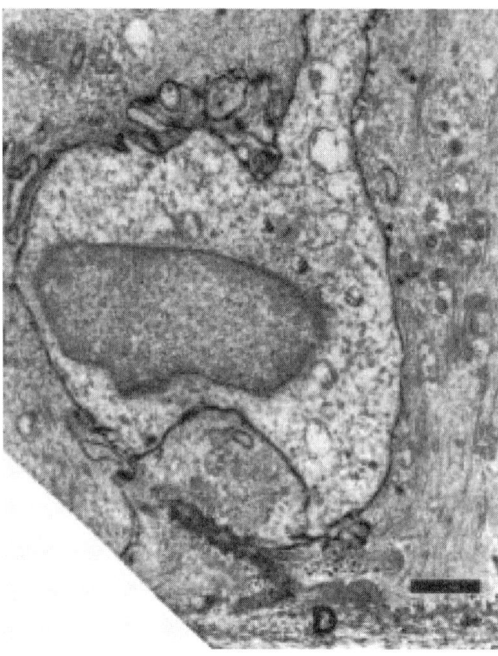


**FIGURE 3.6** Transmission electron micrograph of an ATPase+ LC in the epidermis of the turtle *Kinosternum integrum*. Note the electron-dense reaction product localized in the plasma membrane of this cell characterized by an indented nucleus and clear cytoplasm devoid of tonofilaments, desmosomes, premelanosomes, and melanosomes. D, dermis. Bar: 1 µm. (From Pérez-Torres, A. et al., *Dev. Comp. Immunol.*, 19, 225, 1995. With permission.)

tation studies to ascertain the existence of cell-mediated immunity in insects.[93–96] Thomas and Ratcliffe[93] reported a mean survival time for integumental xenografts transplanted to the American cockroach to be 18 days. According to George et al.[97] the nature of the nonliving cuticle does not lend itself to an accurate assessment of immune reactions taking place inside roaches. To improve on the interpretation, George et al.[97] placed control autografts on the same animals to establish a baseline of reactivity. The relative number of hemocytes in a 100-µm-wide section underneath the transplanted integument was used as a measure of host reactivity against grafts.

Host responses to xenografts were significant by day 3 post-transplantation. George et al.[97] found that this significant difference in cellular infiltration was maintained in xenografts through 70 days post-transplantation and suggested that the assignment of a mean survival time on this basis was not feasible. Jones and Bell[94] found that animals that had received allografts did not show a significant accumulation of hemocytes beneath the donor cuticle. In summary, the American cockroach was found to be capable not only of recognizing allogeneic differences, but also of mounting an effector response that destroyed foreign epidermal tissue. Because 92% of the animals rejected their allografts, apparently there is a great deal of allogeneic polymorphism among roaches.[94] Moreover, the allograft response was found to peak later than the xenograft response. The fact that 7 days is required to mount a maximal allograft reaction leaves open the possibility of devising experiments to test for the existence of cockroach immunological memory. In fact, sensitized roaches reject second-set allografts twice as fast as primary allografts, while third-party allografts are rejected at the same rate as first-set allografts. These results add to mounting information indicating that the ability to detect allogeneic differences is not only evolutionarily conserved among the invertebrates, but also must play an integral role in their continued existence. The transplant rejection work on the cockroaches, an advanced protostome (arthropods), is rather recent. However, research using earthworms (with a well-defined integument) has been performed since the early 1960s and aspects of memory and specificity have been clearly defined recently.[98,99] In addition, similar responses dealing with specificity and memory have been described in a representative deuterostome (the tunicates).[100–102]

### B. Development of Histocompatibility Clones in the Common Carp (*Cyprinus carpio*)

The fate of skin allografts exchanged among heterozygous and homozygous gynogenetic common carp siblings and among newly developed inbred strains and F1 hybrids has been recently described. Heterozygous, gynogenetic offspring have been produced from treating the resulting zygotes with a cold shock (0C, 45 min), which causes retention of the second polar body, thus allowing eggs to develop into normal, diploid fry. Homozygous, gynogenetic offspring can also be produced by heat shock (40C, 2 min), which suppresses the first mitotic division. Skin allografts exchanged among heterozygous, gynogenetic carp exhibited prolonged survival, with some allografts (21.8%) surviving for more than 28 days; a strong histocompatibility locus was observed to segregate in this group. In contrast, skin allografts exchanged among homozygous gynogenetic siblings were all rejected within 14 days (MST 9.4 days). New homozygous inbred strains, designated JJ and MM, were produced by gynogenetic reproduction of homozygous female carps, while F1 hybrids were produced by crossing these homozygous females with homozygous male siblings. All grafts exchanged among members of the same strain were permanently accepted. Likewise, grafts from homozygous strain members were accepted by fish from the related F1 hybrids, while the reverse grafts were rejected. These results provide evidence for the idea that in the carp histocompatibility genes exist at a minimum of one major locus and multiple minor loci, which are codominantly expressed.[103]

### C. Role of Circadian Cycle in the Rejection of Allografts in Fish

The circadian variation of scale allograft rejection has been analyzed in teleost fish maintained on 12-h daily photoperiods (LD 12:12). Immune activity, measured by melanophore breakdown, was two to three times greater during the dark than during the light whether scale allografts were transplanted at light onset or light offset. Because rejection occurred predominantly at night, survival times of both primary and secondary allografts were about 0.4 days longer than when transplants were exchanged at light onset. Immune activity undergoes robust daily variation in teleost fish.[104] These results point to the existence of relationships between the neuroendocrine and immune systems.

### D. Transplantation Immunity in Amphibians

Reference to extensive accounts of this subject may be found in Section IIE.

### E. Graft Rejection in Reptiles

During summer, 33, 52, and 15% of lizards *Chalcides ocellatus* have been shown to reject first set skin allografts, respectively, in an acute (11 to 14 days), subacute (15 to 20 days), and chronic (21 to 24 days) manner (time between day of first sign of rejection and end point). Second set grafts were rejected in an acute fashion (8 to 13 days). Histological examination of samples from grafted areas revealed evident lymphoid cell aggregations in allografts but not in autografts. This suggests that graft rejection results from an immunological reaction against allogeneic cells. In other seasons, all skin allotransplanted lizards rejected grafts in a chronic manner: in 46 to 132 days during autumn, 31 to 79 days in winter, and 40 to 78 days during spring. These data indicate that graft rejection in reptiles is effected by specific adaptive mechanisms and is under the control of seasonal conditions.[105]

## VI. IMMUNOCYTOCHEMICAL EVIDENCE OF TWO TYPES OF POTENTIAL IMMUNOCYTES IN THE SKIN OF RAINBOW TROUT

### A. Introduction

In trout epidermis there are several cell types whose presence underscores the skin's potential as an immunocompetent organ. Trout differs from mammals in possessing few if any antigen-presenting cells in their skin, although soluble antigens have been taken up by an unidentified epidermal cell.[106] Moreover, fish skin epithelial cells can secrete an interleukin-1-like substance.[107] IgM, the only immunoglobulin class in teleosts, has been described in superficial mucous,[108,109] mucous cells, and epidermal interstitium.[110] In addition a lymphocyte-like cell population has been localized in either the superficial mucus[109] or epidermis[110] using polyclonal antisera to IgM.

### B. Skin Lymphocytes Express Immunoglobulin

According to Magor (personal communication), initial observations of trout skin lymphocytes with polyclonal antisera coupled with ultrastructural studies corroborated findings of Peleteiro and Richards[110] who found a poorly vesicularized lymphocyte-like cell, which was distributed primarily above the skin's basal epithelial cells. This distribution of $IgM^+$ cells was also apparent in frozen sections of delaminated epidermis stained with monoclonal antibody 1–14 (Figure 3.7). In uninfected trout, lymphocytes are concentrated most heavily in the basal regions of the epidermis particularly in scale pockets. The morphology and cytoplasmic IgM in these cells is discerned in cytospin preparations of epidermal cell suspensions (Figure 3.8). These cells share gross morphological characteristics of mature, resting B-lymphocytes found in peripheral blood (Figure 3.9). Capping of surface IgM was observed in skin lymphocytes incubated with monoclonal antibody 1–14 (Figure 3.10). The exact role of these resident lymphocytes is unclear.

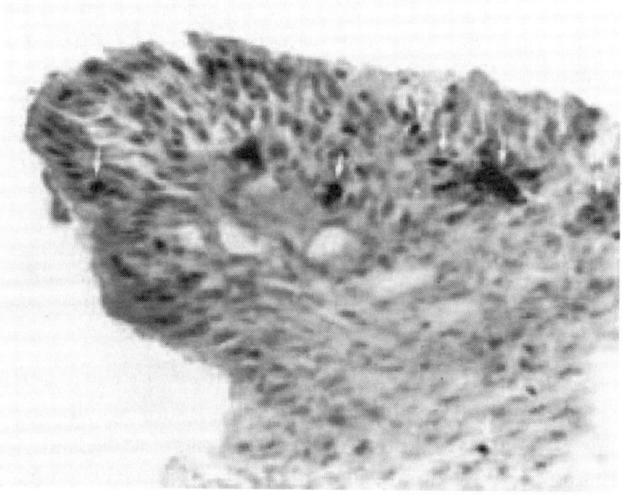

**FIGURE 3.7** Frozen section of epidermis from a scale pocket stained with monoclonal (1–14) antibodies to trout IgM, and counterstained with hematoxylin. This tissue, delaminated from the underlying dermis, has numerous dark-staining lymphocytes (arrows) above the basal epithelial cells. The greatest numbers of lymphocytes are observed in scale pockets and in epidermis surrounding the distal edge of the scale. (Magnification 200×.) (Courtesy of Dr. Bradley Magor.)

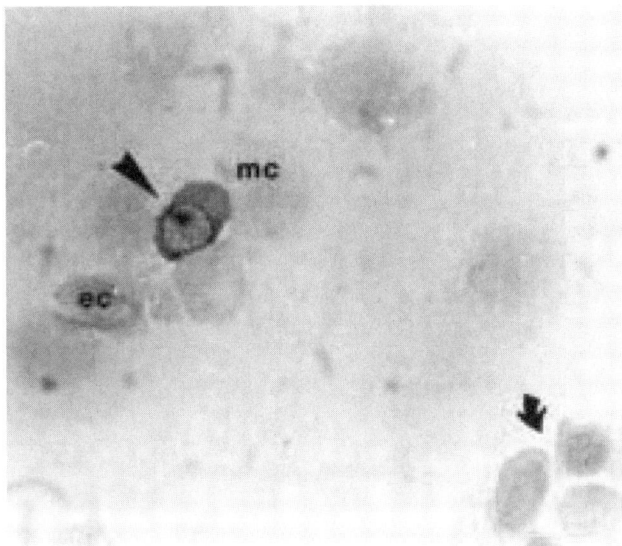


**FIGURE 3.8** Cytoplasmic staining of a B lymphocyte (arrow) from a suspension of epidermal cells. A mucous cell (mc) and epithelial cell (ec) adjacent to the lymphocyte are negative, although there is light surface staining of two epithelial cells in the corner of this photomicrograph (curved arrow). This is stained with monoclonal antibodies to trout IgM and counterstained with hematoxylin. (Magnification 320×.) (Courtesy of Dr. Bradley Magor.)

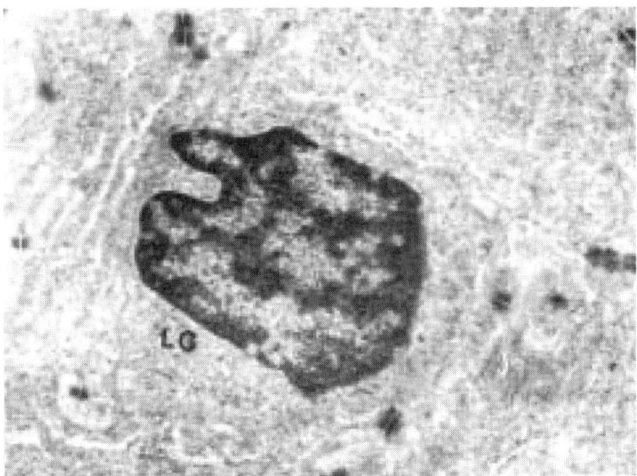


**FIGURE 3.9** Ultrastructure of a trout skin lymphocyte (Lc). Note the absence of any connections (i.e., desmosomes, tight junctions, etc.) between the lymphocyte and adjacent cells, and the absence of rough endoplasmic reticulum in the cytoplasm. Stained with lead citrate and uranyl acetate. (Magnification 14000×.) (Courtesy of Dr. Bradley Magor.)

## C. Surface Immunoglobulin on Epithelial Cells

Preliminary observations on skin sections using polyclonal antisera prompted an examination of cell suspensions for cytoplasmic and surface antigen (Figure 3.11). Using the polyclonal antiserum on unfixed epidermal cytospin preparations indicated that some 20% of epithelial cells (EC) expressed surface antigen (Figure 3.12). Rendering cell membranes permeable with organic solvents (acetone or alcohols) resulted in cells showing cytoplasmic staining after using the polyclonal

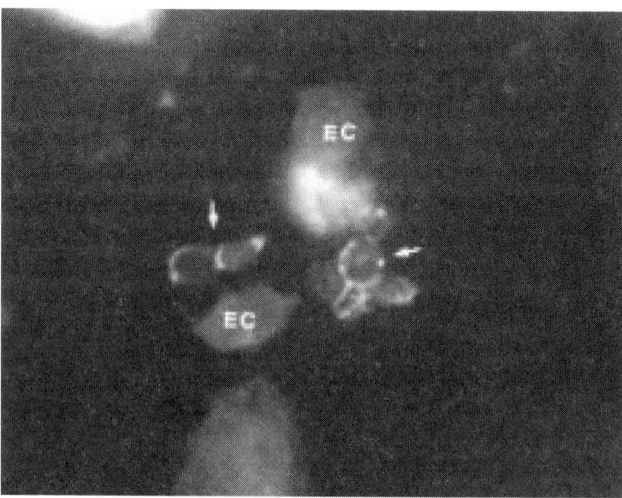


**FIGURE 3.10** Capping of surface IgM on suspended skin lymphocytes (arrows) after incubation for 30 min. In monoclonal (1–14) antibodies to trout IgM. Adjacent epithelian cells (EC) have no surface staining. (Fluorescence microscopy.) (Magnification 320×.) (Courtesy of Dr. Bradley Magor.)

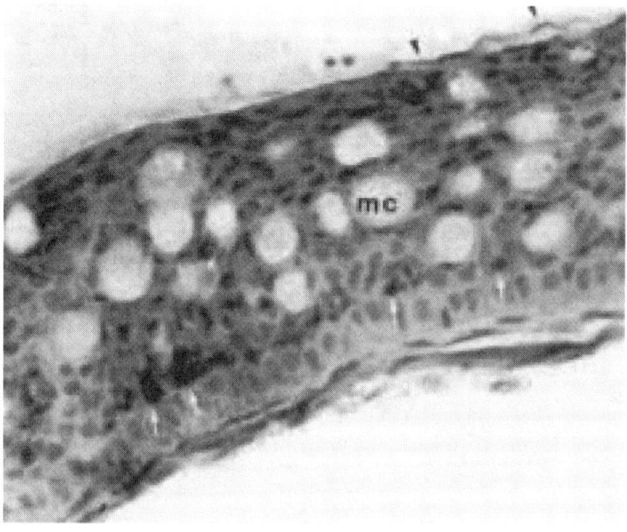


**FIGURE 3.11** Freeze-dried and vapor-fixed section of trout epidermis stained with polyclonal antisera to IgM and counterstained with hematoxylin. Individual or grouped lymphocytes (white arrows) are visible just above the basal epithelial cells. Interstitial IgM is visible in tissue adjacent to the grouped lymphocytes. The apparent cytoplasmic staining of some epithelial cells is due to cross-reactivity of the antisera with cytoplasmic constituents. The lightly counterstained mucous cells (mc) do not express any staining for IgM, although there is limited staining of surficial mucus (black arrows). (Magnification 200×.) (Courtesy of Dr. Bradley Magor.)

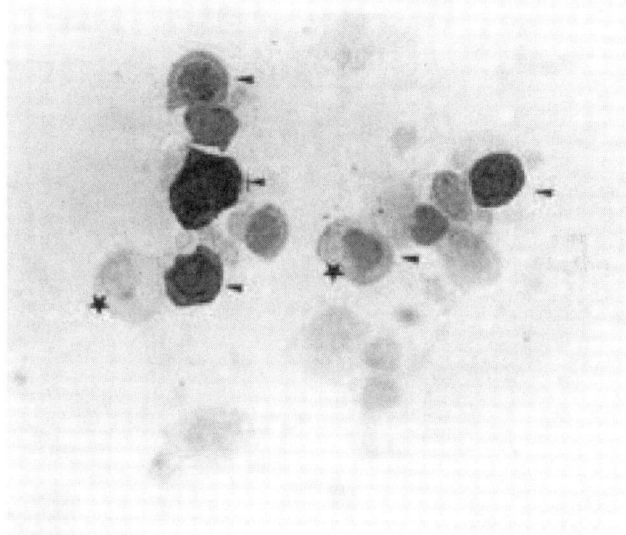

**FIGURE 3.12** Epithelial cells (arrows) express varying amounts of surface IgM. Basal epithelial cells (*) often show less or no surface staining. Epidermal cell suspension cytospin, stained with monoclonal (1–14) antibodies to trout IgM and counterstained with hematoxylin. (Magnification 320×.) (Courtesy of Dr. Bradley Magor.)

antisera, although this was later shown to be attributable to cross-reactivity with another serum protein. Absorption of polyclonal antibodies with purified trout IgM or other serum proteins indicated that the surface staining was due to IgM or a surface antigen with shared epitopes. Surface staining for IgM was confirmed using monoclonal antibodies to IgM. Varying degrees of patching and capping were observed on EC, which had been incubated for 30 min in monoclonal antibody against trout IgM (1–14) (Figure 3.13).

## VII. THE FISH SKIN: IMMUNOPOTENTIAL

### A. Inflammatory Responses

#### 1. Introduction

The question of inflammatory responses in invertebrates and ectothermic vertebrates has a long history. However, with respect to ectotherms it was the work of Fletcher and colleagues[111–113] who resurrected fish skin as a site for immune responses. They studied immediate hypersensitivity reactions in poikilotherms by examining the cutaneous response of flatfish to a variety of extracts known to be allergenic in endothermic vertebrates. Two marine teleosts, the plaice, *Pleuronectes platessa* (L.), and the flounder, *Platichthys flesus* (L.), were selected because of their availability throughout the year, their ease of maintenance, handling, and the clarity with which skin reactions can be observed on their nonpigmented undersurfaces.

According to their results, the erythematous skin reaction described in the plaice, *Pleuronectes platessa* (L.),[114] is caused by the release of pharmacological mediators. The only active material so far identified from *in vitro* studies is prostaglandin $E_2$ ($PGE_2$).[115] Plaice skin is extremely sensitive to $PGE_2$, since 1 g $ml^{-1}$ gives an erythematous response comparable to 10 g $ml^{-1}$ $PGE_1$, compound 48/80; 1 mg $ml^{-1}$ histamine or 5-hydroxy-tryptamine. Although the prostaglandin synthetase inhibitor, indomethacin, completely inhibits *in vitro* release of PG from plaice skin, *in vivo* responses are only completely and consistently inhibited by disodium cromoglycate.[111] Their conclusions suggested that the PG was not the only mediator involved. Carnuccio et al.[116] reported that cortisol (10 g $ml^{-1}$) inhibited PG generation in rat leukocytes by induction of a factor, probably protein or

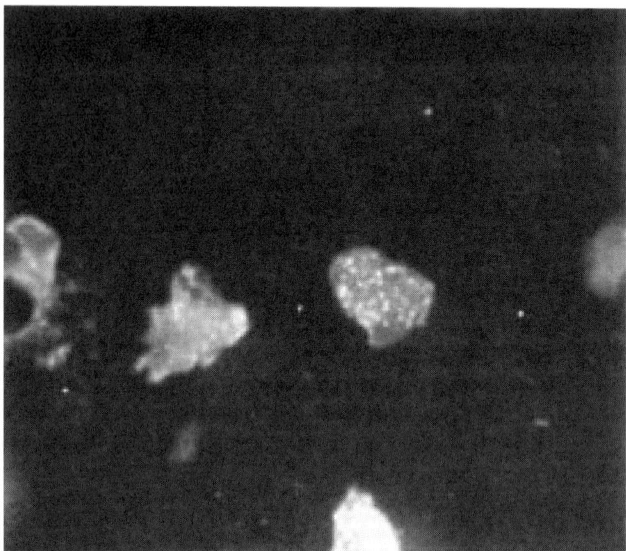

**FIGURE 3.13** Viable epithelial cells showing patching of surface IgM for fluorescence microscopy. The cells were incubated for 30 min in monoclonal (1–14) antibodies to trout IgM. (Magnification 320×.) (Courtesy of Dr. Bradley Magor.)

polypeptide in nature, that inhibits phospholipase $A_2$. Cortisol (1 mg $ml^{-1}$) did not, however, inhibit the *in vitro* release of $PGE_2$ from plaice skin, nor the *in vivo* reaction when given once intravenously (10 mg $kg^{-1}$ fish) or intraperitoneally (5 mg $kg^{-1}$ fish) on 5 consecutive days before challenge. Similarly, chronic dosing with corticosterone did not inhibit the *in vivo* response.

### 2. Immediate Hypersensitivity

Fletcher[114] found that intradermal injections of fungal extracts produce immediate (type 1) skin reactions[116] in some marine teleost species belonging to the order Heterosomata (flatfish). Fungal extracts that precipitate with human C-reactive protein[117] caused immediate erythema on subdermal injection into marine flatfish. Only species with calcium-dependent serum precipitins against these fungi showed skin reactions. Immediate hypersensitivity in a nonreactive species could be induced after injection with serum from reactive species. The transferable serum factor (or factors) was heat sensitive.

### 3. Role of Prostaglandins

Toward the beginning of the 1980s Fletcher and colleagues[118] extended their work on pharmacological substances and succeeded in identifying $PGE_2$. The evidence for systemic anaphylaxis in fish is controversial,[119,120] but the skin reaction was considered to be a hypersensitivity response, because it was transferable to the flounder with plaice serum containing precipitins to the fungal extracts. Flounders normally contained no detectable precipitins and the factor in fungal extracts eliciting responses was C-reactive proteins or C-polysaccharide, which then react with host C-RP.[120]

### 4. Prostaglandin Biosynthesis

To extend this work, experiments were designed to identify pharmacological mediators responsible for erythema. Fletcher and co-workers[115] provided evidence that the fungal extract of *Epidermophyton floccosum* can stimulate PG synthesis in plaice skin both *in vitro* and *in vivo*. A preliminary analysis of the fatty acid composition of plaice skin revealed, however, that arachidonic acid (AA) was not the major PG precursor in the skin, as might have been expected. In an effort to resolve this anomaly, a study was undertaken involving the conversion of synthetic precursor fatty acids into prostaglandins by a particulate enzyme fraction of plaice skin. AA and eicosapentaenoic acid (EPA), the precursors of $PGE_2$ and $PGE_3$, represent 3 and 9%, respectively, of the total fatty acids isolated from plaice skin. A microsomal preparation from plaice skin converted 2% of AA, but only 0.3% of EPA. Microsomal PG synthetase activity was completely inhibited by indomethacin (1 m*M*), whereas hydrocortisone (10 m*M*) was inactive. EPA caused a concentration-dependent inhibition of $PGE_2$ synthesis from AA and could therefore influence the inflammatory response resulting from the release of $PGE_2$ in plaice skin.[121]

### 5. Vasoactive Substances

As mentioned earlier, localized erythematous reactions have been observed in the white undersurface of the plaice following cellular damage and also following the intradermal injection of specific fungal extracts.[114,115] These reactions can be mimicked by injecting vasoactive substances,[122] consistent with the erythema resulting from the release of local mediators affecting the plaice skin vasculature. The demarcation between mediators of anaphylaxis and of inflammation is diffuse.[123] A methanolic extract of plaice skin, from which lipids had been removed, was chromatographed on alumina and eluted with decreasing concentrations of ethanol. Only the 60% ethanol fraction exhibited smooth muscle activity, with bradykinin-like properties. The 20% ethanol fraction increased vascular permeability in rat skin, as measured by dye-leakage. This was not due to the degranulation of mast cells. Intradermal injection of either fraction into plaice caused localized erythema.

## B. Macrophages

Melanin-containing macrophages are prominent within epithelium on the dorsal surface of certain fish at all age groups. They are readily seen, in sections, as black or brown stellate cells, at all levels of epithelium. In electron microscope sections they contain the typical indented macrophage nucleus. The melanin is held in its characteristic granular form, and each granule appears to be within a separate vesicle. The melanin granules are voided at the surface in the same way as mucus. Leukocytes carrying melanin particles have been described in the blood of many mammalian, amphibian, and reptilian species.[124]

## C. Eosinophilic Granule Cells

### 1. General Characteristics

Considerable numbers of cells whose structure have not been described in any skin are found in the basal layers of plaice epidermis, and have been called eosinophilic granular cells (EGC). Probably another, the acidophilic granular cell, is the same as the eosinophilic cell. Acidophilic cells have been described in a wide variety of fish epidermis including South American and Asian freshwater teleosts,[125–132] marine flatfish,[133,134] several members of the *Cottidae*, the ocean sunfish *Nola nola* L., and the selachian *Torpedo ocellata* Raf.[135] However, while all these cells have an affinity for acidic dyes in common, there appear to be marked structural differences between some of them. Because the function of none of these cells has been demonstrated conclusively, it would be premature to speculate on possible homologies.

In view of marked individual and temporal variations in the occurrence of these cells, their often irregular distribution within the epidermis, and the relatively small sample of tissue normally used for histological investigations, it is entirely possible for EGCs not to have been present in the examined material. Pickering[136] has previously reported eosinophilic cells in the epidermis of the char. A possible protective role in the defense mechanisms at the surface has been considered by

Mittal, Banarjee, and co-workers.[128,137] In this respect, it is interesting that as early as 1935, toxicity of certain fish mucus secretions to ectoparasites was demonstrated.[138] More recently, immunoglobulins have been demonstrated in fish mucus.[139] Lysozyme and enzyme with possible antibiotic activity have been isolated from plaice mucus. To date, the cellular sources of these molecules have not been established.

### 2. Antibacterial Activity

Antibacterial activity present in the skin mucus of turbot *Scophthalmus maximus*, seabream *Sparus aurata*, and seabass *Dicentrarchus labrax* against *Pasteurella piscicida* and *Flexibacter maritimus* has been evaluated. Using assays on agar plates, none of the mucus samples from the above fish showed any antibacterial activity against *F. maritimus* isolates. Turbot mucus inhibited the growth of the *P. piscicida* but mucus from seabream and seabass did not. Assays in liquid systems corroborated results obtained by the agar plate method. The bactericidal properties of the mucus were lost after heat treatment at pH 3.5 and all skin mucus samples displayed activity against *Staphylococcus aureus* ATTC 25923, a strain resistant to lysozyme. These findings indicate that thermolabile substances other than lysozyme were responsible for the antibacterial activity in mucus of marine fish. Enzymatic and heat treatments of mucus also showed that factors other than complement were involved and those active components were likely glycoproteins. Regardless of the source of isolation and degree of virulence, all *P. piscicida* and *F. maritimus* strains adhered strongly to skin mucus of the three fish species tested. Taking all of the foregoing results into consideration, it appears that whereas a possible portal of entry for *F. maritimus* into the fish body is the skin; in *P. piscicida* another pathway must be involved.[140]

### 3. Ultrastructure

The ultrastructure of blood eosinophils in fish has only been described earlier for the goldfish.[141] The granules are distinctive, irregular, lamellated structures extremely dissimilar to those of EGC, and the carbol chromotrope method, which failed to stain EGC, is considered specific for eosinophil cells. The Kulchitsky, or argentaffin, cells of the intestine and chromaffin cells of the adrenal medulla have eosinophilic formalin-dependent granules, but these also stain orange green when fixed in dichromate and stained by Giemsa. They are capable of reducing silver, whereas EGC stain red by this method. Because the former cells contain 5-hydroxy-tryptamine, they fluoresce with 300-nm wavelength light, which again fails with EGC.

### 4. Localized Leukocyte Response to Parasites

O-group carp (*Cyprinus carpio*), which had been immunized against *Ichthyophthirius multifilis* by controlled infections, were challenged by topical application of theronts to the caudal fin. Parasites that established were examined ultrastructurally, and host leukocyte responses were compared with those observed in primary infections. In the primary exposure group, eosinophils and to a lesser extent basophils were the predominant cells infiltrating infection sites. In contrast, parasite development in immunized fish initiated localized leukocytic infiltrations, which were dominated by EGCs and basophils. Greater localized phagocytosis was recorded in immunized fish by neutrophils, macrophages, and resident epidermal filament cells. Pronephric leukocytes from immunized fish displayed enhanced nonspecific phagocytosis. In the skin, leukocytes were observed in close proximity to the trophozoite surface in both immunized and primary exposure fish, often undergoing lysis and release of cellular contents. However, there was no evidence of active cell adherence nor of any cell-mediated damage incurred to the parasite in either case. These observations are discussed in relation to the possible role of leukocytes in mediating pathogenesis and immune responses.[142]

### 5. Effects of Copper on Immune Responses

Immunologic responses and stereoscan analysis of the skin and gill surfaces were performed in the air-breathing catfish, *Saccobranchus fossilis* (Bloch), following sublethal exposure to copper. At 0.056, 0.1, and 0.32 mg $l^{-1}$ of Cu, a dose-dependent decrease in red and white blood cell counts, hemoglobin content, and packed cell volume values were observed at the end of the 28-day experiment. Fish exposed to Cu had lower antibody titers, reduced numbers of splenic and kidney plaque-forming cells, and higher counts of splenic lymphocytes when compared to control groups. Cellular immune responses were evaluated by the rejection of eye allografts. Fish exposed to 0.32 mg $l^{-1}$ for 28 days showed a 2- to 3-day delay in eye allograft rejection. Reduced phagocytic activity against sheep red blood cells was observed in Cu-treated fish. Exposure to 0.32 mg $l^{-1}$ of Cu for 7 days causes surface architectural abnormalities in the arrangement of microvilli on the surface of superficial epidermal cells. Hypersecretion of mucus, loss of shape, size, and structural arrangement of epidermal cells, and mucous goblet cells were observed following Cu exposure. Increased numbers of active tubular dilated mucous cells were also noticed. Accumulation of mucus suggests a molecular interaction between mucus glycoproteins and toxic Cu ions. Fish exposed to 0.32 mg $l^{-1}$ for 7 days showed edema, fusion of secondary gill lamellae at many places, and degeneration of epithelial cells. Marked ultrastructural alterations in the arrangement of microridges and intervening grooves of gill lamellae were noted. It is suggested that these degenerative changes in gill lamellae are responsible for respiratory and osmoregulatory dysfunction.[143]

## D. Dendritic Cells and Langerhans Cells

### 1. Fish Skin: An Innate Immunity Organ

The mucosa-associated lymphoid tissues in teleost fishes include the gut, skin, and gills. A common characteristic of these three anatomical sites is their intimate contact to the external environment, which is potentially pathogenic.[144] Fish skin contains several noncellular and nonspecific immunodefense mechanisms that include the mucus, which is continually secreted and sloughed off, acting as an efficient physical and chemical barrier to be crossed. The skin mucus composition includes lysozyme, complement, lectins, proteolytic enzymes[145,146] and antimicrobial peptides and proteins.[146] Even without physical damage to the integument, fish still maintain a healthy state through nonspecific immunodefenses, but also with leukocyte populations responsible for local immune response.

Fish integument is alterable by several toxicants (heavy metals, detergents, nonylphenol), which produce changes in amount, release, physical state, and composition of skin mucus, and can also induce structural lesions like outer epidermal layer by sloughing and to the thinnest of epidermal layer (reviewed in Reference 147). These effects are highly comparable with those observed in the carp (*Cyprinus carpio*) exposed to acidified water[148] or to diluted seawater,[149] and in the trout (*Oncorhynchus mykiss*) exposed to a moderate temperature elevation.[150] Stressors mentioned above can increase fish susceptibility to general and specific infectious agents. Skin infiltration of many leukocytes, mainly lymphocytes, and the penetration of pigment-containing cytoplasmic extensions of melanocytes into the epidermis is probably a common efferent response against infectious agents.[148–150] These responses are immunologically relevant because melanin may possess a bactericidal function[151] and the presence of lymphocytes indicates that innate immunity may lead to acquired immunity.

The sloughing of malpighian cells could be a strategic mechanism for fish immunodefense, as has been observed in the Atlantic salmon *Salmo salar*, after malpighian cells become laden with engulfed bacteria. These epidermal cells appear to be both phagocytic and discriminatory because they phagocytose latex beads and the bacteria *Carnobacterium piscicola, Pseudomona fluorescens,* and *Aeromonas salmonicida,* whereas *Staphylococcus intermedius* were not phagocytosed.[152]

## 2. Fish Skin and Pro-Inflammatory Cytokines

The study of fish skin reactivity against pathogens, particularly monogeneans, has been useful to understand the responsible immune mechanisms that result in the elimination of infectious microorganisms. Rainbow trout *O. mykiss* can respond against infection with *Gyrodactylus salaris*[153] and *G. derjavini*[154] and eliminate these parasites. Based on recent knowledge of skin response mechanisms in mammals, a model was proposed to explain the various immune reactions involved in this host response. The components of the model are the epithelial cells, the mucous cells, leukocytes, and the release of cytokines as interleukin-1 (IL-1).[155] It is well known that this pro-inflammatory cytokine is central for the initiation of host immune reactions, and their involvement in anti-parasitic responses has also been demonstrated.[156] Following mechanical or chemical injury of the epithelial cells, IL-1 is released and this can affect mucus secretion, diapedesis, complement secretion, mast cell degranulation, production of reactive oxygen metabolites and the secretion of other hostile molecules.[155] The demonstration of a clear induction of specific gene expression of IL-1 isoforms during the initial phases of primary *G. derjavini* infections supports this hypothesis.[157]

The exact cellular origin of the *in vivo* IL-1β transcription in fish skin is still to be determined. Epidermal cells could be a good candidate as it has been shown in human epidermis, which represents a reservoir of IL-1α.[158,159] Their release induced by mechanical or chemical injuries could then induce its own trascription.[160] In fish skin, carp epidermis stimulated with human IL-1 secretes an IL-1-like factor.[161] Recently, it has been shown that recombinant trout IL-1β strongly promotes IL-1β expression in trout macrophage cell lines and trout head kidney cell preparations *in vitro* in a dose-dependent manner.[107] A dermal source of fish IL-1β, kidney or spleen-dependent, could be considered. This suggestion is supported by results in IL-1β-deficient mice, which can regain the ability to exhibit hapten-induced IL-1β expression, primarily in the dermis rather than epidermis, after reconstitution with bone marrow from wild-type mice.[162] Therefore, resident as well as infiltrating or migratory leukocytes could be the source of IL-1β in fish skin. This pro-inflammatory cytokine could be relevant in fish skin and act to increase mucus secretion and mucous cell depletion in gyrodactylid infections.[154] This in turn could stimulate T cells and activate neutrophils and macrophages,[163] which could be induced to release reactive oxygen metabolites[164] and complement factors with adverse effects on monogeneas.[165,166]

Vaccination experiments highlight the role of acute phase factors, mainly IL-1β1,[167] in the induction of mucosal (skin)-associated innate and acquired immunity. Vaccination by hyperosmotic immersion greatly enhanced the uptake of soluble, but not particulate, antigens through temporary disruption of the gill and skin epithelial. This activates the innate immune system, characterized by the upregulation of IL-1β1 as soon as 10 min; 3 h after, IL-1β1 expression reached its peak at >70-fold increase over controls, and returns to baseline values between 24 and 48 h after hyperosmotic pretreatment.[168] However, tumor necrosis factor-alpha (TNF-α) expression is not upregulated, despite that it is generally considered a pro-inflammatory cytokine that is often co-stimulated with IL-1β1 and is induced by lipopdysaccharide (LPS).[169] Surprisingly, inducible NO synthase followed similar kinetics as IL-1β1.[168]

IL-1β in fish skin probably represents the first or one of the earliest links in the chain of events initiated by mechanical or chemical injuries or by antigenic challenges that precede ultimate nonspecific and specific mucosal immunity. Obviously, an integral response of fish innate immune system includes other effectors such as chemokines CC and CXC and their receptors, cytokines — IL-8, interferons, transforming growth factor-beta (TGF-β), TNF-α — acute phase proteins (α2M, complement components, etc.), natural killer (NK) cell receptors, and molecules of the Toll signaling pathways (reviewed in Reference 170). Innate immunity also comprises phagocytic cells, such as macrophages and granulocytes, or cytotoxic, such as NK cells.

In addition to providing a first line of immunodefense against pathogens, innate immunity dictates adaptive responses to antigens.[171] The innate response is phylogenetically more ancient than the adaptive response and, for a long time, it has been considered to be broadly directed to microorganisms. However, the discovery of the Toll-like receptor family, involved in recognition of pattern characteristics of groups of microorganisms, has led to a reevaluation of the role of the innate immune system as a discriminating system.[172] The central role of mammalian dendritic cells in the induction and modulation of adaptive immune responses toward infectious agents has been extensively described.[173,174] Following antigen uptake, these cells have been shown to be a cornerstone of antigen-specific T-cell primary and secondary immune responses.[175] In addition, dendritic cells are essential for the development of antibody responses by direct B-cell activation.[176] Dendritic cells are widely distributed, especially in tissues that interface the external environment, such as skin, gut, lung, and other mucosa,[177] where they can perform a sentinel function for incoming pathogens and have the capacity to recruit and activate cells of the innate immune system after inflammation.[178–181] Uptake of pathogens induces a state of activation, which eventually leads to the migration of the antigen-loaded dendritic cells to the lymphoid organs where the cells of the adaptive immune response can be activated.[182–184] Thus, dendritic cells can serve as a bridge or modulator between innate and adaptive immune responses, as it has been proposed recently.[185,186] In the context of skin immunity, epidermal LC and dermal dendritic cells, a subpopulation of immature dendritic cells, have the morphological and functional properties to be the link.

## 3. Fish Dendritic Cells

Histochemical observation of distinctive $Mg^{2+}$-dependent ATPase$^+$ dendritic cells in the spleen associated with ellipsoids and the accumulations of melanomacrophages, and in the head kidney of Atlantic salmon (*Salmo salar* L.)[187] is probably the first demonstration of fish dendritic cells in T-cell areas that could be active in the presentation of antigens to T cells. However, more convincing evidence for the presence of fish dendritic cells was provided from long-term rainbow trout spleen cultures.[188] Trout dendritic cells were irregular in shape and appeared 14 to 16 days after plating of primary cultures and 3 to 5 days after plating of secondary cultures. Their cytoplasmic processes included spiny dendrites, bulbous pseudopods, and thin lamellipodia, which were rapidly and constantly moving; the cells were poorly phagocytic and nonspecific esterase activity was doubtful. These features of trout dendritic cells are identical to mammalian dendritic cells of the spleen.[187–191] Macrophages were identified by their phagocytic ability and positive staining for nonspecific esterase activity, characteristics commonly accepted as criteria for rainbow trout macrophages.[192] These results are important because many functional properties of mammalian dendritic cells, mainly the processing and antigen presentation, can be assayed in common commercial and laboratory species of teleost as it has been examined in catfish.[193]

## 4. Fish Epidermal Langerhans Cells

The hypothesis that fish epidermis contains LC is supported by the finding of dendritic cells in trout spleen, an organ where hemopoiesis take place.[194] These LC could be functionally symbiotic of intraepidermal lymphocytes[110,195] capable of inducing antigen-specific responses. Additionally, the demonstration of LC in amphibian, reptilian (reviewed in this chapter), and avian epidermis[196–199] stimulated the search for LC in fish skin. Recently,[200,201] our laboratory demonstrated the presence of ATPase$^+$ cells in epidermal sheets obtained from the ventral white skin of the juvenile catfish, *Arius seemanii* (Günther, 1864) (Figure 3.14a). Most of these cells had short dendritic processes (Figure 3.14b) but some exhibited a characteristic dendritic appearance and were distributed uniformly, around and beneath clear spaces probably occupied by the so-called large alarm cells. The number of ATPase$^+$ cells of catfish was not quantified because most of them were in close contact. These results were a constant finding, independent of seasonal changes. Epithelial cells had a light brownish color clearly differentiated from the dark brown color of the developed enzymatic product reaction of the epidermal Langerhans-like cells. Pigmented cells were never observed, which was confirmed in control epidermal sheets incubated in a medium without ATP and in sections of epidermal sheets stained with hemotoxylin and eosin (H-E) and Fontana–Masson silver method.

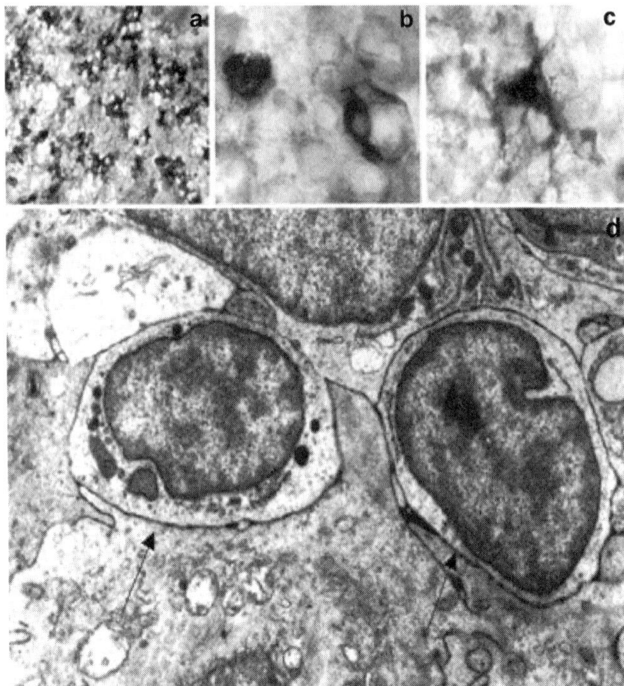


**FIGURE 3.14** ATPase+ cells with short dendritic processes in epidermal sheets from catfish *Arius seemanii* (a, b). At the ultrastructural level (d), an electron-dense deposit of the ATPase reaction delineates the plasma membrane of suprabasal cells (arrows) characterized by indented nuclei and clear cytoplasm devoid of tonofilaments, desmosomes, and melanosomes. Note that nuclear envelope and some organelles were positive to this reaction. (c) ATPase+ dendritic cells that resemble Langerhans cells were also observed in epidermal sheets from ray *Torpedo*. (Original magnification: a = 200×; b, c = 1000×; d = 12,500×.)

Catfish epidermis possesses two distinctive cells that are large suprabasal eosinophilic alarm cells and a population of PAS + rounded cells (probably mucous cells) found in the basal stratum and very near to the surface where they release secretions.

Small fragments of catfish skin have been incubated to demonstrate ATPase activity in the same manner as in epidermal sheets and then processed for electron microscopy. At the ultrastructural level, enzymatic activity was identified as an electron-dense precipitate on the plasma membrane of suprabasally located clear cells, which lacked tonofilaments, desmosomes, and melanosomes but exhibited rounded or indented nuclei (Figure 3.14d). The profile of these cells was irregular, because of the presence of cytoplasmic extensions interdigitating with the keratinocytes. Most epidermal ATPase+ cells of catfish possess well-developed endosomal and lysosomal compartments associated with numerous coated pits and vesicles, which are probably endocytic and exocytic. Ultrastructural analysis also reveals that these catfish epidermal Langerhans-like cells possess rod-shaped structures with a central linear density between two limiting membranes, similar to LC granules or Birbeck granules. No melanocyte-like cells were observed in the epidermis. However, granulocyte-like cells and lymphoid cells were observed in the vicinity of ATPase+ dendritic cells, beneath the alarm cells.

To our knowledge, this is the first evidence concerning the presence of epidermal dendritic cells in teleost skin, which exhibit the classical markers that identify LC in normal mammalian, avian, reptilian, and amphibian skin: pleomorphic or dendritic morphology, intense ATPase activity, and all ultrastructural features including the only reliable criterion to designate a cell as an LC, the typical and unique intracellular organelle termed the Birbeck or LC granules. A perspective for the epidermal LC of catfish described here suggests that they also express MHC class molecules, one of the main elements of the acquired immune system, which can confer functional properties that allow interaction with innate immune responses (reviewed in Reference 202) as antigen-presenting cells. The availability of antibodies to these molecules in teleost fish[203–206] is a promising tool. Finally, we observed that ATPase+ dendritic cells are also present in the epidermis of the ray *Torpedo* (Figure 3.14c). This preliminary result sheds light on the phylogeny of LC in the oldest class of contemporary vertebrates.

## VIII. SUMMARY

The skin is the largest organ of the human body and functions as a general defense system, while the immune system has evolved as a complementary line of defense. Consider how easy it is to contaminate an *in vitro* cell culture, which is a living system lacking skin and an immune system. Now that skin-associated lymphoid tissue is established in mammals, it is highly appropriate to trace its evolutionary origin by comparing its structure and function in representative animal groups. It is becoming increasingly clear that even among the lowest vertebrates (elasmobranchs and fishes) many basic constituents of the mammalian immune system (T and B lymphocytes, lymphokines, leukotrienes, etc.) are found. The changes in the skin immune system are primarily organizational and reflect not only increased specialization of the immune system and its constituents, but also changes in skin morphology that may be dictated by habitat changes. Some of the evolutionary trends in skin, immunity, and skin immune system include (1) increased cornification of the epidermis, particularly following the move from aquatic to terrestrial habitats; (2) increased lymphatic system in the dermis and development of antigen processing or germinal center in the dermis and subcutis; (3) presence of Langerhans-like cells in all groups of vertebrates, and then the shift from lymphocytes to dendritic antigen-presenting cells as the principal immunocytes of epidermis; (4) increased repertoire of antigens to which higher vertebrates can respond;[71] (5) development of delayed hypersensitivity in association with appearance of histamine-releasing mast cells and multiple immunoglobulin classes; and (6) possible decreasing emphasis on nonspecific defensive compounds, which are associated with secretory cells or glands.

Some systems, such as cell-mediated allograft rejection, appear to remain fairly constant, with certain but not all fish differing primarily in the speed at which they respond to allografts, and the apparent complexity with which the response is regulated. Humoral immunity appears to reflect the considerable differences among the vertebrate classes.

In fishes and amphibians, the humoral immune system may operate primarily in the epidermis. The presence of resident epidermal B lymphocytes and absence of regional germinal centers suggest that these cells are activated *in situ*, perhaps under the influence Langerhans-like cells and cytokines from epithelial cells. That these ectothermic vertebrates seen up to now respond to comparatively few antigens may be offset by employing nonspecific defense systems associated with surface secretions.

Among terrestrial vertebrates, the reptiles (also ectothermic and some aquatic), and birds, stratum corneum insulates the stratum germinativum from the external environment by means of extensive cornification and specialized keratin structures; nonetheless, there are epidermal LC and increased dermal lymphoid tissues or follicles. Presumably, any insults sufficient to compromise the integrity of the stratum corneum directly affect the dermis.

In mammals there is a return to large numbers of epidermal immunocytes, concurrent with a partial decrease in epidermal cornification. However, LC, the dendritic antigen-presenting cells, are present in all vertebrate groups without direct relationship with skin cornification and/or cutaneous annexes. We may conclude that LC are the principal epidermal immunocytes throughout the phylogenetic scale. These cells operate through a system of well-organized subcutaneous lymphoid tissue to recruit necessary lymphocytes to the epidermis.

The differences in the skin immune system among the vertebrate classes reflect habitat differences as much as evolutionary advancement. The skin immune system in concert with the respective skin morphologies of the classes is able to provide a large degree of protection against a variety of facultative parasitic microbes with which vertebrates might come in contact in their respective habitats.

## ACKNOWLEDGMENT

The authors express appreciation to Dr. Bradley Magor, Department of Biological Sciences, University of Alberta, Canada, for providing Figures 3.7 to 3.13.

## REFERENCES

1. Bos, J.D. and Kapsenberg, M.L., The skin immune system. Its cellular constituents and their interactions, *Immunol. Today*, 7, 235, 1986.
2. Fichtelius, K.E., Groth, O., and Liden, S., The skin, a first level lymphoid organ? *Int. Arch. Allergy*, 37, 607, 1970.
3. Cooper, E.L., *Comparative Immunology*, Prentice Hall, Englewood Cliffs, NJ, 1976, 336.
4. Cooper, E.L., *General Immunology*, Pergamon Press, New York, 1982, 343.
5. Cooper, E.L., Phylogenetic aspects of transplantation, in *Handbuch der Allgemeinen Pathologie*, Transplantation VI/8, Masshoff, J.W., Ed., Springer-Verlag, Berlin, 1977, 139.
6. Cooper, E.L., Immunity mechanisms, in *Physiology of the Amphibia,* Lofts, B., Ed., Academic Press, New York, 1976, 164.
7. Cooper, E.L., Klempau, A.E., and Zapata, A.G., Reptilian immunity, in *Biology of the Reptilia*, Vol. 14, Gans, C., Ed., John Wiley & Sons, New York, 1985, 599.
8. Streilein, J.W., Skin-associated lymphoid tissue (SALT): origins and functions, *J. Invest. Dermatol.*, 80, 12s, 1983.
9. Bos, J.D. and Kapsenberg, M.L., The skin immune system: progress in cutaneous biology, *Immunol. Today,* 14, 75, 1993.
10. Maurer, D. and Stingl, G., Langerhans cells, in *Dendritic Cells*, Lotze, M.T. and Thomson, A.W., Eds., Academic Press, London, 2001, chap. 5.
11. Mackenzie, I.C. and Squier, C.A., Cytochemical identification of ATPase-positive Langerhans cells in EDTA-separated sheets of mouse epidermis, *Br. J. Dermatol.*, 92, 523, 1975.
12. Robins, P.G. and Brandon, D.R., A modification of the adenosine triphosphatase method to demonstrate epidermal Langerhans cell, *Stain Tech.*, 56, 87, 1981.
13. Maruyama, T., Uda, H., and Yokoyama, M., Localization of non-specific esterase and endogenous peroxidase in the murine Langerhans cells, *Br. J. Dermatol.*, 103, 61, 1980.
14. Hart, D.N.J. et al., Phenotypic characterization of dendritic cells, in *Dendritic Cells*, Lotze, M.T. and Thomson, A.W., Eds., Academic Press, London, 2001, chap. 8.
15. Birbeck, M.S., Breathnach, A.S., and Everall, J.D., An electron microscopic study of basal melanocytes and high level clear cells (Langerhans cells) in vitiligo, *J. Invest. Dermatol.*, 37, 51, 1961.
16. Farqhuar, M. and Palade, G., Adenosine triphosphatase localization in amphibian epidermis, *J. Cell. Biol.*, 30, 359, 1966.
17. Banerjee, T.K. and Hoshino, T., ATPase-positive and metallophilic cells in the skin of frog *Rana catesbeiana, Nagoya J. Med. Sci.*, 47, 83, 1985.
18. Castell, A.E., Caracterización Morfológica de las Células de Langerhans de Anfibios, M.Sci. thesis, Universidad Nacional Autónoma de México, Mexico City, 1989.
19. Carrillo, J. et al., Langerhans like cells in amphibian epidermis, *J. Anat.*, 172, 39, 1990.
20. Du Pasquier, L. and Flajnik, M.F., Expression of MHC class II antigens during *Xenopus* development, *Dev. Immunol.*, 1, 85, 1990.
21. Castell-Rodríguez, A.E. et al., ATPase and MHC class II molecules co-expression in *Rana pipiens* dendritic cells, *Dev. Comp. Immunol.*, 23, 473, 1999.
22. Schuler, G. et al., Subsets of epidermal Langerhans cells as defined by lectin binding profiles, *J. Invest. Dermatol.*, 81, 397, 1983.

23. Dezutter-Dambuyant, C. et al., Quantitative evaluation of two distinct cell populations expressing HLA-DR antigens in normal human epidermis, *Br. J. Dermatol.*, 111, 1, 1984.
24. Romani, N. et al., The thy-1 bearing cell of murine epidermis. A distinctive leukocyte perhaps related to natural killer cells, *J. Exp. Med.*, 161, 1368, 1985.
25. Schmitt, D.A. et al., *In vitro* human epidermal indeterminate cells (CD1a$^+$, 40 kD Fc-gamma-R-) are potent immunostimulatory cells for allogenic lymphocytes, *J. Invest. Dermatol.*, 91, 388, 1988.
26. Cumberbatch, M. et al., MHC class II expression by Langerhans' cells and lymph node dendritic cells: possible evidence for maturation of Langerhans' cells following contact sensitization, *Immunology*, 74, 414, 1991.
27. Castell, A., et al., unpublished data, 2003.
28. Hanau, D. et al., ATPase and morphologic changes in Langerhans cells induced by epicutaneous applications of a sensitizing dose of DNFB, *J. Invest. Dermatol.*, 92, 689, 1989.
29. Hanau, D. et al., La formation des granules de Langerhans semble liee a l'activite ATPasique membranaire de cellules de Langerhans epidermiques, *C.R. Acad. S.C. Paris*, 301, 167, 1985.
30. Picut, C.A., Lee, C.S., and Lewis, R.M., Ultrastructural and phenotypic changes in Langerhans cells induced *in vitro* by contact allergens, *Br. J. Dermatol.*, 116, 773, 1987.
31. Poulter, L.W. et al., Immunohistological analysis of delayed-type hypersensitivity in man, *Cell. Immunol.*, 74, 358, 1982.
32. Scheynius, A. et al., Phenotypic characterization *in situ* of inflammatory cells in allergic and irritant contact dermatitis in man, *Clin. Exp. Immunol.*, 55, 81, 1982.
33. Roberts, L. et al., Correlation between the inducible keratinocyte expression of Ia and the movement of Langerhans cells into the epidermis, *J. Invest. Dermatol.*, 134, 3781, 1985.
34. Breathnach, S.M., Immunologic aspects of contact dermatitis, *Clin. Dermatol.*, 4, 5, 1986.
35. Horton, J.J., Ontogeny of immune system in amphibians, *Am. Zool.*, 11, 219, 1971.
36. Zapata, A.G. and Cooper, E.L., *The Immune System: Comparative Histophysiology*, Wiley, Chichester, U.K., 1990, chap 6.
37. Herrera, M.A., Sampedro, A.E., and Castell, A.E., unpublished data, 2003.
38. Mommaas, M. et al., Functional human epidermal Langerhans cells that lack Birbeck granules, *J. Invest. Dermatol.*, 103, 807, 1994.
39. Drexhage, H.A., et al., A study of cells present in peripheral lymph of pigs with special reference to a type of cell resembling the Langerhans cell, *Cell Tissue Res.*, 202, 407, 1979.
40. Takehana, S. et al., Ultrastructural observations on Langerhans cells in the rat gingival epithelium, *J. Periodont. Res.*, 20, 275, 1985.
41. Romano, J. and Balaguer, R., Ultrastructural identification of Langerhans cells in normal swine epidermis, *J. Anat.*, 179, 43, 1991.
42. Breathnach, A.S. and Wyllie, L.M., Electron microscopy of melanocytes and Langerhans cells in human fetal epidermis at fourteen weeks, *J. Invest. Dermatol.*, 44, 51, 1965.
43. Baculi, B.S. and Cooper, E.L., Lymphoid changes during antibody synthesis in larval *Rana catesbeiana*, *J. Exp. Zool.*, 183, 185, 1970.
44. Jones, S.E. and Ruben, N., Internal histocompatibility during amphibian metamorphosis?, *Immunology*, 43, 741, 1981.
45. Chardonnens, X. and DuPasquier, L., Induction of skin allograft tolerance during metamorphosis of the toad *Xenopus laevis*: a possible model for studying generation of self tolerance to histocompatibility antigens, *J. Immunol.*, 3, 569, 1973.
46. Castell, A.E., et al., Non-specific esterase-positive dendritic cells in epithelia of the frog *Rana pipiens*, *Histochem. J.*, 33, 311, 2001.
47. Li, C.Y., Lam, K.W., and Yam, L.T., Esterases in human leukocytes, *J. Histochem. Cytochem.*, 21, 1, 1973.
48. Havenith, C.E.G. et al., Separation of alveolar macrophages and dendritic cells via autofluorescence: phenotypical and functional characterization, *J. Leukocyte Biol.*, 53, 504, 1993.
49. Holt, P., et al., Function(s) of pulmonary dendritic cells *in vivo* by resident alveolar macrophages, *J. Exp. Med.*, 177, 379, 1993.
50. Austyn, J.M., Lymphoid dendritic cells, *Immunology*, 62, 161, 1987.
51. Steptoe, R.J., O'Connell, P.J., and Thomson A.W., Dendritic cells in the liver, kidney, heart, and pancreas, in *Dendritic Cells*, Lotze, M.T. and Thomson, A.W., Eds., Academic Press, London, 2001, chap. 24.

52. Knight, S.C., et al., Non-adherent, low density cells from human peripheral blood contain dendritic cells and monocytes, both with veiled morphology, *Immunology*, 57, 595, 1986.
53. Cavanagh, L.L. and von Adrian, U.H., Travellers in many guises: the origins and destinations of dendritic cells, *Immunol. Cell Biol.*, 80, 448, 2002.
54. Kamperdijk, E.W.A., Macrophages in different compartments of the non-neoplastic lymph node, *Curr. Topics Pathol.*, 84, 219, 1990.
55. Veerman, A.J.P. and van Ewijk, W., White pulp compartments in the spleen of rats and mice, *Cell Tissue Res.*, 156, 416, 1975.
56. Kamperdijk, E.W.A. et al., Characterization of dendritic cells, isolated from normal and stimulated lymph-nodes of the rat, *Cell Tissue Res.*, 242, 469, 1985.
57. Duijvestijn, A.M. and Kamperdijk, E.W.A., Birbeck granules in interdigitating cells of thymus and lymph node, *Cell Biol. Int. Rep.*, 6, 655, 1982.
58. Plytycz, B. and Bigaj, J., Seasonal cyclic changes in the thymus gland of the adult frog *Rana temporaria*, *Thymus*, 5, 327, 1983.
59. Bigaj, J. and Plytycz, B., Cytoarquitecture of the thymus of the adult frog *Rana temporaria*, *Folia Histochem. Cytobiol.*, 22, 63, 1984.
60. Bigaj, J. and Plytycz, B., Interdigitating cells in the thymus of the frog *Rana temporaria*, *Folia Histochem. Cytobiol.*, 24, 65, 1987.
61. Alvarez, R., Thymus of *Rana perezi*: presence of interdigitating cells, *J. Morphol.*, 204, 305, 1990.
62. Barrutia, M.G. et al., Presence of presumptive interdigitating cells in the spleen of the natterjack *Bufo calamita, Experientia*, 41, 1393, 1985.
63. Castell, A.E., Hernández, A., and Sampedro, E.A., unpublished data, 2003.
64. Barondes, S.H., Soluble lectins: a new class of extracellular proteins, *Science*, 223, 1259, 1984.
65. Dockray, G.J. and Hokins, C.R., Caerulein secretion by dermal glands in *Xenopus laevis*, *J. Cell Biol.*, 64, 1975.
66. Bols, N.C. et al., Secretion of a cytoplasmic lectin from *Xenopus laevis* skin, *J. Cell Biol.*, 102, 492, 1986.
67. Daly, J.W. and Witkop, B., Chemistry and pharmacology of frog venoms, in *Venomous Animals and Their Venoms*, Vol. 2, Bucherl, W. and Buckley, E., Eds., Academic Press, New York, 1971, 497.
68. Erspamer, V. and Melchiorri, P., Active polypeptides: from amphibian skin to gastrointestinal tract and brain of mammals, *Trends Pharmacol. Sci.*, 1, 391, 1975.
69. Gartner, T.K. and Ogilivie, M.L., Isolation and characterization of three $Ca^{2+}$-dependent B-galactoside-specific lectin from snake venoms, *Biochem. J.*, 224, 301, 1984.
70. Ogilivie, M.L. and Gartner, T.K., Identification of lectins in snake venoms, *J. Herpetol.*, 18, 285, 1984.
71. Du Pasquier, L., Antibody diversity in lower vertebrates — why is it so restricted. *Nature*, 296, 311, 1982.
72. Perez-Torres, A., Millán-Aldaco, D.A., and Rondán-Zárate, A., Epidermal Langerhans cells in the terrestrial turtle, *Kinosternum integrum. Dev. Comp. Immunol.*, 19, 225, 1995.
73. Wolff, K. and Winklemann, R.K., Ultrastructural localization of nucleoside triphosphatase in Langerhans cells, *J. Invest. Dermatol.*, 48, 50, 1967.
74. Wolff, K., The fine structure of the Langerhans cell granule, *J. Cell Biol.*, 35, 468, 1967.
75. Hashimoto, K., Langerhans cell granule, *Arch. Dermatol.*, 104, 148, 1971.
76. Takahashi, S. and Hashimoto, K., Derivation of Langerhans cell granules from cytomembrane, *J. Invest. Dermatol.*, 84, 469, 1985.
77. Falck, B., Andersson, A., and Bartosik, J., Some new ultrastructural aspects on human epidermis and its Langerhans cells, *Scand. J. Immunol.*, 21, 409, 1985.
78. Bartosik, J., Cytomembrane-derived Birbeck granules transport horseradish peroxidase to endosomal compartment in the human Langerhans cells, *J. Invest. Dermatol.*, 99, 53, 1992.
79. Hanau, D. et al., Human epidermal Langerhans cells internalize by receptor-mediated endocytosis T-6 (CD1 "NA1/34") surface antigen. Birbeck granules are involved in the intracellular traffic of the T6 antigen, *J. Invest. Dermatol.*, 89, 172, 1987.
80. Hanau, D. et al., Human epidermal Langerhans cells cointernalize by receptor-mediated endocytosis "non-classical" major histocompatibility complex class I molecules (T6 antigens) and class II molecules (HLA-DR antigens), *Proc. Natl. Acad. Sci. U.S.A.*, 84, 2001, 1987.

81. Hanau, D., et al., Appearance of Birbeck granule-like structures in anti-T6-antibody-treated human Langerhans cells, *J. Invest. Dermatol.*, 90, 298, 1988.
82. Hollis, D.E. and Lyne, A.G., Acetylcholinesterase-positive Langerhans cells in the epidermis of wool follicles of the sheep, *J. Invest. Dermatol.*, 58, 211, 1972.
83. Khalil, M.M., Nitiuthai, S., and Allen, J.R., Alkaline phosphatase positive Langerhans cells in the epidermis of cattle, *J. Invest. Dermatol.*, 79, 47, 1982.
84. Monteiro-Riviere, N.A., Ultrastructure of the integument of the domestic pig (*Sus scrofa*) from one through fourteen weeks of age, *Anat. Histol. Embryol.*, 14, 97, 1985.
85. Wolff, K., The Langerhans cell, *Curr. Probl. Dermatol.*, 4, 79, 1972.
86. Böck, P., Fine structure of Langerhans cells in the stratified epithelia of the oesophagus and stomach of mice, *Z. Zellforsch. Mikrosk. Anat.*, 147, 237, 1974
87. Al Yassin, T.M. and Toner, D.G., Langerhans cells in human oesophagus, *J. Anat.*, 122, 435, 1976.
88. Belsito, et al., Effect of glucocorticosteroids on epidermal Langerhans cells, *J. Exp. Med.*, 155, 291, 1982.
89. Berman, B. et al., Modulation of expression of epidermal Langerhans cell properties following *in situ* exposure to glucocorticosteroids, *J. Invest. Dermatol.*, 80, 168, 1983.
90. Koyama, Y. et al., Effect of systemic and topical application of testosterone propionate on the density of epidermal Langerhans cells in the mouse, *J. Invest. Dermatol.*, 92, 86, 1989.
91. Zapata, A.G., Varas, A., and Torroba, M., Seasonal variations in the immune system of the lower vertebrates, *Immunol. Today,* 13, 142, 1992.
92. El Ridi, R. et al., Cyclic changes in the differentiation of lymphoid cells in reptiles, *Cell Differ.*, 24, 1, 1988.
93. Thomas, I.G. and Ratcliffe, N.A., Integumental grafting and immunorecognition in insects, *Dev. Comp. Immunol.*, 6, 643, 1982.
94. Jones, S.E. and Bell, W.J., Cell-mediated immune-type response of the American cockroach, *Dev. Comp. Immunol.*, 6, 35, 1982.
95. Lackie, A.M., Immunological recognition of cuticular transplants in insects, *Dev. Comp. Immunol.*, 7, 41, 1983.
96. George, J.F., Karp, R.D., and Rheins, L.A., Primary integumentary xenograft reactivity in the American cockroach, *Periplenta americana*, *Transplantation*, 37, 478, 1984.
97. George, J.F., Howcroft, T.K., and Karp, R.D., Primary integumentary allograft reactivity in the American cockroach, *Periplanta americana*, *Transplantation*, 43, 524, 1987.
98. Cooper, E.L. and Roch, P., Second set allograft response in the earthworm, *Lumbricus terrestis*: kinetics and characteristics, *Transplantation,* 41, 514, 1986.
99. Cooper, E.L. and Roch, P., Earthworm leukocyte interactions during early stages of graft rejection, *J. Exp. Zool.*, 232, 67, 1984.
100. Raftos, D.A., Tait, N.N., and Briscoe, D.A., Allograft rejection and alloimmune memory in the solitary urochordate, *Styela plicata, Dev. Comp. Immunol.*, 11, 343, 1987.
101. Raftos, D.A., Tait, N.N., and Briscoe, D.A., Cellular basis of allograft rejection in the solitary urochordate, *Styela plicata*, *Dev. Comp. Immunol.*, 11, 713, 1987.
102. Raftos, D.A., Briscoe, D.A., and Tait, N.N., Mode of recognition of allogeneic tissue in the solitary urochordate *Styela plicata*, *Transplantation,* 45, 1123, 1988.
103. Komen, J. et al., Skin grafting in gynogenetic common carp (*Cyprinus carpio,* L.). The development of histocompatible clones, *Transplantation*, 49, 788, 1990.
104. Nevid, N.J. and Meier, A.H., A day-night rhythm of immune activity during scale allograft rejection in the gulf killifish, *Fundulus grandis*, *Dev. Comp. Immunol.*, 17, 221, 1993.
105. Afifi, A., Mohamed, E.R., and El Ridi, R., Seasonal conditions determine the manner of skin rejection in reptiles. *J. Exp. Zool.*, 265, 459, 1993.
106. Hackney, M.J., Investigation of the skin of rainbow trout *Salmo gaidneri* Richards for antigen uptake mechanisms following spray vaccination, in *Fish Immunology*, Manning M.J. and Tatner M.F., Eds., Academic Press, New York, 1958, 195.
107. Sigel, M.M., Hamby, B.A., and Higgins, E.M., Phylogenetic studies on lymphokines. Fish lymphocytes respond to IL-1 and epithelial cells produce an IL-1 like factor, *Vet. Immunol. Immunopathol.*, 12, 47, 1986.

108. Fletcher, T.C. and Grant, T.T., Immunoglobulins in the serum and mucus of the plaice *Pleuronectes platessa*, *Biochem. J.*, 115, 65, 1969.
109. St. Louis Cormier, E.A., Osterland, C.K., and Anderson, P.D., Evidence for a cutaneous secretory immune system in rainbow trout *Salmo gaidneri* Richards, *Dev. Comp. Immunol.*, 8, 77, 1984.
110. Peleteiro, M.C. and Richards, R.H., Identification of lymphocytes in the epidermis of the rainbow trout *Salmo gaidneri* Richards, *J. Fish Dis.*, 8, 161, 1985.
111. Baldo, B.A. and Fletcher, T.C., Phylogenetic aspects of hypersensitivity: immediate hypersensitivity reactions in flatfish, in *Immunologic Phylogeny*, Hildemann, W.H. and Benedict, A.A., Eds., Plenum Press, London, 1975, 365.
112. Fletcher, T.C., Defense mechanisms in fish, in *Biochemical and Biophysical Perspectives in Marine Biology*, Vol. 4, Malins, D.C. and Sargent, R., Eds., Academic Press, New York, 1978, 189.
113. Fletcher, T.C., Non-antibody molecules and the defense mechanisms of fish, in *Stress and Fish*, Pickering, A.D., Ed., Academic Press, New York, 1981, 171.
114. Fletcher, T.C. and Baldo, B.A., Immediate hypersensitivity responses in flatfish, *Science*, 185, 360, 1974.
115. Anderson, A.A., Fletcher, T.C., and Smith, G.M., The release of prostaglandin E2 from the skin of the plaice, *Pleuronectes platessa* L., *Br. J. Pharmacol.*, 66, 547, 1979.
116. Carnuccio, R., Di Rosa, M., and Persico, P., Hydrocortisone-induced inhibitor of prostaglandin biosynthesis in rat leukocytes, *Br. J. Pharmacol.*, 68, 14, 1980.
117. Coombs, R.R.A. and Gell, P.G.H., in *Clinical Aspects of Immunology*, Gell, P.G.H. and Coombs, R.R.A., Eds., Blackwell, Oxford, 1968, 575.
118. Anderson, A.A., Fletcher, T.C., and Smith, G.M., The release of prostaglandin E2 from the skin of the plaice, *Pleuronectes platessa* L., *Br. J. Pharmacol.*, 66, 547, 1979.
119. Dreyer, N.B. and King, J.W., Anaphylaxis in the fish, *J. Immunol.*, 60, 277, 1978.
120. Baldo, B.A., Fletcher, T.C., and Pepys, J., Isolation of a peptido-polysaccharide from the dermatophyte *Epidermophyton floccosum* and a study of its reaction with C-reactive protein and a mouse antiphosphorylcholine myeloma serum, *Immunology*, 32, 831, 1977.
121. Anderson, A.A., Fletcher, T.C., and Smith, G.M., Prostaglandin biosynthesis in the skin of the plaice *Pleuronectes platessa* L., *Comp. Biochem. Physiol.*, 70c, 195, 1981.
122. Ashraf, A.J., Smith, G.M., and Fletcher, T.C., Isolation of substances with vascular permeability-increasing activity from the skin of the plaice (*Pleuronectes platessa* L.), *Comp. Biochem. Physiol.*, 81C, 53, 1985.
123. Bach, M.K., Mediators of anaphylaxis and inflammation, *Annu. Rev. Microbiol.*, 36, 371, 1982.
124. Wasserman, M.P., Leukocytes and melanin pigmentation, *J. Invest. Dermatol.*, 45, 104, 1965.
125. Blackstock, N. and Pickering, A.D., Acidophilic granular cells in the epidermis of the brown trout, *Salmo trutta* L., *Cell Tissue Res.*, 210, 359, 1980.
126. Bhatti, H.K., The integument and dermal skeleton of siluroidea, *Trans. Zool. Soc. Lond.*, 24, 1, 1938.
127. Mittal, A.K. and Munshi, J.S.D., A comparative study of the structure of the skin of certain air-breathing fresh-water teleosts, *J. Zool. Lond.*, 163, 515, 1971.
128. Mittal, A.K. and Munshi, J.S.D., On the regeneration and repair of superficial wounds in the skin of *Rita rita* (Ham) (Bagridae, Pisces), *Acta Anat.*, 88, 424, 1974.
129. Mittal, A.K. and Banerjee, T.K., Histochemistry and the structure of the skin of a murrel, *Channa striata* (Bloch) (Channiformes, Channidae). 1. Epidermis, *Can. J. Zool.*, 53, 833, 1977.
130. Mittal, A.K. and Banerjee, T.K., Functional organization of the skin of the green-puffer-fish *Tetraodon fluviatilis* (Ham.-Buck.) (Tetraodontidae, Pisces), *Zoomorphologie*, 84, 195, 1976.
131. Mittal, A.K., Agarwal, S.K., and Banerjee, T.K., Protein and carbohydrate histochemistry in relation to the keratinization in the epidermis of *Barbus sophur* (Cyprinidae, Pisces), *J. Zool. Lond.*, 179, 1, 1976.
132. Mittal, A.K. and Agarwal, S.K., Histochemistry of the unicellular glands in relation to their physiological significance in the epidermis of *Monopterus cuchia* (Symbranchiformes, Pisces), *J. Zool. Lond.*, 182, 429, 1977.
133. Robert, R.J., Young, H., and Milne, J.A., Studies on the skin of plaice (*Pleuronectes platessa* L.). 1. The structure and ultrastructure of normal plaice skin, *J. Fish Biol.*, 4, 87, 1971.
134. Bullock, A.M. and Roberts, R.J., The dermatology of marine teleost fish. 1. The normal integument, *Oceanogr. Mar. Biol. Annu. Rev.*, 13, 383, 1975.

135. Celada, M. and de Paoli, A.M., Contributo alla conoscenza delle cellu albuminose (Schneider) cutanee di *Torpedo ocellata* Raf., *Riv. Istochim. Norm. Pat.*, 8, 411, 1962.
136. Pickering, A.D., Seasonal changes in the epidermis of the brown trout *Salmo trutta* (L.), *J. Fish Biol.*, 10, 561, 1977.
137. Banerjee, T.K., Agarwal, S.K., and Rai, A.K., Histochemical localization of alkaline phosphatase, acid phosphatase, and succinic dehydrogenase activities in the epidermis of the freshwater teleost *Amphipnous cuchia* (Hamilton) (Symbranchiformes, Pisces), *Mikroskopie*, 3, 294, 1976.
138. Nigrelli, R.F., On the effect of fish mucous on *Epibdella melleni*, a monogenetic trematode of marine fishes, *J. Parasitol.*, 21, 43 1935.
139. Bradshaw, C.M., Richard, A.S., and Sigel, M.M., IgM antibodies fish mucus, *Proc. Soc. Exp. Biol. Med.*, 136, 1122, 1971.
140. Magarinos, B. et al., Response of *Pasteurella piscicida* and *Flexibacter maritimus* to skin mucus of marine fish, *Dis. Aquat. Organ.*, 21, 103, 1995.
141. Weinnels, E.L., Studies on the fine structure of teleost blood cell, *Anat. Rec.*, 147, 219, 1963.
142. Cross, M.L. and Mathews, R.A., Localized leukocyte response to *Ichthyophthirius multifiliis* establishment in immune carp *Cyprinus carpio* L., *Vet. Immunol. Immunopathol.*, 38, 341, 1993.
143. Khangarot, B.S. and Tripathi, D.M., Changes in humoral and cell-mediated immune responses and in skin and respiratory surfaces of catfish, *Saccobranchus fossilis*, following copper exposure, *Ecotoxicol. Environ. Saf.*, 22, 291, 1991.
144. Dalmo, R.A., Ingebrigtsen, K., and Bogwald, J., Non-specific defence mechanisms in fish, with particular reference to the reticuloendothelial system (RES), *J. Fish Dis.*, 20, 241, 1997.
145. Alexander, J.B. and Ingram, G.A., Noncellular nonspecific defence mechanisms of fish, *Annu. Rev. Fish Dis.*, 2, 249, 1992.
146. Ellis, A.E., Non-specific defence mechanisms in fish and their role in disease, *Processes Develop. Biol. Standard.*, 49, 337, 1981.
147. Ebran, N. et al., Pore-forming properties and antibacterial activity of protein extracted from epidermal mucus of fish, *Comp. Biochem. Physiol. A.*, 122, 181, 1999.
148. Bols, N.S. et al., Ecotoxicology and innate immunity in fish, *Dev. Comp. Immunol.*, 25, 853, 2001.
149. Iger, Y. and Wendelaar Bonga, S.E., Cellular responses of the skin of carp (*Cyprinus carpio*) exposed to acidified water, *Cell Tissue Res.*, 275, 481, 1994.
150. Abraham, M., Iger, Y., and Zhang, L., Fine structure of the skin cells of a stenohaline freshwater fish *Cyprinus carpio* exposed to diluted seawater, *Tissue Cell*, 33, 46, 2001.
151. Iger, Y., Jenner, H.A., and Wendelaar Bonga S.E., Cellular responses in skin of the trout (*Oncorhynchus mykiss*) exposed to temperature elevation, *J. Fish Biol.*, 44, 921, 1994.
152. Burkhardt-Holm, P., Escher, M., and Meier W., Waste-water management plant effluents cause cellular alterations in the skin of brown trout, *J. Fish Biol.*, 50, 744, 1997.
153. Asbakk, K., Elimination of foreign material by epidermal malpighian cells during wound healing in fish skin, *J. Fish Biol.*, 58, 953, 2001.
154. Bakke, T.A., Jansen, P.A., and Kennedy, C.R., The host specificity of *Gyrodactylus salaries* Malmberg (Platyhelminthes, Monogenea): susceptibility of *Oncorhynchus mykiis* (Walbaum) under experimental conditions, *J. Fish Biol.*, 39, 45, 1991.
155. Lindenstrøm, T. and Buchmann, K., Acquired resistance in rainbow trout against *Gyrodactylus derjavini, J. Helmintol.*, 74, 155, 2000.
156. Buchmann, K., Immune mechanisms in fish skin against monogeneans — a model, *Folia Parasitol.* (Praha), 46, 1, 1999.
157. Buchmann, K. and Bresciani, J., Microenvironment of *Gyrodactylus derjavini* on rainbow trout *Oncorhynchus mykiis*: association between mucous cell density in skin and site selection, *Parasitol. Res.*, 84, 17, 1998.
158. Lindenstrøm, T., Buchmann, K., and Secombes, C.J., *Gyrodactylus derjavini* infection elicits IL-1 expression in rainbow trout skin, *Fish Shellfish Immunol*, 15, 107, 2003.
159. Hauser, C. et al., Interleukin 1 is present in normal human epidermis, *J. Immunol.*, 136, 3317, 1986.
160. Kupper, T.S., Immune and inflammatory processes in cutaneous tissues — mechanisms and speculations, *J. Clin. Invest.*, 86, 1783, 1990.
161. Lee, R.T. et al., Mechanical deformation promotes secretion of IL-1α and IL-1 receptor antagonist, *J. Immunol.*, 159, 5084, 1997.

162. Hong, S. et al., The production and bioactivity of rainbow trout (*Oncorhynchus mykiis*) recombinant IL-1β, *Vet. Immunol. Immunopathol.*, 81, 1, 2001.
163. Shornick, L.P., Bisarya, A.K., and Chaplin, D.D., IL-1β is essential for Langerhans cell activation and antigen delivery to the lymph nodes during contact sensitization: evidence for a dermal source of IL-1β, *Cell. Immunol.*, 211, 105, 2001.
164. Titus, R.G., Sherry, B., and Cerami, A., The involvement of TNF, IL-1 and IL-6 in the immune response to protozoan parasites, *Immunol. Today*, 12, 13, 1991.
165. Buchmann, K. and Bresciani, J., Rainbow trout leucocyte activity: influence on the ectoparasitic monogenean *Gyrodactylus derjavini, Dis. Aquat. Organ.*, 35, 13, 1999.
166. Buchamann, K., Binding and lethal effect of complement from *Oncorhynchus mykiis* on *Gyrodactylus derjavini* (Platyhelminthes: Monogenea), *Dis. Aquat. Organ.*, 32, 195, 1998.
167. Engelsma, M.Y. et al., Neuroendocrine-immune interactions in fish: a role for interleukin-1, *Vet. Immunol. Immunopathol.*, 87, 467, 2002.
168. Huising, M.O. et al., Increased efficacy of immersion vaccination in fish with hyperosmotic pretreatment, *Vaccine*, 21, 4178, 2003.
169. Saeij, J.P. et al., Molecular and functional characterization of carp TNF: a link between TNF polymorphism and trypanotolerance? *Dev. Comp. Immunol.*, 27, 29, 2003.
170. Magor, B.G. and Magor, K.E., Evolution of effectors and receptors of innate immunity, *Dev. Comp. Immunol.*, 25, 651, 2001.
171. Medzhitov, R. and Janeway, C.A., Jr., Innate immunity: impact on the adaptive immune response, *Curr. Opin. Immunol.*, 9, 4, 1997.
172. Medzhitov, R. and Janeway, C.A., Jr., Innate immunity: the virtues of a nonclonal system of recognition, *Cell*, 91, 295, 1997.
173. Steinman, R.M., The dendritic cell system and its role in immunogenicity, *Annu. Rev. Immunol.*, 9, 271, 1991.
174. Ibrahim, M.A.A., Chain, B.M., and Katz, D.R., The injured cell: the role of the dendritic cells system as a sentinel receptor pathway, *Immunol. Today*, 6, 181, 1995.
175. Banchereau, J. and Steinman, R.M., Dendritic cells and the control of immunity, *Nature*, 392, 245, 1998.
176. Dubois, B. et al., Dendritic cells enhance growth and differentiation of CD-40-activated B lymphocytes, *J. Exp. Med.*, 185, 941, 1997.
177. de Fraissinette, A., Schmitt, D., and Thivolet, J., Langerhans cells of human mucosa, *J. Dermatol.*, 16, 255, 1989.
178. Foti, M. et al., Upon dendritic cells activation chemokines and chemokine receptor expression are rapidly regulated for recruitment and maintenance of dendritic cells at inflammatory site, *Int. Immunol.*, 11, 979, 1998.
179. Sallusto, F. et al., Rapid and coordinated switch in chemokine receptor expression during dendritic cell maturation, *Eur. J. Immunol.*, 28, 2760, 1998.
180. Fernandez, N.C. et al., Dendritic cells directly trigger NK cell functions: cross-talk relevant in innate anti-tumor immune responses *in vivo, Nat. Med.*, 5, 405, 1999.
181. Rescigno, M., et al., Coordinated events during bacteria-induced DC maturation, *Immunol. Today*, 20, 200, 1999.
182. Macatonia, S.E. et al., Localization of antigen in lymph node dendritic cells after exposure to the contact sensitizer fluorescein isothiocyanate, *J. Exp. Med.*, 166, 1654, 1987.
183. Kripke, M.L. et al., Evidence that cutaneous antigen-presenting cells migrate to regional lymph nodes during contact sensitization, *J. Immunol.*, 145, 2833, 1990.
184. Moll, H., Fuchs, H., and Rollinghof, M., Langerhans cells transport leishmania major from the infected skin to the draining lymph node for presentation to antigen-specific T cells, *Eur. J. Immunol.*, 23, 1595, 1993.
185. Fernandez, N.C. et al., NK cells, in *Dendritic Cells: Biology and Clinical Applications*, Lotze, M.T. and Thompson, A.W., Eds., Academic Press, London, 2001, chap. 18.
186. Rescigno, M. et al., Interaction of dendritic cells with bacteria, in *Dendritic Cells: Biology and Clinical Applications*, Lotze, M.T. and Thompson, A.W., Eds., Academic Press, London, 2001, chap. 34.

187. Press, C.McL., Dannevig, B.H., and Landsverk, T., Immune and enzyme histochemical phenotypes of lymphoid and nonlymphoid cells within the spleen and head kidney of Atlantic salmon (*Salmo salar* L.), *Fish Shellfish Immunol.*, 4, 79, 1994.
188. Ganassin, R.C. and Bols, N.C., Development of long-term rainbow trout spleen cultures that are haemopoietic and produce dendritic cells, *Fish Shellfish Immunol.*, 6, 17, 1996.
189. Steinman, R.M. and Cohn, Z.A., Identification of a novel cell type in peripheral lymphoid organs of mice. I. Morphology, quantification, and tissue distribution, *J. Exp. Med.*, 137, 1142, 1973.
190. Steinman, R.M. and Cohn, Z.A., Identification of a novel cell type in peripheral lymphoid organs of mice. II. Functional properties *in vitro, J. Exp. Med.*, 139, 380, 1974.
191. Steinman, R.M., Lustig, D.S., and Cohn, Z.A., Identification of a novel cell type in peripheral lymphoid organs of mice. III. Functional properties *in vivo, J. Exp. Med.*, 139, 1431, 1974.
192. Estepa, A. and Coll, J.M., Properties of blast colonies obtained from trout head-kidney in fibrin clot cultures, *Fish Shellfish Immunol.*, 3, 71, 1993.
193. Vallejo, A.N., Miller, N.W., and Clem, L.W., Cellular pathway(s) of antigen processing in fish APC: effect of varying *in vitro* temperatures on antigen catabolism, *Dev. Comp. Immunol.*, 16, 367, 1992.
194. Zapata, A., Ultrastructural study of the teleost fish kidney, *Dev. Comp. Immunol.*, 3, 55, 1979.
195. Lobb, C.J., Secretory immunity induced in catfish, *Ictalurus punctatus*, following bath immunization, *Dev. Comp. Immunol.*, 11, 727, 1987.
196. Pérez, A., Caracterización morfológica de las células de Langerhans del pollo, M.Sci. thesis, Universidad Nacional Autónoma de México, Mexico City, 1989.
197. Carrillo, J. et al., Adenosine triphospatase-positive Langerhans-like cells in the epidermis of the chicken (*Gallus gallus*), *J. Anat.*, 176, 1, 1991.
198. Pérez, A. and Millán, D.A., Ia antigens are expressed on ATPase-positive dendritic cells in chicken epidermis, *J. Anat.*, 184, 591, 1994.
199. Pérez, A. and Ustarroz, M., Demonstration of Birbeck (Langerhans cells) granules in the normal chicken epidermis, *J. Anat.*, 199, 493, 2001.
200. Aquino, A., Identificación y caracterización morfológica de las células de Langerhans en la piel del bagre *Arius seemanii*, Günther, thesis, Universidad Nacional Autónoma de México, Mexico City, 2003.
201. Pérez, A. et al., unpublished data, 2003.
202. Dixon, B. and Stet, R.J.M., The relationship between major histocompatibility receptors and innate immunity in teleost fish, *Dev. Comp. Immunol.*, 25, 683, 2001.
203. van Erp, S.H.M. et al., Identification and characterization of a novel MHC class I gene from carp (*Cyprinus carpio* L.), *Immunogenetics*, 44, 49, 1996.
204. Rodrigues, P.N. et al., Expression and temperature-dependent regulation of the beta2-microglobulin (*Cyca-B2m*) gene in a cold-blooded vertebrate, the common carp (*Cyprinus carpio* L.), *Dev. Immunol.*, 5, 263, 1998.
205. Antao, A.B. et al., MHC class I genes of the channel catfish: sequence analysis and expression, *Immunogenetics*, 49, 303, 1999.
206. Van Lierop, J.C. et al., Production and characterization of an antiserum raised against recombinant rainbow trout (*Oncorhynchus mykiis*) MHC class II beta-chain (MhcOnmy-DAB), *Fish Shellfish Immunol.*, 8, 231, 1998.

# 4 The Immunogenetics of Inflammatory Skin Disease

*William O.C.M. Cookson, Anne C. Bowcock, John I. Harper, and Miriam F. Moffatt*

## CONTENTS



0-8493-1959-5/05/$0.00+$1.50

# I. INTRODUCTION

Living creatures exist within a hostile environment surrounded by constantly evolving threats from other organisms. As a consequence, the genes and proteins of the immune system are often selected to provide a high level of variation. In the modern environment, in which devastating infection is increasingly rare, variation in genes (genetic polymorphism) of the immune system influences many diseases with an inflammatory etiology.

The study of genetics leads to the identification of polymorphism in genes causing susceptibility to disease. The discovery of disease genes by linkage and association is a structured process that provides an assured means of identifying otherwise unrecognizable disease pathways. The study of complex genetic diseases is becoming steadily more tractable, with the promise of new classifications of disease as well as new means of prevention and treatment.

Genomics describes the global examination of gene function. Typically, this may involve sequence analyses, or gene expression profiling. Genomic studies give large amounts of information about thousands or tens of thousands of genes. These type of results are potentially very powerful, but present a considerable challenge in interpretation.

The two most common inflammatory diseases of the skin are atopic dermatitis (AD: eczema) and psoriasis. Both show a strong familial clustering and are due to the interaction of genetic and environmental factors. Surprisingly, there appears to be considerable overlap between the genetic loci that predispose to both diseases. Although most of the genes causing these illnesses are yet to be discovered, their chromosomal locations are in many cases known, and the results of genetic studies are already showing new insights into the etiology of inflammatory dermatoses.

## A. Atopy and Atopic Dermatitis

The atopic state is recognized by skin prick tests to common allergens, by the presence of allergen-specific IgE in their serum, and by elevations of the total serum IgE.[1]

Approximately 80% of cases of childhood eczema are atopic by these criteria.[2,3] Atopic mechanisms consequently dominate current understanding of the pathogenesis of the disease. However, eczema in the 20% of children without atopic manifestations is clinically indistinguishable from disease in those who are atopic,[3,4] and it is not clear whether disease in non-atopics is the result of different processes.

Twin studies of AD show concordance rates of 0.72 to 0.86 in monozygotic and 0.21 to 0.23 in dizygotic twin pairs.[5,6] Physician-diagnosed asthma exhibits a similar pattern, with concordance of 0.65 in monozygotic twins and 0.25 in dizygotic twins.[7] Total serum IgE levels show a heritability of approximately 50%.[1,8] These results indicate the presence of strong genetic factors underlying the development of atopy and AD.

## B. Psoriasis

Psoriasis has a worldwide distribution with prevalence varying according to race and geographical location. It is commonest in Scandinavia and Northern Europe, where it approaches 3%. In North America and the United Kingdom, its prevalence is about 2%. In Japan, the prevalence is 0.2% of the population, and in native American Indians it is rare.[9]

The concordance of psoriasis in monozygotic twins is 0.65 to 0.72 vs. 0.15 to 0.30 in dizygotic twins. Determination of concordance in older twin pairs from a national twin registry in Denmark revealed nearly 90 to 100% heritability.[10] In an Australian study, the monozygotic twin concordance rate was less (0.35 for monozygotic twins and 0.12 for dizygotic twins), giving an estimated heritability of 80%.[11]

Males and females are equally affected and 75% of patients develop the disease before the age of 40. First manifestations of the disease are most common in the third decade. Two peaks of age of onset have been described; a more severe form at 20 to 30 years and a smaller peak at 50 to 60 years, perhaps indicating different subsets of disease.[12] Psoriatic arthritis occurs in 10 to 30% of patients, possibly forming an additional disease variant.

## II. GENOMIC STUDIES OF AD AND PSORIASIS

Although AD is clinically and pathologically quite distinct from psoriasis, some features are shared by both diseases, including dry, scaly skin and disturbed epidermal differentiation. Psoriasis is characterized by infiltration of inflammatory cells into the dermis and epidermis and is accompanied by hyperproliferation of keratinocytes. The latter is not seen in AD. Some insights into these gross changes can be gained by gene expression profiling, in which the genes actively transcribed in a cell or tissue can be systematically identified by DNA microarrays.

Psoriasis has been more thoroughly studied with microarray techniques than has AD. A global expression study of psoriatic skin biopsies highlighted a large number of dysregulated genes and gene clusters, particularly those involved in epithelial proliferation and in the immune system,[13] but did not determine the primary molecular defects underlying the disease.

A smaller expression study of 12,000 selected transcripts compared psoriasis and AD, and indicated that most genes were similarly expressed in both diseases.[14] However, the study reported that chemokines increased twofold in psoriatic vs. AD skin were CCL-4/MIP-1b, CCL20/MIP-3α, CXCL-2/GRO-β, CXCL-8/IL8, and CXCR2/IL8R, as well as MCP-1 and IP-10.[14] These results are consistent with the global gene profiling of psoriatic skin, which revealed the upregulation of 19 chemokines,[13] including most of those described above.

These immunological findings do not explain the massive hyperproliferation of keratinocytes that is a feature of psoriasis. Increased keratinocyte proliferation in psoriasis may explain the differential expression of genes of the epidermal differentiation complex (EDC; see below) that are not seen in AD such as PRP2C, lipocalin, elafin, and airway trypsin-like protease.[14]

Different chemokines may be increased twofold in AD vs. psoriatic skin, including CCL13/MCP-4, CCL-18/PARC, and CCL-27/CTACK. It has also been proposed that keratinocytes of patients with AD have high RANTES expression in lesions.[15]

Nel-1 like 2 protein is involved in the differentiation of growth factors of sensory nerves in the skin. It is overexpressed in AD, which has been interpreted to result in the increased sensitivity and itching that is characteristic of AD.[14] Elevation of tenascin C, an extracellular matrix protein, and plasminogen activator inhibitor, has also been observed.[14]

Significantly lower levels of antimicrobial peptides such as beta-defensin, LL-37, and other innate immune effector molecules have been observed in AD lesions, and it has been proposed that this may explain the increase in the susceptibility of patients with AD to recurrent skin infections.[16]

## III. MOLECULAR GENETICS

The genetic study of complex diseases is more advanced than their genomic study. Candidate genes of known function can be investigated by comparing the frequency of polymorphisms in individuals with and without disease. This approach is limited by the ability to choose rational candidates. Positional cloning is an alternative strategy, which begins with the finding of co-inheritance of disease with particular chromosomal segments. Once such genetic linkage has been established (typically with a genome screen with markers spaced to cover all chromosomes), it then becomes possible to refine progressively the region of linkage until the underlying disease gene has been identified. Positional cloning is a long and laborious pursuit, but it is particularly powerful because it does not rely on any previous knowledge or hypotheses about the etiology of the disease under investigation.

## A. Molecular Genetics of Atopic Dermatitis

### 1. The MHC

The major histocompatibility complex (MHC) is the longest-studied locus influencing atopy. It is well known that *HLA-DR* alleles restrict the IgE response to particular allergens, usually with a relative risk less than 2.[17–20]. In addition, the MHC class II-associated *TNF-308* promoter single nucleotide polymorphism (SNP) shows robust associations with asthma independently of association to particular allergens.[21–27]

The MHC has, however, been little studied in individuals with AD. Genome screens do not show linkage of AD to the region,[28–30] and no convincing associations with HLA class I or class II alleles have been established. Definitive studies are, however, lacking.

The ability to react to particular allergens has also been linked to the *TCR*-α/δ locus (but not *TCR*-β),[31] and *HLA-DR* and *TCR*-α/δ alleles interact in the susceptibility to house dust mite allergens.[32] The importance of γ/δ T cells in dermal immunity suggests that the *TCR*-α/δ locus should also be explored in individuals with AD.

### 2. FcεRI-β (Chromosome 11q13)

Chromosome 11q13 was originally linked to atopy[33] and was subsequently shown to contain the β chain of the high-affinity receptor for IgE.[34] Polymorphisms in *FcεRI*-β are associated with asthma,[35] allergy,[36] bronchial hyperresponsiveness,[37] and AD.[38] These variations seem to be associated with severe atopic disease.

*FcεRI*-β acts as an approximately sevenfold amplifying element of the high-affinity IgE receptor response to activation[39] and stabilizes the expression of the receptor on the mast cell surface.[40] *FcεRI*-β may therefore modify nonspecifically the strength of the response to allergens. Coding polymorphisms have been identified within the gene, but do not appear to alter its function.[41] The actions of other polymorphisms within regulatory elements of the gene[42, 43] are currently under investigation.[44]

### 3. The IL-4 Cytokine Cluster (Chromosome 5q34)

The cytokine cluster on chromosome 5q34 contains many candidates that might influence atopic processes, including *IL-4*, *IL-13*, *GM-CSF*, and *IL-9*. Polymorphisms in *IL-4* may be weakly associated with asthma,[45] but a far stronger association has been established between *IL-13* polymorphisms and increased serum IgE levels,[46] atopy, and asthma.[47–50] The coding polymorphism Arg130->Gln seems to show the strongest effect.[46]

These polymorphisms have not yet been explored for a role in AD. An association between *GM-CSF* and the severity of AD has been suggested but not yet confirmed.[51]

### 4. Mast Cell Tryptase

Mast cell tryptase (chymase) has chymotrypsin-like specificity and is abundant in skin mast cells. An association between a polymorphism in this gene and AD was reported in a Japanese population,[52] but the results have not been replicated in Japanese[53] or Italian[54] subjects.

### 5. RANTES

Allergic inflammation and atopic diseases are characterized by upregulation of C-C chemokine expression. A functional mutation in the proximal promoter of the RANTES gene has been identified, which results in a new consensus binding site for the GATA transcription factor family. Transfection experiments showed that the mutant promoter altered the expression levels of RANTES by a factor of 8.[55] The mutant allele was associated with atopic dermatitis in children of the German

Multicenter Allergy Study, but not with asthma.[55] These results suggest that the mutation may contribute to the development of AD. RANTES is located on chromosome 17, but is some distance from the region of linkage to AD and psoriasis described below. Its potential role now needs to be explored further.

### 6. Genome Screens

Two genome screens for childhood AD have been carried out.[28,29] Both screens were of modest size and were of comparable power. Both used sophisticated statistics to generate empirical *P* values to show that they had identified regions of real genetic linkage. The first screen, carried out in families of German and Scandinavian children with AD, found linkage to a region on chromosome 3q21.[28] The second screen, of British families recruited through children with AD attending a hospital of tertiary referral, found three regions of linkage to AD or to AD and asthma combined, on chromosomes 1q21, 17q25, and 20p.[29]

The first study found also linkage of the total serum IgE to the 3q21 locus[28] and the second study found linkage of this trait to chromosomes 5q31 and 16qtel.[29] In each case the evidence for linkage to the serum IgE was weaker than the evidence for linkage to AD.

A third genome screen has been reported, in which the subjects were Swedish adults with AD who were identified at hospital outpatient clinics.[30] In general, the results were less conclusive than the screens of children with AD. Suggestive evidence was found for linkage of AD to chromosome 3p24-22. The authors also used a severity score of AD and found suggestive linkage to chromosomes 3q14, 13q14, 15q14-15, and 17q21. It is possible that the 3q14 locus and the 17q21 loci may correspond to the AD loci identified in children. Chromosome 13q14 has been previously linked to children with AD[56] and to atopy and asthma.[57] The other loci may be considered to be novel.

### 7. Atopic Dermatitis and Asthma

In all, 11 full genome screens have been reported for asthma and its associated phenotypes,[58–68] and others have been carried out in industry. Several of these screens have been performed in distinct European populations: German,[61] French,[64] Finnish,[65] Icelandic,[66] Dutch,[67] and Danish.[68] These have consistently identified a limited number of regions containing genes influencing asthma, including chromosomes 2, 4, 5, 6, 7, 11, 12, 13, and 16.[69,70] Three genes underlying asthma have been recently identified by fine mapping and positional cloning in regions of genetic linkage. These include the membrane-anchored zinc-dependent metalloproteinase *ADAM33* from chromosome 20,[71] the putative modulator of transcription *PHF11* from chromosome 13q12,[72] and the prolyl peptidase *DPP10* from chromosome 2q14.[73]

*ADAM33* and *DPP10* do not appear to play major roles in AD. However, chromosome 13q12 does shows linkage to AD,[56] and polymorphisms in *PHF11* are strongly associated with high IgE levels in families containing children with AD.[72] The mode of action of *PHF11* is not yet known, but it encodes protein-binding zinc fingers that may modify both immunoglobulin production and clonal expansion of B cells.[72]

In general, however, the loci identified by asthma genome screens are not shared with the regions of linkage to AD, suggesting that AD and asthma are not simply part of the same spectrum of allergic disorders, but that they result at least in part from distinct mechanisms.

## B. Molecular Genetics of Psoriasis

### 1. HLA Association

In 1980, association of psoriasis with HLA class I alleles was demonstrated, with the most highly associated allele being *HLA-Cw6* (known as *HLA-Cw*0602* when identified with DNA typing).[74] However, the identity of the HLA class I allele driving the association (*PSORS1*) has been controversial. This due to the extensive linkage disequilibrium that exists on either side of *HLA-C*, within an interval of approximately 275 kb between *HLA-B* and a cluster of genes including *HCR* (alpha-helix coiled-coil rod homologue) and *CDSN* (corneodesmosin).

Nair et al.[75] localized *PSORS1* to a 60-kb region telomeric to *HLA-C*. Others have proposed *CDSN* or *HCR* to be the most likely candidate gene at this locus,[76–78] although they lie in a non-overlapping region ~150 kb away from *HLA-C* and they contain no obvious functional variants in subjects with psoriasis. A further study with a dense set of single nucleotide polymorphisms (SNPS) from throughout this region[79] refined *PSORS1* to a 10-kb interval very close to *HLA-C*.

This controversy illustrates the difficulty of differentiating between the effects of genes that are closely grouped together in tight linkage disequilibrium. However, mutations in *CDSN* have recently been shown to cause hypotrichosis simplex of the scalp, suggesting that *CDSN* has its function in scalp hair physiology.[80] This result reduces the probability that *CDSN* is responsible for predisposition to psoriasis.

The most likely possibility is that *HLA-Cw*0602* is itself conferring susceptibility to psoriasis. *HLA-C* is thought to mediate antigen presentation in viral infections such as hepatitis C and human immunodeficiency virus (HIV), but chronic viral infection (as opposed to streptococcal infection) has not been demonstrated in psoriasis. As with many other diseases, the detection of *HLA* associations has not yet informed knowledge of the disease mechanism.

Despite the strength of the association with *HLA-C,* not all affected individuals harbor *HLA-Cw*0602*. In independent sets of affected individuals/families this allele is only found in 40 to 80% of cases. Moreover, only 10% of individuals with *HLA-Cw*0602* develop disease, implicating environmental effects or additional genetic susceptibility factors.

Patients with psoriasis have different clinical features depending on whether they are *HLA-Cw*0602* positive or negative. *HLA-Cw*0602*-positive patients tend to have earlier onset of more severe disease and more extensive plaques on their arms, legs, and trunk (i.e., Type I psoriasis). They may also have a higher incidence of the Koebner's phenomenon, report more often that their psoriasis worsens during or after throat infections and more frequently have a favorable response to sunlight. In contrast, dystrophic nail changes and psoriatic arthritis are more common in the *HLA-Cw*0602*-negative patients.[81]

Allele dosage may play a role in risk of developing psoriasis and its subsequent severity. Homozygotes for *HLA-Cw*0602* from Iceland had a relative risk of developing psoriasis of 23.1 compared to the relative risk for heterozygotes of 8.9.[82] The mean age of onset of disease in homozygotes from the same study was 15.0 vs. 17.8 years for heterozygotes.[82]

It has been observed that large multiplex families with early-onset psoriasis do not always show linkage to the HLA region.[83,84] Although some families may still contain affecteds associated with *HLA-Cw*0602*, linkage to other loci has been demonstrated in some cases.

## 2. Non-HLA Loci

Localization of a second psoriasis susceptibility locus (PSORS2) to chromosome 17q25 was achieved following a genome-wide linkage scan on eight multiply affected families.[84] Linkage of PSORS3 to chromosome 4q35 was reported in a set of Irish families,[85] and families from the Chinese Han population also showed some evidence for linkage to a slightly proximal region (4q32).[86] Additional scans have revealed evidence for linkage to 1q21 (PSORS4) in families from the Lazlo region of Italy[87] and in families from the United States.[88]

In each of the above studies, psoriasis was inherited as an autosomal dominant trait with reduced penetrance, and the two-point LOD scores exceed the conventionally accepted threshold of 3.0. Other genome-wide scans have provided suggestive evidence for linkage, including linkage to 3q21 (PSORS5) in families from southwest Sweden[89] and 19p13 in German families.[90]

The identification of multiple loci for psoriasis susceptibility, therefore, indicates that psoriasis and psoriatic arthritis are genetically heterogeneous.

### 3. Psoriasis Genes at 17q25

Further evidence for linkage of psoriasis to 17q24-q25 has been provided from a variety of different Caucasian populations (U.S., Swedish, and Irish).[91–93] This same locus shows linkage to AD (see below), multiple sclerosis,[94,95] and rheumatoid arthritis (RA).[96]

Closer localization of disease genes has relied on the demonstration of association (linkage disequilibrium, LD) between disease phenotypes and particular polymorphisms.

Family-based association tests have identified two peaks harboring psoriasis susceptibility loci. One peak harbors *SLC9A3R1* and *NAT9*.[97] A second peak harbors *RAPTOR* (p150 target of rapamycin (TOR)-scaffold protein-containing WD-repeats).[97,98] After adjusting for multiple tests, these peaks remained significant, indicating that both are likely to be associated with disease.

*SLC9A3R1* is a PDZ domain-containing phosphoprotein that associates with members of the ezrin-radixin-moesin family. It is implicated in diverse aspects of epithelial membrane biology and immune synapse formation in T cells. Expression of *SLC9A3R1* is highest in the uppermost stratum malpighi of psoriatic and normal skin and in inactive vs. active T cells.[97]

There are five psoriasis-associated variants in the *SLC9A3R1/NAT9* region that drive the association at 17q25. One lies between the two genes and abolishes a putative site for the transcription factor RUNX1.[99] RUNX1 has a restricted pattern of expression, and is essential for hematopoietic cell development.[100] It is also the target of mutations in sporadic and familial myeloid leukemias.[101–103] It is of particular interest that systemic lupus erythematosus (SLE) and RA susceptibility loci have been shown to lie within altered RUNX1 binding sites of the *PD-1* and *SLC22A4* genes, respectively.[104,105]

Loss of a RUNX1 binding site suggests that *SLC9A3R1* or *NAT9* may contribute to psoriasis through their dysregulation in cells of hematopoietic origin. However, *SLC9A3R1* is also expressed in polarized epithelial cells including the keratinocyte, and its dysregulation could be altering keratinocyte homeostasis in response to an immune signal.

Although there is a biologically plausible role for *SLC9A3R1* in psoriasis, the neighboring *NAT9* may not be excluded from involvement in disease. NAT9 is a novel *n*-acetyltransferase of the GNAT family. Glycosylation of NAT9 is known to play a role in MHC class I antigen presentation, T-cell development, and to affect the development of autoimmune disease.[106,107] Experimental evidence in inflammatory diseases such as psoriasis also suggests that glycosylation might regulate organ-specific leukocyte traffic into inflammatory sites.[108]

## C. Overlap between Psoriasis and AD Loci

The chromosome 1q21, 17q25, and 20p loci identified in the U.K. genome screen for AD are closely coincident with some of the regions known to contain psoriasis susceptibility genes.[84,87,109] The conservative probability of this overlap occurring by chance is less than 3 in 100,000.[29] The German AD genome screen locus on chromosome 3q21[28] also closely overlaps another psoriasis locus.[89]

These findings suggest that the shared regions of linkage between AD and psoriasis contain polymorphic genes with general effects on dermal inflammation and immunity. These shared loci show a number of interesting features.

### 1. Epidermal Differentiation Cluster (chromosome 1q21)

The peak of linkage of AD and psoriasis on chromosome 1q21 overlies the human epidermal differentiation complex (EDC) that spans a region of ~2 Mb.[110] The genes of the EDC are expressed late during maturation of epidermal cells.[111]

Several gene families are recognized within the complex: These code for small proline-rich proteins (SPRRs), S100A calcium-binding proteins, and late envelope proteins (LEPs).[110,112] The *SPRR* and *LEP* genes code for precursor proteins of the cornified cell envelope (CE). The expression of these genes is linked to keratinocyte terminal differentiation both *in vivo* and *in vitro*.[112,113]

In the global expression studies of psoriasis described above,[113,114] 203 genes represented in the U95A-3 arrays were identified in the 2-Mb EDC region and its 1-Mb flanking segments. The 30 transcripts, differentially expressed when normal and involved skin, were compared. Many members of the S100 protein family were overexpressed in psoriatic skin and none was downregulated. Upregulated genes included *S100A1, S100A2, S100A7, S100A9, S1000A9, S100A10,* and *S100A12*. Members of the small proline-rich protein family that were overexpressed include *SPRR3, SPRK, SPRR1B,* and *SPRR2A*.[113, 114]

The known functions of some of the EDC gene products indicate that the skin is not functioning as a passive barrier. In particular, the S100 calcium binding proteins are often secreted and have a wide range of immunological actions.[115] S100A2 is chemotactic for eosinophils.[116] S100A7 (Psoriasin) is a potent and selective chemotactic inflammatory protein for CD4$^+$ T lymphocytes and neutrophils.[117] It is upregulated in inflammatory skin disorders.[118] S100A8 and S100A9 form a complex that displays cytostatic[119,120] and antimicrobial activities.[121,122] The S100A8/A9 complex also inhibits macrophage activation[123] and immunoglobulin synthesis by lymphocytes.[124] S100A8 as a homodimer is a potent chemotactic agent for leukocytes.[125–127] S100A12 has pro-inflammatory activity on endothelial cells and inflammatory cells.[128]

Several other proteins from the EDC are involved in CE formation.[129] Among these, involucrin, SPRR and LEPS are characterized by common structural features such as a central region of short tandem peptide repeats. The multifunctional intermediate filament-associated proteins profilaggrin (FLG) and trichohyalin belong to a gene family with multiple tandem repeats of specific peptide motifs. They are thought to represent fused genes of CE precursor protein genes and genes of the S100 family of small calcium-binding proteins.[130,131] The true functions of these genes remains obscure, but unlike the *S100* and *SPRR* genes, *FLG* is downregulated in involved psoriatic skin.[113, 114]

Mutations in *loricrin* underlie the Mendelian skin disorder of Vohwinkel's syndrome,[132] but mutations or variants in other genes of the EDC have not yet been recognized in common skin disease. The genes of this complex are nevertheless prime candidates for polymorphisms affecting eczema and psoriasis.

Association studies in Italian families suggest that PSORS4 lies within the EDC, within a 900-kb region between D1S1664 and D1S2715. This harbors the *SPRR* and *S100* gene clusters. Association was seen with D1S2346, a marker lying close to *loricrin* and between these two clusters.[133]

## 2. Chromosome 3q21

Linkage of chromosome 3q21 has not only been shown to AD[30,90] and psoriasis[89] but also asthma.[68] It may be of interest that three of these four genome screens were carried out in Scandinavians[30,68,89] and the fourth was carried out in a mixture of German and Swedish families.[90] Allele frequencies for the HLA loci and the *CCR5* mutation[134] show distinct differences between European countries and it seems quite possible that a mutation or variant may be found on chromosome 3q21 that is at its highest frequency in Scandinavians.

An examination of 195 psoriasis families from Sweden led to the identification of association with a five-marker haplotype from chromosome 3q21 that spanned the 3′ half of solute carrier family 12, member 8 (*SLC12A8*), a potassium/chloride transporter.[135] However, association of variants of this gene has not been detected in an independent cohort of Northern European psoriasis families (A.C. Bowcock, unpublished results), suggesting that the initial association is stochastic or that the gene's involvement may be particular to the Swedish population. Nevertheless, its possible involvement in psoriasis susceptibility has become more interesting with the observation that a second solute carrier at chromosome 5q31, *SLC22A4* (solute carrier family 22 member 4), an organic cation transporter, is associated with RA.[105]

*SLC22A4* is specific to hematological and immunological tissues and is induced by pro-inflammatory stimuli. It is highly expressed in the inflammatory joints of mice with collagen-induced arthritis. The defect associated with RA results in RUNX1 binding, and it is hypothesized that SLC22A4 functions as a transporter in lymphoid organs or inflammatory milieu.[105] These findings seem to parallel those of *SLC9A3R1* from chromosome 17q25 and psoriasis susceptibility,[97] and *SLC11A1* is associated with susceptibility to pulmonary tuberculosis.[136] It is possible that functional studies on these proteins will identify a common theme associated with alterations in cation transport in inflammatory diseases.

### 3. Chromosome 17q25

Psoriasis genes associated with this locus are described above. Given the overlap with chromosome 17q25 susceptibility loci for psoriasis and AD,[29] the role of these genes in AD susceptibility is currently being investigated.

This same 17q25 region has also been linked to a single gene disorder, epidermodysplasia verruciformis (EV).[137] Individuals with EV suffer from chronic infections with the oncogenic human papillomavirus type V, and half of these patients may eventually develop skin carcinomas. A shared mechanism between EV and AD or psoriasis is not immediately obvious, unless perhaps AD and psoriasis result from chronic infections with as-yet-unrecognized organisms. The linkage of this locus to multiple sclerosis[94,95] and RA[96] also merits further investigation.

### 4. Chromosome 20p

Linkage to chromosome 20p has been reported to the distinctive phenotype of AD and asthma combined.[29] Children with these two diseases together had a serum IgE concentration that was eight times higher than in children with asthma alone and five times higher than in children with AD alone.[29] These results suggest that the combination of AD and asthma may correspond to a genetic subtype of both diseases. Genetic linkage of susceptibility to leprosy has been identified to the same genetic region,[138] as has linkage to SLE.[139]

## IV. SINGLE GENE SKIN DISORDERS AND ATOPY

Positional cloning of novel genes influencing complex diseases can be greatly facilitated by the study of Mendelian (single gene) disorders. Two Mendelian diseases show strong features of atopic dermatitis.

### A. Wiskott–Aldrich Syndrome

Wiscott–Aldrich Syndrome (WAS) is a rare X-linked disorder of T- and B-cell function, which is typified by recurrent infections and thrombocytopenia. Many boys with the disease also develop a rash that is indistinguishable from AD. A study of the *WAS* gene region has been carried out in Swedish families with AD.[140] One marker (MAOB) showed linkage to the severity score of atopic dermatitis ($p < 0.05$), but association to AD was not seen. These results should provoke further study of the gene in AD. In addition, it might be of value to look at the location of mutations in *WAS* and see if particular regions of the gene are affected in boys with the typical WAS rash, when compared to boys with predominately nondermal manifestations of the illness.

### B. Netherton's Disease

Netherton's disease is a rare recessive disorder characterized by generalized erythroderma, symptoms of atopic disease (hay fever, food allergy, urticaria, and asthma), and very high levels of IgE.[141] The gene for Netherton's disease has been identified (*SPINK5*) and encodes a 15-domain serine protease inhibitor called LEKTI, which is expressed in epithelial and mucosal surfaces and in the thymus.[142,143] A subsequent study of coding and noncoding polymorphisms in *SPINK5* showed that the gene modifies the risk of AD, asthma, and elevated serum IgE levels.[144]

Each of the LEKTI/SPINK5 protease inhibitory domains is slightly different from the others,[143] perhaps suggesting a polyvalent action against multiple substrates. The protein is expressed in the outer epidermis, in sebaceous glands, and around the shafts of hair follicles,[145] so that its actions seem directed toward the environment rather than internally.

In this context it is interesting that more than 90% of patients with AD are colonized with *Staphylococcus aureus*[146] and that house dust mite allergens are proteases with activity against epithelial surfaces (see below). It may be relevant that α1-proteinase inhibitor has been reported in a small trial to be effective in the treatment of AD.[147]

## V. GENE–GENE INTERACTIONS

Gene–gene interaction (known as epistasis) indicates that the presence of two genetic susceptibility loci together has a greater (multiplicative) effect than that of either gene alone. Gene–gene interactions are to be expected in complex diseases, and they are likely to exist between predisposing loci for both AD and psoriasis. Identification of these might indicate biologically important and unexpected disease pathways, and will also allow the determination of genetic risk of disease with a greater certainty.

Epistasis can be detected by statistical modeling, or more simply by stratifying subjects according to their genotypes at one locus and then testing for other loci in the subgroups. The first approach has indicated some interactions between HLA and chromosome 1q21 in the genesis of psoriasis,[148] but the biological meaning of this will have to await the discovery of the chromosome 1 psoriasis susceptibility gene or genes.

Stratification works best in the presence of a common allele of strong effect, such as *HLA-Cw*0602* and psoriasis. Stratification by this allele has been used to increase the evidence for linkage of psoriasis to chromosome 16q[149] and to chromosome 15 (*D15S817*) (NPL 2.96, $p = 0.002$).[150]

Gene–gene interactions may also be of importance to AD. However, in the absence of an effect to match *HLA-C* in psoriasis, sample sizes at present are too small to investigate such possibilities by stratification.

## VI. GENE–ENVIRONMENT INTERACTIONS

As with many complex human diseases, environment is as important as genetics in the development of psoriasis and AD.

The Koebner phenomenon may be an indicator of the effects of environmental stress on flare-up of the disease. In addition to mechanical injury, the environmental causes of psoriasis may include ultraviolet and chemical injury; prescription drug use; psychological stress, and smoking.[151] Infections are also important, and Group A streptococcal throat infections frequently precede outbreaks of guttate psoriasis that may progress to chronic plaque psoriasis,[152] and chronic plaque psoriasis may be made worse by infection.[153] Psoriasis also occurs in association with HIV infection.[154]

The mechanisms for these observations are completely mysterious, and show how little is really known about the disease pathophysiology. However, it is possible that gene discovery will eventually elucidate these phenomena.

In the case of AD, the recognition that the Netherton's disease gene *SPINK5* influences disease susceptibility defines a new line of enquiry. As observed above, *SPINK5* is a polyvalent protease inhibitor and it is found in the outermost layer of the skin, suggesting that its actions are directed against external proteases.

A third of patients with AD suffer from frequent serious skin infections, and more than 90% patients with eczema are colonized with *S. aureus*.[146] *Staphylococcus aureus* and staphylococcal enterotoxins play important roles in the exacerbation and prolongation of AD. *Staphylococcus aureus* in eczema lesions are colonized on and in the horny layers of the eczematous skin, and staphylococcal enterotoxins are distributed on the dermal-infiltrated cells, especially on eosinophils.[155]

Nearly all strains of *S. aureus* from skin lesions of AD have been reported to produce proteolytic activity, with 60% producing activity comparable to that of the proteolytically hyperactive reference strain *S. aureus* V8.[156] This was in contrast to control strains isolated from the nose vestibules of 18 healthy carriers, in which proteolytic activity never exceeded 2.5% of the activity of the reference strain.[156]

Toxins from bacteria including *S. aureus*, have been shown to function as superantigens. These antigens bypass the normal control of T-cell activation and activate all T-cell clones bearing certain types of variable chain on the T-cell receptor, which leads to vigorous T-cell activation and cytokine release. *Staphylococcus aureus* from the skin of patients with eczema frequently produce superantigens, and application of a staphylococcal superantigen to human skin induces an eczematoid reaction.[157]

Many children with AD have positive prick skin tests to common allergens. House dust mite (HDM) major allergens are also proteinases that exert profound effects on epithelial cells, including disruption of intercellular adhesion, increased paracellular permeability, and initiation of cell death.[158]

Understanding of the genetic predisposition to AD should therefore also be informed by investigation of the roles of *S. aureus* and HDM proteinases in inducing an immune response in the skin of patients with the disease.

## VII. PARENTAL EFFECTS

The risk of transmission of atopic disease from an affected mother is approximately four times higher than from an affected father.[159] Similar parent of origin effects have been noted in psoriasis[160] and psoriatic arthritis.[149]

These changes may also be reflected in the behavior of particular disease genes. In the case of psoriatic arthritis, a locus has been identified on chromosome 16q that shows a strong paternal effect on susceptibility.[149] It is possible that the disease gene in this region may be *NOD2/CARD15*, mutations which have been implicated in Blau syndrome[161] and Crohn's disease.[162,163] It has been hypothesized that *CARD15* is a psoriatic arthritis gene that is independent of *HLA-Cw*0602*.[164]

Several known genes show parent-of-origin effects on allergic disease. These genes include the *FcεRI-β* locus on chromosome 11q13,[38,165] the *SPINK5* gene from chromosome 5q34[29] and as-yet-undiscovered genes at loci on chromosomes 4 and 16.[58]

The mechanisms for these parent of origin effects are unknown. Maternal effects may be considered a specialized form of immune gene–environment interactions between the fetus and the mother. These are recognized to take place through the placenta as well as through breast milk.[166]

Alternatively, the maternal effect may be the result of genomic imprinting. Genomic imprinting is a process in which the genes from one parent are differentially expressed to the allele derived from the other parent.[167,168] Epigenetic markers of imprinting, such as the variable presence of methylation on CpG residues,[168] now need to be studied in combination with knowledge of parental disease status as well as parental genotype.

## VIII. CONCLUSIONS

Genetic studies of both psoriasis and AD suggest that defects affecting cells of the skin and the skin immune system may be more important in the pathogenesis of disease than defects in adaptive immunity. In evolutionary terms, epithelial surfaces had to cope with infections and other insults long before the appearance of the adaptive immune system. Keratinocytes are very active immunologically, and produce a wide range of cytokines.[169] Although this activity has previously been assumed to be secondary to signaling from classical immune cells,[170] it is becoming increasingly evident that keratinocytes express functional receptors such as CD14 and TLR-4[171] and are capable of inducing inflammatory responses without pre-induction by other cells.

The epidermal differentiation complex (EDC) has been implicated in AD and psoriasis. Even though the disease-causing variants have not yet been identified, it is of interest that the EDC transcribes within terminally differentiating keratinocytes and contains many genes that may modify immune processes in the epithelium.

The polymorphic nature of genes and gene families expressed in the skin suggest a polyvalent response to a number of different stimuli, including infections and other insults. The discovery of all the major genes affecting common inflammatory skin diseases is likely to come within a few years, and the suggestion already is that the skin itself will be found to initiate and control much of the machinery of its own immune responses.

## REFERENCES


1. Gerrard, J., Rao, D., and Morton, N., A genetic study of immunoglobulin E, *Am. J. Hum. Genet.*, 30, 46–58, 1978.
2. Juhlin, L., Johansson, G., Bennich, H., Hogman, C., and Thyresson, N., Immunoglobulin E in dermatoses. Levels in atopic dermatitis and urticaria, *Arch. Dermatol.*, 100, 12–16, 1969.
3. Johansson, S.G., Hourihane, J.O., Bousquet, J. et al., A revised nomenclature for allergy. An EAACI position statement from the EAACI nomenclature task force, *Allergy,* 56, 813–824, 2001.
4. Schmid-Grendelmeier, P., Simon, D., Simon, H.U., Akdis, C.A., and Wuthrich, B., Epidemiology, clinical features, and immunology of the "intrinsic" (non-IgE-mediated) type of atopic dermatitis (constitutional dermatitis), *Allergy,* 56, 841–849, 2001.
5. Larsen, F.S., Holm, N.V., and Henningsen, K., Atopic dermatitis. A genetic-epidemiologic study in a population-based twin sample, *J. Am. Acad. Dermatol.,* 15, 487–494, 1986.
6. Schultz Larsen, F., Atopic dermatitis: a genetic-epidemiologic study in a population-based twin sample, *J. Am. Acad. Dermatol.*, 28, 719–723, 1993.
7. Duffy, D.L., Martin, N.G., Battistutta, D., Hopper, J.L., and Mathews, J.D., Genetics of asthma and hay fever in Australian twins, *Am. Rev. Respir. Dis.* 142, 1351–1358, 1990.
8. Palmer, L.J., Burton, P.R., Faux, J.A., James, A.L., Musk, A.W., and Cookson, W.O., Independent inheritance of serum immunoglobulin E concentrations and airway responsiveness, *Am. J. Respir. Crit. Care Med.,* 161, 1836–1843, 2000.
9. Christophers, E. and Henseler, T., Contrasting disease patterns in psoriasis and atopic dermatitis, *Arch. Dermatol. Res.*, 279(Suppl.), S48–51, 1987.
10. Wuepper, K.D., Coulter, S.N., and Haberman, A., Psoriasis vulgaris: a genetic approach, *J. Invest. Dermatol.*, 95, 2S–4S, 1990.
11. Duffy, D.L., Spelman, L.S., and Martin, N.G., Psoriasis in Australian twins, *J. Am. Acad. Dermatol.,* 29, 428–434, 1993.
12. Henseler, T. and Christophers, E., Psoriasis of early and late onset: characterization of two types of psoriasis vulgaris, *J. Am. Acad. Dermatol.,* 13, 450–456, 1985.
13. Zhou, X., Krueger, J.G., Kao, M.-C. et al., Novel mechanisms of T-cell and dendritic cell activation revealed by profiling of psoriasis on the 63,100-element oligonucleotide array, *Physiol. Genomics*, 13, 69–78, 2003.
14. Nakatani, T., Kaburagi, Y., Shimada, Y. et al., CCR4 memory CD4+ T lymphocytes are increased in peripheral blood and lesional skin from patients with atopic dermatitis, *J. Allergy Clin. Immunol.,* 107, 353–358, 2001.
15. Ackermann, L., Harvima, I.T., Pelkonen, J. et al., Mast cells in psoriatic skin are strongly positive for interferon-gamma, *Br. J. Dermatol.,* 140, 624–633, 1999.
16. Giustizieri, M.L., Mascia, F., Frezzolini, A. et al., Keratinocytes from patients with atopic dermatitis and psoriasis show a distinct chemokine production profile in response to T cell-derived cytokines, *J. Allergy Clin. Immunol.,* 107, 871–877, 2001.
17. Levine, B.B., Stember, R.H., and Fontino, M., Ragweed hayfever: genetic control and linkage to HLA haplotyes, *Science*, 178, 1201–1203, 1972.

18. Marsh, D.G., Meyers, D.A., and Bias, W.B., The epidemiology and genetics of atopic allergy, *N. Engl. J. Med.,* 305, 1551–1559, 1981.
19. Young, R.P., Dekker, J.W., Wordsworth, B.P., and Cookson, W.O.C.M., HLA-DR and HLA-DP genotypes and immunoglobulin E responses to common major allergens, *Clin. Exp. Allergy,* 24, 431–439, 1994.
20. Moffatt, M.F., Schou, C., Faux, J.A. et al., Association between quantitative traits underlying asthma and the HLA-DRB1 locus in a family-based population sample, *Eur. J. Hum. Genet.,* 9, 341–346, 2001.
21. Moffatt, M.F. and Cookson, W.O., Tumour necrosis factor haplotypes and asthma, *Hum. Mol. Genet.,* 6, 551–554, 1997.
22. Albuquerque, R.V., Hayden, C.M., Palmer, L.J. et al., Association of polymorphisms within the tumour necrosis factor (TNF) genes and childhood asthma, *Clin. Exp. Allergy,* 28, 578–654, 1998.
23. Chagani, T., Pare, P.D., Zhu, S. et al., Prevalence of tumor necrosis factor-alpha and angiotensin converting enzyme polymorphisms in mild/moderate and fatal/near-fatal asthma, *Am. J. Respir. Crit. Care Med.,* 160, 278–282, 1999.
24. Li Kam Wa, T.C., Mansur, A.H., Britton, J. et al., Association between 308 tumour necrosis factor promoter polymorphism and bronchial hyperreactivity in asthma, *Clin. Exp. Allergy,* 29, 1204–1208, 1999.
25. Noguchi, E., Yokouchi, Y., Shibasaki, M. et al., Association between TNFA polymorphism and the development of asthma in the Japanese population, *Am. J. Respir. Crit. Care Med.,* 166, 43–46, 2002.
26. Witte, J.S., Palmer, L.J., O'Connor, R.D., Hopkins, P.J., and Hall, J.M., Relation between tumour necrosis factor polymorphism TNFalpha-308 and risk of asthma, *Eur. J. Hum. Genet.,* 10, 82–85, 2002.
27. Winchester, E.C., Millwood, I.Y., Rand, L., Penny, M.A., and Kessling, A.M., Association of the TNF-alpha-308 (G→A) polymorphism with self-reported history of childhood asthma, *Hum. Genet.,* 107, 591–596, 2000.
28. Lee, Y.A., Wahn, U., Kehrt, R. et al., A major susceptibility locus for atopic dermatitis maps to chromosome 3q21, *Nat. Genet.,* 26, 470–473, 2000.
29. Cookson, W.O., Ubhi, B., Lawrence, R. et al., Genetic linkage of childhood atopic dermatitis to psoriasis susceptibility loci, *Nat. Genet.,* 27, 372–373, 2001.
30. Bradley, M., Soderhall, C., Luthman, H., Wahlgren, C.F., Kockum, I., and Nordenskjold, M., Susceptibility loci for atopic dermatitis on chromosomes 3, 13, 15, 17 and 18 in a Swedish population, *Hum. Mol. Genet.,* 11,1539–1548, 2002.
31. Moffatt, M.F., Hill, M.R., Cornelis, F. et al., Genetic linkage of T cell receptor α/δ complex to specific IgE responses, *Lancet,* 343, 1597–1600, 1994.
32. Moffatt, M.F., Schou, C., Faux, J.A., and Cookson, W.O., Germline TCR-A restriction of immunoglobulin E responses to allergen, *Immunogenetics,* 46, 226–230, 1997.
33. Cookson, W.O., Sharp, P.A., Faux, J.A., and Hopkin, J.M., Linkage between immunoglobulin E responses underlying asthma and rhinitis and chromosome 11q, *Lancet,* 1, 1292–1295, 1989.
34. Sandford, A.J., Shirakawa, T., Moffatt, M.F. et al., Localisation of atopy and beta subunit of high-affinity IgE receptor (Fc epsilon RI) on chromosome 11q, *Lancet,* 341, 332–334, 1993.
35. Shirakawa, T., Mao, X.Q., Sasaki, S. et al., Association between atopic asthma and a coding variant of Fc epsilon RI beta in a Japanese population, *Hum. Mol. Genet.,* 5, 1129–1130, 1996.
36. Hill, M.R., James, A.L., Faux, J.A. et al., Fc epsilon RI-beta polymorphism and risk of atopy in a general population sample, *Br. Med. J.,* 311, 776–779, 1995.
37. van Herwerden, L., Harrap, S.B., Wong, Z.Y. et al., Linkage of high-affinity IgE receptor gene with bronchial hyperreactivity, even in absence of atopy, *Lancet,* 346, 1262–1265, 1995.
38. Cox, H.E., Moffatt, M.F., Faux, J.A. et al., Association of atopic dermatitis to the beta subunit of the high affinity immunoglobulin E receptor, *Br. J. Dermatol.,* 138, 182–187, 1998.
39. Lin, S., Cicala, C., Scharenberg, A., and Kinet, J., The Fc(epsilon)RIbeta subunit functions as an amplifier of Fc(epsilon)RIgamma-mediated cell activation signals, *Cell,* 85, 985–995, 1996.
40. Turner, H. and Kinet, J.P., Signalling through the high-affinity IgE receptor Fc epsilonRI, *Nature,* 402, B24–B30, 1999.
41. Donnadieu, E., Cookson, W.O., Jouvin, M.H., and Kinet, J.P., Allergy-associated polymorphisms of the FcepsilonRIbeta subunit do not impact its two amplification functions, *J. Immunol.,* 165, 3917–3922, 2000.
42. Takahashi, K., Nishiyama, C., Hasegawa, M., Akizawa, Y., and Ra, C., Regulation of the human high affinity IgE receptor beta-chain gene expression via an intronic element, *J. Immunol.,* 171, 2478–2484, 2003.

43. Akizawa, Y., Nishiyama, C., Hasegawa, M. et al., Regulation of human FcepsilonRI beta chain gene expression by Oct-1, *Int. Immunol.,* 15, 549–556, 2003.
44. Traherne, J.A., Hill, M.R., Hysi, P. et al., LD mapping of maternally and non-maternally derived alleles and atopy in Fc{varepsilon}RI-{beta}, *Hum. Mol. Genet.*, 12, 2577–2585, 2003.
45. Rosenwasser, L., Klemm, D., Dresback, J. et al., Promoter polymorphisms in the chromosome 5 gene cluster in asthma and atopy, *Clin. Exp. Allergy,* 25(Suppl. 2), 74–78; discussion 95–96, 1995.
46. Graves, P.E., Kabesch, M., Halonen, M. et al., A cluster of seven tightly linked polymorphisms in the IL-13 gene is associated with total serum IgE levels in three populations of white children, *J. Allergy Clin. Immunol.,* 105, 506–513, 2000.
47. Leung, T., Tang, N., Chan, I., Li, A., Ha, G., and Lam, C., A polymorphism in the coding region of interleukin-13 gene is associated with atopy but not asthma in Chinese children, *Clin Exp Allergy,* 31, 1515–1521, 2001.
48. Noguchi, E., Nukaga-Nishio, Y., Jian, Z. et al., Haplotypes of the 5′ region of the IL-4 gene and SNPs in the intergene sequence between the IL-4 and IL-13 genes are associated with atopic asthma, *Hum. Immunol.,* 62, 1251–1257, 2001.
49. Howard, T., Whittaker, P., Zaiman, A. et al., Identification and association of polymorphisms in the interleukin-13 gene with asthma and atopy in a Dutch population, *Am. J. Respir. Cell Mol. Biol.,* 25, 377–384, 2001.
50. van der Pouw Kraan, T.C., van Veen, A., Boeije, L.C. et al., An IL-13 promoter polymorphism associated with increased risk of allergic asthma, *Genes Immun.*, 1, 61–65, 1999.
51. Rafatpanah, H., Bennett, E., Pravica, V. et al., Association between novel GM-CSF gene polymorphisms and the frequency and severity of atopic dermatitis, *J. Allergy Clin. Immunol.,* 112, 593–598, 2003.
52. Mao, X.Q., Shirikawa, T., Yoshikawa, K. et al., Association between genetic variants of mast-cell chymase and eczema, *Lancet,* 348, 581–583, 1996.
53. Kawashima, T., Noguchi, E., Arinami, T., Kobayashi, K., Otsuka, F., and Hamaguchi, H., No evidence for an association between a variant of the mast cell chymase gene and atopic dermatitis based on case-control and haplotype-relative-risk analyses, *Hum. Hered.,* 48, 271–274, 1998.
54. Pascale, E., Tarani, L., Meglio, P. et al., Absence of association between a variant of the mast cell chymase gene and atopic dermatitis in an Italian population, *Hum. Hered.,* 51, 177–179, 2001.
55. Nickel, R.G., Casolaro, V., Wahn, U. et al., Atopic dermatitis is associated with a functional mutation in the promoter of the C-C chemokine RANTES, *J. Immunol.,* 164, 1612–1616, 2000.
56. Beyer, K., Nickel, R., Freidhoff, L. et al., Association and linkage of atopic dermatitis with chromosome 13q12-14 and 5q31-33 markers, *J. Invest. Dermatol.,* 115, 906–908, 2000.
57. Anderson, G.G., Leaves, N.I., Bhattacharyya, S. et al., Positive association to IgE levels and a physical map of the 13q14 atopy locus, *Eur. J. Hum. Genet.,* 10, 266–270, 2002.
58. Daniels, S.E., Bhattacharrya, S., James, A. et al., A genome-wide search for quantitative trait loci underlying asthma, *Nature*, 383, 247–250, 1996.
59. Xu, J., Meyers, D.A., Ober, C. et al., Genomewide screen and identification of gene-gene interactions for asthma-susceptibility loci in three U.S. populations: collaborative study on the genetics of asthma, *Am. J. Hum. Genet.,* 68, 1437–1446, 2001.
60. Ober, C., Tsalenko, A., Parry, R., and Cox, N.J., A second-generation genomewide screen for asthma-susceptibility alleles in a founder population, *Am. J. Hum. Genet.*, 67, 1154–1162, 2000.
61. Wjst, M., Fischer, G., Immervoll, T. et al., A genome-wide search for linkage to asthma. German Asthma Genetics Group, *Genomics,* 58, 1–8, 1999.
62. Hizawa, N., Freidhoff, L., Chiu, Y. et al., Genetic regulation of Dermatophagoides pteronyssinus-specific IgE responsiveness: a genome-wide multipoint linkage analysis in families recruited through 2 asthmatic sibs. Collaborative Study on the Genetics of Asthma (CSGA), *J. Allergy Clin. Immunol.,* 102, 436–442, 1998.
63. Mathias, R.A., Freidhoff, L.R., Blumenthal, M.N. et al., Genome-wide linkage analyses of total serum IgE using variance components analysis in asthmatic families, *Genet. Epidemiol.*, 20, 340–355, 2001.
64. Dizier, M.H., Besse-Schmittler, C., Guilloud-Bataille, M. et al., Genome screen for asthma and related phenotypes in the French EGEA study, *Am. J. Respir. Crit. Care Med.,* 162, 1812–1818, 2000.
65. Laitinen, T., Daly, M.J., Rioux, J.D. et al., A susceptibility locus for asthma-related traits on chromosome 7 revealed by genome-wide scan in a founder population, *Nat. Genet.*, 28, 87–91, 2001.

66. Hakonarson, H., Bjornsdottir, U.S., Halapi, E. et al., A major susceptibility gene for asthma maps to chromosome 14q24, *Am. J. Hum. Genet.,* 71, 483–491, 2002.
67. Koppelman, G.H., Stine, O.C., Xu, J. et al., Genome-wide search for atopy susceptibility genes in Dutch families with asthma, *J. Allergy Clin. Immunol.*, 109, 498–506, 2002.
68. Haagerup, A., Bjerke, T., Schiotz, P.O., Binderup, H.G., Dahl, R., and Kruse, T.A., Asthma and atopy — a total genome scan for susceptibility genes, *Allergy,* 57:680–686, 2002.
69. Ober, C. and Moffatt, M.F., Contributing factors to the pathobiology. The genetics of asthma, *Clin. Chest Med.,* 21, 245–261, 2000.
70. Cookson, W., Genetics and genomics of asthma and allergic diseases, *Immunol. Rev.,* 190, 195–206, 2002.
71. Van Eerdewegh, P., Little, R.D., Dupuis, J. et al., Association of the ADAM33 gene with asthma and bronchial hyperresponsiveness, *Nature*, 418, 426–430, 2002.
72. Zhang, Y., Leaves, N.I., Anderson, G.G. et al., Positional cloning of a quantitative trait locus on chromosome 13q14 that influences immunoglobulin E levels and asthma, *Nat. Genet*., 34, 181–186, 2003.
73. Allen, M., Heinzmann, A., Noguchi, E. et al., Positional cloning of a novel gene influencing asthma from Chromosome 2q14, *Nat. Genet*., 35, 258–263, 2003.
74. Tiilikainen, A., Lassus, A., Karvonen, J., Vartiainen, P., and Julin, M., Psoriasis and HLA-Cw6, *Br. J. Dermatol.*, 102, 179–184, 1980.
75. Nair, R.P., Stuart, P., Henseler, T. et al., Localization of psoriasis-susceptibility locus PSORS1 to a 60-kb interval telomeric to HLA-C, *Am. J. Hum. Genet.*, 66, 1833–1844, 2000.
76. Ahnini, R.T., Camp, N.J., Cork, M.J. et al., Novel genetic association between the corneodesmosin (MHC S) gene and susceptibility to psoriasis, *Hum. Mol. Genet.,* 8, 1135–1140, 1999.
77. Asumalahti, K., Laitinen, T., Itkonen-Vatjus, R. et al., A candidate gene for psoriasis near HLA-C, HCR (Pg8), is highly polymorphic with a disease-associated susceptibility allele, *Hum. Mol. Genet.*. 9, 1533–1542. 2000.
78. Allen, M., Ishida-Yamamoto, A., McGrath, J. et al., Corneodesmosin expression in psoriasis vulgaris differs from normal skin and other inflammatory skin disorders, *Lab. Invest.,* 81, 969–976, 2001.
79. Veal, C.D., Capon, F., Allen, M.H. et al., Family-based analysis using a dense single-nucleotide polymorphism-based map defines genetic variation at PSORS1, the major psoriasis-susceptibility locus, *Am. J. Hum. Genet.*, 71, 554–564, 2002.
80. Levy-Nissenbaum, E., Betz, R.C., Frydman, M. et al., Hypotrichosis simplex of the scalp is associated with nonsense mutations in CDSN encoding corneodesmosin, *Nat. Genet*., 34, 151–153, 2003.
81. Guedjonsson, J.E., Karason, A., Antonsdottir, A.A. et al., HLA-Cw6-positive and HLA-Cw6-negative patients with psoriasis vulgaris have distinct clinical features, *J. Invest. Dermatol.,* 118, 362–365, 2002.
82. Gudjonsson, J.E., Karason, A., Antonsdottir, A. et al., Psoriasis patients who are homozygous for the HLA-Cw*0602 allele have a 2.5-fold increased risk of developing psoriasis compared with Cw6 heterozygotes, *Br. J. Dermatol.,* 148, 233–235, 2003.
83. Lin, J.D., Auerbach, A.D., Auerbach, R. et al., Genetic linkage studies in psoriasis, *J. Invest. Dermatol.*, 96, 535A, 1991.
84. Tomfohrde, J., Silverman, A., Barnes, R. et al., Gene for familial psoriasis susceptibility mapped to the distal end of human chromosome 17q, *Science*, 1264, 1141–1145, 994.
85. Matthews, D., Fry, L., Powles, A. et al., Evidence that a locus for familial psoriasis maps to chromosome 4q, *Nat. Genet.,* 14, 231–233, 1996.
86. Zhang, X.J., He, P.P., Wang, Z.X. et al., Evidence for a major psoriasis susceptibility locus at 6p21(PSORS1) and a novel candidate region at 4q31 by genome-wide scan in Chinese hans, *J. Invest. Dermatol.,* 19, 1361–1366, 2002.
87. Capon, F., Novelli, G., Semprini, S. et al., Searching for psoriasis susceptibility genes in Italy: genome scan and evidence for a new locus on chromosome 1, *J. Invest. Dermatol.,* 112, 32–35, 1999.
88. Bhalerao, J. and Bowcock, A.M., The genetics of psoriasis: a complex disorder of the skin and immune system, *Hum. Mol. Genet.,* 7, 1537–1545, 1998.
89. Enlund, F., Samuelsson, L., Enerback, C. et al., Psoriasis susceptibility locus in chromosome region 3q21 identified in patients from southwest Sweden, *Eur. J. Hum. Genet.,* 7, 783–790, 1999.
90. Lee, Y.A., Ruschendorf, F., Windemuth, C. et al., Genomewide scan in German families reveals evidence for a novel psoriasis-susceptibility locus on chromosome 19p13, *Am. J. Hum. Genet.*, 67, 1020–1024, 2000.

91. Enlund, F., Samuelsson, L., Enerback, C. et al., Analysis of three suggested psoriasis susceptibility loci in a large Swedish set of families: confirmation of linkage to chromosome 6p (HLA region), and to 17q, but not to 4q, *Hum. Hered.*, 49, 2–8, 1999.
92. Nair, R., Henseler, T., Jenisch, S. et al., Evidence for two psoriasis susceptibility loci (HLA and 17q) and two novel candidate regions (16q and 20p) by genome-wide scan, *Hum. Mol. Genet.*, 6, 1349–1356, 1997.
93. Matthews, D., Fry, L., Powles, A., Weissenbach, J., and Williamson, R., Confirmation of genetic heterogeneity in familial psoriasis, *J. Med. Genet.*, 32, 546–548, 1995.
94. Kuokkanen, S., Gschwend, M., Rioux, J.D. et al., Genomewide scan of multiple sclerosis in Finnish multiplex families, *Am. J. Hum. Genet.*, 61, 1379–1387, 1997.
95. Sawcer, S., Jones, H.B., Feakes, R. et al., A genome screen in multiple sclerosis reveals susceptibility loci on chromosome 6p21 and 17q22, *Nat. Genet.*, 13, 464–468, 1996.
96. Jawaheer, D., Seldin, M.F., Amos, C.I. et al., A genomewide screen in multiplex rheumatoid arthritis families suggests genetic overlap with other autoimmune diseases, *Am. J. Hum. Genet.*, 68, 927–936. 2001.
97. Helms, C., Cao, L., Krueger, J.G. et al., A putative RUNX1 binding site variant between SLC9A3R1 and NAT9 is associated with susceptibility to psoriasis, *Nat. Genet.*, 35, 349–356, 2003.
98. Kim, D.H., Sarbassov, D.D., Ali, S.M. et al., mTOR interacts with raptor to form a nutrient-sensitive complex that signals to the cell growth machinery, *Cell*, 110, 163–175, 2002.
99. Erickson, P., Gao, J., Chang, K.S. et al., Identification of breakpoints in t(8;21) acute myelogenous leukemia and isolation of a fusion transcript, AML1/ETO, with similarity to *Drosophila* segmentation gene, runt, *Blood*, 80, 1825–1831, 1992.
100. Lacaud, G., Gore, L., Kennedy, M. et al., Runx1 is essential for hematopoietic commitment at the hemangioblast stage of development *in vitro, Blood*, 100, 458–466, 2002.
101. Barseguian, K., Lutterbach, B., Hiebert, S.W. et al., Multiple subnuclear targeting signals of the leukemia-related AML1/ETO and ETO repressor proteins, *Proc. Natl. Acad. Sci. U.S.A.,* 99, 15434–15439, 2002.
102. Schwieger, M., Lohler, J., Friel, J., Scheller, M., Horak, I., and Stocking, C., AML1-ETO inhibits maturation of multiple lymphohematopoietic lineages and induces myeloblast transformation in synergy with ICSBP deficiency, *J. Exp. Med.*, 196, 1227–1240, 2002.
103. Osato, M., Yanagida, M., Shigesada, K., and Ito, Y., Point mutations of the RUNx1/AML1 gene in sporadic and familial myeloid leukemias, *Int. J. Hematol.*, 74, 245–251, 2001.
104. Prokunina, L., Castillejo-Lopez, C., Oberg, F. et al., A regulatory polymorphism in PDCD1 is associated with susceptibility to systemic lupus erythematosus in humans, *Nat. Genet.*, 32:666–669, 2002.
105. Tokuhiro, S., Yamada, R., Chang, X. et al., An intronic SNP in a RUNX1 binding site of SLC22A4, encoding an organic cation transporter, is associated with rheumatoid arthritis, *Nat. Genet.*, 35, 341–348, 2003.
106. Rudd, P.M., Elliott, T., Cresswell, P., Wilson, I.A., and Dwek, R.A., Glycosylation and the immune system, *Science,* 291, 2370–2376, 2001.
107. Demetriou, M., Granovsky, M., Quaggin, S., and Dennis, J.W., Negative regulation of T-cell activation and autoimmunity by Mgat5 N-glycosylation, *Nature*, 409, 733–739, 2001.
108. Renkonen, J., Tynninen, O., Hayry, P., Paavonen, T., and Renkonen, R., Glycosylation might provide endothelial zip codes for organ-specific leukocyte traffic into inflammatory sites, *Am. J. Pathol.,* 161, 543–550, 2002.
109. Trembath, R., Clough, R., Rosbotham, J. et al., Identification of a major susceptibility locus on chromosome 6p and evidence for further disease loci revealed by a two stage genome-wide search in psoriasis, *Hum. Mol. Genet.*, 6, 813–820, 1997.
110. Mischke, D., Korge, B.P., Marenholz, I., Volz, A., and Ziegler, A., Genes encoding structural proteins of epidermal cornification and S100 calcium-binding proteins form a gene complex ("epidermal differentiation complex") on human chromosome 1q21, *J. Invest. Dermatol.,* 106, 989–992, 1996.
111. Hardas, B., Zhao, X., Zhang, J., Longqing, X., Stoll, S., and Elder, J., Assignment of psoriasin to human chromosomal band 1q21: coordinate overexpression of clustered genes in psoriasis, *J. Invest. Dermatol.,* 106, 753–758, 1996.
112. Marshall, D., Hardman, M.J., Nield, K.M., and Byrne, C., Differentially expressed late constituents of the epidermal cornified envelope, *Proc. Natl. Acad. Sci. U.S.A.,* 98, 13031–13036, 2001.

113. Lohman, F., Medema, J., Gibbs, S., Ponec, M., van de Putte, P., and Backendorf, C., Expression of the SPRR cornification genes is differentially affected by carcinogenic transformation, *Exp. Cell Res.*, 231, 141–148, 1997.
114. Bowcock, A.M., Shannon, W., Du, F. et al., Insights into psoriasis and other inflammatory diseases from large-scale gene expression studies, *Hum. Mol. Genet.*, 10, 1793–1805, 2001.
115. Donato, R., S100: a multigenic family of calcium-modulated proteins of the EF-hand type with intracellular and extracellular functional roles, *Int. J. Biochem. Cell. Biol.*, 33, 637–668, 2001.
116. Komada, T., Araki, R., Nakatani, K., Yada, I., Naka, M., and Tanaka, T., Novel specific chemtactic receptor for S100L protein on guinea pig eosinophils, *Biochem. Biophys. Res. Commun.*, 220, 871–874, 1996.
117. Jinquan, T., Vorum, H., Larsen, C.G. et al., Psoriasin: a novel chemotactic protein, *J. Invest. Dermatol.*, 107, 5–10, 1996.
118. Watson, P.H., Leygue, E.R., and Murphy, L.C., Psoriasin (S100A7), *Int. J. Biochem. Cell. Biol.*, 30, 567–571, 1998.
119. Eue, I., Pietz, B., Storck, J., Klempt, M., and Sorg, C., Transendothelial migration of 27E10$^+$ human monocytes, *Int. Immunol.*, 12, 1593–1604, 2000.
120. Yui, S., Mikami, M., and Yamazaki, M., Purification and characterization of the cytotoxic factor in rat peritoneal exudate cells: its identification as the calcium binding protein complex, calprotectin, *J. Leukocyte Biol.*, 58, 307–316, 1995.
121. Brandtzaeg, P., Gabrielsen, T.O., Dale, I., Muller, F., Steinbakk, M., and Fagerhol, M.K., The leucocyte protein L1 (calprotectin): a putative nonspecific defence factor at epithelial surfaces, *Adv. Exp. Med. Biol.*, 371A, 201–206, 1995.
122. Steinbakk, M., Naess-Andresen, C.F., Lingaas, E., Dale, I., Brandtzaeg, P., Fagerhol, M.K., Antimicrobial actions of calcium binding leucocyte L1 protein, calprotectin, *Lancet*, 336, 763–765, 1990.
123. Aguiar-Passeti, T., Postol, E., Sorg, C., and Mariano, M., Epithelioid cells from foreign-body granuloma selectively express the calcium-binding protein MRP-14, a novel down-regulatory molecule of macrophage activation, *J. Leukocyte Biol.*, 62, 852–858, 1997.
124. Brun, J.G., Ulvestad, E., Fagerhol, M.K., and Jonsson, R., Effects of human calprotectin (L1) on *in vitro* immunoglobulin synthesis, *Scand. J. Immunol.*, 40, 675–680, 1994.
125. Passey, R.J., Xu, K., Hume, D.A., and Geczy, C.L., S100A8: emerging functions and regulation, *J. Leukocyte Biol.*, 66, 549–556, 1999.
126. Lackmann, M., Rajasekariah, P., Iismaa, S.E. et al., Identification of a chemotactic domain of the proinflammatory S100 protein CP-10, *J. Immunol.*, 150, 2981–2991, 1993.
127. Cornish, C.J., Devery, J.M., Poronnik, P., Lackmann, M., Cook, D.I., and Geczy, C.L., S100 protein CP-10 stimulates myeloid cell chemotaxis without activation, *J. Cell. Physiol.*, 166, 427–437, 1996.
128. Hofmann, M.A., Drury, S., Fu, C. et al., RAGE mediates a novel proinflammatory axis: a central cell surface receptor for S100/calgranulin polypeptides, *Cell*, 97, 889–901, 1999.
129. Steinert, P.M. and Marekov, L.N., The proteins elafin, filaggrin, keratin intermediate filaments, loricrin, and small proline-rich proteins 1 and 2 are isodipeptide cross-linked components of the human epidermal cornified cell envelope, *J. Biol. Chem.*, 270, 17702–17711, 1995.
130. Markova, N.G., Marekov, L.N., Chipev, C.C., Gan, S.Q., Idler, W.W., Steinert, P.M., Profilaggrin is a major epidermal calcium-binding protein, *Mol. Cell. Biol.*, 13, 613–625, 1993.
131. Lee, S.C., Wang, M., McBride, O.W., O'Keefe, E.J., Kim, I.G., and Steinert, P.M., Human trichohyalin gene is clustered with the genes for other epidermal structural proteins and calcium-binding proteins at chromosomal locus 1q21, *J. Invest. Dermatol.*, 100, 65–68, 1993.
132. Maestrini, E., Monaco, A., McGrath, J. et al., A molecular defect in loricrin, the major component of the cornified cell envelope, underlies Vohwinkel's syndrome, *Nat. Genet.*, 13, 70–77, 1996.
133. Capon, F., Semprini, S., Chimenti, S. et al., Fine mapping of the PSORS4 psoriasis susceptibility region on chromosome 1q21, *J. Invest. Dermatol.*, 116, 728–730, 2001.
134. Libert, F., Cochaux, P., Beckman, G. et al., The deltaccr5 mutation conferring protection against HIV-1 in Caucasian populations has a single and recent origin in Northeastern Europe, *Hum. Mol. Genet.*, 7, 399–406, 1998.
135. Hewett, D., Samuelsson, L., Polding, J. et al., Identification of a psoriasis susceptibility candidate gene by linkage disequilibrium mapping with a localized single nucleotide polymorphism map, *Genomics*, 79, 305–314, 2002.

136. Bellamy, R., Ruwende, C., Corrah, T., McAdam, K.P., Whittle, H.C., and Hill, A.V., Variations in the NRAMP1 gene and susceptibility to tuberculosis in West Africans, *N. Engl. J. Med.*, 338, 640–644, 1998.
137. Ramoz, N., Rueda, L.A., Bouadjar, B., Favre, M., and Orth, G., A susceptibility locus for epidermodysplasia verruciformis, an abnormal predisposition to infection with the oncogenic human papillomavirus type 5, maps to chromosome 17qter in a region containing a psoriasis locus, *J. Invest. Dermatol.*, 112, 259–263, 1999.
138. Tosh, K., Meisner, S., Siddiqui, M.R. et al., A region of chromosome 20 is linked to leprosy susceptibility in a South Indian population, *J. Infect. Dis.*, 186, 1190–1193, 2002.
139. Gaffney, P.M., Ortmann, W.A., Selby, S.A. et al., Genome screening in human systemic lupus erythematosus: results from a second Minnesota cohort and combined analyses of 187 sib-pair families, *Am. J. Hum. Genet.*, 66, 547–556, 2000.
140. Bradley, M., Soderhall, C., Wahlgren, C.F., Luthman, H., Nordenskjold, M., and Kockum, I., The Wiskott–Aldrich syndrome gene as a candidate gene for atopic dermatitis, *Acta Derm. Venereol.*, 81, 340–342, 2001.
141. Chavanas, S., Garner, C., Bodemer, C. et al., Localization of the Netherton syndrome gene to chromosome 5q32, by linkage analysis and homozygosity mapping, *Am. J. Hum. Genet.*, 66, 914–921, 2000.
142. Chavanas, S., Bodemer, C., Rochat, A. et al., Mutations in SPINK5, encoding a serine protease inhibitor, cause Netherton syndrome, *Nat. Genet.*, 25, 141–142, 2000.
143. Mägert, H.J., Standker, L., Kreutzmann, P. et al., LEKTI, a novel 15-domain type of human serine proteinase inhibitor, *J. Biol. Chem.*, 274, 21499–21502, 1999.
144. Walley, A.J., Chavanas, S., Moffatt, M.F. et al., Gene polymorphism in Netherton and common atopic disease, *Nat. Genet.*, 29, 175–178, 2001.
145. Komatsu, N., Takata, M., Otsuki, N. et al., Elevated stratum corneum hydrolytic activity in Netherton syndrome suggests an inhibitory regulation of desquamation by SPINK5-derived peptides, *J. Invest. Dermatol.*, 118, 436–443, 2002.
146. Leyden, J.J., Marples, R.R., and Kligman, A.M., *Staphylococcus aureus* in the lesions of atopic dermatitis, *Br. J. Dermatol.*, 90, 525–530, 1974.
147. Wachter, A.M. and Lezdey, J., Treatment of atopic dermatitis with alpha 1-proteinase inhibitor, *Ann. Allergy*, 69, 407–414, 1992.
148. Capon, F., Semprini, S., Dallapiccola, B., and Novelli, G., Evidence for interaction between psoriasis-susceptibility loci on chromosomes 6p21 and 1q21, *Am. J. Hum. Genet.*, 65, 1798–1800, 1999.
149. Karason, A., Gudjonsson, J.E., Upmanyu, R. et al., A susceptibility gene for psoriatic arthritis maps to chromosome 16q: evidence for imprinting, *Am. J. Hum. Genet.*, 72, 125–131, 2003.
150. Samuelsson, L., Enlund, F., Torinsson, A. et al., A genome-wide search for genes predisposing to familial psoriasis by using a stratification approach, *Hum. Genet.*, 105, 523–529, 1999.
151. Peters, B.P., Weissman, F.G., and Gill, M.A., Pathophysiology and treatment of psoriasis, *Am. J. Health Syst. Pharm.*, 57, 645–659, 2000.
152. Baker, B.S., Garioch, J.J., Hardman, C., Powles, A., and Fry, L., Induction of cutaneous lymphocyte-associated antigen expression by group A streptococcal antigens in psoriasis, *Arch. Dermatol. Res.*, 289, 671–676, 1997.
153. Mallon, E., Bunce, M., Savoie, H. et al., HLA-C and guttate psoriasis, *Br. J. Dermatol.*, 143, 1177–1182, 2000.
154. Breuer-McHam, J.N., Marshall, G.D., Lewis, D.E., and Duvic, M., Distinct serum cytokines in AIDS-related skin diseases, *Viral Immunol.*, 11, 215–220, 1998.
155. Morishita, Y., Tada, J., Sato, A. et al., Possible influences of Staphylococcus aureus on atopic dermatitis — the colonizing features and the effects of staphylococcal enterotoxins, *Clin. Exp. Allergy*, 29, 1110–1117, 1999.
156. Miedzobrodzki, J., Kaszycki, P., Bialecka, A., and Kasprowicz, A., Proteolytic activity of *Staphylococcus aureus* strains isolated from the colonized skin of patients with acute-phase atopic dermatitis, *Eur. J. Clin. Microbiol. Infect. Dis.*, 21, 269–276, 2002.
157. Skov, L. and Baadsgaard, O., Bacterial superantigens and inflammatory skin diseases, *Clin. Exp. Dermatol.*, 25, 57–61, 2000.

158. Winton, H.L., Wan, H., Cannell, M.B. et al., Cell lines of pulmonary and non-pulmonary origin as tools to study the effects of house dust mite proteinases on the regulation of epithelial permeability, *Clin. Exp. Allergy*, 28, 1273–1285, 1998.
159. Moffatt, M. and Cookson, W., The genetics of asthma. Maternal effects in atopic disease, *Clin. Exp. Allergy*, 28(Suppl. 1), 56–61, 1998.
160. Burden, A., Javed, S., Bailey, M., Hodgins, M., Connor, M., and Tillman, D., Genetics of psoriasis: paternal inheritance and a locus on chromosome 6p [see comments], *J. Invest. Dermatol.*, 110, 958–960, 1998.
161. Miceli-Richard, C., Lesage, S., Rybojad, M. et al., CARD15 mutations in Blau syndrome, *Nat. Genet.*, 29, 19–20, 2001.
162. Ogura, Y., Bonen, D.K., Inohara, N. et al., A frameshift mutation in NOD2 associated with susceptibility to Crohn's disease, *Nature*, 411, 603–606, 2001.
163. Hugot, J.P., Chamaillard, M., Zouali, H. et al., Association of NOD2 leucine-rich repeat variants with susceptibility to Crohn's disease, *Nature*, 411, 599–603, 2001.
164. Rahman, P., Bartlett, S., Siannis, F. et al., CARD15: a pleiotropic autoimmune gene that confers susceptibility to psoriatic arthritis, *Am. J. Hum. Genet.,* 73, 677–681, 2003.
165. Cookson, W.O., Young, R.P., Sandford, A.J. et al., Maternal inheritance of atopic IgE responsiveness on chromosome 11q, *Lancet*, 340, 381–384, 1992.
166. Holt, P.G., Macaubas, C., Stumbles, P.A., and Sly, P.D., The role of allergy in the development of asthma, *Nature*, 402, B12–17, 1999.
167. Hall, J.G., Genomic imprinting, *Arch. Dis. Childhood,* 65, 1013–1016, 1990.
168. Reik, W. and Walter, J., Genomic imprinting: parental influence on the genome, *Natl. Rev. Genet.,* 2, 21–32, 2001.
169. Tomic-Canic, M., Komine, M., Freedberg, I.M., and Blumenberg, M., Epidermal signal transduction and transcription factor activation in activated keratinocytes, *J. Dermatol. Sci.*, 17, 167–181, 1998.
170. Freedberg, I., Tomic-Canic, M., Komine, M., and Blumenberg, M., Keratins and the keratinocyte activation cycle, *J. Invest. Dermatol.*, 116, 633–640, 2001.
171. Song, P.I., Park, Y.M., Abraham, T. et al., Human keratinocytes express functional CD14 and Toll-like receptor 4, *J. Invest. Dermatol.,* 119, 424–432, 2002.

# Part II

## Cellular Constituents of the Skin Immune System

# 5 The Keratinocyte

*Anthony C. Chu and Jenny F. Morris*

## CONTENTS



## I. INTRODUCTION

The concept of the skin simply as an inert barrier to infection and as an organ of temperature control has given way to the modern concept of the skin as an important immunological organ. The keratinocyte, which constitutes the growing epidermal component of the skin, has generated considerable interest because of three important findings. The first is that the keratinocyte expresses or can be induced to express a number of immunologically important surface antigens including the major histocompatability complex (MHC) class II molecule, HLA-DR, intercellular adhesion molecule 1 (ICAM-1)(CD54), and the co-stimulatory molecule B7-H1. These findings have generated enormous interest in the possible role of the keratinocyte as an accessory cell in both allogeneic and antigen-specific T-cell responses. The second major finding was that keratinocytes elaborate a number of cytokines that can influence immunological reactions and that have effects on immunocompetent cells. The third was the finding that keratinocytes express surface Toll-like receptors and produce antimicrobial proteins, which demonstrates that the keratinocyte is important

0-8493-1959-5/05/$0.00+$1.50

in the innate immune response. In this chapter, we examine these three facets of keratinocyte biology and present the current data that are available.

## II. MHC CLASS II MOLECULES

Class II molecules of the MHC play a central role in immune responses.[1] In humans, there are three major expressed classical MHC class II genetic loci — HLA-DR, DP, and DQ. Mice have only two expressed class II loci, I-A and I-E. Class II molecules are formed by the noncovalent association of three polypeptides designated α, β, and the invariant or λ chains, with the subsequent transportation of α:β dimers to the cell surface, where they are expressed. The λ chain is exclusively expressed during cytoplasmic processing of the class II molecules and is thought to be necessary for such processing.

The expression of MHC class II antigens by itself should not be sufficient to generate accessory cell function, but such function will depend on the ability of the cell to process, internalize, digest, and link the antigenic fragment with a suitable agretope to MHC class II antigen, which is then expressed on the cell surface. T-cell response is then dependent on a second signal produced by the accessory cell, which in part involves the secretion of interleukin-1 (IL-1) and association of the antigen-presenting cell to the T cell by adhesion molecules and binding of co-stimulatory molecules to ligands on the T cell.[2]

## III. HLA-DR EXPRESSION BY KERATINOCYTES

In 1981, Lampert and colleagues[3] first reported the expression of HLA-DR on keratinocytes in human graft-vs.-host disease (GVHD). Until that time, the only HLA-DR$^+$ cells recognized in human epidermis were the Langerhans cell[4] and acrosyringeal epithelium.[5] This exciting discovery marked a major extension of our understanding of the skin immune system. Examination of other dermatoses showed that HLA-DR was expressed on keratinocytes in dermatoses in which there was a lymphoid infiltrate within the skin. This included GVHD, mycosis fungoides, eczema, discoid lupus erythematosus, and lichen planus,[6] but HLA-DR was not observed in dermatoses in which a lymphoid infiltrate was not a feature, such as bullous pemphigoid and pemphigus vulgaris. It has long been known that γ interferon (IFN-γ), which is a Th1 cytokine, can induce expression of HLA-DR in cells that do not constitutively express this antigen. Such cells include endothelial cells, fibroblasts, and intestinal epithelial cells.[7] IFN-γ was therefore the prime contender for the agent responsible for the expression of HLA-DR in keratinocytes.

*In vitro* experiments have demonstrated that γ, but not α or β interferon,[8] will induce HLA-DR expression in human and murine keratinocytes. This can be blocked by using an anti-IFN-γ monoclonal antibody.[9] Studies have now established at the transcriptional level that IFN-γ induces the synthesis of MHC class II antigen *in vitro* and *in vivo*. Studies by Albanesi and colleagues[10] have demonstrated that IFN-γ induces both the classical MHC class II antigen HLA-DR and the nonclassical class II antigen HLA-DM, λ chain and two major transcriptional regulatory genes, class II transactivator and RFX5. HLAQ-DM acts as a chaperone, facilitating loading of antigen onto MHC class II molecules. These authors also demonstrated that induced HLA-DR was very resistant to sodium dodecyl sulfate denaturation at room temperature, which is a feature that class II molecules acquire when the groove is properly loaded with peptide.[10]

In addition to normal human keratinocytes in culture, IFN-γ will also induce HLA-DR expression on various keratinocyte lines, including cell lines derived from squamous cell carcinomas and trichilemomas.[11]

Keratinocytes express receptors for IFN-γ and induction of expression of HLA-DR is mediated by these receptors. Studies have shown that resting keratinocytes express high levels of high-affinity IFN-γ receptors but that the density of these receptors is significantly reduced in cells stimulated by epidermal growth factor or somatomedin-C, and consequently cells stimulated by these growth factors show reduced expression of HLA-DR in response to IFN-γ.[12]

In addition to IFN-γ, recent studies have shown that IL-8, produced by keratinocytes, will induce HLA-DR expression on cultured human keratinocytes via specific IL-8 receptors.[13]

As discussed earlier, HLA-DR is usually present on immunocompetent cells and is intimately related to antigen presentation to $CD4^+$ helper T cells and alloreactivity. The ability of keratinocytes to express HLA-DR thus suggests that the keratinocyte may be an immunocompetent cell and may have some activity as an accessory cell in T-cell stimulation. Expression of HLA-DR on a squamous cell carcinoma cell line induced by IFN-γ is inhibited by irradiation with ultraviolet (UV) light.[14] This finding suggests a mechanism by which UV irradiation gives therapeutic benefits in inflammatory dermatoses.

## IV. EXPRESSION OF MHC CLASS II ANTIGENS OTHER THAN HLA-DR ON KERATINOCYTES

Although HLA-DR has been shown to be expressed by human keratinocytes stimulated by IFN-γ *in vitro* and *in vivo*, little attention has been focused on the expression of the MHC class II isotypes DQ and DP.

In a study of MHC class II molecule expression by keratinocytes in various dermatoses, Volc-Plantzer et al.[15] observed HLA-DR, but not HLA-DQ, expression in cutaneous T-cell lymphoma, lichen planus, GVHD, or overlying a PPD response. HLA-DQ expression by keratinocytes has been reported in patients with late skin manifestations of *Borrelia* spirochete infection. In this study, patients with erythema chronicum migrans and acrodermatitis chronica atrophicans, both caused by *Borrelia* infection, were investigated. Keratinocytes in patients with erythema chronicum migrans showed HLA-DR, but no HLA-DQ, expression. However, in acrodermatitis chronica atrophicans, four of five patients who showed strong keratinocyte expression of HLA-DR also showed HLA-DQ.[16] The authors suggested that HLA-DQ expression in this disease was due to an abnormal immunological response of the host to this infection.

In a study of allergic and irritant contact dermatitis, HLA-DQ was observed in established reactions due to irritant dermatitis and in sensitization and challenge phases of contact allergic dermatitis. HLA-DQ expression was only observed in some but not all subjects investigated.[17] In this study, HLA-DP was also observed on keratinocytes in allergic but not irritant dermatitis.

HLA-DQ expression concurrently with HLA-DR is necessary for antigen presentation by macrophages to T cells,[18] and $DQ^+$ macrophages have been shown to be better stimulators of the autologous mixed lymphocyte reaction than their DQ-counterparts.[18] The role of DQ expression by keratinocytes remains obscure.

## V. OTHER BIOLOGICAL EFFECTS OF IFN-γ AND OTHER CYTOKINES ON KERATINOCYTES

In addition to inducing expression of HLA-DR in keratinocytes, IFN-γ has been shown to induce a number of other antigens on the surface of keratinocytes. Simon and Hunyadi[19] demonstrated in 1987 that IFN-γ induced CD36 on keratinocytes. CD36 is an 88-kDa glycoprotein, which is expressed on the membranes of a number of cells: endothelial cells, monocytes, platelets, and the C32 melanoma cell line,[20] and is regarded as a scavenger receptor. CD36 aids in the recognition of apoptotic cells and is important in mediating the uptake of oxidized low-density lipoprotein by monocytes leading to the formation of foam cells.[21]

CD36 is expressed by a subpopulation of monocytes ($CD14^-$ and $CD36^+$), which *in vitro* are potent activators of autoreactive T cells.[22] A similar functional population of accessory cells has been reported in human skin following UV irradiation.[23] This $CD1^-$, $DR^+$, $CD36^+$ population of cells is melanophagocytic, presents alloantigen, soluble antigen, and mitogens to T cells, and stimulates the autologous epidermal cell/lymphocyte reaction.[24] Of interest is the finding that keratinocytes in mycosis fungoides[25] and in allergic intracutaneous tests for delayed-type hypersensitivity[19] *in vivo* express CD36.

The relevance of CD36 expression by keratinocytes is speculative. The fact that CD36 is involved in cell adhesion may suggest a role for keratinocytes in trapping T cells or other leukocytes within the epidermis. Because $CD36^+$ and $CD14^-$ monocytes are potent activators of autoreactive T cells and because such cells express HLA-DQ indicate that keratinocytes, which can be induced to express both CD36 and HLA-DQ, may be involved in similar mechanisms.

Studies have demonstrated that in addition to CD36, keratinocytes can also be induced to express the macrophage marker CD16.[25] Keratinocytes overlying tuberculin tests and also in lichen planus, psoriasis, and mycosis fungoides, but not in normal skin and urticaria, have been shown to express CD13, CD14, and CD68.[25]

In 1988, Dustin et al.[26] demonstrated that IFN-γ and tumor necrosis factor α (TNF-α) could increase the expression of ICAM-1 (CD54) on cultured human keratinocytes. CD54 is usually expressed in very low levels or is absent from keratinocytes, but both IFN-γ and TNF-α increase the expression of this molecule to easily recognized levels. This was associated with an increase in the adhesion of T lymphoblasts to monolayers of cultured keratinocytes, presumably due to binding of lymphocyte function-associated antigen (CD11a) on the lymphocyte to its ligand CD54 on the keratinocyte. Other authors have also demonstrated that TNF-α and IFN-γ will increase binding of peripheral mononuclear cells and $CD4^+$ T-cell clones to cultured keratinocytes and squamous cell carcinoma cell lines.[27] This was blocked by antibodies to CD11a. The expression of CD54 on keratinocytes by IFN-γ and TNF-α may play an important role in the trafficking of T cells through the epidermis in inflammatory dermatoses.

CD54 induction by IFN-γ and TNF-α is variable in keratinocytes from different donors. In a study examining keratinocytes from 55 different donors, the pattern of CD54 induction by UV radiation correlated with the induction of CD54 by TNF-α but not IFN-γ, suggesting that UV radiation induces CD54 expression by upregulating TNF-α production by keratinocytes.[28]

IL-13 receptors have been identified on keratinocytes and stimulation of keratinocytes with IL-13 induces IL-6 production.[29] IL-17 produced by activated $CD4^+$ T cells acts on keratinocytes via the IL-17 receptor, which they constitutively express. IL-17 increases in a dose-dependent manner IFN-γ induced CD54 expression on keratinocytes. Other effects of IL-17 on keratinocytes include reduction of IL-1 receptor antagonist (IL-1Ra), release of growth-regulated oncogene alpha, granulocyte-macrophage colony-stimulating factor (GM-CSF), and IL-6 with synergistic or additive effects when used with IL-4 or IFN-γ. IL-17 and IL-4 increase stem cell factor release, which is inhibited by IFN-γ.[30]

IFN-γ activated keratinocytes have been shown to bind to the T cell ALL cell line HBS, but only poorly bind to the CTCL cell line H9. AD2 is a molecule expressed on the surface of HSB but not H9 that is recognized by the monoclonal antibody 13H12. 13H12 inhibits binding of HSB cells to IFN-γ-activated keratinocytes, suggesting that these cells express the ligand for AD2.[31] AD2 is expressed at low levels by peripheral T cells but at high levels by immature thymocytes.

IFN-γ has been shown to upregulate vascular endothelial growth factor (VEGF) by keratinocytes. VEGF is a mediator of angiogenesis associated with wound healing, inflammation, and tumor invasion and is produced by activated keratinocytes and fibroblasts.[32]

Keratinocytes constitutively express CD40, which is important in collaboration between T and B cells leading to T-cell-dependent activation, proliferation, or differentiation of B cells. CD40 expression is upregulated by IFN-γ but not by TNF-α or IL-1β. Ligation of CD40 to gp39 increases CD54 expression on keratinocytes induced by IFN-γ and leads to IL-8 release by keratinocytes. In psoriasis there is marked expression of CD40 on keratinocytes, suggesting a possible role of CD40 in the pathogenesis of psoriasis.[33]

IFN-γ is known to stimulate production of suppressor of cytokine signaling (SOCS) 1 and 3 by a number of different cell types. SOCS is a negative regulator of IFN-γ signaling. Recent studies have shown that SOCS1, 2, 3, and cytokine-inducible SH2-containing protein mRNA are induced by IFN-γ in human keratinocytes. SOCS1 can also be induced in keratinocytes by TNF-α and SOCS1, and cytokine-inducible SH2-containing protein can be induced in keratinocytes by IL-4. Transfection of SOCS1 and 3 into keratinocytes led to inhibition of IFN-γ-induced phosphorylation of IFN-γR and activation of STAT1 and STAT 3. SOCS1 and to a lesser extent SOCS3 reduced membrane expression of CD54 and HLA-DR and release of IFN-γ-inducible protein 10 by keratinocyte clones in response to IFN-γ.[34] Production of SOCS 1 and 3 may act as a negative feedback for IFN-γ and activation of keratinocytes.

IFN-γ will upregulate production of IL-1α, IL-1ra, GM-CSF, and TNF-α by keratinocytes. Interestingly, keratinocytes from patients with atopic eczema show a hyperresponsiveness to IFN-γ with increased production of IL-1α, IL-1ra, GM-CSF, and TNF-α compared to normal human keratinocytes in response to IFN-γ.[35]

Keratinocytes constitutively produce C3 and factor B. C3 synthesis is upregulated by IL-1α, IFN-γ, and TNF-α, whereas factor B synthesis is increased by IL-1α, IL-6, and IFN-γ.[36]

## VI. CYTOKINE PRODUCTION BY KERATINOCYTES

Keratinocytes constitutively secrete or can be induced by cytokines to secrete a large number of cytokines that can affect the immune response. These include both stimulatory and downregulatory molecules. Cytokine production by keratinocytes is discussed in detail in Chapter 14. In this chapter, we give only a very brief resume of the different cytokines produced by keratinocytes so that their importance in the possible accessory cell function of keratinocytes can be discussed.

### A. Pro-Inflammatory Cytokines (Table 5.1)

One of the most important pro-inflammatory cytokines produced by keratinocytes is IL-1 — initially described as epidermal thymocyte activating factor (ETAF).[37] This cytokine is an important co-stimulatory molecule of T-helper-cell activation, promotes B-cell maturation and clonal expansion, enhances natural killer (NK) cell activity, is chemotactic for neutrophils and macrophages, and increases CD54 expression on endothelial cells. Keratinocytes synthesize IL-1α, IL-1β, and IL-1ra and express both type I and type II IL-1 receptors.[38] Keratinocytes produce IL-1α and IL-1β mRNA *in vitro*, but only IL-1α biological activity has been identified in keratinocyte cultures. IL-1β is produced as a 31-kDa inactive form, which can be cleaved into an 18-kDa active molecule by chymotrypsin. Keratinocytes do not possess the IL-1 convertase enzyme that naturally cleaves the IL-1β precursor and the molecule remains inactive until it is released by the cell.[39] IFN-γ increases production of IL-1α, IL-1β, and IL-1ra by cultured keratinocytes.[40] Keratinocytes appear to elaborate a further IL-1 form distinct from IL-1α and IL-1β but with the same biological properties. Partial cDNA for this factor has been isolated from the human keratinocyte cell line COLO-16.[41]

Keratinocytes express low levels of the type I IL-1 receptor (IL-1RI), which signal transduces. GM-CSF secretion by keratinocytes, induced by IL-1, is mediated by these receptors. Type II IL-1 receptors (IL-2RII) are nonsignal transducing, but are expressed at high levels by keratinocytes and on activation this expression is increased. *In vitro*, IL-1RII receptors are shed into the supernatant, where they avidly bind to IL-1 and may play a biological role as an IL-1 antagonist.[42]

Keratinocytes secrete TNF-α, and this is upregulated by lipopolysaccharide and UV radiation.[43] TNF-α has a cytotoxic effect on tumor cells and induces cytokines involved in the inflammatory response to be secreted by numerous cell types. TNF-α will increase IL-1ra and IL-1α production by keratinocytes.[38] Keratinocytes express the p55 TNF-α receptor.[44] When TNF-α is given intradermally in human volunteers, there is initially a neutrophil infiltrate of the dermis and then a $CD4^+$

**TABLE 5.1**
**Pro-Inflammatory Cytokines Produced by Keratinocytes**

| Cytokine | Also Known As | Function |
|---|---|---|
| IL-1 | Epidermal thymocyte activating factor (ETAF) | Co-stimulatory molecule of T-helper-cell activation; promotes B-cell maturation; enhances NK cell activity; is chemotactic for neutrophils and macrophages; increases ICAM-1 expression on endothelial cells |
| GM-CSF | | Growth factor for monocyte and macrophage precursors, important in Langerhans cell differentiation; stimulates macrophages for antimicrobial and antitumor activity |
| TNF-α | | Cytotoxic effect on tumor cells; induces cytokine secretion my numerous cell types |
| IL-6 | | Increases secretion of antibody by plasma cells; with IL-1 acts as a co-stimulatory molecule for T-cell activation; aids in the differentiation of myeloid stem cells |
| IL-7 | | Increases surface expression of the integrin α3β1, which is involved in the adhesion of T cells, and thus trafficking across the basement membrane zone of the epidermis |
| IL-12 | | Multiple effects on T cells and NK cells, required for optimal Th1 cell development |
| IL-15 | | Induces other cytokine release including TNF-α, IFN-γ, and IL-17; recruits and activates T cells and other inflammatory cells |
| IL-18 | IFN-γ-inducing factor | Enhances IL-12 driven Th1 responses; in the absence of IL-12 can stimulate Th2 responses; enhances cytolysis by NK cells |

T-cell infiltrate with an accumulation of $CD36^+$ macrophages and migration of epidermal Langerhans cells into the dermis. There is also induction of CD54 and VCAM-1 (CD106) on endothelial cells and interstitial dermal dendritic cells and CD54 on keratinocytes.[45]

IL-6 increases secretion of antibody by plasma cells and, together with IL-1, acts as a co-stimulatory molecule for T-cell activation and aids in the differentiation of myeloid stem cells. IL-1 and IL-6 mRNA and protein are increased in keratinocytes in response to TNF-α, GM-CSF, TGF-β, lipopolysaccharide, and phorbol myristate acetate.[46,47] IL-6 but not IL-1 production by keratinocytes is upregulated by IL-17.[48] Keratinocytes have been shown to express IL-6 receptors.

Keratinocytes produce IL-7 in the basal cell layer. IL-7 increases cell surface expression of the integrin alpha3beta1, which is involved in adhesion of T cells to laminin 5. Studies suggest that IL-7 is required for the adhesion of T cells to laminin 5, which may be important in T-cell trafficking across the basement membrane zone of the epidermis.[49]

Recent studies have shown that human keratinocytes express and release IL-12. IL-12 has multiple effects on T cells and NK cells and is required for optimal Th1 cell development.[50] IL-12 is a heterodimer composed of p35 and p40 chains. mRNA for the p35 chain is constitutively produced by keratinocytes, but mRNA for the p40 chain is only detected after contact allergen application to the skin and not by contact irritant application.[51] The p40 chain is also induced in a dose-dependent fashion in response to UVA radiation.[52]

IL-18, previously known as IFN-γ-inducing factor, is a recently described member of the IL-1 cytokine superfamily. It is expressed at sites of chronic inflammation, in autoimmune disease, and in various forms of cancer. It enhances IL-12-mediated IFN-γ production by lymphocytes and Fas/perforin-mediated cytolysis by NK cells.[53] Immunohistochemical studies have identified IL-18 in all living layers of the epidermis with the protein expressed in the cytoplasm and the receptor on the cell membrane. Immunoblotting techniques have shown both the mature 18-kDa and precursor 24-kDa forms.[54] Polymerase chain reaction analysis of cultured human keratinocytes has shown that IL-18 is constitutively transcribed but not increased by IL-1β, TNF-α, IFN-γ,

**TABLE 5.2**
**Growth Factors Produced by Keratinocytes**

| Factor | Also Known As | Function |
|---|---|---|
| GM-CSF | | Growth factor for monocyte and macrophage precursors, important in Langerhans cell differentiation; stimulates macrophages for antimicrobial and antitumor activity |
| IL-7 | | Growth factor for B cells; has a proliferative effect on T-cell progenitors and mature peripheral T cells |
| IL-15 | | T-cell growth factor |
| SCF | Stem cell factor | Induces proliferation of mast cells and other hemopoietic cells; involved in the development and activation of mast cells |
| VEGF | Vascular endothelial growth factor | Induces angiogenesis |

phorbol mystate acetate, or nickel sulfate. In this study only the 24-kDa precursor form was identified in cell lysates.[55] High plasma levels of IL-18 have been identified in patients with psoriasis and in this study, the levels of IL-18 correlated with psoriasis area and severity index (PASI).[56] IL-18 enhances IL-12-driven Th1 immune responses but in the absence of IL-12 can stimulate Th2 responses.[57]

## B. Growth Factors for Immunocompetent Cells (Table 5.2)

Keratinocytes were initially thought to secrete IL-3, but recent studies have shown that mRNA for IL-3 and IL-3 protein cannot be detected in human keratinocytes or culture supernatants. Antibodies to GM-CSF and IL-6 can abrogate the IL-3 biological activity found in keratinocyte supernatants.[58] GM-CSF is produced by keratinocytes and cytokine production is upregulated by IL-1. IL-7 is a growth factor for B cell progenitors and has a proliferative effect on T-cell progenitors and mature peripheral T cells. IL-7 production by keratinocytes has prompted suggestions that it may be involved in the pathogenesis of inflammatory skin diseases and cutaneous T-cell lymphoma. Keratinocytes also produce IL-15,[59] which is a growth factor for T cells but is also a pro-inflammatory cytokine acting early in the inflammatory response, inducing other cytokines including TNF-α, IFN-γ, and IL-17 and recruiting and activating T cells and other inflammatory cells.[60] IL-15 is induced by lipopolysaccharide and plays a crucial role in activation of polymorphonuclear leukocytes.[61] IFN-γ has also been shown in keratinocytes to upregulate vascular endothelial growth factor (VEGF). VEGF is a mediator of angiogenesis associated with wound healing, inflammation, and tumor invasion and is produced by activated keratinocytes and fibroblasts.[32]

Keratinocytes have been shown to produce stem cell factor (SCF), which induces proliferation of mast cells and other hemopoietic cells and is involved in the development and activation of melanocytes.[62] The receptor for SCF is KIT, a class III tyrosine kinase receptor. This growth factor is upregulated in the human epidermal keratinocyte cell line DJM-1 by vasoactive intestinal peptide, IL-4, IL-13, TNF-α, and IFN-γ.[63]

## C. Chemoattractant Cytokines (Table 5.3)

IL-1 is a potent chemokine for neutrophils and macrophages, which has led to speculation on its potential role in neutrophil accumulation in psoriasis. IL-8 is chemotactic for neutrophils and T cells. IL-8 secretion by keratinocytes is induced by TNF-α[64] and by a number of nonspecific stimuli to the skin including contact sensitizers, tolerogens, and irritants.[65]

Keratinocytes produce the chemokine CCL27[66]. The receptor for CCL27, CCR10, is expressed in the skin on melanocytes, dermal fibroblasts, and endothelial cells and is also expressed by $CLA^+CD4^-$ T cells and immature dendritic cells. CCL27 is upregulated by TNF-α and IL-1β but

**TABLE 5.3**
**Chemoattractant Cytokines Produced by Keratinocytes**

| Cytokine | Also Known As | Function |
|---|---|---|
| IL-1 | | Chemokine for neutrophils and macrophages |
| CCL27 | Cutaneous T-cell-attracting chemokine CTACK, ILC | Important in T-cell-mediated skin inflammation and normal trafficking of T cells through the skin |
| CCL5 | RANTES | Chemokine for eosinophils, memory T cells and monocytes |
| CCL17 | TARC | Th2 cell chemokine and ligand for CCR4 |
| CXCL10 | Inducible protein 10 (IP-10) | Chemokine for Th1 type cells and ligand for CXCR3 |
| Mig | Mitogen inducible gene | T-cell chemotractant |
| IP9 | Inducible protein 9, I-TAC, betaR1, H-174 | T-cell chemoattractant |
| CCL20 | Macrophage inflammatory protein 3α | Chemokine for Langerhans cells |

this upregulation is reduced by IL-10. These characteristics suggest that CCL27 is important in T-cell-mediated skin inflammation and possibly in the normal trafficking of T cells through the skin.[67]

Keratinocytes have been shown to produce RANTES/CCL5, a chemokine for eosinophils, memory T cells, and monocytes. Production of CCL5 is increased by TNF-α and IL-1β in a synergistic fashion.[68]

Keratinocytes have been shown to produce the thymus- and activation-regulated chemokine (TARC/CCL17),[69] which is a chemokine for Th2-type cells and a ligand for CCR4. Keratinocytes also produce an interferon-induced protein of 10 kDa (IP-10/CXCL10),[70] a chemokine for Th1-type cells, which is a ligand for CXCR3, following stimulation with TNF-α or IFN-γ. IL-4 has been shown to reduce CCL17 levels induced by TNF-α and IFN-γ in human HaCaT cells (immortalized human keratinocytes) but increased levels of CXCL10 by HaCaT cells stimulated by TNF-α and IFN-γ.[71]

Keratinocytes produce a monokine induced by IFN-γ (mitogen inducible gene, Mig) and IFN-inducible T-cell alpha chemoattractant (I-TAC), also known as inducible protein–9, beta R1, and H-174,[72] which are potent chemoattractants for T cells acting through the CXCR3 receptor. These chemokines are upregulated by INFγ and TNF-α and this is potentiated by IL-4.[73]

Keratinocytes produce CCL20 (macrophage inflammatory protein 3 alpha), which is a chemokine for Langerhans cells. At both protein and message level, CCL20 is upregulated by TNF-α and is mainly expressed by cells in the spinous layer. The receptor for CCL20 is CCR6.[74]

## D. Downregulatory Cytokines (Table 5.4)

IL-1 receptor antagonist (IL-1Ra) was originally described as a secreted molecule that competitively inhibits binding of IL-1 to its surface receptor. In addition to the secreted isoform, three intracellular isoforms — icIL-1Ra1, 2 and 3 — have been characterized. The intracellular isoforms are synthesized in the cytoplasm and are not transported to the nucleus. In keratinocytes, icIL-1Ra2 may be released in some circumstances.[75]

Keratinocytes produce small amounts of active IL-1R1 but produce large amounts of the inactive receptor IL-1RII, which is upregulated on activation of the keratinocyte. IL-1RII is cleaved from expressing cells and avidly binds IL-1β and functions within the milieu of the skin as an IL-1 inhibitor.

IL-10 production by human keratinocytes is controversial. Recent studies suggest that IL-10 is constitutively secreted by human keratinocytes and secretion is upregulated by tape stripping of the skin, in poison ivy reactions,[76] and following UV radiation.[77] IL-10 mRNA is upregulated by UVB and UVA in a time- and dose-dependent manner and is maximal with UVA.[78] Studies

**TABLE 5.4**
**Downregulatory Cytokines Produced by Keratinocytes**

| Cytokine | Also Known As | Function |
|---|---|---|
| IL-1Ra | IL-1 receptor antagonist | Competitively inhibits binding of IL-1 to its surface receptor |
| IL-10 | | Suppresses cytokine production by Th1 cells |
| α-MSH | α Melanocyte-stimulating hormone | Inhibits TNF-α and IL-1β production; increases IL-10 production; inhibits IFN-γ and IL-12; downregulates expression of CD86 and CD40 |
| CXCL10 | IP10 (interferon inducible protein) | Suppresses colony formation by CD34+ cells |
| Contra IL-1 | | Negative feedback in response to excessive IL-1 production |
| PGE2 | Prostaglandin E2 | Promotes keratinocyte growth and downregulates the immune response |

have also suggested that IL-10 mRNA is upregulated in human keratinocytes by alpha melanocyte stimulating hormone (MSH).[79] Other studies, however, have demonstrated that human keratinocytes do not produce IL-10 and that traces of IL-10 identified in epidermal preparations originate from melanocytes contaminating the system.[80] IL-10 receptor (IL-10R) have been identified in keratinocytes and shown to be functionally active.[81] IL-10 suppresses cytokine production by Th 1 cells and thus inhibits IL-2, IFN-γ, and TNF-α production by these cells. IL-10 is thus a potent immunosuppressive agent and may be implicated in the immunosuppression induced by UV radiation.

α-MSH is a 13-amino-acid peptide that is produced in a number of tissues including intermediate lobe of the pituitary, gut, and skin. In addition to its role in pigmentation, it has also been shown to inhibit inflammation and induce immunomodulation.[82] In human skin α-MSH has been identified in keratinocytes as well as in melanocytes[83] and is upregulated by UVB radiation. One of the receptors for α-MSH, MC-1R, is also expressed by keratinocytes as well as dendritic cells, macrophages, and endothelial cells. α-MSH inhibits TNF-α and IL-1β and increases IL-10 production by both monocytes and keratinocytes.[79] α-MSH also inhibits IFN-γ and IL-2 and downregulates expression of CD86 and CD40.[84] The fact that α-MSH is induced in keratinocytes by UVB radiation suggests that it may have a role in reducing inflammatory reaction to UVB and reducing immunological reactions to neoantigens generated in the skin following UV irradiation.

Human interferon inducible protein 10, IP10 (CXCL10), has been shown to be produced by keratinocytes. IP-10 is produced by T cells, monocytes, and endothelial cells, and it suppresses colony formation by CD34+ cells.[85]

Other downregulatory molecules produced by the epidermis include epidermally derived contra IL-1[84] and prostaglandin E2.[86,87] Epidermally derived contra IL-1 is a poorly characterized factor produced by keratinocytes, and the concurrent production of its antagonist may be part of a physiological negative feedback mechanism in response to excessive IL-1 production. Prostaglandin E2 is the major arachadonic acid metabolite produced by keratinocytes. It is a growth-promoting autocoid for keratinocytes,[89] and in culture its production is reduced by contact inhibition. Reduced levels of PGE2 are associated with reduced growth rate of the keratinocytes. PGE2, however, is also an important downregulatory molecule in inflammatory responses. Its association as a keratinocyte growth promoter and as a downregulatory molecule for T-cell responses suggests that it plays a prominent role in healing phases following epidermal injury.[90]

Keratinocytes are thus able to produce a range of cytokines that will provide upregulatory and downregulatory signals to an immune response. The end result will depend on the stimulus used and may involve genetic factors that influence cytokine production in the skin in different individuals (Figure 5.1).

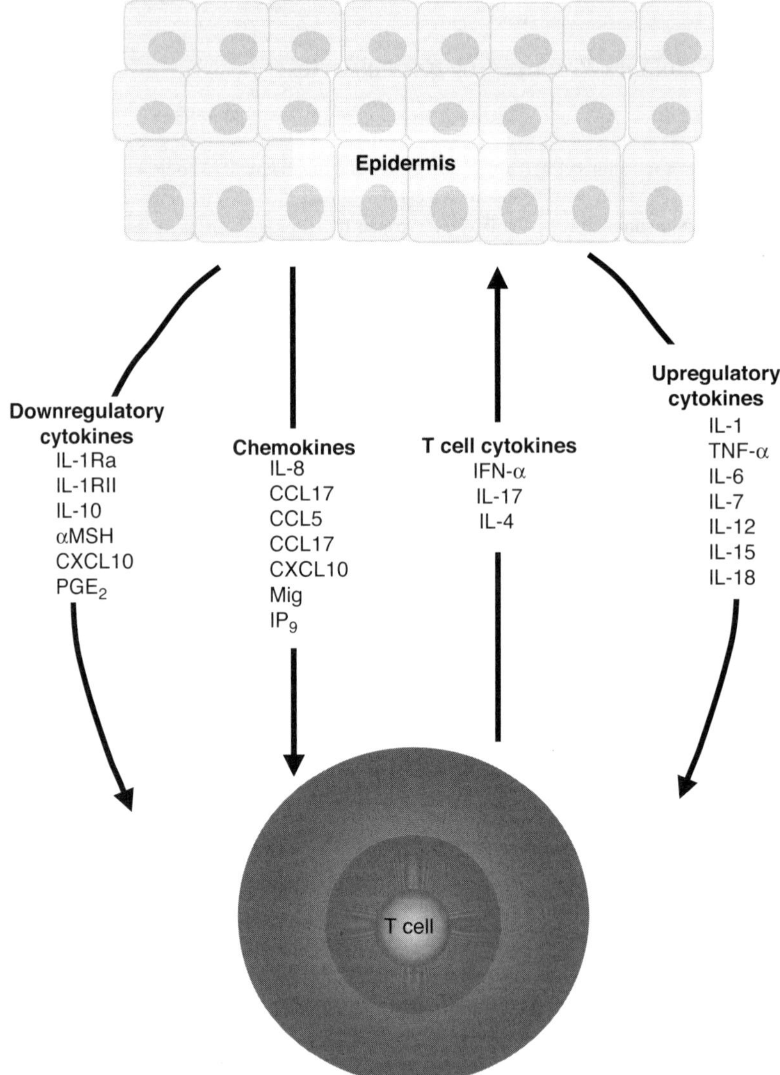


**FIGURE 5.1** Interaction of keratinocytes and T-cell-derived cytokines.

## VII. FUNCTIONAL ACTIVITY OF KERATINOCYTES

### A. Inductive Effect of Keratinocytes on T Cells

The first studies to show that keratinocytes could have an effect on lymphocyte maturation were reported by Rubenfeld et al. in 1981.[91] These authors used both a murine and a human system to examine the effect of co-cultivation of keratinocytes with mature and immature T cells. In the murine system, autologous bone marrow cells were co-cultivated with epidermal cells. These bone marrow cells subsequently demonstrated the expression of the enzyme terminal deoxyribonucleotidyl transferase (TDT), which is an early marker of T-cell differentiation and also the acquisition of the Thy 1 (CD90) antigen on the cell surface. These studies showed that T-cell precursors in bone marrow could be induced along a T-cell maturational pathway by epidermal cells.

In the human system, peripheral blood mononuclear cells were co-cultivated with epidermal cell cultures. These cells were found to express the enzyme TDT following co-cultivation. This was a surprising finding, as TDT is a marker of very immature T cells, and the expression of this enzyme in peripheral blood lymphocytes suggested a downregulation of these cells into a more immature phenotype. The authors suggested that the cells sensitive to this inductive influence might be uncommitted post-thymic precursor T cells. The true nature of these cells remains to be elucidated.

In the human system, Mackie and Hughes[92] demonstrated that human epidermal cell culture supernatants could induce a degree of maturation in human thymocytes. In this assay, the authors found that thymocytes could be induced to modulate CD1a and to express a more mature phenotype. A subsequent study has shown that epidermal cell supernatants and epidermal cell cultures could induce CD1a in leukemic T cells that express the phenotype and functional activity of mature helper T cell, i.e., $CD3^+$, $CD4^+$, $CD8^-$, $CD1a^-$.[93] The epidermis, therefore, appears to be able to significantly affect the maturation of T lymphocytes and may induce a mature phenotype in immature T cells and a less mature phenotype in more mature T cells. Whether IL-12 is a factor involved in these observations is unclear.

## B. Keratinocytes as Accessory Cells

Keratinocytes can be induced to express HLA-DR, CD54, and to a lesser extent, HLA-DQ, and they constitutively secrete IL-1. These cells thus possess some of the major signals necessary for accessory cell function in presenting antigen to T cells and stimulating an allogeneic response.

T-cell receptor recognition of antigen in association with MHC complexes, however, is insufficient to lead to T-cell clonal expansion or effector function. Ligation of CD28/CTLA-4 on T cells to CD80/CD86 on antigen-presenting cells supplies important co-stimulatory signals necessary to allow T-cell activation to proceed.

IFN-γ-stimulated keratinocytes positively stain with monoclonal antibody BB1 but not other antibodies against B7-1 (CD80) or B7-2 (CD86) and do not express mRNA for CD80.[94] CD80 is a low-affinity ligand for CD28 but a high-affinity ligand for CTLA-4.[94] Studies have now demonstrated that monoclonal antibody BB1 recognizes CD74, the MHC class II λ chain, as well as CD80. It is now considered likely that the reactivity with BBI and lack of reactivity with other antibodies to CD80 demonstrates CD74 expression by IFN-γ-stimulated human keratinocytes but not CD80 expression.[95] Lack of CD80 may be responsible for the apparent lack of antigen-presenting activity observed on keratinocytes.

In inflamed skin, keratinocytes have been shown to express a novel member of the B7 family, B7-H1.[96] The ligand for B7-H1 is not CD28 or CLTA-4. B7-H1 will bind to PD-1, a receptor implicated in negative regulation of T and B cells, but it is yet unclear whether co-stimulation of T cells is mediated via these receptors.[97] B7-H1 appears to be involved in induction of tolerance.

## C. Keratinocytes as Accessory Cells for Mitogen-Driven Responses

Normal keratinocytes and IFN-γ-treated keratinocytes have been shown to act as accessory cells for T cells in their response to phytohemagglutinin. Responses were fivefold higher in the IFN-γ-treated keratinocytes. The response requires cell-to-cell contact and could be inhibited by antibodies against CD2 and LFA-3 and to a lesser extent by antibodies to CD18 and CD54.[98]

## D. Keratinocytes as Accessory Cells for Superantigen-Driven Responses

Untreated and IFN-γ-treated keratinocytes are able to provide the co-stimulatory signals necessary for T-cell response to staphylococcal enterotoxins A and B.[98] IFN-γ-treated keratinocytes were significantly more potent accessory cells than untreated keratinocytes. T-cell stimulation was characterized by rosette formation between keratinocytes and T cells. Stimulation by untreated keratinocytes was abrogated by antibodies against CD54 and CD18. In the IFN-γ-treated keratinocytes, antibodies against CD11a, CD18, and CD54 reduced stimulation by 70 to 90%. Antibodies against

CD28, CD80, and CD86 had no effect on this T-cell activation, and antibodies against HLA-DR only inhibited responses by 8 to 28%.

Keratinocytes thus are able to act as accessory cells to T-cell stimulation by superantigens with CD54:CD11a binding a key feature of the keratinocyte/T-cell interaction. This could have implications in psoriasis and atopic dermatitis where superantigens have been shown to have a possible role in the pathogenesis of these diseases.

## E. Keratinocytes as Antigen-Presenting Cells

Studies examining antigen presentation by keratinocytes have given conflicting results. It should be noted that the majority of antigens require processing before they can be presented by an accessory cell. Failure of keratinocytes to act as accessory cells in antigen presentation may thus be due to an absence of antigen processing. Keratinocytes are capable of phagocytosis and endocytosis,[99] but no study has yet investigated the antigen-processing ability of these cells. In studies of HLA-DR$^+$ thymocytes,[100] these cells have been shown to be able to present viral peptide antigen fragments, which require no processing, to T cells, but the cells are unable to process intact virus and present antigen. Processing and presentation may therefore be dissociated in certain cell types.

In studies of keratinocyte antigen-presentation activity, the majority of investigators have used unpurified epidermal cell populations or abnormal cell populations. In the former, the effect of Langerhans cells and in mice of Thy 1$^+$ dendritic cells must be taken into consideration. In the latter, the prior conditioning of epidermal cells may affect the functional activity of the cells.

In a study of a murine model of GVHD, Breathnach et al.[101] demonstrated no antigen-presenting capacity of IA$^+$ keratinocytes. In producing GVHD in C3H/He mice, the animals were first lethally X-irradiated and then injected with allogeneic bone marrow cells. The epidermal cells were used unpurified and tested against T-cell clones specific for 2,3,6-trinitrobenzenesulfonic acid, ovalbumin, pigeon cytochrome C, and the predigested fragment of pigeon cytochrome, 81-104 CytC, which can be presented to T cells without further processing.

These authors showed a decreased capacity of epidermal cells from mice with GVHD to present antigen to T cells compared with normal epidermal cells, despite keratinocyte expression of IA. These cells also showed a reduced capacity in presenting the 81–104 fragment of CytC to T cells. From these results, the authors concluded that IA$^+$ keratinocytes have no antigen-presenting activity. The problems with this study are, first, that the epidermal cells were used unseparated and the effects of other epidermal cells could not be assessed, and second, that the epidermal cells were X-irradiated, which introduced an additional variable that may have influenced the results.

In one study of epidermal cells overlying a PPD response,[102] up to 86% of the epidermal cells were shown to express HLA-DR and there was an amplification of T-cell response by these cells when used as antigen-presenting cells as compared with normal epidermal cells *in vitro*. As with the previous study, the cells were used unseparated, as epidermal cells containing Langerhans cells, keratinocytes, and other possible accessory cells recruited by the PPD response. The authors suggested that the augmentation of T-cell response observed could be due to antigen presentation by keratinocytes or to the release of cytokines such as IL-1 by the keratinocytes.

Using a human system, we have used purified keratinocytes to examine antigen presentation. Keratinocytes were derived from suction blisters overlying a PPD reaction, of which only 10 to 20% of the keratinocytes were DR$^+$ (the skin was taken after a shorter time than in the previous study, when the reaction was at its most pronounced). Langerhans cells were removed using an immunomagnetic technique or sorted using fluorescence-activated cells sorting after labeling the cells with an anti-CD1a monoclonal antibody. HLA-DR$^+$ and DR$^-$ keratinocytes in this study showed no antigen-presenting activity. These cells also had no influence on the functional activity of the Langerhans cells, suggesting that their lack of presentation was not due to the production of downregulatory cytokines. It is possible that the inability of HLA-DR$^+$ keratinocytes to present antigen may be due to the low density levels of HLA-DR molecules expressed on the surface of the keratinocyte, compared with that on conventional antigen-presenting cells.

In a murine system, however, Gaspari and Katz[103] demonstrated that IA+ keratinocytes depleted of Langerhans cells were unable to present native peptide but could present a peptide fragment of pigeon cytochrome C to a hybridoma, suggesting that keratinocytes like thymocytes[104] are unable to process antigen.

In one study, human keratinocytes induced by IFN-γ to express HLA-DR and CD54 were found to stimulate three alloreactive HLA-DR-specific T-cell clones. These keratinocytes could also activate two of four minor histocompatibility antigen-specific T-cell clones derived from the blood of a patient with GVHD. The T-cell-stimulating potential of HLA-DR+ keratinocytes was relatively low compared with conventional antigen-presenting cells and was only seen when keratinocytes were used at low seeding density as adherent cells and was not observed in keratinocytes in suspension.[104]

A possible mechanism of the weak co-stimulatory activity of IFN-γ-stimulated keratinocytes may be due to binding of chondroitin sulfate to CD74. Chondroitin sulfate–modified CD74 has been shown to bind to CD44 on T cells and enhance T-cell responses.[105]

## F. Keratinocytes as Antigen-Presenting Cells for Allogeneic T Cells

The field of alloantigen presentation is controversial. Current theory is that an accessory cell can induce a proliferative response in allogeneic T cells without prior processing of the alloantigen by accessory cells autologous to the responder T cells. This is thought to be due to presentation of self-antigen in association with the HLA-DR molecule on the surface of the accessory cell, which is regarded as foreign by allogeneic T cells with the initiation of a primary response to the antigen. This concept is not entirely accepted within immunology, and some immunologists believe that alloantigen is processed and presented in the same way as conventional soluble antigens.

Alloantigen presentation is, however, used as a measure of accessory cell function with the assumption that the stimulator population needs accessory cell function to be able to elicit a response from responder allogeneic T cells. In their study of IA+ keratinocytes in mice with GVHD, Breathnach et al.[101] showed that epidermal cells from such mice demonstrated decreased alloantigen presentation compared with epidermal cells from normal mice. Responder cells were T cells enriched by passage through sephadex G10 and nylon wool columns. As with their observations of decreased antigen presentation by IA+ keratinocytes from GVHD mice, the stimulator population was not purified, and the keratinocytes may have been modified by X-irradiation.

In a study by Nicholoff et al.[87] using a human system, HLA-DR+ and HLA-DR− cultured keratinocytes were shown to induce RNA synthesis and IFN-γ production by allogeneic peripheral blood mononuclear cells, but did not induce a proliferative response when cultured keratinocytes as a single cell suspension or as a monolayer were added to a conventional mixed lymphocyte reaction. Inhibition of response was seen in a concentration-dependent manner, which did not depend on expression of HLA-DR, induced by IFN-γ on the keratinocytes and was not blocked by indomethacin or anti-IFN-γ antibodies. This inhibition was, however, reduced when epidermal cell monolayers were X-irradiated prior to use. The authors attributed this inhibition to a suppressive factor, keratinocyte-derived lymphocyte inhibitory factor (KLIF).

When cultured epidermal cells were seeded at a low cell density and attached cultures used as stimulators of an allogeneic reaction, a small proliferation response was observed. These authors suggested that the inability of HLA-DR+ keratinocytes to produce mitogenesis of allogeneic peripheral blood mononuclear cells might be due to the following:

1. A low level of HLA-DR expression on the keratinocyte as compared with Langerhans cells and monocytes

2. That other surface markers important in inducing allogenic responses such as HLA-DQ are not induced on keratinocytes by IFN-γ
3. The presence of inhibitory factors such as KLIF

These findings were supported by the findings of Czernielewski[106] that human keratinocytes induced to express HLA-DR by IFN-γ failed to induce an allogeneic response in peripheral blood mononuclear cells. In this assay, a human keratinocyte cell line and epidermal cell cultures were used. The cell line failed to stimulate a reaction and the IFN-γ-treated epidermal cells showed a lower response than untreated epidermal cells, suggesting that HLA-DR expression by keratinocytes provided a downregulatory signal during allogeneic reactions between Langerhans cells and T cells.

The findings that HLA-DR$^+$ and DR$^-$ keratinocytes could induce stimulation of T cells but not mitogenesis was of enormous interest and has been further examined using a murine model.[15] In this study, IA was induced on the Pam 212 murine keratinocyte cell by IFN-γ, and IA$^+$ and IA$^-$ keratinocytes could stimulate syngeneic and allogeneic T cells, although IA$^+$ keratinocytes produced higher stimulation. This stimulation was not inhibited by anti-IA monoclonal antibodies, suggesting that the stimulation of T cells by Pam 212 cells was not due to antigen-presenting functions of Pam 212 cells unless Pam 212 cells were functioning as antigen-presenting cells through I-E antigens. These authors attributed the stimulation of T cells to cytokines produced by the Pam 212 cells.

### G. Keratinocytes in Induction of Tolerance in T Cells

IA$^+$ murine keratinocytes modified with trinitrobenzene sulfonic acid were unable to induce a proliferative response in TNP specific, i.e., κ-restricted Th1 clone SE-4. Following co-cultivation, IL-3 and IFN-γ were detected in culture supernatants but IL-2 was not, and the SE-4 cells remained unresponsive to subsequent stimulation with TNP-modified functional accessory cells.[107]

In a human system, a keratinocyte cell line was immortalized using HPV16 and a Molony murine LTR promoter, stimulated with IFN-γ, and was shown to induce antigen-specific tolerance in an HLA-DR1/4 restricted influenza hemagglutinin specific T-cell clone.[108]

In both these studies, T-cell clones were used and in the human system the keratinocytes were modified by viral immortalization. Further studies using autologous systems in freshly separated cells would confirm that this was a real phenomenon rather than an epiphenomenon.

In a recent study, skin grafting using autologous skin islets inlaid in allogeneic skin sheets was found to delay graft rejection. Using a murine system, autologous keratinocytes were found to suppress lymphocyte responses to allogeneic epidermal cells due to a shift from Th1 to Th2 response mediated by IL-10. The authors suggest that this is due to expression of B7-H1 by keratinocytes, which activates IL-10-secreting lymphocytes.[109]

## VIII. KERATINOCYTE INVOLVEMENT IN INNATE IMMUNE RESPONSES

Keratinocytes are the main constituent of the epidermis and their involvement in the first-line defense against infectious agents is not surprising. The recent demonstration that keratinocytes express Toll-like receptors and produce antimicrobial peptides has helped to elucidate their functional activity in this role.

### A. Toll-Like Receptors

Toll-like receptors were first identified in *Drosophila,* which have no adaptive immune system but are very resistant to microbial infection. The innate immune system in these insects provides protection partly due to the synthesis of antimicrobial peptides induced in response to signaling pathways activated by at least two members of the Toll-like receptor family. dToll induces an antifungal peptide drosomycin and 18-wheeler induces an antibacterial peptide attacin. The first Toll-like receptor identified in humans was initially termed human-Toll and subsequently TLR4. TLR4 was found to induce IL-1, IL-6, and 1L-8 and also members of the B7 molecules required for activation of T cells. Toll-like receptors are transmembrane proteins with an extracellular domain consisting of leucine rich repeats and cytoplasmic domain homologues similar to the IL-1 receptor. To date, nine different mammalian TLRs have been described and the complete sequence of TLR10 has recently been elucidated. TLRs respond to highly conserved motifs on different microorganisms termed pathogen-associated molecular patterns. In the Gram-negative bacteria, these are characterized by lipopolysaccharide (LPS). In Gram-positive bacteria these include peptidoglycan, lipoteichoic acid, and lipopeptides. Lipoarabinomannam is a key pathogen-associated molecular pattern for mycobacteria, and mannans, mannoproteins, and zymosan are keys motifs in yeasts. How these pathogen-associated molecular patterns are recognized by Toll-like receptors is yet unknown. Much work has been done on LPS and it now seems that it is opsonized by its binding protein and the complex is recognized by the opsonic receptor CD14. CD14 is not capable of generating a transmembrane signal but the complex of LPS, its binding protein, and CD14 activates TLR4, eventually leading to induction of immune response genes.[110] Activation of the TLR is via an intracellular domain that is homogenous with that of the IL-1 receptor known as TIR. TIR binds to an adaptor protein MyD88, which in turn interacts with the serine kinase IL-1R-associated kinase (IRAK), which eventually leads to activation of NF-κB in a sequence similar to that used by the IL-1 receptor (Figure 5.2). In normal human skin CD14, TLR1, 2, 4, and 5 have been identified.[111,112] TLR4 is the major Toll-like receptor responding to LPS. TLR2 responds mainly to Gram-positive bacterial products but there is some evidence that it may be involved in recognition of LPS. In normal skin TLR1, 2, and 5 are constitutively expressed whereas TLR3 and 4 are barely detectable. Cytoplasmic TLR1 and 2 are expressed throughout the epidermis with high staining of TLR2 on basal keratinocytes. TLR5 is mainly expressed in the basal cell layer. In inflammatory conditions, such as psoriasis, TLR2 is upregulated on keratinocytes in the upper epidermis and TLR5 is downregulated in basal keratinocytes.[111] Recent studies have suggested that epidermal keratinocytes do not express functional CD14 or TLR4 and that LPS recognition and response is mediated through a TLR2-dependent pathway.[113] These finding are, however, controversial as other studies have demonstrated that keratinocytes constitutively express CD14 and TLR4, and when bound by LPS a rapid intracellular $Ca^{2+}$ response, nuclear factor κβ translocation and the secretion of pro-inflammatory cytokines and chemokines resulted.[114]

## B. Antimicrobial Peptides

Antimicrobial peptides represent a rapid first-line defense against infectious agents. Peptides are of the cathelicidin and defensin gene families.[114] These peptides are multifactorial, acting as natural antibiotics but also signaling activation of host immune cells. These agents are able to directly kill a broad spectrum of microbes including Gram-positive and Gram-negative bacteria, fungi, and some viruses. They have common structural features including a cationic charge and hydrophobic amino acids, which interact with bacterial membranes.

**Cathelicidins.** These are characterized by N-terminal signal peptide, highly conserved prosequence, and structurally variable cationic peptide at the C terminal. The prosequence is similar to cathelin, which is a protein isolated initially from porcine neutrophils as an inhibitor of cathepsin L. The prosequence is highly conserved both inter- and intraspecies. In humans, cathelicidin is limited to a single gene. Stored cathelicidin is present as a larger pre-pro-protein, which is enzymatically digested into two parts: the cathelicidin itself and a cathelin domain, which to date has no clear function. Human cathelicidin (LL-37/hCAP18) was initially cloned as FALL39. It has a broad spectrum of antimicrobial activity and is also a chemoattractant by binding to formyl peptide receptor-like1 for neutrophils, macrophages, and T cells. It has also been shown to be chemotactic for mast cells.

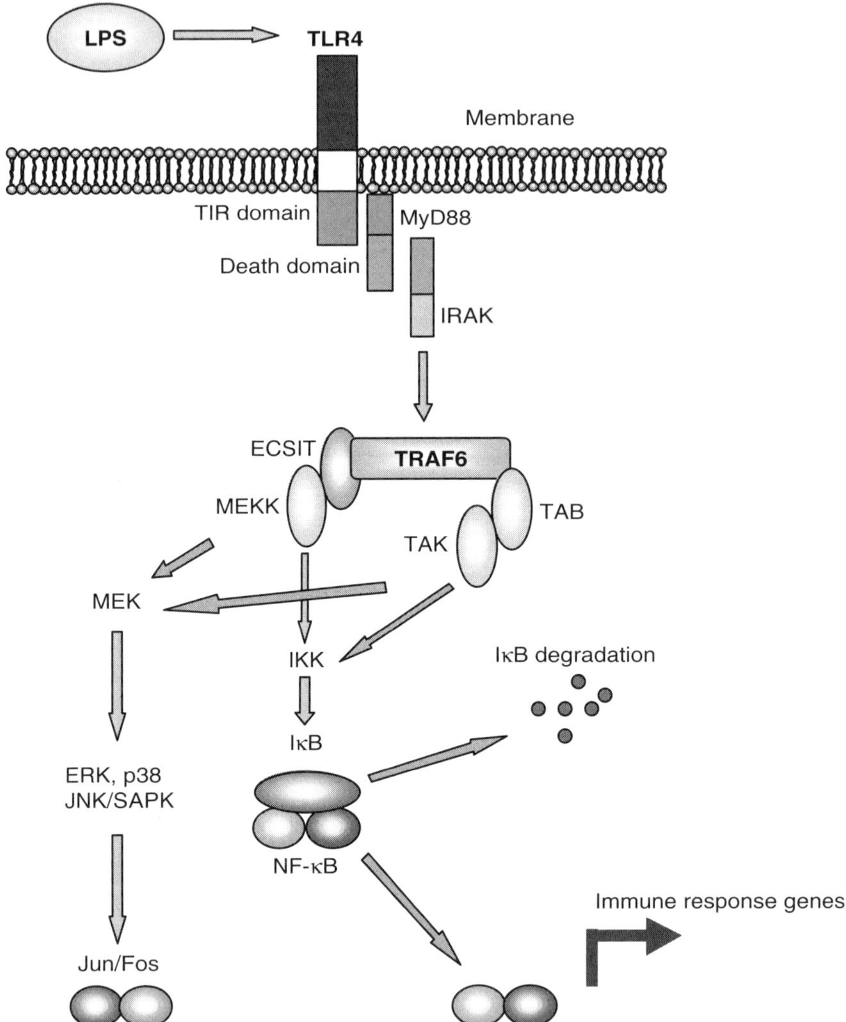


**FIGURE 5.2** Signaling pathways activated via TLR4 on keratinocytes.

**Defensins.** These are small cationic peptides of 28 to 44 amino acid–containing 6-8 cysteine residues that form characteristic intramolecular disulfide bridges. They have broad antimicrobial activity against bacteria, fungi, and some enveloped viruses. The alignment of disulfide bridges is used to classify them into three families, α, β, and O. α defensins consist of 29 to 35 amino acid residues with three disulfide bridges in a 1-6, 2-4, and 3-5 alignment. There are six human α defensins: α defensin 1, 2, 3, and 4, and human defensin 5 and 6. These are stored in azurophilic granules of neutrophils as the fully processed mature peptides. The β defensins contain six cysteine motifs and three disulfide bridges at C1-C5, C2-C4, and C3-C6. There are four β defensins in humans: human β defensins (HBD)1 through 4. They have a broad spectrum of antimicrobial activity comparable with that of the cathelicidins.

HBD bind to CCR6 and are chemotactic for immature dendritic cells and memory T cells. HBD 2 promotes histamine release and prostaglandin D2 production in mast cells. The α defensins 1 to 3 can increase TNF-α and IL-1 production from the human monocytes activated by bacteria such as *Staphylococcus aureus*. They also reduce VCAM1 expression in human umbilical vein endothelial cells activated by TNF-α.

The cathelicidin peptide, LL-37, has been observed in human epidermal keratinocytes under inflammatory conditions, such as, psoriasis and contact allergic dermatitis and is increased after epidermal injury. HBD 2 has been purified from psoriatic scale and HBD 2 and 3 have been shown to be upregulated in psoriasis. HBD 1 has been found in human epidermis but is less abundant than 2 and 3. HBD 1 and 2 are seen within normal epidermis within the epithelium of sweat glands and hair follicles. In resting conditions potential sites of entry by bacteria, i.e., follicular openings and sweat ducts, produce small amounts of antimicrobial peptides providing a chemical barrier to infection where a physical one is missing. After injury or inflammation there is a rapid increase in antimicrobial peptides and deposition from degranulation of recruited neutrophils. The chemotactic activity of LL-37 and HBD 2 increases leukocyte recruitment and, therefore, potentially potentiates the reaction.

A vast number of infectious agents can affect the skin and a major problem posed to the innate immune system is to discriminate these agents from self, using a limited number of receptors. This has been overcome by the evolution of receptors that recognize highly conserved motifs of infectious agents that are critical to their biology and thus not subject to high mutation rates. These motifs include formylated peptides and bacterial cell wall components such as LPS, lipopeptides, peptidoglycan and teichoic acids, lipoarainomannan in mycobacteria, mannans and zymosan in yeasts, and heat shock proteins in prokaryotes and eukaryotes.

## IX. CONCLUSIONS

The keratinocyte represents an important and integral part of the skin immune system. It represents an efficient factory producing a number of cytokines that can influence many immunologically active cells, but the *in vivo* function of these cytokines remains highly speculative. Merely because a cell produces a particular factor does not mean that that factor is of any biological significance and does not necessarily endow that cell with any special functional activity. Considerably more work needs to be performed to properly characterize all the factors that have been described and to make sure that we are not dealing with many functional activities of a very few substances.

The activity of keratinocytes as accessory cells remains controversial. Although the keratinocyte exhibits many of the characteristics of accessory cells, including the expression of class II MHC antigen, phagocytosis, and constitutive production of IL-1, many studies have so far given conflicting and contradictory information about accessory cell function of keratinocytes in antigen presentation or alloantigen presentation. Lack of antigen-presenting function in some studies may well be due to failure of the keratinocyte to process antigen and to lack expression of co-stimulatory signals that are essential for T-cell stimulation. A provocative finding is that keratinocytes may induce a long-lived immune unresponsiveness rather than stimulating a mitogenic T-cell response. Keratinocytes expressing B7-H1 also induce IL-10 and can lead to immune tolerance. This certainly suggests ways in which the skin could be manipulated to enable desensitization of patients from contact allergens.

## REFERENCES

1. Lechler, R., MHC class II molecular structure-permitted pairs, *Immunol. Today*, 9, 76,1988.
2. June, C.H., Bluestone, J.A., Nadler, L.M., and Thompson, C.B., The B7 and CD28 receptor families, *Immunol. Today*, 5, 321, 1994.
3. Lampert, I.A., Smitters, A.J., and Chisholm, P.M., Expression of Ia antigen on epidermal keratinocytes in graft versus host disease, *Nature* (London), 293, 149, 1981.
4. Stingl, G., Katz, S., Clement, C., Green, I., and Shevach, E.M., Immunologic function of Ia bearing epidermal Langerhans cells, *J. Immunol.*, 121, 2005, 1978.

5. Murphy, G.F., Shepard, R.S., Harrist, T.J., Brunstein, B.R., and Bhan, A.K., Ultrastructural documentation of HLA-DR antigen reactivity in normal human acrosyringeal epithelium, *J. Invest. Dermatol.,* 81, 181, 1983.
6. Lampert, I.A., Expression of HLA-DR (Ia like) antigen on epidermal keratinocytes in human dermatoses, *Clin. Exp. Immunol.,* 57, 93, 1984.
7. Geppert, T.D. and Lipsky, P.E., Antigen presentation by interferon treated endothelial cells and fibroblasts: differential ability to function as antigen presenting cells despite comparable Ia expression, *J. Immunol.,* 135, 3750, 1985.
8. Basham. T.Y., Nickoloff, B.J., Merigan, T.C., and Morhenn, V.B., Recombinant gamma interferon differentially regulates class II antigen expression and biosynthesis on cultured normal human keratinocytes, *J. Interferon Res.,* 5, 23, 1985.
9. Czernielewski, J.M. and Bagot, M., Class II MHC antigen expression by human keratinocytes results from lymphoepidermal interactions and interferon production, *Clin. Exp. Immunol.,* 66,295, 1986.
10. Albanesi, C., Cavani, A., and Girolomoni, G., Interferon gamma stimulated human keratinocytes express the genes necessary for the production of peptide loaded MHC class II molecules, *J. Invest. Dermatol.,* 110, 138–142, 1998.
11. Kameyama, K., Tone, T., Eto, H., Takezaki, S., Kanzaki, T., and Nishiyama, S., Recombinant gamma interferon induces HLA-DR expression on squamous cell carcinoma, tichilemomas, adenocarcinoma cell lines and cultured human keratinocytes, *Arch. Dermatol. Res.,* 279, 161, 1987.
12. Mitra, R.S. and Nickoloff, B.J., Epidermal growth factor and transforming growth factor alpha decrease gamma interferon receptors and induction of intercellular adhesion molecule (CD54) on cultured keratinocytes, *J. Cell. Physiol.,* 150, 264, 1992.
13. Kemeny, L., Kenderessy, A.S., Olsovszky, I., Michel, G., Ruzicka, T., and Dobozy, A., Interleukin 8 induces HLA-DR expression on cultured human keratinocytes via specific receptors, *Int. Arch. Allergy Immunol.,* 106, 351, 1995.
14. Khan, I.U., Boehm, K.D., and Elmets, C.A., Modulation of interferon gamma induced HLA-DR expression on the human keratinocyte cell line SCC-13 by ultraviolet radiation, *Photochem. Photobiol.,* 57, 285, 1993
15. Volc-Platzer, B., Majdic, O., Knapp, W., Wolff, H., Hinter Berger, W., Lechner, K., and Stingl, G., Evidence of HLA-DR antigen biosynthesis by human keratinocytes in disease, *J. Exp. Med.,* 159, 1784, 1984.
16. Tjernlund, U., Scheynius, A., Asbrink, E., and Hovmark, A., Expression of HLA-DQ antigens on keratinocytes in *Borrelia* spirochete-induced skin lesions, *Scand. J. Immunol.,* 23, 383, 1986.
17. Gawkroger, D.J., Carr, M.M., McVittie, E., Guy, K., and Hunter, J.A., Keratinocyte expression of MHC Class II antigens in allergic sensitisation and challenge reactions, *J. Invest. Dermatol.,* 88, 11, 1987.
18. Gonwa, T.A., Picker, L.J., Raff, H.V., Goyert, S.M., Silver, J., and Stobo, J.D., Antigen presenting capabilities of human monocytes correlates with their expression of HLA-DS, an Ia determinant distinct from HLA-DR, *J. Immunol.,* 130, 706, 1983.
19. Simon, M. and Hunyadi, J., Expression of OKM5 antigen on human keratinocytes in positive intracutaneous tests for delayed type hypersensitivity, *Dermatologica,* 175, 121, 1987.
20. Bamwell, J.W., Ockenhouse, C.F., and Knowlea, D.M., Monoclonal antibody OKM5 inhibits the *in vitro* binding of *Plasmodium falciparum*-infected erythrocytes to monocytes, endothelial and C32 melanoma cells, *J. Immunol.,* 135, 3494, 1985.
21. Ruiz-Veiasco, N., Dominguez, A., and Vegam, M.A., Statins upregulate CD36 expression in human monocytes, an effect strengthened when combined with PPAR-ligands. Putative contribution of Rho GTPases in statin-induced CD36 expression, *Biochem Pharmacol.*, 67, 303–313, 2004.
22. Shen, H.H., Talle, M.A., Goldstein, G., and Chess, L., Functional subsets of human monocytes defined by monoclonal antibodies: a distinctive subset of monocytes, containing cells capable of inducing the autologous mixed lymphocyte culture, *J. Immunol.,* 130, 698, 1983.
23. Cooper, K.D., Keises, G.R., and Katz, S.I., Antigen presenting OKM5$^+$ melanophages appear in human epidermis after ultraviolet irradiation, *J. Invest. Dermatol.,* 86, 363, 1986.
24. Hunyadi, J., Simon, M., Kenderessy, A.S., and Dobozy, A., Expression of monocyte/macrophage markers (CD13, CD14, CD68) on human keratinocytes in healthy and diseased skin, *J. Dermatol.,* 20, 341, 1993.

25. Lisby, S., Baadsgaard, O., Cooper, K.D., Thomsen, K., and Lange Wantzin, G.R., Expression of OKM5 antigen on epidermal cells in mycosis fungoides plaque stage, *J. Invest. Dermatol.*, 90, 716, 1988.
26. Dustin, M.L., Singer, K.H, Tuck, D.T., and Springer, T.A., Adhesion of T lymphoblasts to epidermal keratinocytes is regulated by interferon gamma and is mediated by intercellular adhesion molecule 1 (CD54), *J. Exp. Med.*, 167, 1323, 1988.
27. Nickoloff, B.J., Lewinsohn, D.M., Butcher, E.C., Krensky, A.M., and Clayberger, C., Recombinant gamma interferon increases the binding of peripheral blood mononuclear leucocytes and a Leu $3^+$ T lymphocyte clone to cultured keratinocytes and to a malignant cutaneous squamous carcinoma cell line that is blocked by antibody against the CD11A molecule, *J. Invest. Dermatol.*, 90, 17, 1988.
28. Middleton, M.A. and Norris, D.A., Cytokine induced CD54 expression in human keratinocytes is highly variable in keratinocyte strains from different donors, *J. Invest. Dermatol.*, 104, 489, 1995.
29. Derocq, J.M., Segui, M., Poinot-Chazel, C., Minty, A., Caput, D., Ferrara, P., and Casellas, P., Interleukin 13 stimulates interleukin 6 production by human keratinocytes. Similarly with interleukin 4. *FEBS Lett.*, 343, 32–36, 1994.
30. Albanesi, C., Scarponi, C., Cavani, A., Federici, M., Nasorri, F., and Girolomoni, G., Interleukin 17 is produced by both Th1 and Th2 lymphocytes and modulates interferon gamma and interleukin 4 induced activation of human keratinocytes, *J. Invest. Dermatol.*, 115, 81-87, 2000.
31. Bruggers, C.S., Patel, D.D., Scearce, R.M., Whichard, L.P., Haynes, B.F., and Singer, K.H., AD2, a human molecule involved in the interaction of T cells with epidermal keratinocytes and thymic epithelium, *J. Immunol.*, 154, 2012, 1995.
32. Trompezinski, S., Denis, A., Vinche, A., Schmitt, D., and Viac, J., IL4 and interferon gamma differentially modulate vascular endothelial growth factor release from normal human keratinocytes and fibroblasts, *Exp. Dermatol.*, 11, 224–231, 2002.
33. Denfield, R.W., Hollenbaugh, D., Fehrenbach, A., Weiss, J.M., von Leoprechting, A., Mai, B., Voith, U., Schopf, E., Aruffo, A., and Simon, J.C., CD40 is functionally expressed on human keratinocytes, *Eur. J. Immunol.*, 26, 2329–2334, 1996.
34. Frederici, M., Giustizieri, M.L., Scarponi, C., Girolomoni, G., and Albanesi, C., Impaired IFN gamma dependant inflammatory response in human keratinocytes over-expressing the suppressor of cytokine signalling 1, *J. Immunol.*, 169, 434–442, 2002.
35. Pastore, S., Cortinti, S., La Placa, M., Didona, B., and Girolomoni, G., Interferon gamma promotes exaggerated cytokine production in keratinocytes cultured from patients with atopic dermatitis, *J. Allergy Clin. Immunol.*, 101, 538–544, 1998.
36. Pasch, M.C., van den Bosch, N.H., Daha, M.R., Bos, J.D., and Asghar, S.S., Synthesis of complement component C3 and factor B in human keratinocytes is differentially regulated by cytokine, *J. Invest. Dermatol.*, 114, 78–82, 2000.
37. Luger, T.A., Stadler, B.M., Katz, S.I., and Oppenheim, J.J., Epidermal cell (keratinocyte) derived thymocyte activating factor (ETAF), *J. Immunol.*, 127, 1493, 1981.
38. Kutsch, C.C., Norris, D.D., and Arend, W.P., Tumor necrosis factor alpha induces interleukin 1 alpha and interleukin 1 receptor antagonist production by cultured human keratinocytes, *J. Invest. Dermatol.*, 101, 79, 1993.
39. Mizutani, H., Black, R., and Kupper, T.S., Human keratinocytes produce but do not process prointerleukin 1 beta. Different strategies of IL1 production and processing in monocytes and keratinocytes, *J. Clin. Invest.*, 87, 1066, 1991.
40. Gueniche, A., Viac, J., Charveron, M., and Schmitt, D., Effect of gamma interferon on IL1 alpha, beta, and receptor antagonist production by normal human keratinocytes, *Exp. Dermatol.*, 3, 113, 1994.
41. Arsenault, T.V., Sauder, D.N., Harley, C.B., and McKenzie, R.C., Identification and characterisation of a partial cDNA expressing interleukin I like activity in keratinocytes, *Mol. Immunol.*, 29, 431, 1992.
42. Groves, R.W., Giri, J., Sims, J., Dower, S., and Kupper, T.S., Inducible expression of type II IL1 receptors by cultured human keratinocytes. Implications for IL1 mediated processes in the epidermis, *J. Immunol.*, 154, 4065, 1995.
43. Kock, A., Schwarz, T., Kirnbauer, R., Urbanski, A., Perry, P., Ansel, J.C., and Luger, T.A., Human keratinocytes are a source for tumour necrosis factor alpha: evidence for synthesis and release upon stimulation with endotoxin or ultraviolet light, *J. Exp. Med.*, 172, 1609, 1990.

44. Kristensen, M., Chu, C.Q., Eedy, D.J., Feldmann, M., Brennan, F.M., and Breathnach, S.M., Localisation of tumour necrosis factor alpha (TNFa) and its receptors in normal and psoriatic skin: epidermal cells express the 55kD but not the 75 kD TNF receptor, *Clin. Exp. Immunol.,* 94, 354, 1993.
45. Groves, R.W., Allen, M.H., Ross, E.L., Barker, J.N., and MacDonald, D.M., Tumour necrosis factor alpha is proinflammatory in normal human skin and modulates cutaneous adhesion molecule expression, *Br. J. Dermatol.,* 132, 345, 1995.
46. Partridge, M., Chantry, D., Turner, M., and Feldmann, M., Production of interleukin 1 and interleukin 6 by human keratinocytes and squamous cell carcinoma cell lines, *J. Invest. Dermatol.,* 96, 771, 1991.
47. Moller, A., Schwarz, A., Neuner, P., Schwarz, T., and Luger, T.A., Regulation of monocyte and keratinocyte interleukin 6 production by transforming growth factor beta, *Exp. Dermatol.,* 3, 314, 1994.
48. Teunissen, M.B., Koomen, C.W., de Waal Malefyt, R., Wierenga, E.A., and Bos, J.D., Interleukin 17 and interferon gamma synergize in the enhancement of proinflammatory cytokine production by human keratinocytes, *J. Invest. Dermatol.,* 111, 645–649, 1998.
49. Wagner, L.A., Brown, T., Gil, S., Frank, I., Carter, W., Tamura, R., and Wayner, E.A., The keratinocyte cytokine IL7 increases adhesion of the epidermal T cell subset to the skin basement membrane protein laminin 5, *Eur. J. Immunol.,* 29, 2530–2538, 1999.
50. Aragane, Y., Riemann, H., Bhardwaj, R.S., Schwarz, A., Sawada, Y., Yamada, H., Luger, T.A., Kubin. M., Trinchieri, G., and Schwarz, T., IL12 is expressed and released by human keratinocytes and epidermoid carcinoma cell lines, *J. Immunol.,* 153, 5366, 1994.
51. Muller, G., Saloga, J., Germann, T., Bellinghausen, I., Mohamadzadeh, H., Knop, J., and Enk, A.H., Identification and induction of human keratinocyte derived IL12, *J. Clin. Invest.,* 94, 1799, 1994.
52. Kondo, S. and Jimbow, K., Dose dependent induction of IL12 but not IL10 from human keratinocytes after exposure to ultraviolet light A, *J. Cell Physiol.,* 177, 493–498, 1998.
53. Dinarello CA. Interleukin 18. Methods 1999; 19: 121-132.
54. Koizumi, H., Sato-Matsumura, K.C., Nakamura, H., Shida, K., Kikkawa, S., Matsumoto, M., Toyoshima, K., and Seya, T., Distribution of IL18 and IL18 receptor in human skin: various forms of IL18 are produced by keratinocytes, *Arch. Dermatol. Res.,* 293, 325–333, 2001.
55. Mee, J.B., Alam, Y., and Groves, R.W., Human keratinocytes constitutively produce but do not process interleukin 18, *Br. J. Dermatol.,* 143, 330–336, 2000.
56. Pietrzak, A., Lecewicz-Torun, B., Choborowska, G., and Rolinski, J., Interleukin 18 levels in the plasma of psoriatic patients correlates with extent of skin lesions and PASI score, *Acta Derm. Venereol.,* 83, 262–265, 2003.
57. Nakanishi, K., Yoshimoto, T., Tsutsui, H., and Okamura, H., Interleukin 18 regulates both Th1 and Th2 responses, *Annu. Rev. Immunol.,* 19, 423–474, 2001.
58. Kondo, S., Ciarletta, A., Turner, K.D., Sauder, D.N., and McKenzie, R.C., Failure to detect interleukin 3 mRNA or protein in human keratinocytes: antibodies to granulocyte-monocyte colony stimulating factor or IL6 (but not IL3) neutralise IL3 bioactivity, *J. Invest. Dermatol.,* 104, 335, 1995.
59. Heufler, C., Topar, G., Gasseger, A., Stanzl, U., Koch, F., Romani, N., Namen, A.E., and Schuler, G., Interleukin 7 is produced by murine and human keratinocytes, *J. Exp. Med.,* 178, 1109, 1993.
60. Villadsen, L.S., Schuurman, J., Beurskens, F., Dam, T.N., Dagnaes-Hansen, F., Skov, L., Rygaard, J., Voorhorst-Ogink, M.M., Gerritsen, A.F., van Dijk, M.A., Parren, P.W., Baagsgaard, O., and van de Winkel, J.G., Resolution of psoriasis upon blockade on IL15 biological activity in a xenograft mouse model, *J. Clin. Invest.,* 112, 1571–1580, 2003.
61. Musso, T., Calossa, L., Zucca, M., Millesimo, M., Puliti, M., Bulfone-Paus, S., Merlino, C., Savioia, D., Cavallo, R., Ponzi, A.N., and Badolato, R., Interleukin-15 activates proinflammatory and antimicrobial functions in polymorphonuclear cells, *Infect. Immun.,* 66, 2640–2647, 1998.
62. Grichnik, J.M., Burch, J.A., Burchette, J., and Shea, C.R., The SCF/KIT pathway plays a critical role in the control of normal human melanocyte homeostasis, *J. Invest. Dermatol.,* 111, 233–239, 1998.
63. Kakurai, M., Fujita, N., Kiyosawa, T., Inoue, T., Ishibashi, S., Furukawa, Y., Demitsu, T., and Nakagawa, H., Vasoactive intestinal peptide and cytokines enhance stem cell factor production from epidermal keratinocytes DJM-1, *J. Invest. Dermatol.,* 119, 1183–1188, 2002.
64. Barker, J.N., Jones, M.L., Mitra, R.S., Crockett-Torabe, E., Fantone, J.C., Kunkel, S.L., Warren, J.S., Dixit, V.M., and Nickoloff, B.J., Modulation of keratinocyte derived interleukin 8 which is chemotactic for neutrophils and T lymphocytes, *Am. J. Pathol.,* 139, 869, 1991.

65. Mohamadzadeh, M., Muller, M., Hultsch, T., Enk, A., Saloga, J., and Knop, J., Enhanced expression of IL8 in normal human keratinocytes and human keratinocyte cell line HaCaT *in vitro* after stimulation with contact sensitisers, tolerogens and irritants, *Exp. Dermatol.*, 3, 298, 1994.
66. Homey, B., Wang, W., Soto, H., Buchanan, M.E., Wiesenborn, A., Catron, D., Muller, A., McClanahan, T.K., Dieu-Nosjean, M.C., Orozco, R., Ruzicka, T., Lehmann, P., Oldham, E., and Zlotnik, A., Cutting edge: the orphan chemokine receptor G protein-coupled receptor-2 (GPR-2, CCR10) binds the skin-associated chemokine CCL27 (CTACK/ALP/ILC), *J. Immunol.*, 164, 3465–3470, 2000.
67. Homey, B., Alenius, H., Muller, A., Soto, H., Bowman, E.P., Yuan, W., McEvoy, L., Lauerma, A.I., Assmann, T., Bunemann, E., Lehto, M., Wolff, H., Yen, D., Marxhausen, H., To, W., Sedgwick, J., Ruzicka, T., Lehmann, P., and Zlotnik, A., CCL27-CCR10 interactions regulate T cell mediated skin inflammation, *Nat. Med.*, 8, 157–165, 2002.
68. Fukuoka, M., Ogino, Y., Sato, H., Ohta, T., Komoriya, K., Nishioka, K., and Katayama, I., RANTES expression in psoriatic skin and regulation of RANTES and IL8 production in cultured epidermal keratinocytes by active vitamin D3 (tacalcitol), *Br. J. Dermatol.*, 138, 63–70, 1998.
69. Vestergaard, C., Bang, K., Gesser, B., Yonyama, H., Matsushimi, K., and Larsen, C.G., A Th2 chemokine, TARC, produced by keratinocytes may recruit $CLA^+CCR4^+$ lymphocytes onto lesional atopic dermatitis skin, *J. Invest. Dermatol.*, 115, 640–646, 2000.
70. Gottlieb, A.B., Luster, A.D., Posnett, D.N., and Carter, D.M., Detection of a gamma interferon-inducing protein IP10 in psoriatic plaques, *J. Exp. Med.*, 168, 941–948, 1988.
71. Kakinuma, T., Nakamura, K., Wakugawa, M., Yano, S., Saeki, H., Torii, H., Komine, M., Asahina, A., and Tamaki, K., IL4 but not IL13 modulates TARC (thymus and activation-regulated chemokine)/CCL17 and IP10 (interferon-induced protein of 10kDa)/CXCL10 release by TNF-alpha and IFN-gamma in HaCaT cell line, *Cytokine*, 20, 1–6, 2002.
72. Tensen, C.P., Flier, J., Van der Raaij-Helmer, E.M., Sampat-Sardjoepersad, S., Van der Schors, R.C., Leurs, R., Scheper, R.J., Boorsma, D.M., and Willemze, R., Human IP9: a keratinocyte derived high affinity CXC chemokine ligand for IP10/Mig receptor (CXCR3), *J. Invest. Dermatol.*, 112, 716–722, 1999.
73. Albanesi, C., Scarponi, C., Sebastiani, S., Cavani, A., Federici, M., de Pita, O., Puddu, P., and Girolomoni, G., IL4 enhances keratinocyte expression of CXCR3 agonistic chemokines, *J. Immunol.*, 165, 1395–1402, 2000.
74. Tohyama, M., Shirakara, Y., Yamasaki, K., Sayama, K., and Hashimoto, K., Differentiated keratinocytes are responsible for TNF-$\alpha$ regulated production of macrophage inflammatory protein $3\alpha$/CCL20, a potent chemokine for Langerhans cells, *J. Dermatol. Sci.*, 27, 130–139, 2001.
75. Arend, W.P. and Guthridge, C.J., Biological role of interleukin 1 receptor antagonist isoforms, *Ann. Rheum. Dis.*, 59(Suppl. 1), 60–64, 2000.
76. Enk, A.H. and Katz, S.I., Identification and induction of keratinocyte derived IL10, *J. Immunol.*, 149, 92, 1992.
77. Enk, C.D., Sredni, D., Blauvelt, A., and Katz, S.I., Induction of IL10 gene expression in human keratinocytes by UVB exposure *in vivo* and *in vitro, J. Immunol.*, 154, 4851, 1995.
78. Grewe, M., Gyufko, K., and Krutmann, J., Interleukin 10 production by cultured human keratinocytes: regulation by ultraviolet B and ultraviolet A1 radiation, *J. Invest. Dermatol.*, 104, 3, 1995.
79. Redondo, P., Garcia-Foncillas, J., Okroujnov, I., and Bandres, E., Alpha-MSH regulates interleukin-10 expression by human keratinocytes, *Arch. Dermatol. Res.*, 290, 425–428, 1998.
80. Teunissen, M.B.M., Koomen, C.W., De Waal Malefyt, R., and Bos, J.D., Inability of human keratinocytes to synthesise interleukin-10, *J. Invest. Dermatol.*, 102, 632, 1994.
81. Michel, G., Mirmohammadsadegh, A., Olasz, E., Jarzebska-Deussen, B., Muschen, A., Kemeny, L., Abts, H.F., and Ruzicka, T., Demonstration and functional Analysis of IL10 receptors in human epidermal cells: decreased expression in psoriatic skin, down modulation by IL8 and upregulation by an antipsoriatic glucocorticosteroid in normal cultured keratinocytes, *J. Immunol.*, 15, 6291–6297, 1997.
82. Hiltz, M.E. and Lipton, J.M., Anti-inflammatory activity of a COOH-terminal fragment of the neuropeptide a-MSH, *FASEB J;* 3, 2282–2284, 1989.
83. Hedley, S.J., Gawkrodger, D.J., Weetman, A.P., and MacNeil, S., a-MSH and melanogenesis in normal human adult melanocytes, *Pigment Cell Res.*, 11, 45–56, 1998.

84. Luger, T.A., Kalden, D., Scholzen, T.E., and Brzoska, T., Alpha melanocyte stimulating hormone as a mediator of tolerance induction, *Pathobiology*, 67, 318–321, 1999.
85. Sarris, A.H., Broxmeyer, H.E., Wirthmuller, U., Karasavuas, N., Cooper, S., Lu, L., Krueger, J., and Ravetch, J.V., Human interferon-inducible protein 10: expression and purification of recombinant protein demonstrate inhibition of early human haemopoetic progenitors, *J. Exp. Med.*, 178, 1127, 1993.
86. Schwarz, T., Urbanska, A., Gschnait, F., and Luger, T., UV-irradiated epithelial cells produce a specific inhibitor of interleukin 1 activity, *J. Immunol.*, 138, 1457, 1987.
87. Nickoloff, B.J., Basham, T.Y., Merigan, T.C., Torseth, J.W., and Morhenn, V.B., Human keratinocyte reaction *in vitro, J. Invest. Dermatol.*, 87, 11, 1986.
88. Henke, D., Danilowciz, R., and Eling, T., Arachinonic acid metabolism by isolated epidermal basal and differentiated keratinocytes from the hairless mouse, *Biochim. Biophys.*, 876, 271, 1986.
89. Pentland, A.P. and Needleman, P., Modulation of keratinocyte proliferation *in vitro* by endogenous prostaglandin synthesis, *J. Clin. Invest.*, 77, 246, 1986.
90. Pentland, A.P., George, J., Moran, C., and Needleman, P., Cellular confluence determines injury induced prostaglandin E2 synthesis by human keratinocyte cultures, *Biochim. Biophys. Acta*, 919, 71, 1987.
91. Rubenfeld, M.R., Silverstone, A.E., Knowles, D.M., Halper, J.P., De Sostoa, A., Fenoglio, C.A., and Edelson, R.L., Induction of lymphocyte differentiation by epidermal cultures, *J. Invest. Dermatol.*, 77, 221, 1981.
92. Mackie, R.M. and Hughes, M.E., Basal cells from human epidermis induce thymocyte maturation, *J. Invest. Dermatol.*, 80, Abstr., 330, 1983.
93. Chu, A.C., Berger, C., Morris, J., and Edelson, R., Induction of immature T cell phenotype in malignant T cells by co-cultivation with epidermal cell cultures, *J. Invest. Dermatol.*, 89, 358, 1987.
94. Linsley, P.S., Clark, E.A., and Ledbetter, J.A., T-cell antigen CD28 mediates adhesion with B cells by interacting with activation antigen B7/BB1, *Proc. Natl. Acad. Sci. U.S.A.*, 87, 5031–5034, 1990.
95. Freeman, G.J., Cardoso, A.A., Boussiotis, V.A., Anumanthan, A., Groves, R.W., Kupper, T.S., Clark, E.A., and Nadler, L.M., The BB1 monoclonal antibody recognises both cell surface CD74 (MHC class II-associated invariant chain) as well as B7-1 (CD80), resolving the question regarding a third CD28/CTLA-4 counterreceptor, *J. Immunol.*, 161, 2708–2715, 1998.
96. Mazanet, M.M. and Hughes, C.C., B7-H1 is expressed by human endothelial cells and suppresses T cell cytokine synthesis, *J. Immunol.*, 169, 3581–3588, 2002.
97. Wang, S., Bajorath, J., Flies, D.B., Ding, H., Honjo, T., and Chen, L., Molecular modeling and functional mapping of B7-H1 and B uncouple costimulatory function from PD-1 interaction, *J. Exp. Med.*, 197, 1083–1091, 2003.
98. Nickoloff, B.J., Mitra, R.S., Green, J., Zheng, X.G., Shimizu, Y., Thompson, C., and Turka, L.A., Accessory cell function of keratinocytes for superantigens, *J. Immunol.*, 150, 2148, 1993.
99. Luger, T.A., Sztein, M.B., Schmidt, J.A., Murphy, P., Grabner, G., and Oppenheim, J.J., Properties of murine and human epidermal cell-derived thymocyte activating factor, *Fed. Proc.*, 42, 2772, 1983.
100. Londei, M., Lamb, J.R., Bottazzo, G.F., and Feldman, M., Epithelial cells expressing abhorrent MHC class II determinants can present antigen to cloned human T cells, *Nature* (London), 312, 679, 1984.
101. Breathnach, S.M., Shimada, S., Kovac, Z., and Katz, S.I., Immunologic aspects of acute graft versus host disease: decreased density and antigen presenting function of Ia+ Langerhans cells and absent antigen presenting capacity of Ia+ keratinocytes, *J. Invest. Dermatol.*, 86, 226, 1986.
102. Tjernlund, U. and Scheynius, A., Amplification of T cells response to PPD by epidermal suspensions containing HLA-DR expressing keratinocytes, *Scand. J. Immunol.*, 26, 1, 1987.
103. Gaspari, A.A. and Katz, S., Induction and functional characterisation of class II MHC (Ia) antigen on murine keratinocytes, *J. Immunol.*, 140, 2956, 1988.
104. De Bueger, M., Bakker, A., and Goulmy, E., Human keratinocytes activate primed major and minor histocompatibiliy antigen Th cells *in vitro, Transpl. Immunol.*, 1, 52, 1993.
105. Naujokas, M.F., Morin, M., Anderson, S., Peterson, M., and Miller, J., The chondroitin sulfate form of invariant chain can enhance stimulation of T cell responses through interaction with CD44, *Cell*, 74, 257–256, 1993.
106. Czernielewski, J.M., Mixed skin cell-lymphocyte reaction (MSLR) as a model for the study of lymphoepidermal interactions, *Br. J. Dermatol.*, 113(Suppl. 28), 17, 1985.

107. Gaspari, A.A., Jenkins, M.K., and Katz, S.I., Class Ii MHC-bearing keratinocytes induce antigen specific unresponsiveness for hapten-specific TH1 cells, *J. Immunol.,* 141, 2216, 1988.
108. Bal, V., McIndoe, A., Denton, G., Hudson, D., Lombardi, G., Lamb, J., and Lechler, R., Antigen presentation by keratinocytes induces tolerance in human T cells, *Eur. J. Immunol.,* 20, 1893, 1990.
109. Cao, Y., Zhou, H., Tao, J., Zheng, Z., Li, N., Shen, B., Shih, T.S., Hing, J., Zhang, J., and Chou, K.Y., Keratinocyte induced local tolerance to skin graft by activating interleukin 10 secreting T cells in context of costimulation molecule B7-H1, *Transplantation*, 75, 1390–1396, 2003.
110. Aderem A. and Ulevich R. Toll-like receptors in the induction of the innate immune response, *Nature*, 406, 782–787, 2000.
111. Baker, B.S., Ovigine, J.M., Powles, A.V., Corcoran, S., and Fry, L., Normal keratinocytes express Toll-like receptors (TLRs) 1,2 and 5: modulation of TLR expression in chronic plaque psoriasis, *Br. J. Dermatol.*, 148, 670–679, 2003.
112. Song, P.I., Young-Min, P., Abraham, T., Harten, B., Zivony, A., Naparidze, N., Armstrong, C., and Ansel, J.C., Human keratinocytes express functional CD14 and Toll-like receptor 4, *J. Invest. Dermatol.,* 119, 424–432. 2002.
113. Kawai, K., Shimura, H., Mingagawa, M., Ito, A., Tomiyama, K., and Ito, M., Expression of functional Toll-like receptor 2 on human epidermal keratinocytes, *J. Dermatol. Sci.,* 30, 185–194, 2002.
114. Gallo, R., Murakami, M., Ohtake, T., and Zaiou, M., Biology and clinical relevance of naturally occurring antimicrobial peptides, *J. Allergy Clin. Immunol.,* 110, 823–831, 2002.

# 6 Lymphocyte Subpopulations of the Skin

*Andrea Cavani, Sergio Di Nuzzo, Giampiero Girolomoni, and Giuseppe De Panfilis*

## CONTENT



## I. INTRODUCTION

T lymphocytes are the effector cells of adaptive immune responses, and continuously patrol the skin (as well as other organs) ready to be activated by antigens collected by antigen-presenting cells (APCs). The great majority of T cells involved in cutaneous immunity display a memory-effector phenotype, and a defined repertoire of homing and chemokine receptors, which are acquired during naive to memory T-cell transition. In primary immune responses, dendritic cells (DCs) pick up antigens at peripheral sites and migrate to regional lymph nodes, where they present the newly formed antigenic determinants to naive T cells. Effective T-cell activation requires not only appropriate T-cell receptor (TCR) triggering, but also the delivery of co-stimulatory signals and cytokines by APCs. Emigration of committed T lymphocytes at peripheral organs is regulated by several integrated signals, including cytokines, chemokines, and adhesion molecules. Finally, skin-recruited T cells can be activated by the antigen, and exploit their effector functions toward disparate targets. Exhaustion of such specific skin T-cell responses is guaranteed by several mechanisms, including activation-induced cell death (AICD) of effector T cells, and intervention of specific T-regulatory

0-8493-1959-5/05/$0.00+$1.50

(Treg) subsets, which either block the APCs or directly damper T-cell activation and proliferation. Skin-homing T cells represent a powerful defensive system against disparate hazardous antigens penetrating the skin, but they are also responsible for a variety of hyperreactive responses, such as allergies or autoimmune diseases, which frequently occur in the cutaneous environment.

## II. T-CELL ORIGIN AND DEVELOPMENT

### A. Intrathymic T-Cell Development

Mature T lymphocytes originate from bone-marrow-derived pluripotent stem cells, which emigrate during fetal life in the thymus. Lymphocyte development requires interactions with major histocompatibility complex-positive ($MHC^+$) thymic epithelial cells, and includes multiple differentiative steps, which can be identified on the basis of membrane receptor and cytoplasmic protein expression.[1,2] Early, double-negative ($CD4^-CD8^-$) T-cell precursors display a pre-TCR constituted by CD3 coupled to a β- and pre-α chain. Signaling through pre-TCR induces proliferation and survival of thymocytes in a ligand-independent manner, and stimulates the transition to the $CD4^+CD8^+$ double positive thymocytes.[3,4] The fate of developing T cells is determined by the avidity of the αβ TCR for self-MHC complexes expressed by DCs and epithelial cells in the thymus.[5,6] T cells bearing TCRs, which are either not triggered, or triggered by high-avidity self-MHC complexes, undergo to death by neglect or negative selection, respectively, and will be eliminated. In contrast, T cells recognizing relatively rare or low-affinity peptides will survive and undergo further differentiation. By downregulating one of the two co-receptors, thymocytes become either $CD4^+$ or $CD8^+$, and then leave the thymus as mature T cells.[7] This process gives rise to functional T cells, which recognize foreign peptides that are generally structurally related to self-peptides, but eliminates most of the autoreactive T cells whose TCR has high affinity for self-determinants. Exceptions to this general rule are the $CD4^+CD25^+$ Treg and the natural killer T (NKT) cells, which both appear positively selected in the thymus by agonistic interactions with self-antigens.[6]

### B. T-Cell Emigration and Positioning in Peripheral Lymphoid Organs

Immunocompetent naive T lymphocytes emigrate from the thymus in the bloodstream and continuously recirculate through secondary lymphoid organs. Lymph node entry of circulating T cells occurs through high endothelial venules (HEVs) in the paracortical area.[8,9] Interaction between naive T cells and high endothelial cells is a complex event regulated by the expression of selectins and chemokine receptors on T cells. L-selectin (CD62L) is specifically expressed on naive T lymphocytes, and allows interaction with the peripheral node addressin (PNAd) and the mucosal addressin cell-adhesion molecule 1 (MAdCAM-1); the latter is specifically exposed on HEVs of Peyer patches.[10,11] Selectin–addressin interaction promotes the tethering and rolling of lymphocytes over HEV endothelial cells and permits the engagement of adhesion molecules, the leukocyte function-associated antigen type 1 (LFA-1) and the α4β1/α4β7 integrins. Proper T-lymphocyte adhesion to the endothelial wall depends on integrin activation, which, in turn, is favored by chemokine receptor interactions with their ligands bound on the luminal surface of endothelial cells. Chemokines are secreted peptides that bind to heparin-like glycosaminoglycans on the cell surface or in the extracellular matrix, and interact with specific membrane receptors coupled with G proteins (for details see Chapter 15). The homeostatic chemokines CCL19 and CCL21 bind to the chemokine receptor CCR7 expressed on naive T lymphocytes and are critically involved in T-cell recruitment and correct positioning in secondary lymphoid organs.[12,13] Mice lacking CCL21 for a spontaneous mutation, named plt (paucity of lymph node T cells), or knocked-down for the CCR7 receptor, have defective T-cell trafficking into secondary lymphoid organs and compromised T-cell responses.[14,15] Continuous circulation through secondary lymphoid organs is essential to enhance naive T-cell encounter with the specific antigen, carried in the paracortical area by DCs.[16]

The prolonged lifespan of naive T cells requires the presence of two signals, namely, self-peptide/MHC complexes on DCs and interleukin 7 (IL-7).[17,18]

# III. T-CELL ACTIVATION AND COMMITMENT

## A. T-Cell Receptor and Antigen Recognition

T cells specifically recognize peptides displayed on MHC molecules of APCs.[19–21] Recently, T cells were also shown to recognize lipid antigens presented in a CD1a-dependent manner by epidermal APCs, namely, Langerhans cells.[22] The outcome of MHC-restricted antigen recognition by T cells varies from clonal expansion and differentiation to anergy and immunological unresponsiveness, according to the signals provided by the APC and the functional status of the T cell.

Most human T lymphocytes bear a $\alpha\beta$ heterodimeric TCR. The disulfide-linked $\alpha$ and $\beta$ chains of the TCR contain a distal variable region (V$\alpha$ and V$\beta$) and a proximal constant region (C$\alpha$ and C$\beta$) immunoglobulin superfamily domains, plus a transmembrane and short cytoplasmic regions. The hypervariable region of the TCR, which contacts the MHC-peptide complex, is constituted by three complementarity-determining regions (CDRs) formed by each V$\alpha$ and V$\beta$ domain.[23] A minor fraction of T cells expresses the $\gamma\delta$ TCR, which has a less well defined antigenic repertoire and antigen recognition modality.[24] Each TCR is associated with the CD3 complex, which includes CD3$\varepsilon\gamma$ and CD3$\varepsilon\delta$ heterodimers and CD3$\zeta$ homodimers. The dynamic interface between T cells and APCs, named immunological synapse, is enriched in MHC-peptide complexes, co-stimulatory molecules, TCRs, as well as molecules involved in the transduction of the signal.[25,26] Spatial organization of immunological synapses is characteristic, with a central area containing TCR-MHC-peptide pairs, CD2-CD58 complexes and CD28-B7s molecules, and a peripheral zone enriched in adhesion molecules. At the immunological synapse, multiple signals delivered by the APC are integrated, ensuring proper T-cell activation. Although TCR–MHC interactions are characterized by a low-affinity binding, the sustained signal required for proper T-cell activation is provided either by a prolonged interaction or through a dynamic process named serial triggering, according to which TCRs are serially engaged and triggered by peptide-MHC complexes.[27–29] TCR occupancy is followed by protein tyrosine kinase (PTK) activation, which is mediated by the Src kinases Lck and Fyn, the 70-kDa chain–associated protein kinase (ZAP-70), and by members of the Tec kinase family, inducible T-cell kinase (Itk) Tec and Txk/Rlk.[30,31] This early wave of protein tyrosine phosphorylation rapidly leads to the activation of downstream signaling pathways, including increases in intracellular calcium flux, protein kinase C (PKC), nuclear factor (NF)-B, and mitogen-activated protein kinase (MAPK) activation. These pathways activate transcription factors that ultimately promote the expression of genes that control specific cellular responses. Src kinases and other signaling components are particularly enriched in membrane domains named lipid rafts, which move toward the immunological synapses and guarantee the refurnishing of signal transducers for T-cell activation.[32] Productive signals delivered by the APC eventually convert naive T lymphocyte into experienced T cells. Conversion is paralleled by changes in the T-cell phenotype, in homing and chemokine receptor expression, as well as in their effector functions and cytokine repertoire.[33–35] Distinct expression of CD45 isoforms allows a rough differentiation between naive and memory/effector T cells, with the first CD45RA$^+$CD45RO$^-$ and the latter CD45RA$^-$CD45RO$^+$. Compared to naive T lymphocytes, memory T cells enter the cell cycle more rapidly, and require less sustained signal for proper activation, which is partially independent from co-stimulation.[36–38] In addition, memory-effector T cells have a broader repertoire of cytokines and a typical asset of chemokine receptors, which allows their recirculation in peripheral tissues.[39]

Antigen presentation in the absence of proper co-stimulatory signals may fail to induce productive T-cell activation, resulting in a long-term state of antigen-specific unresponsiveness, termed anergy. Anergic T lymphocytes, although viable and variably capable of secreting certain cytokines, fail to proliferate and to secrete IL-2 in response to antigenic stimulation.[40] In some, but not all, experimental models, anergy can be reverted *in vitro* by high doses of IL-2 and optimal co-stimulation through CD28. Biochemical events associated with T cell anergy have not been fully elucidated: altered expression of $p27^{kip\ 1}$, defects in activation of AP-1 responsive elements, decreased activation of the Ras/MAP kinase pathways have all been documented.[41–43]

Recently, at least two subsets of memory T lymphocytes have been described: an "effector memory" T cell, which does not express CD62L (L-selectin) and CCR7, and can rapidly secrete interferon-γ(IFN-γ) or IL-4, thus mediating rapid recall responses; and a "central memory" T cell that, due to the expression of L-selectin and CCR7, retains the ability to migrate into secondary lymphoid organs.[44] Central memory T cells can eventually differentiate into effector cells upon secondary antigenic stimulation. It has been proposed that a short TCR stimulation in the presence of TGF-β preserves T cells into the central memory pool, whereas persistent TCR triggering and the presence of IL-12 or IL-4 leads to the development of effector T helper (Th)1 and Th2 T cells.

### B. Requirement and Diversity of Co-Stimulatory Signals for T-Cell Activation

There is a considerable body of evidence indicating that naive T cells challenged with optimal doses of antigen, but in the absence of accessory signals provided by professional APCs, are hardly activated. CD28, the major transducer of co-stimulation for naive T cells, promotes T-cell activation by increasing the amount of thyrosine phosphorylation following TCR engagement, and by recruiting lipid rafts and Lck to the immunological synapse.[36,45–48] CD28 is constitutively expressed on T lymphocytes, and serves as a receptor for two members of the B7 family, B7-1 (CD80) and B7-2 (CD86). CD80 and CD86 are highly expressed on mature DCs and macrophages, and at lower levels on B cells and activated T lymphocytes (Table 6.1). CD28 engagement increases IL-2 transcription and mRNA stability, induces IL-2R expression, and augments the synthesis of the antiapoptotic molecule BCL-$X_L$, thus promoting T-cell proliferation and survival. The cytotoxic T-

**TABLE 6.1**
**Major Co-Stimulatory Molecules in T Cells**

| Receptor | Expression | Ligands | Ligand Expression | Function |
|---|---|---|---|---|
| CD28 | Constitutive | B7-1 (CD80)<br>B7-2 (CD86) | DCs, monocytes, B cells, T cells (activated) | Promotes IL-2 production, IL-2R expression and cell cycle progression |
| CTLA-4 | Induced upon TCR engagement | B7-1 (CD80)<br>B7-2 (CD86) | DCs, monocytes, B cells, T cells (activated) | Inhibit T cell functions and IL-2 release |
| ICOS | Induced by activation on a subpopulation of T cells | ICOS-L (B7RP-1) | IFN-γ-stimulated DCs, monocytes, B cells, peripheral tissues | Promotes IL-10 secretion by T cells |
| PD-1 | Induced by activation | PD-1L (B7-H1),<br>PD-2L (B7-DC) | PD-L1: various peripheral tissues including the skin<br>PD-L2: mature DCs | Negative effects on T-cell activation |
| Unknown | Unknown | B7-H3 | DCs, peripheral tissues | Negative effect on T-cell activation |
| OX40 (CD134) | Induced by TCR stimulation | OX40L | DCs, monocytes, B cells | Promotes cytokine release and T-cell survival by inducing Bcl-xL and Bcl-2 |
| CD40L (CD154) | Induced by TCR stimulation | CD40 | DCs, monocytes, B cells | Induces DCs and B cell maturation and isotype switching |

lymphocyte antigen (CTLA)-4 is a CD28 analogue with high affinity for B7-1 and B7-2. In contrast to CD28, CTLA-4 is a negative regulator for T-cell activation, and its engagement reduces TCR-mediated IL-2 production and blocks cell cycle progression.[45–48] Expression of CTLA-4 is delayed until 24 to 48 h after TCR triggering, depending on both the redistribution of the intracellular pool and *de novo* synthesis of the molecule. The regulatory effect of CTLA-4 on T-cell activation is well documented in CTLA-$4^{-/-}$ mice, which develop a fatal lymphoproliferative disorder characterized by a great increase in circulating and activated T cells. More recently, additional members of the CD28 family and their B7-like ligands have been identified.[46,47] Among these, inducible co-stimulator (ICOS) is expressed on a subpopulation of activated, but not naive or resting, T cells secreting high levels of IL-10.[49] ICOS binds to a B7-related protein, namely, B7RP-1, B7h, or ICOS-L, displayed by DCs, monocytes, resting B cells, and a portion of T lymphocytes. Interestingly, lipopolysaccharide (LPS) or TNF-α-induced maturation of DCs downregulates ICOS-L expression, which is instead augmented by IFN-γ. In addition, ICOS-L can be induced by inflammatory signals at peripheral sites, such as kidney, liver, heart, and brain.[50] Engagement of ICOS has no effect on IL-2 release, but significantly increases IL-10 production, and only slightly augments T-cell proliferation *in vitro*. Programmed death (PD)-1 is a member of the Ig superfamily, which binds two B7 homologue (B7Hs) molecules B7-H1 and B7-DC, also named PD-L1 and PD-L2. PD-1 cytoplasmic tail contains two immunoreceptor tyrosine-based inhibitory motifs (ITIM), responsible for the predominant inhibitory function of this molecule. Engagement of PD-1 attenuates T-cell activation and cytokine secretion.[51,52] The observation that DCs from PD-L2-deficient mice display a reduced stimulatory capacity compared to that from littermate controls suggests the existence of an additional ligand for PD-L2 mediating positive signals to the T cells.[53] Interestingly, PD-L1 and PD-L2 have a distinct expression pattern, being the first expressed by most hematopoietic cells as well as by other tissues, including IFN-γ-stimulated keratinocytes and endothelial cells.[54] In contrast, PD-L2 expression appears mostly restricted to mature DCs. The latter B7-like molecule identified has been named B7-H3 and binds to a still unknown co-stimulatory molecule on activated $CD4^+$ and $CD8^+$ T cells.[55] B7-H3 is expressed by various tissues and can be induced on DCs by inflammatory cytokines. Conflicting results have been provided concerning the role of B7-H3 in T-cell immune responses. Although initial reports indicated that B7-H3 can promotes T-cell proliferation and IFN-γ secretion, APCs from B7-H3-deficient mice display enhanced immunostimulatory capacity, thus suggesting a predominant negative effect of B7-H3 on murine T lymphocytes.[56]

A second group of co-stimulatory receptors belongs to the TNF family. Among these, the better characterized are OX40 (CD134) and CD40L (CD154). OX40 is not constitutively expressed on T cells, but is induced 24 to 48 h after TCR engagement.[57] OX40 ligation by OX40L expressed on APCs promotes T-cell clonal expansion and cytokine release, and regulate T-cell survival by increasing the antiapoptotic proteins Bcl-xL and Bcl-2.[58,59] OX40, acting synergistically with CD28, prevents excessive T-cell death, and may thus be involved in the maintenance of the number of memory T cells generated after antigen encounter. In addition, it has been suggested that OX40 may alter the balance between Th1 and Th2 immune responses by strongly promoting a Th2 switch in differentiating T cells. However, recent evidence has been provided that blocking OX40–OX40L interactions also modulate murine Th1-driven diseases, such as inflammatory bowel disease and experimental allergic encephalomyelitis.[60,61] Finally, CD40L is a member of the TFN family transiently expressed on recently activated T cells, which mediates critical signals for CD40-expressing APCs, such as DCs and B cells.[62,63] CD40L–CD40 interactions are essential for both humoral and cellular immune responses. CD40 engagement induces B-cell activation, immunoglobulin isotype-switching, and promotes germinal center formation. Mutation of CD40L is responsible for a severe immunodeficiency syndrome, the hyper-IgM syndrome, characterized by elevated IgM, low levels of IgG and IgA, and deficient humoral responses. In addition, CD40L–CD40 interaction is the major signal for IL-12 production and terminal maturation of DCs, a critical mechanism for induction of Th1 immune responses.[64,65]

## C. Cytokine Polarization of T Cells: The Th1/Th2 Paradigm

The existence of functionally distinct "effector" T-cell subsets originating from common T-cell precursors has been widely documented.[27,66,67] Type 1 lymphocytes, named Th1 and T cytotoxic (Tc) 1 for $CD4^+$ and $CD8^+$ T cells, respectively, release abundant IL-2, IFN-γ, lymphotoxin, and TNF-β. Th1 and Tc1 cells confer protective immunity against intracellular pathogens and are strongly involved in many autoimmune disorders. Conversely, type 2 cells, named Th2 and Tc2 for $CD4^+$ and $CD8^+$ T cells, respectively, release IL-4, IL-5, IL-13, but not IFN-γ. Th2/Tc2 cells provide help for B cells, are critical in humoral immune responses and in protective immunity against extracellular parasites, and play a key role in IgE-mediated atopic disease. Signals regulating the commitment of T lymphocytes include the type of APC, the dose of antigen, but mainly the cytokine milieu at the moment of antigen encounter. Cytokines are critical orchestrators of T-cell maturation and functional polarization. In particular, IL-12 and IL-18 are dominant cytokines for type 1 polarization, whereas IL-4 and IL-13 strongly promote Th2 development.[68,69] Additionally, in human, but not murine T cells, Th1 development is promoted by type I interferons.[70] Although immature DCs produce little or no IL-12, secretion of bioactive p70 IL-12 is induced by a number of signals, including bacterial and viral products and CD40 ligation.[64,65,71,72] Th1 polarization induced by IL-12 is mediated by signal transducers and activators of transcription (STAT)-4, and is defective in STAT-4-deficient mice.[73] In addition, STAT-4-independent mechanisms for Th1 commitment have been described. IFN-γ, which is incapable of inducing Th1 polarization by itself, assists Th1 development by promoting IL-12Rβ subunit expression on T cells, with a mechanism mediated by STAT-1 and T-bet. The latter is induced early during Th1 polarization through a STAT-4-independent pathway, and promotes IL-12R-β2 and IFN-γ expression.[74] IL-18 augments IL-12-mediated Th1 commitment, by enhancing IL-12Rβ2 expression and AP-1-dependent transactivation of the IFN-γ promoter. The source of IL-4 for Th2 commitment is not completely elucidated; however, it is known that it is not produced by professional APCs. IL-4 induces Th2 polarization by activating the signaling pathway mediated by the transcription factor STAT-6. GATA-3 is selectively induced during Th2 polarization, with a STAT-6 and NF-kB-dependent mechanism. In turn, GATA-3 promotes IL-4, IL-5, and IL-13 gene expression.[75–78] The role of co-stimulatory molecules B7-1 and B7-2 in directing T-cell commitment has received large attention in the past 10 years,[79,80] but these findings did not receive further confirmation. Defects in Th2 polarization has been documented in the absence of OX40 signaling. However, more recent data indicate that blocking OX40–OX40L interactions, both Th1 and Th2 immune responses are impaired, and IFN-γ secretion strongly reduced.[59]

## D. Effector Mechanisms of T Cells: T-Cell-Mediated Cytotoxicity

Lymphocyte-mediated cytotoxicity is the most efficient mechanism for the elimination of cells infected by bacteria or viruses, or altered as a consequence of mutations or chemical injuries. In addition, suicide/fratricide killing among T lymphocytes, i.e., AICD, is an important mechanism to prevent uncontrolled T-cell activation and to terminate immune responses.[81,82] Two major pathways for T-cell cytotoxicity have been identified: the granule exocytotosis and the cell membrane–associated cytolysis, e.g., Fas-ligand (FasL, CD95L)/Fas (CD95) pathway.[83] The granule exocytosis pathway dominates in $CD8^+$ T cells and NK cells, whereas the Fas-mediated mechanism appears more relevant in $CD4^+$ T-cell-mediated cytotoxicity. Cytotoxic granules contain an heterogeneous group of substances, comprising perforin, granzyme A, granzyme B, and other orphan granzymes, that are rapidly synthesized by T cells upon TCR triggering, and then stored in the cytoplasm of the cell.[84] Upon antigen recognition, components of the cytotoxic granules are discharged in the intercellular space between the killer and target cell. In the presence of $Ca^{2+}$, perforin polymerizes and inserts into the plasma membrane, thus promoting the entry of granzymes into the target cell. Granzyme B is a serine protease, which induces target cell apoptosis by activating the caspase cascade. In contrast, granzyme A is a tryptase and induces apoptosis through a caspase-independent mechanism.[85] FasL is a member of the TNF family that can trigger apoptosis in Fas-expressing target cells. Compared to Fas, which has a broad distribution among both hematopoietic and nonhematopoietic cells, FasL expression is restricted to T lymphocytes, which upregulate and transport FasL to the plasma membrane upon TCR stimulation. Fas engagement by its ligand leads to the recruitment of the Fas adaptor protein FADD, which in turn recruits caspase 8. Active caspase-8 promotes cleavage of various downstream caspases (including caspase 3, 6, and 7) with the capacity of degrading cytoskeletal proteins, nuclear lamins, and the inhibitor of caspase-activated DNase (ICAD). ICAD then permits activation of CAD to degrade DNA, leading to apoptosis.[86] Several important differences distinguish the FasL- and the perforin-mediated cytotoxicity. Generally, the granule exocytosis pathway is more rapid, as granules can be stored in the cytoplasm and rapidly released upon TCR triggering. In contrast, only a small amount of FasL is stored in recently activated cells. Consequently, maximal activity of the FasL mechanism requires the induction of newly synthesized molecules. On the other hand, FasL persists for a longer period on the T-cell membrane, because cleavage of FasL by proteolysis occurs in several hours. The long half-life of FasL is responsible for bystander lysis, which means that $Fas^+$ cells approaching the cytotoxic T cell can be killed even if they do not display TCR ligands on their surface.[87] For this reason, Fas-FasL function is not limited to the T-cell killing of target cells, but has a fundamental role in the immune system homeostasis, such as deletion of developing thymocytes and the AICD of peripheral T cells.[82,87]

## E. Regulatory T Cells

Prevention of excessive or undesired immune responses is a necessary duty for the immune system. This task is ensured either by nonspecific mechanisms, for example, AICD, or through the active intervention of specialized Treg (Table 6.2). Most of the Treg identified so far belongs to the $CD4^+$ compartment and suppresses immune responses through two principal pathways: the release of anti-inflammatory cytokines or a cell-to-cell contact-dependent mechanism.[88,89] In the mid-1990s, a regulatory subset of T lymphocytes was identified as Th3 cells.[90,91] The cytokine profile of Th3 cells closely resembles that of Th1 lymphocytes, but with high TGF-β release. Th3 lymphocytes suppress antigen-specific T-cell activation *in vitro* and *in vivo*, and their expansion is promoted by oral feeding with the antigen. However, Th3 intervention in skin immune responses has not been demonstrated so far.

More recently, IL-10 producing Treg, also called Tr1 (T regulatory 1) lymphocytes, has been characterized *in vitro* and isolated from various tissues, including the skin.[92,93] Upon TCR engagement, Tr1 cells release high amounts of IL-10 and little or no IFN-γ and IL-4. Many, but not all studies showed high TGF-β release by Tr1 cells, which may reinforce IL-10-mediated immune

**TABLE 6.2**
**Regulatory T-Cell Subsets**

| T Regulatory Cell | Cell Type | Target Cells | Mechanisms of Suppression | Induction |
|---|---|---|---|---|
| Th3 | $CD4^+$ | APCs | TGF-β | Oral feeding with Ag; TGF-β |
| Tr1 | $CD4^+$, $CD8^+$ | APCs | IL-10, TGF-β | Oral feeding with Ag; UV radiation; IL-10-TGF-β; immature or partially mature DCs |
| $CD25^+$ | $CD4^+$ | T cell | Cell–cell contact | Oral feeding with Ag, UV radiation |
| $CD28^-$ | $CD8^+$ | DCs | Cell–cell contact; IL-T3/IL-T4 induction on DCs | Repetitive stimulation with immature DCs |

suppression. *In vitro,* Tr1 cells poorly proliferate in the presence of the antigen, and suppress immune responses by dampening the APC capacity of DCs and macrophages. The phenotype of Tr1 cells includes the expression of several markers associated with Th1 polarization, such as the IL-12R β2 chain, CD26, and the lymphocyte activation gene (LAG)-3.[93] Importantly, Tr1 cells can be expanded *in vitro* by culturing naive T-cell precursors in the presence of IL-10 and IFN-α,[94] or after stimulation with antigens presented by immature DCs.[95] In addition, Tr1-like $CD8^+$ T cells, releasing high levels of IL-10 but not IFN-γ or IL-4, can be expanded *in vitro* using plasmacytoid DCs as APC, thus indicating that the Tr1 phenotype is not restricted to the $CD4^+$ T-cell population.[96] The importance of IL-10 in the regulation of skin immune responses has been widely documented. In murine contact hypersensitivity, IL-10-producing Treg appears critical cells for the induction of hapten-specific oral tolerance.[97,98] Similarly, hapten sensitization onto ultraviolet B (UV-B)-irradiated skin expands a subset of IL-10-releasing $CD4^+$ T cells, which expresses high levels of CTLA-4 and prevents hapten sensitization when transferred into naive recipients.[99,100] In addition, nickel-reactive Tr1 cells have been isolated from peripheral blood and from lesional skin of patients affected by allergic contact dermatitis.[93,101] In psoriasis, a defective IL-10 release in the skin appears involved in the expression of the chronic inflammation.[102] Finally, IL-10 has been described as a powerful mechanism for melanoma cells to escape from T-cell surveillance.[103]

A second group of Treg, which inhibits T-cell responses in a cytokine-independent, cell-contact-dependent manner, includes the $CD4^+CD25^+$ Treg. $CD25^+$ Treg accounts for 5 to 10% of circulating $CD4^+$ cells, expresses high levels of CTLA-4, and is naturally anergic upon mitogenic stimulation *in vitro.*[89,104] Expression of *Foxp3* gene, which encodes a transcriptional factor named Scurfin, has been positively correlated with the development of $CD25^+$ T cells, both in the thymus and at the periphery.[105] The current view is that $CD25^+$ Treg represents a distinct T-cell lineage arising from the thymus and involved in the maintenance of peripheral tolerance to self-antigens. However, increasing evidence suggests that a subset of $CD25^+$ Treg may also be involved in the regulation of immune responses to environmental antigens. Indeed, $CD4^+CD25^+$ Treg can be expanded following oral feeding with exogenous antigens,[106,107] and regulates immune responses to infectious agents.[108,109] A portion of circulating $CD4^+CD25^+$ T cells expressing the cutaneous lymphocyte associated antigen (CLA) has been recently involved in the regulation of nickel responsiveness in non-allergic individuals,[110] and suppresses contact hypersensitivity reactions in mouse.[111] Although regulatory function appears to prevail among $CD4^+$ T lymphocytes, a subset of $CD8^+CD28^-$ Treg has been recently shown to inhibit allospecific T-cell responses by inducing a tolerogenic phenotype in DCs.[112] Suppressive capacity of $CD8^+CD28^-$ Treg is associated with induction on the DC surface of the inhibitory molecule immunoglobulin-like transcript-3 (ILT3) and ILT4. Tolerogenic $CD80^-CD86^-$, $ILT3^+ILT4^+$ DCs resulting from interaction with $CD8^+CD28^-$ Treg anergize effector $CD4^+$ T cells in an MHC-restricted fashion.

## F. Natural Killer and Natural Killer T Cells

NK cells are a distinct and conserved subpopulation of lymphocytes, which display spontaneous cytolysis *in vitro* against a variety of targets.[113] The outcome of the NK activity depends on a balance between the ligation of activating and inhibitory receptors.[114] Best known among the inhibitory receptors are the members of the killer immunoglobulin-like receptor (KIR) family, which bind various HLA-A, -B, and -C alleles on the target cells, preventing NK-mediated cytotoxicity.[115] In contrast, ligation of activating receptors without inhibitory signals, e.g., when NK cell approach tumor cells with defective or altered MHC class I, induce NK proliferation, cytokine release, and cytotoxicity of the target cells. Among several natural cytotoxic receptors (NCR), NKp46, NKp30, and NKp44 appear to play an important role in NK-mediated cytotoxicity. Cooperation with NKG2D and other co-receptors, such as 2B4 and NKp80, is required for efficient effector function; indeed, experimental models indicate that blocking single NCR results in partial inhibition of cytotoxic activity. However, most of the ligand for these activating receptors remains unknown, except NKG2D, whose ligand has been identified as closely related molecules MICA and MICB, which are stress-inducible molecules expressed by most epithelial tumors.

NK-T cells (NKT) are a distinct lineage of T lymphocytes that co-express several NK receptors (CD56, CD16, CD161) and the CD3-TCR complex.[116,117] Two major subsets of NKT have been identified: NKT cells that are positively selected by the nonconventional MHC molecule CD1d, and those that are CD1d-independent. Most CD1d-restricted NKT displays a conserved V$\alpha$24 V$\beta$11 (V$\alpha$14 V$\beta$8 in mouse) TCR, and can be triggered by the glycopilid $\alpha$-galattosil ceramide (a-GalCer).[118,119] A portion of CD1d-restricted NKT expresses the CD4 or the CD3.

NK and NKT cells actively participate in the pathogenesis of several dermatoses, although their role in skin immune responses has not been completely defined. A high percentage of CD56$^+$ T cells have been detected among the leukocytes infiltrating skin lesions of lichen planus, lupus erythematosus, erythema anulare centrifugum, and psoriasis.[120] NKT cells also appear involved in the pathogenesis of psoriasis.[121]

## IV. T-CELL CIRCULATION IN THE SKIN

Compartmentalization of immune responses has great impact on the capacity of the immune system to ensure proper responses to a large variety of potentially hazardous stimuli and antigens. Selective targeting of leukocytes into peripheral tissues is controlled by their repertoire of homing and chemokine receptors and, on the other side, by the expression of adhesion molecules and the release of chemotactic factors by resident cells (see Chapter 15 for description of chemokine receptor expression on T cells). CLA is a glycosilated form of the P-selectin glicolipid ligand (PSGL)-1 receptor that is expressed by 15% of circulating T cells, and by the majority of T lymphocytes involved in cutaneous immune responses.[122–124] Glicosilation of PSGL-1 is ensured by fucosyltransferase VII and $\beta$-galattosyltranserase IV, whose expression is promoted by IL-12 and downregulated by IL-4.[125,126] Most of CLA$^+$ T cells also express the CCR4, receptor for CCL17/CCL22, and CCR10, which bind to CCL27, a chemokine selectively produced by keratinocytes.[127–129] Finally, CCR6, receptor for CCL20, appears important for T-cell recruitment in psoriatic lesions, although not specifically expressed by skin-homing T cells.[130]

T-cell extravasation is a dynamic process that can be divided in four critical steps: (1) initial tethering and rolling along the vessel wall, (2) activation of leukocyte integrins, (3) firm arrest, and (4) T-cell extravasation.[131,132] T-cell tethering and rolling along the endothelium are primarily mediated by the interaction of CLA and PSGL-1 with E- and P-selectins induced on endothelial cells by inflammatory cytokines, such as IL-1 and TNF-$\alpha$.[133] Rolling leukocytes are subsequently exposed to chemokines bound to heparin-like glycosaminoglycans on the endothelial cell. CCR4 mediates T-cell binding to CCL17, abundantly expressed by skin endothelial cells during inflammation. Chemokine receptor engagement determines conformational change and activation of the leukocyte integrins LFA-1 and $\alpha4\beta1$, which bind to endothelial ICAM-1 and VCAM-1, respectively, and promote T-cell firm adhesion and, finally, extravasation.[134]

## V. T CELLS IN HEALTHY SKIN AND IN COMMON T-CELL-MEDIATED INFLAMMATORY DISEASES

### A. T Cells in Healthy Skin

Normal, healthy skin is continuously inspected by T lymphocytes, which can be easily detected both in the epidermis and in the dermis by common immunohistochemical procedures.[135–137] Most of the skin T cells reside in the dermis, predominantly clustered around the postcapillary venules of the superficial plexus, and within the connective tissue sheaths of adnexal appendages, whereas intraepidermal T lymphocytes account for approximately 2% of the total number of cutaneous CD3$^+$ cells. The vast majority of intraepidermal T cells are CD4$^+$ or CD8$^+$ single positive lymphocytes, and express the αβ TCR, with only a minor portion (1 to 15%) of $\gamma\delta^+$ TCR cells and rare B lymphocytes.[138–145] A skewing toward the $CD8^+$ T cells in the epidermis has been described by several authors, whereas in the dermis the $CD4^+$ component greatly prevails in number.[135,136,143,145] Rare double-negative $CD4^-CD8^-$ T cells, mostly carrying the TCR γδ, have been observed in both the epidermis and dermis.[139,141] In addition, mouse, but not human skin contains a resident γδ T-cell population, called dendritic epidermal T cells (DETC), heavily involved in the regulation of skin immune responses.[146] Most cutaneous T lymphocytes express a memory/effector phenotype, as defined by expression of CD45RO and the absence of CD45RA.[137,138,141,145] In addition, several studies have shown that skin lymphocytes reside in the epidermis in a resting state, as indicated by the $CD25^-$, MHC class $II^-$ phenotype,[138,145] and by the observation that only a few intraepidermal T lymphocytes expressed the HNK-1 epitope (CD57) and the very late activation antigen-1 (VLA-1),[138,141] which are both markers that appear late after activation. Immunohistological studies demonstrated a regional variation of the number of intraepidermal T cells, maximal (43 $CD3^+$ cells/linear centimeter of epidermis) in the thorax and minimal (6 CD3+ cells/linear centimeter of epidermis) in the soles.[138] Regional variability was also found in the $CD4^+/CD8^+$ ratio, with the predominance of $CD8^+$ T cells at most sites (i.e., sole, buttock, and limbs), and of $CD4^+$ T cells in thorax epidermis.[138,141] Additionally, environmental factors, such as sun exposure, may contribute to determine these topographic differences. In particular, it has been observed that a physiological dose of solar-simulated radiation (SSR) induces a rapid decrement of intraepidermal $CD4^+$ and $CD8^+$, cells which persists for a few days and is followed by a selective influx of $CD4^+$ T cells, whose number appears increased compared to that of normal skin at 2 weeks after UV exposure.[145,147] Furthermore, skin areas chronically exposed to UV irradiation contain a lower number of epidermal T cells, predominantly $CD4^+$ T cells, compared to sun-protected skin sites, enriched in $CD8^+$ T cells.

Although most cutaneous T cells may migrate into normal skin as "passenger leukocytes," it cannot be excluded that a population of T cells may localize in the skin environment as "resident cells." CCL27, released at low levels by resting keratinocytes, appears critical for T-cell recruitment in steady-state skin.[128,129] The biological role of such resident epidermal T cells is still unknown; however, it is reasonable to hypothesize that cutaneous T cells perform a local sentinel function by ensuring rapid responses upon encountering recall antigens, or may be involved in the continuous immunosurveillance against the development of cutaneous cancers and persistent infection with intracellular pathogens. Indeed, a population of epidermal T cells isolated from normal human skin expresses FasL, and might be involved in Fas-FasL-mediated cytotoxicity of resident cell populations.[82,148] Renal-transplant recipients provide indirect evidence for the role of cutaneous T cells in the immunosurveillance against skin cancer and skin infections. These patients, usually receiving long-term immunosuppressive therapy to maintain the viability of the transplanted kidney, have an increased risk of acquiring skin tumors, such as squamous cell carcinoma, and viral opportunistic skin infections such as warts.[149] In addition, it was found that skin specimens from renal-transplant recipients, who did not have any skin diseases, had fewer T cells in both the epidermal and the dermal compartments than age-matched healthy volunteers.[150] Moreover, the number of cutaneous T cells decreased during the entire duration of the immunosuppressive therapy, which is in line with the clinical evidence that the longer the immunosuppression is present, the more skin cancers and skin infections develop.

## B. T Cells in Atopic Dermatitis

Inflammatory infiltrate in acute atopic dermatitis (AD) lesions comprises $CLA^+CD4^+$ and $CD8^+$ T lymphocytes, eosinophils, monocytes, and an augmented number of DCs. A characteristic feature of DCs in AD skin is the elevated expression of the high-affinity IgE receptor (FcεRI), which has been shown to function as an efficient antigen-focusing device for allergen capture.[151,152] Although the role of allergen exposure in exacerbating AD has not been not fully elucidated, AD skin bears atopen-specific T cells, and the application of allergens under occlusion (atopy patch test) induces eczematous reactions indistinguishable from naturally occurring AD.[153–156] These findings indicate that local activation of recruited T cells by specific allergens plays a role in AD expression. Despite the overall agreement about the Th2 bias of circulating T lymphocytes from atopic patients, several observations indicate that both IL-4/IL-13/IL-5-producing Th2 cells and the IFN-γ-secreting Th1 lymphocytes contribute to skin inflammation in AD. Initiation of AD lesions is characterized by a predominant Th2 infiltrate, releasing IL-4, IL-13, and IL-5. In more chronic lesions, IL-4 decreases, whereas Th1 cytokines, IFN-γ in particular, increase.[157,158] The switch to a Th1-dominated T-cell infiltrate may depend on the secretion of IL-12 by eosinophils, macrophages, and DCs.[159–162] Skin colonization by *Staphylococcus aureus*, frequently observed in AD patients, may contribute to the activation of resident DCs and monocytes to produce IL-12. In addition, IL-4 participates in keratinocyte activation and release of CXCL10, which, in turn, greatly contributes to the selective Th1 homing in the skin.[163] Tissue damage in AD lesions mostly depends on Fas-FasL-mediated T-cell cytotoxicity against keratinocytes.[164] Induction of keratinocyte apoptosis rapidly leads to cleavage of E-cadherins, molecules involved in the homotypic cellular adhesion, followed by keratinocyte detachment and spongiosis.[165] Keratinocyte susceptibility to apoptosis is augmented by IFN-γ exposure, which increases Fas as well as MHC class I and II and ICAM-1 expression.

An increased number of activated CLA$^+$ T cells spontaneously releasing IL-4 and IL-13 have been described in the peripheral blood of patients with AD, compared to healthy, non-allergic individuals.[166,167] Atopen-specific T-cell clones obtained from peripheral blood of patients with AD revealed a strong Th2 polarization compared to those obtained in the same conditions from non-atopic donors.[168–173] These observations indicated that aberrant cytokine production of specific T cells, rather than an abnormal T-cell repertoire, may be relevant for the disease expression. Alternatively, the predominant Th2 polarization of peripheral T cells in atopic donors has been explained as the consequence of unequal AICD of circulating T cells, with a more pronounced apoptosis of Th1 compared to Th2 cells.[174] A defect in CD8$^+$ T-cell functions has been suggested because of the increased susceptibility to viral infections, and the reduced number of perforin positive CD8$^+$ and NK cells in patients with AD compared to healthy individuals.[175,176] On the other hand, it has been shown that CD8$^+$ T cells participate in AD expression by secreting IL-5 and IL-13. In addition, CD8$^+$ T cells isolated from AD lesions proliferated in the presence of staphylococcal superantigens.[177]

## C. T Cells in Psoriasis

Psoriasis is an immunomediated inflammatory skin disorder characterized by keratinocyte hyperproliferation and altered differentiation, and by an inflammatory infiltrate comprising both CD4$^+$ and CD8$^+$ T cells, neutrophils, and an increased number of mature dendritic cells.[178] A large body of evidence has provided supporting the role of T cells in the pathogenesis of psoriasis. In particular, administration of drugs that block T-cell activation greatly improves psoriasis.[179] Administration of CTLA-4-Ig, a chimeric protein that binds B7-1 and B7-2 and prevents the delivery of co-stimulation to T cells, has been proven as an effective therapeutic approach, with a reduction of activated T lymphocytes in psoriatic plaques and decreased proliferation and HLA-DR, CD40, and CD54 expression in keratinocytes.[180] Alefacept, a LFA-3-IgG fusion protein that binds to CD2 on T cells and NK cells promoting their apoptosis, is also highly effective in the treatment of chronic psoriasis.[181,182] Finally, immunodeficient mice grafted with psoriatic skin develop typical psoriatic lesions only upon transfer of T cells.[183] Most of the T cells infiltrating psoriasis lesions belong to the Th1/Tc1 subset with a predominant release of IFN-γ and TNF-α.[184,185] The role of type 1 cytokines in the pathogenesis of psoriasis received confirmation by the beneficial effects of treatments aimed to reduce or suppress IFN-γ released by T cells, such as fumarate, IL-10, and IL-11 administration.[186–190] In addition, skewing IFN-γ-producing psoriatic T cells to a Th2 phenotype through IL-4 administration greatly improves psoriasis.[191] Finally, the role of infliximab, a mouse/human chimeric antibody that directly binds to TNF-α has been stressed for the treatment of psoriasis.[192]

Although the putative antigen responsible for T-cell activation in the epidermis has remained unidentified, an autoimmune origin of psoriasis has been hypothesized, based on the capacity of T cells from patients with psoriasis to react to cultured psoriatic keratinocytes. In addition, repetitive TCRβ VDJ rearrangement coding for the CDR3 motif of T cells infiltrating psoriatic lesions has been documented, which likely depends on clonal expansion of T cells that have proliferated in response to antigenic stimulation.[193–195] On the other hand, the degree of T-cell activation and proliferation in psoriatic plaques appears low, as indicated by the low percentage of proliferating Ki67$^+$CD8$^+$ T cells in the infiltrate.[196] Altered responsiveness of keratinocytes to T-cell-derived cytokines, IFN-γ in particular, has been proposed as a major mechanism for disease expression, and IFN-γ injection in nonlesional psoriatic skin rapidly leads to clinical manifestation of the disease.[197,198] Association of the disease with bacterial infections has suggested a role of T-cell activation by bacterial superantigens in the initiation of psoriasis plaques. T cells infiltrating both guttate and chronic plaques of psoriasis produce IFN-γ in the presence of streptococcal antigens and superantigens can trigger the disease with a T-cell-dependent mechanism in nonlesional psoriatic skin transplanted onto SCID mice.[199,200]

More recently, the presence of NKT cells in acute and chronic psoriasis lesions and the augmented expression of CD1d on basal psoriatic keratinocytes have driven the attention to the role of innate immunity in psoriasis.[201–203] NKT cell recognition of lipid determinants restricted by CD1d may be an important source of IFN-γ for disease expression, as indicated by *in vitro* experiments.[203] In addition, IFN-γ released by NKT cells strongly augments CD1d expression on psoriatic keratinocytes, thus establishing a positive loop for amplification of the inflammatory reaction.

## D. T Cells in Allergic Contact Dermatitis

Haptens are small, lipophilic chemicals that stimulate T-cell immune responses by virtue of their capacity to generate hapten–peptide complexes displayed on MHC complexes of APCs.[204–207] Hapten–peptide complexes are formed either by direct interaction of the chemical with peptide bound to MHC molecules or after intracellular metabolic transformation of the chemical to generate reactive intermediates with peptide-binding properties.[208–210] Moreover, some haptens may form the antigenic determinants by transiently interacting with peptide–MHC complexes in a noncovalent, labile way.[211,212] For each given hapten, multiple epitopes, either processing dependent or independent, originate following their skin penetration. This heterogeneous generation of antigenic determinants leads to the expansion of a broad repertoire of T cells involved in hapten-specific immune responses, encompassing both CD4$^+$ and CD8$^+$ T lymphocytes.[213,214]

Acute allergic contact dermatitis (ACD) is characterized by intense edema and spongiosis, and an heavy infiltrate in the dermis and epidermis, mostly constituted by T cells, monocytes, and DCs. Although CD4$^+$ T cells outnumber CD8$^+$ lymphocytes in ACD skin, the latter are crucial for disease expression.[215,216] Murine contact hypersensitivity (CH) is reduced in mice depleted of CD8$^+$ T cells or deficient in MHC class I molecules, whereas MHC class II–deficient mice, depleted of functional CD4$^+$ cells, display enhanced CH reactions.[217–219] Expression of human ACD to nickel correlates with the frequency of specific CD8$^+$ T cells in the peripheral blood, which is high in allergic individuals and low or undetectable in healthy individuals. In contrast, peripheral blood of both allergic and non-allergic subjects bears nickel-reactive CD4$^+$ T cells.[101] Altogether, these findings indicate that CD4$^+$ T cells are not essential for ACD expression, and suggest they may rather play a role in its regulation. Most human hapten-specific CD8$^+$ cells display a type 1 cytokine profile, whereas CD4$^+$ T lymphocytes isolated either from ACD lesions or from peripheral blood of allergic donors show a more variable pattern of cytokine release, with a predominance of Th1 cells and a lower number of Th2 lymphocytes.[220,221] A preferential usage of TCR-Vβ17 in peripheral blood and cutaneous T cells in nickel-induced ACD has been shown by several investigators.[222,223] Activation of hapten-specific T cells at the site of hapten challenge is fundamental for amplification of the inflammatory reaction and full expression of ACD. Although crucial for hapten sensitization, DCs may be not be required for ACD expression, and murine CH is augmented in the skin depleted of Langerhans cells.[224] Alternative pathways for T-cell activation could play a role in the rapid amplification of the immune response after hapten challenge. Indeed, fibroblasts and endothelial cells can serve as APCs for memory/effector lymphocytes,[225,226] and about one third of nickel-specific $CD4^+$ T cells, predominantly Th1, can be activated by the hapten through a direct T-T presentation.[227]

IFN-γ and TNF-α released by type 1 cells together with IL-17, secreted by both Th1 and Th2 cells, are the most efficient stimuli for cytokine and chemokine secretion by keratinocytes.[163,228,229] IL-4 contributes to keratinocyte activation by increasing their ICAM-1 expression and CXCL10 secretion.[230] CXCL10 selectively promotes the recruitment of $CXCR3^+$ Th1 and Tc1 lymphocytes, which represent more than 70% of the infiltrating T lymphocytes in ACD.[230,231] IFN-γ released by activated T cells is also crucial for keratinocyte expression of MHC class II, ICAM-1, and Fas. Keratinocyte apoptosis is a major mechanism of tissue damage in ACD. Mice that are deficient in perforin and Fas ligand fail to mount CH to haptens.[232] ACD skin displays numerous apoptotic keratinocytes, as detected by Tunel staining, and high mRNA expression of FasL and perforin.[233,234] Cytotoxicity of resting keratinocytes is predominantly due to the intervention of $CD8^+$ T lymphocytes through a perforin-mediated mechanism. In contrast, $CD4^+$ Th1 cell–mediated cytotoxicity is mostly mediated by the Fas-FasL pathway, and requires IFN-γ pretreatment of keratinocytes, which induces MHC class II and augments Fas expression.[234] The role of Th2 cells in the modulation of immune responses to haptens remains controversial. Evidence has been provided that Th2 cells can regulate murine CH and that IL-4 administration can reverse established murine CH.[235] However, CH is reduced or unmodified in $IL\text{-}4^{-/-}$ mice and decreased in STAT-6-deficient mice, in which Th2 responses are impaired.[236–238]

More recently, the role of specialized subsets of Treg in the control of ACD has been established. In mouse, emergence of IL-10 secreting Treg has been documented after oral feeding with haptens or upon hapten sensitization on UVB irradiated skin.[97–100] In humans, nickel-specific IL-10-releasing Tr1-like cells can be isolated from nickel-allergic individuals and, at higher frequency, in healthy, non-allergic donors.[93] Nickel-specific Tr1 cells block in an IL-10-dependent manner the antigen-presenting function of monocytes and DCs, thus decreasing their capacity to activate specific $CD4^+$ and $CD8^+$ T-cell responses to the metal. The major role of Tr1 cells may be to regulate the magnitude of T-cell responses to skin-applied haptens and to induce the termination of the immune response to avoid destructive inflammation. Chemokine receptor analysis of Tr1 cells revealed the propensity of these cells to respond to a vast array of chemokines, and selectively, together with hapten-specific Th2 cells, but not Th1, to CCL1, which is released late during ACD reactions.[239] Recently, a subset of $CD4^+CD25^+$ Treg has been identified, which expresses the homing receptor CLA and appears to be involved in the regulation of cutaneous immune responses and in the oral tolerance to skin sensitizers.[110,111,240] Indeed, $CLA^+CD25^+$ Treg isolated from peripheral blood of healthy, non-allergic individuals can regulate *in vitro* activation of both naive and effector nickel-specific T cells responses *in vitro*. In addition, hapten application onto the skin of non-allergic individuals determines the rapid recruitment of $CD4^+$ T cells containing about 20% of $CD25^+$ T cells, which, once isolated *in vitro*, are capable of suppressing the activation of nickel-specific T cells. In comparison, $CD25^+$ T cells isolated from nickel-allergic subjects showed a limited or absent capacity to regulate $CD4^+$ and $CD8^+$ nickel-specific activation *in vitro*. These findings strongly support for the hypothesis that development of exaggerated immune responses to environmental haptens may be the consequence of a defective or altered expansion and/or functional suppressive activity of specific Treg.

## REFERENCES

1. MacDonald, H.R., Radtke, F., and Wilson, A., T cell fate specification and alpha-beta/gamma-delta lineage commitment, *Curr. Opin. Immunol.*, 13, 219, 2001.

2. Anderson, G. and Jenkinson, E.J, Lymphostromal interactions in thymic development and function, *Nat. Rev. Immunol.,* 1, 31, 2001.
3. Aifantis, I. et al., Constitutive pre-TCR signaling promotes differentiation through $Ca^{2+}$ mobilization and activation of NF-kB and NFAT, *Nat. Immunol.,* 2, 403, 2001.
4. Borowski, C. et al., On the brink of becoming a T cell, *Curr. Opin. Immunol.*, 14, 200, 2002.
5. Love, P.E. and Chan, A.C., Regulation of thymocyte development: only the meek survive, *Curr. Opin. Immunol.*, 15, 199, 2003.
6. Starr, T.K., Jameson, S.C., and Hogquist, K.A., Positive and negative selection of T cells, *Annu. Rev. Immunol.*, 21, 139, 2003.
7. Singer, A., New perspectives on a developmental dilemma: the kinetic signalling model and the importance of signal duration for the CD4/CD8 lineage decision, *Curr. Opin. Immunol.*, 14, 207, 2002.
8. Butcher, E.C. and Picker, L.J., Lymphocyte homing and homeostasis, *Science*, 272, 60, 1996.
9. Warnock, R.A. et al., Molecular mechanisms of lymphocyte homing to peripheral lymph nodes, *J. Exp. Med.*, 187, 205, 1998.
10. Wagner, N. et al., Critical role for β7 integrins in the formation of the gut-associated lymphoid tissue, *Nature*, 382, 366, 1996.
11. Von Adrian, U.H. and Mackay, C.R., T-cell function and migration, *N. Engl. J. Med.*, 343, 1020, 2001.
12. Cyster, J.G., Chemokines and cell migration in secondary lymphoid organs, *Science*, 286, 2098, 1999.
13. Müller, G. and Lipp, M., Concerted action of the chemokine and lymphotoxin system in secondary lymphoid-organ development, *Curr. Opin. Immunol.*, 15, 217, 2003.
14. Gunn, M.D. et al., Mice lacking expression of secondary lymphoid organ chemokine have defects in lymphocyte homing and dendritic cell localization, *J. Exp. Med.*, 189, 451, 1999.
15. Förster, R. et al., CCR7 coordinates the primary immune responses by establishing functional microenvironment in secondary lymphoid organs, *Cell*, 99, 22, 1999.
16. Bajenoff, M., Granjeaud, S., and Guerder, S., The strategy of T cell antigen-presenting cell encounter in antigen-draining lymph nodes revealed by imaging of initial T cell activation, *J. Exp. Med.*, 198, 715, 2003.
17. Takeda, S. et al., MHC class II molecules are not required for survival of newly generated $CD4^+$ T cells, but affects their long term life-span, *Immunity*, 5, 217, 1996.
18. Tan, J.T. et al., IL-7 is critical for homeostatic proliferation and survival of naïve T cells, *Proc. Natl. Acad. Sci. U.S.A.*, 98, 8732, 2001.
19. Pieters, J., MHC class II-restricted antigen processing and presentation, *Adv. Immunol.*, 75, 159, 2000.
20. Hiltbold, E.M. and Roche, P.A., Trafficking of MHC class II molecules in the late secretory pathway, *Curr. Opin. Immunol.*, 14, 30, 2002.
21. Rudolph, M.G. and Wilson, I.A., The specificity of TCR and pMHC interaction, *Curr. Opin. Immunol.*, 14, 52, 2002.
22. Peña-Cruz, V. et al., Epidermal Langerhans cells efficiently mediate CD1a-dependent presentation of microbial lipid antigens to T cells, *J. Invest. Dermatol.*, 121, 517, 2003.
23. van der Merwe, P.A. and Davis, S.J., Molecular interactions mediating T cell antigen recognition, *Annu. Rev. Immunol.*, 21, 659, 2003.
24. Hayday, A.C., γδ cells: a right time and a right place for conserved third way of protection, *Annu. Rev. Immunol.*, 18, 975, 2000.
25. Bromley, S.K. et al., The immunological synapse, *Annu. Rev. Immunol.*, 19, 375, 2001.
26. van de Merwe, P.A., Formation and function of the immunological synapse, *Curr. Opin. Immunol.*, 14, 293, 2002.
27. Lanzavecchia, A. and Sallusto, F., Antigen decoding by T lymphocytes: from synapse to fate determination, *Nat. Immunol.*, 2, 487, 2001.
28. Valitutti, S. and Lanzavecchia, A., Serial triggering of TCRs: a basis for the sensitivity and specificity of antigen recognition, *Immunol. Today*, 18, 299, 1997.
29. Kalergis, A.M. et al., Efficient T cell activation requires an optimal dwell-time of interaction between the TCR and the pMHC complex, *Nat. Immunol.*, 2, 229, 2001.
30. Germain, R.N. and Stefanova, I., The dynamics of T cell receptor signalling: complex orchestration and the key roles of tempo and cooperation, *Annu. Rev. Immunol.*, 17, 467, 1999.
31. Trautmann, A. and Randriamampita, C., Initiation of TCR signalling revised, *Trends Immunol.*, 24, 425, 2003.

32. Dykstra, M. et al., Location is everything: lipid rafts and immune cell signalling, *Annu. Rev. Immunol.*, 21, 457, 2003.
33. Dutton, R.W., Bradley, L.M, and Swain, S.L., T cell memory, *Annu. Rev. Immunol.*, 16, 201, 1998.
34. Sprent, J. and Surth, C.D., Generation and maintenance of memory T cells, *Curr. Opin. Immunol.*, 13, 248, 2001.
35. Seder, R.A. and Ahmed, R., Similarities and differences in CD4+ and CD8+ effector and memory T cell generation, *Nat. Immunol.*, 4, 835, 2003.
36. Iezzi. G., Karjalainen, K., and Lanzavecchia, A., The duration of antigenic stimulation determines the fate of naïve and effector T cells, *Immunity*, 8, 89, 1998.
37. Cho, B. K. et al., Functional differences between memory and naïve CD8 T cells, *Proc. Natl. Acad. Sci. U.S.A.*, 96, 2976, 1999.
38. Kimachi, K., Sugie, K., and Gray, H.M., Effector T cells have a lower ligand affinity threshold for activation than naïve T cells, *Int. Immunol.*, 15, 885, 2003.
39. Colantonio, L. et al., Modulation of chemokine receptor expression and chemotactic responsiveness during differentiation of human naïve T cells into Th1 or Th2 cells, *Eur. J. Immunol.*, 32, 1264, 2002.
40. Schwartz, R.H., T cell anergy, *Annu. Rev. Immunol.*, 21, 305, 2003.
41. Li, W. et al., Blocked signal transduction to the ERK and JNK protein kinases in anergic CD4$^+$ T cells, *Science*, 271, 1272, 1996.
42. Fields, P.E, Gajewski, T.F., and Fich, F.W., Blocked Ras activation in anergic CD4$^+$ T cells, *Science*, 271, 1276, 1996.
43. Boussiotis, V.A. et al., p27kip 1 functions as an anergic factor inhibiting IL-2 transcription and clonal expansion of alloreactive human and murine helper T lymphocytes, *Nat. Med.*, 6, 290, 2000.
44. Sallusto, F., et al., Two subsets of memory T lymphocytes with distinct homing potentials and effector functions, *Nature*, 401, 708, 1999.
45. Salomon, B. and Bluestone, J.A., Complexities of CD28/B7: CTLA-4 costimulatory pathway in autoimmunity and transplantation, *Annu. Rev. Immunol.*, 19, 225, 2001.
46. Carreno, B.M. and Collins, M., The B7 family of ligands and its receptors: new pathways for costimulation and inhibition of immune responses, *Annu. Rev. Immunol.*, 20, 29, 2002.
47. Coyle, A.J. and Gutierrez-Ramos, J-C., The expanding B7 superfamily: increasing complexity in costimulatory signals regulating T cell function, *Nat. Immunol.*, 2, 203, 2001.
48. Schwartz, J-C.D. et al., Structural mechanisms of costimulation, *Nat. Immunol.*, 3, 427, 2002.
49. Löhning, M. et al., Expression of ICOS *in vivo* defines CD4$^+$ effector T cells with high inflammatory potential and a strong bias for secretion of interleukin 10, *J. Exp. Med.*, 197, 181, 2003.
50. Swallow, M.M., Wallin, J.J., and Sha, W.C., B7h, a novel costimulatory homolog of B7.1 and B7.2 is induced by TNFalpha, *Immunity*, 11, 423, 1999.
51. Freeman, G. et al., Engagement of the PD-1 immunoinhibitory receptor by a novel B7 family member leads to negative regulation of lymphocyte activation, *J. Exp. Med.*, 192, 1027, 2000.
52. Carter, L.L. et al., PD-1: PD-L inhibitory pathway affects both CD4$^+$ and CD8$^+$ T cells and is overcome by IL-2, *Eur. J. Immunol.*, 32, 634, 2002.
53. Shin, T. et al., Cooperative B7-1/2 (CD80/CD86) and B7-DC costimulation of CD4$^+$ T cells independent of the PD-1 receptor, *J. Exp. Med.*, 198, 31, 2003.
54. Mazanet, M.M. and Hughes, C.C.W., B7-H1 is expressed by human endothelial cells and suppresses T cell cytokine synthesis, *J. Immunol.*, 169, 3581, 2002.
55. Chapoval, A.I. et al., B7-H3: a costimulatory molecule for T cell activation and IFN-$\gamma$ production, *Nat. Immunol.*, 2, 261, 2001.
56. Shu, W.-K. et al., The B7 member B7-H3 preferentially down-regulates T helper type-1-mediated immune responses, *Nat. Immunol.*, 4, 899, 2003.
57. Croft, M., Co-stimulatory members of the TNFR family: keys to effective T-cell immunity?, *Nat. Rev. Immunol.*, 3, 609, 2003.
58. Rogers, P.R. et al., OX40 promotes Bcl-xL and Bcl-2 expression and is essential for long-term survival of CD4 T cells, *Immunity*, 15, 445, 2001.
59. De Smedt, T. et al., OX40 costimulation enhances the development of T cell responses induced by dendritic cells *in vivo*, *J. Immunol.*, 168, 661, 2002.
60. Lane, P., Role of OX-40 signals in coordinating CD4 T cell selection, migration, and cytokine differentiation in T helper (Th)1 and Th2 cells, *J. Exp. Med.*, 191, 201, 2000.

61. Higgings, L.M. et al., Regulation of T cell activation *in vitro* and *in vivo* by targeting the OX40-OX40 ligand interaction: amelioration of ongoing inflammatory bowel disease with an OX40-IgG fusion protein, but not with an OX40 ligand-IgG fusion protein, *J. Immunol.*, 162, 486, 1999.
62. Grewal, I.S. and Flavell, R.A., CD40 and CD154 in cell-mediated immunity, *Annu. Rev. Immunol.*, 16, 111, 1998.
63. Lee, B.O. et al., The biological outcome of CD40 signaling is dependent on the duration of CD40 ligand expression: reciprocal regulation by interleukin (IL)-4 and IL-12, *J. Exp. Med.* 196, 693, 2003.
64. Cella, M. et al., Ligation of CD40 on dendritic cells triggers production of high levels of interleukin-12 and enhances T cell stimulatory capacity: T-T help via APC activation, *J. Exp. Med.*, 184, 747, 1996.
65. Koch, F. et al., High level IL-12 production by murine dendritic cells: upregulation via MHC class II and CD40 molecules and downregulation by IL-4 and IL-10, *J. Exp. Med.,* 184, 741, 1996.
66. Constant, S.L. and Bottomly, K., Induction of Th1 and Th2 $CD4^+$ T cell responses: the alternative approaches, *Annu. Rev. Immunol.*, 15, 297, 1997.
67. Grogan, J.L. and Locksley, R.M., T helper cell differentiation: on again, off again, *Curr. Opin. Immunol.*, 14, 366, 2002.
68. Murphy, K.M. et al., Signalling and transcription in T helper development, *Annu. Rev. Immunol.*, 18, 451, 2000.
69. Ferrar, J.D., Asnagli, H., and Murphy, K.M., T helper subset development: role of instruction, selection and transcription, *J. Clin. Invest.*, 109, 431, 2002.
70. Ferrar, J.D. et al., Recruitment of Stat-4 to the human interferon-$\alpha/\beta$ receptor requires activated Stat-2, *J. Biol. Chem.*, 275, 2693, 2000.
71. Moser, M. and Murphy, K.M., Dendritic cell regulation of Th1-Th2 development, *Nat. Immunol.*, 1, 199, 2000.
72. Corinti, S., Human dendritic cells very efficiently present a heterologous antigen expressed on the surface of recombinant gram-positive bacteria to $CD4^+$ T lymphocytes, *J. Immunol.*, 163, 3029, 1999.
73. Kaplan, M.H. et al., Impaired IL-12 responses and enhanced development of Th2 cells in Stat4-deficient mice, *Nature*, 382, 174, 1996.
74. Afkarian, M. et al., T-bet is a STAT-1 induced regulator of IL-12R in naïve $CD4^+$ T cells, *Nat. Immunol.*, 3, 549, 2002.
75. Zhang, D-H. et al., Transcription factor GATA-3 is differentially expressed in murine Th1 and Th2 cells and controls Th2-specific expression of the interleukin-5 gene, *J. Biol. Chem.*, 272, 21597, 1997.
76. Farrar, J.D. et al., An instructive component in T helper cell type 2 (Th2) development mediated by GATA-3, *J. Exp. Med.*, 193, 643, 2001.
77. Das, J. et al., A critical role for NF-kB in GATA-3 expression and Th2 differentiation in allergic airway inflammation, *Nat. Immunol.*, 2, 45, 2001.
78. Lavenu-Bombled, C. et al., Interleukin-13 gene expression is regulated by GATA-3 in T cells, *J. Biol. Chem.*, 277, 18313, 2002.
79. Freeman, G.J. et al., B7-1 and B7-2 do not deliver identical costimulatory signals, since B7-2 but not B7-1 preferentially costimulates the initial production of IL-4, *Immunity*, 2, 523, 1995.
80. De Becker, G. et al., Regulation of T helper cell differentiation *in vivo* by soluble and membrane proteins provided by antigen-presenting cells, *Eur. J. Immunol.*, 28, 3161, 1998.
81. Hildeman, D.A. et al., Molecular mechanisms of activated T cell death *in vivo*, *Curr. Opin. Immunol.*, 14, 354, 2002.
82. De Panfilis, G., "Activation induced cell death": a special program able to preserve the homeostasis of the skin, *Exp. Dermatol.*, 11, 1, 2002.
83. Russel, J.H. and Ley, T.J., Lymphocyte-mediated cytotoxicity, *Annu. Rev. Immunol.,* 20, 323, 2002.
84. Raja, S.M., Metkar, S.S., and Froelich, C.J., Cyotoxic granule-mediated apoptosis: unravelling the complex mechanism, *Curr. Opin. Immunol.*, 15, 528, 2003.
85. Pinkoski, M.J. and Green, D.R., Granzime A: the road less travelled, *Nat. Immunol.*, 4, 106, 2003.
86. Wang, R. et al., CD95-dependent bystander lysis caused by $CD4^+$ T helper 1 effectors, *J. Immunol.*, 157, 2961, 1996.
87. Krammer, P.H., CD95's deadly mission in the immune system, *Nature*, 407, 789, 2000.
88. Curotto de Lafaille, M.A. and Lafaille, J.J., $CD4^+$ regulatory T cells in autoimmunity and allergy, *Curr. Opin. Immunol.*, 14, 771, 2002.

89. Shevach, E.M., CD4+CD25+ suppressor T cells: more question than answers, *Nat. Rev. Immunol.*, 2, 389, 2002.
90. Chen, Y. et al., Regulatory T cell clones induced by oral tolerance: suppression of autoimmune encephalomyelitis. *Science*, 265, 1237, 1994.
91. Fukaura, H. et al., Induction of circulating myelin basic protein and proteolipid protein-specific transforming growth factor-β1-secreting Th3 T cells by oral administration of myelin in multiple sclerosis patients, *J. Clin. Invest.*, 98, 70, 1996.
92. Groux, H. et al., A CD4+ T-cell subset inhibits antigen-specific T-cell responses and prevents colitis, *Nature*, 389, 737, 1997.
93. Cavani, A. et al., Human CD4+ T lymphocytes with remarkable regulatory functions on dendritic cells and nickel-specific Th1 immune responses, *J. Invest. Dermatol.*, 114, 295, 2000.
94. Levings, M.K. et al., IFN-alpha and IL-10 induce the differentiation of human type 1 T regulatory cells, *J. Immunol.*, 166, 5530, 2001.
95. Jonuleit, H., Schmitt, E., and Enk, A.H., Dendritic cells as a tool to induce anergic and regulatory T cells, *Trends Immunol.*, 22, 394, 2001.
96. Gilliet, M. and Liu, Y.-J., Generation of human CD8 T regulatory cells by CD40-ligand activated plasmocytoid dendritic cells, *J. Exp. Med.*, 195, 695, 2002.
97. Desvignes C. et al., Oral administration of haptens inhibits *in vivo* induction of specific cytotoxic CD8+ T cells mediating tissue inflammation: a role for regulatory CD4+ T cells, *J. Immunol.*, 2000, 164, 2515, 2000.
98. Artik, S. et al., Tolerance to nickel: oral nickel administration induces a high frequency of anergic T cells with persistent suppressor activity, *J. Immunol.*, 167, 6794, 2001.
99. Niizeki, H. and Streilein, J.W., Hapten-specific tolerance induced by acute, low-dose ultraviolet B radiation of skin is mediated via interleukin-10, *J. Invest. Dermatol.*, 109, 25, 1997.
100. Schwarz, A. et al., Evidence for functional relevance of CTLA-4 in ultraviolet-radiation-induced tolerance. *J. Immunol.*, 165,1824, 2000.
101. Cavani, A. et al., Patients with allergic contact dermatitis to nickel and nonallergic individuals display different nickel-specific T cell responses: evidence for the presence of effector CD8+ T cells and regulatory CD4+ T cells, *J. Invest. Dermatol.*, 111, 621, 1998.
102. Asadullah, K. et al., IL-10 is a key cytokine in psoriasis. Proof of principle by IL-10 therapy: a new therapeutic approach, *J. Clin. Invest.*, 101, 783, 1998.
103. Steinbrink, K. et al., Interleukin-10-treated dendritic cells induce a melanoma-antigen-specific anergy in CD8+ T cells resulting in a failure to lyse tumor cells, *Blood*, 5, 1634, 1999.
104. Maloy, K.J. and Powrie, F., Regulatory T cells in the control of immune pathology, *Nat. Immunol.*, 2, 816, 2001.
105. Ramsdell, F., Foxp3 and naturally regulatory T cells: key to a cell lineage? *Immunity*, 19, 165, 2003.
106. Thorstenson, K.M. and Khoruts, A., Generation of anergic and potentially immunoregulatory CD25+CD4+ T cells *in vivo* after induction of peripheral tolerance with intravenous or oral antigen, *J. Immunol.*, 167, 188, 2001.
107. Zhang, X. et al., Activation of CD4+CD25+ regulatory T cells by oral antigen administration, *J. Immunol.*, 167, 4245, 2001.
108. Belkaid, J. et al., CD4+CD25+ regulatory T cells control *Leishmania major* persistence and immunity, *Nature*, 420, 502, 2002.
109. Hori, S., Carvalho, T.L., and Demengeot, J., CD25+CD4+ regulatory T cells suppress CD4+ T cell-mediated pulmonary hyperinflammation driven by *Pneumocysis carinii* in immunodeficient mice, *Eur. J. Immunol.*, 32, 1282, 2002.
110. Cavani, A. et al., Human CD25+ regulatory T cells maintain immune tolerance to nickel in healthy, non allergic individuals, *J. Immunol.*, 171, 5760, 2003.
111. Dubois, B. et al., Innate CD4+CD25+ regulatory T cells are required for oral tolerance and inhibition of CD8+ T cells mediating skin inflammation, *Blood*, 102, 3295, 2003.
112. Chang, C.C. et al., Tolerization of dendritic cells by Ts cells: the crucial role of inhibitory receptors ILT3 and ILT4, *Nat. Immunol.*, 3, 237, 2002.
113. Moretta, L. et al., Human natural killer cells: their origin, receptors and function, *Eur. J. Immunol.*, 32, 1205, 2002.

114. Natarajan, K. et al., Structure and function of natural killer cell receptors: multiple molecular solutions to self, nonself discrimination, *Annu. Rev. Immunol.*, 20, 853, 2002.
115. Vilches, C. and Parham, P., KIR: diverse, rapidly evolving receptors of innate and adaptive immunity, *Annu. Rev. Immunol.*, 20, 217, 2002.
116. Gapin, L. et al., NKT cells derive from double-positive thymocytes that are positively selected by CD1d, *Nat. Immunol.*, 2, 971, 2001.
117. Jayawardena-Wolf, J. and Bendelac, A., CD1 and lipid antigens: intracellular pathway for antigen presentation, *Curr. Opin. Immunol.*, 13, 109, 2001.
118. Joyce, S. and Van Kaer, L., CD1-restricted antigen presentation: the oily matter, *Curr. Opin. Immunol.*, 15, 95, 2003.
119. Matsuda, J.L. et al., Tracking the response of natural killer T cells to a glycolipid using CD1d tetramers, *J. Exp. Med.*, 192, 741, 2000.
120. Harvell, J.D., Nowfar-Rad, M., and Sundram, U., an immunohistochemical study of CD4, CD8, TIA-1, and CD56 subsets in inflammatory skin diseases, *J. Cutaneous Pathol.*, 30, 108, 2003.
121. Nickoloff, G.J., Skin innate immune system in psoriasis: friend or foe? *J. Clin. Invest.*, 104, 1161, 1999.
122. Picker, L.J. et al., Control of leukocyte recirculation in man: II. Differential regulation of the cutaneous lymphocyte-associated antigen, a tissue-selective homing receptor for skin-homing T cells, *J. Immunol.*, 150, 1122, 1993.
123. Fuhlbrigge, R.C. et al., Cutaneous lymphocyte antigen is a specialized form of PSGL-1 expressed on skin homing T cells, *Nature*, 389, 978, 1997.
124. Schön, M.P., Zollner, T.M., and Henning Boehncke, W., The molecular basis of lymphocyte recruitment to the skin: clues for pathogenesis and selective therapies of inflammatory disorders, *J. Invest. Dermatol.*, 121, 951, 2003.
125. Wagers, A.J. et al., Interleukin 12 and interleukin 4 control T cell adhesion to endothelial selectins through opposite effects on α1,3-fucosyltransferase VII gene expression, *J. Exp. Med.*, 188, 2225, 1998.
126. Lim, Y-C. et al., Expression of functional selectin ligands on Th cells is differentially regulated by IL-12 and IL-4, *J. Immunol.*, 162, 3193, 1999.
127. Campbell, J.J. et al., The chemokine receptor CCR4 in vascular recognition by cutaneous but not intestinal memory T cells, *Nature*, 400, 776, 1999.
128. Reiss, Y. et al., CC chemokine receptor (CCR)4 and the CCR10 ligand cutaneous T cell-attracting chemokine (CTACK) in lymphocyte trafficking to inflamed skin, *J. Exp. Med.*, 194, 1541, 2001.
129. Homey, B. et al., CCL27-CCR10 interactions regulate T cell-mediated skin inflammation, *Nat. Med.*, 8, 157, 2002.
130. Homey, B. et al., Up-regulation of macrophage inflammatory protein-3α/CCL20and CC chemokine receptor 6 in psoriasis, *J. Immunol.*, 164, 6621, 2000.
131. Springer, T.A., Traffic signals for lymphocyte recirculation and leukocyte emigration: the multistep paradigm, *Cell*, 76, 301, 1994.
132. Butcher, E.C. and Picker, L.J., Lymphocyte homing and homeostasis, *Science*, 272, 60, 1996.
133. Mantovani, A., Bussolino, F., and Introna, M., Cytokine regulation of endothelial cell function: from molecular level to the bedside, *Immunol. Today*, 18, 231, 1997.
134. Laudanna, C, Kim, J.Y., and Butcher, E., Rapid leukocyte integrin activation by chemokines, *Immunol. Rev.*, 186, 37, 2002.
135. Smolle, J. et al., Inflammatory cell types in normal human epidermis: an immunohistochemical and morphometric study, *Acta Derm. Venereol.*, 65, 479, 1985.
136. Bos, J.D. et al., The skin immune system (SIS): distribution and immunophenotype of lymphocyte subpopulations in normal human skin, *J. Invest. Dermatol.*, 88, 569, 1987.
137. Bos, J.D. et al., Predominance of "memory" T cells ($CD4^+$, $CDw29^+$) over "naive" T cells ($CD4^+$, $CD45RA^+$) in both normal and diseased human skin, *Arch. Dermatol. Res.*, 281, 24, 1989.
138. Foster, C.A. et al., Human epidermal T cells predominantly belong to the lineage expressing alpha/beta T cell receptor, *J. Exp. Med.*, 171, 997, 1990.
139. Groh, V. et al., Human lymphocytes bearing T cell receptor gamma/delta are phenotypically diverse and evenly distributed throughout the lymphoid system, *J. Exp. Med.*, 169, 1277, 1989.
140. Bucy, R.P. et al., Tissue localization and CD8 accessory molecule expression of T gamma delta cells in humans, *J. Immunol.*, 142, 3045, 1989.
141. Spetz, A. et al., T cells subsets in normal human epidermis, *Am. J. Pathol.*, 149, 665, 1996.

142. Bos, J.D. et al., T-cell receptor gamma delta bearing cells in normal human skin, *J. Invest. Dermatol.*, 94, 37, 1990.
143. Dupuy, P. et al., T-cell receptor-gamma/delta bearing lymphocytes in normal and inflammatory human skin, *J. Invest. Dermatol.*, 94, 764, 1990.
144. Alaibac, M. et al., T lymphocytes bearing the gamma delta T-cell receptor: a study in normal human skin and pathological skin conditions, *Br. J. Dermatol.*, 127, 458, 1992.
145. Di Nuzzo, S. et al., UVB radiation preferentially induces recruitment of memory $CD4^+$ T cells in normal human skin: long-term effect after a single exposure, *J. Invest. Dermatol.*, 110, 978, 1998.
146. Hayday, A. and Tigelaar, R., Immunoregulation in the tissues by gd T cells, *Nat. Rev. Immunol.*, 3, 233, 2003.
147. Di Nuzzo, S. et al., Solar-stimulated ultraviolet irradiation induces selective influx of CD4+ T lymphocytes in normal human skin, *Photochem. Photobiol.*, 64, 988, 1996.
148. De Panfilis, G. et al., CD95-ligand (Fas-L)-expressing epidermal lymphocytes, *Br. J. Dermatol.*, 143, 892, 2000.
149. Brown, J.H. et al., Dermatologic lesions in a transplant population, *Transplantation*, 46, 65, 1988.
150. Galvao, M.M. et al., Lymphocyte subsets and Langerhans cells in sun-protected and sun-exposed skin of immunosuppressed renal allograft recipients, *J. Am. Acad. Dermatol.*, 38, 38, 1998.
151. von Bubnoff, D., Koch, S., and Bieber., T., Dendritic cells and atopic eczema/dermatitis syndrome, *Curr. Opin. Allergy Clin. Immunol.*, 3, 353, 2003.
152. Maurer, D. et al., Fcε receptor I on dendritic cells delivers IgE-bound multivalent antigens into a cathepsin S-dependent pathway of MHC class II presentation, *J. Immunol.,* 161, 2731, 1998.
153. Abernathy-Carver, K.J. et al., Milk-induced eczema is associated with the expansion of T cells expressing cutaneous lymphocyte antigen, *J. Clin. Invest.*, 95, 913, 1995.
154. van der Hejiden, F.L. et al., High frequency of IL-4-producing $CD4^+$ allergen-specific T lymphocytes in atopic dermatitis lesional skin, *J. Invest. Dermatol.*, 97, 389, 1991.
155. van Rejisen, F.C. et al., Skin-derived aeroallergen-specific T-cell clones of Th2 phenotype in patients with atopic dermatitis, *J. Allergy Clin. Immunol.*, 90, 184, 1992.
156. Sager, N. et al., House dust mite-specific T cells in the skin of subjects with atopic dermatitis: frequency and lymphokine profile in the allergen patch test, *J. Allergy Clin. Immunol.*, 89, 801, 1992.
157. Hamid, Q., Boguniewicz, M., and Leung, D.Y.M., Differential *in situ* cytokine gene expression in acute versus chronic atopic dermatitis, *J. Clin. Invest.,* 94, 870, 1994.
158. Werfel, T. et al., Allergen specificity of skin-infiltrating T cells is not restricted to a type-2 cytokine pattern in chronic skin lesions of atopic dermatitis, *J. Invest. Dermatol.*, 107, 871, 1996.
159. Hamid, Q. et al., *In vivo* expression of IL-12 and IL-13 in atopic dermatitis, *J. Allergy Clin. Immunol.*, 98, 225, 1996.
160. Grewe, M. et al., A role for Th1 and Th2 cells in the immunopathogenesis of atopic dermatitis, *Immunol. Today*, 19, 359, 1998.
161. Brand, U. et al., Allergen-specific immune deviation from a Th2 to a Th1 response induced by dendritic cells and collagen type I, *J. Allergy Clin. Immunol.,* 104, 1052, 1999.
162. Yawalkar N. et al., Down-regulation of IL-12 by topical corticosteroids in chronic atopic dermatitis, *J. Allergy Clin. Immunol.,* 106, 941, 2000.
163. Albanesi, C. et al., A cytokine-to-chemokine axis between T lymphocytes and keratinocytes can favour Th1 cell accumulation in chronic skin diseases, *J. Leukocyte Biol.*, 70, 617, 2001.
164. Trautmann, A. et al., T cell-mediated FAS-induced keratinocyte apoptosis plays a key pathogenetic role in eczematous dermatitis, *J. Clin. Invest.,* 106, 25, 2000.
165. Trautmann, A. et al., The differential fate of cadherins during T-cell-induced keratinocytes apoptosis leads to spongiosis in eczematous dermatitis, *J. Invest. Dermatol.*, 117, 927, 2001.
166. Santamaria Babi, L.F. et al., Circulating allergen-reactive T cells from patients with atopic dermatitis and allergic contact dermatitis express the skin-selective homing receptor, the cutaneous lymphocyte-associated antigen, *J. Exp. Med.*, 181, 1935, 1995.
167. Dworzac, M.N. et al., Skin-associated lymphocytes in the peripheral blood of patients with atopic dermatitis: signs of subset expansion and stimulation, *J. Allergy Clin. Immunol.*, 103, 901, 2001.
168. Akdis, M. et al., Skin-homing, $CLA^+$ memory T cells are activated in atopic dermatitis and regulate IgE by an IL-13-dominated cytokine pattern. IgG4 counter-regulation by $CLA^-$ memory T cells, *J. Immunol.*, 159, 4611, 1997.

169. Wierenga, E.A. et al., Comparison of diversity and function of house dust mite-specific T lymphocyte clones from atopic and non-atopic donors, *Eur. J. Immunol.*, 20, 1519, 1990.
170. Wierenga, E.A. et al., Human atopen-specific types 1 and 2 T helper cell clones, *J. Immunol.*, 147, 2942, 1991.
171. Sallusto, F. et al., T-cell and antibody response to *parietaria judaica* allergenic fraction in atopic and nonatopic individuals, *Allergy*, 48, 37, 1993.
172. Ebner, C. et al., Nonallergic individuals recognize the same T cell epitope of Bet v 1, the major birch pollen allergen, as atopic patients, *J. Immunol.*, 154, 1932, 1995.
173. Parronchi, P. et al., Aberrant interleukin (IL)-4 and IL-5 production *in vitro* by $CD4^+$ helper T cells from atopic subjects, *Eur. J. Immunol.*, 22, 1615, 1990.
174. Akdis, M. et al., T helper (Th) 2 predominance in atopic disease is due to preferential apoptosis of circulating memory/effector Th1 cells, *FASEB J.*, 17, 1026, 2003.
175. Ambach, A., Bonnekoh, B., and Gollnick, H., Perforin hyperreleasability and depletion in cytotoxic T cells from patients with exacerbated atopic dermatitis and asymptomatic rhinoconjunctivitis allergica, *J. Allergy Clin. Immunol.*, 107, 878, 2001.
176. Lonati, A. et al., Reduced production of both Th1 and Tc1 lymphocyte subsets in atopic dermatitis, *Clin. Exp. Immunol.*, 115, 1, 1999.
177. Akdis, M. et al., Skin-homing (cutaneous lymphocyte-associated antigen-positive) $CD8^+$T cells respond to superantigens and contribute to eosinophilia and IgE production in atopic dermatitis, *J. Immunol.*, 163, 466, 1999.
178. Bos, J.D. and De Rie, M.A., The pathogenesis of psoriasis: immunological facts and speculations, *Immunol. Today*, 14, 391, 1999.
179. Gottlieb, S.L. et al., Response of psoriasis to a lymphocyte-selective toxin (DA389IL-2) suggests a primary immune, but not keratinocyte, pathogenic basis, *Nat. Med.*, 1, 442, 1995.
180. Abrams, J.R. et al., Blockade of T lymphocyte costimulation and cytotoxic T lymphocyte-associated antigen 4-immunoglobulin (CTLA-4Ig) reverses the cellular pathology of psoriatic plaques, including the activation of keratinocytes, dendritic cells, and endothelial cells, *J. Exp. Med.*, 192, 681, 2000.
181. Ellis, C.N. and Krueger, G.G., Treatment of chronic plaque psoriasis by selective targeting of memory effector T lymphocytes, *N. Engl. J. Med.*, 345, 248, 2001.
182. Da Silva, A.J., Alefacept, an immunomodulatory recombinant LFA-3/IgG1 fusion protein, induces CD16 signaling and CD2/CD16-dependent apoptosis of $CD2^+$ cells, *J. Immunol.*, 168, 4462, 2002.
183. Nickoloff, B.J. and H. Wrone-Smith, Injection of pre-psoriatic skin with CD4 T cells induces psoriasis, *Am. J. Pathol.*, 155, 145, 1999.
184. Schlaak, J.F. et al., T cells involved in psoriasis vulgaris belong to the Th1 subset, *J. Invest. Dermatol.*, 102, 145, 1994.
185. Austin, L.M. et al., The majority of epidermal T cells in psoriasis vulgaris lesions can produce type 1 cytokines, interferon-$\gamma$, interleukin-2, and tumor necrosis factor-$\alpha$, defining TC1 (cytotoxic T lymphocytes), and TH1 effector populations: a type 1 differentiation basis also measured in circulating blood T cells in psoriatic patients, *J. Invest. Dermatol.*, 113, 752, 1999.
186. Litjens, N.H.R. et al., Beneficial effects of fumarate therapy in psoriasis vulgaris patients coincide with downregulation of type 1 cytokines, *Br. J. Dermatol.*, 148, 444, 2003.
187. Asadullah, K. et al., IL-10 is a key cytokine in psoriasis: proof of principle by IL-10 therapy: a new therapeutic approach, *J. Clin. Invest.*, 101, 783, 1998.
188. Asadullah, K. et al., Effects of systemic interleukin-10 therapy on psoriatic skin lesions: histologic, immunohistologic, and molecular biology findings, *J. Invest. Dermatol.*, 116, 721, 2001.
189. Reich, K. et al., Response of psoriasis to interleukin-10 is associated with suppression of cutaneous type 1 inflammation, downregulation of the epidermal interleukin-8/CXCR2 pathway and normalization of keratinocytes maturation, *J. Invest. Dermatol.*, 116, 319, 2001.
190. Trepicchio, W.L. et al., Interleukin-11 therapy selectively downregulates type I cytokine proinflammatory pathways in psoriasis lesions, *J. Clin. Invest.*, 104, 1527, 1999.
191. Ghoreschi K. et al., Interleukin-4 therapy of psoriasis induces Th2 responses and improves human autoimmune diseases, *Nat. Med.*, 9, 40, 2003.
192. Gottlieb, A.B., Infliximab for psoriasis, *J. Am. Acad. Dermatol.*, 49, 112, 2003.
193. Prinz, J.C. et al., Selection of conserved TCR VDJ rearrangement in chronic psoriatic plaques indicates a common antigen in psoriasis vulgaris, *Eur. J. Immunol.*, 29, 3390, 1999.

194. Vollmer, S., Menssen, A., and Prinz, J.C., Dominant lesional T cell receptor rearrangements persist in relapsing psoriasis but are absent from nonlesional skin: evidence for a stable antigen-specific pathogenic T cell response in psoriasis vulgaris, *J. Invest. Dermatol.*, 117, 1296, 2001.
195. Hwang, H. Y. et al., Identification of a commonly used CDR3 region of infiltrating T cells expressing Vβ13 and Vβ15 derived from psoriasis patients, *J. Invest. Dermatol.*, 120, 359, 2003.
196. Deguchi, M. et al., Proliferative activity of $CD8^+$ T cells as an important clue to analyze T cell-mediated inflammatory disorders, *Arch. Dermatol. Res.*, 293, 442, 2001.
197. Chen, S-H. et al., Response of keratinocytes from normal and psoriatic epidermis to interferon-γ differs in the expression of zinc-α2-glicoprotein and cathepsin D, *FASEB J.*, 14, 565, 2000.
198. Fierlbeck, G., Russner, G., and Muller, C., Psoriasis induced at the injection site of recombinant interferon-γ, results of immunohistologic investigation, *Arch. Dermatol.*, 126, 351, 1990.
199. Brown, D.W. et al., Skin $CD4^+$ T cells produce interferon-γ *in vitro* in response to streptococcal antigens in chronic plaque psoriasis, *J. Invest. Dermatol.*, 114, 576, 2000.
200. Wrone-Smith, T. and Nickoloff, B.J., Dermal injection of immunocytes induces psoriasis, *J. Clin. Invest.*, 98, 1878, 1996.
201. Cameron, A.L. et al., Natural killer and natural killer-T cells in psoriasis, *Arch. Dermatol. Res.*, 294, 363, 2002.
202. Aractingi, S. et al., HLA-G and NK receptors are expressed in psoriatic skin. A possible pathway for regulating infiltrating T cells? *Am. J. Pathol.*, 159, 71, 2001.
203. Bonish, B. et al., Overexpression of CD1d by keratinocytes in psoriasis and CD1d-dependent IFN-γ production by NK-T cells, *J. Immunol.*, 165, 4076, 2000.
204. Weltzien, H.U. et al., T cell immune responses to haptens. Structural models for allergic and autoimmune reactions, *Toxicology*, 107, 141, 1996.
205. Nalefski, E.A. and Rao, A., Nature of the ligand recognized by a hapten- and carrier-specific, MHC-restricted T cell receptor, *J. Immunol.*, 150, 3806, 1993.
206. Cavani, A. et al., Characterization of epitopes recognized by hapten-specific $CD4^+$ T cells, *J. Immunol.*, 154, 1232, 1995.
207. Kohler, J. et al., Carrier-independent hapten recognition and promiscuous MHC restriction by CD4 T cells induced by trinitrophenylated peptides, *J. Immunol.*, 158, 591, 1997.
208. Kalish, R.S., Wood, J.A., and LaPorte, A., Processing of urushiol (poison ivy) hapten by both endogenous and exogenous pathways for presentation to T cells *in vitro*, *J. Clin. Invest.*, 93, 2039, 1994.
209. Wulferink, M., Dierkes, S., and Gleichmann, E., Cross-sensitization to haptens: formation of common haptenic metabolites, T cell recognition of cryptic peptides, and true T cell cross-reactivity, *Eur. J. Immunol.*, 32, 1338, 2002.
210. Sieben, S. et al., Delayed-type hypersensitivity to paraphenylenediamine is mediated by 2 different pathways of antigen recognition by specific alphabeta human T-cell clones, *J. Allergy Clin. Immunol.*, 109, 1005, 2002.
211. Pichler, W.J., Pharmacological interaction of drugs with antigen-specific immune receptors: the p-i concept, *Curr. Opin. Allergy Clin. Immunol.*, 2, 301, 2002.
212. Gamerdinger, K. et al., A new type of metal recognition by human T cells: contact residues for peptide-independent bridging of T cell receptor and major histocompatibility complex by nickel, *J. Exp. Med.*, 197, 1345, 2003.
213. Cavani, A. et al., Effector and regulatory T cells in allergic contact dermatitis, *Trends Immunol.*, 22, 118, 2001.
214. Grabbe, S. and Schwarz, T., Immunoregulatory mechanisms involved in elicitation of allergic contact dermatitis, *Immunol. Today*, 19, 37, 1998.
215. Gocinski, B.L. et al., Roles of $CD4^+$ and $CD8^+$ cells in murine contact sensitivity revealed by *in vivo* monoclonal antibody depletion, *J. Immunol.*, 144, 4121, 1990.
216. Martin, S. et al., Peptide immunization indicates that $CD8^+$ T cells are the dominant effector cells in trinitrophenyl-specific contact hypersensitivity, *J. Invest. Dermatol.*, 115, 260, 2000.
217. Bour, H. et al., Major histocompatibility complex class I-restricted $CD8^+$ T cells and class II-restricted $CD4^+$ T cells, respectively, mediate and regulate contact sensitivity to dinitrofluorobenzene, *Eur. J. Immunol.*, 25, 3006, 1995.
218. Bouloc, A., Cavani, A., and Katz, S.I., Contact hypersensitivity in MHC class II-deficient mice depends on CD8 T lymphocytes primed by immunostimulating Langerhans cells, *J. Invest. Dermatol.*, 111, 44, 1998.

219. Wang, B. et al., CD4+ Th1 and CD8+ type 1 cytotoxic T cells both play a crucial role in the full development of contact hypersensitivity, *J. Immunol.*, 165, 6783, 2000.
220. Kapsenberg, M.L. et al., Th1 lymphokine production profiles of nickel-specific CD4+ T-lymphocyte clones from nickel contact allergic and non-allergic individuals, *J. Invest. Dermatol.*, 98, 59, 1992.
221. Xu, H., Dilulio, N.A., and Fairchild, R.L., T cell populations primed by hapten sensitization in contact sensitivity are distinguished by polarized patterns of cytokine production: interferon gamma-producing (Tc1) effector CD8+ T cells and interleukin (Il) 4/Il-10-producing (Th2) negative regulatory CD4+ T cells, *J. Exp. Med.*, 183, 1001, 1996.
222. Vollmer, J. et al., Dominance of the BV17 element in nickel-specific human T cell receptors relates with the severity of contact sensitivity, *Eur. J. Immunol.*, 27, 1865, 1997.
223. Büdinger, L. et al., Preferential usage of TCR-Vb17 by peripheral and cutaneous T cells in nickel-induced contact dermatitis, *J. Immunol.*, 167, 6038, 2001.
224. Grabbe, S. et al., Removal of the majority of epidermal Langerhans cells by topical or systemic steroid application enhances the effector phase of murine contact hypersensitivity, *J. Immunol.*, 155, 4207, 1995.
225. Kündig, T.M. et al., Fibroblasts as efficient antigen-presenting cells in lymphoid organs, *Science*, 268, 1343, 1995.
226. Ma, W. and Pober, J.S., Human endothelial cells effectively costimulate cytokine production by, but not differentiation of, naive CD4+ T cells, *J. Immunol.*, 161, 2158, 1998.
227. Nasorri, F. et al., Activation of nickel-specific CD4+ T lymphocytes in the absence of professional antigen-presenting cells, *J. Invest. Dermatol.*, 118, 172, 2002.
228. Albanesi, C. et al., Interleukin-17 is produced by both Th1 and Th2 lymphocytes, and modulates interferon-γ- and interleukin-4-induced activation of human keratinocytes, *J. Invest. Dermatol.*, 115, 81, 2000.
229. Teunnisen, M.B.M. et al., Interleukin-17 and interferon-γ synergize in the enhancement of proinflammatory cytokine production by human keratinocytes, *J. Invest. Dermatol.*, 111, 645, 1998.
230. Albanesi, C. et al., IL-4 enhances keratinocyte expression of CXCR3 agonistic chemokines, *J. Immunol.*, 165, 1395, 2000.
231. Sebastiani, S. et al., Nickel-specific CD4+ and CD8+ T cells display distinct migratory responses to chemokines produced during allergic contact dermatitis, *J. Invest. Dermatol.*, 118, 1052, 2002.
232. Kehren, J. et al., Cytotoxicity is mandatory for CD8+ T cell mediated contact hypersensitivity, *J. Exp. Med.*, 189, 779, 1999.
233. Yawalkar, N. et al., A comparative study of the expression of cytotoxic proteins in allergic contact dermatitis and psoriasis. Spongiotic skin lesions in allergic contact dermatitis are highly infiltrated by T cells expressing perforin and granzime B, *Am. J. Pathol.*, 158, 803, 2001.
234. Traidl, C. et al., Disparate cytotoxic activity of nickel-specific CD8+ and CD4+ T cell subsets against keratinocytes, *J. Immunol.*, 165, 3058, 2000.
235. Biederman, T. et al., Reversal of established delayed type hypersensitivity reactions following therapy with IL-4 or antigen-specific Th2 cells, *Eur. J. Immunol.*, 31, 1582, 2001.
236. Berg, D.J. et al., Interleukin 10 but not interleukin 4 is a natural suppressant of cutaneous inflammatory responses, *J. Exp. Med.*, 182, 99, 1995.
237. Traidl, C. et al., Inhibition of allergic contact dermatitis to DNCB but no to oxazolone in interleukin-4 deficient mice, *J. Invest. Dermatol.*, 112, 476, 1999.
238. Yokozeki, H. et al., Signal transducer and activator of transcription 6 is essential in the induction of contact hypersensitivity, *J. Exp. Med.*, 191, 995, 2000.
239. Sebastiani. S. et al., Chemokine receptor expression and function in CD4+ T lymphocytes with regulatory activity, *J. Immunol.*, 166, 996, 2001.
240. Iellem, A. et al., Unique chemotactic response profile and specific expression of chemokine receptors CCR4 and CCR8 by CD4(+)CD25(+) regulatory T cells, *J. Exp. Med.*,194, 847, 2001.

# 7 Langerhans Cells and Other Skin Dendritic Cells

*Marcel B.M. Teunissen*

## CONTENTS



## I. INTRODUCTION

Dendritic cells (DCs) comprise a family of professional antigen-presenting cells (APCs) having the unique capability to stimulate naive T cells, thereby generating protective specific immune responses against infections and cancer. In addition to this adaptive immunity, which is delayed in onset, DCs also participate in the more rapid innate immune response in that they react to invading dangers by immediately generating protecting or pro-inflammatory cytokines. DCs form a sparsely distributed population of leukocytes in most peripheral tissues, particularly at sites of interface with the environment, such as skin or mucosa. The DCs in the peripheral tissues are believed to be in an immature state, and like doorkeepers, attentive for unwanted guests. When DCs sense invaders

0-8493-1959-5/05/$0.00+$1.50

they display pathogen-specific gene expression profiles, indicating that they are able to discriminate different types of infectious insults (viruses, bacteria, and parasites). Upon perceiving and capturing pathogens DCs undergo a process of major phenotypical and functional differentiation, generally referred to as maturation, permitting them to initiate an appropriate type of T-cell response required to eliminate the danger. In recent years it became apparent that DCs are also involved in the induction of tolerance. DCs are part of the skin immune system.[1,2] Under nonpathologic circumstances the skin harbors two types of DCs, namely, the epidermal DCs, better known as Langerhans cells (LCs), and the dermal DCs. In contrast to the countless number of reports on LCs, the information on the dermal DCs is rather limited. In the case of inflammatory conditions of the skin, two other types of DCs appear in the skin, which are discussed in the last sections of this chapter.

Several outstanding reviews on DCs and LCs have been published[3–7] dealing with basic knowledge on their history, origin, ontogeny, morphology, phenotype, and distribution, and their roles in protective immunity and tolerance. To avoid exhaustive repetition on basic facts, this chapter focuses on human LC and DC types present in normal and diseased skin, but to begin with, general characteristics of DCs are described in brief. One should be aware that much of what is described about DCs is also applicable to LCs and the DCs in the dermis.

## II. DENDRITIC CELLS

### A. Origin and Distribution

DCs were discovered and described 30 years ago by Steinman and Cohn.[8,9] They observed in murine spleen cell suspensions a distinct population of low buoyant density, macrophage-like cells with a remarkable dendritic morphology, hence the name dendritic cell. Apart from the typical morphology, DCs could be discriminated from macrophages by means of some other characteristics. In contrast to macrophages, DCs did not firmly adhere to tissue culture surfaces, especially after overnight culture, enabling the isolation of DCs.[10] The DCs also differed from macrophages in that they have no or a very limited capacity for phagocytosis (this initial notion has been revised in later years, see one of the next paragraphs), possess a modest load of lysosomal enzymes, express low levels of Fc receptors, but very high and constitutive levels of major histocompatibility complex (MHC) class II molecules. Further, DCs appeared to be very powerful APC having the extraordinary capability to activate naive T cells in an antigen-specific way.[11] In this respect DCs play a key role in the initiation of primary immune responses, also known as the sensitization phase (discussed later in this chapter). On a per cell basis, DCs are also the most powerful APC and accessory cells for secondary T-cell responses and mitogen-induced T-cell responses.[12,13]

In the same period as the discovery of DCs, evidence was obtained that the *in vitro* defined DCs form the representation of interdigitating cells (IDCs) found *in situ* in the T-cell compartments of lymphoid tissues, such as spleen, lymph node, and Peyer's patch.[14] The term interdigitating was derived from the observation of a typical cell in the lymph node of the rabbit, having an irregularly shaped nucleus and a cell outline characterized by many protrusions and invaginations.[15] The close apposition of IDCs with T cells in the paracortical areas of lymph nodes and the periarterial lymphoid sheets in spleen is in good agreement with their presumed role as specialized APC to activate T cells. DCs not only reside in primary and secondary lymphoid organs, but are present in various other sites of the body as well, in particular in surface tissues such as skin or mucosa. In addition, DCs were identified in various organs, including heart, the portal area of liver and kidney, but not the brain.[16] DCs can also be isolated from peripheral blood (circulating DCs)[17,18] and from lymph (veiled cells).[19,20] In all organs DCs constitute a trace population of cells, approximately 1 to 2% of the total cell numbers. In the T-cell areas of lymphoid organs and in peripheral tissues, DCs form a network with their dendrites spanning almost the entire tissue.[14] In this way they have an ideal anatomic localization to encounter foreign products, but also to select T cells that are specific for the antigen presented by the DCs. From numerous experimental studies with rodents, using contact allergy as model, it became clear that DCs are a dynamic population of migratory cells, which are always on the move. DCs in the blood, veiled cells in the lymph vessels, and DCs in peripheral organs are related to each other and may be regarded as subsequent differentiation or maturation stages. It is currently believed that DCs originate from bone marrow progenitors, which migrate as precursor DCs via the bloodstream to the peripheral nonlymphoid tissues to become resident immature DCs that monitor the environment for danger signals. Then they traffic as veiled cells via the afferent lymphatics to the secondary lymphoid organs to end up as IDCs.

## B. Phenotype and Function

### 1. Endocytotic Activity

Expression of surface molecules on DCs is not steady state but alters along their lifetime when DCs migrate and mature and is consistent with their functional capacities, such as antigen uptake and processing and antigen presentation to T cells. Current knowledge on the phenotype and function of DCs is based on numerous reports on isolated tissue or circulating DCs, as well as on DCs generated *in vitro* from $CD14^+$ monocytes or $CD34^+$ hematopoietic stem cells, using granulocyte-macrophage colony-stimulating factor (GM-CSF) plus interleukin 4 (IL-4) or GM-CSF plus tumor necrosis factor (TNF)-$\alpha$ as differentiation factors, respectively. Although DCs were originally reported to have no phagocytosis activity (likely because a number of the initial experiments were done with mature DCs isolated from lymphoid tissue), we now know that immature DCs are greedy endocytotic,[21] whereas this capture activity is downregulated during maturation.[22,23] By means of macropinocytosis molecules rapidly enter DCs within macropinosomes, both in the fluid phase or attached to the membrane via surface receptors. Macropinosomes are formed from surface ruffles that fold back against the cell or against each other to enclose a vesicle.[24] As a result of macropinocytosis a large volume of fluid is internalized. DCs can dispose internalized fluid via recycling of macropinosomes to the membrane (directly or via the endocytic pathway) and/or via diffusion of water across membranes leading to membrane recycling to the cell surface via smaller vesicles or shrunken multivesicular bodies.[25]

Concerning the receptor-mediated uptake, DCs are equipped with an array of different types of receptor families. DCs express immunoglobulin and complement receptors, including IgG receptors Fc$\gamma$RI (CD64) and Fc$\gamma$RII (CD32),[26] high- and low-affinity IgE receptors Fc$\varepsilon$RI[27] and Fc$\varepsilon$RII (CD23),[28] IgA receptor Fc$\alpha$R (CD89),[29] complement receptors CD11b (trace expression) and CD11c to bind C3b,[30,31] and CD88 to bind C5a.[32] With help of these receptors DCs can bind pathogenic organisms or antigenic compounds that have been opsonized, i.e., covered up with antibodies or complement. Constitutive and conserved products of microbial origin (called pathogen-associated molecular patterns or PAMPs) are detected and bound by pattern recognition receptors (PRRs),[33] which can be present on the cell surface, in intracellular compartments, or secreted. The lipid-A portion of lipopolysaccharide (LPS) representing an invariant pattern in all Gram-negative bacteria, unmethylated CpG motifs of bacterial DNA, double-stranded viral RNA, and yeast zymosan are well-known examples of PAMPs. One group of PRRs comprises the so-called Toll-like receptors (TLRs).[33] There exist at least ten different TLRs and each individual TLR can recognize several, structurally unrelated ligands. Several TLRs can directly interact with the ligands, whereas some TLRs require accessory molecules for this recognition. Subsets of DCs appear to express different TLRs and as a consequence respond to different microbial agents.[34,35] Via receptors of the C-type lectin superfamily interaction takes place with sugar side chains of proteins in a calcium-dependent way using conserved carbohydrate recognition domains (CRDs).[36] Type I C-type lectins have extracellular N termini and multiple CRDs, while type II C-type lectins have cytoplasmatic N termini and one CRD or CRD-like domain.[37] Type I C-type lectins that can be found on DCs are the macrophage mannose receptor (CD206) and DEC-205 (CD205) having mannose binding activity.[38,39] DCs express several DC-associated type II C-type lectins including dectin-1,[40,41] dectin-2,[42] CLEC-1,[43] DC-SIGN,[44] DC-ASGPR,[45] DCIR,[46] DLEC,[47] BDCA-2,[48] and DCAL-1.[49] Some of the type II C-type lectins, such as DC-SIGN and DCAL-1 are not only involved in internalization of antigens, but also contribute to the potency with which DCs activate T cells.[44,49] Concerning the acquired immunodeficiency syndrome, expression of DC-SIGN is of particular interest because this DC-specific molecule is able to capture the HIV-1 envelope glycoprotein gp120 and facilitates transport of this virus to the secondary lymphoid organs, enhancing infection of T cells.[50]

Danger signals arise not only from exogenous compounds or invading microbes, but also from autologous necrotic cells, which release heat shock proteins (HSPs). HSP70, HSP90, and HSP96 all bind to CD91 present on DCs,[51,52] and HSP60 can bind to TLR4.[53] Autologous cells that die through programmed senescence (apoptosis) do not release HSP.[51] Clearance of apoptotic cells is important to prevent inflammation and tissue damage. Several cell surface receptors, present on DCs, have been implicated in the recognition of apoptotic cells. CD36 (thrombospondin receptor), αvβ3integrins, αvβ5-integrins,[54,55] but also other molecules such as lectins and CD91[56] are used by DCs to take up apoptotic material. Opsonization of apoptotic cells by complement and pentraxins may amplify the elimination of apoptotic cells.[57] The nucleotide adenosine is another example of a factor that is released in pathological conditions by many different cell types and that modulates DC function via adenosine receptors on these cells.[58] Adenosine promotes chemotaxis of immature DCs and inhibits the production of IL-12 in mature DCs. Finally, uric acid crystals (but not soluble uric acid) released by damaged cells have recently been put forward as a potent danger signal that activates DCs.[59]

## 2. Antigen Processing

Once ingested by DCs, the engulfed material (molecules, particles, cells, microbes) has to be accurately digested to enable DCs to present small antigenic fragments to T cells in a proper way (Figure 7.1). The exogenous material that is taken up by fluid-phase or receptor-mediated macropinocytosis enters the cell in the early endosomes (or phagosomes), which develop into the late acidic endosomes and finally mature into lysosomes.[60] Degradation of the ingested material takes place by proteolytic enzymes in the latter two compartments. This digestive mechanism in DCs is not abundant as in macrophages that have a well-developed scavenging pathway for complete digestion of substrates to amino acids in lysosomes. Upon digestion, small exogenous peptide fragments will be bound to the peptide-binding groove of MHC class II molecules. This loading of the MHC class II molecules occurs primarily within so-called MIICs (MHC class II-rich compartments), which comprises late endosomes and lysosomes.[60,61] The invariant chain (CD74), associated with newly synthesized MHC class II molecules in the endoplasmic reticulum (ER), protects the protein-binding groove from being prematurely filled with self-proteins and acts as a chaperone to direct these molecules to MIICs.[62,63] After partial proteolytic cleavage of this invariant chain in the MIIC, a small fragment called CLIP is left in the protein-binding groove, which is removed by the molecule HLA-DM allowing the exogenous peptide to take its place.[64] Finally, the MHC class II molecules (HLA-DR, HLA-DP, and HLA-DQ) are loaded with antigenic peptides and travel via exocytic vacuoles to the cell surface for display to CD4 helper T cells.

MHC class I molecules, constitutively expressed on virtually all nucleated cells, are used to display antigenic peptides to CD8 cytotoxic T cells. MHC class I (HLA-A, HLA-B, HLA-C, HLA-E, HLA-F, and HLA-G) molecules are heterodimers consisting of a polymorphic transmembrane heavy chain, which is noncovalently associated with a β2-microglobulin. The antigenic peptides, approximately ten amino acids in length, which bind in the groove of a MHC class I molecule are generated in the cytosol by degradation of cytosolic proteins (endogenous as well as virus derived or tumor specific) in proteasomes, the intracellular digestive machinery for the rapid elimination of highly abnormal (defective, incomplete, or misfolded) proteins.[65] Constitutive proteasomes are multi-subunit complexes distributed evenly throughout the cytoplasm and in the nucleus, but the composition, function, and distribution of the proteasomes is changed by interferon (IFN) leading

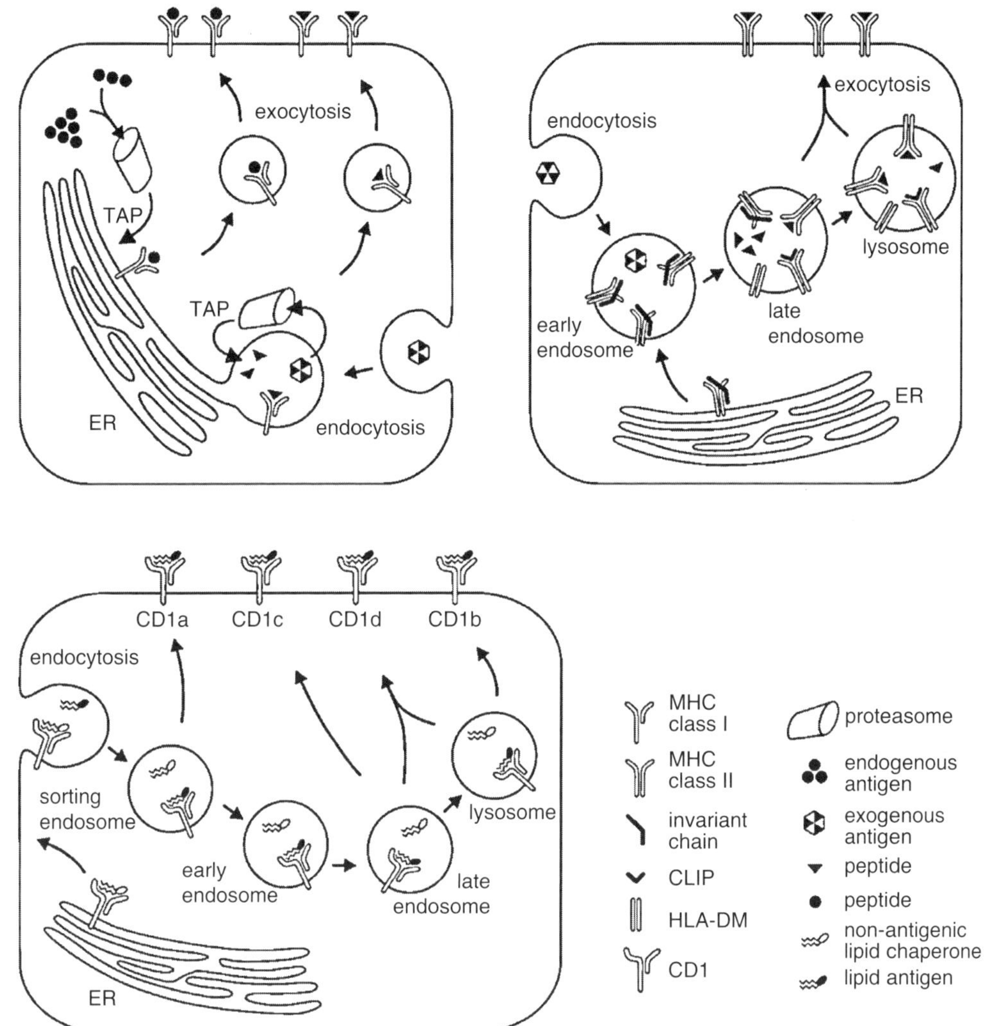


**FIGURE 7.1** Different forms of antigen-processing in DCs. The classical MHC class I pathway and cross-presentation pathway (both in the upper left scheme) and the MHC class II pathway (upper right scheme) are used to process and present peptides, whereas the CD1 pathway (lower left) is used to process and present lipids and glycolipids. Explanation of these figures is given in the text.

to the formation of immunoproteasomes, which are concentrated around the ER.[66,67] The assembly of MHC class I molecules with antigenic peptides takes place in the ER (Figure 7.1) and is a complex process in which several accessory or chaperone molecules are involved.[68–70] The short cytosolic peptides generated in the proteasome are translocated into the ER with help of the heterodimeric molecule TAP (transporter associated with antigen processing). Chaperone molecules calnexin and calreticulin aid in proper folding and stabilizing newly synthesized MHC class I heavy chains and β2 microglobulins in the ER and to retain this "empty" class I intermediates in the ER. Association of TAP with the stabilized class I loading complex, facilitated by the molecule tapasin, finally enables the cytosol-derived antigenic short peptides to bind to the groove of MHC class I molecules. The loaded MHC class I molecules exit the ER via an exocytotic pathway to the cell surface for display to CD8 T cells.

It was originally thought that the MHC class I pathway was only used to present endogenous (synthesized within the cell) peptides. However, DCs have the capacity to direct ingested exogenous antigens via the proteasome- and TAP-dependent pathway toward the binding groove of MHC class I for display to CD8 T cells (Figure 7.1), a process referred to as cross-presentation.[71–73] The resulting primary immune response is called cross-priming. Although peptides to be cross-presented may be degraded and regurgitated by neighboring cells (a proteasome- and TAP-independent pathway[74]), DCs themselves are fully sufficient to perform cross-priming.[75] The cross-presentation of phagocytosed antigens requires a retrotranslocation step of the antigen from the phagosome lumen to the cytoplasm.[76] Soon after or during formation, phagosomes fuse with the ER.[77] The exogenous peptides are degraded by proteasomes, which are associated to the phagosomes at the plasmatic side.[78] Subsequently, the peptide fragments are shuttled back into the lumen of the same phagosomes by a TAP-dependent mechanism enabling the exogenous antigenic fragments to load onto MHC class I molecules within the phagosomes.[77] The phagosome-mediated cross-presentation is a rapid process that takes place within the first few hours upon phagocytosis.[77]

In addition to these protein processing mechanisms, DCs possess intracellular pathways to process lipids and glycolipids of both exogenous and endogenous derivation, which subsequently are loaded in the binding groove of CD1 molecules for display to T cells.[79] In humans the existence of five different nonpolymorphic CD1 molecules, CD1a through CD1e, has been described.[80] Similar to MHC class I, CD1 heavy chains form heterodimeric complexes with β2-microglobulin in the ER using chaperones calnexin and calreticulin. Chaperone lipids block the CD1 groove, analogous to the function of the invariant chain in protecting the groove of MHC class II molecules. The newly synthesized CD1 molecules traffic to the cell surface first, and upon internalization they reach the endosomal compartments to become loaded. The different CD1 molecules are loaded with lipids or glycolipids in distinct compartments of the endocytic pathway (early endosomes, late endosomes, or MIIC)[79] and after recycling they appear on the cell surface again, enabling display of glycolipidic antigens to T cells (Figure 7.1). CD1a, CD1b, CD1c, CD1d, and/or CD1e may be variably present on the DC subsets. The expression can be dependent on the stage of maturation or induced in certain circumstances by environmental factors.[81,82] CD1 molecules may function as antigen-presenting molecules for particular populations of T cells.[83] For example, CD1a- and CD1c-restricted responses of $CD4^-CD8^-$ (double-negative) T-cell clones having αβ-T-cell receptors and CD1c-restricted responses of T-cell clones carrying γδ-T-cell receptors have been described. CD1b is involved in the presentation of mycobacterial-derived lipid antigen to double-negative T cells.[84]

Abundant expression of the cell surface receptors involved in the uptake of exogenous material and exhibition of an antigen-processing machinery in full operation are typical characteristics for immature DCs. During maturation, the expression of these receptors is downregulated and endocytosis activity is switched off.

## 3. Dendritic Cell — T-Cell Interaction

After completion of the maturation process DCs display on their cell surface antigen-loaded MHC class I, MHC class II, and CD1 molecules, which can be recognized by the T-cell antigen receptor of specific T cells. This antigen-specific signal, called "signal 1," on itself is not sufficient to drive activation of naive T cells. Additional triggering termed co-stimulation is required to accomplish full-blown activation. During maturation DCs have gained (upregulated or induced) strong expression on their cell surface of co-stimulatory molecules, which aid in adhesive DC–T-cell clustering and/or provide additional activation signals to the T cell. The interaction of co-stimulatory molecules on DCs with their respective ligands on T cells are referred to as "signal 2." The co-stimulatory molecules present on DCs that next will be mentioned may have an adhesive as well as signaling function. DCs express molecules ICAM-1 (CD54), ICAM-2 (CD102), and ICAM-3 (CD50),[85] which all are receptors for LFA-1 (CD11a) on T cells. Reciprocal interaction can occur as CD11a is also expressed by DCs and can bind to ICAMs on T cells. In addition, DC-SIGN on DCs interacts with ICAM-3 on T cells.[44] LFA-3 (CD58) on DCs can interact with CD2 on T cells.[86] B7-1 (CD80) and B7-2 (CD86) on DCs[87,88] bind to CD28 on naive T cells, which upon activation upregulate expression of CTLA-4 (CD152), being a stronger ligand for CD80 and CD86 and involved in downregulation of immune responses.[89] Other members of the B7 family found on DCs are B7RP-1 and B7-HI, having interaction with inducible immune co-stimulator (ICOS) and programmed cell death 1 (PD-1) receptors on T cells, respectively.[90,91] Of particular interest is the expression of co-stimulator CD40 on DCs, a member of the TNF ligand/receptor family that binds to CD154 on T cells.[92] Interaction between CD40 and CD154 not only stimulates T cells but retrograde signaling takes place as well, causing enhanced expression of CD80 and CD86 and production of cytokine IL-12 by DCs.[92,93]

As a result of stimulation, CD4 helper T cells and CD8 cytotoxic T cells start to proliferate and produce a cytokine cocktail to fulfill their effector function as controllers and directors of the immune response. On the basis of secreted cytokines T cells are roughly divided into two subtypes.[94,95] T cells that produce high levels of IFN-γ are called type 1, which promote cellular immunity by activating macrophages, cytotoxic T cells, and natural killer (NK) cells; whereas T cells that produce high levels of IL-4 are called type 2, which are responsible for strong antibody production, particularly IgE responses. To survive an infection, the character of the host T-cell response has to match the type of invading pathogen. For example, type 1 T-cell responses are important for protection against intracellular parasites, but the optimal reaction against metazoan parasites is provided by type 2 T cells.[94,95] The decision of naive T cells to produce preferentially either type 1 or type 2 cytokines is dependent on signals they receive from the DCs at the moment of activation. These polarizing signals are commonly referred to as "signal 3." It should be noted that immune responses to infections generally comprise involvement of both type 1 and type 2 T cells. During their sentinel phase in the peripheral tissues immature DCs are directly affected by invading microbes they encounter[96] or receive danger signals from pathogen-affected surrounding tissue.[97,98] These experiences of the immature DCs ultimately determine the phenotype and function of these cells upon maturation as well as the nature of polarizing signals transferred to the naive T cells.[99] This signal 3 is heterogeneous and can be mediated by cytokines or membrane-bound molecules. The most powerful inducer of type 1 T-cell responses is IL-12.[100] Other type 1-polarizing molecules are IL-18,[101] IL-23,[102] IL-27,[103] and IFN-α.[104] The last cytokine is a typical product of the plasmacytoid DC subset.[105] DCs which are made IL-12 deficient as a result of $PGE_2$[106] or IL-10[107] treatment promote the development of type 2 T cells. IL-3,[108] IL-11,[109] and IL-25,[110] as well as keratinocyte-derived TSLP[111] have been described to enhance type 2 T cell responses. Interaction of co-stimulatory molecule ICAM-1 on DCs with its ligand LFA-1 on the T cell may favor type 1 development,[112] whereas interaction of co-stimulatory molecule OX40 ligand with its receptor OX40 (CD134) promote type 2 T cells,[113] indicating that some overlap exists between signal 2 and signal 3. Recently, expression of indoleamine-2,3-dioxygenase (IDO) activity by DCs has been put forward as an alternative mechanism to regulate T-cell responses.[114–116] This enzyme causes local degradation of the essential amino acid tryptophan into several metabolites, collectively known as kynurenines. Tryptophan deprivation or exposure to kynurenines can induce apoptosis of terminally differentiated antigen-specific T cells.[117,118] DCs are distinct in their expression of IDO activity. IDO can strongly be induced by IFN-γ plus CD40 ligation, rendering type 1 T cells more susceptible to the IDO-dependent apoptosis.

A close physical contact between T cells and DCs is needed to enable T cells to recognize antigen. This specialized junction between a T cell and an APC is called the immunological synapse, and consists of a central cluster of T-cell receptors surrounded by a ring of adhesion molecules.[119] The amount of signals that a T cell will receive is dependent on the stability of the synapse, the duration of T-cell receptor engagement, the level of antigen-MHC complex, the level and type of co-stimulatory molecules that amplify the activation process, the maturation stage of the DC, and the T cell's maturation stage.[119,120] Only in case of inflammation or upon recognition of pathogens in the peripheral tissue, the immature DCs will transform into strong stimulatory APCs, having high levels of MHC and co-stimulatory molecules, being susceptible to booster-signals from T cells, and able to elicit vigorous triggering of T cells. Under nonpathologic steady-state conditions, however, DCs are supposed not to reach full maturation[121] and, instead of inducing immunity, these partially mature DCs rather induce tolerance of naive T cells specific for self-antigen, by means of promoting anergy or deletion, or alternatively, promoting differentiation of T cells into so-called regulatory T cells, which are hyporesponsive to activation but able to suppress conventional T cells either via cell contact or via IL-10 or TGF-β.[122–124] The immunosuppressive state achieved by these regulatory T cells is called peripheral tolerance.

#### 4. Dendritic Cell–Associated Molecules

A specific unique marker for all DCs, irrespective their stage of maturation, is still lacking. Nevertheless, many DC-associated molecules have been identified. CD83 is generally accepted as one of the best markers for mature DCs.[125] Although the exact role is not clear yet, CD83 seems to promote the activation of T cells during DC–T-cell interaction.[126] Two other molecules, CMRF-44 and CMRF-56 have been described to be useful markers for mature activated DCs,[127,128] having distribution and kinetics overlaps with that of CD83. The aforementioned C-type lectins DEC-205 (CD205), dectin-1, dectin-2, CLEC-1, DC-SIGN, DCIR, DLEC, DCAL-1 have a strong association with immature DCs and are involved in the receptor-mediated uptake of antigen. The four blood DC antigens BDCA-1 (identical to CD1c), BDCA-2 (identical to the lectin DLEC), BDCA-3, and BDCA-4 (identical to neuropilin-1, a receptor for vascular endothelial growth factor) represent a set of DC markers for subpopulations of DCs.[129] BDCA-2 and BDCA-4 are typical cell surface markers for freshly isolated blood plasmacytoid, but not myeloid, DCs.[48,129] However, BDCA-2 expression is lost during culture, whereas BDCA-4 appears on myeloid DCs as well.[129] In addition, BDCA-3 expression, which is present on a subset of freshly isolated blood myeloid DCs, is upregulated on both plasmacytoid and myeloid DCs during culture.[129] The antibody M-DC8 recognizes a cell surface protein of a subpopulation of circulating DCs.[130] The DC-related molecule DC-LAMP (CD208) is a lysosomal associated glycoprotein, which may be involved in the mechanism of antigen processing.[131] The p55 or fascin protein is a DC-related actin-bundling protein having a function in the motility of these cells.[132] DC-CK1 (CCL18) is a C-C chemokine that is abundantly produced by DCs in secondary lymphoid organs and preferentially attracts naive CD4 and CD8 T cells.[133] High production of chemokines MDC (CCL22) and TARC (CCL17) enables DCs to attract memory T cells.[134,135] DC-STAMP is another DC-associated molecule, having an as yet unknown function and that is downregulated upon CD40 ligation.[136] The use of highly sophisticated technologies such as serial analysis of gene expression (SAGE), cDNA microarray, and proteomics, will certainly lead to the generation of more DC-associated or even DC-specific molecules in the next few years.[137,138]

### C. Ontogeny and Subpopulations

In the last few years, it became evident that DCs represent a heterogeneous population of cells. Distinct DC subsets have been demonstrated in blood,[129,139,140] lymphoid, and nonlymphoid tissues in both humans and mice.[141–143] The DC family displays much plasticity as different DC subsets can be generated from the same precursor and different types of progenitor cells can give rise to similar subsets of DCs. The exact interrelationship between these DC subsets, their lineage of origin, their intermediate stages of differentiation, their requirements of different growth factors, and their overall function still needs clarification. According to the current general opinion, essentially three lineages or types of DC can be distinguished in humans.[3,5,144,145] The first type of DC develops from myeloid precursors and can be found in the epithelial layer of the skin and mucosa, having LCs as the prototypes of this lineage. The second type of DC, referred to as interstitial DC, is also of myeloid origin and inhabits connective tissue in most organs (often localized in perivascular region), being represented by the population of dermal DCs. A separate third type of DCs

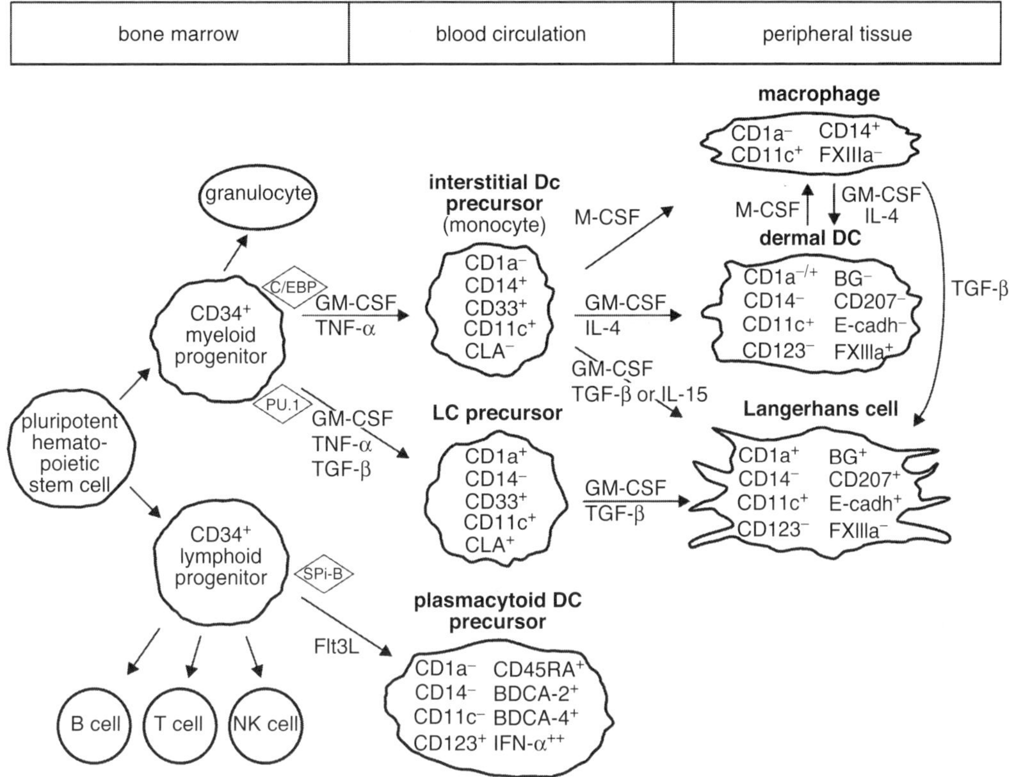


**FIGURE 7.2** Ontogeny of human myeloid and plasmacytoid DC subsets from CD34⁺ progenitors. This scheme summarizes data on DC development from both CD34⁺ stem cells and from CD14⁺ blood monocytes. To be able to connect both experimental systems, the CD14⁺ interstitial DC precursor derived from the CD34⁺ progenitors is arbitrarily made equivalent to CD14⁺ blood monocytes. The diverse populations of blood DCs, as well as the transition of the immature into the mature state, are kept out this figure to make this figure less complicated. Only essential growth factors (adjacent to arrows), characteristic markers (within cells), and crucial transcription factors (within diamonds) are depicted in this flowchart. For additional details and explanation of abbreviations, see text.

arises from lymphoid progenitors and is called plasmacytoid DC, because at the ultrastructural level they resemble plasma cells (i.e., immunoglobulin secreting B cells). A simplified summary of the relationship between the different DC subsets is given in Figure 7.2 and is explained in the text below.

*In vitro* studies indicate that all DC lineages are derived from multipotential CD34⁺ hematopoietic stem cells and that early in the ontogeny a differentiation takes place into common myeloid progenitors and common lymphoid progenitors. The CD34⁺ progenitors can be derived from human bone marrow,[146] cord blood,[147] peripheral blood,[148,149] and thymus,[150] and under certain culture conditions the myeloid or lymphoid DC differentiation pathways can be induced. As concerns the CD34⁺ myeloid DC progenitors, two separate pathways of development from these cells have been reported.[151,152] In CD34⁺ progenitor cultures monocytic CD14⁺CD1a⁻ cells coexist with CD14⁻CD1a⁺ cells, which have restricted DC differentiation potential. When these two types of precursor cells were isolated and placed in subsequent cultures in the presence of GM-CSF and TNF-α, it appeared that both subsets mature into DCs.[151] The CD14⁺ precurors, but not the CD1a⁺ precursors, can be induced to differentiate, in response to M-CSF, into monocyte/macrophage-like cells. Remarkably, the CD1a⁺ precursors give rise to cells with LC characteristics, such as Birbeck granules (BGs), Lag antigen, and E-cadherin, whereas the CD14⁺ precursors differentiate into

CD1a⁺CD14⁻ DCs lacking LC markers but expressing characteristics of dermal DCs, such as coagulation factor XIIIa. The presence of both cytokines GM-CSF and TNF-α in these cultures appeared to be essential for the generation of DCs, but in later studies it was demonstrated that addition of c-kit-ligand or stem cell factor improved the yield of cells without altering cell differentiation,[153,154] and that addition of Flt3 ligand substantially promotes the selective development of DCs from CD34⁺ progenitors[155,156] along both the myeloid and lymphoid developmental pathways.[157] Addition of IL-4 to GM-CSF plus TNF-α supplemented cultures increases the expression of CD1a, while it reduces the expression of CD14.[158,159] Cultures of CD34⁺ progenitor cells are commonly set up with serum-containing medium and it is worthy of note that transforming growth factor-beta 1 (TGF-β1) is a regular component of serum. In case the CD34⁺ progenitors are cultured under serum-free conditions in the presence of survival factor GM-CSF plus TNF-α and stem cell factor, supplementation with TGF-β1 appeared to be not only an essential requirement but also boosts the outgrowth of CD1a⁺ DCs, especially if Flt3 ligand is present as well.[156,160] This enhanced proliferation of CD1a⁺ DCs (up to 64% of the cultured cells) due to the presence of TGF-β1 may be explained by the capacity of this cytokine to protect the DC progenitor cells from apoptosis.[161] Interestingly, approximately one fifth of the DC colonies, generated from single cell cultures of the progenitor cells set up in the presence of TGF-β1, does express the LC-specific marker Lag.[156] In connection to this, it is important to mention that TGF-β1-deficient mice are devoid of epidermal LCs,[162] indicating that this cytokine is a prerequisite for the development of LCs. It has recently been shown that the presence of TNF-α is only important during the first few days of differentiation, when LCs are generated from CD34⁺ progenitors in medium containing GM-CSF, TNF-α, and TGF-β1.[163] Withdrawal of TNF-α after the fifth day of differentiation favors the outgrowth of a highly enriched immature LC population (up to 80%), as characterized by delayed or abrogated expression of CD83, CD86, HLA-DR, and CD208, less efficient capacity to stimulate allogeneic T cells, and retained endocytosis capacity. Presence of TNF-α beyond day 5 would result in a LC population with a higher degree of maturation, indicating that this cytokine acts as a maturation factor. Both GM-CSF and TGF-β appear to be essential for development of LCs. If GM-CSF is replaced by IL-3 in the progenitor cultures, LC-like cells will develop that have a poor expression of Langerin and lack BGs.[164]

Transcription factors seem to play a role in the mechanism controlling the diversification of the pluripotent hematopoietic stem cells into the different myeloid and lymphoid progenitor and precursor cells. Transcription factor PU.1 has been reported to promote LC development from myeloid progenitor cells, whereas factor C/EBP promotes granulocytic differentiation and inhibits PU.1-induced LC commitment, indicating a functional balance between PU.1 and C/EBP.[165] Transcription factor Spi-B is essential for the development of human plasmacytoid DCs, while it impairs T-cell and NK cell development from lymphoid progenitors.[166] IFN consensus sequence binding protein (ICSBP) is another essential transcription factor for plasmacytoid DC (pDC) development, as demonstrated by the lack of these cells in ICSBP-deficient mice.[167] Other studies in mice show that transcription factor STAT3 is required for Flt3 ligand-dependent DC development.[168]

At a certain stage in their development *in vivo* the DC progenitors will leave the bone marrow and enter the bloodstream. Several studies have been performed to determine the various subsets of DCs and DC precursors in peripheral blood. In many of those studies analysis was performed on selected subpopulations of blood leukocytes that lack lineage markers (i.e., CD3 for T cells, CD19 or CD20 for B cells, CD16 or CD56 for NK cells, and CD14 for monocytes) but express high levels of MHC class II molecules. However, interlaboratory variations in the cocktails of lineage antibodies and purification techniques likely resulted in DC preparations with different compositions. Further, fractionation of DCs into different subsets was based on various markers, such as CD11c,[139] CD1a[169] (take notice that the antibody used in this study has been redefined and was shown to recognize CD1b/c rather than CD1a[140]), CD2,[170,171] CD33,[30,172] CD68,[173] CD123,[172] or BDCA-2, -3, and -4,[129] and the panel of monoclonal antibodies to define the individual DC subsets did not overlap, making comparison of these studies difficult. Moreover, evidence suggests that some DC subsets may express lineage markers CD14[30] or CD16,[130,140] whereas traditionally CD14+ and CD16+ cells were excluded from the DC preparations and analysis in most studies. Finally, many of the markers studied are not constitutively expressed by DCs and the levels of expression vary along the process of differentiation from DC precursors via the immature intermediates to mature DCs. In the population of immature blood DCs (defined as CD34−Lineage−HLA-DR+CD4+CD83−CD80−), a distinction can be made between myeloid DCs (CD11c+ CD33+CD68$^{low}$CD123$^{-\text{ or low}}$) and plasmacytoid DCs (CD11c−CD33−CD68$^{hi}$CD123$^{hi}$). The latter population is identical to the natural IFN-α/β-producing cells, which rapidly produce huge amounts of IFN-α/β in response to viral infection.[105] The former population can be subdivided into at least two but perhaps more non-overlapping subsets on the basis of CD2, CD1b/c, CD16, and BDCA-3 expression.[140,169,170] In one study it was claimed that the CD1a+ (later redefined as CD1a−CD1b/c+) DC subset is a direct precursor of LC, because these cells acquire LC characteristics (Lag expression, BGs) upon culture in the presence of GM-CSF, IL-4, and TGF-β.[169] Except for the CD16+ DC subset, all immature blood DCs express to different degrees the skin-homing receptor cutaneous lymphocyte-associated antigen (CLA), indicating that in principle those cells are capable of entering the skin. Even at an earlier stage in the ontogeny a proportion of the CD34+ DC progenitors already show commitment to epithelial tissues, because these cells express CLA.[174] Upon culture *in vitro*, only the CLA+ subset of these CD34+ cells, but not the CD34+CLA− subset, could give rise to LC-like cells as determined by the expression of Lag molecules. As the next step in their development, the different immature myeloid and lymphoid DC subsets will enter the lymphoid or nonlymphoid tissues and indeed these different DC subsets can be observed in the thymus[175] and tonsils.[176] However, in normal human skin under nonpathologic conditions only myeloid-type DCs, but no lymphoid-type DCs can be appreciated.[177]

A giant step forward in DC research was the observation that DCs could be generated from CD14+ peripheral blood monocytes under special culture conditions.[178,179] The presence of GM-CSF is the critical factor to induce CD1a expression,[180] whereas addition of IL-4 is responsible for the loss of CD14 expression.[181] The technique to generate large numbers of immature (CD1a+CD14−CD83−) myeloid DCs *in vitro*, using a 5- to 7-day culture of monocytes in medium supplemented with the combination of GM-CSF and IL-4, was established 10 years ago[182,183] and has been improved since with special regard to clinical applicability.[184,185] These GM-CSF- and IL-4-treated immature CD1a+CD14− DCs are not stable, however, and after removal of the cytokines they will lose their dendritic morphology and become adherent CD1a−CD14+ macrophages. Replacing these macrophages in GM-CSF plus IL-4 converts the cells back to CD1a+CD14− DCs.[186] The immature CD1a+CD14−CD83− monocyte-derived DCs need an additional 2- to 3-day culture with maturating factors, such as LPS, TNF-α, or CD40 ligand, to become stable DCs, expressing the maturation marker CD83. Whereas immature monocyte-derived DCs can transform into macrophages, mature CD83+ monocyte-derived DCs are no longer able to switch, even in the presence of M-CSF.[186] Interestingly, if TGF-β1 is present as well in GM-CSF plus IL-4-treated monocyte cultures, the development of immature LC-like DCs is promoted, having expression of E-cadherin, CLA, BGs, and Lag.[187] In addition, DCs with LC characteristics are also yielded when monocytes are transformed into immature DCs first, and subsequently are treated with the same cytokine triplet. Recently, an alternative approach has been developed to skew monocytes into DCs with features of LCs.[188] Monocytes cultured with GM-CSF and IL-15 also differentiate into immature CD1a+CD14−CD83− DCs, which display E-cadherin and Langerin.

*In vivo* monocytes continuously emigrate from the blood into peripheral tissues, a process called diapedese. To mimic this, an *in vitro* model was set up, in which monocytes were cultured on a monolayer of endothelial cells grown on an endotoxin-free matrix.[189] During 2 days of culture half of the monocytes that transmigrated the endothelial layer were able to reverse transmigrate across the overlying intact endothelium, a migratory process that is reminiscent of the movement of cells from tissues into lymphatic vessels. When phagocytic particles were added to this system, but not in the absence of additional stimuli, about half of the reverse transmigrated cells exhibited features of mature DCs, like expression of CD83, actin-bundling protein p55, and DC-LAMP, but not CD1a.[189] In another model, monocytes are cocultured with fibroblasts to mimic the situation of monocytes that are diapedesed into tissue.[190] Under steady-state conditions fibroblasts direct monocyte differentiation toward macrophages in an M-CSF-dependent fashion, but in case TNF-$\alpha$ is added as a danger signal to simulate a situation of tissue inflammation, CD1a$^+$CD14$^-$ DCs are generated instead, likely due to downregulation of M-CSF receptors. In a different recent study, it is demonstrated that a population of migratory dermal-resident CD1a$^-$CD14$^+$ cells represent a pool of LC precursors, because these cells have the capacity to differentiate into LCs when cultured in the presence of GM-CSF, IL-4 plus TGF-$\beta$.[191] These three examples indicate that CD14$^+$ tissue macrophages presumably serve as an important source for LCs or DCs in case of tissue injury, inflammation, or pathogen invasion.

Concerning the function of the various DC subpopulations, two fundamentally different views have emerged.[3,99,144,145,192] Some investigators favor the hypothesis that each of the separate DC subsets does have distinct immunoregulatory roles, whereas others believe that all that primarily matters for the function of DCs is the environmental influence during their development and the state of maturation, irrespective of origin or subtype.

# III. EPIDERMAL LANGERHANS CELLS

## A. Phenotype of Langerhans Cells

### 1. Definition, Localization, and Distribution

LCs form a special subpopulation of DCs that reside in the stratified squamous epithelia of mammals, e.g., the epidermis and appendages of the skin and in mucosa.[193] The cells are named after Paul Langerhans, who discovered the cells in 1868[194] and considered these dendritic shaped cells to be of neural origin because of their reactivity with gold salts. The absolute feature to designate a cell as LC is the presence of typical and unique intracellular organelles, termed Birbeck granules (BGs),[195] which are rod-shaped structures with a central zipper-like striation and can only be observed by electron microscopy. More information on BGs is presented in following sections. Further observation by electron microscopy reveals that LCs have a lobulated nucleus and clear cytoplasm containing microtubules, microfilaments, lysosomes, and mitochondria, but lacking tonofilaments and desmosomes. BGs can also be observed in so-called veiled cells present in lymph vessels and in IDC present in thymus and lymph nodes, suggesting a relationship with LCs.[196] LCs can also be visualized at light microscopic level in cryostat sections, epidermal sheets, and epidermal cell suspensions by means of immunohistochemical techniques using one of the two unique monoclonal antibodies recognizing molecules Lag[197] and Langerin (CD207),[198] respectively. Lag is a 40-kDa glycoprotein that is located in the membranes of BGs and Langerin is a type II C-type lectin that is present on the cell surface of LCs and involved in the formation of BGs.[199] Thus, both Lag and Langerin are associated to the BG and therefore they are LC specific. Other useful (although not unique for LCs) markers to identify LCs *in situ* are MHC class II[200,201] and CD1a.[202,203] Within normal human epidermis LCs are the only cells expressing these markers, but in case of skin disease, however, MHC class II is not a reliable LC marker, because keratinocytes are induced to express MHC class II (HLA-DR) molecules as well.[204] The demonstration of membrane-bound enzyme adenosine triphosphatase (ATPase) is another way to visualize selectively LCs in the skin.[205] It has recently been demonstrated in mice that CD39 is responsible for this LC-associated ecto-enzymatic activity and that CD39 is expressed exclusively by LCs in the epidermal compartment.[206] This membrane ATPase on LCs provides protection against the permeabilizing/lytic effects of extracellular ATP, a ubiquitous molecule found within all cells and released following cell membrane damage or secreted in a regulated manner by several cell types.[207]

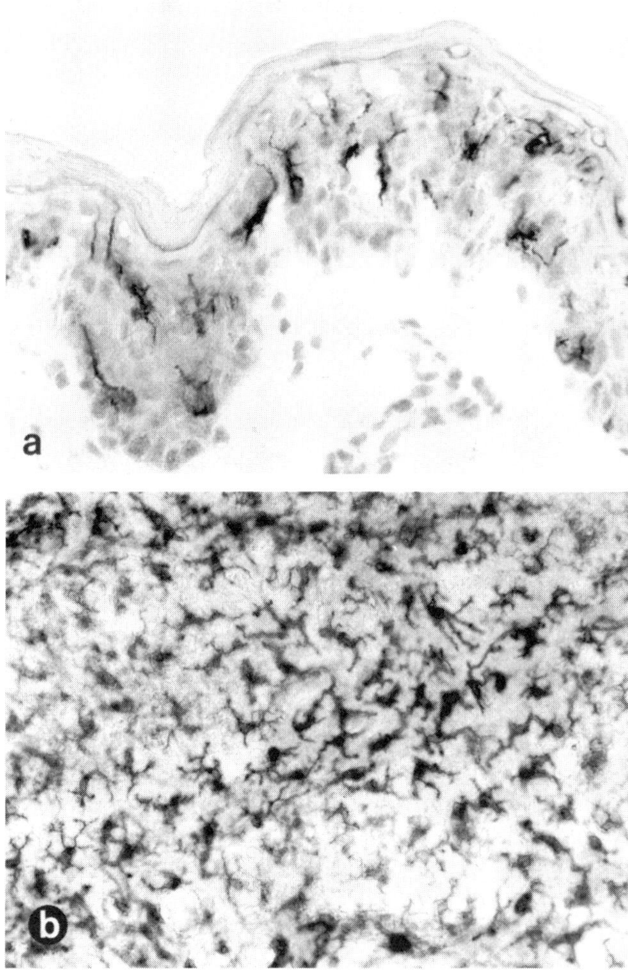

**FIGURE 7.3** Localization of human LCs, stained with an antibody against CD1a, in a transversal section of epidermal skin (a) and in an epidermal sheet after trypsinization (b). With their long protrusions, LCs form a tight network spanning the epidermis.

The dendritic shaped LCs are predominantly located at the suprabasal level of the epidermis as shown in vertical skin sections of normal human skin (Figure 7.3). Keeping in mind that DCs are migratory cells, it is not surprising to see occasional LCs at basal level or even in the dermis as well. Their dendritic shape is best appreciated in epidermal sheet preparations, giving the impression that these cells form a regular, almost interconnected network with their protrusions (Figure 7.3). In sum, LCs can be defined as cutaneous DCs, which express BGs, Lag, and CD207, as well as CD1a and HLA-DR. The "classical" LCs, of course, are found in the epidermis. LCs in the dermis may represent cells that have emigrated upon capturing antigen in the epidermis and are on their way to the lymph node. Lag and CD207 are the easiest and most reliable markers to identify LCs in normal and diseased skin. DCs in other anatomical locations or DCs cultured under certain circumstances, which express BGs, Lag, or CD207, can be designated as LC related. The antibodies against Lag or CD207 are very useful to detect LC-related cells in parts of the body other than skin, even at unexpected places, such as the wall of an atherosclerotic aorta.[208]

Concerning the ontology of LCs, the bone marrow origin has been established,[209] but it is not exactly known what happens between the emigration from bone marrow and their arrival in the skin. Presumed LC precursors, expressing CD1a$^+$, are present at a very low percentage (<1%) in normal peripheral blood,[169,210] but these cells lack BGs. LCs may also develop from peripheral blood monocytes, at least under *in vitro* conditions,[187,188] forming a much larger pool of LC precursors. It is not inconceivable that factor(s) in the epidermal environment are essential for the appearance of BGs and the expression of Lag and CD207. As described in one of the previous sections, these factors may include GM-CSF, TNF-$\alpha$, and in particular TGF-$\beta$ and IL-15, although it is not unlikely that other keratinocyte-derived factors are involved as well. Any role for IL-4 in the generation of LCs *in vivo* seems not likely, because the necessary, relatively high concentrations of IL-4 are neither physiological nor can be found in healthy epidermis.

Multiple studies have focused on the quantification of epidermal LCs yielding a remarkable variety of results.[211–217] This is probably due to differences in the staining technique, the LC marker used, the enumeration method applied (cells per area unit vs. cells per length of basement membrane; how to count LCs that bisect the edge of a calibrated grid; two-dimensional vs. three-dimensional quantification), the use of either vertical sections or epidermal sheets, the origin of the skin specimen (either sun exposed or not), the consideration that tissue may shrink, the age of the skin donor, and certainly some more differences. From all of these studies it can be concluded that (1) LCs constitute approximately 2% of the total epidermal cell population in normal healthy skin; (2) a wide interindividual variation exists for the number of LCs per $mm^2$; (3) on the average there are 1000 to 1200 LCs/$mm^2$ in normal adult human skin; and (4) the density of LCs may vary at different anatomical regions, being the highest in the face and neck and the lowest in the foot sole. In a recent study,[216] in which confocal laser scanning microscopy has been applied to determine LC numbers in epidermal sheets from breast skin and relating these numbers to epidermal nuclei per volume unit, it became clear that a strikingly constant ratio of 1 to 53 exists between LCs and other epidermal cells, irrespective the large interindividual differences. One LC can cover an average area of 554 to 1096 $\mu m^2$ thanks to their dendrites.[216] An adult individual may possess not fewer than 1 billion epidermal LCs, which have an estimated mean stay of 3 weeks in the epidermis.[1] LCs are mobile in nature and continuously leave the epidermis at a low rate and can be detected in the afferent lymph derived from human skin.[218] Local inflammation markedly upregulates the emigration rate (see Section III.B) There is a general belief that LCs are replenished by blood-borne LC precursors. In addition to this concept of repopulation by circulating LC precursors, some investigators indicate alternatively that the population of LCs in the epidermis may be maintained by replication of the LCs themselves.[219–224] Support for this latter concept comes from a recent study,[225] in which it is demonstrated that in lethally X-ray-irradiated mice that had received congenic bone marrow transplants, the LC population of host origin remains stable for at least 18 months, whereas the DC populations in other organs were almost completely replaced by donor cells within 2 months. However, in the case of skin inflammation induced by ultraviolet (UV) radiation, the host LC population disappears and is replaced by circulating donor LC precursors within 2 weeks.[225] In addition, in pairs of parabiotic congenic nonirradiated mice that share a single blood circulation, no mixing of LC populations is detectable after parabiosis maintained for at least 6 months.[225] The results of this study suggest that under steady-state conditions LCs are not replaced by circulating precursors and that the turnover rate of LCs or LC precursors present in the skin is apparently sufficient to keep up LC numbers. In case of inflammatory conditions in the skin, however, this self-reproducing capacity is not sufficient to replenish the enhanced LC emigration, making repopulation by circulating LC precursors necessary.[225]

## 2. Immature Langerhans Cells

To obtain a more detailed description of the phenotype of epidermal LCs, well-defined monoclonal antibodies were applied to stain cryostat skin sections, epidermal sheets, or single cell suspensions obtained after trypsinization of the epidermis. The technique of staining cell suspensions with two or more different fluorescent-labeled antibodies and analyzing these cells by flow cytofluorometry (FACS analysis) is the most sensitive way to determine the presence or absence of a particular marker in a quantitative fashion. However, this technique requires trypsin treatment of the epidermis to obtain single cells, inevitably leading to the loss of trypsin-sensitive markers. Analysis of cryostat sections circumvents this problem and allows one to determine the location of the stained cells in the epidermis and dermis as well. The phenotype of immature human epidermal LCs, as shown in Table 7.1, is the result of a great number of studies performed in many different laboratories. This table contains data yielded by FACS analysis, by immunohistochemistry on skin cryostat sections, epidermal sheets, or cytospins, as well as by reverse transcriptase-polymerase chain reaction (RT-PCR) analysis.

It is generally accepted that resident epidermal LCs represent a population of DCs that are in an immature state. In line with this, LCs do not express DC activation markers CD83 and CMRF-44.[226] The myeloid markers CD14 and CD33 are absent and weakly present on LCs, respectively.[227] Several studies have shown that LCs, like all DCs, express MHC class I molecules,[228,229] composed of a polymorphic heavy chain and the nonpolymorphic β2-microglobulin chain. The latter chain is shared with the group of CD1 molecules that have a structural relationship with MHC class I. The fact that CD1 molecules are nonpolymorphic and coded by chromosome 1 disputes that CD1 are MHC proteins, which are polymorphic and coded by chromosome 6.[80] The CD1 family is subdivided in group 1 (including CD1a, CD1b, CD1c, and CD1e), which are involved in lipid and glycolipid antigen presentation to cytotoxic T cells, and group 2 (including only CD1d), which participate in the activation of NK killer T cells.[79,230] LCs have a strong expression of CD1a and a weak expression of CD1c,[81,231] whereas CD1b and CD1d are not detectable on LCs *in situ* and in cell suspensions.[81,232] Antibodies against CD1e are not available yet. The expression of CD1a is limited to compartments that are dominated by ectodermal epidermal cells as stromal cells (e.g., the epidermis and the thymus cortex) suggesting a critical role for these epidermal cells in the expression of CD1a. *In vitro* culture experiments showed that CD1a expression is enhanced by IL-1 and suppressed by an IL-1 inhibitor.[233] CD1a expression can also be induced by GM-CSF.[180] Both cytokines can be produced by keratinocytes in the epidermis and it remains to be established whether the induction of expression of CD1a may be upregulated by other keratinocyte-derived proteins as well. Recently, formal proof for CD1a-restricted lipid antigen presentation to specific T cells by human epidermal LCs has been published.[234] LCs have a constitutive and strong expression of MHC class II molecules HLA-DR, HLA-DP, and HLA-DQ molecules.[235] Immunoelectron microscopy studies revealed that most of the MHC class II molecules in resident LCs *in situ* are intracellularly localized, in particular in the ER and the MIICs, and that the cell surface MHC class II molecules are predominantly displayed on the dendrites, but not on the cell body.[236,237] Freshly isolated LCs, however, have an even and strong expression on their entire cell surface.[237] The invariant chain (CD74), which associates with newly synthesized MHC class II molecules to prevent premature binding of endogenous antigens and to guide these molecules to MIICs where exogenous antigen is met, is also expressed by LCs.[236,238] In addition, epidermal LCs express HLA-DM,[239] which removes CLIP from the MHC class II molecules, allowing antigenic peptides to take place in the binding groove. LCs have slight and variable expression of RFD1, an HLA-DQ-like determinant with unknown function, which is associated with IDCs.[240] A small fraction of LCs express more brightly HLA-DR and RFD1: approximately 5 to 10% in epidermal sheets[227] and 25% in epidermal cell suspensions.[241] This small fraction of HLA-DR$^{high}$ resident LCs appeared to display receptors for C5a (CD88), which are functionally involved in the migratory properties of these cells.[32] Whereas resident epidermal LCs are considered to be immature DCs, this HLA-DR$^{high}$ LC fraction likely represents that part of the LCs that has switched on their maturation process and is about to leave the epidermis. In addition to the MHC molecules, LCs also have a functional expression of minor histocompatibility antigens, which might play a role in the graft-vs.-host disease in HLA-matched transplantation.[242]

As would be expected of immature DCs, epidermal LCs display an array of different receptors that facilitate the endocytotic activity. Isolated LCs bear low levels of FcγRII (CD32) and CR3 (CD11b/CD18), but not FcγRI (CD64), FcγRIII (CD16), CR1 (CD35), and CR2 (CD21).[227,243,244] The former two receptors are difficult to demonstrate on LCs in skin sections.[245] In addition to cell

**TABLE 7.1**
**Phenotype of Normal Human Epidermal Langerhans Cells[a]**

| Marker | Presence |
|---|---|
| **LC-specific** | |
| Birbeck granule | +[b] |
| Lag antigen | + |
| Langerin (CD207) | + |
| **DC markers** | |
| CD83 | – |
| CMRF44 | – |
| **Molecules for antigen-presentation** | |
| HLA-ABC | + |
| β2-microglobulin | + |
| HLA-DR | + |
| HLA-DP | + |
| HLA-DQ | + |
| HLA-DM | + |
| CD74 (invariant chain) | + |
| RFD1 (DQ-like) | +[c] |
| CD1a | + |
| CD1b | – |
| CD1c | + |
| CD1d | – |
| **Cytokine or chemokine receptors** | |
| GM-CSF Rα (CD116) | + |
| GM-CSF Rβ (CD131) | +[c] |
| TNF R I (CD120a) | – |
| TNF R II (CD120b) | + |
| IL-1R type 1 (CD121a) | +[c] |
| IL-1R type 2 (CD121b) | + |
| IL-2Rα (CD25) | – |
| IL-2Rβ (CD122) | – |
| IL-3Rα (CD123) | – |
| IL-4R (CD124) | – |
| IL-6R (CD126) | +[c] |
| IL-7Rα (CD127) | – |
| IL-8R (CD128) | – |
| IFN-γ R (CD119) | + |
| CD130 | +[c] |
| CCR3 | + |
| CXCR4 (CD184) | – (+[d]) |
| CCR5 (CD195) | + |
| CCR6 | + |
| CCR7 (CD197) | – |
| **Receptors for antigen-uptake** | |
| CD205 | + |
| CD206 | – |
| DC-SIGN (CD209) | – |
| DCIR | – |
| DC-ASGPR | – |
| FcγRI (CD64) | – |
| FcγRII (CD32) | + |
| FcγRIII (CD16) | – |
| FcεRI | + |
| FcεRII (CD23) | – |
| eBP | + |
| CD35 (CR1) | – |
| CD21 (CR2) | – |
| CD11b (CR3) | + |
| CD11c (gp150/95) | + |
| CD18 (β chain of CD11a-c) | + |
| CD88 (C5aR) | – (+[c]) |
| **Migration or homing related** | |
| CLA (HECA-452) | + |
| E-cadherin | + |
| ICAM-2 (CD102) | – |
| CD44 (splice variants) | +[c] |
| CD49a (VLA-1) | +[c] |
| CD49b (VLA-2) | +[c] |
| CD49c (VLA-3) | +[c] |
| CD49d (VLA-4) | +[c] |
| CD49e (VLA-5) | +[c] |
| CD49f (VLA-6) | +[c] |
| CD29 (β chain of CD49a-f) | + |
| CD87 | + |
| MDR1 | + |
| MRP1 | + |
| 12-HETE receptor | + |
| MMP2 | + |
| MMP9 | + |
| fascin (p55) | – |
| **Co-stimulatory molecules** | |
| LFA-1 (CD11a) | – |
| LFA-3 (CD58) | – or +[e] |
| ICAM-1 (CD54) | – or +[e] |
| ICAM-3 (CD50) | + |
| CD40 | +[f] |
| CD80 (B7-1) | – (+) |
| CD86 (B7-2) | – |
| ICOS-ligand (B7RP-1) | + |
| **T-cell or B-cell markers** | |
| CD2 | – |
| CD3 | – |
| CD4 | +[c] |
| CD5 | – |
| CD7 | – |
| CD8 | – |
| αβ T-cell receptor | – |
| γδ T-cell receptor | – |
| CD10 | – |
| CD19 | – |
| CD20 | – |
| CD22 | – |
| CD24 | – |
| **Monocyte/macrophage markers** | |
| CD15 (LeuM1) | – (+[g]) |
| CD15s (sialyl-Lewis$^{x}$) | +[c] |
| LeuM2 | – |
| CD14 (LeuM3) | – |
| CD33 | + |
| CD68 | – (+[h]) |
| CD36 (OKM5) | – |
| **Nervous system-associated markers** | |
| S100 | + |
| POMC-derived | + |
| PGP9.5 | +[c] |
| enolase | + |
| CGRP receptor | + |
| substance P receptor | + |
| GRP receptor | +[c] |
| **Miscellaneous markers** | |
| CD39 (ATPase) | + |
| CD45 (pan-leukocyte) | + |
| CD45RA | – |
| CD45RB | – |
| CD45RO | +[c] |
| CD69 | + |
| FXIIIa | – |
| CD95 | + |
| CD178 | + |
| CD98 | + |
| H1 receptor | – |
| H2 receptor | – |

[a] This table represents the phenotypic profile of human LCs *in situ* and in freshly isolated epidermal cell suspensions and is compiled from a great number of different studies. For details, see text.

[b] Arbitrary units: – absent; + present.

[c] Subset of LCs positive or expression at a variable level.

[d] Intracellular expression.

[e] Trypsin-sensitive molecule; detectable by immunoperoxidase staining (intracellular) or by immunoelectron microscopy (cell surface), but not by flow cytofluorometry.

[f] Trypsin-sensitive molecule; detectable when LCs are isolated by mild trypsinization.

[g] Positive after neuraminidase treatment.

[h] A spot near the nucleus.

surface expression of CD32, LCs are also able to secrete a soluble form of this receptor.[246] The observation that IgE molecules were present on LCs in clinically involved skin from patients with atopic dermatitis,[247] indicating the presence of receptors for IgE (FcεR), preceded the final proof that LCs carry these receptors. This IgE-binding capacity of LCs is due to the high-affinity receptor FcεRI,[248,249] which consists of one α chain and two γ chains, while the β chain is lacking. Ligation of this receptor by IgE induces the activation of LCs, but the expression of FcεRI and the induced response differ between LCs from normal individuals and individuals with atopic dermatitis.[250,251] The low-affinity receptor for IgE (FcεRII or CD23) is absent on normal LCs, but can be induced by stimulation with IL-4 and/or IFN-γ.[28] A third type of IgE-binding structure, called IgE-binding protein or eBP, has been found on the cell surface of LCs.[252] This eBP, which is distinct from FcεRI and FcεRII, is produced and secreted by keratinocytes and subsequently binds to LCs by virtue of its lectin property.[252] The IgE receptors enable LCs to trap allergen complexed to IgE in a highly efficient way, thereby contributing to the continuing of allergic responses to minute doses of encountered allergens.[253,254] As concerns the lectin receptors, resident LCs have a very high expression of Langerin (CD207), which is as discussed above, an excellent marker for the identification of LCs.[198] Epidermal LCs express low but significant functional levels of the multilectin receptor CD205,[39] but lack the macrophage mannose receptor CD206,[239] DC-SIGN (CD209),[44] DCIR,[46] and the asialoglycoprotein receptor DC-ASGPR.[45] Expression of other type II C-type lectins as well as TLRs by epidermal LCs is not reported yet.

Epidermal LCs express a number of adhesion molecules that are involved in the interaction with T cells. Freshly isolated LCs weakly express ICAM-1 (CD54) and LFA-3 (CD58), as tested by immunohistochemical staining of cytospin preparations.[243] However, by means of FACS analysis, these two molecules could not be detected on fresh LCs.[227,255,256] LCs do not express ICAM-2 (CD102),[256] but have a strong constitutive expression of ICAM-3 (CD50).[257,258] In contrast to other DC subsets, human LCs do not express LFA-1 (CD11a) protein and mRNA.[256,258,259] They have a cell surface expression of CD11c.[243,259] The presence of B7-1 (CD80) on LCs *in situ* is controversial.[260,261] B7-1 proteins are not detectable on freshly isolated LCs, whereas weak expression of cell surface B7-2 (CD86) may be observed; however, mRNA for both proteins is present.[260,262] The presence of ICOS-ligand (B7RP-1), another member of the B7 family, has been demonstrated on LCs.[263] CD40 expression by LCs is weak and best detectable on the subset of epidermal LCs that have a bright expression of HLA-DR and RFD1.[227,264] Approximately 10% of LCs bear variable levels of CD4 molecules: always low in normal skin of different individuals, but enhanced on LCs in diseased skin.[265–267] LCs *in situ* and in cell suspensions express CD4 both as monomers and as covalently linked homodimers, with the latter predominant.[267] CD4 on LCs may act as receptor for chemotactic factor IL-16.[268,269] In addition, CD4 is also used as receptor by the AIDS-inducing human immunodeficiency virus (HIV) to infect LCs.[270] In connection to this, freshly isolated LCs express chemokine receptor CCR5, but not CXCR4, on their surfaces, which are two other co-receptors for HIV.[271] However, CXCR4 is present intracellularly in the LCs and is transported to the cell surface upon culture. LCs carry receptors for GM-CSF, TNF-α (TNF receptor II, but not TNF receptor I), IL-1, IL-6, and IFN-γ, enabling these cells to respond to these cytokines, but lack receptors for IL-2, IL-4, IL-7, and IL-8.[272] Human LCs also lack both histamine H1 and H2 receptors.[273]

Epidermal LCs express several molecules that play a role in migration and/or homing. LCs express E-cadherin, a $Ca^{2+}$-dependent homophilic molecule that mediates LC-keratinocyte binding.[274] LCs in epidermal sheets *in situ* have a heterogeneous expression of sialyl Lewis$^X$ (CD15s),[275,276] the ligand of E-selectin (CD62E) expressed by endothelial cells. The antibody HECA-452 directed against CLA, recognizes a neuraminidase sensitive determinant on CD15s and binds to virtually all LCs in freshly prepared epidermal cell suspensions.[276] In a more recent study, however, it has been reported that CLA is an inducible modification of PSGL-1 (CD162), switching this P-selectin ligand into a ligand for E-selectin as well.[277] A peculiar finding is that LCs can be stained with the CD15 antibody LeuM1 provided that the skin specimen or the single cells were pretreated with the enzyme neuraminidase to eliminate the sialic acid decoration from the CD15 (Lewis$^X$) carbohydrate backbone.[227] The very late antigen (VLA) molecules 1 through 6 belong to the group of integrins. They are composed of a unique $\alpha$ chain (CD49a through f) and a shared common $\beta$1 chain (CD29) and function as receptors for extracellular matrix components, such as collagen, fibronectin, and laminin. All LCs express CD29, but the expression of the CD49 subtypes is heterogenous.[278,279] CD44, as a cell surface receptor for the extracellular matrix-component hyaluronan, is involved in cell migration and adhesion. LCs express several CD44 splice variants that have an essential function in trafficking of these cells.[280] LCs express receptors for the arachidonic acid metabolite 12-hydroxyeicosatetraenoic acid (12-HETE), the main eicosanoid produced by keratinocytes and assumed to play a role in LC migration.[281] Finally, expression of CD87 (urokinase plasminogen activator receptor) on LCs has been noted.[282] The enzymatic activity of this molecule may be important for the penetration of collagenous barriers such as the basement membrane.

All epidermal LCs react with a pan-CD45 antibody.[283,284] Due to alternate splicing, several isoforms of CD45 (a protein tyrosine phosphatase; also known as T200 antigen or leukocyte common antigen) exist. It appeared that 85% of freshly isolated LCs are reactive with CD45RO, while CD45RA and CD45RB are not detectable.[284] The CD45RO on LCs differs from the CD45RO expressed by memory T cells and monocytes/macrophages, probably due to lineage-specific post-translational glycosylation.[285] CD68, a marker of lysosomal glycoproteins, is not detectable by FACS analysis,[227] but a positive reacting spot near the nucleus of LCs can be observed by staining of cytospin preparations.[286] Expression of CD69 on LCs has been documented,[287] but the significance of this finding is, as yet, not clear. LCs have a low expression of the molecule Fas (CD95),[288] which can mediate apoptosis-inducing signals upon ligation. By means of immunoelectron microscopy the presence of CD178 (CD95 ligand) is detected on the cell surface of LCs in fresh crude epidermal cell suspensions, but not on LCs *in situ*, which show only a weak signal for this marker in the cytoplasm.[289] LCs in normal human skin have been reported to express S-100 antigen,[290] a $Ca^{2+}$-binding protein that is usually encountered in cells of the nervous system. LCs, which are intimately associated with epidermal neurons,[291] are also able to express neuronal peptides, such as proopiomelanocortin (POMC)-derived proteins,[292] neuron-specific enolase,[293] PGP9.5 (carboxy-terminal ubiquitin hydrolase),[294] and receptors for neuromediators, such as calcitonin gene-related peptide (CGRP),[291] gastrin-releasing peptide (GRP),[295] and substance P.[296] Studies in mice revealed that neuropeptides can enhance the LC migration, affect the T-cell-stimulatory function of LCs, and modulate inflammatory responses in the skin, such as allergic contact dermatitis.[297–299]

## 3. Mature Langerhans Cells

The phenotype of LCs is not fixed but rather dynamic and likely dependent on the environment in which they reside. The former section describes the phenotype of LCs that reside in normal human epidermis and when they are freshly isolated. Upon short-term culture, with or without the presence of cytokines, they undergo considerable changes (Table 7.2) and transform into extraordinarily powerful APCs. These alterations are considered similar to those *in vivo* when LCs migrate from the skin to the skin-draining lymph node to become IDC. Therefore, cultured LC can be considered as the *in vitro* equivalent of IDC. During *in vitro* culture, epidermal LCs tend to downregulate their characteristic BGs and CD1a expression,[243] as well as molecules involved in antigen uptake like Fc$\gamma$RII (CD32), CD11b, CD11c.[227,243] Expression of several cell surface molecules that are required for the stimulation of T cells remains high, like ICAM-3 (CD50),[258] or are strongly upregulated, like MHC class I and II, ICAM-1 (CD54), LFA-3 (CD58), B7-1 (CD80), B7-2 (CD86), and CD40.[227,243,255,256,260,262] The expression of CD80 and CD86 on human LCs can be enhanced by IFN-$\gamma$.[300,301] In addition, all cultured human LCs acquire strong expression of the IDC-marker RFD-1.[243] Other molecules that emerge upon culture are the $\alpha$ chain (CD25) and the $\beta$ chain (CD122) of the receptor for IL-2,[272] which were originally thought to be exclusively expressed and functional on

**TABLE 7.2**
**Phenotypical Comparison between Immature and Mature Human Langerhans Cells[a]**

| Marker | Fresh LCs | Cultured LCs |
|---|---|---|
| Lag (Birbeck granule) | ++[b] | –/+ |
| Langerin (CD207) | +++ | + |
| ATPase | ++ | –/+ |
| MHC class I | ++ | +++ |
| MHC class II (DR, DP, DQ) | ++ | +++ |
| RFD1 (DQ-like) | + | +++ |
| CD1a | ++ | –/+ |
| CD1c | + | –/+ |
| CD83 | – | + |
| CMRF44 | – | + |
| FcγRII (CD32) | + | – |
| FcεRI | + | – |
| FcεRII (CD23) | – | – (+[c]) |
| CD11b (C3biR) | + | – |
| CD11c (gp 150/95) | + | – |
| CD18 (β chain of CD11a,b,c) | + | – |
| ICAM-1 (CD54) | – or +[d] | ++ |
| ICAM-3 | ++ | ++ |
| LFA-1 (CD11a) | – | – |
| LFA-3 (CD58) | – or +[d] | ++ |
| CD40 | +[e] | ++ |
| CD80 (B7-1) | – | ++ |
| CD86 (B7-2) | – | ++ |
| GM-CSF Rα (CD116) | + | ++ |
| GM-CSF Rβ (CD131) | +[f] | + |
| TNF R II (CD120b) | ++ | + |
| IL-1R type 1 (CD121a) | + | – |
| IL-1R type 2 (CD121b) | + | ++ |
| IL-6R (CD126) | +[f] | + |
| CD130 | +[f] | + |
| CD25 (IL-2Rα) | – | + |
| CD122 (IL-2Rβ) | – | + |
| CCR6 | + | – |
| CCR7 | – | + |
| CD24 | – | + |
| CD45RO | + | –/+ |
| CD45RB | – | + |
| CD69 | + | – (+[g]) |
| fascin (p55) | – | + |

[a] This table was compiled from various different studies as stated in the text.
[b] Arbitrary units: – absent; + weak to moderate; ++ strong; +++ very strong.
[c] Induced by IFN-γ or IL-4.
[d] Trypsin-sensitive molecule; detectable by immunoperoxidase staining (intracellular) or immunoelectron microscopy (cell surface), but not by flow cytofluorometry.
[e] Detectable when LCs are isolated by mild trypsinization.
[f] Subset of LCs positive.
[g] Sustained by IFN-γ.

T lymphocytes. The expression of GM-CSF receptors, IL-1R type 2 (CD121b), IL-6R, and its signal transducer CD130 are upregulated during culture of LCs, TNF-α receptors and IL-1R type 1 (CD121a) are downregulated, whereas IFN-γ receptor expression is not affected.[272] CD69 expression is lost during culture, but this loss can be prevented by the addition of IFN-γ.[287] As concerns the expression of the protein tyrosine phosphatase, CD45RO expression decreases whereas CD45RB emerges.[284] CD24, the ligand of P-selectin (CD62P), is absent on resident LCs, but appears on all cultured LCs. Studies in mice indicated that the actin-bundling protein fascin (p55), which is involved in the formation of dendritic processes, is highly expressed in cultured LCs, but not in freshly isolated LCs.[302] Preliminary (unpublished observation) studies on human LCs revealed absence of p55 staining of LCs *in situ*, but increased expression of fascin on isolated LCs after culture.[303]

LCs can attract leukocytes through the production of chemokines like CXCL8 (IL-8),[288] CCL3 (MIP-1α),[304] CCL17 (TARC),[305] and CCL22 (MDC).[305] In addition to the strongly upregulated cell surface co-stimulatory molecules, they also provide co-stimulatory signals to T cells via the production of cytokines, such as IL-1α and β,[306,307] IL-1 receptor antagonist,[307] IL-6,[308] IL-12,[309] IL-15,[310] IL-16,[311] IL-18,[288] TNF-α.[312] IL-12 and IL-18 are important for the induction/upregulation of the IFN-γ production and the generation of type 1 T-helper cells,[313,314] which are associated with cell-mediated immunity, including contact allergy reactions. The mRNA expression for the two subunits of the biological active p70 IL-12 heterodimer is clearly detectable in isolated LCs, but remarkably the amount of secreted IL-12 from stimulated LCs *in vitro* appears not to be detectable.[288]

*In vitro* differentiation of murine LCs by a 3-day culture resulted in a considerably enhanced (up to 100-fold) T-cell stimulatory capacity.[315] In contrast, a 3-day culture of human LCs showed a less pronounced (up to tenfold) enhancement of this capacity to stimulate memory T cells.[255] Further, during *in vitro* culture LCs acquire the capacity to induce primary responses of naive T cells.[22,23,316] The potent antigen-presenting function of human LCs is also reflected by the finding that newly cloned antigen-specific T cells can show a selective requirement for human LCs as APCs.[317] Numerous reports demonstrate the potent stimulatory function of LCs, but only a few are cited here. On a per cell basis, human LCs tend to be more potent than monocytes to induce responses to contact allergens, *Candida albicans,* tetanus toxoid, or protein antigens from *Mycobacteria*.[318–320] This superiority of human LCs is most obvious in the responses of T cells from nickel-allergic donors to nickel sulfate. Patients with a positive patch test to nickel can have peripheral blood T cells that show no or low proliferative responses with peripheral blood monocytes as APC, but the use of LCs, instead, results in restoration of the responsiveness to nickel.[320] Further striking evidence for an essential role of DCs (such as LCs) in the induction of T-cell activation, is that hapten-modified DCs injected subcutaneously without adjuvant in tolerized mice can break the tolerant state.[321,322] LCs not only act as APCs but also as extremely potent stimulator cells in the autologous and allogeneic mixed leukocyte reaction and in the generation of cytotoxic cells.[323] Because LCs are strong stimulators of allogeneic responses, they are considered crucial inducers of skin transplant rejection.[324] Prolonged survival of skin transplants can be achieved by depletion of LCs from the allogeneic graft.[325] As few as ten LCs can effectively allosensitize a recipient mouse, stressing the powerful stimulator function of LCs.[326]

## 4. Birbeck Granules

More than 40 years ago it was discovered that LCs express unique rod-shaped structures with a central, periodically striated lamella, giving this central part a zipper-like appearance (Figure 7.4).[195] These structures, named after their discoverer, can only be observed by electron microscopy. LCs possess a varying number of BGs of variable size, occasionally having a vesicular dilatation at one end, giving them a racket-like appearance. Three-dimensional models of individual BGs revealed that they are flat, disc-, or cup-shaped organelles.[327] The racket-like structures, showing the transition from vesicle membrane into BGs, led to the assumption that BGs are constituted of two layers of membrane that are closely associated (Figure 7.4). A racket-shaped BG may be interpreted either

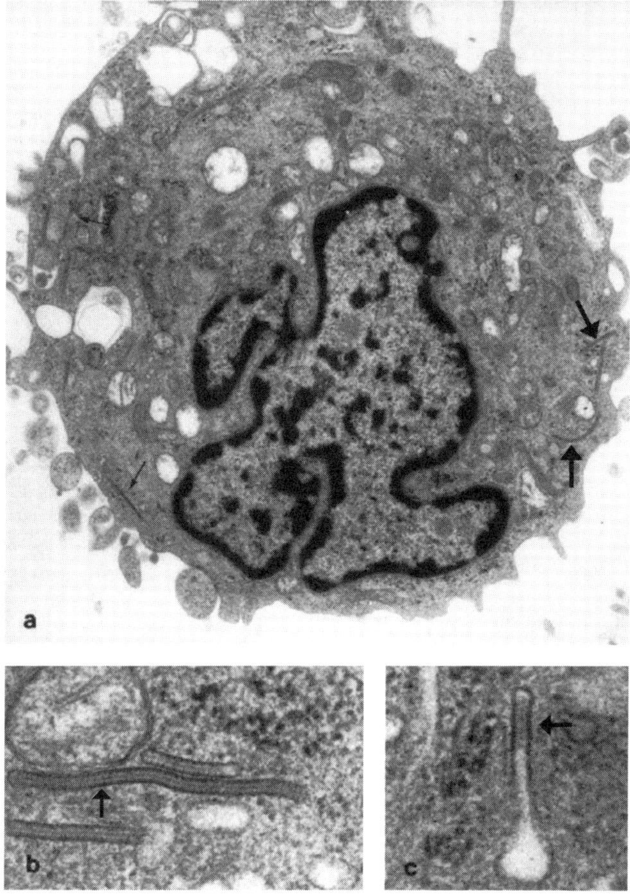

**FIGURE 7.4** Electron microscopic representation of an LC with BGs indicated by arrows (a). Higher magnification of BGs (b and c), which consist of two membranes in close apposition. This assumption was originally born from the observation of BGs in association with small vesicles, thereby forming a racket-like structure (c). A regular pattern of electron-dense material is frequently observed between the membranes (arrows).

as a process of unzipping, which may reflect a first step in the degradation of a BG, or as the result of fusion between a BG and a lysosomal vesicle. The formation of BGs as a result of sandwiching of villi and the cell body can be observed in normal LCs (Figure 7.5). Electron microscopic studies further suggest that BG formation is initiated by cross-linking of cell surface structures, because the sandwiching of the plasma membrane is associated with the formation of repeating electron-dense structures (Figure 7.5), similar to the zipper-like structure observed in intracellularly located BGs. Most reports support the view that BGs develop from cell membrane invaginations or from folding of villi, in this way making contact with the cytomembrane. The formation of BGs seems to be $Ca^{2+}$ dependent, but the nature of the signals that trigger BG formation is still unknown. Some BGs are continuous with the external compartment, as shown by lanthanum, osmium, ferritin particles, or horseradish peroxidase, indicating that LCs capture extracellular material.[328,329] By short-term incubation of living LCs with CD1a antibodies coupled to gold beads, it was demonstrated that the first gold particles appeared in BGs following a process resembling receptor-mediated endocytosis.[330] Anti-MHC class II antibodies coupled to gold beads of different size are simultaneously co-internalized with these CD1a-labeled antibodies.[331] Using cationized horseradish peroxidase as a tracer compound, it was demonstrated that after 10 min of incubation the tracer was mainly found in BGs and in MHC class II negative vesicles, whereas at later time points (30

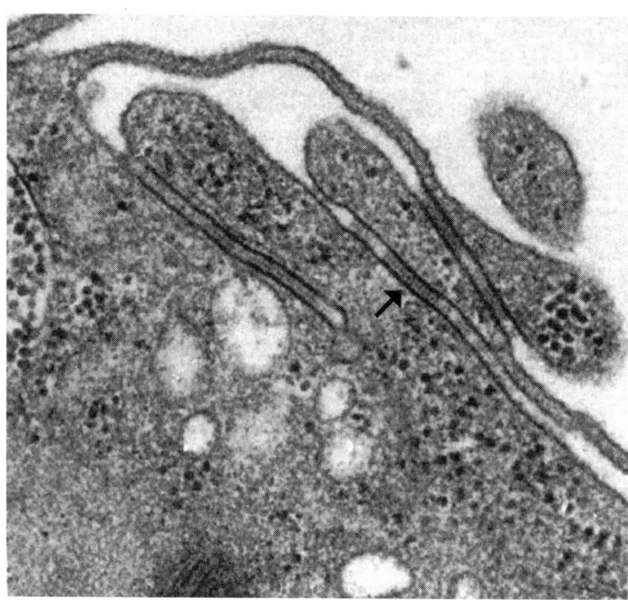

**FIGURE 7.5** Detail of a Langerhans cell showing sandwiching of the plasma membrane. Villi that touch the cell body or adjacent villi tend to form BG structures, characterized by repeating electron-dense material between the membranes (arrow).

to 60 min) the tracer reached the MIICs.[236] Thus, receptors on the LC cell membrane, as well as exogenous proteins (either pinocytosis or receptor-bound), appear in BGs, indicating that these granules likely represent early endocytic structures. The molecule Langerin is essentially involved in the development of BGs.[199] It still must be discovered whether BGs arise through the interaction of Langerin molecules with one another or with other, as-yet-unknown ligands. Transfection of Langerin cDNA into fibroblasts induces BG formation in these cells, indicating that this single gene is sufficient for the occurrence of BGs.[199] In addition to the presence of Langerin molecules on the cell surface of LCs, Langerin molecules are present in membranes of clathrin-coated pits, the endosomal recycling compartment, and in BGs, to a lesser extent in early/sorting endosomes, but not in lysosomes and MIICs.[199,332] Temperature-dependent time-lap studies with freshly isolated LCs show that Langerin behaves as a recycling molecule, in a similar manner to CD1a molecules, and suggest that BGs could be part of the endosomal recycling compartment, involved in the recycling of transmembrane proteins from early endosomes to the cell surface.[332,333] In maturated LCs (i.e., cultured LCs) the intracellular Langerin content is markedly reduced or lost, which coincides with the depletion of BGs.[332]

The exact function of BGs is unknown thus far, but one may believe that BGs represent a unique antigen-trapping mechanism. It may be speculated that BGs form a reservoir of exogenous antigens and that BGs prevent an early loss or early extensive degradation of antigen in the lysosomal compartment in the time required to transport the antigen from skin to the draining lymph node. Antigen-pulsed B lymphocytes, for example, have no BGs and lose their ability to stimulate T cells after an additional culture period longer than 4 h.[334] Surprisingly, however, the occurrence of an individual was reported whose LCs were devoid of BGs, but expressed all other LC-characteristic features, e.g., CD1a and MHC class II.[335] Unfortunately, no information is available on the (possible lack of) expression of Langerin by these LCs. Nevertheless, these BG-negative LCs exhibit normal antigen-presenting function *in vivo* and *in vitro*. This strongly indicates that BGs are not a prerequisite for the function of LCs to stimulate T cells. Ultrastructural elements similar to BGs can be induced in the non-APC population of human blood platelets upon treatment with the chelating agent EDTA (i.e., binds $Ca^{2+}$), apparently as a result of cross-linking of EDTA-induced dissociated membrane glycoproteins.[336] Remarkably, treatment of LCs with EDTA leads to unzipping of BGs and transition of BG rods into vesicles. This is in concordance with the notion that Langerin is a $Ca^{2+}$-dependent lectin.[199] It is well known that LC precursors lack BGs and that this granule is induced once the LCs have entered the epidermis, possibly upon interaction of an epidermal factor with a membrane receptor of LCs. When LCs are taken out of the epidermal microenvironment (for example, by culturing purified LCs *in vitro*), they lose the BG expression.[243] Development of BGs thus seems to be linked to the epidermal micromilieu. Taken all together, it is clear that BGs represent a special form of endocytosis, but the reason LCs display such a different way of endocytosis, as compared to the other members of the DC family, remains still unclear.

Recently, the presence of additional specific ultrastructural organelles, called cored tubules,[337] has been reported in human LCs.[338] Like BGs, these organelles are rod-shaped structures of variable length, but they may be tortuous in shape. Whereas BGs have a periodically striated center, the cored tubules have an inner central line that lacks periodicity and when sectioned transversely these structures appear as circles with a central dot. The cored tubules can branch off and form a network or can be continuous with early endosomes. Temperature-dependent immunogold-labeling experiments revealed that CD1a and Langerin molecules are present in the inner central line of cored tubules and indicate that these organelles, just like BGs, belong to the endosomal recycling compartment of LCs.[338] Cored tubules and BGs can separately coexist in the cytoplasm of LCs, but occasionally continuity between these two structures can be observed. It cannot be excluded that cored tubules represent a developmental stage of BGs. The relationship between the BGs and cored tubules remains to be solved.

## B. Migration of Langerhans Cells

Current knowledge on the migration of LCs is mainly derived from experiments with rodents, but most of these findings are probably also applicable to human LCs. Migration of cells is the result of a coordinated interplay of regulated expression of functional integrin/adhesion molecules and chemokine receptors on the cell surface with their respective ligands, i.e., downregulation of these molecules and receptors involved in homing of the cells (enabling departure) and, concurrently, upregulation of other integrin/adhesion molecules and chemokine receptors, relevant for the target organ and guiding the cells to this tissue. The following is known about the mechanism regulating the traffic of LC precursors from the bone marrow via the bloodstream to the epidermis. LC precursors in blood can tether and roll constitutively along non-inflamed endothelium of cutaneous postcapillary venules, a prerequisite for extravasation into tissues.[339] The skin-homing receptor CLA (recognized by antibody HECA-452) and PSGL-1 (CD162) on LC precursors and their respective ligands E-selectin (CD62E) and P-selectin (CD62P) on endothelial cells are involved in this interaction (Figure 7.6).[339] LC precursors and freshly isolated LCs, which express chemokine receptor CCR6,[340] are selectively attracted to and retained in the epidermis by the keratinocyte-derived chemokine CCL20 (MIP-3α, also known as LARC or exodus-1).[341–343] A new classification system of chemokines and their receptors has been established at the beginning of this millennium.[344] This attraction by CCL20 appears to be dependent on the presence of TGF-β1.[340] In addition, β defensins produced by keratinocytes may also mediate recruitment of LCs through CCR6.[345] Chemokine receptors CCR1 (binds, among others, CCL3/MIP-1α, CCL4/MIP-1β, and CCL5/RANTES), CCR2 (binds CCL2/MCP-1, CCL7/MCP-3, CCL8/MCP-2, and CCL13/MCP-4), and CCR5 (binds CCL3/MIP-1α, CCL4/MIP-1β, and CCL5/RANTES) on immature DCs recognizing inflammatory chemokines would be responsible for the recruitment of these cells into inflamed tissues, including skin.[346,347] Experiments with $CD34^+$ DC progenitors revealed that the $CD14^+$ DC precursor subset has a transient sequential expression of CCR2 and CCR6 during their development and are sequentially responsive to CCL13 and CCL20.[348] This is consonant with the model that, during inflammation, different chemokines are produced by different tissue compartments: CCL13 produced by basal epithelial cells recruits $CD11c^+$ blood DC or DC precursors

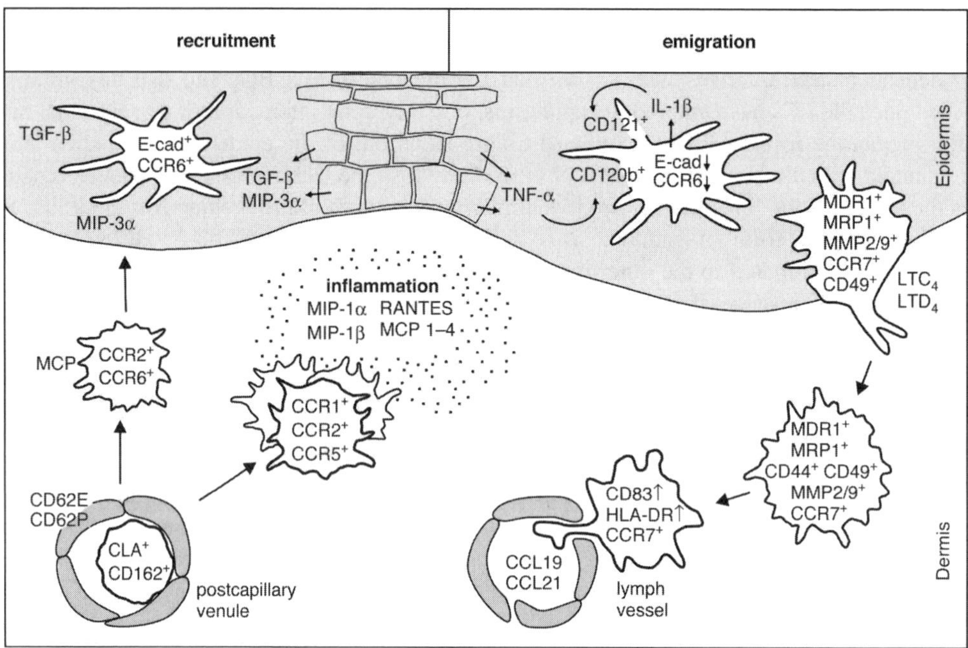


**FIGURE 7.6** Model of Langerhans cell trafficking. This scheme depicts essential factors and their respective receptors involved in the recruitment of LC precursors to the epidermis, in the homing in the epidermis, as well as in the emigration from the epidermis to the draining lymph node. In case of inflammation, additional chemokines and receptors are involved in the attraction of dendritic cells to the affected tissue. Extensive explanation of this figure is given in the text.

(including monocytes) from the blood into the tissue (e.g., dermis), whereupon the recruited cells acquire CCR6 and lose CCR2 enabling them to reach the epidermis in response to CCL20.[348] Transgenic mice with selective overexpression of CCL2/MCP-1 in their basal keratinocytes have local accumulation of DCs/LCs in the epidermis.[349] Once they arrive in the epidermis, LCs make physical contact with surrounding keratinocytes via homophilic interactions of E-cadherin molecules,[274,350] appearing as adherens junctions by electron microscopy.[351] This ligation of E-cadherin on the newly arrived immature LCs, but also the presence of TGF-β in the epidermis, prevents premature maturation.[352,353]

The exit of LCs from the epidermis is supposed to take place under steady-state conditions as well, but can be strongly augmented by inflammatory or danger signals provided by microbes, contact allergens, cytokines, UVB radiation, and many others. The LCs do not leave the epidermis *en masse*, likely because a heterogeneity exists in the LC population with regard to the maturational stage and functional responsiveness.[354] The initiation of LC mobilization coincides with the onset of the maturation of these cells. Crucial early signals for the induction of these two processes are both cytokines TNF-α, derived from keratinocytes, and IL-1β, derived from LCs or from dermal macrophages and DDC.[355–358] The TNF receptor II (CD120b) on LCs, but not TNF receptor I (CD120a), appears to be critical in this respect.[359,360] Another critical molecule required for migration is caspase-1 (previously known as IL-1-converting enzyme, which is responsible for cleavage of the precursor IL-1β molecule prior to the release of the biologically active mature IL-1β) as demonstrated with caspase-1-deficient mice and caspase-1 inhibitors.[361] In response to the application of contact sensitizers, LCs downregulate E-cadherin expression, in a TNF-α/IL-1β-dependent way, which enables dissociation from surrounding keratinocytes.[350,362] In addition, LCs need to downregulate the expression of chemokine receptors CCR1, CCR5, and CCR6 that encourage retention of LCs in the epidermis. Quick disappearance of these receptors from the cell surface has been shown for monocyte-derived DCs upon maturation induced by TNF-α or LPS,[347,363] but for human epidermal LCs this still remains to be established. At the same time, LCs start to express CCR7, making these cells responsive to chemokines CCL19 (MIP3-β, also known as ELC or exodus-3) and CCL21 (6Ckine, also known as SLC or exodus-2).[341,364–366] In mice different forms of CCL21 exist that differ from each other by one amino acid (either serine or leucine) at position 65.[367] The serine form is termed CCL21a and the leucine form comprises CCL21b and CCL21c.[368] CCL21a is predominantly expressed in lymphoid organs and CCL21b in the nonlymphoid tissues.[368] Despite extensive research, in humans only the leucine form of CCL21 has been identified thus far.[367] CCL21 is expressed by lymphatic endothelium in murine nonlymphoid tissues and may recruit CCR7$^+$ cells into the draining lymphatics.[369] In addition, lymphatic endothelial cells in chronically inflamed human skin, but not in normal skin, express CCL21.[370] CCL19 and CCL21 are selectively co-expressed in the T-cell zones in lymphoid organs, predominantly by the stromal cells,[371] guiding CCR7$^+$ LCs/DCs to this tissue, bringing these cells in contact with naive T cells for the initiation of immune responses. In CCR7-deficient mice[372] as well as in *plt* mice lacking both CCL19 and CCL21-serine (although expressing CCL21-leucine in their nonlymphoid tissues)[367,373] LCs fail to migrate to the draining lymph nodes. In addition, neutralizing polyclonal antibodies to CCL19 can cause a profound retention of LCs in the epidermis.[374] Cysteinyl leukotrienes $LTC_4$ and $LTD_4$ are critically involved in chemotaxis to CCL19, but not to CCL21.[374] Multidrug resistance–related protein 1 (MRP1) is known to mediate the secretion of eicosanoid $LTC_4$, which following secretion is converted to $LTD_4$ and $LTE_4$. LC mobilization from the epidermis and trafficking into lymphatic vessels are greatly reduced in MRP1-deficient mice, but migration was restored by exogenous $LTC_4$ and $LTD_4$. In normal human epidermis, LCs are the major, and possibly sole, producers of $LTC_4$.[375] Another member of the multidrug resistance family, MDR1, is also involved in the LC migration.[376] Anti-MDR1 antibody or MDR1 antagonist verapamil present in human skin explant cultures is able to block the emigration out of the explants. The exact mechanism by which MDR1 acts to facilitate migration remains unclear. MDR1,[377] but also MRP1,[378] can translocate sphingolipid analogues across the plasma membrane. Metabolism of sphingolipids leads to the production of ceramide, which can trigger the phospholipase $A_2$-mediated generation of arachidonic acid, the initial substrate in the production of leukotrienes and prostaglandins. It has been suggested[379] that perturbation of MDR1 or MRP1 activity may lead to intracellular accumulation of ceramide and arachidonic acid metabolites, which are known to participate in signaling for cytokine transcription, and lead to altered phospholipase $A_2$ activity, which has been shown to regulate chemotactic responses.

In a recent study, employing melanin granules as an easily traceable, naturally occurring antigen in special mouse strains, it is demonstrated that in the steady state (i.e., a non-inflammatory condition) melanin granule-laden cutaneous DCs accumulate in the regional lymph nodes, but not in other tissues.[380] This indicates that even in the steady state LCs continuously emigrate and are loaded up with antigens (e.g., apoptotic cells, melanin granules) encountered in the skin. This melanin granule transport to the regional lymph node is lacking in TGF-β1-deficient mice, which are devoid of LCs. Interestingly, in CCL19 plus CCL21-serine-deficient *plt* mice, in which LCs fail to migrate to the draining lymph nodes upon application of contact sensitizers (as described above), normal steady-state transport of melanin granules to the regional lymph nodes does take place.[381] This finding indicates that under non-inflammatory conditions the LC trafficking is utilizing a different mechanism, independent of the CCR7–CCL19/CCL21 pathway used in the inflammatory state. This constitutive LC migration in the steady state might be important in the regulation of immunity against self-antigens (e.g., apoptotic cells, melanin granules) and peripheral tolerance.

Functional expression of CCR2 is likely needed for LC migration to local lymph nodes. Mice deficient in CCR2 show normal epidermal LC density and intact ability of LCs to migrate into the dermis; however, their migration to the draining lymph nodes was markedly impaired.[382] As is the case for other DC subsets, human LCs have a functional CCR3 expression, which is independent on the state of maturation, giving them the opportunity to respond to eotaxins CCL11, CCL24, and

CCL26,[383] which play a role in allergic inflammation. Other groups of molecules have been identified to play a role in LC migration. CD40-ligand-deficient mice have normal numbers of LCs with normal morphology, but upon contact sensitization LCs fail to migrate out of the skin.[384] This defect in migration is associated with impaired epidermal production of TNF-α and can be corrected by recombinant TNF-α or an agonistic anti-CD40 antibody, indicating that CD40–CD40 ligand interaction is involved in LC migration.[384] Experiments with ICAM-1-deficient mice revealed that expression of adhesion molecule ICAM-1 (CD54) on lymphatic endothelium rather than on LCs is responsible for the reduced migration of LCs into the draining lymph nodes.[385] Emigration of LCs out of the skin and recruitment of new LCs to the epidermis appears to be normal in these mice. Blocking laminin/invasion-receptor α6 integrin (CD49f) with antibodies causes a marked inhibition of LC migration from skin explants and *in vivo*.[386] Upon anti-α6 treatment, the LCs become rounded, retract their dendrites, but the LC number hardly reduces, indicating that these LCs are about to leave the epidermis although are not able to pass the basement membrane. Similar results can be obtained with blocking antibodies to a common N-terminal epitope of CD44, a receptor for hyaluronic acid, which is a component of the dermal matrix.[280] LC activation/maturation is accompanied by increased expression of CD44 and a switch of CD44 variant isoform expression. Intraepidermal LCs and freshly isolated LCs display pan-CD44 and CD44 variants v7 and v8, while LCs that have migrated into the dermis and cultured LCs display enhanced levels of pan-CD44 and CD44 variants v4, v5, v6, and v9, but lost v7 and v8.[280] Osteopontin, a secreted phosphoprotein containing an integrin-binding domain, has been identified as a ligand for several integrins as well as for CD44.[387,388] Osteopontin can function as a chemokine and is regarded as an early component of type 1 immune responses.[389] Further, this molecule can bind to extracellular matrix components fibronectin and collagen, thereby promoting interactions of cells with the extracellular matrix.[390] It is demonstrated that intradermal osteopontin injection induces LC emigration and that LCs leaving the epidermis predominantly traffic toward osteopontin-rich areas in the papillary dermis, which are especially located in the vicinity of endothelial cells of the microvascular plexus where endothelial cells of the lymphatics are located as well.[391] The osteopontin-induced emigration from the epidermis can be inhibited by blocking antibodies against integrin αv (CD51) and the common CD44 epitope.[391] CD44 variants cooperate with β1 (CD29)-containing integrins to bind to osteopontin facilitating motility and chemotaxis of tumor cells,[392] but it is as yet not known whether this holds true for LC migration. A reduced migration of LCs to the lymph node is found in osteopontin-deficient mice in response to application of contact allergen FITC.[391]

Several cytokines can influence the migration process of LCs. As earlier mentioned, inflammatory factors TNF-α and IL-1β induce and amplify the migration of LCs out of the epidermis.[355,357] GM-CSF, when administered intradermally in healthy volunteers, causes a reduction of LCs in the epidermis, whereas the number of $CD1a^+HLA\text{-}DR^+$ cells in the dermis increases, indicating that GM-CSF can recruit LCs in this skin compartment.[393] Interestingly, enhanced elicitation responses occur when subjects are immunized through GM-CSF-treated skin sites.[393] It is also reported that GM-CSF may promote the chemokinesis of LCs, probably as a result of rendering them more susceptible to chemotactic signals.[394] IL-4 can inhibit the migratory activity of LCs by means of downregulation of TNF receptor II (CD120b) expression,[395] an essential prerequisite for LC migration.[359,360] Enhanced migration of LCs from the skin of IL-10-deficient mice is observed.[396] Using the skin explant model, it is demonstrated that IL-10 enhances LC migration from the cultured skin, while in contrast TGF-1 inhibits this phenomenon.[397] Systemic treatment of mice with Flt3 ligand results in a significant increase of mature DCs preferentially in the dermis, whereas IL-12 promoted a significant increase of immature LCs.[398] The mechanism for these increased DC numbers in skin is not known, but may be due to accelerated development of DCs from bone marrow progenitors rather than to altered local synthesis of chemotactic factors. Fibroblast-conditioned medium contains chemotactic factors for LCs but these have not yet been defined.[399] Extracellular ATP (e.g., released from damaged cells) can upregulate CCR7 expression, strongly induce CXCR4, but reduce CCR5 expression by immature DCs and stimulate their migration to stromal-derived factor 1 (CXCL12) and CCL19, whereas the response to CCL4 reduces.[400] In addition, ATP-treated DCs are less efficient in attracting type 1 T cells and have a diminished capacity to initiate type 1 T-cell responses, favoring the outcome of type 2 immune responses.[400,401] The neurotransmitter norepinephrine can amplify migration of LCs in mice *in vivo* and from skin explants *ex vivo*.[402] Norepinephrine exerts its effect on chemotactic and chemokinetic activity of these DCs via $\alpha_{1b}$-adrenergic receptors, which are expressed by immature DCs, but not by mature DCs.[402] Complement cleavage product C5a is a chemotactic factor for monocytes and monocyte-derived immature DCs[403] (and perhaps also for LC precursors). C5a not only attracts these cells in case of inflammation but also induces differentiation of these cells into mature DCs via TNF-$\alpha$- and $PGE_2$-dependent mechanisms.[404]

On their way from the epidermis to the draining lymph nodes LCs have to cross several physical barriers, such as the basement membrane, the extracellular dermal matrix, and the lymphatic vascular endothelium. LCs are able to make temporary holes in the basement membrane, allowing the cells to pass through this obstacle *in vivo*,[405] *ex vivo*,[406] as well as through artificially reconstituted basement membranes *in vitro*.[399] Important tools in this respect are matrix metalloproteinases (MMP)-2 and MMP-9, enzymes that can degrade collagen IV, which is a main constituent of the basement membrane, but that can also degrade extracellular matrix components.[407] Both MMP-2 and MMP-9 are expressed on the surface of human LCs enabling these cells to perform localized proteolysis to create a path for migration.[408] Inhibition of MMP-2 and MMP-9 function by specific MMP-inhibiting drugs, by antibodies against MMP-2 and MMP-9, or by naturally occurring tissue inhibitor of metalloproteinase (TIMP)-1 and TIMP-2 strongly decreases the migration of LCs from the epidermis *in vivo* and from skin explants in culture.[408–410] After reaching the dermal lymphatics, the migrating LCs have to transmigrate through the lymphatic endothelium to proceed on their journey. Electron microscopic studies with human and murine skin explant cultures reveal that the lymphatic endothelium contains interruptions and that LCs may reach the lumen of the lymph vessels via these gaps.[406,411]

## C. Role of Langerhans Cells in Contact Hypersensitivity

### 1. The Sensitization Phase

In the early 1970s it was discovered that a close apposition occurs between lymphocytes and LCs (i.e., peripolesis) at sites of allergic contact dermatitis (a type IV delayed hypersensitivity reaction). It was hypothesized that LCs may play a crucial role as APC in contact hypersensitivity (CHS).[412,413] LCs can function as antigen-trapping cells because they are able to accumulate selectively contact sensitizers, but not irritants, on the cell surface.[414,415] Macropinocytosis and the multilectin receptor DEC-205 are probably involved in this process.[21,38] Contact sensitizers are relatively small chemicals, usually below 500 Da in size, and by virtue of this they are able to pass the epidermal barrier.[416] These small molecules (haptens) must bind to a protein carrier, forming a hapten–carrier complex, to become immunogenic. The carrier molecules are probably components within the epidermis. Notorious contact sensitizers, like TNBS or nickel ions, can also directly bind to MHC class II molecules of APC with high affinity.[417,418] Induction of CHS, also referred to as sensitization, is commonly achieved by painting contact sensitizers onto the skin of naive recipient animals. The success of sensitization appears to be largely dependent on the density of LCs. Induction of CHS fails or is strongly reduced in skin areas with naturally low densities of LCs (i.e., the murine tail) or in skin areas with low functional LC densities induced by either UVB irradiation, stripping of epidermal tissue by adhesive tape, or chemicals.[419–422] However, application of hapten on tape-stripped skin (i.e., LC-depleted) still permits the development of CHS indicating that dermal DCs may also participate in this process.[423] In addition, subcutaneous injection of hapten (circumventing cutaneous DC involvement) can also result in the induction of CHS, suggesting that cutaneous DCs are sufficient but not obligatory for the sensitization process.[423]

During the last 30 years, numerous reports, most on contact sensitizers in experimental animal models, support the prominent role of LCs in the sensitization stage of CHS.[20,196,424–426] According

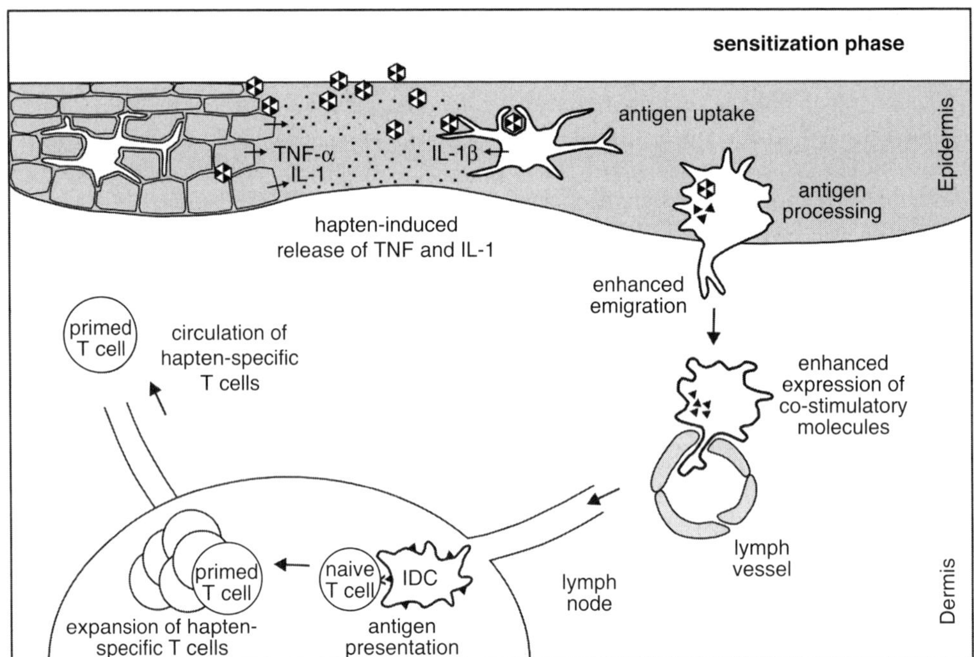


**FIGURE 7.7** Sensitization phase of allergic contact dermatitis. Langerhans cells take up contact allergens (haptens) they encounter in the skin. Haptens induce the release of TNF-α and IL-1β, both inducing and enhancing the emigration and maturation of the Langerhans cells. Once arrived in the skin-draining lymph node, Langerhans cells are transformed into interdigitating cells, which present the hapten to naive T cells. This leads to the activation and clonal expansion of hapten-specific T cells and subsequent distribution of these cells via the blood circulation. Further explanation of this figure is given in the text.

to a generally supported classical concept, LCs harvest antigens they encounter in the epidermis (Figure 7.7). Antigen-laden LCs migrate subsequently via dermal lymph vessels to the draining lymph node. This concept is supported by the observation that contact sensitizer DNCB can be detected intracellularly in $CD1a^+$ DCs in human afferent lymph approximately 20 h after epicutaneous application of the sensitizing agent.[427] During their traffic in the lymph vessels the LCs acquire flattened protrusions or membrane flaps (hence they are called veiled cells) and on arrival in the skin-draining lymph nodes they acquire the IDC phenotype. Veiled cells and IDCs that bear LC-specific BGs have been observed at 6 to 72 h after antigen exposure of skin, indicating that these cells originate from LCs. Only veiled cells and IDCs, but not macrophages, B cells, or T cells, carry the contact sensitizing antigen, which was applied to the skin, providing further evidence for the concept that LCs migrate to draining lymph nodes to become IDCs.

The exact mechanisms triggering and controlling the emigration of LCs from the epidermis in the sensitization phase are still unclear. There is a common belief that contact sensitizers, but not irritants or tolerogens, are able to convert the LCs and keratinocytes from a resting to an activated state.[428] Epicutaneous allergen application induces a rapid (already noticeable after 15 min) induction of IL-1β in LCs and, among others, TNF-α in keratinocytes.[355,429] Even a dermal source of IL-1β, presumably DDC or dermal macrophages, has been suggested to play a role.[358] As outlined above in the section on migration of LCs, these two pro-inflammatory cytokines are not only essential for LC migration but are also capable of accelerating this function.[355,357] This hapten-induced enhanced emigration of epidermal LCs correlates nicely with the increased number of veiled cells in the skin-draining lymph and the observed gradual reduction of LC numbers in the hapten-treated skin during the first 24 h after application of the contact sensitizer.[430–432] Epicutaneous application of contact sensitizers also leads to a loss of ATPase and enhanced endocytosis activity in LCs, as determined at the ultrastructural level.[431,433]

Once they arrive in the draining lymph node, the hapten-laden LCs are supposed to activate naive ($CD45RA^+$) T cells via a hapten-specific signal along with co-stimulatory and type 1 or type 2 polarizing signals. This activation leads to the generation of hapten-specific memory ($CD45RO^+$) T cells that leave the lymph node and begin to circulate through peripheral tissues. It seems very likely that the hapten-laden LCs generate both $CD4^+$ and $CD8^+$ memory T cells containing effector and suppressor subsets. *In vivo* antibody-depletion and adoptive transfer experiments reveal that both $CD4^+$ and $CD8^+$ T cells are involved in CHS.[434] It has to be noted that, although dispensable for the activation of $CD8^+$ T cells, $CD4^+$ T cells are required for the differentiation of $CD8^+$ T cells into memory cells.[435] Human skin is daily exposed to an array of environmental haptens, but it rarely results in CHS. Taking this into account, it can be assumed that tolerance induction must be the default setting of the T-cell response against encountered haptens. How the skin immune system can reach this state of unresponsiveness is still an enigma. One may hypothesize that the balance between hapten-specific effector and suppressor T cells induced by contact sensitizers is normally in favor of the latter. This suppression may be exerted by anergic T cells or regulatory T cells, which are generated if T cells receive insufficient co-stimulation while being activated.[122,124] The dose of contact sensitizer itself appears also to affect the outcome of the T-cell response. It has been demonstrated that application of subsensitizing doses of hapten results in the generation of type 2-like $CD8^+$ T cells that give rise to hapten-specific tolerance in mice.[436] In humans, hapten-specific $CD4^+$ regulatory T cells, displaying inhibitory effects on DC and T-cell function through release of IL-10, have been documented.[437] Many cytokines are induced during the course of CHS and will affect the development of this process, but the contribution of each of the various cytokines is not clear. Some cytokines, such as IL-12[438] and IL-16,[269] amplify the CHS response, whereas other cytokines, such as IL-10[396] and IL-21,[439] downmodulate the induction of CHS. In addition, the neural factor Slit 2 can mediate inhibition of LC migration and suppression of CHS responses.[440]

The characteristics and distribution of human LCs within the epidermis can be preserved in skin biopsies during 3 to 4 days of *in vitro* culture.[441] Epicutaneous treatment of skin explants with contact sensitizers, but not irritants or tolerogens, induces migration of LCs to the dermis 24 h after application.[442] In addition, a critical role for IL-1β in LC emigration in this model has been shown.[443] These studies indicate that this *ex vivo* skin organ culture model is useful in unraveling the mechanism of LC migration upon application of contact allergens. Moreover, this model of organotypic skin explant cultures might also be used as assay to predict potential allergenicity of newly synthesized chemical compounds.[442]

## 2. The Elicitation Phase

After being primed for a certain contact sensitizer, renewed epicutaneous contact will lead to elicitation of CHS, which clinically manifests as allergic contact dermatitis. The earliest signs of a CHS response are mast cell degranulation, vasodilatation, and infiltration of neutrophils, followed by monocytes/macrophages and T cells. The development of allergic contact dermatitis is a T-cell-dependent process, as illustrated by the fact that T-cell-deficient mice cannot generate CHS. Memory T cells, especially the ones expressing skin-homing receptor CLA, selectively patrol through the skin.[444,445] There is a general belief that a full-blown CHS response will occur in case hapten-specific memory T cells within the skin encounter their relevant allergen presented by LCs. Although this classical concept can not be excluded, it is hard to believe that at any given time point sufficient hapten-specific T cells are present in that particular part of the skin that is in contact with the allergen, to generate a CHS response. Few T cells are present in the epidermis and the number of LCs diminishes upon epicutaneous contact with hapten through upregulation of IL-1β and TNF-α production.

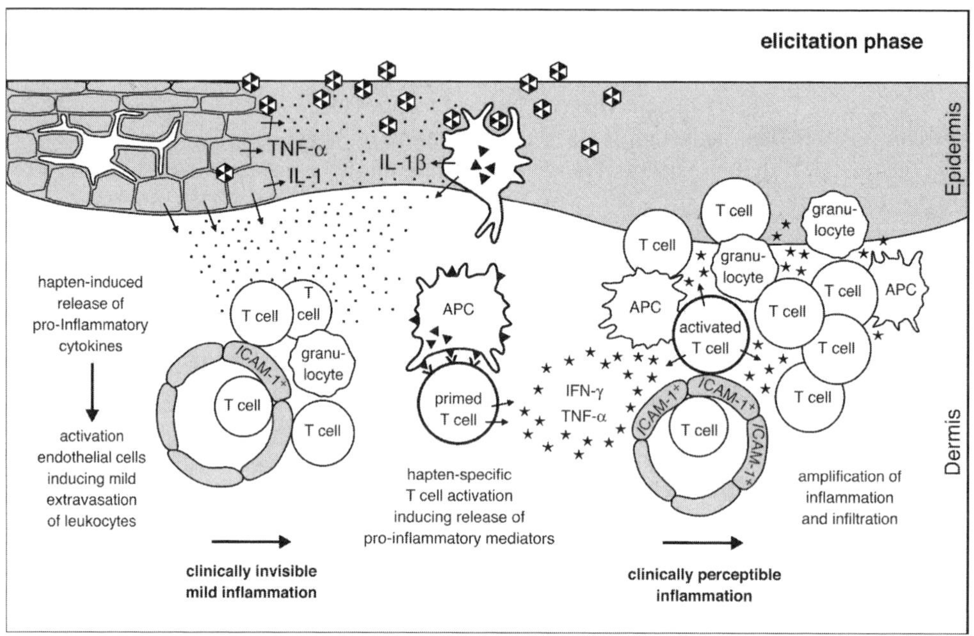


**FIGURE 7.8** Elicitation phase of contact dermatitis. Contact with haptens stimulates keratinocytes and Langerhans cells to release pro-inflammatory cytokines (TNF-α and IL-1), which induce the activation of endothelial cells and facilitate the infiltration of leukocytes. This inflammation is mild and clinically not perceptible. Infiltration of leukocytes at the site of hapten contact increases the change that hapten-specific T cells are recruited. Only in case such hapten-specific T cells are present, hapten-specific T-cell activation by local APCs occurs inducing the release of pro-inflammatory factors from these activated T cells. This will boost the inflammatory process and enhance the recruitment of leukocytes, ultimately (48 to 72 h after contact of the skin with hapten) leading to the clinically perceptible allergic contact dermatitis in sensitized individuals. Further explanation is given in the text.

An alternative concept for the elicitation of CHS has been proposed (Figure 7.8).[428] Haptens themselves can initiate local inflammatory processes in the epidermis and superficial dermis. This induction of inflammation is an important aspect and appears to be dependent on the amount of applied sensitizer. Challenging the skin of a sensitized mouse with very low doses of hapten fails to elicit CHS, but co-administration of an irritant or an irrelevant hapten (to provoke some inflammation) together with the low dose of hapten resulted in a full CHS response.[446] A similar effect has been found in humans.[447] This illustrates that the mere recognition of hapten is not enough to elicit CHS, but that concurrent nonspecific pro-inflammatory signals are required. Keratinocytes are regarded as important signal transducers in this respect, converting environmental stimuli into antigen-independent cutaneous inflammation through the secretion of pro-inflammatory cytokines.[448] The activation of keratinocytes initiates a cascade of events, among others, local induction and upregulation of adhesion molecule ICAM-1 (CD54) on keratinocytes and on endothelial cells.[449,450] Interaction between ICAM-1 and its ligand LFA-1 is clearly involved in the elicitation phase of CHS, because blocking antibodies against these adhesion molecules markedly reduce the CHS response and ICAM-1-deficient mice show impaired CHS.[451,452] The local increased expression of adhesion molecules facilitates and promotes the influx of memory T cells into those sites where skin contacts hapten. These infiltrating T cells will receive some activation signals. However, this activation is assumed to be mild and not sufficient to cause clinically visible contact dermatitis, explaining why no response is elicited in nonsensitized individuals.[428] But, if hapten-specific memory T cells are present in the initial infiltrate, these will be hapten-specifically activated by local APC, and massive amplification of the inflammatory process will occur following cytokine release by these T cells. The activated

CD4+ and CD8+ T cells produce, among others, IFN-γ and TNF-α,[453,454] which boosts the inflammation response, ultimately resulting in a clinical perceptible allergic contact dermatitis.

Memory T cells (in contrast to naive T cells) can be activated by a wide range of professional and nonprofessional APC. The hapten-challenged skin harbors several different kinds of APC, i.e., LCs, LC-precursors, dermal dendritic cells, inflammatory dendritic epidermal cells, and plasmacytoid DCs, but also macrophages, keratinocytes, and fibroblasts, which have acquired MHC class II expression due to the local inflammatory condition of the skin. According to this view, LCs are not necessarily required for the elicitation of CHS. This notion is stressed by the observation that depletion of LCs prior to the elicitation of CHS enhances rather than diminishes the CHS response.[455] The memory T cells, either resident or in the early infiltrate, comprise CD4+ and CD8+ T cells exhibiting a type 1 or type 2 cytokine profile. They can be hapten specific or have irrelevant specificity, and they can have effector or suppressor functions.[437,453,456–459] It is clear that the interplay of all these cells in the early infiltrate in the hapten-challenged skin represents a melting pot of activation and suppression and the ultimate outcome of the immune response is dependent on the delicate balance of stimulatory and inhibitory signals. Lack of sufficient suppression by hapten-specific regulatory T cells may result in the development of allergic contact dermatitis.[437,456] In addition, natural killer cells may also participate in the regulation of immune responses by mutual interaction with DCs.[460,461] Close contact of NK cells with CD1a+ DCs[462] and with plasmacytoid DCs[456] within inflamed skin *in situ* has been observed.

To summarize all in one sentence: The nonspecific pro-inflammatory effects of hapten application enhance the probability for hapten-specific memory T cells to encounter the relevant allergen presented by cutaneous APC and also lower the threshold for induction of a self-amplifying CHS response. Still, the question remains why the skin immune system of CHS-prone individuals overreacts to one or few contact sensitizers but can resist the provocative effects of so many other haptens.

## IV. INDETERMINATE CELLS

At the end of the 1960s a group of LC-like cells in the skin were described, designated indeterminate cells, that display a morphology resembling LCs, but lack the typical BGs.[463] Like LCs, indeterminate cells express CD1a and MHC class II molecules,[464,465] although CD1a− indeterminate cells have been reported as well.[466] In these "early" studies the presence of BGs detected by (immuno)electron microscopy formed the definite proof for the determination of LCs, whereas LC-like cells devoid of BGs were not definable, hence the name indeterminate. However, one has to perform appropriate serial sections of the total intermediate cell to prove that the cell is completely devoid of BGs. In addition, the angle of the electron beam toward the ultrathin section is of crucial importance to detect BGs, and it has been demonstrated that by means of tilting the preparations in the electron microscope it is possible to find BGs in indeterminate cells.[467] It may be concluded that indeterminate cells represent either LC precursors that just arrived in the epidermis and still have to develop BGs or LCs that contain very few numbers of BGs. Alternatively, the indeterminate cell may represent a member of the interstitial DC subset. The designation indeterminate cell emerged in the old days because of ignorance of current knowledge on DCs. At present, as described in this chapter, a good understanding and definition of the myeloid and plasmacytoid DC subsets has developed. In view of this it would be better to disregard indeterminate cell as a separate cell type and to abandon this term.

## V. DERMAL DENDRITIC CELLS

The dermis represents a connective tissue, which is composed of vascularized extracellular matrix and is rich in cutaneous adnexae. In addition, the dermis harbors several different cell types, including members of the DC family. The population of HLA-DR+ DCs in the human dermis is rather heterogeneous,[468] in contrast to the normal epidermis, which is populated by a homologous population of HLA-DR+ LCs. Dermal HLA-DR+ DCs are usually located around capillary vessels in the stratum papillare. A minority of the DCs in the dermis *in situ* stain with either the LC-marker CD1a and/or with IDC-marker RFD1.[240,469] These cells can be observed in the vicinity of dermal lymphatics and may be considered LCs that have left the epidermis and are on their way to the regional lymph node. Of course, the dermis also contains LC precursors that are moving from circulation toward the epidermis. It is not clear whether these LC precursors already express CD1a or whether they obtain this expression after arrival in the epidermal microenvironment. The LC-related cells ($CD1a^{low}CD1c^{+}HLA\text{-}DR^{+}$) in freshly isolated dermal cell suspensions comprise 2.7% ± 1% of the total dermal cells.[468]

On the basis of the intracellular expression of bloodclotting enzyme factor XIII subunit a (FXIIIa), a distinct subset of DCs in the dermis has been identified, the so-called dermal dendrocytes or dermal dendritic cells (DDCs).[470–472] The FXIIIa+ DDCs are mainly found in the papillary dermis and in the upper part of the reticular dermis, predominantly around the superficial blood vessels. By means of double-staining of cryostat sections it is found that the FXIIIa+ DDCs co-express HLA-DR, HLA-DQ (45%), CD11a (LFA-1), CD14 (22%), CD36 (OKM5), and CD45, but not CD11b, CD11c, RFD1, and CD54 (ICAM-1), although the last can be induced by IFN-γ.[471] In addition, MS-1 sinusoidal endothelial antigen can be detected in FXIIIa+ DDC,[473] as well as GPIbα, a Von Willebrand factor receptor and component of the GPIb-IX-V complex.[474] Further, the FXIIIa is not expressed by fibroblasts, endothelial cells, dermal LCs, and T cells *in situ*.[471]

In fresh dermal cell suspensions, four different HLA-DR+ cell subpopulations have been described,[468] indicating that different DC subsets in the dermis may exist. One of these subsets lacks the leukocyte marker CD45 and the typical CD11c expression present on DCs. The remaining three HLA-DR+ subsets all expressed CD45, CD11b, CD11c, and CD32, but can be discriminated by the presence of either CD1a-c or CD36, or by the absence of both markers. Intracellular expression of FXIIIa is present in virtually all CD1a+ cells, but is also present to a lesser extent in the other subsets.[468] These *in vitro* findings differ from the *in situ* observations described in the previous paragraph. The $CD1a^{+}CD1b^{+}CD1c^{+}$ cells are the most powerful HLA-DR+ subset in the dermis to stimulate allogeneic T cells *in vitro*.[468,475] In other investigations, DDCs that migrated from dermal tissue during *in vivo* culture have been studied.[468,476] The DDCs obtained in this way have undergone a process of maturation and therefore may differ from the above-described phenotypes of DDCs *in situ* and in freshly prepared dermal cell suspensions. In one study three subsets of migrated HLA-DR+ DDCs are found that are classified on the expression of CD1a and CD14. In this study all three DDC subsets have FXIIIa expression, but surprisingly, in a different study using the same technique, no DDC subsets are found and no FXIIIa is detected in the migrated DDCs.[476] In both studies the migrated DDCs appear as motile cells, which continually retract and extend or wave their dendritic protrusions, carrying the following markers: HLA-DR (high), HLA-DQ (high), CD1a (low or absent), CD1c, CD11a-c, CD18, CD36 (low, variable), CD40, CD45, CD54 CD58, CD80, IDC marker RFD1, and myeloid markers CD13 and CD33, but lack BGs and CD34. In a recent study, migratory cells from full skin explants were characterized, thus avoiding separation of epidermis and dermis, although yielding a mix of DCs from both epidermal and dermal origin. This makes it complicated to compare this investigation to the aforementioned studies, in which only dermal tissue is used. Nevertheless, in the full skin migratory cells again three DDC populations are identified, but having a different subdivision, i.e., $CD1a^{+}CD14^{-}$ (2 to 5% of total DDC), $CD1a^{-}CD14^{+}$ (25 to 35%), and $CD1a^{-}CD14^{-}$ (55 to 75%).[191] Both CD14+ and CD14− populations express CD45RO, CD116 (GM-CSF receptor), and CD123 (IL-3 receptor), have myeloid markers CD13 and CD33, and carry MHC class I, HLA-DR, CD11b, CD11c, and co-stimulatory molecules CD40, CD54, CD80, and CD86. Other cytokine receptors expressed by DCs migrated from skin explants are IL-1R type 1 and type 2, IL-2R a and γ chains, IL-4R, IL-6 and its signal transducer CD130, IL-7R, GM-CSF receptor α and β chains, TNF receptor II, and IFN-γR, whereas these cells are negative for IL-8R, TNF receptor I, G-CSF

**TABLE 7.3**
**Phenotypical Comparison between Resident Epidermal LCs and Dermal DCs[a]**

| Marker | LCs | DDCs |
|---|---|---|
| Lag (Birbeck granule) | +[b] | – |
| Langerin (CD207) | + | – |
| MHC class I | + | + |
| MHC class II (DR, DP, DQ) | + | + |
| CD1a | + | –/+[c] |
| CD1b | – | + |
| CD1c | + | + |
| CD1d | – | + |
| LFA-1 (CD11a) | – | + |
| CD14 | – | +[c] |
| CD36 | – | + |
| FXIIIa | – | + |
| CD11b | + | + |
| CD11c | + | + |
| CD205 | + | + |
| CD206 | – | + |
| DC-SIGN (CD209) | – | + |
| DCIR | – | + |
| DC-ASGPR | – | + |
| H1 receptor | – | + |
| H2 receptor | – | + |

[a] This table was compiled from various different studies as stated in the text.
[b] Arbitrary units: – absent; + present.
[c] Subset positive.

receptor, and M-CSF receptor.[477] Only CD14$^+$, but not CD14$^-$ DDCs are CD207$^+$ and CD36$^+$ (subset). Conversely, only CD14$^-$, but not CD14$^+$ DDCs express CD83 and FXIIIa. The CD14$^-$ DDCs display mature features, like CD83, bean-shaped nuclei, and abundant surface prolongations, whereas CD14$^+$ DDCs have more immature features, such as oval nuclei, lack of veils or dendrites, and capability of macropinocytosis and receptor-mediated endocytosis. In connection to this, DDCs have been reported to express the C-type lectins CD206,[239] DC-SIGN (CD209),[44] DCIR,[46] and DC-ASGPR,[45] which all are absent on LCs (Table 7.3). The same holds true for both the two histamine receptors H1 and H2.[273]

At electron microscopic level, interaction of FXIIIa$^+$ DDC with the extracellular matrix can be appreciated as transmembrane associations of intracellular actin filaments and extracellular fibronectin microfibrils.[478] In addition, a close anatomical association between DDCs and mast cells has been noted.[478] About 70% of the mast cells are spatially related to DDCs and conversely, 20 to 40% of the DDCs are closely associated with mast cells.[479] Three-dimensional reconstruction of electron microscopic images reveals that the thin elongated dendrites of DDCs (as observed in two-dimensional photographs) are in fact thin membrane flaps.[479] These membrane flaps enshroud mast cell membranes for 50 to 90% of their perimeter, giving the impression of a ball (mast cell) in a baseball glove (DDC). Induced degranulation of mast cells in cultured skin explants enhances the expression of FXIIIa.[478] This process can be mimicked by TNF-α,[478] a predominant cytokine in the granules of dermal mast cells.[480] Blocking mast cell degranulation or anti-TNF-α abrogates this FXIIIa induction, indicating that this process is TNF-α dependent. The GPIbα expression by DDCs is transiently upregulated after mast cell degranulation, but in contrast, this increase likely appears to be TNF-α independent.[474] The functional relationship between DDCs and mast cells may be relevant *in vivo* in case of damage to dermal blood capillaries. Mast cells degranulate soon after injury or during the early stages of inflammation and stimulate the local DDCs to produce FXIIIa, a fibrin- and fibronectin-stabilizing factor, the last enzyme in the coagulation cascade, as well as to increase GPIbα expression, enforcing interaction with Von Willebrand factor on endothelial cells and possibly thrombin in the extracellular matrix.

Distinct from the FXIIIa$^+$ DDCs, another type of cell with dendritic morphology has been described in the human dermis, which is identified by the expression of hematopoietic progenitor antigen CD34.[481] These CD34$^+$ cells are located in the reticular and deep dermis rather than in the papillary dermis. The CD34$^+$ cells express antigens common to mesenchymal cells (e.g., vimentin), indicating a mesodermal derivation.[482] Only 2% of the CD34$^+$ cells co-express HLA-DR, but none of the CD34$^+$ cells exhibits markers that are displayed by other cutaneous DCs, such as CD1a, BGs, FXIIIa, CD11a, CD14, CD36, and CD54.[482] Apart from their dendritic morphology, these CD34$^+$ cells are likely not immunologically active and have nothing in common with the DC family that possesses a high antigen-presenting potential to stimulate naive T cells. Therefore, the dendritic CD34$^+$ cells observed in the dermis are beyond the scope of this chapter.

## VI. INFLAMMATORY DENDRITIC EPIDERMAL CELLS

In inflammatory skin conditions (e.g., in lesional skin of atopic eczema, psoriasis, allergic contact dermatitis, and mycosis fungoides), two phenotypical different coexisting CD1a$^+$ subpopulations can be distinguished in the epidermis by means of FACS analysis.[483,484] The first subset comprises the classical LC with the phenotype CD1a$^{bright}$CD1b$^{neg}$FcεRI$^{dim}$CD36$^{dim}$ and a strong staining with the BG-specific antibody Lag, whereas the second population of CD1a$^+$ cells, present in variable numbers, can be recognized as CD1a$^{dim}$CD1b$^{dim}$FcεRI$^{bright}$CD36$^{bright}$ and the absence of reactivity with the Lag antibody. Both epidermal CD1a$^+$ populations have a high expression of HLA-DR and a low expression of CD32. Based on the different phenotype and the clear-cut presence or absence of BGs, it was postulated that these Lag-negative cells represent an entirely distinct cell population rather than a differentiation stage of LCs. Because the manifestation of this distinct population is most clear in inflamed skin, it was proposed to call these cells inflammatory dendritic epidermal cells (IDECs).[483] However, the markers CD1b and CD36 are typically expressed by DCs in the dermis. Therefore, on the other hand, it may also be hypothesized that IDECs represent an interstitial type of DCs, which under nonpathologic circumstances occupy the dermis, but are relocated to the epidermis due to the inflammatory condition of the skin. The CD1a expression on these cells, albeit lower than on LCs, is induced by the epidermal microenvironment. Remarkably, the LC population in inflamed skin exhibited a low expression of CD36,[483] whereas the classical LC is CD36 negative. This finding suggests that CD36 might be inducible on LCs by factor(s) present in inflamed skin, such as IFN-γ, which has been demonstrated to upregulate CD36 expression on human dermal-derived, but not umbilical-derived, endothelial cells.[485]

IDECs have a LC-like distribution pattern and can be found at a suprabasal and basal level in the epidermis. There exists a substantial interindividual variation in the percentage of the IDECs in the entire epidermal CD1a$^+$ cell population.[483,486] Whereas LCs are normal residents of the epidermis, IDECs are considered to migrate *de novo* into this compartment during skin inflammation. The IDECs in lesional skin of various inflammatory skin diseases express different levels of FcεRI, FcγRII (CD32), CD36.[483,486] This may be explained by differences in the local cytokine pattern, which of course vary from one skin disease to one other, but which are also affected by the gravity of the disease. It has been suggested that the expression ratio of the receptors FcεRI and FcγRII can be used as a diagnostic tool to differentiate atopic eczema (ratio exceeding 3) from other inflammatory skin diseases (ratios 1 or less).[486] In addition, the level of CD36 expression is shown to be related to the inflammatory activity inside the epidermal compartment.[486] IDECs in lesional epidermis of patients with atopic eczema display the highest expression of FcεRI, reaching levels surpassing markedly those appreciated on IDECs in other inflammatory skin diseases.[483] The FcεRI expression on CD1a+ cells from any inflammatory skin disease correlates significantly with the serum IgE level in these patients, but this correlation is the strongest in the group of atopic eczema patients.[486] In this skin disease the high expression of FcεRI is assumed to play an important role in the pathogenesis of atopic eczema through the IgE-mediated uptake and focusing of environmental allergens leading to amplification of the activation of allergen-specific T cells.[487]

Apart from the differential expression of CD1a, CD1b, FcεRI, and CD36, IDECs can also be discriminated from LCs in fresh epidermal cell suspensions by the strong expression of the integrins CD11a and CD11b[488] and the mannose receptor CD206,[489] which all are absent on LCs. In addition, IDECs, but not LCs, do display the low-affinity receptor for IgE (FcεRII/CD23).[490] These receptors can be removed by acid stripping, indicating that the CD23 molecules are not membrane anchored, but rather are soluble FcεRII, which are attached to the IDECs via as-yet-unidentified binding sites.[490] Likely candidates for this binding are CD11b and CD11c, because it has been reported that CD11b and CD11c on monocytes can bind soluble FcεRII, leading to FcεRII-mediated activation of the monocytes.[491] The finding that FcεRII expression on IDECs correlates with both CD11b and CD11c surface staining supports this speculation.[490] The IDECs have a higher expression of CD80 and CD86 than LCs from inflammatory skin.[492] The level of CD80 and CD86 appears to be correlated to the expression level of CD36. The enhanced expression of CD80, CD86, and CD36 in atopic dermatitis lesions may be due to locally produced IFN-γ, a stimulatory cytokine known to be expressed in chronic but not in acute atopic dermatitis lesions.[493] Recently, an *in vitro* model has been established to generate IDECs from peripheral blood monocytes.[494] IL-4 plus GM-CSF-treated monocytes from exclusively atopic but not non-atopic individuals differentiate into IDECs if the culture is performed in the presence of reducing agents, such as 2-mercaptoethanol or dithiothreitol. These *in vitro* generated IDECs have all the aforementioned characteristics of lesional atopic dermatitis skin-derived IDECs, including the typical high surface expression of FcεRI. Because cultures supplemented with GM-CSF plus IL-4 usually generate the interstitial type of DCs, the outcome of this study suggests that IDECs belong to the interstitial branch of the DC family. Activation of *in vitro* generated IDECs through engagement of FcεRI induces the production and release of pro-inflammatory cytokines IL-1α and IL-1β and chemokines CCL3, CCL5, and IL-16.[494,495]

## VII. CUTANEOUS PLASMACYTOID DENDRITIC CELLS

Although plasmacytoid DCs (PDCs) have been described just since the late 1990s,[176,496] this cell has in fact been known for a much longer time under different identities. A rare cell type with plasma cell-like morphology occurring mostly in clusters in the paracortical area (the T-cell zones) of reactive lymph nodes was already discovered in 1958.[497] In Giemsa-stained sections the cytoplasm is gray-blue and not dark blue as in typical plasma cells. Electron microscopic studies on this so-called lymphoblast have shown the presence of well-developed concentric rough endoplasmatic reticulum, resembling the morphology of a plasma cell.[498] In 1975, this unique cell was designated T-associated plasma cell, because of the close association of this cell type with T cells and T-cell-dependent areas of lymphoid tissue.[499] In the 1980s, it became apparent that these plasma cell-like cells display both T-cell (CD4 and CD62L, but not CD2, CD3, CD5, CD7, and CD8) and monocyte markers (CD36, CD68, and HLA-DR), but lack B-cell markers (intracellular immunoglobulins, CD19, and CD20); hence they are renamed into plasmacytoid T cells and subsequently into plasmacytoid monocytes.[500–503] In the same period, HLA-DR+ IFN-α-producing leucocytes have been described.[504,505] The real identity and function of this peculiar cell with so many different names remained enigmatic for a long time. In 1997, the mystery was elucidated as it was demonstrated that this HLA-DR+ cell represents a special type of DC, having a typically high expression of the IL-3 receptor α chain (CD123),[496] which can develop into mature DCs during culture in the presence of IL-3 and CD40-ligand.[176] Dependent on the presence or absence of viral molecules during the maturation step, the mature PDCs can stimulate naive T cells to produce type 1 cytokines[506] or type 2 cytokines,[192] respectively. In their precursor state the PDCs can produce huge amounts of IFN-α/β in response to certain viruses.[105] PDCs display a different migration behavior and chemokine production profile, as compared to myeloid DCs, and they localize predominantly in secondary lymphoid organs.[507]

Long before their final designation as PDCs, dermatopathologists were already aware of these special plasmacytoid cells, which can be appreciated in affected skin of certain disorders, but not in normal human skin. The PDCs can be recognized in Giemsa- or hematoxylin–eosin-stained sections in lesional skin as medium-sized (10 to 12 μm) cells that are markedly larger than surrounding small lymphocytes. They have relatively pale nuclei with condensation of the chromatin along the clearly demarcated nuclear membrane and with a prominent nucleolus, and the relatively abundant cytoplasm stains weakly. The characteristic parallel-oriented profiles of rough endoplasmatic reticulum curved around the nucleus can be appreciated by means of electron microscopy (Figure 7.9). The nuclei are round to oval and have mostly a single deep slit-like indention. It is important to note that the fixation method is critical to enable the recognition of PDCs in fixed tissue: the generally applied 10% formalin fixation disables the recognition of PDCs.[500] The plasmacytoid cells have been identified in cutaneous lymphoid hyperplasia[508,509] and in mycosis fungoides.[510] PDCs are present in single or multiple small or large clusters within the perivascular and periadnexal infiltrates in approximately 60% of the biopsy specimens from patients suffering from Jessner-Kanof's disease (Figure 7.10).[511,512] PDCs can also be observed in biopsies from lesional skin of patients with discoid lupus erythematosus and systemic lupus erythematosus,[512,513] whereas these cells do not occur in lesional skin of patients with polymorphic light eruption.[512] The dermal endothelium in cutaneous lupus erythematosus lesions, but not in normal skin, expresses the L-selectin ligand PNAd (peripheral lymph node adressin),[513] which is normally expressed by high endothelial venules in secondary lymphoid organs. This PNAd expression on the dermal capillaries enables the circulating PDCs, having a high L-selectin (CD62L) expression, to extravasate in the skin. Increased expression of IFN-α/β-inducible intracellular protein MxA in cutaneous lupus erythematosus lesions correlates well with the density of PDCs, suggesting that these cells produce IFN-α/β locally.[513] PDCs can also be detected in cutaneous lesions caused by varicella zoster virus[514] and in the peritumoral area in primary cutaneous melanomas.[515] In skin sections PDCs can be identified by the co-expression of CD123, CD45RA, CD68, and HLA-DR (Table 7.4).[513] Immunophenotyping of PDCs in lesional skin in case of cutaneous lymphoid hyperplasia, Jessner-Kanof's disease, and lupus erythematosus reveals that these cells also express CD4, CD36, CD43, CD74, CD62L, and CLA (HECA452), but are devoid of CD1a, CD11b, CD11c, CD14, CD15, and S-100 antigen.[508,509,511,512,515] Surprisingly, PDCs have recently been found in the epidermis of inflamed skin of patients with atopic dermatitis, contact dermatitis, and psoriasis,[177] as well as in the (epi)dermis of epicutaneous patch test reactions[456] on the basis of expression of CD123 and PDC-marker BDCA-2. As yet, it is not clear whether PDCs play a role in the pathogenesis of these skin disorders or whether these cells simply represent an item of the inflammatory process.

## VIII. FINAL REMARKS

Over the past several years a considerable increase in the knowledge on LCs and DCs has emerged, especially due to improved methods to generate large numbers of DCs from $CD14^+$ blood monocytes or $CD34^+$ hematopoietic stem cells. It is now clear that the family of DCs can be classified into three separate lineages, i.e., the epithelial DC (or LC), the interstitial DC, and the plasmacytoid DC. Apart from these three populations, the existence of other subsets has been suggested (among others, the IDEC[483] and the $CD11c^{low}CD45RB^{high}$ PDC-like tolerance-inducing DC[516]), but further

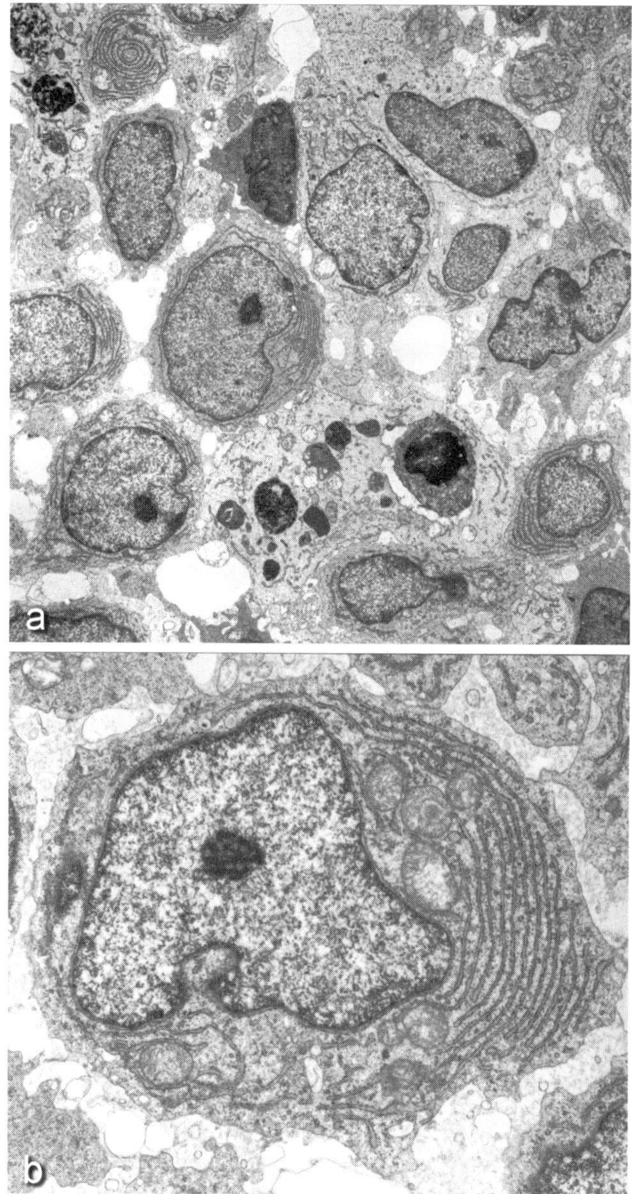


**FIGURE 7.9** Low-power electron micrograph of a Jessner's infiltration of the skin containing PDCs, which display their characteristic parallel strands of ER (a). Higher magnification of a single PDC (b). For details, see text. (Courtesy of Dr. J. Toonstra, University Medical Center Utrecht, the Netherlands. From Toonstra, J. and van der Putte, S.C., *Am. J. Dermatopathol.*, 13, 321, 1991. With permission.)

proof is needed to assess whether this concerns genuine separate lineages or just represents differentiation or maturation stages of one of the established DCs lineages. As concerns normal human skin, this tissue contains only immature epithelial and interstitial types of DCs (LCs and DDCs, respectively). However, in the case of infection or inflammatory skin disorders the situation is different. Altered numbers and distribution of LCs and DDCs, as well as mature intracutaneous DCs can be observed (expression of maturation marker CD83), and, in addition, IDECs and PDCs can also be detected in the diseased skin.

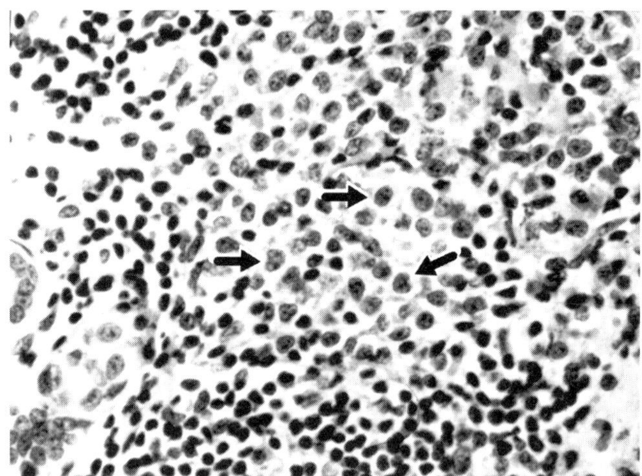

**FIGURE 7.10** Jessner's infiltration of the skin containing PDCs indicated by arrows. For details, see text. (Courtesy of Dr. J. Toonstra, University Medical Center Utrecht, the Netherlands. From Toonstra, J. and van der Putte, S.C., *Am. J. Dermatopathol.,* 13, 321, 1991. With permission.)

**TABLE 7.4**
**DC Subsets Present in Diseased Human Skin**[a]

| Marker | LCs | DDCs | IDECs | PDCs |
|---|---|---|---|---|
| HLA-DR | ++[b] | ++ | ++ | ++ |
| Lag (Birbeck granule) | ++ | – | – | – |
| CD1a | ++ | – | + | – |
| Langerin (CD207) | ++ | – | – | – |
| CD11b | + | + | + | – |
| CD11c | + | + | + | – |
| CD33 | + | + | + | – |
| CD36 | –/+[c] | ++ | + | + |
| FXIIIa | – | ++ | – | – |
| CD45RO | + | + | + | – |
| CD45RA | – | – | – | + |
| CD123 | – | – | – | ++ |
| BDCA-2 | – | – | – | + |

[a] This table was compiled from various different studies as stated in the text.
[b] Arbitrary units: – absent; + present.
[c] Weak expression, negative in normal skin.

There is a general belief that immature DCs have the primary task to take up and process pathogens or foreign antigens they encounter in the peripheral tissues. For this purpose DCs are equipped with an array of receptors, which like sensory organs make it possible to discriminate different pathogens resulting in pathogen-specific gene expression profiles.[517] In addition, the immature DCs also sense antigen- or pathogen-induced changes (e.g., inflammatory cytokines) or the lack of such changes (e.g., when taking up apoptotic cells in absence of inflammation) in the surrounding tissue. These two experiences (danger and inflammation) in the periphery likely determine the process of DC maturation and eventually the stimulatory potential as well as the polarizing signals of these APCs leading to the activation of relevant T-cell repertoires in the draining lymphoid tissue. This strategy enables an organism in case of infection to generate DCs endowed with powerful co-stimulatory potential, provoking vigorous type 1 or type 2 T-cell responses, dependent of the pathogen species. In the absence of danger (in the steady state), however, the maturation process will be suboptimal and the semimature DCs that arrive in the lymph nodes have low or no co-stimulatory properties, giving rise to regulatory T cells responsible for peripheral tolerance. This view corresponds with the observation that lymphoid organs harbor a large cohort of phenotypical and functional immature DCs in the steady state.[518] Inflammatory skin diseases may arise from disturbance of the subtle balance between DC-derived activation and tolerance-generating signals. The determination of alterations in number and distribution of the different DC subsets in diseased skin, as well as changes in phenotype and function of these cells, may provide insight into which role the different cutaneous DCs play in the development and perpetuation of inflammatory skin diseases.

The recognition of DCs as potent inducers of either antigen-specific immunity or tolerance has led to the challenge to exploit DCs as tools for vaccination. Although several small clinical DC vaccination studies have been performed in humans, the therapeutic application of DCs is still in its infancy. A variable rate of success is reported after vaccination of patients with melanoma with peptide- or tumor lysate-pulsed DCs.[519–521] The observation that the majority of the intracutaneously injected DCs remains at the injection site, whereas a small fraction could reach the lymph node,[522] indicates that this therapy in humans is far from efficient and emphasizes the necessity to further improve our understanding of the regulation of DC migration. The injected mature DCs remaining in the inoculation site nevertheless seem to be involved in specific immune modulation.[523] Studies in mice indicate that co-administration of pro-inflammatory cytokine TNF-$\alpha$ can increase the number of injected antigen-pulsed DCs that reach the lymph node.[524] The way to pulse DCs *in vitro* or *in vivo* with the relevant antigen appears to be important, because some of the receptors on DCs are able to induce signals that render DCs tolerogenic instead of inducers of protective immunity.[525] An alternative way to deliver antigen to DCs is to transfect these cells with DNA encoding for the relevant antigen. LCs transfected *in situ* with plasmids containing melanoma antigen MART-1 are able to migrate and to activate MART-1-specific cytotoxic T cells.[526] Mature DCs are believed to induce long-lasting T-cell-mediated specific immunity, whereas immature DCs are associated with the induction of regulatory T cells or deletion of effector T cells resulting in tolerance. In relation to the latter aspect, vaccination with immature DCs would be an interesting tool to treat unwanted immune responses, such as allergic contact dermatitis. However, one should be aware that the administered antigen-laden immature DCs do not act like Trojan horses, because maturation of these cells upon injection would exacerbate rather than ameliorate the disease. Therefore, insight into how to control the stability of the immature state of the DCs after injection is highly important. In the years that lie ahead, knowledge on DC biology will further increase and may eventually lead to the development of safe, sophisticated immunotherapies for different kinds of skin disorders, using DCs either as powerful vaccine adjuvants to treat skin cancer and infections or as potent blocking agents to intercept useless autoimmune inflammatory skin diseases.

## REFERENCES

1. Bos, J.D. and Kapsenberg, M.L., The skin immune system: its cellular constituents and their interactions, *Immunol. Today*, 7, 235, 1986.
2. Bos, J.D. and Kapsenberg, M.L., The skin immune system: progress in cutaneous biology, *Immunol. Today*, 14, 75, 1993.
3. Shortman, K. and Liu, Y.J., Mouse and human dendritic cell subtypes, *Nat. Rev. Immunol.*, 2, 151, 2002.
4. Hart, D.N., Dendritic cells: unique leukocyte populations which control the primary immune response, *Blood*, 90, 3245, 1997.
5. Banchereau, J. et al., Immunobiology of dendritic cells, *Annu. Rev. Immunol.*, 18, 767, 2000.

6. Guermonprez, P. et al., Antigen presentation and T cell stimulation by dendritic cells, *Annu. Rev. Immunol.*, 20, 621, 2002.
7. Banchereau, J. and Steinman, R.M., Dendritic cells and the control of immunity, *Nature*, 392, 245, 1998.
8. Steinman, R.M. and Cohn, Z.A., Identification of a novel cell type in peripheral lymphoid organs of mice. I. Morphology, quantitation, tissue distribution, *J. Exp. Med.*, 137, 1142, 1973.
9. Steinman, R.M. et al., Identification of a novel cell type in peripheral lymphoid organs of mice. V. Purification of spleen dendritic cells, new surface markers, and maintenance *in vitro*, *J. Exp. Med.*, 149, 1, 1979.
10. Teunissen, M.B.M. et al., Dendritic cells as accessory cells in antigen-specific murine T lymphocyte proliferation *in vitro*, *J. Immunol. Methods*, 77, 131, 1985.
11. Steinman, R.M., The dendritic cell system and its role in immunogenicity, *Annu. Rev. Immunol.*, 9, 271, 1991.
12. Van Voorhis, W.C. et al., Relative efficacy of human monocytes and dendritic cells as accessory cells for T cell replication, *J. Exp. Med.*, 158, 174, 1983.
13. Bjercke, S. and Gaudernack, G., Dendritic cells and monocytes as accessory cells in T-cell responses in man. II. Function as antigen-presenting cells, *Scand. J. Immunol.*, 21, 501, 1985.
14. Steinman, R.M., Pack, M., and Inaba, K., Dendritic cells in the T-cell areas of lymphoid organs, *Immunol. Rev.*, 156, 25, 1997.
15. Veldman, J.E., Histophysiology and Electron Microscopy of the Immune Response, thesis, N.V. Boekdrukkerij Dijkstra Niemeyer, Groningen, 1970.
16. Hart, D.N. and Fabre, J.W., Demonstration and characterization of Ia-positive dendritic cells in the interstitial connective tissues of rat heart and other tissues, but not brain, *J. Exp. Med.*, 154, 347, 1981.
17. Van Voorhis, W.C. et al., Human dendritic cells. Enrichment and characterization from peripheral blood, *J. Exp. Med.*, 155, 1172, 1982.
18. Knight, S.C. et al., Non-adherent, low-density cells from human peripheral blood contain dendritic cells and monocytes, both with veiled morphology, *Immunology*, 57, 595, 1986.
19. Drexhage, H.A. et al., A study of cells present in peripheral lymph of pigs with special reference to a type of cell resembling the Langerhans cell, *Cell Tissue Res.*, 202, 407, 1979.
20. Knight, S.C., Veiled cells — "dendritic cells" of the peripheral lymph, *Immunobiology*, 168, 349, 1984.
21. Sallusto, F. et al., Dendritic cells use macropinocytosis and the mannose receptor to concentrate macromolecules in the major histocompatibility complex class II compartment: downregulation by cytokines and bacterial products, *J. Exp. Med.*, 182, 389, 1995.
22. Romani, N. et al., Presentation of exogenous protein antigens by dendritic cells to T cell clones. Intact protein is presented best by immature, epidermal Langerhans cells, *J. Exp. Med.*, 169, 1169, 1989.
23. Streilein, J.W. et al., Functional dichotomy between Langerhans cells that present antigen to naive and to memory/effector T lymphocytes, *Immunol. Rev.*, 117, 159, 1990.
24. Swanson, J.A., Phorbol esters stimulate macropinocytosis and solute flow through macrophages, *J. Cell Sci.*, 94, 135, 1989.
25. Steinman, R.M. and Swanson, J., The endocytic activity of dendritic cells, *J. Exp. Med.*, 182, 283, 1995.
26. Fanger, N.A. et al., Type I (CD64) and type II (CD32) Fcγ receptor-mediated phagocytosis by human blood dendritic cells, *J. Immunol.*, 157, 541, 1996.
27. Maurer, D. et al., Peripheral blood dendritic cells express FcεRI as a complex composed of FcεRIα- and FcεRI γ-chains and can use this receptor for IgE-mediated allergen presentation, *J. Immunol.*, 157, 607, 1996.
28. Bieber, T. et al., Induction of FcεR2/CD23 on human epidermal Langerhans cells by human recombinant interleukin 4 and γ interferon, *J. Exp. Med.*, 170, 309, 1989.
29. Geissmann, F. et al., A subset of human dendritic cells expresses IgA Fc receptor (CD89), which mediates internalization and activation upon cross-linking by IgA complexes, *J. Immunol.*, 166, 346, 2001.
30. Thomas, R. and Lipsky, P.E., Human peripheral blood dendritic cell subsets. Isolation and characterization of precursor and mature antigen-presenting cells, *J. Immunol.*, 153, 4016, 1994.
31. O'Doherty, U. et al., Dendritic cells freshly isolated from human blood express CD4 and mature into typical immunostimulatory dendritic cells after culture in monocyte-conditioned medium, *J. Exp. Med.*, 178, 1067, 1993.

32. Morelli, A. et al., Expression and modulation of C5a receptor (CD88) on skin dendritic cells. Chemotactic effect of C5a on skin migratory dendritic cells, *Immunology*, 89, 126, 1996.
33. Medzhitov, R., Toll-like receptors and innate immunity, *Nat. Rev. Immunol.*, 1, 135, 2001.
34. Kadowaki, N. et al., Subsets of human dendritic cell precursors express different Toll-like receptors and respond to different microbial antigens, *J. Exp. Med.*, 194, 863, 2001.
35. Jarrossay, D. et al., Specialization and complementarity in microbial molecule recognition by human myeloid and plasmacytoid dendritic cells, *Eur. J. Immunol.*, 31, 3388, 2001.
36. Weis, W.I., Taylor, M.E., and Drickamer, K., The C-type lectin superfamily in the immune system, *Immunol. Rev.*, 163, 19, 1998.
37. Kogelberg, H. and Feizi, T., New structural insights into lectin-type proteins of the immune system, *Curr. Opin. Struct. Biol.*, 11, 635, 2001.
38. Jiang, W. et al., The receptor DEC-205 expressed by dendritic cells and thymic epithelial cells is involved in antigen processing, *Nature*, 375, 151, 1995.
39. Kato, M. et al., Expression of multilectin receptors and comparative FITC-dextran uptake by human dendritic cells, *Int. Immunol.*, 12, 1511, 2000.
40. Ariizumi, K. et al., Identification of a novel, dendritic cell-associated molecule, dectin-1, by subtractive cDNA cloning, *J. Biol. Chem.*, 275, 20157, 2000.
41. Yokota, K. et al., Identification of a human homologue of the dendritic cell-associated C-type lectin-1, dectin-1, *Gene*, 272, 51, 2001.
42. Ariizumi, K. et al., Cloning of a second dendritic cell-associated C-type lectin (dectin-2) and its alternatively spliced isoforms, *J. Biol. Chem.*, 275, 11957, 2000.
43. Colonna, M., Samaridis, J., and Angman, L., Molecular characterization of two novel C-type lectin-like receptors, one of which is selectively expressed in human dendritic cells, *Eur. J. Immunol.*, 30, 697, 2000.
44. Geijtenbeek, T.B. et al., Identification of DC-SIGN, a novel dendritic cell-specific ICAM-3 receptor that supports primary immune responses, *Cell*, 100, 575, 2000.
45. Valladeau, J. et al., Immature human dendritic cells express asialoglycoprotein receptor isoforms for efficient receptor-mediated endocytosis, *J. Immunol.*, 167, 5767, 2001.
46. Bates, E.E. et al., APCs express DCIR, a novel C-type lectin surface receptor containing an immunoreceptor tyrosine-based inhibitory motif, *J. Immunol.*, 163, 1973, 1999.
47. Arce, I. et al., Molecular and genomic characterization of human DLEC, a novel member of the C-type lectin receptor gene family preferentially expressed on monocyte-derived dendritic cells, *Eur. J. Immunol.*, 31, 2733, 2001.
48. Dzionek, A. et al., BDCA-2, a novel plasmacytoid dendritic cell-specific type II C-type lectin, mediates antigen capture and is a potent inhibitor of interferon $\alpha/\beta$ induction, *J. Exp. Med.*, 194, 1823, 2001.
49. Ryan, E.J. et al., Dendritic cell-associated lectin-1: a novel dendritic cell-associated, C-type lectin-like molecule enhances T cell secretion of IL-4, *J. Immunol.*, 169, 5638, 2002.
50. Geijtenbeek, T.B. et al., DC-SIGN, a dendritic cell-specific HIV-1-binding protein that enhances trans-infection of T cells, *Cell*, 100, 587, 2000.
51. Basu, S. et al., Necrotic but not apoptotic cell death releases heat shock proteins, which deliver a partial maturation signal to dendritic cells and activate the NF-kappa B pathway, *Int. Immunol.*, 12, 1539, 2000.
52. Basu, S. et al., CD91 is a common receptor for heat shock proteins gp96, hsp90, hsp70, and calreticulin, *Immunity*, 14, 303, 2001.
53. Ohashi, K. et al., Cutting edge: heat shock protein 60 is a putative endogenous ligand of the Toll-like receptor-4 complex, *J. Immunol.*, 164, 558, 2000.
54. Rubartelli, A., Poggi, A., and Zocchi, M.R., The selective engulfment of apoptotic bodies by dendritic cells is mediated by the $\alpha(v)\beta3$ integrin and requires intracellular and extracellular calcium, *Eur. J. Immunol.*, 27, 1893, 1997.
55. Albert, M.L. et al., Immature dendritic cells phagocytose apoptotic cells via $\alpha v\beta 5$ and CD36, and cross-present antigens to cytotoxic T lymphocytes, *J. Exp. Med.*, 188, 1359, 1998.
56. Ogden, C.A. et al., C1q and mannose binding lectin engagement of cell surface calreticulin and CD91 initiates macropinocytosis and uptake of apoptotic cells, *J. Exp. Med.*, 194, 781, 2001.
57. Nauta, A.J. et al., Recognition and clearance of apoptotic cells: a role for complement and pentraxins, *Trends Immunol.*, 24, 148, 2003.

58. Panther, E. et al., Expression and function of adenosine receptors in human dendritic cells, *FASEB J.*, 15, 1963, 2001.
59. Shi, Y., Evans, J.E., and Rock, K.L., Molecular identification of a danger signal that alerts the immune system to dying cells, *Nature*, 425, 516, 2003.
60. Geuze, H.J., The role of endosomes and lysosomes in MHC class II functioning, *Immunol. Today*, 19, 282, 1998.
61. Neefjes, J.J. and Ploegh, H.L., Intracellular transport of MHC class II molecules, *Immunol. Today*, 13, 179, 1992.
62. Roche, P.A. and Cresswell, P., Invariant chain association with HLA-DR molecules inhibits immunogenic peptide binding, *Nature*, 345, 615, 1990.
63. Lamb, C.A. et al., Invariant chain targets HLA class II molecules to acidic endosomes containing internalized influenza virus, *Proc. Natl. Acad. Sci. U.S.A*, 88, 5998, 1991.
64. Morris, P. et al., An essential role for HLA-DM in antigen presentation by class II major histocompatibility molecules, *Nature*, 368, 551, 1994.
65. Coux, O., Tanaka, K., and Goldberg, A.L., Structure and functions of the 20S and 26S proteasomes, *Annu. Rev. Biochem.*, 65, 801, 1996.
66. Brooks, P. et al., Association of immunoproteasomes with the endoplasmic reticulum, *Biochem. J.*, 352, 611, 2000.
67. Hwang, L.Y. et al., Functional regulation of immunoproteasomes and transporter associated with antigen processing, *Immunol. Res.*, 24, 245, 2001.
68. Pamer, E. and Cresswell, P., Mechanisms of MHC class I–restricted antigen processing, *Annu. Rev. Immunol.*, 16, 323, 1998.
69. Cresswell, P. et al., The nature of the MHC class I peptide loading complex, *Immunol. Rev.*, 172, 21, 1999.
70. Bouvier, M., Accessory proteins and the assembly of human class I MHC molecules: a molecular and structural perspective, *Mol. Immunol.*, 39, 697, 2003.
71. Reis e Sousa and Germain, R.N., Major histocompatibility complex class I presentation of peptides derived from soluble exogenous antigen by a subset of cells engaged in phagocytosis, *J. Exp. Med.*, 182, 841, 1995.
72. Norbury, C.C. et al., Constitutive macropinocytosis allows TAP-dependent major histocompatibility complex class I presentation of exogenous soluble antigen by bone marrow-derived dendritic cells, *Eur. J. Immunol.*, 27, 280, 1997.
73. Shen, Z. et al., Cloned dendritic cells can present exogenous antigens on both MHC class I and class II molecules, *J. Immunol.*, 158, 2723, 1997.
74. Pfeifer, J.D. et al., Phagocytic processing of bacterial antigens for class I MHC presentation to T cells, *Nature*, 361, 359, 1993.
75. Kurts, C. et al., Dendritic cells are sufficient to cross-present self-antigens to CD8 T cells *in vivo*, *J. Immunol.*, 166, 1439, 2001.
76. Rodriguez, A. et al., Selective transport of internalized antigens to the cytosol for MHC class I presentation in dendritic cells, *Nat. Cell Biol.*, 1, 362, 1999.
77. Guermonprez, P. et al., ER-phagosome fusion defines an MHC class I cross-presentation compartment in dendritic cells, *Nature*, 425, 397, 2003.
78. Houde, M. et al., Phagosomes are competent organelles for antigen cross-presentation, *Nature*, 425, 402, 2003.
79. Moody, D.B. and Porcelli, S.A., Intracellular pathways of CD1 antigen presentation, *Nat. Rev. Immunol.*, 3, 11, 2003.
80. Calabi, F. and Milstein, C., A novel family of human major histocompatibility complex-related genes not mapping to chromosome 6, *Nature*, 323, 540, 1986.
81. Gerlini, G. et al., Cd1d is expressed on dermal dendritic cells and monocyte-derived dendritic cells, *J. Invest. Dermatol.*, 117, 576, 2001.
82. Angenieux, C. et al., Characterization of CD1e, a third type of CD1 molecule expressed in dendritic cells, *J. Biol. Chem.*, 275, 37757, 2000.
83. Blumberg, R.S. et al., Structure and function of the CD1 family of MHC-like cell surface proteins, *Immunol. Rev.*, 147, 5, 1995.

84. Beckman, E.M. et al., Recognition of a lipid antigen by CD1-restricted $\alpha$ $\beta^+$ T cells, *Nature*, 372, 691, 1994.
85. Starling, G.C. et al., Intercellular adhesion molecule-3 is the predominant co-stimulatory ligand for leukocyte function antigen-1 on human blood dendritic cells, *Eur. J. Immunol.*, 25, 2528, 1995.
86. Prickett, T.C., McKenzie, J.L., and Hart, D.N., Adhesion molecules on human tonsil dendritic cells, *Transplantation*, 53, 483, 1992.
87. McLellan, A.D. et al., Activation of human peripheral blood dendritic cells induces the CD86 co-stimulatory molecule, *Eur. J. Immunol.*, 25, 2064, 1995.
88. Fagnoni, F.F. et al., Role of B70/B7-2 in CD4+ T-cell immune responses induced by dendritic cells, *Immunology*, 85, 467, 1995.
89. Walunas, T.L. et al., CTLA-4 can function as a negative regulator of T cell activation, *Immunity*, 1, 405, 1994.
90. Yoshinaga, S.K. et al., T-cell co-stimulation through B7RP-1 and ICOS, *Nature*, 402, 827, 1999.
91. Coyle, A.J. and Gutierrez-Ramos, J.C., The expanding B7 superfamily: increasing complexity in costimulatory signals regulating T cell function, *Nat. Immunol.*, 2, 203, 2001.
92. McLellan, A.D. et al., Human dendritic cells activate T lymphocytes via a CD40: CD40 ligand-dependent pathway, *Eur. J. Immunol.*, 26, 1204, 1996.
93. Caux, C. et al., Activation of human dendritic cells through CD40 cross-linking, *J. Exp. Med.*, 180, 1263, 1994.
94. Romagnani, S., The Th1/Th2 paradigm, *Immunol. Today*, 18, 263, 1997.
95. Mosmann, T.R. and Sad, S., The expanding universe of T-cell subsets: Th1, Th2 and more, *Immunol. Today*, 17, 138, 1996.
96. de Jong, E.C. et al., Microbial compounds selectively induce Th1 cell-promoting or Th2 cell-promoting dendritic cells *in vitro* with diverse Th cell-polarizing signals, *J. Immunol.*, 168, 1704, 2002.
97. Matzinger, P., Tolerance, danger, and the extended family, *Annu. Rev. Immunol.*, 12, 991, 1994.
98. Vieira, P.L. et al., Development of Th1-inducing capacity in myeloid dendritic cells requires environmental instruction, *J. Immunol.*, 164, 4507, 2000.
99. Kalinski, P. et al., T-cell priming by type-1 and type-2 polarized dendritic cells: the concept of a third signal, *Immunol. Today*, 20, 561, 1999.
100. Heufler, C. et al., Interleukin-12 is produced by dendritic cells and mediates T helper 1 development as well as interferon-$\gamma$ production by T helper 1 cells, *Eur. J. Immunol.*, 26, 659, 1996.
101. Micallef, M.J. et al., Interferon-$\gamma$-inducing factor enhances T helper 1 cytokine production by stimulated human T cells: synergism with interleukin-12 for interferon-$\gamma$ production, *Eur. J. Immunol.*, 26, 1647, 1996.
102. Oppmann, B. et al., Novel p19 protein engages IL-12p40 to form a cytokine, IL-23, with biological activities similar as well as distinct from IL-12, *Immunity*, 13, 715, 2000.
103. Pflanz, S. et al., IL-27, a heterodimeric cytokine composed of EBI3 and p28 protein, induces proliferation of naive CD4(+) T cells, *Immunity*, 16, 779, 2002.
104. Sareneva, T. et al., Influenza A virus-induced IFN-$\alpha/\beta$ and IL-18 synergistically enhance IFN-$\gamma$ gene expression in human T cells, *J. Immunol.*, 160, 6032, 1998.
105. Siegal, F.P. et al., The nature of the principal type 1 interferon-producing cells in human blood, *Science*, 284, 1835, 1999.
106. Kalinski, P. et al., Prostaglandin E2 induces the final maturation of IL-12-deficient CD1a+CD83+ dendritic cells: the levels of IL-12 are determined during the final dendritic cell maturation and are resistant to further modulation, *J. Immunol.*, 161, 2804, 1998.
107. Liu, L. et al., Induction of Th2 cell differentiation in the primary immune response: dendritic cells isolated from adherent cell culture treated with IL-10 prime naive CD4+ T cells to secrete IL-4, *Int. Immunol.*, 10, 1017, 1998.
108. Ebner, S. et al., A novel role for IL-3: human monocytes cultured in the presence of IL-3 and IL-4 differentiate into dendritic cells that produce less IL-12 and shift Th cell responses toward a Th2 cytokine pattern, *J. Immunol.*, 168, 6199, 2002.
109. Curti, A. et al., Interleukin-11 induces Th2 polarization of human CD4(+) T cells, *Blood*, 97, 2758, 2001.
110. Fort, M.M. et al., IL-25 induces IL-4, IL-5, and IL-13 and Th2-associated pathologies *in vivo*, *Immunity*, 15, 985, 2001.

111. Soumelis, V. et al., Human epithelial cells trigger dendritic cell mediated allergic inflammation by producing TSLP, *Nat. Immunol.*, 3, 673, 2002.
112. Smits, H.H. et al., Intercellular adhesion molecule-1/LFA-1 ligation favors human Th1 development, *J. Immunol.*, 168, 1710, 2002.
113. Flynn, S. et al., CD4 T cell cytokine differentiation: the B cell activation molecule, OX40 ligand, instructs CD4 T cells to express interleukin 4 and upregulates expression of the chemokine receptor, Blr-1, *J. Exp. Med.*, 188, 297, 1998.
114. Hwu, P. et al., Indoleamine 2,3-dioxygenase production by human dendritic cells results in the inhibition of T cell proliferation, *J. Immunol.*, 164, 3596, 2000.
115. Munn, D.H. et al., Potential regulatory function of human dendritic cells expressing indoleamine 2,3-dioxygenase, *Science*, 297, 1867, 2002.
116. Grohmann, U., Fallarino, F., and Puccetti, P., Tolerance, DCs and tryptophan: much ado about IDO, *Trends Immunol.*, 24, 242, 2003.
117. Lee, G.K. et al., Tryptophan deprivation sensitizes activated T cells to apoptosis prior to cell division, *Immunology*, 107, 452, 2002.
118. Fallarino, F. et al., T cell apoptosis by tryptophan catabolism, *Cell Death. Differ.*, 9, 1069, 2002.
119. Grakoui, A. et al., The immunological synapse: a molecular machine controlling T cell activation, *Science*, 285, 221, 1999.
120. Lanzavecchia, A. and Sallusto, F., Antigen decoding by T lymphocytes: from synapses to fate determination, *Nat. Immunol.*, 2, 487, 2001.
121. Lutz, M.B. and Schuler, G., Immature, semi-mature and fully mature dendritic cells: which signals induce tolerance or immunity?, *Trends Immunol.*, 23, 445, 2002.
122. Jonuleit, H. et al., Dendritic cells as a tool to induce anergic and regulatory T cells, *Trends Immunol.*, 22, 394, 2001.
123. Dhodapkar, M.V. and Steinman, R.M., Antigen-bearing immature dendritic cells induce peptide-specific CD8(+) regulatory T cells *in vivo* in humans, *Blood*, 100, 174, 2002.
124. Steinman, R.M. and Nussenzweig, M.C., Avoiding horror autotoxicus: the importance of dendritic cells in peripheral T cell tolerance, *Proc. Natl. Acad. Sci. U.S.A*, 99, 351, 2002.
125. Zhou, L.J. et al., A novel cell-surface molecule expressed by human interdigitating reticulum cells, Langerhans cells, and activated lymphocytes is a new member of the Ig superfamily, *J. Immunol.*, 149, 735, 1992.
126. Lechmann, M. et al., The extracellular domain of CD83 inhibits dendritic cell-mediated T cell stimulation and binds to a ligand on dendritic cells, *J. Exp. Med.*, 194, 1813, 2001.
127. Hock, B.D. et al., Characterization of CMRF-44, a novel monoclonal antibody to an activation antigen expressed by the allostimulatory cells within peripheral blood, including dendritic cells, *Immunology*, 83, 573, 1994.
128. Hock, B.D. et al., Human dendritic cells express a 95 kDa activation/differentiation antigen defined by CMRF-56, *Tissue Antigens*, 53, 320, 1999.
129. Dzionek, A. et al., BDCA-2, BDCA-3, and BDCA-4: three markers for distinct subsets of dendritic cells in human peripheral blood, *J. Immunol.*, 165, 6037, 2000.
130. Schakel, K. et al., A novel dendritic cell population in human blood: one-step immunomagnetic isolation by a specific mAb (M-DC8) and *in vitro* priming of cytotoxic T lymphocytes, *Eur. J. Immunol.*, 28, 4084, 1998.
131. Saint-Vis, B. et al., A novel lysosome-associated membrane glycoprotein, DC-LAMP, induced upon DC maturation, is transiently expressed in MHC class II compartment, *Immunity*, 9, 325, 1998.
132. Mosialos, G. et al., Circulating human dendritic cells differentially express high levels of a 55-kd actin-bundling protein, *Am. J. Pathol.*, 148, 593, 1996.
133. Adema, G.J. et al., A dendritic-cell-derived C-C chemokine that preferentially attracts naive T cells, *Nature*, 387, 713, 1997.
134. Godiska, R. et al., Human macrophage-derived chemokine (MDC), a novel chemoattractant for monocytes, monocyte-derived dendritic cells, and natural killer cells, *J. Exp. Med.*, 185, 1595, 1997.
135. Lieberam, I. and Forster, I., The murine β-chemokine TARC is expressed by subsets of dendritic cells and attracts primed $CD4^+$ T cells, *Eur. J. Immunol.*, 29, 2684, 1999.
136. Hartgers, F.C. et al., DC-STAMP, a novel multimembrane-spanning molecule preferentially expressed by dendritic cells, *Eur. J. Immunol.*, 30, 3585, 2000.

137. Hashimoto, S.I. et al., Identification of genes specifically expressed in human activated and mature dendritic cells through serial analysis of gene expression, *Blood*, 96, 2206, 2000.
138. Le Naour, F. et al., Profiling changes in gene expression during differentiation and maturation of monocyte-derived dendritic cells using both oligonucleotide microarrays and proteomics, *J. Biol. Chem.*, 276, 17920, 2001.
139. Robinson, S.P. et al., Human peripheral blood contains two distinct lineages of dendritic cells, *Eur. J. Immunol.*, 29, 2769, 1999.
140. MacDonald, K.P. et al., Characterization of human blood dendritic cell subsets, *Blood*, 100, 4512, 2002.
141. Nestle, F.O. et al., Characterization of dermal dendritic cells obtained from normal human skin reveals phenotypic and functionally distinctive subsets, *J. Immunol.*, 151, 6535, 1993.
142. Leenen, P.J. et al., Heterogeneity of mouse spleen dendritic cells: *in vivo* phagocytic activity, expression of macrophage markers, and subpopulation turnover, *J. Immunol.*, 160, 2166, 1998.
143. Vremec, D. et al., CD4 and CD8 expression by dendritic cell subtypes in mouse thymus and spleen, *J. Immunol.*, 164, 2978, 2000.
144. Grabbe, S., Kampgen, E., and Schuler, G., Dendritic cells: multi-lineal and multi-functional, *Immunol. Today*, 21, 431, 2000.
145. Liu, Y.J., Dendritic cell subsets and lineages, and their functions in innate and adaptive immunity, *Cell*, 106, 259, 2001.
146. Reid, C.D. et al., Interactions of tumor necrosis factor with granulocyte-macrophage colony-stimulating factor and other cytokines in the regulation of dendritic cell growth *in vitro* from early bipotent $CD34^+$ progenitors in human bone marrow, *J. Immunol.*, 149, 2681, 1992.
147. Caux, C. et al., GM-CSF and TNF-$\alpha$ cooperate in the generation of dendritic Langerhans cells, *Nature*, 360, 258, 1992.
148. Reid, C.D. et al., Identification of hematopoietic progenitors of macrophages and dendritic Langerhans cells (DL-CFU) in human bone marrow and peripheral blood, *Blood*, 76, 1139, 1990.
149. Mackensen, A. et al., Delineation of the dendritic cell lineage by generating large numbers of Birbeck granule-positive Langerhans cells from human peripheral blood progenitor cells *in vitro*, *Blood*, 86, 2699, 1995.
150. Res, P. et al., $CD34^+$CD38dim cells in the human thymus can differentiate into T, natural killer, and dendritic cells but are distinct from pluripotent stem cells, *Blood*, 87, 5196, 1996.
151. Caux, C. et al., $CD34^+$ hematopoietic progenitors from human cord blood differentiate along two independent dendritic cell pathways in response to GM-CSF+TNF $\alpha$, *J. Exp. Med.*, 184, 695, 1996.
152. Szabolcs, P. et al., Dendritic cells and macrophages can mature independently from a human bone marrow-derived, post-colony-forming unit intermediate, *Blood*, 87, 4520, 1996.
153. Young, J.W., Szabolcs, P., and Moore, M.A., Identification of dendritic cell colony-forming units among normal human $CD34^+$ bone marrow progenitors that are expanded by c-kit-ligand and yield pure dendritic cell colonies in the presence of granulocyte/macrophage colony-stimulating factor and tumor necrosis factor $\alpha$, *J. Exp. Med.*, 182, 1111, 1995.
154. Szabolcs, P., Moore, M.A., and Young, J.W., Expansion of immunostimulatory dendritic cells among the myeloid progeny of human $CD34^+$ bone marrow precursors cultured with c-kit ligand, granulocyte-macrophage colony-stimulating factor, and TNF-$\alpha$, *J. Immunol.*, 154, 5851, 1995.
155. Siena, S. et al., Massive *ex vivo* generation of functional dendritic cells from mobilized $CD34^+$ blood progenitors for anticancer therapy, *Exp. Hematol.*, 23, 1463, 1995.
156. Strobl, H. et al., flt3 ligand in cooperation with transforming growth factor-$\beta$1 potentiates *in vitro* development of Langerhans-type dendritic cells and allows single-cell dendritic cell cluster formation under serum-free conditions, *Blood*, 90, 1425, 1997.
157. Karsunky, H. et al., Flt3 ligand regulates dendritic cell development from $Flt3^+$ lymphoid and myeloid-committed progenitors to $Flt3^+$ dendritic cells *in vivo*, *J. Exp. Med.*, 198, 305, 2003.
158. Strunk, D. et al., Generation of human dendritic cells/Langerhans cells from circulating $CD34^+$ hematopoietic progenitor cells, *Blood*, 87, 1292, 1996.
159. Rosenzwajg, M., Canque, B., and Gluckman, J.C., Human dendritic cell differentiation pathway from $CD34^+$ hematopoietic precursor cells, *Blood*, 87, 535, 1996.
160. Strobl, H. et al., TGF-$\beta$ 1 promotes *in vitro* development of dendritic cells from $CD34^+$ hematopoietic progenitors, *J. Immunol.*, 157, 1499, 1996.

161. Riedl, E. et al., TGF-β 1 promotes *in vitro* generation of dendritic cells by protecting progenitor cells from apoptosis, *J. Immunol.*, 158, 1591, 1997.
162. Borkowski, T.A. et al., A role for endogenous transforming growth factor β1 in Langerhans cell biology: the skin of transforming growth factor β1 null mice is devoid of epidermal Langerhans cells, *J. Exp. Med.*, 184, 2417, 1996.
163. Noirey, N. et al., Withdrawal of TNF-α after the fifth day of differentiation of $CD34^+$ cord blood progenitors generates a homogeneous population of Langerhans cells and delays their maturation, *Exp. Dermatol.*, 12, 96, 2003.
164. Mollah, Z.U. et al., Interleukin-3 in cooperation with transforming growth factor β induces granulocyte macrophage colony stimulating factor independent differentiation of human $CD34^+$ hematopoietic progenitor cells into dendritic cells with features of Langerhans cells, *J. Invest. Dermatol.*, 121, 1397, 2003.
165. Iwama, A. et al., Reciprocal roles for CCAAT/enhancer binding protein (C/EBP) and PU.1 transcription factors in Langerhans cell commitment, *J. Exp. Med.*, 195, 547, 2002.
166. Schotte, R. et al., The transcription factor Spi-B is expressed in plasmacytoid DC precursors and inhibits T-, B-, and NK-cell development, *Blood*, 101, 1015, 2003.
167. Schiavoni, G. et al., ICSBP is essential for the development of mouse type I interferon-producing cells and for the generation and activation of CD8α(+) dendritic cells, *J. Exp. Med.*, 196, 1415, 2002.
168. Laouar, Y. et al., STAT3 is required for Flt3L-dependent dendritic cell differentiation, *Immunity*, 19, 903, 2003.
169. Ito, T. et al., A $CD1a^+/CD11c^+$ subset of human blood dendritic cells is a direct precursor of Langerhans cells, *J. Immunol.*, 163, 1409, 1999.
170. Takamizawa, M. et al., Dendritic cells that process and present nominal antigens to naive T lymphocytes are derived from $CD2^+$ precursors, *J. Immunol.*, 158, 2134, 1997.
171. Crawford, K. et al., Circulating $CD2^+$ monocytes are dendritic cells, *J. Immunol.*, 163, 5920, 1999.
172. Almeida, J. et al., Extensive characterization of the immunophenotype and pattern of cytokine production by distinct subpopulations of normal human peripheral blood MHC $II^+$/lineage$^-$ cells, *Clin. Exp. Immunol.*, 118, 392, 1999.
173. Strobl, H. et al., Identification of $CD68^+lin^-$ peripheral blood cells with dendritic precursor characteristics, *J. Immunol.*, 161, 740, 1998.
174. Strunk, D. et al., A skin homing molecule defines the Langerhans cell progenitor in human peripheral blood, *J. Exp. Med.*, 185, 1131, 1997.
175. Bendriss-Vermare, N. et al., Human thymus contains IFN-α-producing CD11c(–), myeloid CD11c(+), and mature interdigitating dendritic cells, *J. Clin. Invest*, 107, 835, 2001.
176. Grouard, G. et al., The enigmatic plasmacytoid T cells develop into dendritic cells with interleukin (IL)-3 and CD40-ligand, *J. Exp. Med.*, 185, 1101, 1997.
177. Wollenberg, A. et al., Plasmacytoid dendritic cells: a new cutaneous dendritic cell subset with distinct role in inflammatory skin diseases, *J. Invest. Dermatol.*, 119, 1096, 2002.
178. Peters, J.H., Ruhl, S., and Friedrichs, D., Veiled accessory cells deduced from monocytes, *Immunobiology*, 176, 154, 1987.
179. Peters, J.H. et al., Differentiation of human monocytes into CD14 negative accessory cells: do dendritic cells derive from the monocytic lineage?, *Pathobiology*, 59, 122, 1991.
180. Kasinrerk, W. et al., CD1 molecule expression on human monocytes induced by granulocyte-macrophage colony-stimulating factor, *J. Immunol.*, 150, 579, 1993.
181. Ruppert, J. et al., Down-regulation and release of CD14 on human monocytes by IL-4 depends on the presence of serum or GM-CSF, *Adv. Exp. Med. Biol.*, 329, 281, 1993.
182. Romani, N. et al., Proliferating dendritic cell progenitors in human blood, *J. Exp. Med.*, 180, 83, 1994.
183. Sallusto, F. and Lanzavecchia, A., Efficient presentation of soluble antigen by cultured human dendritic cells is maintained by granulocyte/macrophage colony-stimulating factor plus interleukin 4 and downregulated by tumor necrosis factor α, *J. Exp. Med.*, 179, 1109, 1994.
184. Bender, A. et al., Improved methods for the generation of dendritic cells from nonproliferating progenitors in human blood, *J. Immunol. Methods*, 196, 121, 1996.
185. Romani, N. et al., Generation of mature dendritic cells from human blood. An improved method with special regard to clinical applicability, *J. Immunol. Methods*, 196, 137, 1996.

186. Palucka, K.A. et al., Dendritic cells as the terminal stage of monocyte differentiation, *J. Immunol.*, 160, 4587, 1998.
187. Geissmann, F. et al., Transforming growth factor β1, in the presence of granulocyte/macrophage colony-stimulating factor and interleukin 4, induces differentiation of human peripheral blood monocytes into dendritic Langerhans cells, *J. Exp. Med.*, 187, 961, 1998.
188. Mohamadzadeh, M. et al., Interleukin 15 skews monocyte differentiation into dendritic cells with features of Langerhans cells, *J. Exp. Med.*, 194, 1013, 2001.
189. Randolph, G.J. et al., Differentiation of monocytes into dendritic cells in a model of transendothelial trafficking, *Science*, 282, 480, 1998.
190. Chomarat, P. et al., TNF skews monocyte differentiation from macrophages to dendritic cells, *J. Immunol.*, 171, 2262, 2003.
191. Larregina, A.T. et al., Dermal-resident $CD14^+$ cells differentiate into Langerhans cells, *Nat. Immunol.*, 2, 1151, 2001.
192. Rissoan, M.C. et al., Reciprocal control of T helper cell and dendritic cell differentiation, *Science*, 283, 1183, 1999.
193. Teunissen, M.B., Dynamic nature and function of epidermal Langerhans cells *in vivo* and *in vitro*: a review, with emphasis on human Langerhans cells, *Histochem. J.*, 24, 697, 1992.
194. Langerhans, P., Ueber die Nerven der menschlichen Haut, *Virchows Arch. Pathol. Anat.*, 44, 325, 1868.
195. Birbeck, M.S., An electron microscopic study of basal melanocytes and high level clear cells (Langerhans cells) in vitiligo, *J. Invest. Dermatol.*, 37, 51, 1961.
196. Hoefsmit, E.C., Duijvestijn, A.M., and Kamperdijk, E.W., Relation between Langerhans cells, veiled cells, and interdigitating cells, *Immunobiology*, 161, 255, 1982.
197. Kashihara, M. et al., A monoclonal antibody specifically reactive to human Langerhans cells, *J. Invest. Dermatol.*, 87, 602, 1986.
198. Valladeau, J. et al., The monoclonal antibody DCGM4 recognizes Langerin, a protein specific of Langerhans cells, and is rapidly internalized from the cell surface, *Eur. J. Immunol.*, 29, 2695, 1999.
199. Valladeau, J. et al., Langerin, a novel C-type lectin specific to Langerhans cells, is an endocytic receptor that induces the formation of Birbeck granules, *Immunity*, 12, 71, 2000.
200. Klareskog, L. et al., Epidermal Langerhans cells express Ia antigens, *Nature*, 268, 248, 1977.
201. Rowden, G., Lewis, M.G., and Sullivan, A.K., Ia antigen expression on human epidermal Langerhans cells, *Nature*, 268, 247, 1977.
202. Fithian, E. et al., Reactivity of Langerhans cells with hybridoma antibody, *Proc. Natl. Acad. Sci. U.S.A.*, 78, 2541, 1981.
203. Murphy, G.F. et al., Characterization of Langerhans cells by the use of monoclonal antibodies, *Lab. Invest.*, 45, 465, 1981.
204. Aubock, J. et al., HLA-DR expression on keratinocytes is a common feature of diseased skin, *Br. J. Dermatol.*, 114, 465, 1986.
205. Wolff, K. and Winkelmann, R.K., Ultrastructural localization of nucleoside triphosphatase in Langerhans cells, *J. Invest. Dermatol.*, 48, 50, 1967.
206. Mizumoto, N. et al., CD39 is the dominant Langerhans cell-associated ecto-NTPDase: modulatory roles in inflammation and immune responsiveness, *Nat. Med.*, 8, 358, 2002.
207. Girolomoni, G. et al., Epidermal Langerhans cells are resistant to the permeabilizing effects of extracellular ATP: *in vitro* evidence supporting a protective role of membrane ATPase, *J. Invest. Dermatol.*, 100, 282, 1993.
208. Bobryshev, Y.V., Ikezawa, T., and Watanabe, T., Formation of Birbeck granule-like structures in vascular dendritic cells in human atherosclerotic aorta. Lag-antibody to epidermal Langerhans cells recognizes cells in the aortic wall, *Atherosclerosis*, 133, 193, 1997.
209. Katz, S.I., Tamaki, K., and Sachs, D.H., Epidermal Langerhans cells are derived from cells originating in bone marrow, *Nature*, 282, 324, 1979.
210. Dezutter-Dambuyant, C. et al., Detection of OKT6-positive cells (without visible Birbeck granules) in normal peripheral blood, *Immunol. Lett.*, 8, 121, 1984.
211. Berman, B. et al., Anatomical mapping of epidermal Langerhans cell densities in adults, *Br. J. Dermatol.*, 109, 553, 1983.
212. Chen, H. et al., Distribution of ATPase-positive Langerhans cells in normal adult human skin, *Br. J. Dermatol.*, 113, 707, 1985.

213. Bieber, T., Ring, J., and Braun-Falco, O., Comparison of different methods for enumeration of Langerhans cells in vertical cryosections of human skin, *Br. J. Dermatol.*, 118, 385, 1988.
214. Emilson, A. et al., Quantitative and 3-dimensional analysis of Langerhans' cells following occlusion with patch tests using confocal laser scanning microscopy, *Acta Derm. Venereol.*, 73, 323, 1993.
215. Bacci, S., Romagnoli, P., and Streilein, J.W., Reduction in number and morphologic alterations of Langerhans cells after UVB radiation *in vivo* are accompanied by an influx of monocytoid cells into the epidermis, *J. Invest. Dermatol.*, 111, 1134, 1998.
216. Bauer, J. et al., A strikingly constant ratio exists between Langerhans cells and other epidermal cells in human skin. A stereologic study using the optical disector method and the confocal laser scanning microscope, *J. Invest. Dermatol.*, 116, 313, 2001.
217. Bhushan, M. et al., Tumour necrosis factor-α-induced migration of human Langerhans cells: the influence of ageing, *Br. J. Dermatol.*, 146, 32, 2002.
218. Brand, C.U. et al., Characterization of human skin-derived CD1a-positive lymph cells, *Arch. Dermatol. Res.*, 291, 65, 1999.
219. Konrad, K. and Honigsmann, H., [Electron microscopic demonstration of a mitotic Langerhans cell in the normal human epidermis], *Arch. Dermatol. Forsch.*, 246, 70, 1973.
220. Kumakiri, M. et al., A Langerhans cell in mitosis within the epidermis of a case of lichen amyloidosus, *Am. J. Dermatopathol.*, 6, 195, 1984.
221. Miyauchi, S. and Hashimoto, K., Epidermal Langerhans cells undergo mitosis during the early recovery phase after ultraviolet-B irradiation, *J. Invest. Dermatol.*, 88, 703, 1987.
222. Czernielewski, J.M. and Demarchez, M., Further evidence for the self-reproducing capacity of Langerhans cells in human skin, *J. Invest. Dermatol.*, 88, 17, 1987.
223. Gilliam, A.C. et al., The human hair follicle: a reservoir of $CD40^+$ B7-deficient Langerhans cells that repopulate epidermis after UVB exposure, *J. Invest. Dermatol.*, 110, 422, 1998.
224. de Fraissinette, A. et al., Langerhans cells in S-phase in normal skin detected by simultaneous analysis of cell surface antigen and BrdU incorporation, *J. Invest. Dermatol.*, 91, 603, 1988.
225. Merad, M. et al., Langerhans cells renew in the skin throughout life under steady-state conditions, *Nat. Immunol.*, 3, 1135, 2002.
226. McLellan, A.D. et al., Dermal dendritic cells associated with T lymphocytes in normal human skin display an activated phenotype, *J. Invest. Dermatol.*, 111, 841, 1998.
227. Romani, N. et al., Cultured human Langerhans cells resemble lymphoid dendritic cells in phenotype and function, *J. Invest. Dermatol.*, 93, 600, 1989.
228. Bronstein, B.R. et al., Location of HLA-A,B,C antigens in dendritic cells of normal human skin: an immunoelectron microscopic study, *J. Invest. Dermatol.*, 80, 481, 1983.
229. Gielen, V., Schmitt, D., and Thivolet, J., HLA class I antigen (heavy and light chain) expression by Langerhans cells and keratinocytes of the normal human epidermis: ultrastructural quantitation using immunogold labelling procedure, *Arch. Dermatol. Res.*, 280, 131, 1988.
230. Park, S.H. and Bendelac, A., CD1-restricted T-cell responses and microbial infection, *Nature*, 406, 788, 2000.
231. Schmitt, D. et al., Subclustering of CD1 monoclonal antibodies based on the reactivity on human Langerhans cells, *Immunol. Lett.*, 12, 231, 1986.
232. Bonish, B. et al., Overexpression of CD1d by keratinocytes in psoriasis and CD1d-dependent IFN-γ production by NK-T cells, *J. Immunol.*, 165, 4076, 2000.
233. Walsh, L.J. and Seymour, G.J., Interleukin 1 induces CD1 antigen expression on human gingival epithelial cells, *J. Invest. Dermatol.*, 90, 13, 1988.
234. Pena-Cruz, V. et al., Epidermal Langerhans cells efficiently mediate CD1a-dependent presentation of microbial lipid antigens to T cells, *J. Invest. Dermatol.*, 121, 517, 2003.
235. Sontheimer, R.D., Stastny, P., and Nunez, G., HLA-D region antigen expression by human epidermal Langerhans cells, *J. Invest. Dermatol.*, 87, 707, 1986.
236. Kleijmeer, M.J., Oorschot, V.M., and Geuze, H.J., Human resident Langerhans cells display a lysosomal compartment enriched in MHC class II, *J. Invest. Dermatol.*, 103, 516, 1994.
237. Mommaas, A.M. et al., Distribution of HLA class II molecules in epidermal Langerhans cells *in situ*, *Eur. J. Immunol.*, 25, 520, 1995.
238. Claesson-Welsh, L. et al., Cell surface expression of invariant γ-chain of class II histocompatibility antigens in human skin, *J. Immunol.*, 136, 484, 1986.

239. Mommaas, A.M. et al., Human epidermal Langerhans cells lack functional mannose receptors and a fully developed endosomal/lysosomal compartment for loading of HLA class II molecules, *Eur. J. Immunol.*, 29, 571, 1999.
240. Poulter, L.W. et al., Discrimination of human macrophages and dendritic cells by means of monoclonal antibodies, *Scand. J. Immunol.*, 24, 351, 1986.
241. Dezutter-Dambuyant, C. et al., Quantitative evaluation of two distinct cell populations expressing HLA-DR antigens in normal human epidermis, *Br. J. Dermatol.*, 111, 1, 1984.
242. van Lochem, E. et al., Functional expression of minor histocompatibility antigens on human peripheral blood dendritic cells and epidermal Langerhans cells, *Transplant. Immunol.*, 4, 151, 1996.
243. Teunissen, M.B.M. et al., Human epidermal Langerhans cells undergo profound morphologic and phenotypical changes during *in vitro* culture, *J. Invest. Dermatol.*, 94, 166, 1990.
244. Schmitt, D.A. et al., Human epidermal Langerhans cells express only the 40-kilodalton Fcγ receptor (FcRII), *J. Immunol.*, 144, 4284, 1990.
245. Wood, G.S. et al., Human dendritic cells and macrophages. *In situ* immunophenotypic definition of subsets that exhibit specific morphologic and microenvironmental characteristics, *Am. J. Pathol.*, 119, 73, 1985.
246. Astier, A. et al., Human epidermal Langerhans cells secrete a soluble receptor for IgG (Fcγ RII/CD32) that inhibits the binding of immune complexes to Fcγ $R^+$ cells, *J. Immunol.*, 152, 201, 1994.
247. Bruynzeel-Koomen, C. et al., The presence of IgE molecules on epidermal Langerhans cells in patients with atopic dermatitis, *Arch. Dermatol. Res.*, 278, 199, 1986.
248. Bieber, T. et al., Human epidermal Langerhans cells express the high affinity receptor for immunoglobulin E (FcεRI), *J. Exp. Med.*, 175, 1285, 1992.
249. Grabbe, J. et al., Demonstration of the high-affinity IgE receptor on human Langerhans cells in normal and diseased skin, *Br. J. Dermatol.*, 129, 120, 1993.
250. Jurgens, M. et al., Activation of human epidermal Langerhans cells by engagement of the high affinity receptor for IgE, FcεRI, *J. Immunol.*, 155, 5184, 1995.
251. Novak, N. et al., Evidence for a differential expression of the FcεRIγ chain in dendritic cells of atopic and nonatopic donors, *J. Clin. Invest*, 111, 1047, 2003.
252. Wollenberg, A. et al., Human keratinocytes release the endogenous β-galactoside-binding soluble lectin immunoglobulin E (IgE-binding protein) which binds to Langerhans cells where it modulates their binding capacity for IgE glycoforms, *J. Exp. Med.*, 178, 777, 1993.
253. Mudde, G.C., Bheekha, R., and Bruijnzeel-Koomen, C.A., Consequences of IgE/CD23-mediated antigen presentation in allergy, *Immunol. Today*, 16, 380, 1995.
254. van der Heijden, F.L. et al., Serum-IgE-facilitated allergen presentation in atopic disease, *J. Immunol.*, 150, 3643, 1993.
255. Teunissen, M.B.M. et al., Conversion of human epidermal Langerhans cells into interdigitating cells *in vitro* is not associated with functional maturation, *Eur. J. Dermatol.*, 1, 45, 1991.
256. Teunissen, M.B.M., Rongen, H.A., and Bos, J.D., Function of adhesion molecules lymphocyte function-associated antigen-3 and intercellular adhesion molecule-1 on human epidermal Langerhans cells in antigen-specific T cell activation, *J. Immunol.*, 152, 3400, 1994.
257. Acevedo, A. et al., Distribution of ICAM-3-bearing cells in normal human tissues. Expression of a novel counter-receptor for LFA-1 in epidermal Langerhans cells, *Am. J. Pathol.*, 143, 774, 1993.
258. Teunissen, M.B.M., Koomen, C.W., and Bos, J.D., Intercellular adhesion molecule-3 (CD50) on human epidermal Langerhans cells participates in T-cell activation, *J. Invest. Dermatol.*, 104, 995, 1995.
259. De Panfilis, G. et al., Adhesion molecules on the plasma membrane of epidermal cells. I. Human resting Langerhans cells express two members of the adherence-promoting CD11/CD18 family, namely, H-Mac-1 (CD11b/CD18) and gp 150,95 (CD11c/CD18), *J. Invest. Dermatol.*, 93, 60, 1989.
260. Girolomoni, G. et al., Expression of B7 costimulatory molecule in cultured human epidermal Langerhans cells is regulated at the mRNA level, *J. Invest. Dermatol.*, 103, 54, 1994.
261. Vandenberghe, P. et al., *In situ* expression of B7/BB1 on antigen-presenting cells and activated B cells: an immunohistochemical study, *Int. Immunol.*, 5, 317, 1993.
262. Symington, F.W., Brady, W., and Linsley, P.S., Expression and function of B7 on human epidermal Langerhans cells, *J. Immunol.*, 150, 1286, 1993.
263. Witsch, E.J. et al., ICOS and CD28 reversely regulate IL-10 on re-activation of human effector T cells with mature dendritic cells, *Eur. J. Immunol.*, 32, 2680, 2002.

264. Peguet-Navarro, J. et al., Functional expression of CD40 antigen on human epidermal Langerhans cells, *J. Immunol.*, 155, 4241, 1995.
265. Groh, V. et al., Leu-3/T4 expression on epidermal Langerhans cells in normal and diseased skin, *J. Invest. Dermatol.*, 86, 115, 1986.
266. De Panfilis, G. et al., Simultaneous colloidal gold immunoelectron microscopy labeling of CD1a, HLA-DR, and CD4 surface antigens of human epidermal Langerhans cells, *J. Invest. Dermatol.*, 91, 547, 1988.
267. Lynch, G.W. et al., CD4 is expressed by epidermal Langerhans' cells predominantly as covalent dimers, *Exp. Dermatol.*, 12, 700, 2003.
268. Center, D.M., Kornfeld, H., and Cruikshank, W.W., Interleukin 16 and its function as a CD4 ligand, *Immunol. Today*, 17, 476, 1996.
269. Stoitzner, P. et al., Interleukin-16 supports the migration of Langerhans cells, partly in a CD4-independent way, *J. Invest. Dermatol.*, 116, 641, 2001.
270. Zambruno, G. et al., Langerhans cells and HIV infection, *Immunol. Today*, 16, 520, 1995.
271. Zaitseva, M. et al., Expression and function of CCR5 and CXCR4 on human Langerhans cells and macrophages: implications for HIV primary infection, *Nat. Med.*, 3, 1369, 1997.
272. Larregina, A. et al., Flow cytometric analysis of cytokine receptors on human Langerhans' cells. Changes observed after short-term culture, *Immunology*, 87, 317, 1996.
273. Ohtani, T. et al., H1 and H2 histamine receptors are absent on Langerhans cells and present on dermal dendritic cells, *J. Invest. Dermatol.*, 121, 1073, 2003.
274. Blauvelt, A., Katz, S.I., and Udey, M.C., Human Langerhans cells express E-cadherin, *J. Invest. Dermatol.*, 104, 293, 1995.
275. Tabata, N. et al., Sialyl LewisX expression on human Langerhans cells, *J. Invest. Dermatol.*, 101, 175, 1993.
276. Koszik, F. et al., Expression of monoclonal antibody HECA-452-defined E-selectin ligands on Langerhans cells in normal and diseased skin, *J. Invest. Dermatol.*, 102, 773, 1994.
277. Fuhlbrigge, R.C. et al., Cutaneous lymphocyte antigen is a specialized form of PSGL-1 expressed on skin-homing T cells, *Nature*, 389, 978, 1997.
278. Staquet, M.J. et al., A surface glycoprotein complex related to the adhesive receptors of the VLA family, shared by epidermal Langerhans cells and basal keratinocytes, *J. Invest. Dermatol.*, 92, 739, 1989.
279. Le Varlet, B. et al., Human epidermal Langerhans cells express integrins of the β-1 subfamily, *J. Invest. Dermatol.*, 96, 518, 1991.
280. Weiss, J.M. et al., An essential role for CD44 variant isoforms in epidermal Langerhans cell and blood dendritic cell function, *J. Cell Biol.*, 137, 1137, 1997.
281. Arenberger, P. et al., Langerhans cells of the human skin possess high-affinity 12(S)-hydroxyeicosa tetraenoic acid receptors, *Eur. J. Immunol.*, 22, 2469, 1992.
282. Ebner, S. et al., Expression of maturation-/migration-related molecules on human dendritic cells from blood and skin, *Immunobiology*, 198, 568, 1998.
283. Wood, G.S. et al., Langerhans cells react with pan-leukocyte monoclonal antibody: ultrastructural documentation using a live cell suspension immunoperoxidase technique, *J. Invest. Dermatol.*, 82, 322, 1984.
284. Bieber, T. et al., Characterization of the protein tyrosine phosphatase CD45 on human epidermal Langerhans cells, *Eur. J. Immunol.*, 25, 317, 1995.
285. Wood, G.S., Szwejbka, P., and Schwandt, A., Human Langerhans cells express a novel form of the leukocyte common antigen (CD45), *J. Invest. Dermatol.*, 111, 668, 1998.
286. Richters, C.D. et al., Isolation and characterization of migratory human skin dendritic cells, *Clin. Exp. Immunol.*, 98, 330, 1994.
287. Bieber, T. et al., CD69, an early activation antigen on lymphocytes, is constitutively expressed by human epidermal Langerhans cells, *J. Invest. Dermatol.*, 98, 771, 1992.
288. Nakagawa, S. et al., Differential modulation of human epidermal Langerhans cell maturation by ultraviolet B radiation, *J. Immunol.*, 163, 5192, 1999.
289. De Panfilis, G. et al., The tolerogenic molecule CD95-L is expressed on the plasma membrane of human activated, but not resting, Langerhans' cells, *Exp. Dermatol.*, 12, 692, 2003.

290. Cocchia, D., Michetti, F., and Donato, R., Immunochemical and immuno-cytochemical localization of S-100 antigen in normal human skin, *Nature*, 294, 85, 1981.
291. Hosoi, J. et al., Regulation of Langerhans cell function by nerves containing calcitonin gene-related peptide, *Nature*, 363, 159, 1993.
292. Morhenn, V.B., The physiology of scratching: involvement of proopiomelanocortin gene-related proteins in Langerhans cells, *Prog. Neurol. Endol. Immunol.*, 4, 265, 1991.
293. Fantini, F. et al., Langerhans cells can express neuron-specific enolase immunoreactivity, *Arch. Dermatol. Res.*, 283, 10, 1991.
294. Hamzeh, H. et al., Expression of PGP9.5 on Langerhans' cells and their precursors, *Acta Derm. Venereol.*, 80, 14, 2000.
295. Staniek, V. et al., Expression of gastrin-releasing peptide receptor in human skin, *Acta Derm. Venereol.*, 76, 282, 1996.
296. Staniek, V. et al., Binding and *in vitro* modulation of human epidermal Langerhans cell functions by substance P, *Arch. Dermatol. Res.*, 289, 285, 1997.
297. Torii, H., Tamaki, K., and Granstein, R.D., The effect of neuropeptides/hormones on Langerhans cells, *J. Dermatol. Sci.*, 20, 21, 1998.
298. Luger, T.A., Neuromediators — a crucial component of the skin immune system, *J. Dermatol. Sci.*, 30, 87, 2002.
299. Maestroni, G.J. and Mazzola, P., Langerhans cells β2-adrenoceptors: role in migration, cytokine production, Th priming and contact hypersensitivity, *J. Neuroimmunol.*, 144, 91, 2003.
300. Yokozeki, H. et al., Interferon-γ differentially regulates CD80 (B7-1) and CD86 (B7-2/B70) expression on human Langerhans cells, *Br. J. Dermatol.*, 136, 831, 1997.
301. Kremer, I.B. et al., Low expression of CD40 and B7 on macrophages infiltrating UV-exposed human skin; role in IL-2Rα-T cell activation, *Eur. J. Immunol.*, 28, 2936, 1998.
302. Ross, R. et al., The actin-bundling protein fascin is involved in the formation of dendritic processes in maturing epidermal Langerhans cells, *J. Immunol.*, 160, 3776, 1998.
303. Sonderbye, L. et al., Selective expression of human fascin (p55) by dendritic leukocytes, *Adv. Exp. Med. Biol.*, 417, 41, 1997.
304. Parkinson, E.K. et al., Hematopoietic stem cell inhibitor (SCI/MIP-1 α) also inhibits clonogenic epidermal keratinocyte proliferation, *J. Invest. Dermatol.*, 101, 113, 1993.
305. Vissers, J.L. et al., Quantitative analysis of chemokine expression by dendritic cell subsets *in vitro* and *in vivo*, *J. Leukocyte Biol.*, 69, 785, 2001.
306. Sauder, D.N., Dinarello, C.A., and Morhenn, V.B., Langerhans cell production of interleukin-1, *J. Invest. Dermatol.*, 82, 605, 1984.
307. Lore, K. et al., Erratum to "Immunocytochemical detection of cytokines and chemokines in Langerhans cells and *in vitro* derived dendritic cells," *J. Immunol. Methods*, 218, 173, 1998.
308. Schreiber, S. et al., Cytokine pattern of Langerhans cells isolated from murine epidermal cell cultures, *J. Immunol.*, 149, 3524, 1992.
309. Kang, K. et al., IL-12 synthesis by human Langerhans cells, *J. Immunol.*, 156, 1402, 1996.
310. Blauvelt, A. et al., Interleukin-15 mRNA is expressed by human keratinocytes Langerhans cells, and blood-derived dendritic cells and is downregulated by ultraviolet B radiation, *J. Invest. Dermatol.*, 106, 1047, 1996.
311. Reich, K. et al., Evidence for a role of Langerhans cell-derived IL-16 in atopic dermatitis, *J. Allergy Clin. Immunol.*, 109, 681, 2002.
312. Larrick, J.W. et al., Activated Langerhans cells release tumor necrosis factor, *J. Leukocyte Biol.*, 45, 429, 1989.
313. Trinchieri, G., Interleukin-12 and its role in the generation of TH1 cells, *Immunol. Today*, 14, 335, 1993.
314. Okamura, H. et al., Cloning of a new cytokine that induces IFN-γ production by T cells, *Nature*, 378, 88, 1995.
315. Schuler, G. and Steinman, R.M., Murine epidermal Langerhans cells mature into potent immunostimulatory dendritic cells *in vitro*, *J. Exp. Med.*, 161, 526, 1985.
316. Moulon, C. et al., In vitro primary sensitization and restimulation of hapten-specific T cells by fresh and cultured human epidermal Langerhans' cells, *Immunology*, 80, 373, 1993.

317. Kapsenberg, M.L. et al., Nickel-specific T lymphocyte clones derived from allergic nickel-contact dermatitis lesions in man: heterogeneity based on requirement of dendritic antigen-presenting cell subsets, *Eur. J. Immunol.*, 17, 861, 1987.
318. Braathen, L.R. and Thorsby, E., Human epidermal Langerhans cells are more potent than blood monocytes in inducing some antigen-specific T-cell responses, *Br. J. Dermatol.*, 108, 139, 1983.
319. Bjercke, S. et al., Enriched epidermal Langerhans cells are potent antigen-presenting cells for T cells, *J. Invest. Dermatol.*, 83, 286, 1984.
320. Res, P. et al., The crucial role of human dendritic antigen-presenting cell subsets in nickel-specific T-cell proliferation, *J. Invest. Dermatol.*, 88, 550, 1987.
321. Ptak, W. et al., Role of antigen-presenting cells in the development and persistence of contact hypersensitivity, *J. Exp. Med.*, 151, 362, 1980.
322. Britz, J.S. et al., Specialized antigen-presenting cells. Splenic dendritic cells and peritoneal-exudate cells induced by mycobacteria activate effector T cells that are resistant to suppression, *J. Exp. Med.*, 155, 1344, 1982.
323. Pehamberger, H. et al., Epidermal cell-induced generation of cytotoxic T-lymphocyte responses against alloantigens or TNP-modified syngeneic cells: requirement for Ia-positive Langerhans cells, *J. Invest. Dermatol.*, 81, 208, 1983.
324. Rico, M.J. and Streilein, J.W., Comparison of alloimmunogenicity of Langerhans cells and keratinocytes from mouse epidermis, *J. Invest. Dermatol.*, 89, 607, 1987.
325. Rae, V. et al., An ultraviolet B radiation protocol for complete depletion of human epidermal Langerhans cells, *J. Dermatol. Surg. Oncol.*, 15, 1199, 1989.
326. McKinney, E.C. and Streilein, J.W., On the extraordinary capacity of allogeneic epidermal Langerhans cells to prime cytotoxic T cells *in vivo*, *J. Immunol.*, 143, 1560, 1989.
327. Sagebiel, R.W. and Reed, T.H., Serial reconstruction of the characteristic granule of the Langerhans cell, *J. Cell Biol.*, 36, 595, 1968.
328. Hashimoto, K., Lanthanum staining of Langerhans' cell. Communication of Langerhans cell granules with extracellular space, *Arch. Dermatol.*, 102, 280, 1970.
329. Bartosik, J., Cytomembrane-derived Birbeck granules transport horseradish peroxidase to the endosomal compartment in the human Langerhans cells, *J. Invest. Dermatol.*, 99, 53, 1992.
330. Hanau, D. et al., Human epidermal Langerhans cells internalize by receptor-mediated endocytosis T6 (CD1 "NA1/34") surface antigen. Birbeck granules are involved in the intracellular traffic of the T6 antigen, *J. Invest. Dermatol.*, 89, 172, 1987.
331. Hanau, D. et al., Human epidermal Langerhans cells cointernalize by receptor-mediated endocytosis "nonclassical" major histocompatibility complex class I molecules (T6 antigens) and class II molecules (HLA-DR antigens), *Proc. Natl. Acad. Sci. U.S.A.*, 84, 2901, 1987.
332. McDermott, R., et al., Birbeck granules are subdomains of endosomal recycling compartment in human epidermal Langerhans cells, which form where Langerin accumulates, *Mol. Biol. Cell*, 13, 317, 2002.
333. Salamero, J. et al., CD1a molecules traffic through the early recycling endosomal pathway in human Langerhans cells, *J. Invest. Dermatol.*, 116, 401, 2001.
334. Lakey, E.K. et al., Time dependence of B cell processing and presentation of peptide and native protein antigens, *J. Immunol.*, 140, 3309, 1988.
335. Mommaas, M. et al., Functional human epidermal Langerhans cells that lack Birbeck granules, *J. Invest. Dermatol.*, 103, 807, 1994.
336. Hanau, D. et al., Ultrastructural similarities between epidermal Langerhans cell Birbeck granules and the surface-connected canalicular system of EDTA-treated human blood platelets, *J. Invest. Dermatol.*, 97, 756, 1991.
337. Kobayashi, M. and Hoshino, T., Occurrence of "cored tubule" in the Birbeck granule-containing cells of mice, *J. Electron Microsc.* (Tokyo), 27, 199, 1978.
338. Lipsker, D. et al., Cored tubules are present in human epidermal Langerhans cells, *J. Invest. Dermatol.*, 120, 407, 2003.
339. Robert, C. et al., Interaction of dendritic cells with skin endothelium: A new perspective on immunosurveillance, *J. Exp. Med.*, 189, 627, 1999.
340. Godefroy, S. et al., A combination of MIP-3α and TGF-β1 is required for the attraction of human Langerhans precursor cells through a dermal-epidermal barrier, *Eur. J. Cell Biol.*, 80, 335, 2001.

341. Dieu, M.C. et al., Selective recruitment of immature and mature dendritic cells by distinct chemokines expressed in different anatomic sites, *J. Exp. Med.*, 188, 373, 1998.
342. Charbonnier, A.S. et al., Macrophage inflammatory protein 3α is involved in the constitutive trafficking of epidermal Langerhans cells, *J. Exp. Med.*, 190, 1755, 1999.
343. Dieu-Nosjean, M.C. et al., Macrophage inflammatory protein 3α is expressed at inflamed epithelial surfaces and is the most potent chemokine known in attracting Langerhans cell precursors, *J. Exp. Med.*, 192, 705, 2000.
344. Zlotnik, A. and Yoshie, O., Chemokines: a new classification system and their role in immunity, *Immunity*, 12, 121, 2000.
345. Yang, D. et al., Beta-defensins: linking innate and adaptive immunity through dendritic and T cell CCR6, *Science*, 286, 525, 1999.
346. Sozzani, S. et al., Receptor expression and responsiveness of human dendritic cells to a defined set of CC and CXC chemokines, *J. Immunol.*, 159, 1993, 1997.
347. Sallusto, F. et al., Rapid and coordinated switch in chemokine receptor expression during dendritic cell maturation, *Eur. J. Immunol.*, 28, 2760, 1998.
348. Vanbervliet, B. et al., Sequential involvement of CCR2 and CCR6 ligands for immature dendritic cell recruitment: possible role at inflamed epithelial surfaces, *Eur. J. Immunol.*, 32, 231, 2002.
349. Nakamura, K., Williams, I.R., and Kupper, T.S., Keratinocyte-derived monocyte chemoattractant protein 1 (MCP-1): analysis in a transgenic model demonstrates MCP-1 can recruit dendritic and Langerhans cells to skin, *J. Invest. Dermatol.*, 105, 635, 1995.
350. Tang, A. et al., Adhesion of epidermal Langerhans cells to keratinocytes mediated by E-cadherin, *Nature*, 361, 82, 1993.
351. Jakob, T., Brown, M.J., and Udey, M.C., Characterization of E-cadherin-containing junctions involving skin-derived dendritic cells, *J. Invest. Dermatol.*, 112, 102, 1999.
352. Riedl, E. et al., Ligation of E-cadherin on *in vitro*-generated immature Langerhans-type dendritic cells inhibits their maturation, *Blood*, 96, 4276, 2000.
353. Geissmann, F. et al., TGF-β1 prevents the noncognate maturation of human dendritic Langerhans cells, *J. Immunol.*, 162, 4567, 1999.
354. Shibaki, A. et al., Differential responsiveness of Langerhans cell subsets of varying phenotypic states in normal human epidermis, *J. Invest. Dermatol.*, 104, 42, 1995.
355. Enk, A.H. et al., An essential role for Langerhans cell-derived IL-1β in the initiation of primary immune responses in skin, *J. Immunol.*, 150, 3698, 1993.
356. Cumberbatch, M. and Kimber, I., Tumour necrosis factor-α is required for accumulation of dendritic cells in draining lymph nodes and for optimal contact sensitization, *Immunology*, 84, 31, 1995.
357. Cumberbatch, M., Dearman, R.J., and Kimber, I., Langerhans cells require signals from both tumour necrosis factor-α and interleukin-1β for migration, *Immunology*, 92, 388, 1997.
358. Shornick, L.P., Bisarya, A.K., and Chaplin, D.D., IL-1β is essential for Langerhans cell activation and antigen delivery to the lymph nodes during contact sensitization: evidence for a dermal source of IL-1β, *Cell Immunol.*, 211, 105, 2001.
359. Wang, B. et al., Tumour necrosis factor receptor II (p75) signalling is required for the migration of Langerhans' cells, *Immunology*, 88, 284, 1996.
360. Wang, B. et al., Depressed Langerhans cell migration and reduced contact hypersensitivity response in mice lacking TNF receptor p75, *J. Immunol.*, 159, 6148, 1997.
361. Antonopoulos, C. et al., Functional caspase-1 is required for Langerhans cell migration and optimal contact sensitization in mice, *J. Immunol.*, 166, 3672, 2001.
362. Schwarzenberger, K. and Udey, M.C., Contact allergens and epidermal proinflammatory cytokines modulate Langerhans cell E-cadherin expression *in situ*, *J. Invest. Dermatol.*, 106, 553, 1996.
363. Carramolino, L. et al., Down-regulation of the β-chemokine receptor CCR6 in dendritic cells mediated by TNF-α and IL-4, *J. Leukocyte Biol.*, 66, 837, 1999.
364. Yanagihara, S. et al., EBI1/CCR7 is a new member of dendritic cell chemokine receptor that is up-regulated upon maturation, *J. Immunol.*, 161, 3096, 1998.
365. Saeki, H. et al., Cutting edge: secondary lymphoid-tissue chemokine (SLC) and CC chemokine receptor 7 (CCR7) participate in the emigration pathway of mature dendritic cells from the skin to regional lymph nodes, *J. Immunol.*, 162, 2472, 1999.

366. Kellermann, S.A. et al., The CC chemokine receptor-7 ligands 6Ckine and macrophage inflammatory protein-3β are potent chemoattractants for *in vitro*- and *in vivo*-derived dendritic cells, *J. Immunol.*, 162, 3859, 1999.
367. Vassileva, G. et al., The reduced expression of 6Ckine in the *plt* mouse results from the deletion of one of two 6Ckine genes, *J. Exp. Med.*, 190, 1183, 1999.
368. Chen, S.C. et al., Ectopic expression of the murine chemokines CCL21a and CCL21b induces the formation of lymph node-like structures in pancreas, but not skin, of transgenic mice, *J. Immunol.*, 168, 1001, 2002.
369. Gunn, M.D. et al., A chemokine expressed in lymphoid high endothelial venules promotes the adhesion and chemotaxis of naive T lymphocytes, *Proc. Natl. Acad. Sci. U.S.A.*, 95, 258, 1998.
370. Katou, F. et al., Differential expression of CCL19 by DC-Lamp$^+$ mature dendritic cells in human lymph node versus chronically inflamed skin, *J. Pathol.*, 199, 98, 2003.
371. Luther, S.A. et al., Coexpression of the chemokines ELC and SLC by T zone stromal cells and deletion of the ELC gene in the plt/plt mouse, *Proc. Natl. Acad. Sci. U.S.A.*, 97, 12694, 2000.
372. Forster, R. et al., CCR7 coordinates the primary immune response by establishing functional microenvironments in secondary lymphoid organs, *Cell*, 99, 23, 1999.
373. Gunn, M.D. et al., Mice lacking expression of secondary lymphoid organ chemokine have defects in lymphocyte homing and dendritic cell localization, *J. Exp. Med.*, 189, 451, 1999.
374. Robbiani, D.F. et al., The leukotriene C(4) transporter MRP1 regulates CCL19 (MIP-3β, ELC)-dependent mobilization of dendritic cells to lymph nodes, *Cell*, 103, 757, 2000.
375. Spanbroek, R. et al., 5-Lipoxygenase expression in Langerhans cells of normal human epidermis, *Proc. Natl. Acad. Sci. U.S.A.*, 95, 663, 1998.
376. Randolph, G.J. et al., A physiologic function for *p*-glycoprotein (MDR-1) during the migration of dendritic cells from skin via afferent lymphatic vessels, *Proc. Natl. Acad. Sci. U.S.A.*, 95, 6924, 1998.
377. van Helvoort, A. et al., MDR1 P-glycoprotein is a lipid translocase of broad specificity, while MDR3 P-glycoprotein specifically translocates phosphatidylcholine, *Cell*, 87, 507, 1996.
378. Raggers, R.J. et al., The human multidrug resistance protein MRP1 translocates sphingolipid analogs across the plasma membrane, *J. Cell Sci.*, 112(3), 415, 1999.
379. Randolph, G.J., Dendritic cell migration to lymph nodes: cytokines, chemokines, and lipid mediators, *Semin. Immunol.*, 13, 267, 2001.
380. Hemmi, H. et al., Skin antigens in the steady state are trafficked to regional lymph nodes by transforming growth factor-β1-dependent cells, *Int. Immunol.*, 13, 695, 2001.
381. Yoshino, M. et al., Distinct antigen trafficking from skin in the steady and active states, *Int. Immunol.*, 15, 773, 2003.
382. Sato, N. et al., CC chemokine receptor (CCR)2 is required for Langerhans cell migration and localization of T helper cell type 1 (Th1)-inducing dendritic cells. Absence of CCR2 shifts the *Leishmania* major-resistant phenotype to a susceptible state dominated by Th2 cytokines, β cell outgrowth, and sustained neutrophilic inflammation, *J. Exp. Med.*, 192, 205, 2000.
383. Beaulieu, S. et al., Expression of a functional eotaxin (CC chemokine ligand 11) receptor CCR3 by human dendritic cells, *J. Immunol.*, 169, 2925, 2002.
384. Moodycliffe, A.M. et al., CD40-CD40 ligand interactions *in vivo* regulate migration of antigen-bearing dendritic cells from the skin to draining lymph nodes, *J. Exp. Med.*, 191, 2011, 2000.
385. Xu, H. et al., The role of ICAM-1 molecule in the migration of Langerhans cells in the skin and regional lymph node, *Eur. J. Immunol.*, 31, 3085, 2001.
386. Price, A.A. et al., Alpha 6 integrins are required for Langerhans cell migration from the epidermis, *J. Exp. Med.*, 186, 1725, 1997.
387. Liaw, L. et al., The adhesive and migratory effects of osteopontin are mediated via distinct cell surface integrins. Role of α v β 3 in smooth muscle cell migration to osteopontin *in vitro*, *J. Clin. Invest*, 95, 713, 1995.
388. Weber, G.F. et al., Receptor-ligand interaction between CD44 and osteopontin (Eta-1), *Science*, 271, 509, 1996.
389. Ashkar, S. et al., Eta-1 (osteopontin): an early component of type-1 (cell-mediated) immunity, *Science*, 287, 860, 2000.
390. Kaartinen, M.T. et al., Cross-linking of osteopontin by tissue transglutaminase increases its collagen binding properties, *J. Biol. Chem.*, 274, 1729, 1999.

391. Weiss, J.M. et al., Osteopontin is involved in the initiation of cutaneous contact hypersensitivity by inducing Langerhans and dendritic cell migration to lymph nodes, *J. Exp. Med.*, 194, 1219, 2001.
392. Katagiri, Y.U. et al., CD44 variants but not CD44s cooperate with β1-containing integrins to permit cells to bind to osteopontin independently of arginine-glycine-aspartic acid, thereby stimulating cell motility and chemotaxis, *Cancer Res.*, 59, 219, 1999.
393. Kremer, I.B. et al., Intradermal granulocyte-macrophage colony-stimulating factor alters cutaneous antigen-presenting cells and differentially affects local versus distant immunization in humans, *Clin. Immunol.*, 96, 29, 2000.
394. Rupec, R. et al., Granulocyte/macrophage-colony-stimulating factor induces the migration of human epidermal Langerhans cells *in vitro*, *Exp. Dermatol.*, 5, 115, 1996.
395. Takayama, K. et al., IL-4 inhibits the migration of human Langerhans cells through the downregulation of TNF receptor II expression, *J. Invest. Dermatol.*, 113, 541, 1999.
396. Wang, B. et al., Enhanced epidermal Langerhans cell migration in IL-10 knockout mice, *J. Immunol.*, 162, 277, 1999.
397. Halliday, G.M. and Le, S., Transforming growth factor-β produced by progressor tumors inhibits, while IL-10 produced by regressor tumors enhances, Langerhans cell migration from skin, *Int. Immunol.*, 13, 1147, 2001.
398. Esche, C. et al., Differential regulation of epidermal and dermal dendritic cells by IL-12 and Flt3 ligand, *J. Invest. Dermatol.*, 113, 1028, 1999.
399. Kobayashi, Y. et al., Development of motility of Langerhans cell through extracellular matrix by *in vitro* hapten contact, *Eur. J. Immunol.*, 24, 2254, 1994.
400. la Sala, A. et al., Dendritic cells exposed to extracellular adenosine triphosphate acquire the migratory properties of mature cells and show a reduced capacity to attract type 1 T lymphocytes, *Blood*, 99, 1715, 2002.
401. Panther, E. et al., Adenosine affects expression of membrane molecules, cytokine and chemokine release, and the T-cell stimulatory capacity of human dendritic cells, *Blood*, 101, 3985, 2003.
402. Maestroni, G.J., Dendritic cell migration controlled by α 1b-adrenergic receptors, *J. Immunol.*, 165, 6743, 2000.
403. Sozzani, S. et al., Migration of dendritic cells in response to formyl peptides, C5a, and a distinct set of chemokines, *J. Immunol.*, 155, 3292, 1995.
404. Soruri, A. et al., Anaphylatoxin C5a induces monocyte recruitment and differentiation into dendritic cells by TNF-α and prostaglandin E2-dependent mechanisms, *J. Immunol.*, 171, 2631, 2003.
405. Murphy, G.F. et al., Association of basal-lamina defects with epidermal and dermal T6-positive cells: evidence of Langerhans-cell migration, *Arch. Dermatol. Res.*, 278, 126, 1985.
406. Stoitzner, P. et al., A close-up view of migrating Langerhans cells in the skin, *J. Invest. Dermatol.*, 118, 117, 2002.
407. Shapiro, S.D., Matrix metalloproteinase degradation of extracellular matrix: biological consequences, *Curr. Opin. Cell Biol.*, 10, 602, 1998.
408. Ratzinger, G. et al., Matrix metalloproteinases 9 and 2 are necessary for the migration of Langerhans cells and dermal dendritic cells from human and murine skin, *J. Immunol.*, 168, 4361, 2002.
409. Kobayashi, Y. et al., Possible involvement of matrix metalloproteinase-9 in Langerhans cell migration and maturation, *J. Immunol.*, 163, 5989, 1999.
410. Lebre, M.C. et al., Inhibition of contact sensitizer-induced migration of human Langerhans cells by matrix metalloproteinase inhibitors, *Arch. Dermatol. Res.*, 291, 447, 1999.
411. Lukas, M. et al., Human cutaneous dendritic cells migrate through dermal lymphatic vessels in a skin organ culture model, *J. Invest. Dermatol.*, 106, 1293, 1996.
412. Silberberg, I., Apposition of mononuclear cells to Langerhans cells in contact allergic reactions. An ultrastructural study, *Acta Derm. Venereol.*, 53, 1, 1973.
413. Silberberg, I., Baer, R.L., and Rosenthal, S.A., The role of Langerhans cells in allergic contact hypersensitivity. A review of findings in man and guinea pigs, *J. Invest. Dermatol.*, 66, 210, 1976.
414. Shelley, W.B. and Juhlin, L., Selective uptake of contact allergens by the Langerhans cell, *Arch. Dermatol.*, 113, 187, 1977.
415. Botham, P.A. et al., Control of the immune response to contact sensitizing chemicals by cutaneous antigen-presenting cells, *Br. J. Dermatol.*, 117, 1, 1987.

416. Bos, J.D. and Meinardi, M.M., The 500 Dalton rule for the skin penetration of chemical compounds and drugs, *Exp. Dermatol.*, 9, 165, 2000.
417. Clement, L.T. and Shevach, E.M., Characterization of major histocompatibility antigens on trinitrophenyl-modified cells, *Mol. Immunol.*, 16, 67, 1979.
418. Sinigaglia, F., The molecular basis of metal recognition by T cells, *J. Invest. Dermatol.*, 102, 398, 1994.
419. Toews, G.B., Bergstresser, P.R., and Streilein, J.W., Langerhans cells: sentinels of skin associated lymphoid tissue, *J. Invest. Dermatol.*, 75, 78, 1980.
420. Stingl, G. et al., Antigen presentation by murine epidermal Langerhans cells and its alteration by ultraviolet B light, *J. Immunol.*, 127, 1707, 1981.
421. Sauder, D.N. et al., Induction of tolerance to topically applied TNCB using TNP-conjugated ultraviolet light-irradiated epidermal cells, *J. Immunol.*, 127, 261, 1981.
422. Rheins, L.A. and Nordlund, J.J., Modulation of the population density of identifiable epidermal Langerhans cells associated with enhancement or suppression of cutaneous immune reactivity, *J. Immunol.*, 136, 867, 1986.
423. Streilein, J.W., Antigen-presenting cells in the induction of contact hypersensitivity in mice: evidence that Langerhans cells are sufficient but not required, *J. Invest. Dermatol.*, 93, 443, 1989.
424. Silberberg-Sinakin, I. et al., Langerhans cells: role in contact hypersensitivity and relationship to lymphoid dendritic cells and to macrophages, *Immunol. Rev.*, 53, 203, 1980.
425. Macatonia, S.E. et al., Localization of antigen on lymph node dendritic cells after exposure to the contact sensitizer fluorescein isothiocyanate. Functional and morphological studies, *J. Exp. Med.*, 166, 1654, 1987.
426. Kripke, M.L. et al., Evidence that cutaneous antigen-presenting cells migrate to regional lymph nodes during contact sensitization, *J. Immunol.*, 145, 2833, 1990.
427. Hunger, R.E. et al., CD1a-positive dendritic cells transport the antigen DNCB intracellularly from the skin to the regional lymph nodes in the induction phase of allergic contact dermatitis, *Arch. Dermatol. Res.*, 293, 420, 2001.
428. Grabbe, S. and Schwarz, T., Immunoregulatory mechanisms involved in elicitation of allergic contact hypersensitivity, *Immunol. Today*, 19, 37, 1998.
429. Enk, A.H. and Katz, S.I., Early molecular events in the induction phase of contact sensitivity, *Proc. Natl. Acad. Sci. U.S.A.*, 89, 1398, 1992.
430. Zhao, B. and Wang, B.H., Cytochemical and ultrastructural studies of the Langerhans cells. Sequential observations in experimental contact allergic reaction, *Int. J. Dermatol.*, 24, 653, 1985.
431. Hanau, D. et al., ATPase and morphologic changes in Langerhans cells induced by epicutaneous application of a sensitizing dose of DNFB, *J. Invest. Dermatol.*, 92, 689, 1989.
432. Weinlich, G. et al., Entry into afferent lymphatics and maturation *in situ* of migrating murine cutaneous dendritic cells, *J. Invest. Dermatol.*, 110, 441, 1998.
433. Kolde, G. and Knop, J., Different cellular reaction patterns of epidermal Langerhans cells after application of contact sensitizing, toxic, and tolerogenic compounds. A comparative ultrastructural and morphometric time-course analysis, *J. Invest. Dermatol.*, 89, 19, 1987.
434. Gocinski, B.L. and Tigelaar, R.E., Roles of $CD4^+$ and $CD8^+$ T cells in murine contact sensitivity revealed by *in vivo* monoclonal antibody depletion, *J. Immunol.*, 144, 4121, 1990.
435. Bourgeois, C. and Tanchot, C., Mini-review CD4 T cells are required for CD8 T cell memory generation, *Eur. J. Immunol.*, 33, 3225, 2003.
436. Steinbrink, K., Sorg, C., and Macher, E., Low zone tolerance to contact allergens in mice: a functional role for $CD8^+$ T helper type 2 cells, *J. Exp. Med.*, 183, 759, 1996.
437. Cavani, A. et al., Human $CD4^+$ T lymphocytes with remarkable regulatory functions on dendritic cells and nickel-specific Th1 immune responses, *J. Invest. Dermatol.*, 114, 295, 2000.
438. Riemann, H. et al., Neutralization of IL-12 *in vivo* prevents induction of contact hypersensitivity and induces hapten-specific tolerance, *J. Immunol.*, 156, 1799, 1996.
439. Brandt, K. et al., Interleukin-21 inhibits dendritic cell-mediated T cell activation and induction of contact hypersensitivity *in vivo*, *J. Invest. Dermatol.*, 121, 1379, 2003.
440. Guan, H. et al., Neuronal repellent Slit2 inhibits dendritic cell migration and the development of immune responses, *J. Immunol.*, 171, 6519, 2003.
441. Rambukkana, A. et al., *In situ* behavior of human Langerhans cells in skin organ culture, *Lab. Invest.*, 73, 521, 1995.

442. Pistoor, F.H. et al., Novel predictive assay for contact allergens using human skin explant cultures, *Am. J. Pathol.*, 149, 337, 1996.
443. Rambukkana, A. et al., Effects of contact allergens on human Langerhans cells in skin organ culture: migration, modulation of cell surface molecules, and early expression of interleukin-1β protein, *Lab. Invest.*, 74, 422, 1996.
444. Bos, J.D. et al., Skin-homing T lymphocytes: detection of cutaneous lymphocyte-associated antigen (CLA) by HECA-452 in normal human skin, *Arch. Dermatol. Res.*, 285, 179, 1993.
445. Picker, L.J. et al., Control of lymphocyte recirculation in man. II. Differential regulation of the cutaneous lymphocyte-associated antigen, a tissue-selective homing receptor for skin-homing T cells, *J. Immunol.*, 150, 1122, 1993.
446. Grabbe, S. et al., Dissection of antigenic and irritative effects of epicutaneously applied haptens in mice. Evidence that not the antigenic component but nonspecific proinflammatory effects of haptens determine the concentration-dependent elicitation of allergic contact dermatitis, *J. Clin. Invest*, 98, 1158, 1996.
447. McLelland, J., Shuster, S., and Matthews, J.N., "'Irritants" increase the response to an allergen in allergic contact dermatitis, *Arch. Dermatol.*, 127, 1016, 1991.
448. Barker, J.N. et al., Keratinocytes as initiators of inflammation, *Lancet*, 337, 211, 1991.
449. Griffiths, C.E. and Nickoloff, B.J., Keratinocyte intercellular adhesion molecule-1 (ICAM-1) expression precedes dermal T lymphocytic infiltration in allergic contact dermatitis (Rhus dermatitis), *Am. J. Pathol.*, 135, 1045, 1989.
450. Wildner, O., Lipkow, T., and Knop, J., Increased expression of ICAM-1, E-selectin, and VCAM-1 by cultured human endothelial cells upon exposure to haptens, *Exp. Dermatol.*, 1, 191, 1992.
451. Scheynius, A., Camp, R.L., and Pure, E., Reduced contact sensitivity reactions in mice treated with monoclonal antibodies to leukocyte function-associated molecule-1 and intercellular adhesion molecule-1, *J. Immunol.*, 150, 655, 1993.
452. Sligh, J.E., Jr. et al., Inflammatory and immune responses are impaired in mice deficient in intercellular adhesion molecule 1, *Proc. Natl. Acad. Sci. U.S.A.*, 90, 8529, 1993.
453. Kapsenberg, M.L. et al., Th1 lymphokine production profiles of nickel-specific $CD4^+$ T-lymphocyte clones from nickel contact allergic and non-allergic individuals, *J. Invest. Dermatol.*, 98, 59, 1992.
454. Cavani, A. et al., Patients with allergic contact dermatitis to nickel and nonallergic individuals display different nickel-specific T cell responses. Evidence for the presence of effector $CD8^+$ and regulatory $CD4^+$ T cells, *J. Invest. Dermatol.*, 111, 621, 1998.
455. Grabbe, S. et al., Removal of the majority of epidermal Langerhans cells by topical or systemic steroid application enhances the effector phase of murine contact hypersensitivity, *J. Immunol.*, 155, 4207, 1995.
456. Bangert, C. et al., Immunopathologic features of allergic contact dermatitis in humans: participation of plasmacytoid dendritic cells in the pathogenesis of the disease? *J. Invest. Dermatol.*, 121, 1409, 2003.
457. Probst, P., Kuntzlin, D., and Fleischer, B., TH2-type infiltrating T cells in nickel-induced contact dermatitis, *Cell Immunol.*, 165, 134, 1995.
458. Wang, B. et al., $CD4^+$ Th1 and $CD8^+$ type 1 cytotoxic T cells both play a crucial role in the full development of contact hypersensitivity, *J. Immunol.*, 165, 6783, 2000.
459. Xu, H., DiIulio, N.A., and Fairchild, R.L., T cell populations primed by hapten sensitization in contact sensitivity are distinguished by polarized patterns of cytokine production: interferon-γ-producing (Tc1) effector $CD8^+$ T cells and interleukin (Il) 4/Il-10-producing (Th2) negative regulatory $CD4^+$ T cells, *J. Exp. Med.*, 183, 1001, 1996.
460. Fernandez, N.C. et al., Dendritic cells directly trigger NK cell functions: cross-talk relevant in innate anti-tumor immune responses *in vivo*, *Nat. Med.*, 5, 405, 1999.
461. Piccioli, D. et al., Contact-dependent stimulation and inhibition of dendritic cells by natural killer cells, *J. Exp. Med.*, 195, 335, 2002.
462. Buentke, E. et al., Natural killer and dendritic cell contact in lesional atopic dermatitis skin — Malassezia-influenced cell interaction, *J. Invest. Dermatol.*, 119, 850, 2002.
463. Zelickson, A.S. and Mottaz, J.H., Epidermal dendritic cells. A quantitative study, *Arch. Dermatol.*, 98, 652, 1968.
464. Chu, A. et al., Immunoelectron microscopic identification of Langerhans cells using a new antigenic marker, *J. Invest. Dermatol.*, 78, 177, 1982.

465. Rowden, G., Phillips, T.M., and Lewis, M.G., Ia antigens on indeterminate cells of the epidermis: immunoelectron microscopic studies of surface antigens, *Br. J. Dermatol.*, 100, 531, 1979.
466. Czernielewski, J.M. et al., Functional and phenotypic analysis of isolated human Langerhans cells and indeterminate cells, *Br. J. Dermatol.*, 108, 129, 1983.
467. Andersson, A. et al., The epidermal indeterminate cell — a special cell type? *Acta Dermatovener.* (Stockholm), 99, 41s, 1981.
468. Meunier, L., Gonzalez-Ramos, A., and Cooper, K.D., Heterogeneous populations of class II MHC$^+$ cells in human dermal cell suspensions. Identification of a small subset responsible for potent dermal antigen-presenting cell activity with features analogous to Langerhans cells, *J. Immunol.*, 151, 4067, 1993.
469. Murphy, G.F. et al., *In situ* identification of T6-positive cells in normal human dermis by immunoelectron microscopy, *Br. J. Dermatol.*, 108, 423, 1983.
470. Headington, J.T., The dermal dendrocyte, *Adv. Dermatol.*, 1, 159, 1986.
471. Cerio, R. et al., Characterization of factor XIIIa positive dermal dendritic cells in normal and inflamed skin, *Br. J. Dermatol.*, 121, 421, 1989.
472. Narvaez, D., Kanitakis, J., and Claudy, A., Dendritic cells of human dermis, *Eur. J. Dermatol.*, 5, 69, 1995.
473. Walsh, L.J. et al., MS-1 sinusoidal endothelial antigen is expressed by factor XIIIa$^+$, HLA-DR$^+$ dermal perivascular dendritic cells, *Lab. Invest.*, 65, 732, 1991.
474. Monteiro, M.R. et al., Von Willebrand factor receptor GPIb $\alpha$ is expressed by human factor XIIIa-positive dermal dendrocytes and is upregulated by mast cell degranulation, *J. Invest. Dermatol.*, 113, 272, 1999.
475. Sepulveda-Merrill, C. et al., Antigen-presenting capacity in normal human dermis is mainly subserved by CD1a$^+$ cells, *Br. J. Dermatol.*, 131, 15, 1994.
476. Lenz, A. et al., Human and murine dermis contain dendritic cells. Isolation by means of a novel method and phenotypical and functional characterization, *J. Clin. Invest*, 92, 2587, 1993.
477. Larregina, A.T. et al., Pattern of cytokine receptors expressed by human dendritic cells migrated from dermal explants, *Immunology*, 91, 303, 1997.
478. Sueki, H. et al., Novel interactions between dermal dendrocytes and mast cells in human skin. Implications for hemostasis and matrix repair, *Lab. Invest.*, 69, 160, 1993.
479. Sueki, H., Telegan, B., and Murphy, G.F., Computer-assisted three-dimensional reconstruction of human dermal dendrocytes, *J. Invest. Dermatol.*, 105, 704, 1995.
480. Walsh, L.J. et al., Human dermal mast cells contain and release tumor necrosis factor $\alpha$, which induces endothelial leukocyte adhesion molecule 1, *Proc. Natl. Acad. Sci. U.S.A.*, 88, 4220, 1991.
481. Nickoloff, B.J., The human progenitor cell antigen (CD34) is localized on endothelial cells, dermal dendritic cells, and perifollicular cells in formalin-fixed normal skin, and on proliferating endothelial cells and stromal spindle-shaped cells in Kaposi's sarcoma, *Arch. Dermatol.*, 127, 523, 1991.
482. Narvaez, D. et al., Immunohistochemical study of CD34-positive dendritic cells of human dermis, *Am. J. Dermatopathol.*, 18, 283, 1996.
483. Wollenberg, A. et al., Immunomorphological and ultrastructural characterization of Langerhans cells and a novel, inflammatory dendritic epidermal cell (IDEC) population in lesional skin of atopic eczema, *J. Invest. Dermatol.*, 106, 446, 1996.
484. Taylor, R.S. et al., Hyperstimulatory CD1a$^+$CD1b$^+$CD36$^+$ Langerhans cells are responsible for increased autologous T lymphocyte reactivity to lesional epidermal cells of patients with atopic dermatitis, *J. Immunol.*, 147, 3794, 1991.
485. Swerlick, R.A. et al., Human dermal microvascular endothelial but not human umbilical vein endothelial cells express CD36 *in vivo* and *in vitro*, *J. Immunol.*, 148, 78, 1992.
486. Wollenberg, A., Wen, S., and Bieber, T., Phenotyping of epidermal dendritic cells: clinical applications of a flow cytometric micromethod, *Cytometry*, 37, 147, 1999.
487. Bieber, T., Fc$\varepsilon$RI-expressing antigen-presenting cells: new players in the atopic game, *Immunol. Today*, 18, 311, 1997.
488. Haberstok, J. et al., The phenotype of human Langerhans cells and inflammatory dendritic epidermal cells reflects the disease specific microenvironment of cutaneous inflammation., *Arch. Dermatol. Res.*, 288, 334, 1996.

489. Wollenberg, A. et al., Expression and function of the mannose receptor CD206 on epidermal dendritic cells in inflammatory skin diseases, *J. Invest. Dermatol.*, 118, 327, 2002.
490. Wollenberg, A. et al., Demonstration of the low-affinity IgE receptor FcεRII/CD23 in psoriatic epidermis: inflammatory dendritic epidermal cells (IDEC) but not Langerhans cells are the relevant CD1a-positive cell population, *Arch. Dermatol. Res.*, 290, 517, 1998.
491. Lecoanet-Henchoz, S. et al., CD23 regulates monocyte activation through a novel interaction with the adhesion molecules CD11b-CD18 and CD11c-CD18, *Immunity*, 3, 119, 1995.
492. Schuller, E. et al., *In situ* expression of the costimulatory molecules CD80 and CD86 on Langerhans cells and inflammatory dendritic epidermal cells (IDEC) in atopic dermatitis, *Arch. Dermatol. Res.*, 293, 448, 2001.
493. Grewe, M. et al., Lesional expression of interferon-γ in atopic eczema, *Lancet*, 343, 25, 1994.
494. Novak, N. et al., A reducing microenvironment leads to the generation of FcεRIhigh inflammatory dendritic epidermal cells (IDEC), *J. Invest. Dermatol.*, 119, 842, 2002.
495. Reich, K. et al., Engagement of the FcεRI stimulates the production of IL-16 in Langerhans cell-like dendritic cells, *J. Immunol.*, 167, 6321, 2001.
496. Olweus, J. et al., Dendritic cell ontogeny: a human dendritic cell lineage of myeloid origin, *Proc. Natl. Acad. Sci. U.S.A.*, 94, 12551, 1997.
497. Lennert, K. and Remmele, W., Karyometrische Untersuchungen und Lymphknotenzellen des Menschen. I. Mitt Germinoblasten, Lymphoblasten und Lymphozyten, *Acta Haematol.*, 19, 99, 1958.
498. Muller-Hermelink, H.K., Kaiserling, E., and Lennert, K., [Pseudofollicular nests of plasmacells (of a special type?) in paracortical pulp of human lymph nodes (author's translation)], *Virchows Arch. B Cell Pathol.*, 14, 47, 1973.
499. Lennert, K., Kaiserling, E., and Muller-Hermelink, H.K., T-associated plasma-cells, *Lancet*, 1, 1031, 1975.
500. Muller-Hermelink, H.K. et al., Malignant lymphoma of plasmacytoid T-cells. Morphologic and immunologic studies characterizing a special type of T-cell, *Am. J. Surg. Pathol.*, 7, 849, 1983.
501. Beiske, K. et al., Single cell studies on the immunological marker profile of plasmacytoid T-zone cells, *Lab. Invest.*, 56, 381, 1987.
502. Horny, H.P. et al., Immunocytology of plasmacytoid T cells: marker analysis indicates a unique phenotype of this enigmatic cell, *Hum. Pathol.*, 18, 28, 1987.
503. Facchetti, F. et al., Plasmacytoid T cells: a cell population normally present in the reactive lymph node. An immunohistochemical and electron microscopic study, *Hum. Pathol.*, 19, 1085, 1988.
504. Abb, J., Abb, H., and Deinhardt, F., Phenotype of human α-interferon producing leucocytes identified by monoclonal antibodies, *Clin. Exp. Immunol.*, 52, 179, 1983.
505. Chehimi, J. et al., Dendritic cells and IFN-α-producing cells are two functionally distinct non-B, non-monocytic HLA-DR$^+$ cell subsets in human peripheral blood, *Immunology*, 68, 488, 1989.
506. Kadowaki, N. et al., Natural interferon α/β-producing cells link innate and adaptive immunity, *J. Exp. Med.*, 192, 219, 2000.
507. Penna, G. et al., Differential migration behavior and chemokine production by myeloid and plasmacytoid dendritic cells, *Hum. Immunol.*, 63, 1164, 2002.
508. Eckert, F. and Schmid, U., Identification of plasmacytoid T cells in lymphoid hyperplasia of the skin, *Arch. Dermatol.*, 125, 1518, 1989.
509. Facchetti, F. et al., Plasmacytoid T cells in a case of lymphocytic infiltration of skin. A component of the skin-associated lymphoid tissue? *J. Pathol.*, 155, 295, 1988.
510. Vollenweider, R. and Lennert, K., Plasmacytoid T-cell clusters in non-specific lymphadenitis, *Virchows Arch. B Cell Pathol. Incl. Mol. Pathol.*, 44, 1, 1983.
511. Facchetti, F. et al., Plasmacytoid monocytes in Jessner's lymphocytic infiltration of the skin, *Am. J. Dermatopathol.*, 12, 363, 1990.
512. Toonstra, J. and van der Putte, S.C., Plasmacytoid monocytes in Jessner's lymphocytic infiltration of the skin. A valuable clue for the diagnosis, *Am. J. Dermatopathol.*, 13, 321, 1991.
513. Farkas, L. et al., Plasmacytoid dendritic cells (natural interferon- α/β-producing cells) accumulate in cutaneous lupus erythematosus lesions, *Am. J. Pathol.*, 159, 237, 2001.
514. Jahnsen, F.L. et al., Involvement of plasmacytoid dendritic cells in human diseases, *Hum. Immunol.*, 63, 1201, 2002.

515. Vermi, W. et al., Recruitment of immature plasmacytoid dendritic cells (plasmacytoid monocytes) and myeloid dendritic cells in primary cutaneous melanomas, *J. Pathol.*, 200, 255, 2003.
516. Wakkach, A. et al., Characterization of dendritic cells that induce tolerance and T regulatory 1 cell differentiation *in vivo*, *Immunity*, 18, 605, 2003.
517. Huang, Q. et al., The plasticity of dendritic cell responses to pathogens and their components, *Science*, 294, 870, 2001.
518. Wilson, N.S. et al., Most lymphoid organ dendritic cell types are phenotypically and functionally immature, *Blood*, 102, 2187, 2003.
519. Nestle, F.O. et al., Vaccination of melanoma patients with peptide- or tumor lysate-pulsed dendritic cells, *Nat. Med.*, 4, 328, 1998.
520. Thurner, B. et al., Vaccination with mage-3A1 peptide-pulsed mature, monocyte-derived dendritic cells expands specific cytotoxic T cells and induces regression of some metastases in advanced stage IV melanoma, *J. Exp. Med.*, 190, 1669, 1999.
521. Banchereau, J. et al., Immune and clinical responses in patients with metastatic melanoma to CD34(+) progenitor-derived dendritic cell vaccine, *Cancer Res.*, 61, 6451, 2001.
522. Morse, M.A. et al., Migration of human dendritic cells after injection in patients with metastatic malignancies, *Cancer Res.*, 59, 56, 1999.
523. Schrama, D. et al., Aggregation of antigen-specific T cells at the inoculation site of mature dendritic cells, *J. Invest. Dermatol.*, 119, 1443, 2002.
524. Martin-Fontecha, A. et al., Regulation of dendritic cell migration to the draining lymph node: impact on T lymphocyte traffic and priming, *J. Exp. Med.*, 198, 615, 2003.
525. Mahnke, K. et al., Induction of $CD4^+/CD25^+$ regulatory T cells by targeting of antigens to immature dendritic cells, *Blood*, 101, 4862, 2003.
526. Larregina, A.T. et al., Direct transfection and activation of human cutaneous dendritic cells, *Gene Ther.*, 8, 608, 2001.

# 8 Monocytes and Macrophages in Human Skin

*Kurt Q. Lu, Thomas S. McCormick, Anita C. Gilliam, Kefei Kang, and Kevin D. Cooper*

## CONTENTS



## I. INTRODUCTION

Classic immunology has demonstrated that the interaction of antigen-presenting cells (APCs) and T cells can lead to inflammation. There has recently been renewed interest in the innate immune system in which primitive pathways of defense against foreign agents occur. Some of this excitement is attributable to the explosion in the study of Toll-like receptors (TLR), chemokines, defensins, and integrins. These modulators have helped establish a greater appreciation for how monocytes and macrophages (Mo/Macs) initiate and orchestrate specific vital signals for adaptive immunity and for regulating cellular homeostasis. As with any cell type, the process of unraveling the complex

0-8493-1959-5/05/$0.00+$1.50

Mo/Mac functions have benefited from ongoing development of techniques for their isolation. The ability to isolate distinct cells has allowed for study of events in cellular differentiation and for observations of cellular function. Mo/Macs are recognized as complex modulators of immunity as they are observed to be vital in different models of skin and immunologic diseases. This chapter highlights key roles that Mo/Mac play in immunosuppression and autoimmunity through models of ultraviolet (UV) irradiation, contact hypersensitivity, and inflammation.

Mo/Macs also act as crucial effector cells mediating the generation of inflammation in response to infection by the innate immune system. The discussion at large focuses on their role as phagocytes in conjunction with their polymorphonuclear counterparts. Attention often placed on neutrophils as key responder phagocytes is due to their higher cell numbers and ability to mobilize at a rapid pace. The perceived slower responding Mo/Macs bring an additional function to the microenvironment following activation. Following engulfment of foreign bodies, Mo/Macs are able to act as APCs in the context of MHC. Although they are often compared to their counterpart dendritic cells (DCs), Mo/Macs are generally viewed as less potent stimulators of naive T cells. However, in several instances in the skin Mo/Macs function effectively as alternative APCs, such as in the post-UV dermal microenvironment, or for maintaining inflammatory disease such as psoriasis, as well as for handling infection. Thus, Mo/Macs represent a critical bridge cell between innate and adaptive immunity, and participate in a wide variety of antimicrobial defense mechanisms as well as pathogenic chronic inflammatory conditions.

## II. CHARACTERIZATION OF MONOCYTES/MACROPHAGES

### A. Morphology and Lineage Relationships

Resting precursor monocytes with eccentric nuclei are the largest leukocytes that circulate in the peripheral bloodstream (Figure 8.1a). They are derived from myeloid precursors that originate in the bone marrow. They comprise 2 to 10% of peripheral blood leukocytes and can be marginated in response to chemotactic factors released from systemic events. Monocytes can enter most tissue where they transform into activated macrophages (Figure 8.1b). Their appearance in dermal and epidermal areas of the skin has been well documented.[1] Cutaneous macrophages are also known as histiocytes.[2]

Macrophages, along with their related resident tissue-specific myeloid derived cells, comprise a network called the mononuclear phagocyte system (MPS) (Figure 8.2).[3] Driven by local microanatomic and systemic environmental factors, dynamic modification of cell function is the cornerstone of the Mo/Mac response to acute inflammation or infection. Unlike thymocytes, which typically show no difference from tissue to tissue, macrophages in lung have different properties from those in skin or peritoneum. Functionally, Mo/Macs occupy a unique niche in the inflammatory response. Following extravasation of neutrophils, macrophages become the dominant cells in inflammation in many organs where they function primarily to transition the host from inflammation to restoration of homeostasis. An active role in restoring homeostasis is also observed in complex reparative processes such as wound healing, where Mo/Macs functions as important sources of growth factors and regulatory mediators.[4,5] Acute and chronic inflammation may result in tissue wounding, in which Mo/Macs participate in damage, cleanup, and repair. Furthermore, one bystander effect of inflammation is apoptosis, requiring swift and efficient engulfment by Mo/Macs without inciting further inflammation or allowing leakage of potentially immunogenic material.

### B. Phenotype and Functional/Effector Repertoire of Monocytes/Macrophages

#### 1. Functional Repertoire in Relation to Cell Surface Molecules

The skin and epithelia together with many leukocytes comprise the innate immune system. The cells of the innate immune system have evolved receptors that can distinguish foreign and patho-

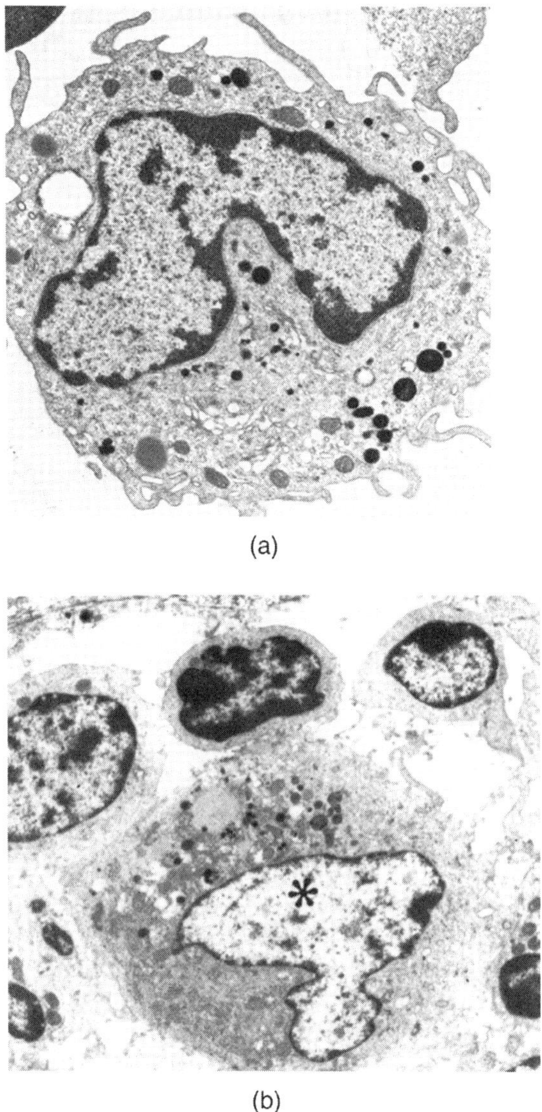


**FIGURE 8.1** (a) Peripheral blood monocyte (human) showing typical nuclear and cytoplasmic features. Transmission EM (TEM). (Original magnification × 7000.) (b) Marginal sinus of a lymph node (human) showing a macrophage (marked *) and other mononuclear cells. TEM. (Original magnification × 5000.)

genic antigens triggering the initiation of inflammation. The Mo/Macs bear multiple cell surface molecules that mediate pathogen recognition and processing as well as those that mediate recruitment and trafficking of inflammatory cells to the site of infection in combination with host cell ligand expression. The cells also express receptors that recognize apoptotic bodies and mediate removal of debris, which may be important in controlling the extent of inflammatory response. Certain broad classes of cell surface molecules can be attributed specific cellular function, while others demonstrate multiple overlapping functions. The reader is referred to several recent reviews of innate immune membrane surface molecules.[6,7]

### a. *Pathogen Recognition*

Pathogen recognition followed by delivery of selective and regulated responses is the hallmark of host defense. One strategy evolved by the innate immune system is the recognition of conserved

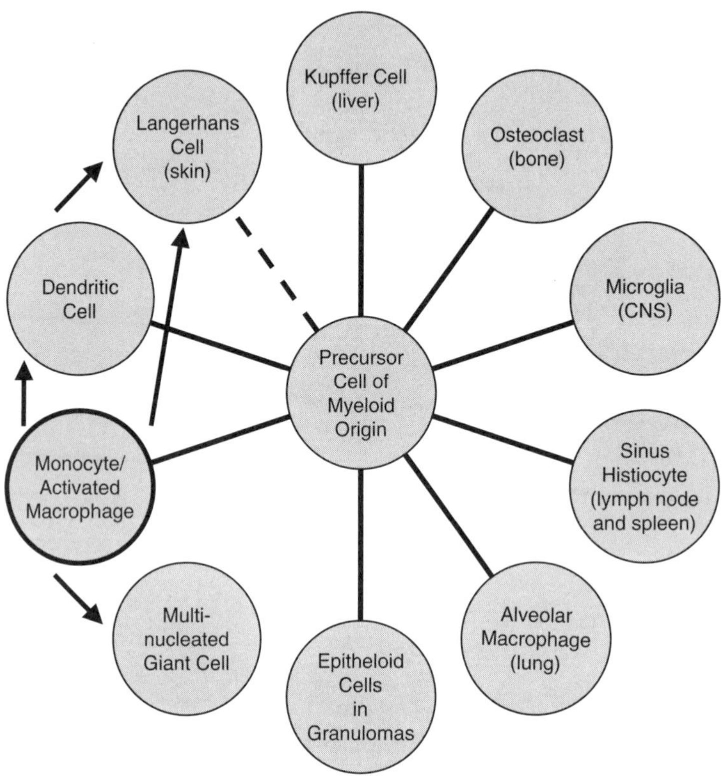


**FIGURE 8.2** Mononuclear phagocyte system (MPS). The classification of cells shares the common bone marrow myeloid precursor. The differentiated tissue-specific cell types share certain morphological and functional features.

microbial structures and sequences, coined pathogen-associated molecular patterns (PAMPs) and their pattern recognition receptors (PRRs).[8] PAMPs represent a variety of products unique to microbial but not necessarily pathogenic organisms and include such molecules as lipopolysaccharide (LPS), peptidoglycan (PTD), and bacterial CpG DNA.

Mo/Macs express several classes of receptors such as TLRs, CD14, complement receptor 3 (CR3), and scavenger receptors that recognize PAMPs. An important class of receptors central to innate immunity and macrophage function is the TLRs, in which binding induces inflammation and effector responses, including initiation of adaptive immune responses. There have been several significant reviews of the TLR family and their ligands.[9–13] The TLR family to date consists of ten type I transmembrane receptor proteins with diverse structural recognition of microbial motifs ranging from lipids to proteins to nucleic acids. Interest in the receptors emerged as they were demonstrated to signal through a NF-κB-dependent pathway,[14,15] triggering specific transcription of cytokines such as tumor necrosis factor-alpha (TNF-α), interleukin-1 (IL-1), IL-6, and IL-12.[16,17] Although TLRs are expressed in a variety of cells including endothelial cells and DCs, numerous studies of TLRs have helped to establish the macrophage as an important effector cell at the interface of early innate immune responses.

The most-studied member of the TLR family is TLR4, a PRR that recognizes LPS, an important PAMP for which the innate immune system has evolved many receptors. TLR4 engagement is an important step toward initiating LPS-induced signaling, although controversy remains regarding how the actual binding and contact occurs. Evidence demonstrates that TLR members may work synergistically with redundancy in ligand recognition while maintaining activation of distinct intracellular mechanisms following receptor engagement.[18,19]

TLRs may serve as co-receptors with various innate immune receptors, such as CD14, to potentiate inflammatory reactions.[20,21] CD14 is a receptor for multiple microbial antigens including LPS, soluble PTD, lipoteichoic acid, Gram-positive cell walls, yeast, and spirochetal antigens.[22] The mechanism mediating such broad specificity remains to be elucidated. Some antigens are facilitated by additional binding proteins, for example, LPS-binding protein (LBP) required for LPS.[23,24] Different factors may trigger changes in the level of expression of membrane vs. soluble CD14. Both the antigen itself and the microenvironment can modify CD14 expression on Mo/Macs, as observed in downregulation elicited by the Th2 cytokines, IL-4, and IL-10, and upregulation elicited by TNF-$\alpha$ and interferon-gamma (IFN-$\gamma$)[25,26] The skin microenvironment is no exception in modulating CD14 expression on cutaneous Mo/Macs, whether in response to injury or in disease pathogenic states. Additionally, CD14 expression is used for immunohistologic confirmation of the presence of macrophages in tissue such as skin and is accepted as the common epitope expressed on the surface of both monocytes and macrophages but not on DCs.

In addition to TLRs and CD14, Mo/Macs express a number of proteins that aid in pathogen recognition and processing, as well as mediating cell localization to the site of infection. One class of molecules called integrins is a family of receptor proteins that have enhanced our understanding of inflammation and Mo/Mac biology, particularly $\beta$1 and $\beta$2 integrins. They have a heterodimeric structure consisting of an $\alpha$ and $\beta$ chain, which are classified according to their $\beta$ subunit. The $\beta$1 integrin subfamily is involved in assembly and recognition of extracellular matrix (ECM), which includes fibronectin, collagen, laminin, and vitronectin.[27–29] They are also involved in adhesion and migration of Mo/Mac through the skin along ECM structures.[30,31] $\beta$1 integrins are observed to activate inflammatory cytokines through NF-$\kappa$B-dependent and -independent mechanisms and may be important in effecting the dermal cytokine milieu that directs monocyte differentiation.[32] $\beta$1 integrins, also known as very late antigen proteins (VLA), expressed by Mo/Macs include high VLA-6, moderate VLA-2, VLA-4 ($\alpha_4\beta_1$), VLA-5 ($\alpha_5\beta_1$), and low VLA-1 and VLA-3.[33]

Although $\beta$1 integrins are expressed by many cell types, the $\beta$2 integrin subfamily is expressed only in leukocytes. $\beta$2 integrins expressed in Mo/Macs include LFA-1 (CD11a/CD18), CR3 (CD11b/CD18), CR4 (CD11c/CD18), and $\alpha_D\beta_2$ (CD11d/CD18). CR3, also known as Mac-1, Mo-1, CD11b/CD18, and $\alpha_M\beta_2$, functions as a receptor for the complement activation product of C3b called iC3b. The receptor is also involved in several leukocyte functions, such as phagocytosis and phagocyte adhesion and migration. CR3 is a receptor that has a remarkably diverse recognition of ligands, endogenous and microbial.[34] For example, it can recognize carbohydrate moieties not only on the complement C3 product iC3b, but also LPS and several other bacterial particulates. Working in concert with other receptors, such as CD14, it cooperates in host innate responses. Additionally, CR3 plays a role in monocyte differentiation, as well as regulating IL-10 and IL-12 counterbalance. This wide range of binding partners helps to reinforce the classification of CR3 as a PRR.

### *b. Apoptotic Cell Recognition*

The response to infection produces inflammation and the release of numerous cell products that may be detrimental locally and systemically if not contained. Cells exposed to the cascades of soluble products may become damaged and directed toward apoptosis. Once committed to apoptosis, cells express various markers as well as released products that are recognized by phagocytes for clearance, thus preventing leakage of potentially toxic substances from cell degradation. While neighboring cells in the microenvironment can aid in phagocytosis, the macrophage's role as a professional phagocyte is critical to this process. Clearing of unwanted potentially immunogenic substances can bring resolution to inflammatory processes as well as critically influencing further immune responses. Several families of receptors have been described in the process of macrophage-mediated clearance of apoptotic bodies.[35] A family of receptors expressed on macrophages called scavenger receptors (SRs), important in atherogenesis via uptake of low-density lipoproteins (LDLs), has increasingly been observed to mediate other host functions.[36] The class A receptors (SR-A), with a collagenous domain, are constitutively expressed in resident and migrating macrophages and are nearly undetectable in epidermal Langerhans cells (LCs). In addition to binding to modified LDLs, the type I and II SR-A receptors are important in mediating phagocytosis of apoptotic cellular debris as well as mediating the early phase of cell adhesion.[37] There are reports of type I and II receptors binding bacterial endotoxin without activation of signaling, possibly to absorb excess antigens thereby limiting TNF-$\alpha$ release and acting to potentially prevent sepsis. The class B SRs includes CD36 and the lesser-known SR-B1. CD36 expression appears to be regulated by MCSF and IL-4[38] and functions in uptake of oxidized LDLs. Additionally CD36 mediates phagocytosis of infected erythrocytes[39] and has been demonstrated to recognize and mediate phagocytosis via $\alpha_v\beta_3$ and phosphatidylserine (PS) on apoptotic cells.[40] Although the evidence for SR participation in skin diseases is limited, the recognition of several macromolecules and oxidized species by these receptors has important implication in the skin microenvironment. Environmental insults such as UV radiation to the skin produce reactive oxygen species and subsequent cutaneous cell apoptosis that may require cleanup by macrophages through their SRs.

In addition to the SRs, several macrophage molecules are emerging as important participants in the removal of apoptotic cells by macrophages. This redundancy underscores the vital significance of the clearance process in the immune response. The macrophage receptor CD14, described above as a receptor for LPS, was demonstrated to also mediate binding and phagocytosis of apoptotic cells in the region closely associated with the LPS binding site without triggering the release of pro-inflammatory cytokines.[41–43] Several subsequent reports have helped to confirm the role of membrane bound CD14-dependent phagocytosis of apoptotic cells in macrophages. Further work is needed to examine the contribution of the soluble form of CD14 and the monocyte membrane-bound CD14.[40,44]

## 2. Functional Repertoire in Relation to Secreted Products

Upon Mo/Mac activation, cell size increases in conjunction with enhanced phagocytic and killing capabilities. One of the most important effector functions of macrophages is their potent ability to secrete a wide range of mediators in response to agents in the surrounding microenvironment. They contain a cadre of enzymatic and metabolic mediators, some as preformed stores that can be quickly distributed and then regenerated, and some as inducible agents. Thus, both resident skin histiocytes and monocytes newly recruited to the skin can amplify and regulate inflammation in the skin.

Mo/Macs, in response to inflammatory signals, release pro-inflammatory and cytotoxic cytokines including TNF-$\alpha$, IL-1, IFN-$\gamma$, IFN-$\alpha$, IL-6, and numerous other cytokines (Table 8.1).[45–47] The Mo/Macs secrete various chemokines known to activate other leukocytes and lymphocytes such as IL-8, GRO-$\alpha$, IP-10, MIG, and RANTES.[48] They also secrete chemokines that function in an autocrine manner such as MIP-1$\alpha$, -1$\beta$, MCP-1, -3.

Mo/Macs secrete components of two important classes of plasma proteins, namely, the complement proteins and coagulation factors. Activation of complement cascades results in diverse functions such as clearance of immune complexes, enhancement of phagocytosis, chemotaxis of inflammatory cells, and formation of the membrane attack complex. Furthermore, complement is also important in regulating cells that participate in adaptive responses.[49] Once believed to be serum factors synthesized exclusively by the liver, it has since been well documented that Mo/Macs can synthesize all components of complement.[50–53] Thus, in addition to ensuring that sufficient complement components are available in the local site of infection, Mo/Macs may be a significant contributing source of plasma C1.[54,55]

In a variety of inflammatory conditions, Mo/Macs secrete factors that activate the coagulation cascade. The release of procoagulant factors (PCFs) varies according to the stimulant and also by the state of differentiation of the Mo/Mac cell itself. Mo/Macs can be induced to express tissue factor (TF), a membrane-bound glycoprotein capable of initiating procoagulant activity.[56,57] In addition to blood coagulation, TF expressed by Mo/Macs is involved in acute and chronic inflammatory processes, stimulated by bacterial products, and regulated by various inflammatory medi-

**TABLE 8.1**
**Secretory Products of Mo/Mac Effector Function**

**Cytokines and Chemokine** (see references 45–48)
TNF-α, IL-1, IFN-γ, IFN-α,
TGF-β, IL-1ra, IL-10, IL-12,
IL-6, LIF, OSM, MIF,
M-CSF, G-CSF, GM-CSF,
IL-8, GRO-α,
IP-10, MIG, MCP-1,-3,
MIP-1α, -1β, RANTES
**Complement Components** (see reference 51)
Classical: C1q, r/s, C4, C2, C1-INH, C4bp
Alternative: C3, B, D, P, H, I
Terminal: C5-C9
**Coagulation Factors** (see reference 60)
Tissue Factor
Factors V/Va, VII/VIIa, and X/Xa
**Growth Factors** (see reference 68)
TGF-α
FGFs 1, 2, and 4
PDGF, VEGF, HB-EGF
TGF-β1, -β2, -β3
**Reactive Metabolites** (see references 84, 88)
Reactive oxygen species — superoxide and hydrogen peroxide
Nitric oxide
**Enzymes** (see references 71–74)
Matrix metalloproteinases (MMPs)
Elastase (MMP-12), Collagenase 1(MMP-1), stromelysin (MMP-3), Gelatinase B (MMP-9)
**Urokinase-Type Plasminogen activator** (see reference 78)
Phosphatases
Lipases
**Bioactive Lipids** (see reference 80)
Prostaglandins (PGE2)
Thromboxanes (TXA2)

*Note:* Mo/Mac have potent capability to secrete a wide range of mediators in response to agents in the surrounding microenvironment.

ators, including complement and cytokines.[58,59] Except for factor IX/IXa and factor X in unstimulated human blood monocytes,[60] Mo/Macs have been demonstrated to express various factors of the extrinsic coagulation pathway including factors V/Va,[61,62] VII/VIIa,[63,64] and X/Xa.[65,66] The role of activation of coagulation by Mo/Macs is unclear. The presence of a microthrombus may serve to enhance clearance of infection by inducing additional release of inflammatory mediators and platelet-derived chemotactic factors, thereby recruiting more immune cells, a process that, when uncontrolled, may lead to disease pathogenesis, such as vasculitic infarcts of the skin, disseminated intravascular coagulation (DIC), and multiorgan failure.[67]

Coagulated blood contains many cytokines and growth factors particularly in injured skin, and may serve to initiate the wound-healing process.[68] The blood clot also contains many chemotactic signals for granulocytes and Mo/Macs. After the initial influx of inflammatory cells, Mo/Macs become the predominate cells at wound sites. They are capable of releasing numerous growth factors (Table 8.1) that provide further signals for wound repair[68,69] and play fundamental roles in stimulating angiogenesis and collagen synthesis.[70]

In the skin Mo/Macs secrete a variety of enzymes that participate in host defense and tissue repair, remodeling, and photoaging. One class of enzymes is the matrix metalloproteinases (MMPs), which include elastase, collagenase 1, gelatinase B, and stromelysin.[71–76] Other enzymes produced by Mo/Macs in cutaneous wound healing include urokinase-type plasminogen activator.[76–78]

Mo/Macs also produce bioactive lipid mediators, such as the prostanoids, consisting of prostaglandins (PGs) and thromboxanes (TXs), in response to various growth factors and cytokines.[79] Profiles of prostanoid generation vary according to cell type and their activation state, but are highly active in regulating the skin microvasculature vasoconstriction and dilation. Macrophages predominately generate PGE2 and TXA2 in a ratio that changes with cell activation.[80] The compounds are synthesized from arachidonic acid, by multiple enzymes, including cyclooxygenases (COXs). While most cells express COX-1 constitutively, COX-2 is inducible in leukocytes. In macrophages COX-2 is regulated by multiple transcription factors including NF-κB and C/EBPβ.[81-83] Prostanoid involvement in immune function is complex, leading to both promotion and inhibition of inflammation. The consequence depends on factors such as the stimuli, the specific prostanoid(s) generated, and specific prostanoid receptor(s) used. Several prostanoid/prostanoid receptor gene-targeted mouse strains may aid in unraveling the complex role of these compounds.[80]

It is widely recognized that Mo/Macs can generate reactive oxygen species (ROS), such as superoxide anion via NADPH-oxidase, to aid in bactericidal action.[84] Furthermore, there is increasing evidence that ROS may participate in cell signaling including the activation of NF-κB.[85,86] Although beneficial in killing microbes, ROS are also thought to result in tissue damage associated with both chronologic aging and photoaging.

The discovery of nitric oxide (NO) and its antimicrobial properties has been a controversial complex story for the last two decades with numerous reviews dedicated to the subject. NO collectively represents several reactive intermediates of nitric oxide, a lipid- and water-soluble radical gas, with oxygen.[87] The generation of NO from L-arginine results from the catalytic action of NO synthases (NOSs). While isoforms of NOS exist, NOS2, also known as iNOS, is of particular interest to innate immune function. The expression of NOS2/iNOS is inducible in activated macrophages in response to IFN-γ, or to combination of various cytokines and bacterial products such as TNF-α, IFN-α/β, and LPS. There are non-cytokine agents that have been described to induce NOS2/iNOS including UV and ozone, possibly via cytokine intermediates. Several studies have helped to confirm the antimicrobial action of NO produced by macrophages in connection with expression of NOS2/iNOS,[88,89] through studies demonstrating correlation of NOS2 expression and host resistance to infection and, conversely, decreased host resistance with NOS2 alleleic disruption, and exacerbation of infection with NOS inhibitors. Additionally, there is increasing evidence that NO, produced in small amounts in the early phase of cellular response, may serve to regulate innate immune responses.[90]

## C. Challenges to the Isolation of Monocytes/Macrophages

A number of caveats may affect both interpretation of Mo/Mac biology and extrapolation of their function in human physiology. Human *in vivo* studies provide the gold standard, but are often limited by obvious experimental constraints, and only limited murine models are available. Because Mo/Mac function is closely linked to morphological features and highly localized functional activities in tissues, it is desirable to obtain *in situ* data that has minimal manipulation with maximal preservation of microanatomical structures. Studies of human skin *ex vivo* are limited because Mo/Macs are not easily accessible. Extraction from tissue samples for cutaneous-Mo/Macs for the establishment of cell culture presents a challenge in yielding a useful number of cells that have not been activated by the extraction process. As depicted in the scanning electron microscopic (EM) photograph (Figure 8.3), psoriatic skin macrophages (labeled LC for "lining cell") in disease are wedged in a unique microanatomic compartment that is immediately adjacent to the epidermal layer and is elongated in morphology.[91] Keratome samples often require significant physical manip-

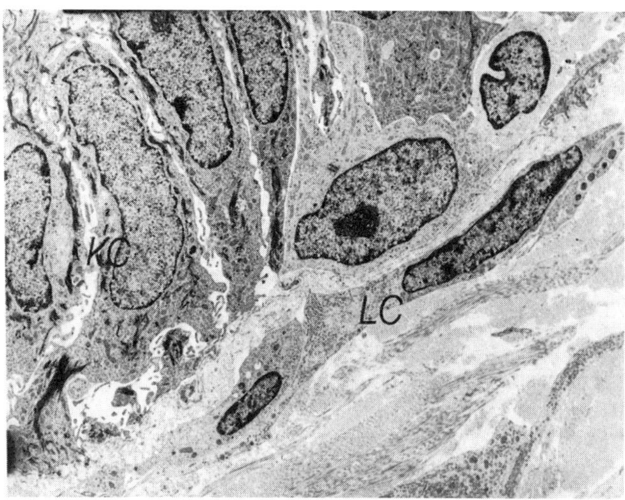


**FIGURE 8.3** Scanning EM photograph of psoriatic skin macrophages (labeled LC) in disease wedged in a unique microanatomic compartment that is immediately adjacent to the epidermal layer and is elongated in morphology. LC = lining cell, KC = keratinocytes. (From Boehncke, W.H. et al., *Am. J. Dermatopathol.*, 17(2), 139–144, 1995. Permission granted from Lippincott, Williams & Wilkins Press.)

ulation and enzymatic digestion to yield single-cell suspensions. These treatments will undoubtedly have effect on cell surface expression as well as alterations of functional molecules. Indeed, separation of the skin by enzymatic methods such as dispase or trypsin is known to result in the altered expression of cell surface molecules such as CD14.

For the reasons stated above, parallel *in vitro* studies are more abundant. As with the study of any tissue, a common goal is attainment of particular cell populations with high purity. Peripheral blood provides an accessible source of monocytes. Monocyte isolation commonly relies on separation by cell density followed by exploiting adhesive properties to further purify the population.[92] The continuing development of antibody-directed cell separation in conjunction with column separation may improve yield and purity with less manipulation.[93,94] While purity with the use of a monoclonal antibody (mAB), typically anti-CD14, to select for the Mo/Mac population may be high, there is concern that positive selection assays may induce cell activation. Hence, a negative selection approach is preferable, using an antibody cocktail to deplete unwanted leukocyte populations from total peripheral blood mononuclear cells (PBMCs) starting material. This does not obviate the problem completely, since there may be manipulation of the cells at some level because use of an antibody cocktail requires blocking the Fc$\gamma$RII (anti-CD32 mAB) on Mo/Mac. Following collection, culturing cells in media often necessitates the addition of fetal bovine serum, an opportunity for introduction of potential antigenic sources. Steps are needed to ensure that media are free of contamination especially from stimulants such as endotoxin. Appropriate treatment controls are essential as treatment and mere handling of the cells might alter their activation states and, in turn, affect relevant cell markers.

## III. MONOCYTE/MACROPHAGE DIFFERENTIATION IN THE SKIN

### A. Stimulus for Cellular Differentiation

The interest in generating monocyte-derived DCs for use in human DC-based immunotherapies has greatly enhanced our understanding of monocyte differentiation. Cellular proteins involved in signaling are continually being implicated and classified dichotomously as either influencing a cell toward a dendritic or macrophage differentiation phenotype. A survey of the literature demonstrates

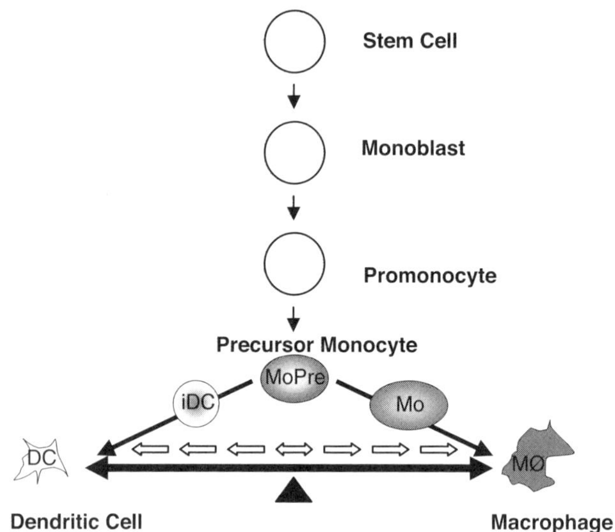


**FIGURE 8.4** Schematic of cell differentiation. Dynamic balance between DC-like vs. Mac-like phenotypes.

that classification of different stimuli can be challenging and may even have different outcomes following the same molecule stimulation in both classifications. Several factors impinge on the differentiation of the precursor cells. First, what is the profile of the starting cell type? Is it a precursor monocyte vs. a partially activated or differentiated cell, either Mac-like or DC-like? Second, what is the profile of the resulting cell? Are classifications based on cell surface molecule expression, assessed by FACS analysis, or via soluble cytokine production, and/or functional assays, such as engulfment? A schematic to consider is a dynamic profile of cell phenotypes that can be influenced in either polar direction (Figure 8.4). It can be postulated that precursor monocytes encounter many signals upon their respective differentiation pathway. This is especially true in skin, where Mo migration into inflammatory tissue encounters a number of soluble molecules within the microenvironment that may ultimately influence differentiation.

DCs or Macs generated by different laboratories have been reported to possess a dominant DC-like or Mac-like phenotype with variation in profile with respect to expression of additional phenotypic markers and co-stimulatory molecules, and/or abilities to function in a mixed leukocyte reaction (MLR). The observation of a spectrum of phenotypes rather than a single defining phenotype is indicative of the involvement of multiple signaling pathways.

### B. Monocyte Differentiation Utilized in Skin Disease Therapeutic Model

In the realm of cancer therapeutics, numerous strategies exploit the immune system's power of surveillance against neoplasms. One approach that uses blood monocyte differentiation *ex vivo* is being utilized in the treatment of cutaneous T-cell lymphoma (CTCL), a clonal epidermotropic neoplasm of $CD4^+$ memory T cells. Edelson and associates[95] use whole tumor cells as targets for induction of host immune responses as a modification of the clinically successful extracorporeal photophoresis (ECP). Like ECP, mononuclear cells, containing both leukemic T cells and monocytes, are removed from the blood and are treated with 8-methoxypsoralen and UVA. In the modification termed *transimmunization* (TI), treated cells are cultured overnight before re-infusion into the patient. The extra incubation time allows for blood monocytes and DC precursors to differentiate and phagocytize apoptotic CTCL cells more efficiently than they may do once they are re-infused and dilute *in vivo*.

The immature $CD83^+$ DCs and not the $CD14^+$ monocytes were observed to have increased phagocytosis of the CTCL cells.[95] Furthermore, the APC-functioning mature DCs generated by TI differ from the immunosuppressive-functioning Mo/Mac-derived APCs generated by ECP. The immunosuppressive action of the Mo/Mac-derived APCs is exploited in the use of conventional ECP in treatment of disorders related to autoimmune disease, graft-vs.-host disease (GVHD), and transplantation rejection. The mechanisms involved in monocyte differentiation in these disease models remain speculative, but monocyte activation along differentiation pathways can be considerably influenced by the cytokines, chemokines, and growth factors in the micromilieu. Manipulation to control immune response outcomes is a desired goal of clinical immunology.

## C. *In Vivo* and *In Vitro* Immunobiology of Monocytes in the Skin — UV Model

### 1. Role of Mo/Mac in UV-Induced Immunosuppression

UV irradiation, particularly the biologically relevant UVB spectrum (290 to 320 nm), is a significant environmental factor that acts via skin mediators, in a dose-dependent manner, to exert multiple local cutaneous and systemic effects. UVB is heavily absorbed in the epidermis and is advantageous from a cellular research point of view for *ex vivo* and *in situ* study of UVB-mediated effects in epidermal skin. Additionally, UVB effects can be studied *in vivo* in murine models as well as in humans. In the majority of humans and certain strains of mice, UV causes dosage-dependent UV-induced local or systemic immunosuppression. This is studied by inducing contact hypersensitivity (CHS) by topical application of a contact sensitizer. Induction of local tolerance is observed as suppression of CHS if sensitization is applied through a low-dose UV-irradiated cutaneous site. Furthermore, if higher doses of UV are applied to the single site, suppression of CHS is observed after a rechallenge with the given contact sensitizer at distant non-irradiated sites, demonstrating systemic immunosuppression.

Multiple mechanisms have been proposed for the alteration of the contact sensitization response at the site of UV irradiation (Figure 8.5), indicating an evolutionary need for redundancy. Using the CHS-UVB system, maximal tolerance induction is observed between 48 and 72 h post-UV exposure.[96] Following UV irradiation, perhaps the most striking observation is the sweeping reduction in CD1a$^+$ LCs in the epidermis[97] and the appearance of a distinct CD11b$^+$ Mo/Mac population

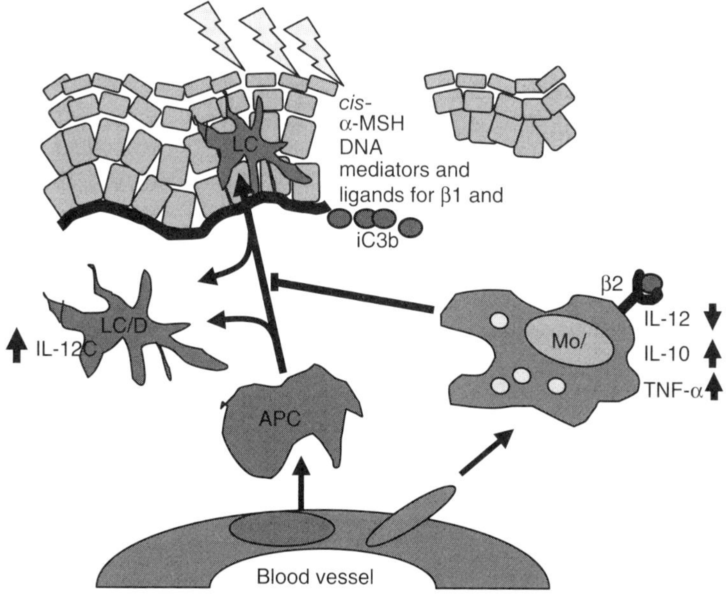


**FIGURE 8.5** Model of UV effect on skin APCs.

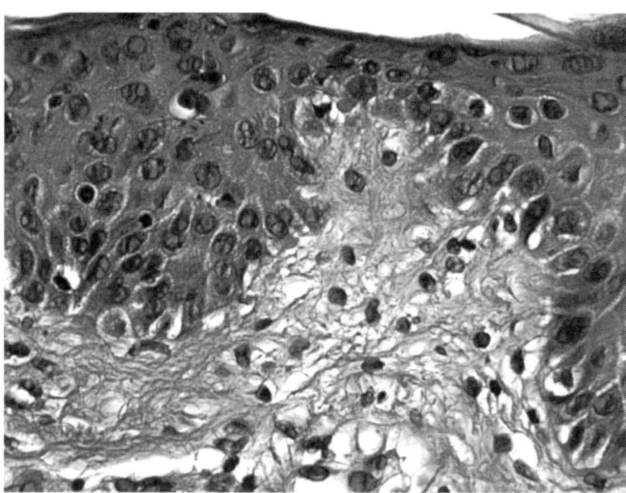

**FIGURE 8.6 (See color insert following page 304.)** UV-light-induced macrophages infiltration into skin after 4 MED UV irradiation, macrophages in papillary dermis and epidermis.

that produce immunosuppressive IL-10.[98,99] LCs are APCs that are normally responsible for the majority of antigen presentation that occurs with contact-sensitizing agents through the skin through their migration to draining lymph nodes (DLNs), upregulation of co-stimulatory APC molecules for activating naïve T cells, and production of IL-12 to facilitate T cell activation and differentiation [100]. UV irradiation leads to a sharp decline in the numbers of LC and peak in Mo/Macs within the epidermis and dermis by 48 to 72 h (Figure 8.6) following irradiation.[101,102]

However, as LCs are depleted, they are replaced as intracutaneous APCs by a Mo/Mac population that expresses class II MHC and CD11b, and in humans, CD36. Tolerance induction, in murine *in vivo* models, can be blocked via anti-CD11b antibody treatment.[103] Microanatomic localization of the CD11b cells demonstrates that they are the source for increased levels of IL-10 that occur following UVB exposure, and that a spike of IL-10 that occurs in the DLN of UV-exposed skin after immunization is due to macrophages.[99,102] The connection between IL-10 upregulation and CD11b cells appears to be that the CD11b$^+$ cells are stimulated to produce IL-10 due to the interaction of keratinocyte-derived complement fragment iC3b, which interacts with the CD11b ligand on the Mo/Mac cell surface.[104] In post-UV-exposed skin, iC3b deposits are observed at the dermal–epidermal junction in intimate apposition to CD11b$^+$ Mo/Macs. Studies have also demonstrated that prevention of iC3b deposition through C3 depletion, C3 knockout, or treatment with soluble CR1, can block immunosuppression and tolerance normally associated with UVB treatment.[105] At the same time, as IL-10 is increased, IL-12 is decreased through binding of the iC3b fragment, and the expected increase of DC-derived IL-12 in the DLN associated with successful immunization through normal skin is not seen under tolerogenic UV conditions.[104]

Therefore, UV produces a quite different immune cell, cytokine, and an inflammatory mediator environment compared to normal skin, with a prominent role played by Mo/Macs that transiently populate the skin in the acute post-injury period.

## 2. Role of Mo/Mac in UV Tumorigenesis

Excessive exposure to solar UV radiation, an environmental carcinogen, as well as a potent inducer of skin leukocyte infiltration, is responsible for immune suppression and damage to the epidermis. Based on studies by several research teams, a model for UV tumorigenesis is proposed in which each episode of acute UV exposure causes at least two injurious signaling events to the epidermal

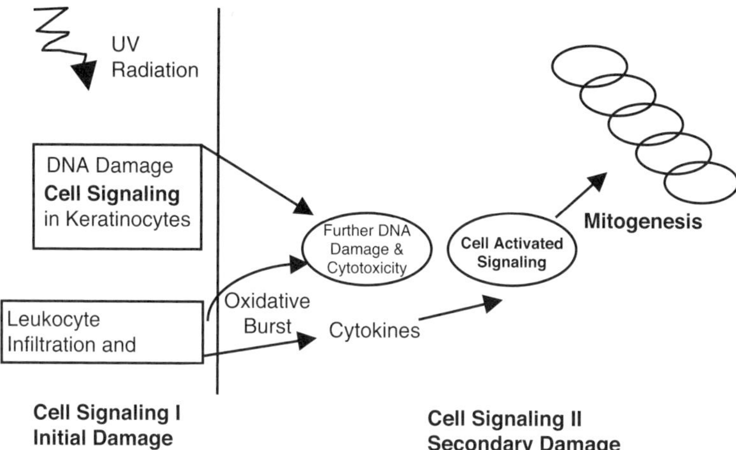


**FIGURE 8.7** A model of UV-induced tumorigenesis. Acute UV exposure causes at least two injurious signaling events to the epidermal keratinocytes.

keratinocytes (Figure 8.7). Regarding the first signal in this model, many studies have shown that UV causes DNA damage and activation of cell signaling, specifically through receptor tyrosine kinase epidermal growth factor receptor (EGFR), protein kinase C (PKC), mitogen-activated protein kinase (MAPK/ERK), and stress-activated protein kinase (SAPK/JNK).

Although solar UV contains both tumor-initiating and tumor-promoting effects, it is not clear to what degree UV-induced somatic changes and signaling are attributable to direct photophysical damage vs. indirect (e.g., oxidative burst) effects via inflammatory leukocytes or other constitutive cell types. For example, blockade of CD11b after UV injury greatly reduces the amount of epidermal keratinocyte injury.[103]

Thus, a hypothesis is that an important and substantial component of UV injury is mediated through oxidative burst, which is critically dependent on CD11b$^+$ leukocytes that infiltrate the epidermis following UV-induced damage. UV is strongly absorbed by cellular DNA in skin resulting in several different types of DNA alterations, including cyclobutane pyrimidine dimers and photoproducts, which ultimately lead to mutations in target genes in long-lived keratinocytic stem cells. A second phase of damage derives from induction of leukocyte infiltration and activation resulting in the generation of skin reactive oxidative moieties (Figure 8.8), causing further DNA damage as well as lipid peroxidation reactions that trigger growth-promoting cell-signaling pathways. As a result of UV exposure, important antioxidant defenses are depleted after responding to the first signaling events. Consequently, moieties such as free radicals, ROS, and reactive nitrogen species (e.g., NO) are elevated in the skin following the second respiratory burst. Anti-CD11b blockade reduces $H_2O_2$ production in the UV-exposed skin. Thus, blockade of macrophage and neutrophil infiltration and activation after UV results in the reversal of immune suppression and epidermal damage, likely due to blocked oxidative burst, and may support a role for these cells in causing additional oxidative DNA damage and, ultimately, UV tumorigenicity.

## IV. MONOCYTE/MACROPHAGE IN SKIN DISEASES AND SKIN INFLAMMATION

### A. Infection

The most investigated area of research regarding Mo/Mac function is clearly their role in infection. In the skin, infection with fungi and treponemes produces a spectrum of clinical manifestations depending on the strain of organism. *Leishmania* is one of the best studied of the cutaneous

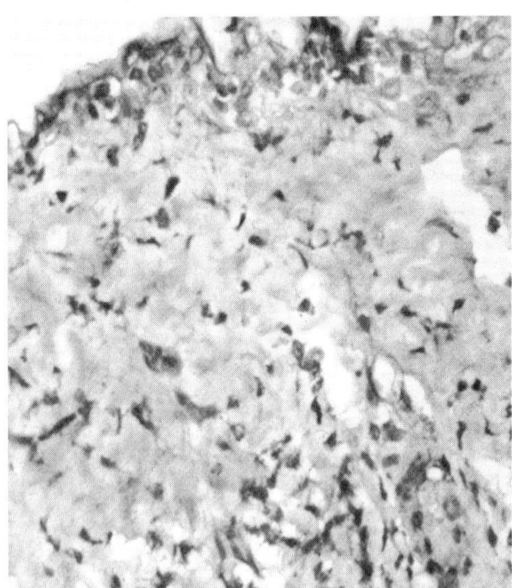

**FIGURE 8.8 (See color insert following page 304.)** Highly significant staining for $H_2O_2$ was observed in UVB-exposed sample. Numerous cells in the dermis and the epidermis exhibit positive staining. Intense staining was observed in cells with large cytoplasm, most likely representing macrophages in the perivascular and epidermal compartments.

pathogens that results in parasitized histiocytes. Others include histoplasmosis, the opportunistic *Penicillium marneffei,*[106,107] a rare dimorphic fungus, and mycobacteria. Deep fungal infection can induce cutaneous granulomas seen in blastomycosis and sporotrichosis.

## 1. Cutaneous Leishmaniasis

Immunobiologic differences exist between the *Leishmania* spp. In a simplified overview, the flagellated form of *Leishmania,* the promastigote, expresses lipophosphoglycan (LPG) and the 63-kDa glycoprotein (gp63) on its entire surface. Upon entering the bloodstream, the parasite encounters host serum and binds C3 via these two identified structures, causing activation of the alternative complement pathway. In addition to mediating lysis via the complement cascade, C3 serves as a ligand for macrophage receptors and subsequent opsinization. The receptors implicated in this process are CR3, CR1, and potentially CR4. However, macrophages may also directly recognize parasitic ligands and mediate phagocytosis via this stimulation. There is some evidence to suggest that LPG and gp63 can directly interact with β2 integrin receptors and additionally with fibronectin receptors. Once intracellular, the promastigote undergoes transformation into the amastigote form that can evade innate immune processes. Both self-healing and chronic leishmaniasis are associated with infiltrates of cutaneous macrophages that are parasitized with *Leishmania* amastigotes (Figure 8.9a).

The murine experimental system of *Leishmania* infection, whereby the parasite is injected subcutaneously, is a useful model for the study of human cutaneous leishmaniasis. While certain strains of mice are more susceptible than others, mice that do succumb to infection have parasitized macrophages that become selectively hyporesponsive to treatment with inflammatory stimuli. One example is the failure to induce IL-12 production.[108] Evidence points to Th1 responses, IL-12 and IFN-γ production, as well as NO production as important to confer resistance and to limit the progression of disease.[109,110] Modification of the APC function of Mo/Macs, DCs, and monocytes entering the tissue by PAMPs, iC3b, and other CD11b ligands on the organism may lead to escape of the organism from the effective Th1 lytic response.

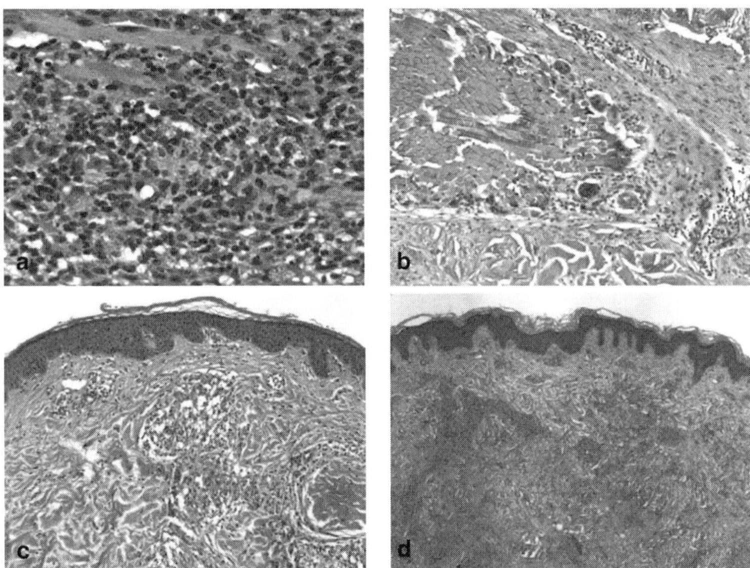


**FIGURE 8.9 (See color insert following page 304.)** Different patterns of macrophage infiltration in skin. (a) Infectious granuloma. Dense infiltrates of histiocytes, some of which contain *Leishmania* organisms. (b) Foreign body granuloma. Collections of macrophages and foreign body giant cells around suture fragments. (c) Sarcoidosis. An epitheloid cell granuloma. (d) Granuloma annulare. A palisaded granuloma with collections of histiocytes around central area of clearing.

## 2. Deep Fungal Infection

*Blastomyces dermatitidis* is a dimorphic saprophyte that is capable of growing intracellularly after being phagocytized by macrophages. The disease is often of pulmonary origin with the skin and bones as the most common site of dissemination. Primary inoculation of the skin has been described, often relating to trauma.[111] The yeast antigen WI-1, a 120-kDa protein, has been associated with adhesion promotion through interaction with the macrophage receptors CD14 and CD11b/CD18 (CR3).[112] The WI-1 knockout strain had impaired binding and entry into macrophages and also poorly multiplied in murine lung infection studies. Additionally, the WI-1 knockout yeast strain was contained in organized granulomata while their wild-type counterpart demonstrated overgrowth.[113] The virulence conferred by WI-1 to date has been linked to its ability to interfere with host macrophage TNF-α production.[114]

Sporotrichosis caused by *Sporothrix schenkii* is often inoculated into the skin by injury. The disease may progress with nodule enlargement and ulceration in a chain pattern reflecting lymphatic drainage. The less common fixed infection variant may form granulomas. The disease severity depends on the size of the inoculum and the virulence of the strain. Systemic dissemination is rare. Extracutaneous manifestations can be seen in immunocompromised individuals. Virulence has been associated with a lipid compound of the cell wall conferring the ability of the organism to evade phagocytosis by macrophages.[115] Histologically, the lesions are macrophage granulomas with an admixture of lymphocytes and neutrophils.

## B. Granulomatous Diseases

One subset of cutaneous diseases where Mo/Macs clearly play a role in their own recruitment and activation is in the formation of granulomas. The inciting events, crucial receptors, and orchestrated release of cytokines and chemokines during granuloma formation are being mapped out. Macrophages accumulate and undergo several activation and transformation steps during this process.

Morphologically, these are visible by histological examination as striking epitheloid cells and giant-multinucleated cells and can further progress into dramatic gross structures.

Granulomas are often classified as either immunologic, involving T-cell-mediated processes, or non-immunologic.[116] While both groupings involve activated macrophages and possibly a mixture of leukocytes at the initiation of formation, the major distinction made in immunologic granulomas is the presence and persistence of lymphocytes engaged in cell-mediated reaction. Non-immunologic granulomas often involve introduction of large amounts of insoluble material (Figure 8.9b). While immunologic granulomas may result from introduction of a small amount of substances ranging from pathogenic stimuli, such as bacteria, fungi, mycobacteria, or certain virus and molds, to chemical initiators. In some cases such as sarcoidosis, the initiating source is unknown but is thought to be processed and presented by monocytes to helper $CD4^+$ T cells that produce IFN-$\gamma$ and monocyte chemokines (Figure 8.9c).[117] A cycle is formed when activated T cells secrete factors that attract monocytes. There are also granulomatous diseases that do not fall into either classification. In granuloma annulare (Figure 8.9d), necrobiosis lipoidica, and rheumatoid nodules, inflammation is the main feature, although no microorganisms are thought to be involved. Release of substances from vascular injury has been proposed as an initiating event for the palisaded granulomas.[118] In exceedingly rare cases associated with CTCL, such as granulomatous slack skin, granulomatous infiltrates with destruction of elastic tissue have been described, indicating the ability of T cells in the skin to activate macrophages that destroy the extracellular matrix, resulting in clinically lax, inelastic skin.[118]

One approach to the study of granuloma formation is the use of a persistent infection model, to which there are several generalized visceral granuloma formation models. Although there is no doubt that macrophages are crucial in the development of granulomas, there are few models for the development of granulomas. Using a knockout mouse deficient of mast cells, investigators observed that cutaneous granuloma formation depended on neutrophil recruitment by mast cell TNF-$\alpha$ release. Restoration could be achieved by supplying neutrophil supernatants, containing Mo/Mac chemotactic factors such as MIP-1$\alpha$/$\beta$.[119]

## C. Autoimmune Disorders

Although antigen presentation by dendritic cells to T cells is thought to trigger a classic immune reaction, in autoimmune diseases, the antigens may not always be known, and other downstream effector cells such as monocytes and macrophages may be as important as T cells in the manifestation and presentation of disease.

### 1. Scleroderma – GVHD

The hallmark of scleroderma is thickened skin, resulting from excessive deposition of collagen. The process can be confined to the skin or may involve other organs, resulting in vascular damage and visceral fibrosis as in systemic sclerosis.[120,121] The etiology of scleroderma is unknown, but autoimmune disease, exposure to organic chemicals, silica, and drugs are the most common associations. Chronic GVHD can be a sclerodermatous-like process, as well.[122] The disease pathogenesis involves multiple components with a complex network of signaling events. While evidence suggests that T cells are essential in mediating disease in involved tissue, the pro-inflammatory cytokine and chemokine microenvironment supports the recruitment of macrophages, which have been demonstrated both in human and mouse models for scleroderma.[123]

One murine model for scleroderma, in which allogeneic bone marrow and spleen cells are used to reconstitute lethally irradiated mice, produces sclerodermatous GVHD.[124] In early active disease, the involved skin contains numerous monocytes, macrophages, and T cells, preceded by a cytokine- and chemokine-rich microenvironment that includes TGF-$\beta$1, IFN-$\gamma$, MCP-1, MIP-1$\alpha$, and RANTES. This influx of immune cells can be prevented with the addition of anti-TGF-$\beta$ antibodies, limiting further progression of disease. It was observed that cutaneous macrophages themselves can produce TGF-β1 at the very earliest time point.[122] It remains to be determined if the macrophages serve as principal cells that amplify the TGF-β1 signaling to further disease progression, or if they are merely effector cells responding to a T-cell-controlled autoimmune process.

### 2. Psoriasis

Two of the major features in early psoriasis are the hyperproliferation of keratinocytes and the infiltration of mononuclear cells to the papillary dermis. This mononuclear cell population comprises macrophages and activated, proliferating T cells secreting IL-2 and IFN-γ.[125–127] which can be inhibited by cyclosporin A.[128]

Microanatomic localization of macrophages in psoriatic tissue has demonstrated a restricted class of macrophages termed lining macrophages.[129,130] that lie immediately adjacent to the basal keratinocyte layer. The precise role of this class of macrophages in psoriasis has not been defined. However, the microanatomic space occupied by lining macrophages is concurrent with the cutaneous area where EDA fibronectin has been demonstrated to be overexpressed in patients with psoriasis.[131] EDA fibronectin is one type of cellular fibronectin.[132] Cellular fibronectin exhibits the splice variant inclusion of either the extra domain A (EDA) or extra domain B (EDB), or a combination of both. It has been previously demonstrated that fibronectin can exacerbate the proliferation of psoriatic keratinocytes driven by T-cell lymphokines.[133] The ability of macrophages to both synthesize and assemble fibronectin suggested that macrophages may colocalize with EDA fibronectin in psoriatic tissue. Stimulation of cellular proliferation has also been demonstrated to occur following interaction of cells with EDA fibronectin, as shown in wound healing[134,135] and cell cycle studies.[136,137] As shown in Figure 8.10, psoriasis-involved tissue contains bone marrow–derived ($CD45RO^+$ $RB^+$) lining macrophages that colocalize with EDA fibronectin.

In addition to their participation with ECM products that are unique to psoriatic tissue, macrophages have also been reported to produce high levels of the cytokine IL-18, a potent inducer of both TNF-α and IFN-γ. Although it has not been examined, one potential role for "lining macrophage"-derived IL-18 in psoriatic tissue would be to induce T-cell lymphokines that exacerbate psoriasis in a very localized manner. In involved psoriatic skin, EDA fibronectin is significantly more often expressed on $CD11c^+$ macrophages than in uninvolved skin. This finding together with the potential of EDA fibronectin to regulate cell cycle progression suggests cell maturation and differentiation of bone marrow–derived cells to a macrophage phenotype as part of the psoriatic lesional evolutionary process. If the interaction of T cells with macrophage and associated EDA fibronectin is a crucial part of this process, targeting of the cell types involved in EDA mRNA induction, production, assembly, and responsiveness may represent a novel approach to psoriasis therapy.

## D. Aggressive Macrophage Tumors

Although the existence of a "malignant macrophage" is not known, there are several aggressive tumors of mononuclear cell/macrophages in skin disorders. A group of diseases called cutaneous xanthomatoses, varied in clinical and pathological presentation, share the feature of accumulation of lipids in involved macrophages, known as "foam" cells. The second entity referred to as non-Langerhans cell histiocytosis (NLCH) is a group of diverse disorders with proliferative histiocytes of the mononuclear/macrophage phenotype.

### 1. Cutaneous Xanthomatoses

The etiology of cutaneous xanthomatoses is not known. However, drawn from models of atherogenesis, the mechanism is thought to involve cellular uptake of modified LDLs.[138] While most cells

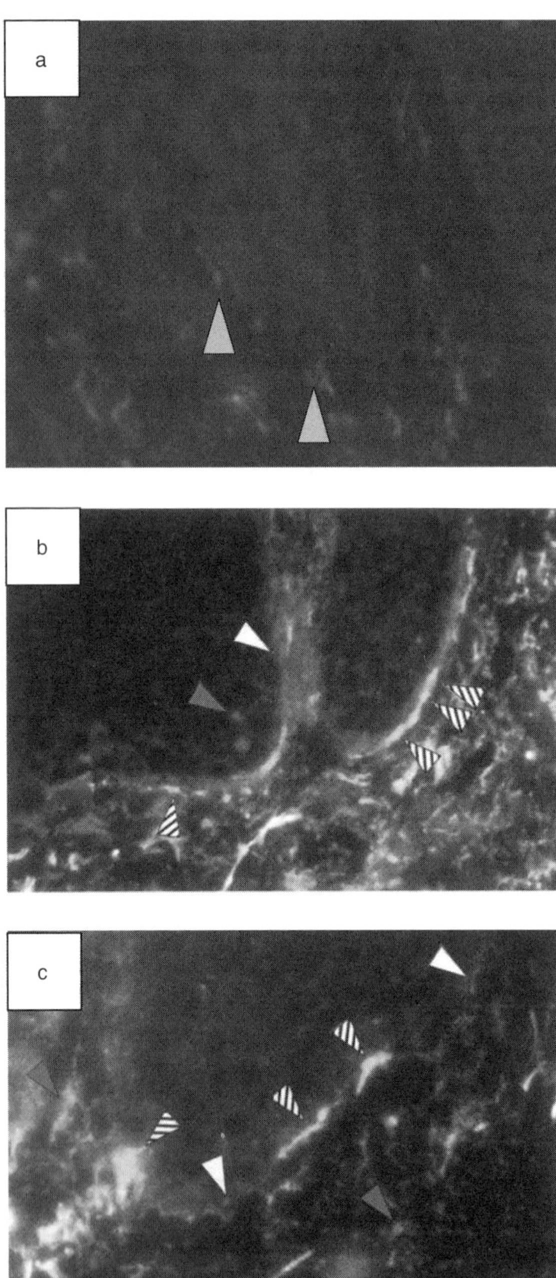


**FIGURE 8.10 (See color insert following page 304.)** CD68+ cells along the DEJ of involved psoriasis tissue are also CD45+ and colocalize with extradomain A (EDA) fibronectin. (a) CD68 expression was detected using a FITC-conjugated anti-CD68-specific antibody. CD68+ cells can be seen lining the DEJ, as well as in the papillary dermis (gray arrows). Double immunohistochemistry staining was performed on involved skin sections. CD45RO (b) or RB (c) and EDA fibronectin antibodies were detected by a FITC-conjugated antibody and a biotinylated antibody, respectively, plus Streptavidin-Rhodamine. Double staining resulted in yellow fluorescence (striped arrows) was present in elongate cells along the DEJ (BandC). EDA fibronectin deposition along the DEJ without CD45+ cell association is noted in red (white arrow). CD45RO+ cells and CD45RB+ cells without EDA fibronectin co-expression is noted in b and c, respectively (gray arrows).

do not accumulate cholesterol because of the downregulated expression of LDL receptors by intracellular sterols, macrophages express SRs, which are not regulated by sterols[139] and can uptake modified LDL. Xanthomas often occur in the setting of hypertriglyceridemia, hypercholesteremia, dyslipoproteinemia, or apolipoproteinemia, and this also includes xanthelasma, eruptive xanthomas, tuberous/tuberoeruptive xanthomas, tendinous xanthomas, plane xanthoma. A rare variant of xanthoma, which can develop in normo-lipidemic individuals is verruciform xanthoma. Characterized by accumulation of foam cells in the papillary dermis with verrucous epidermal acanthosis and hyperkeratosis in mucosal regions, the foam cells co-express CD68 and an intense intracytoplasmic-vacuolar pattern of SRs.[140]

Extensive xanthomas and xanthelasmas in the absence of any known lipid abnormality have been reported in two siblings.[141] Analysis of the patients' monocytes and macrophages reveals an overexpression of SR type I and II receptor mRNA and protein. Peculiarly, the remaining unaffected siblings of this family shared a monocyte phenotype characterized by increased adhesion and rapid maturation into large macrophages with high accumulation of lipids. Further comparison of the monocytes from the affected vs. non-affected siblings by differential display reveals the expression of the molecules, signal transducer and activator of transcription (STAT1$\alpha$) and IP-10, a STAT1$\alpha$ responsive gene.[142] The association of xanthomatosis and inflammatory mediators is consistent with a proposed mechanism of macrophage foam cells in atherogenesis. While native LDL is believed to be the main source of cholesterol in foam cells, co-incubation with resting macrophages does not lead to cholesterol accumulation.[143] Yet, PMA-activated macrophages can accumulate large amounts of cholesterol via macropinocytosis. This suggests that inflammatory mediators may play a role as prerequisites for macrophage-mediated lipid uptake.

### 2. Non-Langerhans Cell Histiocytosis

The NLCH is a group of rare diseases with poorly understood etiologies. The common feature is the presence of a histiocytic infiltrate with positive immunophenotyping of Mo/Mac markers and a negative immunophenotyping with the LC markers such as CD1. There is variation in Mo/Mac antigen profiles among the clinical entities as well from lesions of the same patient, representing a disease spectrum. NLCH consists of benign cephalic histiocytosis, generalized eruptive histiocytoma, indeterminate cell histiocytosis, juvenile xanthogranuloma, necrobiotic xanthogranuloma, reticulohistiocytoma, multicentric reticulohistiocytosis, Rosai-Dorfman disease, and xanthoma disseminatum.[144]

Necrobiotic xanthogranuloma (NXG) is a rare variant of xanthomatosis seen in normo-lipidemic patients with an increased risk of plasma cell dyscrasia and an association with paraproteinemia. The disease is characterized by destructive dermal and subcutaneous inflamed lesions with predilection for periorbital margins[145] with a tendency for ulcerations in the cutaneous lesions. The pathogenesis of disease is uncertain. The distinguishing histologic feature is the presence of collagen necrosis with clusters of foam cells, macrophages, and giant cells.[146] One description of an NXG patient did not reveal differences in monocyte SR-A and CD36 expression.[147] Another description observes the presence of paraprotein–LDL complexes within foam cells surrounded by mast cells.[148] This is consistent with *in vitro* foam cell formation of macrophage uptake of mast cell enzymatically modified LDL aggregates.[149]

## V. CONCLUDING REMARKS AND PERSPECTIVES

Macrophage infiltration has become synonymous with chronic inflammation, especially in the skin. Although a macrophage response is normally a favorable event in the course of an infection, quite often macrophages can mediate chronic inflammation, such as is seen in several inflammatory dermatoses including psoriasis, atopic dermatitis, and chronic contact dermatitis. Several lines of investigation have concentrated on limiting the macrophage response as a means of eliminating the inflammatory response. They demonstrate that clearance of the inflammatory macrophages subsequently leads to the diminution of both T cells and DCs, thus allowing the inflammation to become quiescent.

Macrophages are very plastic cells found in most tissues, where they can direct or participate in a variety of biological processes that include, but are not limited to: wound healing, immune response to pathogens (parasites, fungi), phagocytosis, and antigen presentation. Additionally, the responses of macrophages are tailored to the microenvironment in which they are located; macrophage response and differentiation is dependent on tissue specificity. In the cutaneous setting, macrophages participate in the immune response to such diverse stimuli as UV irradiation and contact-sensitizing agents and are involved in psoriasis, granulomas, histiocytes, and skin cancers. Because of the central pathway that macrophages occupy in the immune response route, investigators propose that elimination of the macrophage would greatly facilitate clearing an inflammatory response. Two paths are generally taken to regulation of macrophages. One path is to block the downstream effector molecules (cytokines, chemokines) produced by the macrophage thereby downregulating the subsequent responses to macrophage products (i.e., anti-TNF-α antibodies or soluble TNF-α receptors). The alternative approach is to block the macrophage from acting, either by altering the ability of the macrophage to reach its target (i.e., anti-LFA-1) or by eliminating the macrophage physically with such agents as liposomes carrying macrophagocidal agents.

Many researchers have taken advantage of the selective uptake of liposomes by macrophages and have designed liposomes that encapsulate toxins, liposome-encapsulated dichloromethylene bisphosphonate (L-$Cl_2$MBP), for example, and demonstrate selective deletion of macrophage populations via this approach.[150,151] As a systemic therapy, this has proved effective at eliminating macrophage populations, but may eliminate necessary macrophage responses, thereby rendering the host immune system compromised.

Macrophages can also be targeted via their receptors and unique functional capabilities. For example, ricin-A conjugated to an anti-FcγRII receptor (CD 32), and administered *in vivo*, reduced inflammation.[152]

Tissue macrophages play a role in a variety of cutaneous diseases and are therefore targets for macrophage-specific therapy. Potential disorders would include cutaneous GVHD (sclerodermatous), granuloma annulare, sarcoid, chronic contact dermatitis, psoriasis, UV injury,[104] atopic dermatitis, cutaneous T-cell lymphoma, and photoaging. All of these diseases have macrophages implicated in disease progression, and elimination or modification of the macrophage response may be of potential benefit following local cutaneous therapy with immunotoxins. However, the degree to which macrophages play a critical role in driving lesion appearance and persistence is not fully understood in some of these diseases. Agents that limit the macrophage response may play an important role in understanding the pathophysiology of these dermatoses, particularly the relative importance of macrophages.

Clinically, reducing macrophage numbers correlates with impressive immunologic responses in murine models of cutaneous disease, and may hold promise for human therapeutics. The novel biological findings on the role of macrophages in chronic cutaneous inflammation are also quite interesting. There are promising approaches to the treatment of chronic dermatoses by alteration of cutaneous macrophages.

## REFERENCES

1. van Furth, R., Nibbering, P.H., van Dissel, J.T., and Diesselhoff-den Dulk, M.M., The characterization, origin, and kinetics of skin macrophages during inflammation,, *J. Invest. Dermatol.*, 85, 398–402, 1985.
2. Headington, J.T., The histiocyte, In memoriam. *Arch. Dermatol.*, 122, 532–533, 1986.

3. van Furth, R. et al., The mononuclear phagocyte system: a new classification of macrophages, monocytes, and their precursor cells, *Bull. World Health Organ.*, 46, 845–852, 1972.
4. Lingen, M.W., Role of leukocytes and endothelial cells in the development of angiogenesis in inflammation and wound healing, *Arch. Pathol. Lab. Med.*, 125, 67–71, 2001.
5. DiPietro, L.A., Wound healing: the role of the macrophage and other immune cells, *Shock*, 4, 233–240, 1995.
6. Janeway, C.A., Jr. and Medzhitov, R., Innate immune recognition, *Annu. Rev. Immunol.*, 20, 197–216, 2002.
7. Gordon, S., Pattern recognition receptors: doubling up for the innate immune response, *Cell*, 111, 927–930, 2002.
8. Medzhitov, R. and Janeway, C.A., Jr., Innate immune recognition and control of adaptive immune responses, *Semin. Immunol.*, 10, 351–353, 1998.
9. Hacker, G., Redecke, V. and Hacker, H., Activation of the immune system by bacterial CpG–DNA, *Immunology*, 105, 245–251, 2002.
10. Akira, S. and Sato, S., Toll-like receptors and their signaling mechanisms, *Scand. J. Infect. Dis.*, 35, 555–562, 2003.
11. Barton, G.M. and Medzhitov, R., Toll-like receptor signaling pathways, *Science*, 300, 1524–1525, 2003.
12. Dobrovolskaia, M.A. and Vogel, S.N., Toll receptors, CD14, and macrophage activation and deactivation by LPS, *Microbes Infect.*, 4, 903–914, 2002.
13. Underhill, D.M., Toll-like receptors: networking for success, *Eur. J. Immunol.*, 33, 1767–1775, 2003.
14. Chaudhary, P.M. et al., Cloning and characterization of two Toll/interleukin-1 receptor-like genes TIL3 and TIL4: evidence for a multi-gene receptor family in humans, *Blood*, 91, 4020–4027, 1998.
15. Medzhitov, R., Preston-Hurlburt, P., and Janeway, C.A., Jr., A human homologue of the *Drosophila* Toll protein signals activation of adaptive immunity, *Nature*, 388, 394–397, 1997.
16. Means, T.K., Golenbock, D.T., and Fenton, M.J., Structure and function of Toll-like receptor proteins, *Life Sci.*, 68, 241–258, 2000.
17. Underhill, D.M. and Ozinsky, A., Toll-like receptors: key mediators of microbe detection, *Curr. Opin. Immunol.*, 14, 103–110, 2002.
18. Pinhal-Enfield, G. et al., An angiogenic switch in macrophages involving synergy between Toll-like receptors 2, 4, 7, and 9 and adenosine A(2A) receptors, *Am. J. Pathol.*, 163, 711–721, 2003.
19. Rhee, S.H., Jones, B.W., Toshchakov, V., Vogel, S.N., and Fenton, M.J., Toll-like receptors 2 and 4 activate STAT1 serine phosphorylation by distinct mechanisms in macrophages, *J. Biol. Chem.*, 278, 22506–22512, 2003.
20. Vogel, S., Hirschfeld, M.J., and Perera, P.Y., Signal integration in lipopolysaccharide (LPS)-stimulated murine macrophages, *J. Endotoxin Res.*, 7, 237–241, 2001.
21. Perera, P.Y. et al., CD11b/CD18 acts in concert with CD14 and Toll-like receptor (TLR) 4 to elicit full lipopolysaccharide and taxol-inducible gene expression, *J. Immunol.*, 166, 574–581, 2001.
22. Landmann, R., Muller, B., and Zimmerli, W., CD14, new aspects of ligand and signal diversity, *Microbes Infect.*, 2, 295–304, 2000.
23. Schumann, R.R. et al., Structure and function of lipopolysaccharide binding protein, *Science*, 249, 1429–1431, 1990.
24. Tobias, P.S., Soldau, K., Gegner, J.A., Mintz, D., and Ulevitch, R.J., Lipopolysaccharide binding protein-mediated complexation of lipopolysaccharide with soluble CD14, *J. Biol. Chem.*, 270, 10482–10488, 1995.
25. Hart, P.H., Jones, C.A., and Finlay-Jones, J.J., Monocytes cultured in cytokine-defined environments differ from freshly isolated monocytes in their responses to IL-4 and IL-10,, *J. Leukocyte Biol.*, 57, 909–918, 1995.
26. Tamai, R., Sugawara, S., Takeuchi, O., Akira, S., and Takada, H., Synergistic effects of lipopolysaccharide and interferon-gamma in inducing interleukin-8 production in human monocytic THP-1 cells is accompanied by up-regulation of CD14, Toll-like receptor 4, MD-2 and MyD88 expression, *J. Endotoxin Res.*, 9, 145–153, 2003.
27. Watt, F.M., Role of integrins in regulating epidermal adhesion, growth and differentiation, *Embo J.*, 21, 3919–3926, 2002.

28. Danen, E.H. and Sonnenberg, A., Integrins in regulation of tissue development and function, *J. Pathol.*, 200, 471–480, 2003.
29. Hynes, R.O., Integrins: versatility, modulation, and signaling in cell adhesion, *Cell*, 69, 11–25, 1992.
30. Shang, X.Z., Lang, B.J., and Issekutz, A.C., Adhesion molecule mechanisms mediating monocyte migration through synovial fibroblast and endothelium barriers: role for CD11/CD18, very late antigen-4 (CD49d/CD29), very late antigen-5 (CD49e/CD29), and vascular cell adhesion molecule-1 (CD106), *J. Immunol.*, 160, 467–474, 1998.
31. Meerschaert, J. and Furie, M.B., The adhesion molecules used by monocytes for migration across endothelium include CD11a/CD18, CD11b/CD18, and VLA-4 on monocytes and ICAM-1, VCAM-1, and other ligands on endothelium, *J. Immunol.*, 154, 4099–4112, 1995.
32. Reyes-Reyes, M., Mora, N., Gonzalez, G., and Rosales, C., Beta1 and beta2 integrins activate different signalling pathways in monocytes, *Biochem. J.*, 363, 273–280, 2002.
33. Hemler, M.E., VLA proteins in the integrin family: structures, functions, and their role on leukocytes, *Annu. Rev. Immunol.*, 8, 365–400, 1990.
34. Ehlers, M.R., CR3: a general purpose adhesion-recognition receptor essential for innate immunity, *Microbes Infect.*, 2, 289–294, 2000.
35. Savill, J. and Fadok, V., Corpse clearance defines the meaning of cell death, *Nature*, 407, 784–788, 2000.
36. Yamada, Y., Doi, T., Hamakubo, T., and Kodama, T., Scavenger receptor family proteins: roles for atherosclerosis, host defence and disorders of the central nervous system, *Cell Mol. Life Sci.*, 54, 628–640, 1998.
37. Naito, M., Kodama, T., Matsumoto, A., Doi, T., and Takahashi, K., Tissue distribution, intracellular localization, and *in vitro* expression of bovine macrophage scavenger receptors, *Am. J. Pathol.*, 139, 1411–1423, 1991.
38. Yesner, L.M., Huh, H.Y., Pearce, S.F., and Silverstein, R.L., Regulation of monocyte CD36 and thrombospondin-1 expression by soluble mediators, *Arterioscler. Thromb. Vasc. Biol.*, 16, 1019–1025, 1996.
39. Ockenhouse, C.F., Magowan, C., and Chulay, J.D., Activation of monocytes and platelets by monoclonal antibodies or malaria-infected erythrocytes binding to the CD36 surface receptor *in vitro*, *J. Clin. Invest.*, 84, 468–475, 1989.
40. Fadok, V.A., Warner, M.L., Bratton, D.L., and Henson, P.M., CD36 is required for phagocytosis of apoptotic cells by human macrophages that use either a phosphatidylserine receptor or the vitronectin receptor (alpha v beta 3), *J. Immunol.*, 161, 6250–6257, 1998.
41. Gregory, C.D., CD14-dependent clearance of apoptotic cells: relevance to the immune system, *Curr. Opin. Immunol.*, 12, 27–34, 2000.
42. Devitt, A. et al., Human CD14 mediates recognition and phagocytosis of apoptotic cells, *Nature*, 392, 505–509, 1998.
43. Heidenreich, S., Monocyte CD14: a multifunctional receptor engaged in apoptosis from both sides, *J. Leukocyte Biol.*, 65, 737–743, 1999.
44. Schlegel, R.A., Krahling, S., Callahan, M.K., and Williamson, P., CD14 is a component of multiple recognition systems used by macrophages to phagocytose apoptotic lymphocytes, *Cell Death Differ.*, 6, 583–592, 1999.
45. Belardelli, F., Role of interferons and other cytokines in the regulation of the immune response, *Apmis*, 103, 161–179, 1995.
46. Ma, J. et al., Regulation of macrophage activation, *Cell Mol. Life Sci.*, 60, 2334–2346, 2003.
47. Kedzierska, K., Crowe, S.M., Turville, S., and Cunningham, A.L., The influence of cytokines, chemokines and their receptors on HIV-1 replication in monocytes and macrophages, *Rev. Med. Virol.*, 13, 39–56, 2003.
48. Rollins, B.J., Chemokines. *Blood*, 90, 909–928, 1997.
49. Carroll, M.C., The role of complement and complement receptors in induction and regulation of immunity, *Annu. Rev. Immunol.*, 16, 545–568, 1998.
50. Laufer, J., Katz, Y., and Passwell, J.H., Extrahepatic synthesis of complement proteins in inflammation, *Mol. Immunol.*, 38, 221–229, 2001.
51. Morgan, B.P. and Gasque, P., Extrahepatic complement biosynthesis: where, when and why? *Clin. Exp. Immunol.*, 107, 1–7, 1997.

52. Hetland, G., Johnson, E., and Aasebo, U., Human alveolar macrophages synthesize the functional alternative pathway of complement and active C5 and C9 *in vitro*, *Scand. J. Immunol.,* 24, 603–608, 1986.
53. McPhaden, A.R. and Whaley, K., Complement biosynthesis by mononuclear phagocytes, *Immunol. Res.,* 12, 213–232, 1993.
54. Gulati, P., Lemercier, C., Guc, D., Lappin, D., and Whaley, K., Regulation of the synthesis of C1 subcomponents and C1-inhibitor, *Behring Inst. Mitt,* 196–203, 1993.
55. Tenner, A.J. and Volkin, D.B., Complement subcomponent C1q secreted by cultured human monocytes has subunit structure identical with that of serum C1q, *Biochem. J.,* 233, 451–458, 1986.
56. Osterud, B., Tissue factor expression by monocytes: regulation and pathophysiological roles, *Blood Coagul. Fibrinolysis,* 9(Suppl. 1), S9–14, 1998.
57. Gregory, S.A., Morrissey, J.H., and Edgington, T.S., Regulation of tissue factor gene expression in the monocyte procoagulant response to endotoxin, *Mol. Cell. Biol.,* 9, 2752–2755, 1989.
58. Tenno, T., Botling, J., Oberg, F., Nilsson, K., and Siegbahn, A., Tissue factor expression in human monocytic cell lines, *Thromb. Res.,* 88, 215–228, 1997.
59. Brand, K., Fowler, B.J., Edgington, T.S., and Mackman, N., Tissue factor mRNA in THP-1 monocytic cells is regulated at both transcriptional and posttranscriptional levels in response to lipopolysaccharide, *Mol. Cell. Biol.,* 11, 4732–4738, 1991.
60. Pejler, G. and Geczy, C.L., Human peripheral blood mononuclear cells require factor X and platelets for expression of prothrombinase activity in response to bacterial lipopolysaccharide, *Ann. Hematol.,* 80, 278–283, 2001.
61. Altieri, D.C. and Edgington, T.S., Sequential receptor cascade for coagulation proteins on monocytes. Constitutive biosynthesis and functional prothrombinase activity of a membrane form of factor V/Va, *J. Biol. Chem.,* 264, 2969–2972, 1989.
62. Osterud, B., Bogwald, J., Lindahl, U., and Seljelid, R., Production of blood coagulation factor V and tissue thromboplastin by macrophages *in vitro*, *FEBS Lett.,* 127, 154–160, 1981.
63. Chapman, H.A., Jr., Allen, C.L., Stone, O.L. and Fair, D.S., Human alveolar macrophages synthesize factor VII *in vitro*. Possible role in interstitial lung disease, *J. Clin. Invest.,* 75, 2030–2037, 1985.
64. McGee, M.P., Wallin, R., Devlin, R., and Rothberger, H., Identification of mRNA coding for factor VII protein in human alveolar macrophages — coagulant expression may be limited due to deficient postribosomal processing, *Thromb. Haemost.,* 61, 170–174, 1989.
65. Pejler, G., Lunderius, C., and Tomasini-Johansson, B., Macrophages synthesize factor X and secrete factor X/Xa-containing prothrombinase activity into the surrounding medium,. *Thromb. Haemost.,* 84, 429–435, 2000.
66. Osterud, B., Lindahl, U., and Seljelid, R., Macrophages produce blood coagulation factors, *FEBS Lett.,* 120, 41–43, 1980.
67. Levi, M., Keller, T.T., van Gorp, E., and ten Cate, H., Infection and inflammation and the coagulation system, *Cardiovasc. Res.,* 60, 26–39, 2003.
68. Martin, P., Wound healing — aiming for perfect skin regeneration, *Science,* 276, 75–81, 1997.
69. Leibovich, S.J. and Ross, R., The role of the macrophage in wound repair. A study with hydrocortisone and antimacrophage serum, *Am. J. Pathol.,* 78, 71–100, 1975.
70. Hunt, T.K., Knighton, D.R., Thakral, K.K., Goodson, W.H., III, and Andrews, W.S., Studies on inflammation and wound healing: angiogenesis and collagen synthesis stimulated *in vivo* by resident and activated wound macrophages, *Surgery,* 96, 48–54, 1984.
71. Campbell, E.J., Cury, J.D., Shapiro, S.D., Goldberg, G.I., and Welgus, H.G., Neutral proteinases of human mononuclear phagocytes. Cellular differentiation markedly alters cell phenotype for serine proteinases, metalloproteinases, and tissue inhibitor of metalloproteinases, *J. Immunol.,* 146, 1286–1293, 1991.
72. Cury, J.D., Campbell, E.J., Lazarus, C.J., Albin, R.J., and Welgus, H.G., Selective up-regulation of human alveolar macrophage collagenase production by lipopolysaccharide and comparison to collagenase production by fibroblasts, *J. Immunol.,* 141, 4306–4312, 1988.
73. Shapiro, S.D., Elastolytic metalloproteinases produced by human mononuclear phagocytes. Potential roles in destructive lung disease, *Am. J. Respir. Crit. Care Med.,* 150, S160–164, 1994.
74. Welgus, H.G. et al., Neutral metalloproteinases produced by human mononuclear phagocytes. Enzyme profile, regulation, and expression during cellular development, *J. Clin. Invest.,* 86, 1496–1502, 1990.

75. Vaalamo, M., Kariniemi, A.L., Shapiro, S.D. and Saarialho-Kere, U., Enhanced expression of human metalloelastase (MMP-12) in cutaneous granulomas and macrophage migration, *J. Invest. Dermatol.*, 112, 499–505, 1999.
76. Lepidi, S. et al., MMP9 production by human monocyte-derived macrophages is decreased on polymerized type I collagen, *J. Vasc. Surg.*, 34, 1111–1118, 2001.
77. Schafer, B.M., Maier, K., Eickhoff, U., Todd, R.F., and Kramer, M.D., Plasminogen activation in healing human wounds, *Am. J. Pathol.*, 144, 1269–1280, 1994.
78. Romer, J. et al., Differential expression of urokinase-type plasminogen activator and its type-1 inhibitor during healing of mouse skin wounds, *J, Invest. Dermatol.*, 97, 803–811, 1991.
79. Lin, W.W., Chen, B.C., Hsu, Y.W., Lee, C.M., and Shyue, S.K., Modulation of inducible nitric oxide synthase induction by prostaglandin E2 in macrophages: distinct susceptibility in murine J774 and RAW 264.7 macrophages, *Prostaglandins Other Lipid Mediat.*, 58, 87–101, 1999.
80. Tilley, S.L., Coffman, T.M., and Koller, B.H., Mixed messages: modulation of inflammation and immune responses by prostaglandins and thromboxanes, *J. Clin. Invest.*, 108, 15–23, 2001.
81. D'Acquisto, F. et al., Involvement of NF-kappaB in the regulation of cyclooxygenase-2 protein expression in LPS-stimulated J774 macrophages, *FEBS Lett.*, 418, 175–178, 1997.
82. Gorgoni, B., Caivano, M., Arizmendi, C., and Poli, V., The transcription factor C/EBPβ is essential for inducible expression of the cox-2 gene in macrophages but not in fibroblasts, *J. Biol. Chem.*, 276, 40769–40777, 2001.
83. Caivano, M., Gorgoni, B., Cohen, P., and Poli, V., The induction of cyclooxygenase-2 mRNA in macrophages is biphasic and requires both CCAAT enhancer-binding protein beta (C/EBP beta) and C/EBP delta transcription factors, *J. Biol. Chem.*, 276, 48693–48701, 2001.
84. Mastroeni, P. et al., Antimicrobial actions of the NADPH phagocyte oxidase and inducible nitric oxide synthase in experimental salmonellosis. II. Effects on microbial proliferation and host survival *in vivo*, *J. Exp. Med.*, 192, 237–248, 2000.
85. Forman, H.J. and Torres, M., Reactive oxygen species and cell signaling: respiratory burst in macrophage signaling, *Am. J. Respir. Crit. Care Med.*, 166, S4–8, 2002.
86. Janssen-Heininger, Y.M., Poynter, M.E., and Baeuerle, P.A., Recent advances towards understanding redox mechanisms in the activation of nuclear factor κB, *Free Radical Biol. Med.*, 28, 1317–1327, 2000.
87. Moncada, S., Palmer, R.M., and Higgs, E.A., Nitric oxide: physiology, pathophysiology, and pharmacology, *Pharmacol. Rev.*, 43, 109–142, 1991.
88. Nathan, C.F. and Hibbs, J.B., Jr., Role of nitric oxide synthesis in macrophage antimicrobial activity, *Curr. Opin. Immunol.*, 3, 65–70, 1991.
89. MacMicking, J., Xie, Q.W., and Nathan, C., Nitric oxide and macrophage function, *Annu. Rev. Immunol.*, 15, 323–350, 1997.
90. Bogdan, C., Rollinghoff, M., and Diefenbach, A., The role of nitric oxide in innate immunity, *Immunol. Rev.*, 173, 17–26, 2000.
91. Boehncke, W.H., Wortmann, S., Kaufmann, R., Mielke, V., and Sterry, W., A subset of macrophages located along the basement membrane ("lining cells") is a characteristic histopathological feature of psoriasis, *Am. J. Dermatopathol.*, 17, 139–144, 1995.
92. Davies, D.E. and Lloyd, J.B., Monocyte-to-macrophage transition *in vitro*. A systematic study using human cells isolated by fractionation on Percoll, *J. Immunol. Methods*, 118, 9–16, 1989.
93. Thomas, T.E., Sutherland, H.J., and Lansdorp, P.M., Specific binding and release of cells from beads using cleavable tetrameric antibody complexes, *J. Immunol. Methods*, 120, 221–231, 1989.
94. Miltenyi, S., Muller, W., Weichel, W., and Radbruch, A., High gradient magnetic cell separation with MACS, *Cytometry*, 11, 231–238, 1990.
95. Berger, C.L., Hanlon, D., Kanada, D., Girardi, M., and Edelson, R.L., Transimmunization, a novel approach for tumor immunotherapy, *Transfus Apheresis Sci.*, 26, 205–216, 2002.
96. Hammerberg, C., Duraiswamy, N., and Cooper, K.D., Active induction of unresponsiveness (tolerance) to DNFB by *in vivo* ultraviolet-exposed epidermal cells is dependent upon infiltrating class II MHC+ CD11b(bright) monocytic/macrophagic cells, *J. Immunol.*, 153, 4915–4924, 1994.
97. Cooper, K.D. et al., UV exposure reduces immunization rates and promotes tolerance to epicutaneous antigens in humans: Relationship to dose, CD1a-DR$^{+}$ epidermal macrophage induction, and Langerhans cell depletion, *Proc. Natl. Acad. Sci. U.S.A.*, 89, 8497–8501, 1992.

98. Meunier, L., Bata-Csorgo, Z., and Cooper, K.D., In human dermis, UV induces expansion of a CD36+CD11b+CD1− macrophage subset by infiltration and proliferation; CD1+ Langerhans-like dendritic antigen-presenting cells are concomitantly depleted, *J. Invest. Dermatol.*, 105, 782–788, 1995.
99. Kang, K., Hammerberg, C., Meunier, L., and Cooper, K.D., CD11b+ macrophages that infiltrate human epidermis after *in vivo* ultraviolet exposure potently produce IL-10 and represent the major secretory source of epidermal IL-10 protein, *J. Immunol.*, 153, 5256–5264, 1994.
100. Toichi, E., McCormick, T.S., and Cooper, K.D., Cell surface and cytokine phenotypes of skin immunocompetent cells involved in ultraviolet-induced immunosuppression, *Methods*, 28, 104–110, 2002.
101. Hammerberg, C., Duraiswamy, N., and Cooper, K.D., Temporal correlation between UV radiation locally-inducible tolerance and the sequential appearance of dermal, then epidermal, class II MHC+ CD11b+ monocytic/macrophagic cells, *J. Invest. Dermatol.*, 107, 755–763, 1996.
102. Kang, K., Gilliam, A.C., Chen, G., Tootell, E., and Cooper, K.D., In human skin, UVB initiates early induction of IL-10 over IL-12 preferentially in the expanding dermal monocytic/macrophagic population, *J. Invest. Dermatol.*, 111, 31–38, 1998.
103. Hammerberg, C., Duraiswamy, N., and Cooper, K.D., Reversal of immunosuppression inducible through ultraviolet-exposed skin by *in vivo* anti-CD11b treatment, *J. Immunol.*, 157, 5254–5261, 1996.
104. Yoshida, Y. et al., Monocyte induction of IL-10 and down-regulation of IL-12 by iC3b deposited in ultraviolet-exposed human skin, *J. Immunol.*, 161, 5873–5879, 1998.
105. Hammerberg, C., Katiyar, S.K., Carroll, M.C., and Cooper, K.D., Activated complement component 3(C3) is required for UV induction of immunosuppression and antigenic tolerance, *J. Exp. Med.*, 187, 1133–1138, 1998.
106. Piehl, M.R., Kaplan, R.L., and Haber, M.H., Disseminated penicilliosis in a patient with acquired immunodeficiency syndrome, *Arch. Pathol. Lab. Med.*, 112, 1262–1264, 1988.
107. Chiewchanvit, S., Mahanupab, P., Hirunsri, P., and Vanittanakom, N., Cutaneous manifestations of disseminated *Penicillium marneffei* mycosis in five HIV-infected patients, *Mycoses*, 34, 245–249, 1991.
108. Carrera, L. et al., Leishmania promastigotes selectively inhibit interleukin 12 induction in bone marrow-derived macrophages from susceptible and resistant mice, *J. Exp. Med.*, 183, 515–526, 1996.
109. Scott, K.D., Stafford, J.L., Galvez, F., Belosevic, M., and Goss, G.G., Plasma membrane depolarization reduces nitric oxide (NO) production in P388D.1 macrophage-like cells during *Leishmania major* infection, *Cell. Immunol.*, 222, 58–68, 2003.
110. von Stebut, E. et al., Skin-derived macrophages from *Leishmania major*-susceptible mice exhibit interleukin-12- and interferon-gamma-independent nitric oxide production and parasite killing after treatment with immunostimulatory DNA, *J. Invest. Dermatol.*, 119, 621–628, 2002.
111. Helm, T.N., in *Topics in Clinical Dermatology: Cutaneous Fungal Infections*, Elewski, B., Ed., Igaku-Shoin Medical Publishers, New York, 1992.
112. Newman, S.L., Chaturvedi, S., and Klein, B.S., The WI-1 antigen of *Blastomyces dermatitidis* yeasts mediates binding to human macrophage CD11b/CD18 (CR3) and CD14, *J. Immunol.*, 154, 753–761, 1995.
113. Brandhorst, T.T., Wuthrich, M., Warner, T., and Klein, B., Targeted gene disruption reveals an adhesin indispensable for pathogenicity of *Blastomyces dermatitidis*, *J. Exp. Med.*, 189, 1207–1216, 1999.
114. Finkel-Jimenez, B., Wuthrich, M., Brandhorst, T., and Klein, B.S., The WI-1 adhesin blocks phagocyte TNF-α production, imparting pathogenicity on *Blastomyces dermatitidis*, *J. Immunol.*, 166, 2665–2673, 2001.
115. Carlos, I.Z., Sgarbi, D.B., Santos, G.C., and Placeres, M.C., *Sporothrix schenckii* lipid inhibits macrophage phagocytosis: involvement of nitric oxide and tumour necrosis factor-α, *Scand. J. Immunol.*, 57, 214–220, 2003.
116. Dahl, M.V., *Clinical Immunodermatology*, Mosby-Year Book, St. Louis, MO, 1996.
117. Okamoto, H., Mizuno, K., and Horio, T., Monocyte-derived multinucleated giant cells and sarcoidosis, *J. Dermatol. Sci.*, 31, 119–128, 2003.
118. Howard, A. and White, C.R., Jr., in *Dermatology*, Bolognia, J.L., Jorizzo, J.L., and Rapini, R.P., Eds., Elsevier Limited/Mosby, St. Louis, MO, 2003, 1455–1469.
119. von Stebut, E., Metz, M., Milon, G., Knop, J., and Maurer, M., Early macrophage influx to sites of cutaneous granuloma formation is dependent on MIP-1α/β released from neutrophils recruited by mast cell-derived TNFα, *Blood*, 101, 210–205, 2003.

120. Steen, V.D., Clinical manifestations of systemic sclerosis, *Semin. Cutaneous Med. Surg.*, 17, 48–54, 1998.
121. Mitchell, H., Bolster, M.B., and LeRoy, E.C., Scleroderma and related conditions, *Med. Clin. North Am.*, 81, 129–149, 1997.
122. Zhang, Y., McCormick, L.L., Desai, S.R., Wu, C., and Gilliam, A.C., Murine sclerodermatous graft-versus-host disease, a model for human scleroderma: cutaneous cytokines, chemokines, and immune cell activation, *J. Immunol.*, 168, 3088–3098, 2002.
123. Atamas, S.P. and White, B., The role of chemokines in the pathogenesis of scleroderma, *Curr. Opin. Rheumatol.*, 15, 772–777, 2003.
124. McCormick, L.L., Zhang, Y., Tootell, E., and Gilliam, A.C., Anti-TGF-β treatment prevents skin and lung fibrosis in murine sclerodermatous graft-versus-host disease: a model for human scleroderma, *J. Immunol.*, 163, 5693–5699, 1999.
125. Austin, L.M., Coven, T.R., Bhardwaj, N., Steinman, R., and Krueger, J.G., Intraepidermal lymphocytes in psoriatic lesions are activated GMP-17(TIA-1)$^+$CD8$^+$CD3$^+$ CTLs as determined by phenotypic analysis, *J. Cutaneous Pathol.*, 25, 79–88, 1998.
126. Morganroth, G.S., Chan, L.S., Weinstein, G.D., Voorhees, J.J., and Cooper, K.D., Proliferating cells in psoriatic dermis are comprised primarily of T cells, endothelial cells, and factor XIIIa$^+$ perivascular dendritic cells, *J. Invest. Dermatol.*, 96, 333-340., 1991.
127. Szabo, S., Hammerberg, C., Bata-Csorgo, Z., and Cooper, K., The mechanism of action of UVB in psoriasis: rapidly decreased T cell numbers and preferential reduction of interferon gamma (IFN gamma) production, *J. Invest. Dermatol.*, 108, 558, 1997.
128. Gupta, S., Fass, D., Shimizu, M., and Vayuvegula, B., Potentiation of immunosuppressive effects of cyclosporin A by 1a, 25-dihydroxyvitamin D3, *Cell. Immunol.*, 121, 290–297, 1989.
129. Van Den Oord, J.J. and De Wolf-Peeters, C., Epithelium-lining macrophages in psoriasis, *Br. J. Dermatol.*, 130, 589–594, 1994.
130. Boehncke, W.H., Wortmann, S., Kaufmann, R., Mielke, V., and Sterry, W., A subset of macrophages located along the basement membrane ("lining cells") is a characteristic histopathological feature of psoriasis, *Am. J. Dermatopathol.*, 17, 139–144, 1995.
131. Ting, K.M. et al., Overexpression of the oncofetal Fn variant containing the eda splice-in segment in the dermal-epidermal junction of psoriatic uninvolved skin, *J. Invest. Dermatol.*, 114, 706–711, 2000.
132. Manabe, R.-I., Oh-e, N., Maeda, T., Fukada, T., and Sekiguchi, K., Modulation of cell-adhesive activity of fibronectin by the alternatively spliced EDA segment, *J. Cell Biol.*, 139, 295–307, 1997.
133. Bata-Csorgo, Z., Cooper, K.D., Ting, K.M., Voorhees, J.J., and Hammerberg, C., Fibronectin and α5 integrin regulate keratinocyte cell cycling. A mechanism for increased fibronectin potentiation of T cell lymphokine-driven keratinocyte hyperproliferation in psoriasis, *J. Clin. Invest.*, 101, 1509–1518, 1998.
134. Brown, L.F. et al., Macrophages and fibroblasts express embryonic fibronectins during cutaneous wound healing, *Am. J. Pathol.*, 142, 793–801, 1993.
135. Juhasz, I., Murphy, G.F., Yan, H.C., Herlyn, M., and Albelda, S.M., Regulation of extracellular matrix proteins and integrin cell substratum adhesion receptors on epithelium during cutaneous human wound healing *in vivo*, *Am. J. Pathol.*, 143, 1458–1469, 1993.
136. Garcia, A.J., Vega, M.D., and Boettiger, D., Modulation of cell proliferation and differentiation through substrate-dependent changes in fibronectin conformation, *Mol. Biol. Cell*, 10, 785–798, 1999.
137. Manabe, R., Oh-e, N., and Sekiguchi, K., Alternatively spliced EDA segment regulates fibronectin-dependent cell cycle progression and mitogenic signal transduction, *J. Biol. Chem.*, 274, 5919–5924, 1999.
138. Glass, C.K. and Witztum, J.L., Atherosclerosis. the road ahead, *Cell*, 104, 503–516, 2001.
139. Goldstein, J.L., Ho, Y.K., Basu, S.K., and Brown, M.S., Binding site on macrophages that mediates uptake and degradation of acetylated low density lipoprotein, producing massive cholesterol deposition, *Proc. Natl. Acad. Sci. U.S.A.*, 76, 333–337, 1979.
140. Furue, M. et al., Colocalization of scavenger receptor in CD68 positive foam cells in verruciform xanthoma, *J. Dermatol. Sci.*, 10, 213–219, 1995.
141. Giry, C., Giroux, L.M., Roy, M., Davignon, J., and Minnich, A., Characterization of inherited scavenger receptor overexpression and abnormal macrophage phenotype in a normolipidemic subject with planar xanthomas, *J. Lipid Res.*, 37, 1422–1435, 1996.

142. Grewal, T. et al., Expression of γ-IFN responsive genes in scavenger receptor over-expressing monocytes is associated with xanthomatosis, *Atherosclerosis,* 138, 335–345, 1998.
143. Kruth, H.S., Huang, W., Ishii, I., and Zhang, W.Y., Macrophage foam cell formation with native low density lipoprotein, *J. Biol. Chem.,* 277, 34573–34580, 2002.
144. Goodman, W.T. and Barrett, T.L., in *Dermatology,* Bolognia, J.L., Jorizzo, J.L., and Rapini, R.P., Eds., Elsevier Limited/Mosby, St. Louis, MO, 2003, 1429–1445.
145. Mehregan, D.A. and Winkelmann, R.K., Necrobiotic xanthogranuloma, *Arch. Dermatol.,* 128, 94–100, 1992.
146. Winkelmann, R.K. and McEvoy, M.T., Diffuse-plane normolipaemic xanthoma with aortic-valve xanthoma, *Clin. Exp. Dermatol.,* 16, 38–40, 1991.
147. Matsuura, F. et al., Activation of monocytes *in vivo* causes intracellular accumulation of lipoprotein-derived lipids and marked hypocholesterolemia — a possible pathogenesis of necrobiotic xanthogranuloma, *Atherosclerosis,* 142, 355–365, 1999.
148. Jeziorska, M. et al., Clinical, biochemical, and immunohistochemical features of necrobiotic xanthogranulomatosis, *J. Clin. Pathol.,* 56, 64–68, 2003.
149. Kovanen, P.T., Role of mast cells in atherosclerosis, *Chem. Immunol.,* 62, 132–170, 1995.
150. Hoch, J.R. et al., Macrophage depletion alters vein graft intimal hyperplasia, *Surgery,* 126, 428–437, 1999.
151. Richards, P.J., Williams, A.S., Goodfellow, R.M., and Williams, B.D., Liposomal clodronate eliminates synovial macrophages, reduces inflammation and ameliorates joint destruction in antigen-induced arthritis, *Rheumatology* (Oxford), 38, 818–825, 1999.
152. Thepen, T. et al., Resolution of cutaneous inflammation after local elimination of macrophages, *Nat. Biotechnol.,* 18, 48–51, 2000.

# 9 Endothelial Cells of Blood and Lymphatic Vessels

*Krystyna A. Pasyk, George W. Cherry, and Barbara A. Jakobczak*

## CONTENTS



## I. INTRODUCTION

Vascular endothelium forms a continuous monolayer of endothelial cells (ECs) that line the circulatory system and constitute an anatomical barrier between blood and all extravascular tissues of the body. Since the time of Rudolf Virchow[1] in the 19th century, a theory has persisted that endothelium is important in supporting normal blood fluidity and that it plays a passive role in the transfer of nutrients from the bloodstream to various tissues. It was also thought that endothelium functions as an insulation barrier separating platelets from the thrombogenic subendothelial connective tissue.

At present, vascular endothelium is considered a dynamic "widespread organ" with immense secretory properties. It is well known that the endothelium has a wide range of vital functions in the body.[2–8] Communication between blood and tissues is a crucial process and occurs across ECs. The endothelium is active in numerous complex interactions of macromolecular and cellular intravascular components of blood, smooth muscle, and extracellular matrix of the vessel wall.[9] Furthermore, ECs are involved in multiple physiological and pathological processes. The vascular endothelium has a variety of biosynthetic and metabolic capabilities and is involved in immune, inflammatory, tissue growth and repair processes, as well as in coagulation.[7] The list of vital functions of ECs is rapidly increasing with the application of new research techniques.

Intense studies performed on EC culture,[2,4,10–13] physiology,[14–18] and ultrastucture[19,20] allow investigators to learn about EC properties and understand their numerous functions.[21] Anatomical integrity, as well as proper functional status of the endothelium, are important in multiple physiological processes of this widespread organ. This chapter reviews EC morphology, function, and pathophysiology, and focuses on the roles of ECs in the immune response. Apoptosis of ECs and EC survival factors are also discussed.

0-8493-1959-5/05/$0.00+$1.50

## II. MORPHOLOGY AND PHYSIOLOGY: VASCULAR ENDOTHELIAL CELL RECEPTORS

ECs form a monolayer over a vessel basal lamina (basement membrane). ECs have three surfaces: cohesive, adhesive (abluminal or basal), and luminal (apical).[22] The cohesive surface adjoins ECs to one another and facilitates transport processes. This adjoining surface consists of miscellaneous intercellular junctions that vary in different vascular segments.[23,24] Gap junctions (communicating junctions), for example, are involved in the intercellular exchange of ions and low-molecular-weight metabolites. Gap junctions are present in arteries and arterioles. Main venules and veins have tight junctions (occluding junctions or zonula occludens), as well as gap junctions that are fewer in number than in the arteries. Capillaries have clefts between ECs interrupted by tight junctions.[25] However, gap junctions are absent from capillary and postcapillary venular endothelium.[26] Myoendothelial junctions, i.e., foot or finger-like EC projections toward the smooth muscle cell, are present in the arterioles and are particularly prominent in precapillary segments.[27,28] These endothelial–smooth muscle contacts are involved in intercellular exchange of information through ionic, metabolic, or electrotonic coupling.[29,30] The intercellular junctions and their significance in permeability, especially in capillary endothelium, is still a subject of research.[30] Very flat ECs of lymphatic vessels are connected by zonula-like plaque possessing desmoplakin and the calcium-dependent transmembrane glycoproteins, V-cadherin and cadherin-5.[31] The adhesive (abluminal or basal) surface of ECs adheres to the basal lamina and connective tissue of the vascular wall. The luminal (apical) side of the endothelium contains important adhesion molecules and specific binding proteins, which are involved in attachment and migration of leukocytes, lymphocytes, and monocytes to tissues during inflammation.[30] Studies of the luminal surface of ECs of small vessels in the Gasserian ganglion, and in the testis in rats, indicate the presence of microvilli and microfolds.[32,33] Microvilli and microfolds have also been found in several human diseases such as angiofibromas,[34] diabetes mellitus,[35] adiponecrosis subcutanea neonatorum,[36] and in the skin after treatment with hydrocortisone butyrate.[37] The role of these microvilli is not completely understood.

Depending on the functions of various organs and tissues, the vascular endothelium may be continuous (arteries, veins, arterioles, venules, and capillaries of somatic tissues, lung, and nervous system), fenestrated (renal glomeruli, visceral capillaries), and discontinuous (sinusoids of liver, spleen, and bone marrow).[38] In normal human dermis, the blood vessels are lined by continuous and fenestrated endothelium. Fenestrae are present at tips of capillary loops adjacent to the epidermis,[39,40] in capillaries in hair bulbs, and in close proximity to eccrine sweat glands.[41,42] Fenestration of endothelium is necessary for rapid exchange of molecules between circulating blood and perivascular tissues.[41,43]

Morphology and function of ECs and their surface molecule expression differ with vessel size and vessel type in various organs, as well as in different states of disease. Microvascular ECs cultured from different organs express distinct patterns of cell surface markers, protein transporters, and intracellular enzymes.[44] Every tissue, including the dermis and subcutis, has characteristic endothelium that has adapted to specific environmental stimuli.[7,45] Thus, the microenvironment can regulate EC phenotype through the process of transdifferentiation.[46] In the past, differences in microvascular endothelium of various organs were recognized in numerous morphological, physiological, and pharmacological studies. The recent explosion in monoclonal antibody and molecular cloning techniques allows for the distinction and recognition of unique characteristics of the vascular endothelium in different locations of the vascular system.[47,48]

The major ultrastructural differences between ECs in dermal vasculature and other organs are the greater thickness of ECs in dermal vasculature and the presence of large bundles of very fine filaments in their cytoplasm.[49,50] ECs also differ in macro- and microvasculature, in arterial and venous vessels in superficial, middle, and lower dermis, as well as in the subcutaneous tissue.[41] The superficial dermal vascular plexus cytoplasm of ECs in the smallest arterioles is more electron dense and has more pinocytotic vesicles than the cytoplasm of venous ECs.[27,51] In the deep dermis and adipose tissue, ECs of the arterioles possess intracellular myofilamentous bundles that form a complex (fibronexus) with the extracellular filaments.[41] Ultrastructural examination of normal human dermal microvasculature has shown elongated nuclei of the ECs in the arterial vessels, giving them a smooth luminal surface.[39] In the larger ascending arteries of mid-dermis, the endothelial nuclei are often rounded. The venous vessels, however, contain round, indented endothelial nuclei that bulge into the lumen and form an irregular surface. This nuclear shape in venular ECs is probably associated with the ability of these cells to contract.[32] In enzyme histochemistry testing, ECs of postcapillary venules, in contrast to other small vessels, exhibit high levels of nonspecific esterase, β-glucuronidase, acid phosphatase, and succinic dehydrogenase.[52]

ECs have developed an extensive pinocytotic transport system and unique cytoplasmic storage granules, such as Weibel–Palade bodies. The Weibel–Palade bodies, rod-shaped tubular inclusions with 3-μm length and 0.1-μm diameter,[53] are derived from the Golgi apparatus.[54] In human dermal microvasculature, the Weibel–Palade bodies are more common in ECs of the venular than in the arterial segments of capillaries.[39] In addition, these bodies are more numerous in ECs obtained from animals maintained on an atherogenic diet (cholesterol-fed) than in the control group.[55,56] The Weibel–Palade bodies are organelles with important storage and secretory functions; they contain von Willebrand factor VIII, granule-membrane protein-140 (GMP-140) or P-selectin,[57–59] interleukin-8 (IL-8),[60,61] α1,3-fucosyltransferase VI,[62] and tetraspanin CD63/lamp3 molecules.[63]

Crystalloid bodies (shown in Figure 9.1) have been identified within the cytoplasm of ECs. The size of crystalloids ranges from 0.5 to 2.0 μm. In substructure, crystalloids show parallel lamellar bands with a periodicity of 180 to 300 Å. These unique cytoplasmic structures have been observed in the vascular endothelium of human fetuses,[64] in the vein of the human umbilical cord,[65] and in small blood vessels in normal human skin,[66] as well as in cellular and capillary hemangiomas,[67–69] angioblastoma (Nakagawa or tufted angioma),[70] and hemangioblastoma.[71] The nature and function of these cytoplasmic crystalloids are unknown. Crystalloid inclusions may be a sign of immaturity of endothelial cells in humans.

Pinocytotic vesicles, first described by Palade[19] in 1953, remain the object of numerous studies focusing on their substructure, distribution, and function in ECs.[72,73] It has been noted that the number of these vesicles opening on the luminal surface of dermal venules is larger than in arterioles.[39,51] A single pinocytotic vesicle (or several vesicles linked together) can form transendothelial channels that open on two sides of the EC. Pinocytotic vesicles are involved in molecular transport by endocytosis and exocytosis at both the luminal and abluminal surface of the endothelium. An endo- and exocytotic vesicular system is characteristic in ECs of both blood and lymphatic vessels. Various polyanionic molecules (i.e., sialoglycoproteins and heparan sulfate) are present in specific domains on the luminal surface of the endothelium.[74] These anionic sites play a role in vascular permeability by repelling anionic molecules and facilitating transport of cationic proteins.

The cytoplasm of ECs in dermal blood vessels and lymphatics contains thin 5-nm actin filaments, which have a contractile function.[41] They are oriented parallel to the vessel axis, and are located in the abluminal and junctional areas of ECs.[39,75] The thicker intermediate filaments (10 nm) form a cytoskeleton of the EC, which keeps the nucleus and other organelles in place.[27,51,75] Intermediate filaments are dispersed throughout the cytoplasm, and are concentrated in the perinuclear region; they play a role in mitosis. Occludin is an important molecule that regulates the actin cytoskeleton in ECs.[76] In the arterioles located in the deep dermis and in the adipose tissue, the extracellular filaments (10 to 20 nm) form a connection (fibronexus) with thin intracellular filaments of two adjacent ECs. They are probably fibronectin-coated elastic microfibrils that anchor the basal lamina of the vascular wall.[41] Microfilaments and microtubules in ECs provide structural support and maintain endothelial integrity.[75,77]

The endothelium of all blood vessels is supported externally by a tightly attached basal lamina. The basal lamina of terminal arterioles of human dermal microvasculature has a homogenous appearance and envelops both the ECs and pericytes. In venular segments, as well as at the tips of capillary loops, the basal lamina is multilaminated and interspersed with collagen fibrils between

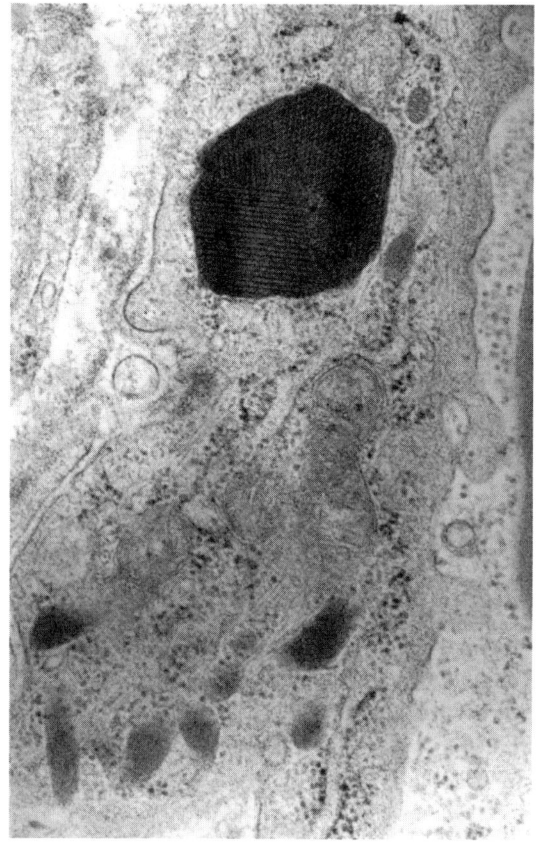

**FIGURE 9.1** Electron micrograph showing Weibel–Palade bodies and crystalloid structure in an endothelial cell of newborn foreskin venule. (Original magnification × 38,280.)

laminations.[27,39,51] Differences in the structure of the basal lamina between the arteriolar and venular segments may reflect differences in controlling blood vessel permeability, especially for plasma proteins. Alternately, the wall of lymphatic capillaries consists of ECs only; here the basal lamina is absent. Furthermore, the lymphatic endothelium is supported by fine collagenous and reticular fibrils on the abluminal surface.[78]

Human ECs have important physiological functions and undergo a wide variety of biosynthetic and metabolic processes. ECs synthesize and release several peptides and biologically active molecules, which take part in vascular tone regulation, vessel contraction, and permeability. ECs play a role in regulation of blood pressure and blood flow by releasing both vasodilatators — nitric oxide (NO), endothelium-derived hyperpolarizing factor (EDHF), prostacyclin ($PGI_2$) — and vasoconstrictors — endothelin-1 (ET), endoperoxides, thromboxane $A_2$, superoxide anions, platelet-activating factor (PAF).[7,79] NO is not only an important homeostatic regulator of the vascular tone, but also acts in other physiological processes such as platelet aggregation, leukocyte adhesion, and vascular smooth muscle cell proliferation.[80] Various pathological conditions such as hypercholesterolemia, hypertension, and reperfusion injury are connected with suppressed NO production in the EC.[81,82]

The vascular endothelium is a source of arachidonate metabolites, tissue factors, and numerous cytokines, such as IL-1α and β, IL-6, IL-8, FGF, G- and GM-CSF, gamma IP-10, IFG gamma, MCP-1, 2, and 3, M-CSF, MIF, MIP-2, OSM, PDGF, and TNF-α.[99–102] ECs synthesize a platelet α-granule membrane protein (GMP 140), which are stored in the Weibel–Palade bodies.[57] Vascular ECs also synthesize connective tissue components of the extracellular matrix such as fibronectin,[83] collagen IV, and proteoglycans that constitute the basal lamina.[84] Two newly recognized laminins, 8 and 10, are also produced by dermal microvascular ECs. These laminins are involved during wound angiogenesis.[85]

A primary function of ECs is to maintain thromboresistance under normal conditions. This is mediated by factors synthesized and secreted by ECs. ECs produce factors involved in blood clotting, such as: von Willebrand factor VIII,[86] von Willebrand antigen II (which forms a soluble complex with von Willebrand factor within ECs),[87] plasminogen activator and factors that control its activity,[88] factor V,[89] and heparin-like molecules (with anticoagulant properties),[90] as well as thrombospondin,[91] thrombomodulin, protein C,[92] and protein S.[13] Furthermore, ECs are capable of binding thrombin molecules,[93] factor Va,[94] and factor Xa,[95] and provide an effective surface for prothrombin activation. The possible EC receptors for thrombin are heparan sulfate and the specific protein receptor thrombomodulin.[16] Antithrombotic EC properties are maintained by the balance between plasminogen activators (PAs) and PA inhibitors (PAIs).[96] Plasminogen-activator inhibitor type 1 (PAI-1) plays a main role in the plasmin/plasminogen activator cascade that regulates vascular fibrinolysis and extravascular generation of plasmin.[80] Increased PAI-1 synthesis and secretion can be induced by cytokines synthesized by endothelial cells in plaque, and during immune or inflammatory reactions. PAI-1, localized on the luminal surface of ECs, can reduce endothelial fibrinolytic activity and cause formation of intravascular thrombi.[80] PAI-1 is also involved in control of migration of ECs[97] and vascular smooth muscle cells, which occur during vascular remodeling and atherogenesis.[98]

Several physiological functions of ECs are mediated through receptors located on the cell membrane (IL-1, IL-4, IL-8, G- and GM-CSF, IFN-$\gamma$, MIP-2, PDGF, and VEGF).[100,101] Activated receptors increase the intracellular $Ca^{2+}$ concentration, which triggers the synthesis and release of vasodilators ($PGI_2$, endothelium-derived relaxing factor, or EDRF),[103] and vasoconstrictors (endothelium-derived constriction factor, endothelin-1, prostanoids, prostaglandin $H_2$, angiotensin, and thromboxane $A_2$).[104–106] Activation of specific EC receptors may lead to a release of EDRF, a regulator of the vascular tone.[107,108] The endothelium of lymphatic vessels also releases vasoactive agents such as EDRF, similar to the ones identified in blood vessels.[109] Protease receptors are essential cofactors in hemostasis and are important in EC function.[110]

ECs are the only cells of the body that have direct contact with the bloodstream; because of this unique location, they are able to bind specific circulating hormones which may change EC function. ECs contain several receptors for different hormones and vasoactive agents. Both $\alpha$- and $\beta$-adrenergic muscarine, angiotensin, histamine, and 5-hydroxytryptamine receptors are present in ECs.[111] In addition, ECs play a role in the activation of angiotensin I and the repression of norepinephrine, serotonin, bradykinin, and adenosine 5′-diphosphate. The presence of specific cell surface receptors for steroid hormones, neurotransmitters, and polypeptides provides evidence for the potential hormone responsiveness of the vascular endothelium.[112] Estrogens play a protective role in cardiovascular disease and act in modulation of lipid metabolism, expression of leukocyte adhesion molecules, and migration of vascular smooth muscle cells in the vascular wall.[113] Estrogens operate as vasodilatators and testosterone functions as a vasorelaxant. An increase in glucocorticoid level causes vasoconstriction through subsequent increase in $\alpha$-adrenoreceptor numbers, decrease in prostacyclin production, and inhibition of NO synthase. Aldosterone, however, causes vascular smooth muscle cell hypertrophy and perivascular fibrosis, and is involved in vascular electrolyte permeability.[113]

The vascular endothelium also synthesizes basic fibroblast growth factor (bFGF), EC-derived growth factors (ECDGF),[114,115] platelet-derived growth factors (PDGF),[116,117] and granulocyte-macrophage colony-stimulating factor (GMCSF).[118] ECs produce a heparin-like growth inhibitor, as well as distinct growth factors and a mitogenic factor, which regulate the growth of vascular smooth muscle cells.[119–121] Two plasma membrane glycoproteins, GPIIb and GPIIIa, form a large heterodimer complex identical to the vitronectin receptor in the EC.[120,122–126] As in platelets, glycoproteins on the EC surface may function as specific receptors for three proteins: fibrinogen, von

Willebrand factor VIII, and fibronectin.[123,127] Endothelial GPIIIa also bears the human platelet alloantigen[128] $PI^{A1}$, that has been localized to a 17-kDa region of GPIIIa.[129] This finding suggests that endothelial GPIIIa may be involved in the etiology of alloimmunological disorders such as post-transfusion purpura, neonatal alloimmune thrombocytopenia, and autoimmune thrombocytopenia. In these conditions, antibodies directed against GPIIb or GPIIIa, or both, participate in the immune destruction of circulating platelets.[124] Angiopoietins are identified as the major ligands of the endothelial-specific receptor Tie2. Upregulation of angiopoietin 1, angiopoietin 2, and Tie2 receptor may be associated with the development of microvascular proliferation in psoriasis.[130]

The principal function of ECs in circulation is mediation and control of transendothelial exchanges of materials between the blood plasma and the interstitial fluid, including gas exchange in the lungs. The transendothelial exchange involves membrane transport of selected amines[131,132] and prostaglandin.[133] Macromolecules such as metabolite carriers (albumin, low-density lipoproteins), metal carriers (transferrin), and hormones (insulin) are transported through cytoplasmic vesicles[24,134] via a two-receptor system.[135] Large particles, on the other hand, are taken up by micropinocytosis[136,137] or phagocytosis.[138,139] According to Simionescu,[140] ECs are able to regulate vascular permeability through three groups of receptors: (1) vasomediator receptors (mediating the impulses to the endothelial cytoskeleton), (2) endocytotic receptors (securing metabolic requirements of the cell), and (3) transcytotic receptors (acting as transporters across the cell). ECs in some tissues express a transcytotic receptor of low affinity for LDL and β-VLDL, and/or a high affinity for albumin, transferrin, insulin, and ceruloplasmin. Moreover, ECs not only regulate the movement of compounds in their microenvironment, but also express cell surface molecules that regulate trafficking of circulating blood cells.[7]

The balance between endothelium-derived relaxing and constricting factors is very important in maintaining vascular homeostasis. Disruption of this balance may cause vasoconstriction, leukocyte adherence, platelet activation, mitogenesis, prooxidation, thrombosis, impaired coagulation, vascular inflammation, and atherosclerosis.[17] Recent studies focus on the complexity of EC functions, as well as on genetic and molecular regulation of their dysfunction.[17,18,141,142] Development of the endothelial cell lines from embryonic stem cells is also a method used in studies involving genetically manipulated ECs *in vitro*.[7,143]

Currently, vascular endothelium is recognized as an immunologically active tissue and can activate T lymphocytes in animal models. Research studies have shown that ECs, after activation with IFN-γ, express high levels of upregulated class I and class II major histocompatibility complex (MHC) molecules.[144] Alloreactive $CD4^+$ and $CD8^+$ T lymphocyte demonstrate proliferation in culture with activated ECs. This indicates that vascular endothelium can activate unprimed $CD4^+$ and $CD8^+$ T lymphocytes *in vitro*.[144] ECs are permanently exposed to circulating antibodies, antigens, and immune complexes, and due to this they may regulate the transport of these agents into the extravascular tissues. In this way, ECs are involved in initiation of immune reactions and play a pivotal role in immunological diseases.[145,146] The presence of receptors for the Fc-part of IgG molecules (FcR) and HLA-DR antigens on ECs proves that ECs mediate immune reactions in the skin.[147]

Apoptosis occurs in all multicellular organisms and also affects ECs.[148] Cells in the apoptotic process have morphological and biochemical characteristics distinctive from ordinary necrosis.[149] Typical morphological changes observed during programmed cell death include loss of cell volume, detachment from cellular matrices (anoikes), nuclear and plasma membrane blebs, or formation of apoptotic bodies, concentration of chromatin, and structural changes in organelles.[150,151] ECs contain all factors necessary for apoptotic cell death, which is crucial during fetal development and plays an important role in cellular homeostasis. Balance of apoptosis and EC proliferation is a major factor in angiogenesis.[152,153] Apoptosis regulates cell elimination during vessel regression. In contrast, angiogenesis involves EC detachment from the extracellular matrix and pericytes, their proliferation, migration, and formation of new capillary tubes.[152,154] It is known that several molecules, such as growth factors and cytokines, synthesized by ECs and other cells located close to the capillaries, regulate apoptosis and angiogenesis.[155] Some hormones and endocrine peptides, mediated by endothelial cell receptors, are able to regulate these two antagonistic processes, i.e., capillary formation and regression of vasculature.[156]

Recently, several studies were performed on angiogenic factors that not only induce angiogenesis, but also prevent ECs from undergoing programmed cell death.[152] The following angiogenic factors have been discovered: vascular endothelial growth factor (VEGF), basic fibroblast growth factor (bFGF), IL-8, platelet-derived endothelial cell growth factor (PDECGF), tumor necrosis factor-alpha (TNF-$\alpha$), hepatocyte growth factor, angiogenin, transforming growth factor-alpha (TGF-$\alpha$), and transforming growth factor-beta (TGF-$\beta$).[142,157] VEGF is not only a strong angiogenic factor, but is also an EC survival factor that is important in embryogenic vasculogenesis and tumor angiogenesis. Integrins (cell adhesion receptors) act as EC survival factors and prevent anoikes through stronger adhesion to the extracellular matrix. Together with VEGF, integrins support EC survival.[152] Angiopoietin (Ang-1) acts in conjunction with VEGF and inhibits EC apoptosis.[158,159] Similarly, pericytes act as EC survival factors through close contacts with ECs, as well as through the releasing of survival factors.[159] In normal skin, the vascular quiescence is maintained by a balance between endogenous angiogenesis inhibitors (thrombospondin-1, thrombospondin-2, endostatin) and a potent proangiogenic factor (VEGF-A).[160,161] Control of angiogenesis in tumor growth inhibition, tumor invasion, and metastasis is a recent research topic.[162]

## III. PATHOLOGY

ECs are involved in all types of vascular pathological processes, such as inflammation, tissue repair, tumor growth and metastasis, transplant rejection, atherogenesis, immunity, etc.[163] Vascular ECs can exhibit two different programs of function. Under normal conditions, ECs that are non-stimulated and non-activated have anticoagulant and nonthrombogenic properties. However, after injurious stimuli, ECs will undergo perturbation. Antithrombotic surface of ECs may create a protrombotic and antifibrinolytic microenvironment and promote blood coagulation. This condition may occur during high hydrodynamic shear stress[7] or at sites of inflammation, and may initiate a variety of vascular disorders such as disseminated intravascular coagulation, atherosclerosis, and immune vasculitis.[164]

Injury of the endothelium can arise from various causes, including mechanical or thermal trauma,[165] hemodynamic stress,[166] hypercholesterolemia,[167] oxygen free radicals,[103] chemical agents such as homocysteine,[168] nicotine,[169,170] immune/inflammatory mediators,[6] bacterial and viral infections,[171] and bacterial toxins.[172,173] Infection with viruses such as herpes simplex virus type 1, influenza, and cytomegalovirus has shown to induce Fc receptors and C3 receptors on ECs. These receptors serve as sites of attachment for immune complexes and may initiate cell injury.[174,175] Cultured human ECs, after being exposed to bacterial endotoxins, can synthesize a tissue factor procoagulant — a potent trigger of blood coagulation.[176] IL-1 and TNF may induce the synthesis and expression of a procoagulant molecule on the EC surface and alter EC functions.[177,178] Circulating alloantibodies produced after transplantation may injure ECs.[179] Moreover, certain stimuli can cause ECs to synthesize substances that stimulate the growth of fibroblasts and smooth muscle cells.[180]

There are three general types of EC responses to various kinds of injury:

1. *The immediate-transient response.* Mild injuries, including mild thermal injury of the endothelium, cause an immediate increase in permeability of ECs due to release of histamine, serotonin, bradykinin, and other chemical mediators. This response begins immediately after injury and lasts 15 to 30 min. Increased vascular permeability is observed clinically as edema. In type I hypersensitivity, the allergic wheal is an example of this immediate- transient response. Primary contraction of ECs causes widening of the cell junctions. Leakage predominantly occurs from small- and medium-sized venules through

gap junctions between ECs. The capillaries are unaffected because venular ECs have a greater number of receptors for histamine than arteriolar and capillary endothelium.[181]

2. *The immediate-sustained response (also called the immediate-prolonged reaction).* This response occurs after severe injury and is usually associated with necrosis of ECs. Leakage starts immediately after injury in all levels of microcirculation, including venules, capillaries, and arterioles. Here, increased vascular permeability is observed after direct damage of ECs, for example, during a severe burn. Leakage in the immediate-sustained response may last for several days.[182]
3. *The delayed-prolonged response*. In this response, vascular leakage takes place in both venules and capillaries after direct injury of ECs caused by mild-to-moderate thermal exposure, X-ray or ultraviolet (UV) irradiation, contact with certain bacterial toxins, and delayed type IV hypersensitivity reactions. Leakage is predominantly intercellular without EC contraction, is delayed, and lasts for several hours or days.[183] It is not known how gaps are formed between ECs in this type of injury and why cellular leakage is delayed.

In addition to disturbances in vascular permeability after injurious stimuli, morphologic changes in ECs have been observed in light and electron microscopy.[28,184,185] Ultrastructural observations have shown an increased number of biosynthetic organelles (i.e., endoplasmic reticulum and Golgi apparatus), changes in the cellular size, as well as in the luminal and abluminal EC membranes. Fluid shear stress can cause not only cytoskeletal rearrangement and alter morphology, but also may change endothelial gene expression.[186,187] Almost four decades ago, altered plump ECs containing an increased number of organelles in delayed type IV hypersensitivity and contact dermatitis were called "activated cells" by Willms-Kretschmer and colleagues.[188] The name mostly emphasized morphologic changes in ECs; however, the nature of the activation process was unknown at that time. Results of EC research during the last two decades indicated that "vascular endothelium responds to various stimuli, not simply as a target for injury, but by undergoing specific alterations in function, metabolism, and structure that may directly influence the evolution and outcome of the response to injury."[189] Alteration of ECs may cause either fluctuations in normal cellular activity or initiation of new EC functions and formation of new molecules that take part in coagulation, inflammation, and immunity.[190] The term *endothelial activation* (similar to macrophage, lymphocyte, and neutrophil activation) was introduced by Cotran and Pober.[191] This concept of "endothelial activation" has a precise cell biology meaning. Pober[192] defined EC activation as "quantitative changes in the expression of specific gene products (i.e., proteins) which in turn endow ECs with new capabilities that cumulatively allow ECs to perform new functions." Many of these functional and morphological effects are induced by activating factors such as cytokines and other stimuli.[193,194] Cytokines such as IL-1, TNF, LT, IFN-α, β, and γ, act as adhesion molecules on the EC surface and increase the affinity of leukocytes for the cytokine-activated endothelium. They also change the morphology of the ECs, including their membrane, cytoskeletal, and matrix organization. ECs become hypertrophied and retract, leaving dentrite-like projections within intercellular gaps. The TNF and IL-1 are implicated in chronic immune reactions and acute inflammations.[195] Moreover, IFN-γ appears to be uniquely involved in immune inflammation and probably is the "signal that converts acute inflammation to immune inflammation."[192]

The ECs that line the postcapillary venules are responsible for local recruitment of leukocytes. This is possible upon signal-induced changes in ECs, since quiescent endothelium cannot interact with circulating leukocytes.[59] Histamine (autacoid mediator) causes rapid production of vasodilators and increases leukocyte migration to surrounding tissues. Histamine is also responsible for increased adhesion of leukocytes to the cell surface (caused by translocation of P-selectin and intercellular adhesion molecule-1, or ICAM-1), activation of leukocytes (resulting from the synthesis of platelet-activating factor, or PAF), and formation of matrix in tissues that support leukocyte trafficking (through EC contraction, which causes leakage of plasma proteins such as fibronectin and fibrinogen).[59]

Endothelial cell response to inflammatory cytokines (TNF or IL-1) leads to an inflammatory reaction. In the skin helper T lymphocytes, antigen-presenting cells (APC), and keratinocytes are the source of these inflammatory cytokines.[59] They increase the EC's capacity to secrete vasodilators, leukocyte-activating chemokines, or leukocyte-adhesion molecules.[196] Vascular ECs can also lead to T-cell recruitment into tissues, by antigen presentation and through cytokine-inducible antigen-dependent responses.[59]

After EC activation, T cells are tethered, by selectins, to the luminal EC surface through low-affinity interactions. Leukocytes are also attached, and are propelled in the direction of blood flow, which rolls them along the EC surface. Three selectin proteins are involved in this process: L-selectin, E-selectin, and P-selectin.[59] L-selectin is expressed on leukocytes, and binds to ligands on (1) high endothelial venules of lymphoid tissues, (2) endothelium at inflammation sites, and (3) other leukocytes.[7] E-selectin is particularly important in cutaneous inflammatory reactions and is exclusively expressed on ECs and leukocytes. Synthesis of E-selectin by ECs is transient (onset 20 min, peak 2 to 4 h); however, expression of E-selectin on cell surfaces may persist for hours or days. E-selectin acts in the selective recruitment of lymphocytes to areas of inflamed skin through binding to the cutaneous lymphocyte antigen-1 (CLA-1).[197] Expression of E-selectin indicates EC activation. E-selectin on cutaneous microvessels appears to play a significant role in the immediate hypersensitivity reaction in atopic individuals.[59] P-selectin is rapidly redistributed from secretory granules to the surface of platelets and stimulated ECs, and binds to ligands on leukocytes.[7] Adhesion of the leukocytes to the endothelium is also mediated by integrins, such as $\beta_2$ integrin LFA-1, which binds to ICAM-1. After exposure to inflammatory factors, ICAM-1 synthesis in ECs is upregulated about 20-fold (onset 4 h, plateau at 24 h).[198,199] Adhesion-mediated recognition by LFA-1 recognition of ICAM-1 is much stronger than that of selectins. Once complexed with ICAM-1, leukocytes spread out and crawl along the EC surface, reach a cell junction, and migrate through the vessel wall into tissues. The $\beta_2$ integrins and ICAM-1 have a main contribution in the adhesion of leukocytes to the endothelium and their subsequent recruitment.[200]

Micromolecular research studies of several diseases explain related pathological symptoms as alterations in normal EC activity. Increased number of circulating activated ECs, as well as increased levels of TNF-$\alpha$ and VEGF, and decreased levels of protein C and protein S in the circulation of patients with thalassemia may indicate the propensity of vascular perturbation in these conditions.[201] Inflammation-induced angiogenesis is the main site of leukocyte–EC interaction, which causes inflammatory infiltrates in giant cell arteritis.[202] Endothelial dysfunction was found in early stages of Alzheimer's disease. Significant increases in plasma levels of thrombomodulin (a marker of endothelial activation) and E-selectin (an endothelial leukocyte-adhesion molecule) were found in these patients.[203] Vascular adhesion molecules play a physiological role in inflammatory skin disease. In normal skin, the expression of E-selectin and ICAM-1 is at low level and can hardly be detected. In pathological conditions, however, presence of vascular adhesion molecules is detected along the whole length of the dermal capillary loop.[204] This leads T cells to exit the vessels, and allows them to be closer to the epidermis.[205]

Microvascular endothelium *in vivo* may respond to cytokines in three ways. (1) ECs may be injured from cytokine binding to EC receptors. This takes place, for example, during transplant rejection[206] as a result of an immune response against foreign endothelium. (2) ECs may migrate, proliferate, and form new capillaries (angiogenesis). (3) Activated ECs may perform new functions.[207]

Usually endothelial activation is beneficial, especially in host defense, because it can cause development of cell-mediated immune reactions. On the other hand, activation of ECs can cause their dysfunction (with or without injury) and contribute to diseases. Endothelial activation can lead to pathological processes such as the vascular leak syndrome and development of vasculitis in Kawasaki syndrome.[189,191–193,208] Diseases with proliferation of ECs, which may result from infection, immunologic disturbances, trauma, or other etiologies, include bacillary angiomatosis, verruga peruana (Carrion's disease), papillary endothelial hyperplasia, benigne (reactive) angioendotheliomatosis, angiolymphoid hyperplasia with eosinophilia (ALHE, also called Kimura's disease), and some hemangiomas.[171,209] The concept of endothelial activation is useful in understanding EC function and its molecular metabolic processes. This concept stimulates a search for the active role of ECs in local response to injury and in pathogenesis of some diseases.[189]

During skin inflammation, ECs may take part in antigen-dependent and cytokine-mediated processes. Human dermal microvascular endothelium may initiate immune responses by presenting antigens to T cells (memory T cells).[7] Cytokines derived from activated T lymphocytes activate ECs and lead to recruitment and activation of effector lymphocytes. Cutaneous microvascular ECs strongly express class I and class II MHC molecules *in vivo.* The function of class I and class II MHC molecules is to present peptides to T cells.[210] The ability to activate memory T cells can differentiate ECs from other cells that also express class I and class II MHC molecules *in vitro,* but cannot activate memory T cells.[211,212] ECs can co-stimulate memory and naive T cells. This kind of co-stimulation is mediated by co-stimulatory molecule LFA-3 (CD58). This demonstrates the importance of the LFA-3 signal pathway in antigen presentation by human ECs.[7,213] The use of vascular ECs as APCs would increase the efficiency of peripheral immune surveillance by memory T cells. Antigen presentation on EC surface could therefore increase the rate of antigen being recognized.[214]

Recent research studies on apoptosis have shown that this programmed physiological cell death is induced by various stimuli, e.g., death factors, stress stimuli, bacterial and viral infections,[173,215,216] as well as by several cellular molecules, including caspases, Bel-2-like proteins, mitochondrial factors, stress-activated protein kinases, sphingomyelinases, etc.[217] Some anti-endothelial cell antibodies activate ECs, others trigger apoptosis.[218,219] Functional Fas ligand (FasL) induces apoptotic cell death.[220] *Staphylococcus aureus,* for example, induces rapid apoptosis of human ECs and causes a break of the endothelial barrier, permitting the bacterium to attack organs.[221] This process suggests that EC apoptosis may be important in bacterial invasions of the body. It was recently shown that high concentration of homocysteine-thiolactone induces EC apoptosis.[222] It was also shown that mammalian cells respond to low or zero oxygen concentrations by undergoing apoptosis, but not necrosis.[223] Oxidative damage to ECs during reoxygenation initiates apoptosis.[224] Similarly, hyperbaric oxygenation of hematopoietic cells enhances apoptosis of these cells by increasing the intracellular accumulation of $H_2O_2$.[225] Increased oxygen tension causes inhibition of EC proliferation and decreases the synthesis of PECAM-1, a major surface protein, and type IV collagen.[226] Hypoxia, however, stimulates angiogenesis and enhances VEGF mRNA.[227–230] The expression of platelet-derived growth factor (PDGF) and TGF-β1 is also increased in this condition.[231–233] Acidosis, which occurs in various physiological and pathological conditions, may protect ECs from apoptosis and inhibit their proangiogenic tendency, but it can induce the expression of VEGF mRNA and FGF mRNA.[12] Dysregulation of apoptotic process may be associated with pathological conditions such as cancer, AIDS, neurodegeneration, heart disease, autoimmunity disorders like systemic lupus erythematosus, and allergy.[234,235] Apoptotic cell death is increasingly better understood. Research studies on proapoptotic markers (bax and p53), antiapoptotic markers (bcl-2), and the proliferation marker (ki-67) in various human cells are developing very rapidly. In the near future, these markers might be helpful in early detection of dysregulation of apoptosis.[236–238]

## IV. VASCULAR ENDOTHELIAL CELL MARKERS

In normal or neoplastic vasculature, basal lamina or endothelium can be detected using immunohistochemical or immunofluorescence techniques. These techniques are used to localize cellular markers in the cytoplasm or in the membrane of ECs.[239] The basal lamina of small blood vessels is visible in the presence of antibodies against the basal lamina components — laminin, type IV collagen, and perlecan.[240] However, because ECs of lymphatic capillaries are supported by fine collagenous and reticular fibrils instead of the true basal lamina, they give a negative or very weak reaction to antigens such as laminin or type IV collagen in immunologic staining.[52] The larger lymphatic vessels, including those in lymphangiomas, stain with laminin.

The ECs in ultrastructural studies of human and animal vasculature can be identified by the presence of Weibel–Palade bodies in the endothelial cell cytoplasm. These structures have been regarded as a morphologic marker for ECs with an exception[53,54] — the endothelium of mouse, where Weibel–Palade bodies are absent.[241]

Recognition of the ECs in blood vessels and in lymphatic vessels is very important for proper diagnosis and treatment of numerous diseases. Pathological conditions such as vascular malformations, tumors, and inflammatory diseases of the skin very often involve both blood vessels and lymphatics. However, morphological characteristics of ECs in these conditions do not allow a clear distinction between blood vessel ECs (BEC) and lymphatic vessel ECs (LEC). Molecular markers for ECs, which may allow precise diagnosis of such diseases, currently are in the developing stage.

Detection and study of LECs is equivalently important in understanding immunological processes. The lymph is filtered through lymph nodes, which may trap various antigens by attracting APCs, i.e., Langerhans cells (LCs) in the epidermis and dendritic cells in epithelia. These cells can monitor the extracellular environment, detect antigens, and lead T-cell activation.[242] The lymphatic vessels in the skin, located near the surface, provide an important transport route for antigen-presenting LCs. They may enter the afferent lymphatic vessels and be taken to the lymph nodes. Chemokines and their receptors are also involved in this process. A recent study has shown that β-chemokine receptor D6 is expressed only in the lymphatic vessels of the skin and in lymph nodes.[243]

The commonly used factor VIII-related antigen (FVIII-RA)[244] is not a very reliable marker for vascular endothelium because it is not expressed uniformly on ECs of all types of vessels.[245,246] The ECs of small normal cutaneous vessels and well-formed blood vessels in Kaposi's sarcoma, stained for FVIII-RA using peroxidase-antiperoxidase technique, give the strongest reaction.[247] ECs of hemangioma and angiokeratoma react with FVIII-RA less consistently. The ECs in tufted angioma (angioblastoma) do not, or only weakly, express FVIII-RA.[248] In lymphangioma, pyogenic granuloma, and pigmented dermatosis, endothelial positivity for FVIII-RA is less intense. The ECs of angiosarcoma stain negatively with this antigen.[247]

Ulex europaeus-I lectin (UEA-I) staining is another method used in recognition of ECs. UEA-I stains are more visible in small vessels than the previously mentioned FVIII-RA antigen. Capillaries in tufted angioma exhibit strong positivity for UEA-I.[249] However, UEA-I shows variable staining of angiosarcoma. Because UEA-I also binds to squamous cell carcinomas and other epithelial neoplasms, it therefore is not specific for ECs.[250]

Monoclonal antibodies (B721, E431) recognize EC surface antigens, and together with other known endothelial markers (F8rAg, Ia, HCL-1), they are used in the study of Kaposi's sarcoma in patients with AIDS.[251] Monoclonal antibodies (E92, OKM5, HCL-1) react with ECs of normal blood vessels, but not with lymphatic vessel endothelium.[252] The monoclonal antibody BMA 120 recognizes a 200-kDa endothelial antigen and shows stronger staining in angiosarcoma than UEA-I and FVIII-RA. Monoclonal antibodies to ICAM-1, used in frozen sections, are excellent markers of the vascular endothelium. Staining with anti-CD-34 (a glycosilated transmembrane protein) may be used to differentiate Kaposi's sarcoma from hemosiderotic dermatofibromas.[253] Similarly, tumor cells in tufted angioma can be detected with this technique because they are positive for CD-34.[248] Monoclonal antibody CD-31, an adhesion molecule (JC70 or ENDOCAM), is also a reliable EC marker.[52,240,250,254] CD-36 (thrombospondin and collagen receptor) is present on endothelium, monocytes, and platelets.[8] The use of a new monoclonal antibody (S-Endo-1), which recognizes CD-146 (a molecule expressed on all human ECs), allows detection of high numbers of circulating ECs in thrombotic, infectious, or immunologic disorders. It is a useful marker for vascular wall injury because it allows diagnosis of infectious diseases that involve intraendothelial microbial agents.[255]

Other possible markers for ECs are cytokeratin 8, 18, 19, and vimentin, cytoskeletal proteins that are present on microvascular ECs.[8] EN 7/44 is present on the apical part of growing capillaries, but is negative on differentiated ECs. 1F10 is a membrane protein located on endothelial cells of capillaries in vascular tumors.[8] ELAM-1, VCAM, E-selectin, and P-selectin (adhesion molecules for leukocytes) appear on postcapillary venules after stimulation with inflammatory mediators.[8] E-selectin was found in proliferating ECs in hemangiomas.[256,257]

VEGF is predominantly localized within the cytoplasm of pericytes and ECs only during the proliferative phase of hemangioma.[240] bFGF staining is positive within ECs in the proliferative and early involuting phases of hemangioma, but not in the late involuting phase of this vascular tumor.[240,258] For distinguishing infantile hemangiomas from vascular malformations, the glucose transporter protein-1 (Glut-1) has been recently used.[259] Glut-1, however, is also highly expressed in normal ECs at sites of blood–tissue barriers, i.e., brain, eye, nerve, and placenta.[260]

Some of the more significant markers for ECs cells are as follows. Alkaline phosphatase (ALPase) is used as a marker for blood vessel endothelium as well as lymphatics; however, adenylate and guanylate cyclase (AC and GC) are specific for the ECs of blood vessels only.[261] Angiotensin-converting enzyme (ACE) or kininase II may also be used as a marker for murine, bovine, and human ECs.[262,263] Human fms-like tyrosine kinase 4 gene (Flt-4) and 5′-nucleotidase (5′Nase) are expressed on lymphatic vessels of endothelial cells (LEC).[261,264] Flt-4 marker is also present on blood vessel endothelial cells (BEC).[230] Vascular endothelial growth factor receptor-3 (VEGFR-3) is the first cloned molecular marker and is an important regulator of lymphatic vessel endothelium.[265] VEGFR-3 is abundant in lymphatic vessels, but is also present in some endocrine glands and fenestrated venules.[264] VEGF-C and VEGF-D bind to and activate VEGFR-3 on the lymphatic endothelium. The expression pattern of VEGF-3, VEGF-C, and VEGF-D suggests that lymphatic vessel growth is regulated by VEGFR-3.[266–270] Podoplanin is a marker for ECs of the lymphatic vessels. It is expressed in the endothelium of lymphatic capillaries, but not in blood vasculature. In the skin, podoplanin colocalizes with VEGFR-3. The function of podoplanin is not known.[271–273] LYVE-1 (type I integral membrane glycoprotein) is a major receptor for hyaluronan on lymphatic vessels, but also reacts with blood vasculature in lung and ECs of umbilical veins.[273,274]

Recent research studies identified integrin $\alpha_v\beta_3$, a cell surface receptor, as a marker for activated and proliferating ECs, and is specific for newly formed blood vessels during angiogenesis.[275] Matrix metalloproteinases (MMPs) and tissue inhibitors of metalloproteinases (TIMPs) are markers for new vessel formation.[230] Neuropilin (NRP)-2 was identified as a coreceptor for VEGF-C expressed in the subset of lymphatic vessels. This marker was detected only in the intestinal lymphatic endothelium, not in the skin. This suggests that the VEGF-C receptor expression is different in various organs.[276] Recently, endomucin (endothelial sialomucin) was identified on the endothelium of each tissue. This novel molecule is a new endothelial-specific marker.[279]

Prox-1 is a homologue of *Drosophila melanogaster* homeobox gene prospero used as a marker for LEC[273] in both normal and diseased tissue. It was suggested that Prox-1 is better than VEGFR-3. Prox-1 is co-expressed with CD31 and VEGFR-3, but not with CD34 and PAL-E.[277] Poc-1 is strongly expressed in the nuclei of Kaposi's sarcoma cells, for this reason it is not a specific marker for lymphatic ECs.[273]

Guanylate-binding protein-1 (GPB-1) is a cytoplasmic protein not present in ECs of normal skin. However, in skin diseases with an inflammatory component (psoriasis, adverse drug reaction, and Kaposi's sarcoma) GPB-1 is strongly expressed. GPB-1 expression in ECs can be highly induced by inflammatory cytokines such as INF-$\gamma$, INF-1$\alpha$, INF-1$\beta$, TNF-$\alpha$, but is not induced by other cytokines, chemokines, or growth factors. Therefore, GPB-1 is a novel molecular marker that indicates inflammatory cytokine-activated phenotype of ECs *in vivo* and *in vitro*.[278]

Anionic phospholipids were classified as potential markers for blood vessels in tumors because they are expressed on ECs in tumor vasculature, but not on ECs of normal blood vessels.[280] Anionic phospholipids are abundant not only on the luminal surface of ECs in tumors, but also on the cell surface during apoptosis, necrosis, cell injury, cell activation, and malignant cells. For this reason, anionic phospholipids can be used as receptors for vascular target substances during cancer treatment.[280] Investigations on this subject are intensively ongoing.

Further studies on molecular markers for ECs might allow differentiation of ECs of blood vessels from lymphatic ECs and explanation of the differences in the mechanism of gene and protein expression between BEC and LEC. These studies will aid understanding of the immunological and pathological processes of various diseases that involve blood vessels and lymphatics.

## V. CONCLUSIONS

This chapter has reviewed information about vascular EC morphology, physiology, and pathology, focusing on ECs in the skin. Because of its importance, widespread location, and innumerable vital functions, the vascular endothelium remains the subject of many research studies in medicine. Throughout several decades, much has been discovered about this dynamic organ. ECs can be stimulated by signals from blood and migratory leukocytes, as well as from cells of the surrounding tissue. As a result of these stimuli, ECs may respond by (1) vasodilatation and increased permeability, (2) production of cytokines and cell mediators, (3) endothelial activation, (4) converting adherent leukocytes into mobile cells migrating to the inflammatory sites, (5) antigen presentation, (6) angiogenesis and apoptosis. The number of discoveries of new EC functions and their biosynthetic and metabolic activities is still growing. Current research on programmed cell death and proliferation and expanded discussions on the mechanisms that maintain EC stability allow understanding of the nature of angiogenesis and vessel regression. Furthermore, differences between the ECs of blood vessels and lymphatics have been discussed, including new markers for their differentiation. Application of new techniques in future research on ECs of the vascular system will help to discover new possibilities for diagnosis and treatment of diseases involving blood vessels and the lymphatic system, and will further explain the immune functions of ECs.

## ACKNOWLEDGMENT

We thank Dr. Juntao Han for a valuable contribution to this chapter.

## REFERENCES

1. Virchow, R., Phlogose and Thrombose in Gefessystem, in *Gesammelte Abhandlungen zur wissenschaftlichen Medicine,* Meidinger Sohn, Frankfurt-am-Main, 1856, 458.
2. Gimbrone. M.A., Jr., Culture of vascular endothelium, in *Progress in Hemostasis and Thrombosis,* Vol. III, Speat, T.H., Ed., Grune & Stratton, New York, 1976.
3. Fishman, A.P., Endothelium, *Ann. N.Y. Acad. Sci.,* 401, 1982.
4. Jaffe, E.A., Ed., *Biology of Endothelial Cells,* Martinus Nijhoff, The Hague, 1984.
5. Shepro, D. and D'Amore, P.A., Physiology and biochemistry of the vascular wall endothelium, in *Handbook of Physiology in the Cardiovascular System,* Vol. 6, Renkin, E.M. and Michael, C.C., Eds., American Physiological Society, Washington, D.C., 1984, 103.
6. Gimbrone, M.A. and Nevilacqua, M.P., Vascular endothelium, functional modulation at the Blood interface, in *Endothelial Cell Biology in Health and Disease,* Simionescu, N. and Simionescu, M., Eds., Plenum Press, New York, 1988, 255.
7. Cines, D.B., Pollak, E.S., Buck, C.A., Loscalzo, J., Zimmerman, G.A., McEver, R.P., Pober, J.S., Wick, T.M., Konkle, B.A., Schwartz, B.S., Barnathan, E.S., McCrae, K.R., Hug, B.A., Schmidt, A.-M., and Stern, D.M., Endothelial cells in physiology and in the pathophysiology of vascular disorders, *Blood,* 91, 3527, 1998.
8. Bachetti, T. and Morbidelli, L., Endothelial cells in culture: a model for studying vascular functions, *Pharmacol. Res.,* 42, 9, 2000.
9. Gimbrone, M.A., Jr., Vascular endothelium: Nature's blood container, in *Vascular Endothelium in Hemostasis and Thrombosis,* Gimbrone, M.A., Ed., Churchill Livingstone, London, 1986, 1.
10. Jaffe, E.A., Nachman, R.L., Becker, C.G., and Minick, C.R., Culture of human endothelial cells derived from umbilical veins. Identification of morphologic and immunologic criteria. *J. Clin. Invest.,* 52, 1745, 1978.

11. Thompson, R.W. and D'Amore, P.A., Growth control of cultured endothelial cells, in *Endothelialization of Vascular Grafts,* Zilla, P.P., Falol, R.D., and Deutsch, M., Eds., S. Karger, Basel, Switzerland, 1987, 100.
12. D'Arcangelo, D., Facchiano, F, Barlucchi, L.M., Melillo, G., Illi, B., Testolin, L., Gaetano, C., and Capogrossi, M.C., Acidosis inhibits endothelial cell apoptosis and function and induces basic fibroblast growth factor and vascular endothelial growth factor expression, *Circ. Res.*, 86, 312, 2000.
13. Brett, J.G., Steinberg, S.F., deGroot, P.G., Nawroth, P.P., and Stern, D.M., Norepinephrine down-regulates the activity of protein S on endothelial cells, *J. Cell. Biol.,* 106, 2109, 1988.
14. Renkin, E.M., Multiple pathways of capillary permeability. *Circ. Res.,* 41, 735, 1977.
15. Libby, P. and Birinyi, L.K., The dynamic nature of vascular endothelial functions, in *Endothelialization of Vascular Grafts,* Zilla, P. P., Fasol, R. D., and Deutsch, M., Eds., S. Karger, Basel, 1987, 80.
16. Machovich, R., Biology of endothelial cells, in *Blood Vessel Walls and Thrombosis,* Vol. 1, Machovich, R., Ed., CRC Press, Boca Raton, FL., 1988, 115.
17. Butany, J.W., Verma, S., Leask, R.L., Mohsen, B., and Asa, S.L., Genetic abnormalities of the endothelium, *Microsc. Res. Tech.* 60, 30, 2003.
18. Mawji, I.A. and Marsden, P.A., Perturbations in paracrine control of the circulation: role of the endothelial-derived vasomediators, endothelin-1 and nitric oxide, *Microsc. Res. Tech.*, 60, 46, 2003.
19. Palade, G.E., Fine structure of blood capillaries, *J. Appl. Physiol.,* 24, 1424, 1953.
20. Hammersen, F. and Lewis, D.H., *Endothelial Cell Vesicles,* S. Karger, Basel, 1985.
21. Sato, V., Current understanding of the biology of vascular endothelium, *Cell Struct. Funct.,* 26, 9, 2001.
22. Muller, W.A. and Gimbrone, M.A., Plasmalemmal proteins of cultured vascular endothelial cells exhibit apical-basal polarity: analysis by surface-selective iodination, *J. Cell Biol.,* 103, 2389, 1986.
23. Yee, A.G. and Revel, J.P., Endothelial cell junctions, *J. Cell. Biol.,* 66, 200, 1975.
24. Simionescu, N., Simionescu, M., and Palade, G.E., Recent studies on vascular endothelium, *Ann. N.Y. Acad. Sci.,* 275, 64, 1976.
25. Simionescu, M., Simionescu, N., and Palade, G.E., Segmental differentiations of cell junctions in the vascular endothelium: the microvasculature, *J. Cell. Biol.,* 67, 863, 1975.
26. Simionescu, M., Simionescu, N., and Palade, G.E., Characteristic endothelial junctions in different segments of the vascular system, *Thromb. Res.,* 8(Suppl. 2), 247, 1976.
27. Yen, A. and Braverman, I.M., Ultrastructure of the human dermal microcirculation: the horizontal plexus of the papillary dermis, *J. Invest. Dermatol.,* 66, 131, 1976.
28. Hammersen, F. and Hammersen, E., The structural reaction of endothelial cells to injurious stimuli, *Agents Actions,* 13, 442, 1983.
29. Rhodin, J.A.G., The ultrastructure of mammalian arterioles and precapillary sphincters, *J. Ultrastruct. Res.,* 19, 181, 1967.
30. Davies, P.F., Olesen, S.-P., Clapham, D.E., Morrel, E.M., and Schoen, F.J., Endothelial communication. State of the art lecture, *Hypertension,* 11, 563, 1988.
31. Schmelz, M., Moll, R., Kuhn, C., and Franke, W.W., Complexus adhaerentes, a new group of desmoplakin-containing junctions in endothelial cells: II. Different types of lymphatic vessels, *Differentiation,* 57, 97, 1994.
32. Majno, G., Shea, S.M., and Leventhal, M., Endothelial contraction induced by histamine-type mediators. An electron microscope study, *J Cell Biol.*, 43, 647, 1969.
33. Gabbiani, G. and Majno, G., Endothelial microvilli in the vessels of the rat Gasserian ganglion and testis, *Z. Zellforsch, Mikroskop. Anat.,* 97, 111, 1969.
34. Bhavan, J. and Edelstein, L., Angiofibromas in tuberous sclerosis: a light and electron microscopic study, *J. Cutaneous Pathol.,* 4, 300, 1977.
35. Łukaszyk, I., Sarankiewicz-Konopka, B., and Motowski, T., Badania ultrastructury naczyń wtosowatych skóry w cukrzycy, *Przegl. Dermatol.,* 65, 137, 1978.
36. Pasyk, K., Studies on subcutaneous fat necrosis of the newborn, *Virchows Arch. A.,* 379, 243, 1978.
37. Groniowska, M., Dabrowski, J., Koczyk, E., and Bojar, B., Badania kliniczne i mikroskopowo-elektronowe dziatania malanu hydrokortizonu, *Przegl. Dermatol.,* 64, 605, 1977.
38. Majno, G. and Jones, I., Endothelium: a review, in *The Thrombotic Process in Atherogenesis,* Chadler, A.B., Eugenius, K., McMillan, G.C., Nelson, C.B., Schwartz, C.J., and Wessler, S., Eds., Plenum Press, New York, 1978, 169.

39. Higgins, J.C. and Eady, R.A.J., Human dermal microvasculature. I. Its segmental differentiation. Light and electron microscopic study, *Br. J. Dermatol.*, 104, 117, 1981.
40. Seifert, H.W. and Klingmuller, G., Elektronenmikroskopische Struktur normaler Hautkapillaren und das verhalten alkalischer Phosphatase, *Arch. Dermatol. Forschung.*, 242, 97, 1972.
41. Braverman, L.M. and Keh-Yen, A., Ultrastructure of the human dermal microcirculation. III. The vessels in the mid- and lower dermis and subcutaneous fat, *J. Invest. Dermatol.*, 77, 297, 1981.
42. McLeod, W.A., Observations of fenestrated capillaries in the human scalp, *J. Invest Dermatol.*, 55, 354, 1970.
43. Clementi, F. and Palade, G.E., Intestinal capillaries. I. Permeability to peroxidase and ferritin, *J. Cell. Biol.*, 41, 33, 1969.
44. Owman, C. and Hardbeo, J.E., Functional heterogeneity of cerebrovascular endothelium. *Brain Behav. Evol.*, 32, 65, 1988.
45. Majno, G., Ultrastructure of the vascular membrane, in *Handbook of Physiology — Circulation*, Hamilton, W.F. and Dow, P., Eds., Waverly Press, Baltimore, MD, 2293.
46. Augustin, H.G., Kozian, D.H., and Johnson, R.C., Differentiation of endothelial cells: analysis of the constitutive and activated endothelial cell phenotypes, *Bioessays*, 16, 901, 1994.
47. Thorpe, P.E. and Ran, S., Mapping zip codes in human vasculature, *Pharmacogenomics J.*, 2, 205, 2002.
48. Ghitescu, L. and Robert, M., Diversity in unity: the biochemical composition of the endothelial cell surface varies between the vascular beds, *Microsc. Res. Tech.*, 57, 381, 2002.
49. Hibbs, R.G., Burch., G.E., and Phillips, J.H., The fine structure of the small blood vessels of normal human dermis and subcutis, *Am. Heart J.*, 56, 662, 1958.
50. Odland, G.F., The fine structure of cutaneous capillaries, in *Advances in the Biology of Skin*, Vol. 2, Montagna, W. and Ellis, R.A., Eds., Pergamon Press, New York, 1961, 57.
51. Braverman, I.M. and Yen, A., Ultrastructure of the human dermal microcirculation. II. The capillary loops of the dermal papillae, *J. Invest. Dermatol.*, 68, 44, 1977.
52. Gallager, P.J., Blood vessels, in *Histology for Pathologists*, Sternberg, S.S., Ed., Raven Press, New York, 1992, 195.
53. Weibel, E.R. and Palade, G.E., New cytoplasmic components in arterial endothelia, *J. Cell. Biol.*, 23, 101, 1964.
54. Sengel, A. and Stoebner, P., Golgi origin of tubular inclusions in endothelial cells, *J. Cell. Biol.*, 44, 223, 1970.
55. Daoud, A.S., Jones, R., and Scott, R.F., Dietary-induced atherosclerosis in miniature swine. II. Electron microscopic observations: characteristics of endothelial and smooth muscle cells in the proliferative lesion and elsewhere in the aorta, *Exp. Mol. Pathol.*, 8, 263, 1968.
56. Trillo, A.A. and Prichard, R.W., Early endothelial changes in experimental primate atherosclerosis, *Lab. Invest.*, 41, 294, 1979.
57. McEver, R., Beckstead, J.H., Moore, K., Marshal-Carlson, L., and Bainton, D., GMP 140, a platelet alpha-granule membrane protein is also synthesized by vascular endothelial cells and is localized in Weibel-Palade bodies, *J. Clin. Invest.*, 84, 92, 1989.
58. Heckmann, M., Karasek, M.A., and Braun-Falco, O., Neueres zur Physiologie und Pathologie von Endothelzellen in der Haut, *Hautarzt*, 42, 677, 1991.
59. Pober, J.S., Kluger, M.S., and Schechner, J.S., Human endothelial cell presentation of antigen and the homing of memory/effector T cells to skin, *Ann. N.Y. Acad. Sci.*, 941, 12, 2001.
60. Utgaard, J.O., Jahnsen, F.L., Bakka, A., Brandtzaeg, P., and Haraldsen, G., Rapid secretion of prestored interleukin 8 from Weibel-Palade bodies of microvascular endothelial cells, *J. Exp. Med.*, 188, 1751, 1998.
61. Wolff, B., Burns, A.R., Middleton, J., and Rot, A., Endothelial cell "memory" of inflammatory stimulation: human venular endothelial cells store interleukin 8 in Weibel-Palade bodies, *J. Exp. Med.*, 188, 1757, 1998.
62. Schnyder-Candrian, S., Borsig, L., Moser, R., and Berger, E.G., Localization of $\alpha$1,3-fucosyltransferase VI in Weibel-Palade bodies of human endothelial cells, *PNAS*, 97, 8369, 2000.
63. Kobayashi, T., Vischer, U.M., Rosnoblet, C., Lebrand, C., Lindsay, M., Parton, R.G., Kruithof, E.K.O., and Gruenberg, J., The tetraspanin CD63/lamp3 cycles between endocytic and secretory compartments in human endothelial cells, *Mol. Biol. Cell*, 11, 1829, 2000.

64. Spear, G.S., Slusser, R.J., Garvin, A.J., Horger, E.O., III., Bailey, R.P., and Schneider, J.A., A cytoplasmic body in human fetal endothelium, *Am. J. Pathol.,* 78, 333, 1975.
65. Hammersen, F. and Osterkamp-Baust, U., A paracrystalline inclusions body in normal human vascular endothelial cells, *Int. J. Microcirc. Clin. Exp.,* 1, 135, 1982.
66. Pasyk, K.A., Hassett, C.A., Cherry, G.W., and Argenta, L.C., Endothelial cell crystalloids in newborn human foreskin, *J. Cutaneous Pathol.,* 15, 84, 1988.
67. Pasyk, K.A., Grabb, W.C., and Cherry, G.W., Cellular hemangioma light and electron microscopic studies of two cases, *Virchows Arch. A.,* 396, 103, 1982.
68. Pasyk, K.A., Grabb, W.C., and Cherry, G.W., Crystalloid inclusions of endothelial cells in cellular and capillary hemangiomas — a possible sign of cellular immaturity, *Arch. Dermatol.,* 119, 134, 1983.
69. Luzi, P., Miracco, C., and Fimiani., M., Intracytoplasmic crystals in endothelial cells, *Ultrastr. Pathol.,*11, 473, 1987.
70. Kumakiri, M., Muramoto, F., Tsukinaga, I., Yoshida, T., and Miura, Y., Crystalline lamellae in the endothelial cells of a type of hemangioma characterized by the proliferation of immature endothelial cells and pericytes — angioblastoma (Nakagawa), *J. Am. Acad. Dermatol.,* 8, 68, 1983.
71. Ho, K.L., Ultrastructure of cerebellar capillary hemangioblastoma. III. Crystalloid bodies in endothelial cells, *Acta Neuropathol.,* 66, 117, 1985.
72. Rippe, B., Kamiya, A.., and Folkow, B., Is capillary micropinocytosis of any significance for the transcapillary transfer of plasma proteins, *Acta Physiol. Scand.,* 100, 258, 1977.
73. Frokjaer-Jensen, J., The vesicle controversy, in *Endothelial Cell Vesicles,* Hammersen, F. and Lewis, D.H., Eds., S. Karger, Basel, 1985, 21.
74. Simionescu, M., Simionescu, N., Silbert, J.E., and Palade, G.E., Differentiated microdomains on the luminal surface of capillary endothelium. II. Partial characterization of their anionic sites, *J. Cell. Biol.,* 90, 614, 1981.
75. Hammersen, F. and Hammersen, E., Some structural aspects of precapillary vessels, *J. Cardiovasc. Pharmacol.,* 2(Suppl. 6), S289, 1984.
76. Kuwabara, H., Kokai, Y., Kojima, T., Takakuwa, R., and Sawada, N., Occludin regulates actin cytoskeleton in endothelial cells, *Cell Struct. Funct.,* 26, 109, 2001.
77. Lee, T.-Y.J. and Gotlieb, A.I., Microfilaments and microtubules maintain endothelial integrity, *Microsc. Res. Tech.,* 60, 115, 2003.
78. Rhodin, J.A.G., *Histology,* Oxford University Press, Oxford, 1974, 372.
79. Vanhoutte, P.M., Say NO to ET, *J. Auton. Nerv. System,* 81, 271, 2000.
80. Światkowska, M., Cierniewska-Cieślak, A., Pawtowska, Z., and Cierniewski, C.S., Dual regulatory effects of nitric oxide on plasminogen activator inhibitor type 1 expression in endothelial cells, *Eur. J. Biochem.,* 267, 1001, 2000.
81. Flavahan, N.A., Atherosclerosis or lipoprotein-induced endothelial dysfunction. Potential mechanisms underlying reduction in EDRF/nitric oxide activity, *Circulation,* 85, 1927, 1992.
82. Lefer, A.M., Tsao, P.S., Lefer, D.J., and Ma, X., Role of endothelial dysfunction in the pathogenesis of reperfusion injury after myocardial ischemia, *FASEB J.,* 5, 2029, 1991.
83. Jaffe, E.A. and Mosher, D.F., Synthesis of fibronectin by cultured human endothelial cells, *J. Exp. Med.,* 147, 1777, 1978.
84. Sage, H., Pritzl, P., and Bornstein, P., Secretory phenotypes of endothelial cells in culture: Comparison of aortic, venous, capillary and corneal endothelium, *Arteriosclerosis,* 1, 427, 1981.
85. Li, J., Zhang, Y.-P., and Kirsner, R.S., Angiogenesis in wound repair: angiogenic growth factors and the extracellular matrix, *Microsc. Res. Tech.,* 60, 107, 2003.
86. Wagner, D.D. and Marden, V.J., Biosynthesis of von Willebrand protein by human endothelial cells: processing steps and their intracellular localization, *J. Cell. Biol.,* 99, 2123, 1984.
87. McCarroll, D.R., Levin, E.G., and Montgomery, R.R., Endothelial cell synthesis of von Willebrand Antigen II, von Willebrand factor, and von Willebrand factor/von Willebrand Antigen II complex, *J. Clin. Invest.,* 75, 1089, 1985.
88. Loskutoff, D.J., Levin, E., and Mussoni, L., Fibrinolytic components of cultured endothelial cells, in *Pathology of the Endothelial Cell,* Nossel, H.L., and Vogel, H.J., Eds., Academic Press, New York, 1982, 167.
89. Cerveny, T.J., Fass, D.N., and Mann, K.G., Coagulation factor V synthesis by cultured endothelium, *Blood,* 63, 1467, 1984.

90. Marcum, J.A. and Rosenberg, R.D., Heparin-like molecules with anticoagulant activity are synthesized by cultured endothelial cells, *Biochem. Biophys. Res. Commun.,* 126, 365, 1985.
91. Mosher, D.F., Doyle, M.J., and Jaffe, E.A., Synthesis and secretion of thrombospondin by cultured human endothelial cells, *J. Cell. Biol.,* 93, 343, 1982.
92. Clouse, L.H. and Comp, P.C., The regulation of hemostasis. The protein C system, *N. Engl. J. Med.,* 314, 1298, 1986.
93. Awbrey, B.J., Hoak, J.C., and Owen, W.G., Binding of human thrombin to cultured human endothelial cells, *J. Biol. Chem.,* 254, 4092, 1979.
94. Maruyama, I., Salem, H.H., and Majerus, P.W., Coagulation factor Va binds to human umbilical vein endothelial cells and accelerates protein C activation, *J. Clin. Invest.,* 74, 224, 1984.
95. Rodgers, G.M. and Shuman, M.A., Prothrombin is activated on vascular endothelial cells by factor Xa and calcium, *Proc. Natl. Acad. Sci. U.S.A.,* 80, 7001, 1983.
96. Ueshima, S., Matsumoto, H., Izaki, S., Mitsui, Y., Fukao, H., Okada, K., and Matsuo, O., Co-localization of urokinase and its receptor on established human umbilical vein endothelial cell, *Cell Struct. Funct.*, 24, 71, 1999.
97. Bajou, K., Noel, A., Gerard, R.D., Masson, V., Brunner, N., Holst-Hanen, C., Dobe, M., Fusening, N.E., Carmeliet, P., Collen, D., and Foidart, J.M., Absence of host plasminogen activator inhibitor 1 prevents cancer invasion and vascularization, *Nat. Med.,* 8, 923, 1998.
98. Stefansson, S. and Lawrence, D.A., The serpin PAI-1 inhibits cell migration by blocking integrin $\alpha_v\beta_3$ binding to vitronectin. *Nature*, 383, 441, 1996.
99. Mantovani, A. and Dejana, E., Functional responses elicited in endothelial cells by cytokines, in *Cytokines in Health and Disease,* Kunkel, S.L., and Resnick, D.G., Eds., Marcel Dekker, New York, 1992, 297.
100. Callard, R.E. and Gearing, A.J.H., *The Cytokine Facts Book,* Academic Press/Harcourt Brace, London, 1994.
101. Hamblin, A.S., *Cytokines and Cytokine Receptors*, Oxford University Press, Oxford, 1993.
102. Kater, L. and Baart de la Faille, H., *Multi-Systemic Auto-Immune Diseases: An Integrated Approach Dermatological and Internal Aspects,* Elsevier, Amsterdam, 1995.
103. Gryglewski, R.J. and Moncada, S., Secretory function of vascular endothelium, *Adv. Prostaglandin Thromb. Leukotriene Res.* 17, 397, 1987.
104. Lüscher, T. F., *Endothelial Vasoactive Substances and Cardiovascular Disease,* S. Karger, Basel, 1988.
105. Yanagisawa, M., Kurihara, H., Kimura, S., Tomobe, Y., Kobayashi, M., Mitsui, Y., Yazaki, Y., Goto, K., and Masaki, T., A novel potent vasoconstrictor peptide produced by vascular endothelial cells, *Nature* (London), 332, 411, 1988.
106. Lüscher, T., Noll, G., and Wenzel, R.R., Systemic hypertension and related vascular diseases. Section A: Pathophysiology vascular causes and clinical manifestations and complications of hypertension, in *Vascular Pathology,* Stehbens, W.E. and Lie, J.T., Eds., Chapman & Hall Medical, London, 1995, 553.
107. Virag, L., Szabo, E., Baknodi, E., Bai, P., Gergey, P., Hunyadi, J., and Szabo, C., Nitric oxide-peroxynitric-poly (ADP-ribose) polymerase pathway in the skin, *Exp Dermatol,* 11, 189–202, 2002.
108. Nicosa, R.F., What is the role of vascular endothelial growth factor-related molecules in tumor angiogenesis? *Am. J. Pathol.,* 135, 11–16, 1998.
109. Ferguson, M.K. and DeFilippi, V.J., Nitric oxide and endothelium-dependent relaxation in tracheo-bronchial lymph vessels, *Microvasc. Res.,* 47, 308, 1994.
110. Preissner, K.T., Nawroth, P.P., and Kanse, S.M., Vascular protease receptors: integrating haemostasis and endothelial cell functions, *J. Pathol*., 190, 360, 2000.
111. Buonassisi, V. and Venter, J.C., Hormone and neurotransmitter receptor in an established vascular endothelial cell line, *Proc. Natl. Acad. Sci. U.S.A.,* 73, 1612, 1976.
112. Schafer, A.I., Gimbrone, M.A., and Handin, R.I., Regulation of endothelial cell function by cyclic nucleotides, in *Biology of Endothelial Cells,* Jaffe, E.A., Ed., Martinus Nijhoff, The Hague, 1984, 248.
113. Suzuki, T., Nakamura, Y., Moriya, T., and Sasano, H., Effects of steroid hormones on vascular functions, *Microsc. Res. Tech*., 60, 76, 2003.
114. Schweigerer, L., Neufeld, G., Friedman, J., Abraham, J.A., Fiddes, J.C., and Gospodarowicz, D., Capillary endothelial cells express basic fibroblast growth factor that promotes their own growth. *Nature* (London), 352, 257, 1987.

115. Vladavsky, L., Folkman, J., Sullivan, R., Friedman, R., Ishai-Michaeli, R., Sasse, J., and Klagsbrun, M., Endothelial cell-derived basic fibroblast growth factor: synthesis and deposition into subendothelial extracellular matrix, *Proc. Natl. Acad. Sci. U.S.A.,* 84, 2292, 1987.
116. Collins, T., Ginsburg, D., Boss, J.M., Orkin, S., and Pober, J.S., Cultured human endothelial cells express platelet-derived growth factor B chain: cDNA cloning and structural analysis, *Nature* (London), 316, 748, 1985.
117. Collins, T., Pober, J.S., Gimbrone, M.A., Jr., Hammacher, A., Betsholtz, C., Westermark, B., and Heldin, C.H., Cultured human endothelial cells express platelet-derived growth factor A chain, *Am. J. Pathol.,* 126, 7, 1987.
118. Sieff, C.A., Tsai, S., and Faller, D.V., Interleukin I induces cultured human endothelial cell production of granulocyte-macrophage colony-stimulating factor, *J. Clin. Invest.,* 79, 48, 1987.
119. Gajdusek, C., DiCorleto, P., Ross, R., and Schwartz, S.M., An endothelial cell-derived growth factor, *J. Cell. Biol.,* 85, 467, 1980.
120. Castellot, J.J., Addonizio, M.L., Rosenberg, R., and Karnovsky, M.J., Cultured endothelial cells produce a heparin-like inhibitor of smooth muscle cell growth, *J. Clin. Invest.,* 90, 372, 1981.
121. DiCorleto, P.E. and Bowen-Pope, D.F., Cultured endothelial cells produce a platelet-derived growth factor-like protein, *Proc. Natl. Acad. Sci. U.S.A.,* 80, 1919, 1983.
122. Alles, J.U. and Bosslet, K., Immunohistochemical and immunochemical characterization of a new endothelial cell specific antigen, *J. Histochem. Cytochem.,* 34, 209, 1986.
123. Fitzgerald, L.A., Charo, L.F., and Phillips, D.R., Human and bovine endothelial cells synthesize membrane proteins similar to human platelet glycoproteins IIb and IIIa, *J. Biol. Chem.,* 260, 10893, 1985.
124. Newman, P.J., Kawai, Y., Montgomery, R.R., and Kunicki, T.J., Synthesis by cultured human umbilical vein endothelial cells of two proteins structurally and immunologically related to platelet membrane glycoproteins IIb and IIIa, *J. Cell. Biol.,* 103, 81, 1986.
125. Suzuki, S., Scott Argraves, A., Arai, H., Languino, L.R., Pierschbacher, M.D., and Ruoslahti, E., Aminoacid sequence of the vitronectin receptor alpha subunit and comparative expression of the receptor mRNAs, *J. Biol. Chem.,* 262, 14080, 1987.
126. Fitzgerald, L., Poncz, M., Steiner, B., Rall, S.C., Jr., Bennett, J.S., and Phillips, D.R., Comparison of cDNA-derived protein sequences of the human fibronectin and vitronectin receptor alpha-subunits and platelet glycoprotein IIb, *Biochemistry,* 26, 8158, 1987.
127. Leeksma, O.C., Zandbergen-Spaargaren, J.C., Giltay, J.C., and van Mourik, J.A., Cultured human endothelial cells synthesize a plasma membrane protein complex immunologically related to the platelet glycoprotein IIb/IIIa complex, *Blood,* 67, 1176, 1986.
128. Kawai, Y., Newman, P.J., Furihata, K., Kunicki, T.J., and Montgomery, R.R., The $P1^{A1}$ alloantigen is expressed on human endothelial cells, *Clin. Res.,* 34, 460A, 1986.
129. Newman, P.J., Martin, L.S., Knipp, M.A., and Kahn, R.A., Studies on the nature of the human platelet alloantigen, $P1^{A1}$ localization to a 17,000 dalton polypeptide, *Mol. Immunol.,* 22, 719, 1985.
130. Kuroda, K., Sapadin, A., Shoji, T., Fleischmajer, R., and Lebwohl, M., Altered expression of angiopoietins and Tie2 endothelium receptor in psoriasis, *J. Invest. Dermatol.,* 116, 713, 2001.
131. Junod, A.J., Uptake, metabolism and reflux of $^{14}$C-5 hydroxytryptamine in isolated perfused rat lungs, *J. Pharmacol. Exp. Ther.,* 183, 341, 1972.
132. Junod, A.J. and Ody, C., Amine uptake and metabolism by endothelium of pig pulmonary artery and aorta, *Am. J. Physiol.,* 232, C88, 1977.
133. Anderson, M.W. and Eling, T.E., Prostaglandin removal and metabolism by isolated perfused rat lung, *Prostaglandins,* 11, 645, 1976.
134. Bruns, R.R. and Palade, G.E., Studies on blood capillaries. II. Transport of ferritin molecules across the wall of muscle capillaries, *J. Cell. Biol.,* 37, 277, 1968.
135. Palade, G.E., The microvascular endothelium revisited, in *Endothelial Cell Biology in Health and Disease,* Simionescu, N. and Simionescu, M., Eds., Plenum Press, New York, 1988, 3.
136. Widmann, J.-J., Cotran, R.S., and Fahimi, H.D., Mononuclear phagocytes (Kupffer cells) and endothelial cells, *J. Cell. Biol.,* 52, 159, 1972.
137. Wagner, R.C., Andrews, S.B., and Matthews, M.A., A fluorescent assay for micropinocytosis in isolated capillary endothelium, *Microvasc. Res.,* 14, 67, 1977.
138. Shimamoto, T., Hidaka, H., Moriya, K., Kobayashi, M., Takahashi, T., and Numano, F., Hyperactive arterial endothelial cells: a clue for the treatment of arteriosclerosis, *Ann. N.Y. Acad. Sci.,* 275, 266, 1976.

139. Cho, Y. and De Bruyn, P.H., Destruction of circulating leukemia cells by phagocytosis in rats with myelogenous leukemia, *J. Natl. Cancer Inst.,* 60, 185, 1978.
140. Simionescu, M., Receptor-mediated transcytosis of plasma molecules by vascular endothelium, in *Endothelial Cell Biology in Health and Disease,* Simionescu, N. and Simionescu, M., Eds., Plenum Press, New York, 1988, 69.
141. Del Mar Yllera, M., Alexandre-Pires, G.M., and Cifuentes, J.M., Placenta: regularization of neovascularization. Microvascularization pattern of the rabbit term placenta. *Microsc. Res. Tech.,* 60, 38, 2003.
142. Suhardja, A. and Hoffman, H., Role of growth factors and their receptors in proliferation of microvascular endothelial cells. *Microsc. Res. Tech.*, 60, 70, 2003.
143. Balconi, G., Spagnuolo, R., and Dejana, E., Development of endothelial cell lines from embryonic stem cells. A tool for studying genetically manipulated endothelial cells *in vitro, Arterioscler. Thromb. Vasc. Biol.*, 20, 1443, 2000.
144. Riha, M., Kreisel, D., Krupnick, A.S., Balsara, K.R., and Rosengard, B.R., Immunology properties of rat vascular endothelium, *J. Heart Lung Transplant.,* 22, S107, 2001.
145. Burger, D.R., Vettp, R., Hamblin, A., and Dumonde, D.C., T-lymphocyte activation by antigen presented by HLA-DR compatible endothelial cells, in *Pathobiology of the Endothelial Cells,* Nossel, H.L. and Vogel, H.J., Eds., Academic Press, New York, 1982, 387.
146. Shingu, M., Hashimoto, Y., Johnson, A.R., and Hurd, E.R., The search for Fc receptors on human tissues and human endothelial cells in culture (41140), *Proc. Soc. Exp. Biol. Med.,* 167, 147, 1981.
147. Bjerke, J.R., Livden, J.K., and Matre, R., Fc gamma-receptors and HLA-DR antigen on endothelial cells in psoriasis skin lesions, *Acta Derm. Venereol.* (Stockholm), 68, 306, 1988.
148. Ekert, P.G. and Vaux, D.L., Apoptosis and the immune system, *Br. Med. Bull.*, 53, 591, 1997.
149. Vidal, S., Horvath, E., Kovacs, K., Scheithauer, B.W., Lloyd, R.V., and Kontogeorgos, G., Ultrastructural features of apoptosis in human pituitary adenomas, *Ultrastruct. Pathol.*, 25, 85, 2001.
150. Kothakota, S., Azuma, T., Reinhard, C., Klippel, A., Tang, J., Chu, K., McGarry, T.J., Kirschner, M.W., Koths, K., Kwiatkowski, D.J., and Williams, L.T., Caspase-3-generated fragment of gelsolin: effector of morphological change in apoptosis, *Science,* 278, 294, 1997.
151. Maruyama, W., Irie, S., and Sato, T.A., Morphological changes in the nucleus and actin cytoskeleton in the process of Fas-induced apoptosis in Jurkat T cells, *Histochem. J.,* 32, 495, 2000.
152. Liu, W., Ahmad, S.A., Reinmuth, N., Shaheen, R.M., Jung, Y.D., Fan, F., and Ellis, L.M., Endothelial cell survival and apoptosis in the tumor vasculature, *Apoptosis.*, 5, 323, 2000.
153. Jekunen, A. and Kairemo, K., Inhibition of angiogenesis at endothelial cell level, *Microsc. Res. Tech.*, 60, 85, 2003.
154. Folkman, J., Tumor angiogenesis: therapeutic implications, *N. Engl. J. Med.,* 285, 1182, 1971.
155. Clapp, C., Lopez-Gomes, F.J., Nava, G., Corbacho, A., Toner, I., Macotela, Y., Duenas, Z., and Martinez de la Escalera, G., Expression of prolactin mRNA and prolactin-like proteins in endothelial cells: evidence for autocrine effects, *J. Endocrinol.*, 158, 137, 1998.
156. Kontogeorgos, G. and Kontogeorgou, C.N., Hormone regulation of endothelial apoptosis and proliferation in vessel regression and angiogenesis, *Microsc. Res. Tech.* 60, 59, 2003.
157. Folkman, J., Angiogenesis in cancer, vascular, rheumatoid and other disease, *Nat. Med.,* 1, 27, 1995.
158. Kwak, H.J., So, J.-N., Lee, S.J., Kim, I., and Koh, G.Y., Angiogenesis-1 is an apoptosis survival factor for endothelial cells, *FEBS Lett.,* 448, 249, 1999.
159. Benjamin, L.E., Hemo, I., and Kesher, E., A plasticity window for blood vessel remodeling is defined by pericyte coverage of the preformed endothelial network and is regulated by PDGF-B and VEGF, *Development*, 125, 1591, 1998.
160. Velasco, P. and Lange-Asschenfeldt, B., Dermatological aspects of angiogenesis, *Br. J. Dermatol.*, 147, 841, 2002.
161. Zatterstrom, U.K., Felbor, U., Fukai, N., and Olsen, B.R., Collagen XVIII/endostatin structure and functional role in angiogenesis, *Cell Struct. Funct.*, 25, 97, 2000.
162. Kerckhaert, O.A.J. and Voest, E.E., The prognostic and diagnostic value of circulating angiogenic factors in cancer patients, in *Tumor Angiogenesis and Microcirculation*, Voest, E.E. and D'Amore, P.A., Eds., Marcel Dekker, New York, 2001, 487.
163. Thorgeirsson, G. and Robertson, A.L. Jr., The vascular endothelium — pathologic significance. A review, *Am. J. Pathol.,* 93, 803, 1978.

164. Rosenberg, J.C., Hawkins, E., and Rector, F., Mechanism of immunological injury during antibody-mediated hyperacute rejection of renal heterografts, *Transplantation,* 11, 151, 1971.
165. Stemerman, M., Spact, T.H., Pitlick, F., Cintron, J., Lejnicks, L., and Tiell, M.L., Intimal healing: The pattern of re-endothelialization and intimal thickening, *Am. J. Pathol.,* 87, 125, 1977.
166. Stehbens, W.E., Hemodynamic production of lipid deposition, intimal tears, mural dissection and thrombosis of blood vessel walls, *Proc. R. Soc. London Ser. B.,*185, 357, 1976.
167. Ross, R. and Harker, L., Hyperlipidemia and atherosclerosis: chronic hyperlipidemia initiates and maintains lesions by endothelial cell desquamation and lipid accumulation, *Science,* 193, 1094, 1976.
168. Wall, R.T., Harlan, J.M., Harker, L.A., and Striker, G.E., Homocysteine-induced endothelial cell injury *in vitro.* A model for the study of vascular injury, *Thromb. Res.,* 18, 113, 1980.
169. Higman, D.J., Powell, J.T., and Greenhalgh, R.M., Smoking and vascular disease, in *Current Therapy in Vascular Surgery,* 3rd ed., Ernst, C.B. and Stanley, J.C., Eds., Mosby, St. Louis, 1995, 333.
170. Bull, H.A., Pittila, R.M., Woolf, N., and Machin, S.J., The effect of nicotine on human endothelial cell release of prostaglandins and ultrastructure, *Br. J. Exp. Pathol.,* 69, 413, 1988.
171. Verma, A., Davis, G.E., and Ihler, G.M., Formation of stress fibers in human endothelial cells infected with *Bartonella bacilliformis* is associated with altered morphology, impaired migration and defects in cell morphogenesis, *Cell. Microbiol.*, 3, 169, 2001.
172. Friedman, H.M., Viral infection of endothelium and the induction of Fc and C3 receptors, in *Biology of Endothelial Cells,* Jaffe, E.A., Ed., Martinus Nijhoff, The Hague, 1984, 268.
173. Braithwaite, A.W. and Russel, I.A., Induction of cell death by adenoviruses, *Apoptosis*, 6, 359, 2001.
174. Ryan, U.S., Schultz, D.R., and Ryan, J.W., Fc and C3b receptors on pulmonary endothelial cells, induction by injury, *Science,* 214, 557, 1981.
175. Cines, D.B., Lyss, A.P., Bina, M., Corkey, R., Kefalides, N.A. and Friedman, H.M., Fc and C3 receptors induced by herpes simplex virus on cultured human endothelial cells, *J. Clin. Invest.,* 69, 123, 1982.
176. Colucci, M., Balcon, G.I., Lorenzet, R., Pietra, A., Locati, D., Donati, M.B., and Semeraro, N., Cultured human endothelial cells generate tissue factor in response to endotoxin, *J. Clin. Invest.,* 71, 1893, 1983.
177. Bevilacqua, M.P., Pober, J.S., Majeau, G.R., Cotran, R.S., and Gimbrone, M.A., Jr., Interleukin-1 (IL-1) induces biosynthesis and cell surface expression of procoagulant activity in human vascular endothelial cells, *J. Exp. Med.,*160, 618, 1984.
178. Bevilacqua, M.P., Pober, J.S., Majeau, G.R., Fiers, W., Cotran, R.S., and Gimbrone, M.A., Jr., Recombinant tumor necrosis factor induces procoagulant activity in cultured human vascular endothelium. Characterization and comparison with the actions of interleukin-1, *Proc. Natl. Acad. Sci. USA.,* 83, 4533, 1986.
179. Vos, I.H. and Briscoe, D.M., Endothelial injury: cause and effect of alloimmune inflammation, *Transplant. Infect. Dis.*, 4, 152, 2002.
180. Libby, P. and Birinyi, L.K., The dynamic nature of vascular endothelial functions, in *Endothelialization of Vascular Grafts*, Zilla, P.P., Fasol, R.D., and Deutsch, M., Eds., Karger, New York, 1987, 80–99.
181. Heltianu, C., Simionescu, M., and Simionescu, N., Histidine receptors of the microvascular endothelium revealed in situ with a histamine-ferritin conjugat: characteristic high-affinity binding sites in venules, *J. Cell. Biol.,* 93, 357, 1982.
182. Cotran, R.S. and Remensynder, J.P., The structural basis of increased vascular permeability after graded thermal injury: light and electron microscopic studies, *Ann. N.Y. Acad. Sci.,* 150, 495, 1968.
183. Cotran, R.S. and Majno, G., A light and electron microscopic analysis of vascular injury, *Ann. N.Y. Acad. Sci.,* 116, 750, 1964.
184. Barnhart, M.I. and Baechler, C.A., Endothelial cell physiology, perturbations and responses, *Semin. Thromb. Hemost.,* 5, 50, 1978.
185. Phillips, P.G., Higgins, P.J., Malik, A.B., and Tsan, M.-F., Effect of hypoxia on the cytoarchitecture of cultured endothelial cells, *Am. J. Pathol.,* 132, 59, 1988.
186. Davies, P., Flow-mediated endothelial mechanotransduction, *Physiol. Rev.,* 75, 519, 1995.
187. Malek, A.M. and Izumo, S., Control of endothelial cell gene expression by flow, *J. Biomech.,* 28, 1515, 1995.
188. Willms-Kretschmer, K., Flax, M.H., and Cotran, R.S., The fine structure of the vascular response in hapten-specific delayed hypersensitivity and contact dermatitis, *Lab. Invest.,* 17, 334, 1967.
189. Cotran, R.S., New roles for the endothelium in inflammation and immunity, *Am. J. Pathol.* 129, 407, 1987.

190. Wallis, W.J. and Harlan, J.M., Effector functions of endothelium in inflammatory and immunologic reactions, *Pathol. Immunopathol. Res.*, 5, 73, 1986.
191. Cotran, R.S. and Pober, J.S., Endothelial activation: its role in inflammatory and immune reactions, in *Endothelial Cell Biology in Health and Disease,* Simionescu, N. and Simionescu, M., Eds., Plenum Press, New York, 1988, 335.
192. Pober, J.S., Cytokine-mediated activation of vascular endothelium — physiology and pathology, *Am. J. Pathol.,* 133, 426, 1988.
193. Kennedy, G., Khan, F., McLaren, M., and Belch, J.J., Endothelial activation and response in patient with hand arm vibration syndrome, *Eur. J. Clin. Invest.*, 29, 577, 1999.
194. de Assis, M.C., Da Costa, A.O., Barja-Fidalgo, T.C., and Plotkowski, M.C., Human endothelial cells are activated by interferon-γ plus tumour necrosis factor-α to kill intracellular *Pseudomonas aeruginosa, Immunology.* 101, 271, 2000.
195. Kunkel, S.L., Standiford, T.J., Chensue, S.W., Strieter, R.M., and Westwick, J., Interleukin-8 and the inflammatory response, in *Cytokine in Health and Disease,* Kunkel, S.L. and Resnick, D.G., Eds., Marcel Dekker, New York, 1992, 121.
196. Pober, J.S. and Cotran, R.S., Cytokines and endothelial cell biology, *Physiol. Rev.,* 70, 427, 1990.
197. Berg, E.L., McEvoy, L.M., Berlin, C., Bargatze, R.F., and Butcher, E.C., L-selectin-mediated lymphocyte rolling on MAdCAM-1, *Nature*, 366, 695, 1993.
198. Bevilacqua, M.P., Endothelial-leukocyte adhesion molecules, *Annu. Rev. Immunol.* 11, 767, 1993.
199. Dustin, M.L., Rothlein, R., Bhan, A.K., Dinarello, C.A., and Springer, T.A., Induction by IL-1 and interferon, tissue distribution, biochemistry and function of a natural adherence molecule (ICAM-l), *J. Immunol.*, 137, 245, 1986.
200. Albelda, S.M., Smith, C.W., and Ward, P.A., Adhesion molecules and inflammatory injury, *FASEB J.*, 8, 504, 1994.
201. Butthep, P., Rummavas, S., Wisedpanichkij, R., Jindadamrongwech, S., Fucharoen, S., and Bunyaratvej, A., Increased circulating activated endothelial cells, vascular endothelial growth factor, and tumor necrosis factor in thalassemia., *Am. J. Hematol.*, 70, 100, 2002.
202. Cid, M.C., Cebrián, M., Font, C., Coll-Vinent, B., Hernández-Rodríguez, J., Esparza, J., Urbano-Márquez, A., and Grau, J.M., Cell adhesion molecules in the development of inflammatory infiltrates in giant cell arteritis: inflammation-induced angiogenesis as the preferential site of leukocyte-endothelial cell interactions, *Arthritis Rheum.,* 43, 184, 2000.
203. Borroni, B., Volpi, R., and Martini, G., Peripheral blood abnormalities in Alzheimer disease: evidence for early endothelial dysfunction, *Alzheimer Dis. Assoc. Disord.,* 16, 150, 2002.
204. Petzelbauer, P., Pober, J.S., Keh, A., and Braverman, I.M., Inducibility and expression of microvascular endothelial adhesion molecules in lesional, perilesional, and uninvolved skin of psoriatic patients, *J. Invest. Dermatol.*, 103, 300, 1994.
205. Campbell, J.J. and Butcher, E.C., Chemokines in tissue-specific and microenvironment-specific lymphocyte homing, *Curr. Opin. Immunol.*, 12, 336, 2000.
206. Clesca, P.T., Endothelial cells and acute rejection in organ transplantation: a review with emphasis on adhesion molecules, *Int. Cong. Ser.,* 1237, 181, 2002.
207. Pober, J.S. and Cotran, R.S., Cytokines and endothelial cell biology, *Physiol. Rev.,* 76, 427, 1990.
208. Grunebaum, E., Blank, M., Cohen, S., Afek, A., Kopolovic, J., Meroni, P.L., Youinou, P., and Shoenfeld, Y, The role of anti-endothelial cell antibodies in Kawasaki disease — *in vitro* and *in vivo* studies, *Clin. Exp. Immunol.,* 130, 233, 2002.
209. Montgomery, E.A. and Fetsch, J.F., Tumors and tumefactions of peripheral vessels, in *Vascular Pathology,* Stehbens, W.E. and Lie, J.T., Eds., Chapman & Hall Medical, London, 1995, 739.
210. Page, C., Rose, M., Yacoub, M., and Pigott, R., Antigenic heterogeneity of vascular endothelium, *Am. J. Pathol.*, 141, 673, 1992.
211. Epperson, D.E. and Pober, J.S., Antigen-presenting function of human endothelial cells. Direct activation of resting CD8 T cells, *J. Immunol.*, 153, 5402, 1994.
212. Pober, J.S., Collins, T., Gimbrone, M.A., Jr., Cotran, R.S., Gittin, J.D., Friers, W., Clayberger, C., Krensky, A.M., Burakoff, S.J., and Reiss, C.S., Lymphocytes recognize human vascular endothelial and dermal fibroblast Ia antigens induced by recombinant immune interferon, *Nature*, 305, 726, 1983.
213. Ma, W. and Pober, J.S., Human endothelial cells effectively costimulate cytokine production by, but not differentiation of, naïve $CD4^+$ T cells, *J. Immunol.*, 161, 2158, 1998.

214. Murray, A.G., Libby, P., and Pober, J.S., Human vascular smooth muscle cells poorly co-stimulate and actively inhibit allogeneic CD4+ T cell proliferation *in vitro, J. Immunol.,* 154, 151, 1995.
215. Thompson, C.B., Apoptosis in the pathogenesis and treatment of disease, *Science*, 267, 1456, 1995.
216. Grassmé, H., Jendrossek, V., and Gulbins, E., Molecular mechanisms of bacteria induced apoptosis, *Apoptosis*, 6, 441, 2001.
217. Takahashi, A., Caspase: executioner and undertaker of apoptosis, *Int. J. Hematol.,* 70, 226, 1999.
218. Bordron, A., Revelen, R., D'Arbonneau, F., Dueymes, M., Renaudineau, Y., Jamin, C., and Youinou, P., Functional heterogeneity of anti-endothelial cell antibodies, *Clin. Exp. Immunol*., 124, 492, 2001.
219. Carvalho, D., Savage, C.O., Black, C.M., and Pearson, J.D., IgG antiendothelial cell autoantibodies from scleroderma patients induce leukocyte adhesion to human vascular endothelial cells *in vitro.* Induction of adhesion molecule expression and involvement of endothelium-derived cytokines, *J. Clin. Invest.,* 97, 111, 1996.
220. Walsh, K. and Sata, M., Is extravasation a Fas-regulated process? *Mol. Med. Today*, 5, 61, 1999.
221. Esen, M., Schreiner, B., Jendrossek, V., Lang, F., Fassbender, K., Grassmé, H., and Gulbins, E., Mechanisms of *Staphylococcus aureus* induced apoptosis of human endothelial cells, *Apoptosis*, 6, 431, 2001.
222. Mercie, P., Garnier, O., Lascoste, L., Renard, M., Closse, C., Durrieu, F., Marit, G., Boisseau, R.M., and Belloc, F., Homocysteine-thiolactone induces caspase-independent vascular endothelial cell death with apoptotic features, *Apoptosis*, 5, 403, 2000.
223. Brunelle, J.K. and Chandel, N.S., Oxygen deprivation induced cell death: an update, *Apoptosis*, 7, 475, 2002.
224. Mold, C. and Morris, C.A., Complement activation by apoptotic endothelial cells following hypoxia/reoxygenation, *Immunology*, 102, 356, 2001.
225. Ganguly, B.J., Tonomura, N., Osborne, B.A., and Granowith, E.V., Hyperbaric oxygen enhances apoptosis in hematopoietic cells, *Apoptosis*, 7, 499, 2002.
226. Zhou, L., Dosanjh, A., Chen, H., and Karasek, M., Divergent effects of extracellular oxygen on the growth, morphology, and function of human skin microvascular endothelial cells, *J. Cell. Physiol*., 182, 134, 2000.
227. Clauss, M. and Schaper, W., Vascular endothelial growth factor. A Jack-of-all-trades or nonspecific stress gene? *Circ. Res*., 86, 251, 2000.
228. Shima, D.T., Deutsch, U., and D'Amore, P.A., Hypoxic induction of vascular endothelial growth factor (VEGF) in human epithelial cells is mediated by increases in mRNA stability, *FEBS Lett*., 370, 203, 1995.
229. Fukumura, D., Xu, L., Chen, Y., Gohongi, T., Seed, B., and Jain, R.K., Hypoxia and acidosis independently up-regulate vascular endothelial growth factor transcription in brain tumors *in vivo*, *Cancer Res*., 61, 6020, 2001.
230. Vidal, S., Horvath, E., Kovacs, K., Scheithauer, B.W., and Lloyd, R.V., Morphologic approaches to the assessment of angiogenesis, *Microsc. Anal.* (The Americas), 57, 9, 2002.
231. Detmar, M., Brown, L. F., Berse, B., Jackman, R.W., Elicker, B. M., Dvorak, H. F., and Claffey, K. P., Hypoxia regulates the expression of vascular permeability factor/vascular endothelial growth factor (VPF/VEGF) and its receptors in human skin, *J. Invest. Dermatol*., 108, 263, 1997.
232. Gleadle, J.M., Ebert, B.L., Firth, J.D., and Ratckliffe, P.J., Regulation of angiogenic growth factor expression by hypoxia, transition metals, and chelating agents, *Am. J. Physiol*., 268, C1362, 1995.
233. Kourembanas, S., Hannan, R.L., and Faller, D.V., Oxygen tension regulates the expression on the platelet-derived growth factor-B chain gene in human endothelial cells, *J. Clin. Invest*., 86, 670, 1990.
234. Wagner, A.J., Kokontis, J.M., and Hay, N., Myc-mediated apoptosis requires wild-type p53 in a manner independent of cell cycle arrest and the ability of p53 to induce p21 wafl/cipl, *Genes. Dev.,* 8, 2817, 1994.
235. Lorenz, H.-M., Role of apoptosis in autoimmunity, *Apoptosis*, 5, 443, 2000.
236. Feinmesser, M., Tsabari, C., Fichman, S., Hodak, E., Sulkes, J., and Okon, E., Differential expression of proliferation- and apoptosis-related markers in lentigo maligna and solar keratosis keratinocytes, *Am. J. Dermatopathol.,* 25, 300, 2003.
237. Maxwell, S.A., Acosta, S.A., Tombusch, K., and Davis, G.E., Expression of Bax, Bcl-2, Waf-1, and PCNA gene productions in an immortalized human endothelial cell line undergoing p53-mediated apoptosis, *Apoptosis*, 2, 442, 1997.

238. Maxwell, S.A., Acosta, S.A., and Davis, G.E., Induction and alternative splicing of the Bax gene mediated by p53 in a transformed endothelial cell line, *Apoptosis,* 4, 109, 1999.
239. Garlanda, C. and Dejana, E., Heterogeneity of endothelial cells. Specific markers. *Arterioscler. Throm. Vasc. Biol.,* 17, 1193, 1997.
240. Tan, S.T., Velickovic, M., Ruger, B.M., and Davis, P.F., Cellular and extracellular markers of hemangioma, *Plast. Reconstr. Surg.*, 106, 529, 2000.
241. Murray, A.B., Weibel–Palade bodies are not reliable ultrastructural markers for mouse endothelial cells, *Lab. Anim. Sci.,* 37, 483, 1987.
242. Skobe, M. and Detmar, M., Structure, function, and molecular control of the skin lymphatic system, *J. Invest. Dermatol. Symp. Proc.*, 5, 14, 2000.
243. Nibbs, R.J., Kriehuber, E., Ponath, P.D., Parent, D., Qin, S., Campbell, J.D.M., Henderson, A., Kerjaschki, D., Maurer, D., Graham, G.J., and Rit, A., The beta-chemokine receptor D6 is expressed by lymphatic endothelium and a subset of vascular tumors, *Am. J. Pathol.*, 158, 867, 2001.
244. Vinter, D.W., Factor VIII and the vascular endothelium, *Diss. Abstr. Int.,* 44-10B, 2962, 1983.
245. Kumar, S., West, D.C., and Ager, A., Heterogeneity in endothelial cells from large vessels and microvessels, *Differentiation*, 36, 57, 1987.
246. Turner, R.R., Beckstead, J.H., Warnke, R.A., and Wood, G.A., Endothelial cell phenotypic diversity. *In situ* demonstration of immunologic and enzymatic heterogeneity that correlates with specific morphologic subtypes, *Am. J. Clin. Pathol.,* 87, 569, 1985.
247. Burgdorf, W.C., Mukai, K., and Rosai, J., Immunohistochemical identification of Factor VIII-related antigen in endothelial cells of cutaneous lesions of alleged vascular nature, *Am. J. Clin. Pathol.,* 75, 167, 1981.
248. Okada, E., Tamura, A., Ishikawa, O., and Miyachi, Y., Tufted angioma (angioblastoma): case report and review of 41 cases in the Japanese literature, *Clin. Exp. Dermatol.,* 25, 627, 2000.
249. Wilson Jones, E. and Orkin, M., Tufted angioma (angioblastoma): a benign progressive angioma not to be confused with Kaposi's sarcoma or low-grade angiosarcoma, *J. Am. Acad. Dermatol.,* 20, 214, 1989.
250. Parums, D.V., Histochemistry and immunochemistry of vascular disease, in *Vascular Pathology,* Stehbens, W.E. and Lie, J.T., Eds., Chapman & Hall Medical, London, 1995, 313.
251. Scully, P.A., Steinman, H.K., Kennedy, C., Trueblood, K., Frisman, D.M., and Voland, J.R., AIDS-related Kaposi's sarcoma displays differential expression of endothelial surface antigens, *Am. J. Pathol.,* 130, 244, 1988.
252. Rutgers, J.L., Wieczorek, R., Bonetti, F., Kaplan, K.L., Posnett, D.N., Friedman-Kien, A.E., and Knowles II, D.M., The expression of endothelial cell surface antigens by AIDS-associated Kaposi's sarcoma: evidence for a vascular endothelial cell origin, *Am. J. Pathol.,* 122, 493, 1986.
253. Cohen, P.R., Rapini, R.P., and Farhood, A.I., Expression of the human hematopoietic progenitor cell antigen CD34 in dermatofibrosarcoma protuberans, other spindle cell tumors, and vascular lesions, *J. Am. Acad. Dermatol.,* 30, 147, 1994.
254. Satter, E.K., Graham, B.S., and Gibbs, N.F., Congenital tufted angioma, *Ped. Dermatol.,* 19, 445, 2002.
255. Dignat-Gorge, F. and Sampol, J., Circulating endothelial cells in vascular disorders: new insights into an old concept, *Eur. J. Haematol.*, 65, 215, 2000.
256. Kraling, B.M., Razon, M.J., Boon, L.M., Zurakowski, D., Seachord, C., Darveau, R.P., Mulliken, J.B., Corless, C.L., and Bischoff, J., E-selectin is present in proliferating endothelial cells in human hemangiomas, *Am. J. Pathol.*, 148, 1181, 1996.
257. Bell, C.D., Endothelial cell tumors, *Microsc. Res. Tech.*, 60, 165, 2003.
258. Takahashi, K., Mulliken, J.B., Kozakewich, H.P., Rogers, R.A., Folkman, J., and Ezekowitz, R.A., Cellular markers that distinguish the phases of hemangioma during infancy and childhood, *J. Clin. Invest.*, 93, 2357, 1994.
259. North, P.E., Waner, M., Mizeracki, A., and Mihm, M.C., GLUT1: a newly discovered immunohistochemical marker for juvenile hemangiomas, *Hum. Pathol.,* 31, 11, 2000.
260. North, P.E., Waner, M., Mizeracki, A., Mrak, R.E., Nicholas, R., Kincannon, J., Suen, J.Y., and Mihm, M.C., A unique microvascular phenotype shared by juvenile hemangiomas and human placenta, *Arch. Dermatol.,* 137, 559, 2001.

261. Weber, E., Lorenzoni, P., Lozzi, G., and Sacchi, G., Cytochemical differentiation between blood and lymphatic endothelium: bovine blood and lymphatic large vessels and endothelial cells in culture, *J. Histochem. Cytochem.*, 42, 1109, 1994.
262. Ryan, U.S., Ryan, J.W., Whitaker, C., and Chiu, A., Localization of angiotensin converting enzyme (kininase II). II. Immunocytochemistry and immunofluorescence, *Tissue Cell.*, 8, 125, 1976.
263. Auerbach, R., Alby, L., Grieves, J., Joseph, J., Lindgren, C., Morrissey, L.W., Sidky, Y.A., Tu, M., and Watt, S.L., Monoclonal antibody against angiotensin-convertin enzyme: its use as a marker for murine, bovine and human endothelial cells, *Proc. Natl. Acad. Sci. U.S.A.*, 79, 7891, 1982.
264. Kaipainen, A., Korhonen, J., Mustonen, T., van Hinsbergh, W., Fang, G.H., Dumont, D., Breitman, M., and Alitalo, K., Expression of the fms-like tyrosine kinase 4 gene becomes restricted to lymphatic endothelium during development, *Proc. Natl. Acad. Sci. U.S.A.*, 92, 3566, 1995.
265. Galland, F., Karamysheva, A., Mattei, M.-G., Rosnet, O., Marchetto, S., and Birnbaum, D., Chromosomal localization of FLT4, a novel receptor-type tyrosine kinase gene, *Genomics*, 13, 475, 1992.
266. Hamada, K., Oike, Y., Takakura, N., Ito, Y., Jussila, L., Dumont, D.J., Alitalo, K., and Suda, T., VEGF-C signaling pathway through VEGFR-2 and VEGFR-3 in vasculoangiogenesis and hematopoiesis, *Blood*, 96, 3793, 2000.
267. Achen, M., Jeltsch, M., Kukk, E., Mäkinen, T., Vitali, A, Wilks, A.F., Alitalo, K., and Stacker, S.A., Vascular endothelial growth factor D (VEGF-D) is a ligand for the tyrosinase kinases VEGF receptor 2 (Flk1) and VEGF receptor 3 (Flt4), *Proc. Natl. Acad. Sci. U.S.A.*, 95, 548, 1998.
268. Mäkinen, T., Veikkola, T., Mustjoki, S., Karpanen, T., Catimel, B., Nice, E.C., Wise, L., Mercer, A., Kowalski, H., Kerjaschki, D., Stacker, S.A., Achen, M.G., and Alitalo, K., Isolated lymphatic endothelial cells transducer growth, survival and migratory signals via the VEGF-C/D receptor VEGFR-3, *EMBO J.*, 20, 4762, 2001.
269. Partanen, T.A., Arola, J., Saaristo, A., Jussila, L., Ora, A., Miettinen, M., Stacker, S.A., Achen, M.G., and Alitalo, K., VEGF-C and VEGF-D expression in neuroendocrine cells and their receptor, VEGFR-3, in fenestrated blood vessel in human tissues, *FASEB J.*, 14, 2087, 2000.
270. Valtola, R., Salven, P., Heikkila, P. et al., VEGFR-3 and its ligand VEGF-C are associated with angiogenesis in breast cancer, *Am. J. Pathol.*, 154, 1381, 1999.
271. Breiteneder-Geleff, S., Matsui, K., Soleiman, A., Kowalski, H., Horvat, R., Amann, G., Krichuber, E., Diem, K., Weninger, W., Tschachler, E., Alitalo, K., and Kerjaschki, D., Podoplanin, novel 43-kD membrane protein of glomerular epithelial cells, is down-regulated in puromycin nephrosis, *Am. J. Pathol.*, 151, 1141, 1997.
272. Breiteneder-Geleff, S., Soleiman, A., Kowalski, H., Hovart, R., Amann, G., Kriehuber, E., Diem, K., Weninger, W., Tschachler, E., Alitalo, K., and Keerjaschki, D., Angiosarcomas express mixed endothelial phenotypes of blood and lymphatic capillaries: podoplanin as a specific marker for lymphatic endothelium, *Am. J. Pathol.*, 154, 385, 1999.
273. Reis-Filho, J.S. and Schmitt, F.C., Lymphangiogenesis in tumors: what do we know? *Microsc. Res. Tech.*, 60, 171, 2003.
274. Banerji, S., Ni, J., Wang, S.X., Clasper, S., Su, J., Tammi, R., Jones, M., and Jackson, D.G., LYVE-1, a new homologue of the CD44 glycoprotein, is a lymph-specific receptor for hyaluronan, *J. Cell. Biol.*, 144, 789, 1999.
275. Karkkainen, M.J. and Alitalo, K., Lymphatic endothelial regulation, lymphedema, and lymph node metastasis, *Semin. Cell. Dev. Biol.*, 13, 9, 2002.
276. Karkkainen, M., Saaristo, A., Jussila, L., Karila, K., Lawrence, E.C., Pajusola, K., Bueler, H., Eichmann, A., Kauppinen, R., Kettunen, M.I., Yia-Herttuaja, S., Fenegorld, D.N., Ferrell, R.E., and Alitalo, K., A model for gene therapy of human hereditary lymphedema, *Proc. Natl. Acad. Sci. U.S.A.*, 98, 12677, 2001.
277. Wilting, J., Papoutsi, M., Christ, B., Nicolaides, K.H., von Keisenberg, C.S., Borges, J., Stark, G-B., Alitalo, K., Tomarev, S.I., Niemeyer, C., and Rössler, J., The transcription factor Prox1 is a marker for lymphatic endothelial cells in normal and diseased human tissues, *FASEB J.*, 16, 1271, 2002.
278. Lubeseder-Martellato, C., Guenzi, E., Jörg, A., Töpolt, K., Naschberger, E., Kremmer, E., Zietz, C., Tschachler, E., Hutzler, P., Schwemmle, M., Matzen, K., Grimm, T., Ensoli, B., and Stürzl, M., Guanylate-binding protein-1 expression is selectively induced by inflammatory cytokines and is an activation marker of endothelial cells during inflammatory diseases, *Am. J. Pathol.*, 161, 1749, 2002.

279. Kuhn, A., Brachtendorf, G., Kurth, F., Sonntag, M., Samulowitz, U., Metze, D., and Vestweber, D., Expression of endomucin, a novel endothelial sialomucin, in normal and diseased human skin, *J. Invest. Dermatol.,* 119, 1388, 2002.
280. Ran, S.D., Downes, A., and Thorpe, P.E., Increased exposure of anionic phospholipids on the surface of tumor blood vessels, *Cancer Res.,* 62, 6132, 2002.

# 10 Mast Cells

*Maurice W. van der Heijden, Hanneke P.M. van der Kleij, Martin Röcken, and Frank A. Redegeld*

## CONTENTS



## I. INTRODUCTION

Mast cells are granular cells widely distributed in tissues of many species including humans.[1,2] They are important effector cells in allergic diseases, but also in other immunologic and nonimmunologic disorders.[3–6] Mast cell activation can be induced by various ways both antigen-specific

0-8493-1959-5/05/$0.00+$1.50

and nonspecific and results in release of a plethora of mediators with, e.g., vasoactive, constrictive, proteolytic, and inflammatory activity. By means of these mediators, mast cells participate in a wide variety of physiological and pathophysiological events in the body.

Much of our present knowledge on mast cell activation and its (patho)physiological role has been obtained using mast cell cultures (primary cultures and stable lines) and animal models. Therefore, the first part of this chapter deals with mast cells in general rather than with the human skin mast cell in particular.

## II. MORPHOLOGY AND HETEROGENEITY

Mast cells are found in nearly all vascularized tissues such as the skin, thymus, lymphoid tissue, tongue, synovia, urogenital tract, and upper and lower respiratory airways, and in the serosal and submucosal layers of the gastrointestinal tract[1,2,7] Mast cells reside mostly in loose connective tissue compartments surrounding blood vessels, nerves, and glandular ducts and in epithelial, serous, and synovial membranes. In the skin, approximately 10,000 mast cells/mm$^3$ can be found mainly near blood vessels, hair follicles, and sebaceous and sweat glands.[8] Histologically, mast cells appear as rounded, ovoid, or elongated, and in dermal fibers they can be spindle shaped, stellate or filiform.[2] Mast cells are about 10 to 30 μm in diameter. For example, rat peritoneal mast cells have a diameter of 12.6 to 13.5 μm.[2] The nucleus is relatively large, measuring 4 to 7 μm in diameter with varying amounts of chromatin. Mast cells are characterized by the presence of secretory granules in the cytoplasm. Typically, mature mast cells contain about 1000 granules with a diameter of 0.5 to 0.7 μm and an average volume of 0.3 μm$^3$.[9] In human mast cells, granules contain lattice and scroll-like structures. Granules stain metachromatically with basic dyes like toluidine blue and azure A, or alcian blue/safranin staining sequences. It was recognized that based on differences in fixation and dye binding properties different subpopulations of mast cells could be distinguished in rodents.[10] Two major subtypes were defined: (1) connective tissue mast cells (CTMC), present in the skin, serosal cavities, and intestinal submucosa containing heparin in their granules and (2) mucosal mast cells (MMC) lying in the epithelium of mucosal surfaces containing lower sulfated proteoglycans as chondroitin sulfate. It now appears that a subdivision between these subpopulations is not adequate, because many more phenotypes can be distinguished based on expression of granular mast cell proteases and differences in functionality (e.g., mediator content, mediator production and differences in response to mast cell activators).[11–16] Murine mast cells contain different neutral proteases: α-chymase (mouse mast cell protease-5, or mMCP-5), -chymases (mMCP-1, 2, 4, 9), tryptases (mMCP-6, 7), carboxypeptidase, and cathepsin G. mMCP-1 is uniquely expressed in MMCs. Expression of the protease phenotype is under the influence of intracellular (strain-dependent expression of transcription factors) and extracellular factors (cytokines, infections, extracellular matrix components). Rat granule chymases rMCP-1 and 2 are expressed in CTMC and MMC, respectively. Rat MMC may also express rMCP-3, 4, 8, 9, and 10, but lack tryptase.[17]

All human mast cells contain heparin and therefore differential staining properties could not be used to classify different subpopulations. Human mast cells can be subdivided into two major populations based on the expression of tryptase (T) and α-chymase (C). A site-dependent presence of both subtypes occurs: tryptase- and chymase-containing mast cells ($MC_{TC}$) predominate in skin and small bowel submucosa, while sole tryptase-containing mast cells ($MC_T$) predominate in normal airways and mucosal layers of the intestine. Both subtypes also contain carboxypeptidase and cathepsin G.[17–21] Human mast cells can be further characterized by the expression of the high-affinity IgE receptor (FcεRI) and c-kit (CD117) among other membrane molecules such as cytokine, chemokine, and complement receptors, and IgG receptors FcγRI (CD64) and FcγRII (CD32), but expression of cell surface molecules is strongly influenced by tissue source, state of differentiation, and cytokine milieu.[22]

# III. ONTOGENY

## A. Mast Cell Precursors

Mast cells develop from CD34+ hematopoietic progenitor cells found in cord blood,[23,24] fetal liver,[25] peripheral blood,[26] and bone marrow.[27,28] A committed mast cell precursor from murine fetal blood has been defined by the phenotype Thy-1$^{lo}$ and c-kit$^{hi}$.[29] Human mast cell precursor cells express CD34, CD117, and CD13. Progenitor cells differentiated into mast cells stay strongly CD117 positive, but the expression of CD13 is diminished.[27] Unlike other granulated hematopoietic cells (e.g., basophils), mast cells exit the bone marrow as committed progenitors and complete differentiation and maturation in the peripheral tissues.

## B. Mast Cell Growth and Development

Mast cell growth and development can be influenced by many cytokines. Of eminent importance in the development and survival of mast cells is the c-kit/stem cell factor (SCF) interaction. SCF is the natural ligand for the mast cell membrane-associated receptor tyrosine kinase c-kit. SCF is expressed by endothelial cells, fibroblasts, and stromal cells.[30,31] Mutant mice lacking a functional c-kit (W/W$^v$)[34] or deficient in expression of SCF (Sl/Sl$^d$)[33] are virtually mast cell–deficient in all organs. Mast cell populations can be restored by injection of congenic bone marrow cells (or bone marrow–derived mast cells) from control animals into W/W$^v$ mice or injection of SCF into Sl/Sl$^d$ mice, respectively.[34] During an inflammation, mast cell numbers in gastrointestinal, genitourinary, and respiratory tract can increase markedly under the influence of locally produced Th2-associated cytokines interleukin-3 (IL-3), IL-4, or IL-9.[35–37] This mast cell proliferation is T-cell dependent. For example, athymic nude mice, lacking functional T lymphocytes, are not able to respond to, e.g., helminth infection with a mast cell hyperplasia in the gut.[38] Proliferated mast cells can be found in mucosal epithelial surfaces and are of mucosal phenotype (MMC). Under normal conditions, only few mast cells can found in these areas, but increases found after mucosal inflammation are important for the elimination of infections. The concentration of mast cells in the skin and peritoneal cavity of athymic nude mice is comparable to that in normal littermates, which suggests that connective tissue-type mast cells are controlled by growth distinct from T-cell-derived cytokines.[39]

*In vitro* proliferation and differentiation of murine or human mast cells are supported by various cytokines such as SCF IL-3, 4, 6, 9, 10, and nerve growth factor.[8,34,40–46] When murine bone marrow cells are cultured in the presence of IL-3 after 3 to 4 weeks a virtually homogeneous population of mast cells (bone marrow–derived mast cell; BMMC) with an immature mucosal phenotype will grow out. Coculture of immature BMMC with SCF, IL-4, nerve growth factor (NGF), or fibroblasts results in further maturation with or without a phenotypic change into CTMCs. Combination of SCF and IL-4 supports direct outgrowth of mast cells of CTMC phenotype from bone marrow cells.[47] Human mast cells develop from hematopoietic progenitors found in cord blood, fetal liver, peripheral blood, and bone marrow.

SCF is the pivotal growth factor for development of human mast cells from CD34+ progenitor cells *in vitro*. For cultures in serum containing medium, a combination of SCF with IL-6 seems requisite to grow sufficient numbers of pure mast cells from cord blood, while in serum free medium SCF alone will suffice.[48]

# IV. ACTIVATION FOR MEDIATOR RELEASE

## A. Mediators Released

Upon activation, mast cells secrete a heterogeneous group of mediators, which are either preformed and stored in secretory granules or newly synthesized. Among the released compounds are vasoactive substances, chemotactic factors, proteolytic enzymes, cytokines, and proteoglycans.

### 1. Preformed Mediators

Preformed mediators include the biogenic amines histamines and serotonin, neutral proteases (tryptase, chymotryptic proteases), acid hydrolases (arylsulfatases, -glucuronidase, and -hexosaminidase), proteoglycans (heparin, chondroitin sulfate), and inflammatory and chemotactic factors (tumor necrosis factor-alpha; TNF-α).[49–55] Human mast cells contain approximately 2 to 5 pg histamine per cell and in contrast to rodent mast cells store no serotonin.[22] In the granules, histamine is bound to proteoglycans and other proteins, and after secretion it is released from its binding sites by cation exchange. A differential release of both biogenic amines form mast cells after pretreatment with certain drugs has been described and may also occur *in vivo* in delayed-type hypersensitivity (DTH) responses.[56] Both serotonin and histamine cause smooth muscle contraction and an increase in vascular permeability, leading to leakage of serum and migration of leukocytes to extravascular tissue. A major component of the granule constituents are the neutral proteases. These proteases have effects on several structural proteins in the microenvironment such as extracellular matrix proteins, complement, myelin sheets of nerves, and also on the core proteins of the proteoglycans of exocytosed granules. The proteoglycan heparin is a potent anticoagulant; it inhibits activation of the alternative complement pathway, stimulates angiogenesis, and has many other effects. Chondroitin sulfate has similar bioactivities as heparin, although it has only weak anti-coagulatory activity.

Mast cells are unique in their ability to release preformed TNF-α upon activation. TNF-α is a multifunctional cytokine promoting, e.g., leukocyte infiltration through upregulation of adhesion molecules.[4]

### 2. Newly Generated Mediators

After receiving an appropriate stimulus, mast cells are able to generate vasoactive (dilating and constricting) and smooth muscle contraction-modulating lipid mediators (prostaglandin $D_2$, $E_2$, $I_2$, and leukotrienes C4, D4, E4). Platelet activating factor is another newly generated lipid mediator with numerous biological effects, e.g., neutrophil and platelet activation, induction of hypotension, and increase in vasopermeability.

Mast cells are also a source of multifunctional cytokines. After stimulation *in vitro*, mast cells have been shown to express numerous cytokines and growth factors. Stimulated mast cells were shown to have increased levels of mRNA and/or to secrete *de novo* synthesized protein of, for example, IL-1, 3, 4, 5, 6, 10, 13, 16, 25, transforming growth factor-β, SCF, granulocyte-macrophage colony-stimulating factor, interferon-γ, microphage inflammatory protein-1α and 1β, and TNF-α.[54,55,57]

## B. Stimulation and Inhibition Regulate Mast Cell Activation

Stimulation of mast cells via the high-affinity IgE-receptors (FcεRI) is the most well studied route for activation at present. IgE binds to the FcεRI ($K_a$ = $10^9$ to $10^{10}$ $M^{-1}$) with the Fc portion of this molecule.[58–60] The high affinity and slow dissociation, combined with an IgE-mediated stabilization effect on FcεRI receptor and mast cell life, enable mast cells to acquire antigen specificity and maintain memory for a long period.[61,62] Mast cell activation is initiated by cross-linking of the FcεRI by, e.g., multivalent antigen, or antibodies against IgE or the FcεRI. In addition to IgE, various immunological and non-immunological stimuli are able to stimulate mast cells or, on the contrary, inhibit mast cell activation (Table 10.1). Certain mast cell populations express IgG receptors, such as FcγRI on human mast cells that were cultured in the presence of IFN-γ, FcγRIIA and B, and FcγRIII on mouse mast cells. IgG-mediated mast cell degranulation has been shown for the human FcγRI and the murine FcγRIII.[63,64] Co-aggregation of FcγRIIB with FcεRI induces activation of FcγRIIB and subsequent inhibition of FcεRI-dependent signaling.[65] FcγRIIB is probably also suppressing the activatory signals of other receptors, such as that of c-kit.[66] Recently,

**TABLE 10.1**
**The Main Activating and Inhibitory Receptors on Mast Cells**

| Activating Receptors | Ligand |
|---|---|
| FcεRI | IgE |
| FcγRI (human)/RIII (rodent) | IgG |
| c-Kit | SCF |
| Adenosine receptor (AR) | Adenosine |
| Toll-like receptors (TLR) 2, 4, 6, 8 | Bacterial components (lipopolysaccharides, lipoproteins, mannans, lectin, peptidoglycan) |
| Paired immunoglobulin-like receptor A (PIR-A) | ? |
| gp49A | ? |
| C3aR, C5aR (CD88) | C3a/C4a, C5a |
| Protease activated receptors (PAR) 1/3/4, 2 | Thrombin, factor Xa/trypsin/tryptase |
| Neurokinin receptor-1 (NK-1) | Substance P |
| **Inhibiting Receptors** | **Ligand** |
| FcγRIIb | IgG |
| AR | Adenosine |
| PIR-B | ? |
| Mast cell function-associated antigen (MAFA) | ? |
| gp49B1 | Integrin αv3 |

cross-linking of free Ig kappa light chains has been shown to activate mast cells in an antigen specific way in addition to the repertoire of the adaptive immune system.[67]

Several activatory mast cell receptors are involved in another essential task of mast cells as a participator in certain innate immune responses. These receptors either directly recognize bacterial components, such as the Toll-like receptors (TLR) and CD48, or recognize components of complement system, such as C3a-receptor (C3aR) and C5a-receptor (C5aR).

Numerous other activating receptors are expressed on mast cells, including adenosine receptors, cytokine and chemokine receptors, c-kit (CD117, receptor for stem cell factor), protease-activated receptors (PAR), receptors for neurokinins, and CD63 (LAMP-3), which has a proposed function in cell adhesion. Inhibitory receptors on mast cells include gp49-B1, with a proposed function in cell adhesion, and signal regulatory protein α (SIRPα1, SHPS-1, BIT, P84), which binds IAP/CD47 with a proposed function in cell migration and adhesion.

Important differences in the susceptibility for different stimuli exist between mucosal (MMC) and connective tissue (CTMC) type mast cells. Also, the optimal temperatures for stimulation of MMC and CTMC are different, i.e., 37°C and 30°C, respectively.[68] The molecular basis for this heterogeneity is not well understood.

## C. Signal Transduction in Mast Cell Activation

As stated in Table 10.1, mast cells can be activated by a myriad of stimuli. Although most knowledge concerning receptor signaling has been gained by studying the FcεRI receptor, much is known about the activation pathways of several other receptors as they often coincide largely with those of the FcεRI receptor. The FcεRI is a member of the family of multichain immune system receptors, which includes the T-cell receptors, B-cell receptor, and the Fc receptors.[69] The FcεRI of mast cells is composed of three subunits: an α-chain, a β-chain, and a homodimer of γ-chains.[61] An alternative $\alpha_2$-conformation exists in other cell types.[70] The α-chain is involved in binding of the IgE molecule. The β-chain and γ-chain have intracellular tails containing a common motif termed immunoreceptor tyrosine-based activation motif (ITAM) of the general sequence $D/EX_2YX_2L/IX_{6/7}YX_2L/I$, which are of critical importance for coupling the receptor to the intracellular signal transduction cascade.[71–73] Binding of monomeric IgE to FcεRI has recently been shown to have signaling functions in mast cells leading to enhanced expression of surface FcεRI and cell survival (reviewed in Reference 74). In addition, some monoclonal IgEs have been found to induce moderate mast cell activation.[75] However, complete activation is only achieved after aggregation of FcεRI by IgE cross-linking, which sets off numerous biochemical events eventually leading to the secretion of preformed and *de novo* synthesized mast cell mediators (Figure 10.1). A great deal of the information described below on signal transduction stems from work done with the rat leukemia cell line RBL-2H3, a very useful experimental model for investigating mast cell activation.

### 1. Protein Tyrosine Phosphorylation

Protein tyrosine phosphorylation is one of the earliest detectable events after cross-linking of the IgE receptor, FcεRI, in mast cells.[76] The receptor lacks intrinsic kinase activity, but the ITAMs of the β- and γ-chain become phosphorylated within seconds after activation by the Src family protein tyrosine kinases (PTK) Lyn,[77] which constitutively binds to the β-chain.[78,79] The phosphorylated ITAMs of the β- and γ-chains serve as docking sites for additional Lyn molecules and kinases belonging to the Syk family, respectively, which bind through their Src homology 2 (SH2) domains.[80–85] Syk bound to the receptor γ-chains is then activated via tyrosine phosphorylation by the receptor β-chain-associated Lyn.[86–88] Activation of Syk is important for transmitting and amplifying downstream signals in the mast cell, as it phosphorylates multiple proteins, including LAT (linker for activation of T cells), SLP-76 (SH2-domain-containing leukocyte protein of 76 kDa) and Vav. A second Src kinase, Fyn, which is activated by cross-linked FcεRI independently from Lyn, phosphorylates Gab2 (Grb2-associated binding protein 2).[89] LAT, SLP-76, Vav, and Gab2 initiate a number of activation cascades. Upon FcεRI aggregation, LAT associates with the adaptors Grb2 and SLP-76, the guanidine nucleotide exchange factor Vav1, and both phospholipase Cγ1 (PLCγ1) and PLCγ2.[90,91] LAT-Grb2-Sos triggers the conversion of Ras-GDP to Ras-GTP, which starts the Ras/ERK pathway leading to the production of phospholipase $A_2$ (see Section C.3) and transcription of cytokine genes. Vav1 binds LAT via association with SLP-76. Vav1 activates Rho family GTPases, in particular Rac proteins, that govern actin cytoskeletal organization, cell proliferation and survival, and cytokine gene transcription regulation.[92–94] Several studies indicate that Vav proteins also control the $Ca^{2+}$ flux by means of the regulation of PLCγ activation.[91,95] PLCγ is a key component that initiates the PKC/$Ca^{2+}$ activation cascade that leads to degranulation (see Section C.2). SLP-76 has also been proposed a critical molecule in the regulation of calcium and degranulation in the LAT-organized signaling complex.[96] The proteins of the LAT/Gads/SLP-76/Vav/PLCγ complex all appear to influence the signaling functions of the complete complex, which is further regulated by other proteins, such as the Tec-like Bruton's tyrosine kinase (Btk). Btk binds to phosphatidylinositol 3,4,5-triphosphate ($PtdInsP_3$) and then becomes activated through phosphorylation by Lyn and Syk.[97] LAT-bound PLCγ becomes a target for Btk after interacting with $PtdInsP_3$.[98,99] Btk also influences other pathways, such as the Rac1 and JNK signaling.[100,101]

Phosphatidylinositol 3-kinase (PI3K), which is regulated by Gab2 and $G_i$ proteins, is another key enzyme in mast cell activation. PI3K converts $PtdInsP_2$ to $PtdInsP_3$, which is a regulator of Btk and Vav activity. Furthermore, PI3K is capable of activating mast cells independently from calcium signaling, probably via a PKC isotype,[89,102] and PI3K and PtdInsP3 together activate the Rac signaling pathway.[103] PI3K plays a crucial role in mast cell survival, c-kit-mediated activation, and adhesion, although it is not always known which of the different PI3K isoforms is involved.[104]

Phosphorylation and activation of the proteins in different signaling routes leads to numerous cellular responses as increased PtdIns turnover, $Ca^{2+}$ mobilization, synthesis, and secretion of lipid mediators, actin polymerization, membrane ruffling, and increased cell spreading and cell–substrate adhesion. Studies using tyrosine kinase-specific inhibitors, like genistein and piceatannol,[105,106] demonstrated a critical dependence of tyrosine phosphorylation in IgE-receptor-mediated granule secretion.

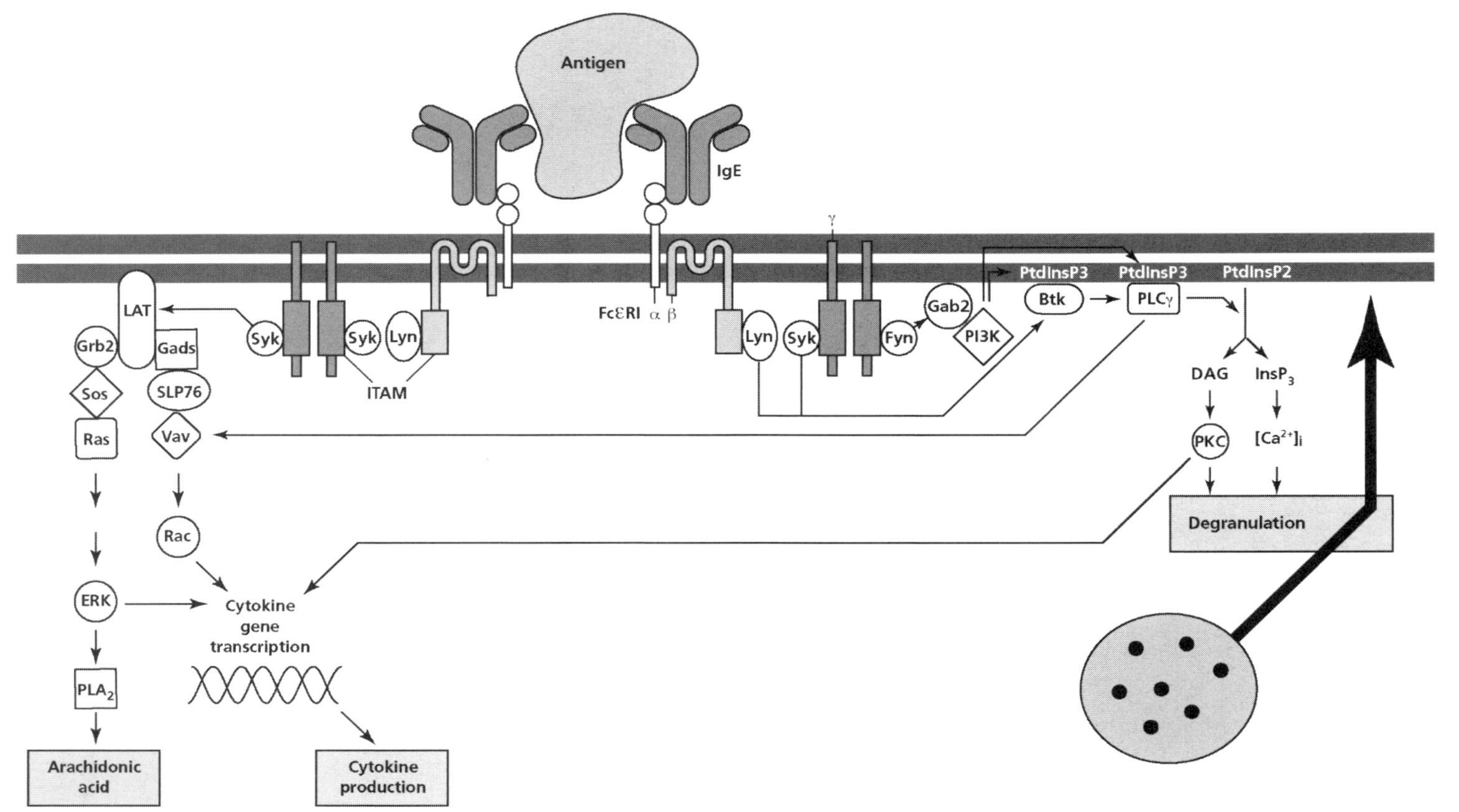


**FIGURE 10.1** Schematic representation of signal transduction pathways activated by cross-linking of the high-affinity IgE receptor on mast cells.

Protein tyrosine phosphatases also play an important role in signaling via the IgE receptor. Src homology 2 domain-containing inositol 5′ phosphatase (SHIP) catalyzes the hydrolysis of PtdInsP3, which inhibits the FcεRI-induced membrane recruitment and activation of Btk and PLCγ. SHIP associates with the adaptor protein Shc and the tyrosine phosphatase SHP-2.[107] SHIP is also recruited to the phosphorylated ITIMs of inhibitory receptors such as FcγRIIB and inhibits FcεRI-induced degranulation.[108,109] The presence of SHIP creates a threshold that prevents mast cells from degranulating at low IgE/antigen concentrations or even in the presence of IgE alone, and this threshold becomes even higher when inhibitory co-receptors are activated.[110,111] Furthermore, SHIP reduces the total activated time.[110] Common leukocyte antigen (CD45), a cell surface protein with tyrosine phosphatase activity, has been found to act on Lyn and determines its activation status,[112] probably together with the opposing action of Src family kinases, such as Csk.[113] Mast cells from CD45-deficient mice are not able to degranulate upon receptor cross-linking.[114]

### 2. Phosphatidylinositol Turnover and $Ca^{2+}$ Mobilization

PtdIns turnover is rapidly increased after mast cell activation via the FcεRI.[115] This is due to Btk-mediated activation of PtdIns-specific PLCγ1,[116] resulting in the hydrolysis of PtdIns into 1,2-diacylglycerol (DAG) and inositol 1,4,5-triphosphate ($IP_3$). Together with the activation of phospholipase D,[117,118] which converts phosphatidylcholine into DAG, this results in a sustained elevation of the cellular level of diglycerides. DAG activates various isoforms of protein kinase C[119] and inositol phosphates release $Ca^{2+}$ from the endoplasmic reticulum.[120] Using permeabilized RBL-2H3 cells, isozymes PKC-β and δ were shown to be important for FcεRI-mediated degranulation,[121,122] whereas other isozymes PKC-α and ε[122] and PKC-β and ε[123] modulate PLC activity and proto-oncogene expression, respectively. Phosphorylation by PKC can be inhibited by staurosporine and this compound completely blocks degranulation.

It is generally acknowledged that $Ca^{2+}$ is essential for the secretion of mast cells. Following IgE-receptor cross-linking, there is a dramatic increase in the cytosolic $Ca^{2+}$ concentration $[Ca^{2+}]_i$.[124–128] The initial rise is due to the binding of $IP_3$ to specific receptors on the endoplasmic reticulum and release of $Ca^{2+}$ from this intracellular store. This initial rise is followed by an influx from $Ca^{2+}$ from the extracellular space by opening of a plasma membrane channel. This influx of extracellular $Ca^{2+}$ leads to sustained elevation of $[Ca^{2+}]_i$, which is essential for triggering the granule exocytosis.

### 3. Stimulation of Phospholipase $A_2$

Release of arachidonic acid by mast cells occurs shortly after activation, and it is likely that it is independent of degranulation.[129] Arachidonic acid can be derived from DAG by DAG lipase and through the hydrolysis of phospholipids after activation of phospholipase $A_2$ ($PLA_2$). Two forms of $PLA_2$ are described: a low molecular weight (m.w.) secreted form and a cytosolic form of high m.w. The latter enzyme contains a $Ca^{2+}$-dependent phospholipid-binding domain and a single serine-containing consensus site for phosphorylation by mitogen-activated protein kinase (MAPK). Both a rise in $[Ca^{2+}]$ and activation of the Ras/ERK pathway have been shown to be required for the release of arachidonic acid,[130] which is further metabolized into the inflammatory eicosanoid lipids.

### 4. Involvement of G Proteins

Although mast cell exocytosis can be triggered by stable GTP analogues or direct stimulation of G proteins and depletion of intracellular GTP inhibits IgE-receptor-mediated mast cell activation,[131,132] G proteins linking the FcεRI to intracellular signal transduction pathways have not been identified. However, FcεRI-mediated degranulation is enhanced by co-stimulation of mast cells with adenosine, which acts primarily by the G protein–coupled $A_{2B}$ and $A_3$ adenosine receptors.[133–137]

C3aR and C5aR belong to the rhodopsin subfamily of G protein–coupled receptors. Also, the members of the PAR family are coupled to G proteins.[138]

Cationic secretagogues, such as compound 48/80, and neuropeptide Y directly activate a pertussis toxin-sensitive G protein coupled to phospholipase C. These compounds most likely directly interact with a C-terminal sequence of the G protein $\alpha$ subunit after insertion of the molecule into the membrane lipids of the mast cell (reviewed in Reference 139). Recently, neuropeptide substance P was found to activate mast cells via the neurokinin receptor 1 (NK1; see Section V).

Most $G_i$-coupled receptors use the $\beta$ subunits of G protein to activate MAPK via a mechanism involving Src and the "classical" Ras/ERK cascade.[140] In addition, some $G_i$-coupled receptors induce activation of $PI_3K$, which produces $PIP_3$,[141] enhancing the release of histamine containing granules.

### 5. Involvement of Lipid Rafts

Ligand engagement of antigen receptors causes their partitioning to specialized regions of the plasma membrane, commonly referred to as lipid rafts.[142] These microdomains are enriched in glycosphingolipids and cholesterol, which render them insoluble in non-ionic detergents.[143] Extensive studies have been performed on the behavior of lipid rafts and associated proteins after activation of RBL-2H3 cells, both by biochemical analysis of detergent-insoluble proteins and by microscopy. Lipid rafts appear to facilitate the engagement of FcεRI with the downstream signaling apparatus. Furthermore, the existence of different raft types suggests an important role in signaling regulation.

Although FcεRI in resting cells is not associated with lipid rafts, cross-linking causes its movement into lipid rafts where there is an enhanced presence of Lyn (reviewed in References 144 and 145). The formation of larger aggregates leads to exclusion of Lyn, which requires actin polymerization, and attraction of Syk to form functional signaling domains.[146] The scaffolding protein LAT is known to be constitutively attached to lipid rafts. However, LAT and FcεRI are not present at the same site either in resting cells or after activation of RBL-2H3 cells. Instead, LAT forms large clusters adjacent to the FcεRI-containing rafts, suggesting that LAT rafts function as topographically distinct secondary sites of active signaling.[147] Lipid raft dynamics are controlled by the cell by means of actin polymerization. However, different types of lipid rafts require different regulatory proteins. Several proteins have been proposed to link signaling to the cytoskeleton, such as Dok-1 and 2 for FcεRI[148] and Vav1 for LAT.[149]

## D. Inhibitors of Mast Cell Activation

Although no selective inhibitors of mast cell activation are at present available, numerous agents are known to affect mediator release from mast cells (Table 10.2). Other compounds (e.g., nonsteroidal anti-inflammatory drugs) can also be used to selectively inhibit generation and release of inflammatory mediators by mast cells. Importantly, mast cells from different origins show differential susceptibility for inhibition by some compounds. For example, cromolyn and nedocromil

**TABLE 10.2**
**Inhibitors of Mast Cell Activation**

| Type | Compound |
|---|---|
| Immunosuppressive | Cyclosporine A, FK506 |
| Glucocorticoids | Dexamethasone |
| Miscellaneous | Doxantrozole, cromolyn sodium, nedocromil sodium |
| β-Adrenoreceptor agonists | Sameterol, salbutamol |
| H1-antagonists | Loratidine, terfenadine |

inhibit CTMC but not MMC from rat; however, CTMC from mouse or humans show refractoriness to inhibition by these drugs.

## V. NEUROPEPTIDES AND MAST CELLS

Mast cells are often found in the proximity of nerve endings.[150–152] In humans and other mammals, the dermis is richly innervated by primary efferent sensory nerves, postganglionic cholinergic parasympathetic nerves, and postganglionic adrenergic and cholinergic sympathetic nerves.[153] Botchkarev and co-workers[152] showed, using *in situ* histochemistry, that these nerve fibers form close contacts with mast cells in the mouse skin. Close proximity to nerves, mostly of sensory origin, allows a bidirectional communication between mast cells and the nervous system. Other than an anatomical and morphological link between the two, this proximity represents a functional link between the immune and nervous systems, whereby mast cells appear to act as bidirectional carriers of information.[154,155]

Neuropeptides released by cutaneous nerves have been shown to activate a number of target cells, including mast cells.[156] Furthermore, topical application of capsaicin results in a significant reduction in the number of mast cells and the appearance of degranulated mast cells in the skin.[157] Because capsaicin does not degranulate mast cells by itself,[158] these data suggest that capsaicin-induced release of peptides from neurons could cause mast cell degranulation, again pointing to a nerve–mast cell communication in the skin.

Neuropeptides, such as substance P and CGRP, exhibit a variety of pro-inflammatory effects. In the skin, they are released in response to nociceptive stimulation by pain and mechanical and chemical irritants to mediate skin responses to infection, injury, and wound healing.[159,160] Skin mast cells can respond to trauma, releasing a variety of inflammatory mediators through an immediate sensory nerve-stimulated response or via an axon reflex, inducing the release of substance P from peripheral nerve endings, in turn leading to more mast cell degranulation (Figure 10.2). Substance P is one of main neuropeptides responsible for the skin reaction characterized by erythema, pain, and swelling.[160] In addition, substance P can cause the release of histamine[161] and TNF-$\alpha$[162] from skin mast cells, which in turn leads to vasodilation.

### A. Neurogenic Inflammation

Sensory neurons play a role in neurogenic inflammation in the skin.[163,164] Aside from the generation of action potentials, the C-fiber terminal is a secretory system, releasing tachykinins to cause neurogenic inflammation. Stimulation of these C-fibers by a range of chemical and physical factors results in afferent neuronal condition eliciting parasympathetic reflexes and antidromic impulses traveling along the peripheral nerve terminal. Such communication from one nerve to another, the axon reflex, results in local release of tachykinins and CGRP from C-fiber terminals.[165]

It has become apparent that in addition to sensory neurons, the mast cell and its mediators also can play a role in neurogenic inflammation.[166,167] Association with the nervous system allows mast cells to act as sensory receptors for a variety of potentially noxious and newly encountered substances.[168] They are therefore ideal to act in these ways to pass information on through afferent nerves to local tissues by axon reflexes (Figure 10.2). Axon reflexes account for many of the local physiological responses to antigen and have long been recognized to be involved in local vasodilatation in the skin.[169]

A multitude of studies have suggested a role for mast cells in the development and maintenance of neurogenic inflammation in the skin.[166,167] First, sensory nerve transmitters can cause the release of histamine from mast cells, which contributes substantially to plasma leakage in the skin.[170] Second, the key signs of neurogenic inflammation in rodent skin, plasma extravasation and vasodilation, are significantly reduced by antihistamines. Third, neuropeptide-induced cutaneous inflammation is markedly reduced in mast cell–deficient mice. Finally, topical capsaicin inhibited plasma

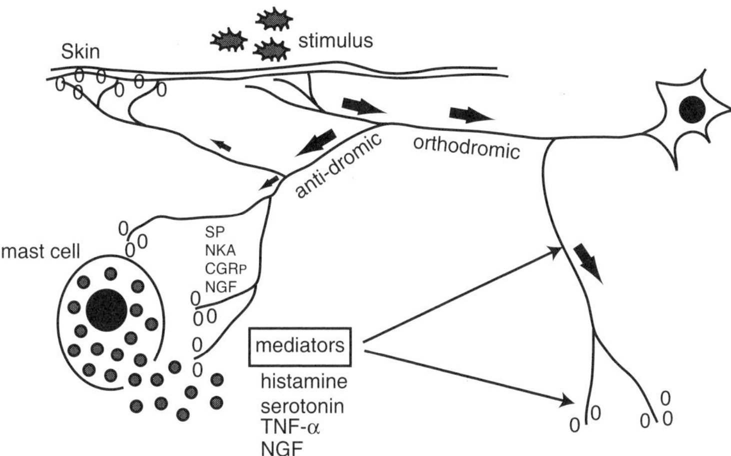


**FIGURE 10.2** Schematic drawing of possible mechanisms involved in dermal neurogenic inflammation. Noxious stimulation of the skin results in the generation of action potentials in nociceptors inducing the release of neuropeptides from the nerve terminals. This will induce mediator release from adjacent mast cells, leading to further activation of other sensory nerve endings.

extravasation and reflex vasodilation to thermal provocation in patients with heat and cold urticaria.[171] However, there are a number of findings showing no role for mast cells in neurogenic vasodilation. The involvement of mast cell mediators in vasodilation and protein extravasation in neurogenic inflammation is still controversial. Therefore, further research is needed to study the activation of skin mast cells by endogenously released neurotransmitters.

## B. Mast Cell Activation

Sensory neurons are characterized by their expression of a certain group of neuropeptides, the tachykinins. Three distinct tachykinin receptor subtypes have been identified and denoted as neurokinin 1 ($NK_1$), neurokinin 2 ($NK_2$), and neurokinin 3 ($NK_3$), which have the highest affinity for substance P, neurokinin A and B, respectively.[172–174]

There are different opinions about the pathways involved in mast cell activation by non-immunological stimuli like tachykinins. Most investigators support nonreceptor-mediated activation induced via direct interaction with pertussis toxin-sensitive G proteins through the N-terminal domain of substance P located in the inner surface of the plasma membrane.[139,175,176] Stimulation of G proteins will activate a signal transduction pathway, eventually leading to mast cell mediator production and release. However, neurokinin A and B have a dissimilar N-terminal domain, and evidence suggests that they are not capable of activating mast cells via a nonreceptor-mediated mechanism.

The cell environment has been suggested as a critical regulatory factor in the responsiveness of mast cells to neuropeptides.[46,177] *In vivo*, several investigators have discussed the increased expression of the $NK_1$ receptor in inflamed tissue.[178,179] Recently, it has been shown that functional tachykinin receptors are expressed on mast cells in the presence of IL-4 and SCF.[180] Therefore, it can be proposed that $NK_1$ receptor expression on immune cells such as mast cells is influenced by environmental inflammatory factors such as cytokines. In conclusion, activation of mast cells by tachykinins can either be receptor or nonreceptor mediated. This process is highly influenced by their microenvironment, which is affected by pathological inflammatory conditions.

## C. Priming

Although relatively high levels of substance P are necessary on a single challenge to induce mast cell degranulation ($>10^{-5}\,M$), it has been demonstrated that repeated doses of very low concentrations (picomolar) of substance P can induce mast cell degranulation. Janiszewski and co-workers[181] reported that mast cells do not respond electrophysiologically to very low concentrations of substance P without degranulation, but that degranulation occurred after repeated triggering. In other words, very low concentrations of substance P showed to be able to prime mast cells and lower their thresholds to subsequent activation. It has been proposed that this electrical stimulation is the functional correlate of priming. If mast cells are, indeed, primed by exposure to substance P, it would enable a lesser stimulus to initiate mast cell activation. However, the relevance of priming in mast cell function has not yet been fully explored and requires further research.

### D. Sensory Nerve Stimulation

Many studies have shown that mast cell–derived mediators, such as histamine, serotonin, and cytokines, modulate NANC neurotransmission.[182–184] Mast cell activation is able to increase the excitability of sensory nerves and neuropeptide production and secretion. NANC nerve endings express receptors for histamine ($H_1$ and $H_3$) and serotonin (5-$HT_{2A}$).[185,186] Under inflammatory-like conditions, it has been shown that primary NANC nerves show an upregulation of at least histamine $H_1$ receptor expression.[187] A recent report by Shubabey and Myers[188] provides evidence of TNF-α receptor expression TNF-R1 and TNF-R2 in DRG neutrons in adult rat. Both receptor subtypes were upregulated in DRG neurons during inflammation. TNF-α can, in this way, cause the direct release of substance P and CGRP from unmyelinated fibers. Thus, sensory nerves altered in this way could result in an increased release of neuropeptides. Allergen/hapten challenge can also lead to substance P production in a subset of sensory nerve fibers that are typically devoid of neuropeptides. In other words, allergen/hapten challenge leads to a phenotypic switch in the sensory neuropeptide innervation, probably via mast cell activation,[189,190] increasing the interaction between mast cells and substance P–immunoreactive nerves.

In summary, mast cell–nerve communication may amplify and spread the inflammatory response that may contribute to the pathogenesis of, for example, skin diseases.

### E. Growth Factors

Immune cells could represent an additional source of tachykinins in inflamed tissues, providing a non-neurogenic tachykininergic contribution to the local inflammatory process.[191] However, classical mediators of inflammation are not alone in their ability to influence the interaction between mast cells and nerves. Nerve and mast cell growth factors are thought to play prominent regulatory roles as well. One such factor, NGF, acts as a chemoattractant, thereby causing an increase in the number of mast cells as well their degranulation.[192–194] NGF receptors on mast cells act as autoreceptors, regulating mast cell NGF synthesis and release, while being sensitive to NGF from the environment. Inflammation can lead to an enhanced production and release of NGF. In turn, NGF induces the expression of neuropeptides and lowers the threshold of neurons for firing.[195] The concentration of NGF is elevated in a number of inflammatory and autoimmune states in conjunction with an increased accumulation of mast cells, suggesting its involvement in neuroimmune interactions and tissue inflammation.

## VI. MAST CELLS IN IMMEDIATE-TYPE HYPERSENSITIVITY RESPONSES

Immediate anaphylactic hypersensitivity (type I) responses are principally due to tissue mast cells sensitized with IgE antibodies. Exposure of these mast cells to antigen results in mast cell activation. In mice, anaphylactic responses can also be induced by $IgG_1$ interacting with FcγRIII.[196] Anaphylactic release of mast cell mediators results in increased local vascular permeability and consequently edema, which can be monitored in laboratory animals as tissue swelling (e.g., of the ear) or local Evans blue accumulation.

In humans, allergic responses are monitored in skin prick or patch tests. In the first test, small amounts of antigen (e.g., environmental allergens) are injected into the skin of individuals resulting in wheal (from vascular permeability and resulting tissue edema) and erythematous flare (from vasodilatation due to an axon reflex) in sensitive/allergic subjects. In the patch test, antigen is supplied in a standardized form on the skin and an eczematous reaction at the site of application 48 to 72 h later will develop in sensitized persons.

## VII. MAST CELLS IN CONTACT HYPERSENSITIVITY AND DELAYED-TYPE HYPERSENSITIVITY REACTIONS

Delayed-type hypersensitivity reactions (DTHR) and, more specifically, contact hypersensitivity reactions (CHSR), are adaptive immune reactions that critically depend on the presence of type I memory T cells, which are defined by their capacity to produce interferon gamma (IFN-γ) but little or no IL-4. Conventional DTHR are normally directed against peptide antigens that are presented inside tissues; CHSR are directed against haptens applied to the skin. In experimental animals deletion of either $CD4^+$ or $CD8^+$ T cells with antibodies, knockout (ko) mice devoid of either $CD4^+$ or $CD8^+$ T cells as well as adoptive transfer of *in vitro* generated T-cell lines have demonstrated that, under most conditions, some DTHR depend primarily on $CD4^+$ Th1 cells, while others are dominated by $CD8^+$ Tc1 cells. *In vivo,* activation of such memory T cells occurs most likely in the draining lymph node. Even though the T-cell pathway during DTHR has well been reconstituted, from the initiation of antigen-presenting cells (APC) through their migration to the priming of T cells,[197–199] recent data show that the final effector phase of DTHR is still less understood. Thus, study of ko-mice unraveled that efficient effector phases of DTHR depend not only on T cells, but also on B cells,[200] complement, and mast cells.[201,202] While T-cell priming seems to be entirely normal in these mice, they are deficient in developing strong DTHR, such as CHSR, but also others, such as allergic encephalitis. Redegeld et al.[67,131] demonstrated that Ig free light chains produced by B lymphocytes are of crucial importance in the development of contact sensitivity responses in mice. Ig free light chains were shown to sensitize mast cells and subsequent cross-linking with antigen-induced mast cell activation.[67]

Askenase and co-workers[201] were the first who showed that mast cells are needed in the development of DTHR, analyzing CHSR in mast cell–deficient mice. This concept was debated for a long period of time because the mast cell–deficient mouse strains also have other immune defects and because at very high doses of hapten the need of mast cells could be overcome in this model.[203] This discrepancy could be resolved once mast cells could be cultured *in vitro* and selectively transplanted to the site of interest in mast cell–deficient mice. This technique allowed investigators to establish that mast cells are essential in the full manifestation of various DTHR, such as experimental allergic encephalitis,[204] protective cutaneous immune responses to infections by microbes such as *Leishmania major*[205] or *Mycobacterium leprae*,[206] responses to foreign bodies such as polyacrylamine gel (PAG),[207] or in CHSR.[198]

Mast cells are a major source of a large spectrum of biologically active substances that modulate inflammation, such as histamine, prostaglandins, cytokines, growth factors, angiogenesis modulating factors, chemokines, or proteases (see Section IV). Importantly in contrast to many other cell types, mast cells not only can synthesize and release these factors, but they are also capable of storing them in large quantities and therefore rapidly creating high local concentrations of these factors. In view of this, it became important to determine exactly which key mediators mast cells use to steer DTHR.

Comparative mRNA analysis of T-cell-independent hapten-induced irritant reactions and of T-cell-dependent CHSR to identical hapten concentration revealed surprisingly close qualitative and

**TABLE 10.3**
**Division of Th1 Cell-Mediated Diseases According to Their Capacity for Recruiting PMN into the Site of Inflammation**

| Without Neutrophils |
|---|
| Experimental allergic encephalitis/multiple sclerosis |
| Autoimmune diabetes |
| Autoimmune thyroiditis |
| **With Neutrophils** |
| Autoimmune arthritis |
| Inflammatory bowel disease |
| Psoriasis |

quantitative similarities in the chemokine and cytokine pattern of both reaction types, even though only CHSR result in severe ear swelling and tissue damage. Only two factors showed relatively clear differences: macrophages inflammatory protein 1 (MIP1), the mouse equivalent of the human chemokine IL-8, and, to a lesser extent, TNF. This was of interest because many DTHR are strongly attenuated in TNF-ko mice and because, in addition, MIP1/IL-8 had been identified as the most important chemoattractant for polymorphonuclear neutrophils (PMN). To determine the role of mast cell–derived IL-8 and TNF in CHSR, IL-8 protein concentrations were analyzed in the presence or absence of reconstituted mast cells and with blocking antibodies. The role of mast TNF was characterized by reconstituting mast cell–deficient mice with mast cells from either wild-type or TNF-ko mice. The data revealed that both mast cell–derived IL-8 and TNF are essential in the establishment of T-cell-mediated CHSR.[198] This was confirmed by studies on granuloma formation in the skin, where again this type of DTHR failed to develop in mast cell–deficient mice and where mast cells from wild-type but not from TNF-ko mice restored this defective T-cell response.[207]

As TNF is very potent in inducing adhesion molecules such as E-selectin, P-selectin, intercellular adhesion molecule 1 (ICAM-1), and vascular cell adhesion molecule 1 (VCAM-1) on endothelial cells, which are required for attachment of lymphocytes and PMN,[208,209] it is likely that mast cell TNF is primarily involved in preparing endothelial cells for the recruitment of mononuclear cells and PMN. As in addition, mast cells produce MIP1/IL-8, the most important of these cells do not induce the expression of the adhesion molecules required for leukocyte rolling and attachment, but also establish the chemotactic gradient for PMN recruitment during Th1 responses. Even though this concept is currently very dominant, several important questions remain to be resolved. Thus, some Th1 responses are associated with PMN recruitment, while others are not (Table 10.3).

Even though the capacity to attract PMN is associated with the induction of MIP2/IL-8, the origin of stimuli that activate Th1 cells during DTHR/CHSR remains enigmatic. Similarly, the signals that induce IL-8 production by mast cells are unknown. The only aspect that seems definitive is that this type of mast cell activation and IL-8 induction is critically dependent on Th1 cells, as hapten-specific, IL-4-producing Th2 cells are not only incapable of inducing this type of pathology, but they can even suppress Th1-mediated tissue damage and PMN recruitment.[210,211]

## VIII. MAST CELLS IN AUTOIMMUNE DISEASES

Numerous studies show that in various autoimmune diseases mast cell numbers and mast cell mediators accumulate in affected tissues (reviewed in References 212 through 214). In murine models for multiple sclerosis, rheumatoid arthritis, and bullous pemphigoid no expression of disease was noticed in genetically mast cell–deficient animals, indicating a direct role for mast cells in the pathogenesis of these diseases. In other diseases, such as Sjögren's syndrome, experimental vasculitis, chronic idiopathic urticaria, and thyroid eye disease, a role for mast cells has been suggested, but definite evidence is still lacking. Because of the multipotency of its released mediators, it remains to be established at what stage mast cells are crucial in the pathogenesis of autoimmune diseases.

## IX. MAST CELLS IN SKIN DISEASES

A central role of mast cells is well established in wheal reactions, whether they are of allergic, pseudo-allergic, or traumatic origin.[8,215–218] This major function became evident through data showing that mast cells are a major source of histamine and leukotrienes that are released upon IgE-signaling through FcεRI.[34,219,220] Similarly, these reactants can be released upon drug-induced mast cell activation or in response to physical trauma. Histamine is involved in vasodilation and serum exudation. In consequence, drugs were developed that impair histamine release to suppress and prevent wheal reaction. These drugs are efficient in suppressing urticaria, allergic rhinitis, bronchial constriction, or vasodilation during immediate-type allergic reactions.[221–224]

In addition, mast cells may proliferate in a controlled, benign fashion and form either localized mastocytomas or disseminated mastocytosis.[225–229] Very rarely, this proliferation turns into malignant leukemia.[230] Serum levels of an enzyme, tryptase, correlate closely with the degree of mast cell expansion. Together with the clinical examination of the skin and tissue biopsies from the gastrointestinal tract or bone marrow cytology, serum tryptase is the most predictable parameter of mastocytosis.[231,232]

These are currently the major "mast cell-associated" pathologies in humans. Increasing data from basic research suggest that mast cells are not only involved in histamine release and wheal formation, but also may be involved much more broadly in the physiological regulation of skin physiology and the development of skin diseases of inflammatory or malignant origin. Thus, mast cell distribution is not random, but follows a clear pattern that is independent of age and sex: mast cell density is highest in the upper dermis and around superficial small vessels. In addition, mast cells are relatively scarce at the trunk and their density increases strongly in the periphery, especially face, hands, and feet.[233]

Relative little attention has been given to a large body of histological and immunohistological analyses of skin tumors,[232,234,235] T-cell-mediated skin diseases such as eczema[236,237] or psoriasis,[238,239] or immunoglobulin-mediated diseases such as bullous pemphigoid,[240,241] where activated and cytokine-producing mast cells are enriched. As antihistamines have largely failed in the therapy of eczema,[237] the enrichment of mast cells in these pathologies was considered as rather coincidental. The availability of mast cell–deficient mice that can selectively be reconstituted with mast cells at distinct sites now allowed experimental testing of the role of mast cells in various disease conditions. These data revealed that mast cells are one, or perhaps the essential, player in the amplification of T-cell-mediated skin inflammation.[242] This is valid in models of CHSR,[198] cutaneous granuloma formation,[207] or adoptively transferred bullous pemphigoid.[243] Based on these data, reevaluation of mast cells and mast cell inhibitors in skin diseases of humans is indicated. One disease that may open such discussion is psoriasis: experiments with mice have shown that mast cells respond to Th1 cells during DTHR and start to release the MIP-2/IL-8 required for neutrophil recruitment during Th1-cell-mediated inflammation. Importantly, IL-4-producing Th2 cells are not capable of such a reaction. Intriguingly, therapeutic deviation of the skin cytokine profile of psoriasis plaques from a Th1-response toward a Th2-response improves not only psoriasis and suppresses neutrophil recruitment, but also blocks IL-8 expression in the skin,[244] the major source of which is the mast cells stimulated by Th1 cells.[210] It has been more than 30 years since activated mast cells were first described in the progressing margins of psoriasis. Together with the animal experiments available, the current data suggest that mast cells are not simple bystanders, but the critical cells translating the specific T-cell message into skin inflammation. Once the mode of T cell–mast cell interactions has been defined, new studies must be designed to develop mast cell–based therapies that may either improve or, more likely, prevent diseases such as psoriasis, eczema, bullous pemphigoid, and possibly also skin tumors.

## REFERENCES

1. Galli, S.J., New insights into "the riddle of the mast cells": microenvironmental regulation of mast cell development and phenotypic heterogeneity. *Lab. Invest.*, 62, 5–33, 1990.
2. Yong, L.C., The mast cell: origin, morphology, distribution, and function. *Exp. Toxicol. Pathol.*, 49, 409–424, 1997.
3. Marone, G., The role of mast cell and basophil activation in human allergic reactions. *Eur. Respir. J. Suppl.*, 6, 446s–455s, 1989.
4. Galli, S.J., New concepts about the mast cell. *N. Engl. J. Med.*, 328, 257–265, 1993.
5. Marshall, J.S. and Bienenstock, J., The role of mast cells in inflammatory reactions of the airways, skin and intestine. *Curr. Opin. Immunol.*, 6, 853–9, 1994.
6. Schwartz, L.B., Mast cells: function and contents. *Curr. Opin. Immunol.*, 6, 91–97, 1994.
7. Marshall, J.S. and Bienenstock, J., Mast cells. *Springer Semin. Immunopathol.*, 12, 191–202, 1990.
8. Metcalfe, D.D. et al., Mast cells. *Physiol. Rev.*, 77, 1033–1079, 1997.
9. Helander, H.F. and Bloom, G.D., Quantitative analysis of mast cell structure. *J. Microsc.*, 100, 315–321, 1974.
10. Enerback, L., Methods for the identification of mast cells by light microscopy, in *Mast Cell Differentiation and Heterogeneity,* Befus, A.D.B.J. and Denburg, J.A., Eds., Raven Press, New York, 1986.
11. Beil, W.J. et al., Mast cell granule composition and tissue location — a close correlation. *Histol. Histopathol.*, 15, 937–946, 2000.
12. Gurish, M.F. and Austen, K.F., The diverse roles of mast cells. *J. Exp. Med.*, 194, F1–5, 2001.
13. Forsythe, P. and Ennis, M., Clinical consequences of mast cell heterogeneity. *Inflamm. Res.*, 49, 147–154, 2000.
14. Okuda, M., Functional heterogeneity of airway mast cells. *Allergy*, 54(Suppl. 57), 50–62, 1999.
15. Welle, M., Development, significance, and heterogeneity of mast cells with particular regard to the mast cell-specific proteases chymase and tryptase. *J. Leukocyte Biol.*, 61, 233–245, 1997.
16. Stevens, R.L. et al., Strain-specific and tissue-specific expression of mouse mast cell secretory granule proteases. *Proc. Natl. Acad. Sci. U.S.A.*, 91, 128–132, 1994.
17. Caughey, G.H., New developments in the genetics and activation of mast cell proteases. *Mol. Immunol.*, 38, 1353–1357, 2002.
18. Irani, A.A. et al., Two types of human mast cells that have distinct neutral protease compositions. *Proc. Natl. Acad. Sci. U.S.A.*, 83, 4464–4468, 1986.
19. Craig, S.S. et al., Ultrastructural analysis of human T and TC mast cells identified by immunoelectron microscopy. *Lab. Invest.*, 58, 682–691, 1988.
20. Craig, S.S. and Schwartz, L.B., Human MCTC type of mast cell granule: the uncommon occurrence of discrete scrolls associated with focal absence of chymase. *Lab. Invest.*, 63, 581–585, 1990.
21. Miller, H.R. and Pemberton, A.D., Tissue-specific expression of mast cell granule serine proteinases and their role in inflammation in the lung and gut. *Immunology*, 105, 375–390, 2002.
22. Prussin, C. and Metcalfe, D.D., 4. IgE, mast cells, basophils, and eosinophils. *J. Allergy Clin. Immunol.*, 111, S486–494, 2003.
23. Saito, H. et al., Selective growth of human mast cells induced by Steel factor, IL-6, and prostaglandin E2 from cord blood mononuclear cells. *J. Immunol.*, 157, 343–350, 1996.
24. Kanbe, N. et al., Cord-blood-derived human cultured mast cells produce interleukin 13 in the presence of stem cell factor. *Int. Arch. Allergy Immunol.*, 119, 138–142, 1999.
25. Irani, A.M. et al., Recombinant human stem cell factor stimulates differentiation of mast cells from dispersed human fetal liver cells. *Blood*, 80, 3009–3021, 1992.
26. Iida, M. et al., Selective down-regulation of high-affinity IgE receptor (FcεRI) α-chain messenger RNA among transcriptome in cord blood-derived versus adult peripheral blood-derived cultured human mast cells. *Blood*, 97, 1016–1022, 2001.

27. Shimizu, Y. et al., Characterization of "adult-type" mast cells derived from human bone marrow CD34(+) cells cultured in the presence of stem cell factor and interleukin-6. Interleukin-4 is not required for constitutive expression of CD54, FcεRIα and chymase, and CD13 expression is reduced during differentiation. *Clin. Exp. Allergy*, 32, 872–880, 2002.
28. Kirshenbaum, A.S. et al., Demonstration of the origin of human mast cells from CD34+ bone marrow progenitor cells. *J. Immunol.*, 146, 1410–1415, 1991.
29. Rodewald, H.R. et al., Identification of a committed precursor for the mast cell lineage. *Science*, 271, 818–822, 1996.
30. Huang, E. et al., The hematopoietic growth factor KL is encoded by the Sl locus and is the ligand of the c-kit receptor, the gene product of the W locus. *Cell*, 63, 225–233, 1990.
31. Galli, S.J. et al., The kit ligand, stem cell factor. *Adv. Immunol.*, 55, 1–96, 1994.
32. Kitamura, Y. et al., Decrease of mast cells in W/Wv mice and their increase by bone marrow transplantation. *Blood*, 52, 447–452, 1978.
33. Kitamura, Y. and Go, S., Decreased production of mast cells in S1/S1d anemic mice. *Blood*, 53, 492–497, 1979.
34. Galli, S.J., Mast cells and basophils. *Curr. Opin. Hematol.*, 7, 32–39, 2000.
35. Lantz, C.S. et al., Role for interleukin-3 in mast-cell and basophil development and in immunity to parasites. *Nature*, 392, 90–93, 1998.
36. Madden, K.B. et al., Antibodies to IL-3 and IL-4 suppress helminth-induced intestinal mastocytosis. *J. Immunol.*, 147, 1387–1391, 1991.
37. Temann, U.A. et al., Expression of interleukin 9 in the lungs of transgenic mice causes airway inflammation, mast cell hyperplasia, and bronchial hyperresponsiveness. *J. Exp. Med.*, 188, 1307–1320, 1998.
38. Ruitenberg, E.J. and Elgersma, A., Absence of intestinal mast cell response in congenitally athymic mice during *Trichinella spiralis* infection. *Nature*, 264, 258–260, 1976.
39. Keller, R. et al., Mast cells in the skin of normal, hairless and athymic mice. *Experientia*, 32, 171–172, 1976.
40. Schmitt, E. et al., Characterization of a T cell-derived lymphokine that acts synergistically with IL 3 on the growth of murine mast cells and is identical with IL 4. *Immunobiology*, 174, 406–419, 1987.
41. Hamaguchi, Y. et al., Interleukin 4 as an essential factor for *in vitro* clonal growth of murine connective tissue-type mast cells. *J. Exp. Med.*, 165, 268–273, 1987.
42. Tsuji, K. et al., Effects of interleukin-3 and interleukin-4 on the development of "connective tissue-type" mast cells: interleukin-3 supports their survival and interleukin-4 triggers and supports their proliferation synergistically with interleukin-3. *Blood*, 75, 421–427, 1990.
43. Hultner, L. et al., Mast cell growth-enhancing activity (MEA) is structurally related and functionally identical to the novel mouse T cell growth factor P40/TCGFIII (interleukin 9). *Eur. J. Immunol.*, 20, 1413–1416, 1990.
44. Thompson-Snipes, L. et al., Interleukin 10: a novel stimulatory factor for mast cells and their progenitors. *J. Exp. Med.*, 173, 507–510, 1991.
45. Matsuda, H. et al., Nerve growth factor promotes human hemopoietic colony growth and differentiation. *Proc. Natl. Acad. Sci. U.S.A.*, 85, 6508–6512, 1988.
46. Karimi, K. et al., Stem cell factor and interleukin-4 increase responsiveness of mast cells to substance P. *Exp. Hematol.*, 28, 626–634, 2000.
47. Karimi, K. et al., Stem cell factor and interleukin-4 induce murine bone marrow cells to develop into mast cells with connective tissue type characteristics *in vitro*. *Exp. Hematol.*, 27, 654–662, 1999.
48. Kinoshita, T. et al., Interleukin-6 directly modulates stem cell factor-dependent development of human mast cells derived from CD34(+) cord blood cells. *Blood*, 94, 496–508, 1999.
49. Marone, G. et al., Molecular and cellular biology of mast cells and basophils. *Int. Arch. Allergy Immunol.*, 114, 207–217, 1997.
50. Hiromatsu, Y. and Toda, S., Mast cells and angiogenesis. *Microsc. Res. Tech.*, 60, 64–69, 2003.
51. Marshall, J.S. et al., Mast cell cytokine and chemokine responses to bacterial and viral infection. *Curr. Pharm. Des.*, 9, 11–24, 2003.
52. Kulka, M. and Befus, A.D., The dynamic and complex role of mast cells in allergic disease. *Arch. Immunol. Ther. Exp.* (Warsaw), 51, 111–120, 2003.
53. Hines, C., The diverse effects of mast cell mediators. *Clin. Rev. Allergy Immunol.*, 22, 149–160, 2002.

54. Puxeddu, I. et al., Mast cells in allergy and beyond. *Int. J. Biochem. Cell. Biol*, 35, 1601–1607, 2003.
55. Kawakami, T. and Galli, S.J., Regulation of mast-cell and basophil function and survival by IgE. *Nat. Rev. Immunol.*, 2, 773–786, 2002.
56. Theoharides, T.C. et al., Differential release of serotonin and histamine from mast cells. *Nature*, 297, 229–231, 1982.
57. Ikeda, K. et al., Mast cells produce interleukin-25 upon FcεRI-mediated activation. *Blood*, 101, 3594–3596, 2003.
58. Kulczycki, A., Jr. and Metzger, H., The interaction of IgE with rat basophilic leukemia cells. II. Quantitative aspects of the binding reaction. *J. Exp. Med.*, 140, 1676–1695, 1974.
59. Helm, B. et al., The mast cell binding site on human immunoglobulin E. *Nature*, 331, 180–183, 1988.
60. Kawakami, T. et al., Tyrosine phosphorylation is required for mast cell activation by FcεRI cross-linking. *J. Immunol.*, 148, 3513, 1992.
61. Metzger, H., The receptor with high affinity for IgE. *Immunol. Rev.*, 125, 37–48, 1992.
62. Kubo, S. et al., Long term maintenance of IgE-mediated memory in mast cells in the absence of detectable serum IgE. *J. Immunol.*, 170, 775–780, 2003.
63. Okayama, Y. et al., Expression of a functional high-affinity IgG receptor, FcγRI, on human mast cells: up-regulation by IFN-γ. *J. Immunol.*, 164, 4332–4339, 2000.
64. Katz, H.R. and Lobell, R.B., Expression and function of FcγR in mouse mast cells. *Int. Arch. Allergy Immunol.*, 107, 76–78, 1995.
65. Daeron, M. et al., Regulation of high-affinity IgE receptor-mediated mast cell activation by murine low-affinity IgG receptors. *J. Clin. Invest.*, 95, 577–585, 1995.
66. Malbec, O. et al., Negative regulation of c-kit-mediated cell proliferation by FcγRIIB. *J. Immunol.*, 162, 4424–4429, 1999.
67. Redegeld, F.A. et al., Immunoglobulin-free light chains elicit immediate hypersensitivity-like responses. *Nat. Med.*, 8, 694–701, 2002.
68. Galli, S.J., New concepts about the mast cell. *N. Engl. J. Med.*, 328, 257–265, 1993.
69. Ravetch, J.V., Fc receptors: rubor redux. *Cell*, 78, 553–560, 1994.
70. Suzuki, K. et al., The Fc receptor (FcR) γ subunit is essential for IgE-binding activity of cell-surface expressed chimeric receptor molecules constructed from human high-affinity IgE receptor (FcεRI) α and FcR γ subunits. *Mol. Immunol.*, 35, 259–270, 1998.
71. Reth, M., Antigen receptor tail clue. *Nature*, 338, 383–384, 1989.
72. Wilson, B.S. et al., Distinct functions of the FcεRIγ and β subunits in the control of FcεRI-mediated tyrosine kinase activation and signaling responses in RBL-2H3 mast cells. *J. Biol. Chem.*, 270, 4013, 1995.
73. Benhamou, M. et al., Protein-tyrosine kinase $p72^{syk}$ in high affinity IgE receptor signaling. Identification as a component of pp72 and association with the receptor γ chain after receptor aggregation. *J. Biol. Chem.*, 268, 23318, 1993.
74. Kawakami, T. and Galli, S.J., Regulation of mast-cell and basophil function and survival by IgE. *Nat. Rev. Immunol.*, 2, 773–786, 2002.
75. Kalesnikoff, J. et al., Monomeric IgE stimulates signaling pathways in mast cells that lead to cytokine production and cell survival. *Immunity.*, 14, 801–811, 2001.
76. Paolini, R. et al., Phosphorylation and dephosphorylation of the high-affinity receptor for immunoglobulin E immediately after receptor engagement and disengagement. *Nature*, 353, 855–858, 1991.
77. Li, W. et al., FcεR1-mediated tyrosine phosphorylation of multiple proteins, including phospholipase Cγ1 and the receptor βγ2 complex, in RBL-2H3 rat basophilic leukemia cells. *Mol. Cell Biol*, 12, 3176–3182, 1992.
78. Vonakis, B.M. et al., The unique domain as the site on Lyn kinase for its constitutive association with the high affinity receptor for IgE. *J. Biol. Chem.*, 272, 24072–24080, 1997.
79. van Houwelingen, A. et al., Hapten-induced hypersensitivity reactions in the airways: atopic versus non-atopic. *Environ. Toxicol. Pharmacol.*, 2002.
80. Songyang, Z. et al., SH2 domains recognize specific phosphopeptide sequences. *Cell*, 72, 767–778, 1993.
81. Pawson, T. and Gish, G.D., SH2 and SH3 domains: from structure to function. *Cell*, 71, 359–362, 1992.
82. Minoguchi, K. et al., Activation of protein tyrosine kinase $p72^{syk}$ by FcεRI aggregation in rat basophilic leukemia cells. $p72^{syk}$ is a minor component but the major protein tyrosine kinase of pp72. *J. Biol. Chem.*, 269, 16902, 1994.

83. Shiue, L. et al., Interaction of p72$^{syk}$ with the $\gamma$ and $\beta$ subunits of the high-affinity receptor for immunoglobulin E, Fc$\varepsilon$RI. *Mol. Cell. Biol.*, 15, 272, 1995.
84. Razin, E. et al., Signal transduction in the activation of mast cells and basophils. *Immunol. Today*, 16, 370–373, 1995.
85. Benhamou, M. and Siraganian, R.P., Protein-tyrosine phosphorylation: an essential component of Fc$\varepsilon$RI signaling. *Immunol. Today*, 13, 195–197, 1992.
86. Yanagi, S. et al., The structure and function of nonreceptor tyrosine kinase p72$^{SYK}$ expressed in hematopoietic cells. *Cell. Signal.*, 7, 185–193, 1995.
87. El Hillal, O. et al., syk kinase activation by a src kinase-initiated activation loop phosphorylation chain reaction. *Proc. Natl. Acad. Sci. U.S.A*, 94, 1919–1924, 1997.
88. Rivera, V.M. and Brugge, J.S., Clustering of Syk is sufficient to induce tyrosine phosphorylation and release of allergic mediators from rat basophilic leukemia cells. *Mol. Cell. Biol.*, 15, 1582–1590, 1995.
89. Parravicini, V. et al., Fyn kinase initiates complementary signals required for IgE-dependent mast cell degranulation. *Nat. Immunol.*, 3, 741–748, 2002.
90. Arudchandran, R. et al., The Src homology 2 domain of Vav is required for its compartmentation to the plasma membrane and activation of c-Jun NH2-terminal kinase 1. *J. Exp. Med.*, 191, 47, 2000.
91. Manetz, T.S. et al., Vav1 regulates phospholipase C$\gamma$ activation and calcium responses in mast cells. *Mol. Cell. Biol.*, 21, 3763, 2001.
92. Crespo, P. et al., Phosphotyrosine-dependent activation of Rac-1 GDP/GTP exchange by the *vav* proto-oncogene product. *Nature*, 385, 169–172, 1997.
93. Crespo, P. et al., Rac-1 dependent stimulation of the JNK/SAPK signaling pathway by Vav. *Oncogene*, 13, 455–460, 1996.
94. Westwick, J.K. et al., Rac regulation of transformation, gene expression, and actin organization by multiple, PAK-independent pathways. *Mol. Cell. Biol.*, 17, 1324–1335, 1997.
95. Inabe, K. et al., Vav3 modulates B cell receptor responses by regulating phosphoinositide 3-kinase activation. *J. Exp. Med.*, 195, 189–200, 2002.
96. Pivniouk, V.I. et al., SLP-76 deficiency impairs signaling via the high-affinity IgE receptor in mast cells. *J. Clin. Invest*, 103, 1737, 1999.
97. Rawlings, D.J. et al., Activation of BTK by a phosphorylation mechanism initiated by SRC family kinases. *Science*, 271, 822–825, 1996.
98. Scharenberg, A.M. et al., Phosphatidylinositol-3,4,5-trisphosphate (PtdIns-3,4,5-P3)/Tec kinase-dependent calcium signaling pathway: a target for SHIP-mediated inhibitory signals. *EMBO J.*, 17, 1961–1972, 1998.
99. Saitoh, S. et al., LAT is essential for Fc$\varepsilon$RI-mediated mast cell activation. *Immunity.*, 12, 525–535, 2000.
100. Kawakami, Y. et al., Bruton's tyrosine kinase regulates apoptosis and JNK/SAPK kinase activity. *Proc. Natl. Acad. Sci. U.S.A*, 94, 3938–3942, 1997.
101. Inabe, K. et al., Bruton's tyrosine kinase regulates B cell antigen receptor-mediated JNK1 response through Rac1 and phospholipase C-$\gamma$2 activation. *FEBS Lett.*, 514, 260–262, 2002.
102. Le Good, J.A. et al., Protein kinase C isotypes controlled by phosphoinositide 3-kinase through the protein kinase PDK1. *Science*, 281, 2042–2045, 1998.
103. Innocenti, M. et al., Phosphoinositide 3-kinase activates Rac by entering in a complex with Eps8, Abi1, and Sos-1. *J. Cell. Biol.*, 160, 17–23, 2003.
104. Lu-Kuo, J.M. et al., Impaired kit- but not Fc$\varepsilon$RI-initiated mast cell activation in the absence of phosphoinositide 3-kinase p85$\alpha$ gene products. *J. Biol. Chem.*, 275, 6022–6029, 2000.
105. Gruchalla, R.S. et al., An indirect pathway of receptor-mediated 1,2-diacylglycerol formation in mast cells. I. IgE receptor-mediated activation of phospholipase D. *J. Immunol.*, 144, 2334, 1990.
106. Oliver, J.M. et al., Inhibition of mast cell Fc$\varepsilon$R1-mediated signaling and effector function by the Syk-selective inhibitor, piceatannol. *J. Biol. Chem.*, 269, 29697–29703, 1994.
107. Liu, L. et al., Interleukin-3 induces the association of the inositol 5-phosphatase SHIP with SHP2. *J. Biol. Chem.*, 272, 10998–11001, 1997.
108. Ono, M. et al., Role of the inositol phosphatase SHIP in negative regulation of the immune system by the receptor Fc$\gamma$RIIB. *Nature*, 383, 263–266, 1996.
109. Vely, F. et al., Differential association of phosphatases with hematopoietic co-receptors bearing immunoreceptor tyrosine-based inhibition motifs. *Eur. J. Immunol.*, 27, 1994–2000, 1997.

110. Huber, M. et al., The src homology 2-containing inositol phosphatase (SHIP) is the gatekeeper of mast cell degranulation. *Proc. Natl. Acad. Sci. U.S.A*, 95, 11330–11335, 1998.
111. Huber, M. et al., The role of SHIP in mast cell degranulation and IgE-induced mast cell survival. *Immunol. Lett.*, 82, 17–21, 2002.
112. Harashima, A. et al., CD45 tyrosine phosphatase inhibits erythroid differentiation of umbilical cord blood CD34$^+$ cells associated with selective inactivation of Lyn. *Blood*, 100, 4440–4445, 2002.
113. Adamczewski, M. et al., Regulation by CD45 of the tyrosine phosphorylation of high affinity IgE receptor β- and γ-chains. *J. Immunol.*, 154, 3047–3055, 1995.
114. Wank, S.A. et al., Analysis of the rate-limiting step in a ligand-cell receptor interaction: the immunoglobulin E system. *Biochemistry*, 22, 954–959, 1983.
115. Fridriksson, E.K. et al., Quantitative analysis of phospholipids in functionally important membrane domains from RBL-2H3 mast cells using tandem high-resolution mass spectrometry. *Biochemistry*, 38, 8056–8063, 1999.
116. Schneider, H. et al., Tyrosine phosphorylation of phospholipase C gamma 1 couples the Fc epsilon receptor mediated signal to mast cells secretion. *Int. Immunol*, 4, 447–453, 1992.
117. Lin, P.Y. et al., Activation of phospholipase D in a rat mast (RBL 2H3) cell line. A possible unifying mechanism for IgE-dependent degranulation and arachidonic acid metabolite release. *J. Immunol.*, 146, 1609, 1991.
118. Kanner, B.I. and Metzger, H., Initial characterization of the calcium channel activated by the cross-linking of the receptors for immunoglobulin E. *J. Biol. Chem.*, 259, 10188, 1984.
119. Sando, J.J. et al., Role of cofactors in protein kinase C activation. *Cell Signal.*, 4, 595–609, 1992.
120. Yoshii, N. et al., Role of endoplasmic reticulum, an intracellular $Ca^{2+}$ store, in histamine release from rat peritoneal mast cell. *Immunopharmacology*, 21, 13–21, 1991.
121. Okazaki, H. et al., Activation of protein-tyrosine kinase Pyk2 is downstream of Syk in Fcepsilon RI signaling. *J. Biol. Chem.*, 272, 32443, 1997.
122. Berger, S.A. et al., Leukocyte common antigen (CD45) is required for immunoglobulin E- mediated degranulation of mast cells. *J. Exp. Med.*, 180, 471, 1994.
123. Malaviya, R. et al., The mast cell tumor necrosis factor alpha response to FimH-expressing *Escherichia coli* is mediated by the glycosylphosphatidylinositol-anchored molecule CD48. *Proc. Natl. Acad. Sci. U.S.A*, 96, 8110–8115, 1999.
124. Sagi-Eisenberg, R. et al., Protein kinase C regulation of the receptor-coupled calcium signal in histamine-secreting rat basophilic leukaemia cells. *Nature*, 313, 59–60, 1985.
125. Penner, R. et al., Regulation of calcium influx by second messengers in rat mast cells. *Nature*, 334, 499–504, 1988.
126. Niyonsaba, F. et al., A cathelicidin family of human antibacterial peptide LL-37 induces mast cell chemotaxis. *Immunology*, 106, 20–26, 2002.
127. Razin, E. et al., Protein kinases C-β and C-ε link the mast cell high-affinity receptor for IgE to the expression of c-fos and c-jun. *Proc. Natl. Acad. Sci. U.S.A*, 91, 7722–7726, 1994.
128. Wofsy, C. et al., Exploiting the difference between intrinsic and extrinsic kinases: implications for regulation of signaling by immunoreceptors. *J. Immunol.*, 159, 5984–5992, 1997.
129. Hirasawa, N. et al., Activation of the mitogen-activated protein kinase/cytosolic phospholipase A2 pathway in a rat mast cell line. Indications of different pathways for release of arachidonic acid and secretory granules. *J. Immunol.*, 154, 5391, 1995.
130. Wilson, B.S. et al., Depletion of guanine nucleotides with mycophenolic acid suppresses IgE receptor-mediated degranulation in rat basophilic leukemia cells. *J. Immunol.*, 143, 259, 1989.
131. Redegeld, F.A. and Nijkamp, F.P., Immunoglobulin free light chains and mast cells: pivotal role in T-cell-mediated immune reactions? *Trends Immunol.*, 24, 181–185, 2003.
132. Ali, H. et al., Receptor-mediated release of inositol 1,4,5-trisphosphate and inositol 1,4-bisphosphate in rat basophilic leukemia RBL-2H3 cells permeabilized with streptolysin O. *Biochim. Biophys. Acta*, 1010, 88–99, 1989.
133. Ramkumar, V. et al., The A3 adenosine receptor is the unique adenosine receptor which facilitates release of allergic mediators in mast cells. *J. Biol. Chem.*, 268, 16887–16890, 1993.
134. Li, L. et al., Mast cells in airway hyporesponsive C3H/HeJ mice express a unique isoform of the signaling protein Ras guanine nucleotide releasing protein 4 that is unresponsive to diacylglycerol and phorbol esters. *J. Immunol.*, 171, 390, 2003.

135. Tilley, S.L. et al., Adenosine and inosine increase cutaneous vasopermeability by activating A(3) receptors on mast cells. *J. Clin. Invest.*, 105, 361–367, 2000.
136. Auchampach, J.A. et al., Canine mast cell adenosine receptors: cloning and expression of the A3 receptor and evidence that degranulation is mediated by the A2B receptor. *Mol. Pharmacol.*, 52, 846–860, 1997.
137. Feoktistov, I. and Biaggioni, I., Adenosine A2b receptors evoke interleukin-8 secretion in human mast cells. An enprofylline-sensitive mechanism with implications for asthma. *J. Clin. Invest*, 96, 1979–1986, 1995.
138. Dery, O. et al., Proteinase-activated receptors: novel mechanisms of signaling by serine proteases. *Am. J. Physiol.*, 274, C1429–C1452, 1998.
139. Mousli, M. et al., Peptidergic pathway in human skin and rat peritoneal mast cell activation. *Immunopharmacology*, 27, 1–11, 1994.
140. van Biesen, T. et al., Mitogenic signaling via G protein-coupled receptors. *Endocr. Rev.*, 17, 698–714, 1996.
141. Laffargue, M. et al., Phosphoinositide 3-kinase $\gamma$ is an essential amplifier of mast cell function. *Immunity.*, 16, 441–451, 2002.
142. Trieselmann, N.Z. et al., Mast cells stimulated by membrane-bound, but not soluble, steel factor are dependent on phospholipase C activation. *Cell Mol. Life Sci.*, 60, 759–766, 2003.
143. Brown, D.A. and London, E., Functions of lipid rafts in biological membranes. *Annu. Rev. Cell Dev. Biol*, 14, 111–136, 1998.
144. Dráber, P. and Dráberová, L., Lipid rafts in mast cell signaling. *Mol. Immunol*, 38, 1247, 2002.
145. Wilson, B. et al., Fc$\varepsilon$RI signaling observed from the inside of the mast cell membrane. *Mol. Immunol*, 38, 1259, 2002.
146. Wilson, B.S. et al., Observing Fc$\varepsilon$RI signaling from the inside of the mast cell membrane. *J. Cell. Biol.*, 149, 1131–1142, 2000.
147. Davidson, A. and Diamond, B., Autoimmune diseases. *N. Engl. J. Med.*, 345, 340–350, 2001.
148. Abramson, J. et al., Dok protein family members are involved in signaling mediated by the type 1 Fc$\varepsilon$ receptor. *Eur. J. Immunol.*, 33, 85–91, 2003.
149. Rivera, J. et al., The architecture of IgE-dependent mast cell signaling — a complex story. *Allergy Clin. Immunol. Int.*, 14, 25–36, 2002.
150. Purcell, W.M. and Atterwill, C.K., Mast cells in neuroimmune function: neurotoxicological and neuropharmacological perspectives. *Neurochem. Res.*, 20, 521–532, 1995.
151. Undem, B.J. et al., Neurophysiology of mast cell-nerve interactions in the airways. *Int. Arch. Allergy Immunol.*, 107, 199–201, 1995.
152. Botchkarev, V.A. et al., A simple immunofluorescence technique for simultaneous visualization of mast cells and nerve fibers reveals selectivity and hair cycle-dependent changes in mast cell–nerve fiber contacts in murine skin. *Arch. Dermatol. Res.*, 289, 292–302, 1997.
153. Rossi, R. and Johansson, O., Cutaneous innervation and the role of neuronal peptides in cutaneous inflammation: a minireview. *Eur. J. Dermatol.*, 8, 299–306, 1998.
154. Bienenstock, J. et al., Nerves and neuropeptides in the regulation of mucosal immunity. *Adv. Exp. Med. Biol.*, 257, 19–26, 1989.
155. Bauer, O. and Razin, E., Mast cell–nerve interactions. *News Physiol. Sci.*, 15, 213–218, 2000.
156. Ansel, J.C. et al., Interactions of the skin and nervous system. *J. Invest. Dermatol. Symp. Proc.*, 2, 23–26, 1997.
157. Bunker, C.B. et al., The effect of capsaicin application on mast cells in normal human skin. *Agents Actions*, 33, 195–196, 1991.
158. Biro, T. et al., Characterization of functional vanilloid receptors expressed by mast cells. *Blood*, 91, 1332–1340, 1998.
159. Grady, E.F. et al., Characterization of antisera specific to NK1, NK2, and NK3 neurokinin receptors and their utilization to localize receptors in the rat gastrointestinal tract. *J. Neurosci.*, 16, 6975–6986, 1996.
160. Scholzen, T. et al., Neuropeptides in the skin: interactions between the neuroendocrine and the skin immune systems. *Exp. Dermatol.*, 7, 81–96, 1998.
161. Church, M.K. et al., Neuropeptide-induced secretion from human skin mast cells. *Int. Arch. Allergy Appl. Immunol.*, 94, 310–318, 1991.

162. Ansel, J.C. et al., Substance P selectively activates TNF-alpha gene expression in murine mast cells. *J. Immunol.*, 150, 4478–4485, 1993.
163. Jarvikallio, A. et al., Mast cells, nerves and neuropeptides in atopic dermatitis and nummular eczema. *Arch. Dermatol. Res.*, 295, 2–7, 2003.
164. Schmelz, M. and Petersen, L.J., Neurogenic inflammation in human and rodent skin. *News Physiol. Sci.*, 16, 33–37, 2001.
165. Solway, J. and Leff, A.R., Sensory neuropeptides and airway function. *J. Appl. Physiol.*, 71, 2077–2087, 1991.
166. Marshall. J.S. and Waserman. S., Mast cells and the nerves — potential interactions in the context of chronic disease. *Clin. Exp. Allergy*, 25, 102–110, 1995.
167. Baraniuk, J.N. et al., Relationships between permeable vessels, nerves, and mast cells in rat cutaneous neurogenic inflammation. *J. Appl. Physiol.*, 68, 2305–2311, 1990.
168. Bienenstock, J., Cellular communication networks. Implications for our understanding of gastrointestinal physiology. *Ann. N.Y. Acad. Sci.*, 664, 1–9, 1992.
169. Westerman, R.A. et al., Electrically evoked skin vasodilatation: a quantitative test of nociceptor function in man. *Clin. Exp. Neurol.*, 23, 81–89, 1987.
170. Baluk, P., Neurogenic inflammation in skin and airways. *J. Invest. Dermatol. Symp. Proc.*, 2, 76–81, 1997.
171. Del Bianco, E. et al., The effects of repeated dermal application of capsaicin to the human skin on pain and vasodilatation induced by intradermal injection of acid and hypertonic solutions. *Br. J. Clin. Pharmacol.*, 41, 1–6, 1996.
172. Severini, C. et al., The tachykinin peptide family. *Pharmacol. Rev.*, 54, 285–322, 2002.
173. Nakanishi, S., Mammalian tachykinin receptors. *Annu. Rev. Neurosci.*, 14, 123–136, 1991.
174. Regoli, D. et al., Receptors and antagonists for substance P and related peptides. *Pharmacol. Rev.*, 46, 551–599, 1994.
175. Kops, S.K. et al., Mast cell activation and vascular alterations in immediate hypersensitivity-like reactions induced by a T cell-derived antigen-binding factor. *Lab. Invest.*, 50, 421–434, 1984.
176. Bueb, J.L. et al., A pertussis toxin-sensitive G protein is required to induce histamine release from rat peritoneal mast cells by bradykinin. *Agents Actions*, 30, 98–101, 1990.
177. Swieter, M. et al., Mast cells and their microenvironment: the influence of fibronectin and fibroblasts on the functional repertoire of rat basophilic leukemia cells. *J. Periodontol.*, 64, 492–496, 1993.
178. Kaltreider, H.B. et al., Upregulation of neuropeptides and neuropeptide receptors in a murine model of immune inflammation in lung parenchyma. *Am. J. Respir. Cell. Mol. Biol.*, 16, 133–144, 1997.
179. Mantyh, C.R. et al., Differential expression of substance P receptors in patients with Crohn's disease and ulcerative colitis. *Gastroenterology*, 109, 850–860, 1995.
180. Van Der Kleij, H.P. et al., Functional expression of neurokinin 1 receptors on mast cells induced by IL-4 and stem cell factor. *J. Immunol.*, 171, 2074–2079, 2003.
181. Janiszewski J. et al., Picomolar doses of substance P trigger electrical responses in mast cells without degranulation. *Am. J. Physiol.*, 267, C138–145, 1994.
182. Hua, X.Y. and Yaksh, T.L., Pharmacology of the effects of bradykinin, serotonin, and histamine on the release of calcitonin gene-related peptide from C-fiber terminals in the rat trachea. *J. Neurosci.*, 13, 1947–1953, 1993.
183. Levi-Montalcini, R. et al., Nerve growth factor: from neurotrophin to neurokine. *Trends Neurosci.*, 19, 514–520, 1996.
184. Michaelis, M. et al., Inflammatory mediators sensitize acutely axotomized nerve fibers to mechanical stimulation in the rat. *J. Neurosci.*, 18, 7581–7587, 1998.
185. Nemmar, A. et al., Modulatory effect of imetit, a histamine H3 receptor agonist, on C-fibers, cholinergic fibers and mast cells in rabbit lungs *in vitro*. *Eur. J. Pharmacol.*, 371, 23–30, 1999.
186. Hu, Z.Q. et al., Down-regulation by IL-4 and up-regulation by IFN-gamma of mast cell induction from mouse spleen cells. *J. Immunol.*, 156, 3925–3931, 1996.
187. Kashiba, H. et al., Gene expression of histamine H1 receptor in guinea pig primary sensory neurons: a relationship between H1 receptor mRNA-expressing neurons and peptidergic neurons. *Brain Res. Mol. Brain Res.*, 66, 24–34., 1999.
188. Shubayev, V.I. and Myers, R.R., Axonal transport of TNF-alpha in painful neuropathy: distribution of ligand tracer and TNF receptors. *J. Neuroimmunol.*, 114, 48–56, 2001.

189. Undem, B.J. et al., Immunologically induced neuromodulation of guinea pig nodose ganglion neurons. *J. Auton. Nerv. Syst.*, 44, 35–44, 1993.
190. Fischer, A. et al., Induction of tachykinin gene and peptide expression in guinea pig nodose primary afferent neurons by allergic airway inflammation. *J. Clin. Invest.*, 98, 2284–2291, 1996.
191. Maggi, C.A., The effects of tachykinins on inflammatory and immune cells. *Regul. Pept.*, 70, 75–90, 1997.
192. Marshall, J.S. et al., Nerve growth factor modifies the expression of inflammatory cytokines by mast cells via a prostanoid-dependent mechanism. *J. Immunol.*, 162, 4271–4276, 1999.
193. Marshall, J.S. et al., The role of mast cell degranulation products in mast cell hyperplasia. I. Mechanism of action of nerve growth factor. *J. Immunol.*, 144, 1886–1892, 1990.
194. Horigome, K. et al., Mediator release from mast cells by nerve growth factor. Neurotrophin specificity and receptor mediation. *J. Biol. Chem.*, 268, 14881–14887, 1993.
195. Lindsay, R.M. and Harmar, A.J., Nerve growth factor regulates expression of neuropeptide genes in adult sensory neurons. *Nature*, 337, 362–364, 1989.
196. Miyajima, I. et al., Systemic anaphylaxis in the mouse can be mediated largely through IgG1 and FcγRIII. Assessment of the cardiopulmonary changes, mast cell degranulation, and death associated with active or IgE- or IgG1-dependent passive anaphylaxis. *J. Clin. Invest.*, 99, 901–914, 1997.
197. Grabbe, S. and Schwarz, T., Immunoregulatory mechanisms involved in elicitation of allergic contact hypersensitivity. *Immunol. Today*, 19, 37–44, 1998.
198. Biedermann, T. et al., Mast cells control neutrophil recruitment during T cell-mediated delayed-type hypersensitivity reactions through tumor necrosis factor and macrophage inflammatory protein 2. *J. Exp. Med.*, 192, 1441–1452, 2000.
199. Krasteva, M. et al., Contact dermatitis I. Pathophysiology of contact sensitivity. *Eur. J. Dermatol.*, 9, 65–77, 1999.
200. Tsuji, R.F. et al., B cell-dependent T cell responses: IgM antibodies are required to elicit contact sensitivity. *J. Exp. Med.*, 196, 1277–1290, 2002.
201. Askenase, P.W. et al., Defective elicitation of delayed-type hypersensitivity in W/Wv and SI/SId mast cell-deficient mice. *J. Immunol.*, 131, 2687–2694, 1983.
202. Paliwal, V. et al., Subunits of IgM reconstitute defective contact sensitivity in B-1 cell-deficient xid mice: kappa light chains recruit T cells independent of complement. *J. Immunol.*, 169, 4113–4123, 2002.
203. Williams, C.M. and Galli, S.J., Mast cells can amplify airway reactivity and features of chronic inflammation in an asthma model in mice. *J. Exp. Med.*, 192, 455–462, 2000.
204. Secor, V.H. et al., Mast cells are essential for early onset and severe disease in a murine model of multiple sclerosis. *J. Exp. Med.*, 191, 813–822, 2000.
205. Louis, J.A. et al., The use of the murine model of infection with Leishmania major to reveal the antagonistic effects that IL-4 can exert on T helper cell development and demonstrate that these opposite effects depend upon the nature of the cells targeted for IL-4 signaling. *Pathol. Biol.* (Paris), 51, 71–73, 2003.
206. Wershil, B.K. et al., Mast cells augment lesion size and persistence during experimental *Leishmania major* infection in the mouse. *J. Immunol.*, 152, 4563–4571, 1994.
207. von Stebut, E. et al., Early macrophage influx to sites of cutaneous granuloma formation is dependent on MIP-1alpha/beta released from neutrophils recruited by mast cell-derived TNFalpha. *Blood*, 101, 210–215, 2003.
208. Staite, N.D. et al., Inhibition of delayed-type contact hypersensitivity in mice deficient in both E-selectin and P-selectin. *Blood*, 88, 2973–2979, 1996.
209. McHale, J.F. et al., Vascular endothelial cell expression of ICAM-1 and VCAM-1 at the onset of eliciting contact hypersensitivity in mice: evidence for a dominant role of TNF-alpha. *J. Immunol.*, 162, 1648–1655, 1999.
210. Biedermann, T. et al., Reversal of established delayed type hypersensitivity reactions following therapy with IL-4 or antigen-specific Th2 cells. *Eur J. Immunol.*, 31, 1582–1591, 2001.
211. Racke, M.K. et al., Cytokine-induced immune deviation as a therapy for inflammatory autoimmune disease. *J. Exp. Med.*, 180, 1961–1966, 1994.
212. Benoist, C. and Mathis, D., Mast cells in autoimmune disease. *Nature*, 420, 875–878, 2002.

213. Pedotti, R. et al., Involvement of both "allergic" and "autoimmune" mechanisms in EAE, MS and other autoimmune diseases. *Trends Immunol.*, 24, 479–484, 2003.
214. Zappulla, J.P. et al., Mast cells: new targets for multiple sclerosis therapy? *J. Neuroimmunol.*, 131, 5–20, 2002.
215. Zuberbier, T. et al., Aromatic components of food as novel eliciting factors of pseudoallergic reactions in chronic urticaria. *J. Allergy Clin. Immunol.*, 109, 343–348, 2002.
216. Edston, E. and van Hage-Hamsten, M., Mast cell tryptase and hemolysis after trauma. *Forensic Sci. Int.*, 131, 8–13, 2003.
217. Kakurai, M. et al., Activation of mast cells by silver particles in a patient with localized argyria due to implantation of acupuncture needles. *Br. J. Dermatol.*, 148, 822, 2003.
218. Durham, S.R., The inflammatory nature of allergic disease. *Clin. Exp. Allergy*, 28(Suppl. 6), 20–24, 1998.
219. Yamaguchi, M. et al., IgE enhances Fc epsilon receptor I expression and IgE-dependent release of histamine and lipid mediators from human umbilical cord blood-derived mast cells: synergistic effect of IL-4 and IgE on human mast cell Fc epsilon receptor I expression and mediator release. *J. Immunol.*, 162, 5455–5465, 1999.
220. Vercelli, D. and Geha, R.S., The IgE system. *Ann. Allergy*, 63, 4–11, 1989.
221. Baroody, F.M. and Naclerio, R.M., Antiallergic effects of H1-receptor antagonists. *Allergy*, 55(Suppl. 64), 17–27, 2000.
222. Gronneberg, R. and Zetterstrom, O., Effect of disodium cromoglycate on anti-IgE induced early and late skin response in humans. *Clin. Allergy*, 15, 167–171, 1985.
223. Ring, J. et al., Antihistamines in urticaria. *Clin. Exp. Allergy*, 29(Suppl. 1), 31–37, 1999.
224. Ciprandi, G. et al., Terfenadine exerts antiallergic activity reducing ICAM-1 expression on nasal epithelial cells in patients with pollen allergy. *Clin. Exp. Allergy*, 25, 871–878, 1995.
225. Katsuda, S. et al., Systemic mastocytosis without cutaneous involvement. *Acta Pathol. Jpn.*, 37, 167–177, 1987.
226. Horny, H.P. et al., Bone marrow mastocytosis associated with an undifferentiated extramedullary tumor of hemopoietic origin. *Arch. Pathol. Lab. Med.*, 121, 423–426, 1997.
227. Delsignore, J.L. et al., Mastocytosis presenting as a skeletal disorder. *Iowa Orthop. J.*, 16, 126–134, 1996.
228. Valent, P. et al., Diagnostic criteria and classification of mastocytosis: a consensus proposal. *Leukocyte Res.*, 25, 603–625, 2001.
229. Mirowski, G. et al., Characterization of cellular dermal infiltrates in human cutaneous mastocytosis. *Lab. Invest.*, 63, 52–62, 1990.
230. Maslak, P., Mast cell leukemia. *Blood*, 101, 789, 2003.
231. Biedermann, T. et al., Mastocytosis associated with severe wasp sting anaphylaxis detected by elevated serum mast cell tryptase levels. *Br. J. Dermatol.*, 141, 1110–1112, 1999.
232. Ludolph-Hauser, D. et al., Mast cells in an angiosarcoma complicating xeroderma pigmentosum in a 13-year-old girl. *J. Am. Acad. Dermatol.*, 43, 900–002, 2000.
233. Weber, A. et al., Pattern analysis of human cutaneous mast cell populations by total body surface mapping. *Br. J. Dermatol.*, 148, 224–228, 2003.
234. Yamamoto, T. et al., Expression of stem cell factor in basal cell carcinoma. *Br. J. Dermatol.*, 137, 709–713, 1997.
235. Grimbaldeston, M.A. et al., Communications: high dermal mast cell prevalence is a predisposing factor for basal cell carcinoma in humans. *J. Invest. Dermatol.*, 115, 317–320, 2000.
236. Steinhoff, M. et al., Proteinase-activated receptor-2 in human skin: tissue distribution and activation of keratinocytes by mast cell tryptase. *Exp. Dermatol.*, 8, 282–294, 1999.
237. Rukwied, R. et al., Mast cell mediators other than histamine induce pruritus in atopic dermatitis patients: a dermal microdialysis study. *Br. J. Dermatol.*, 142, 1114–1120, 2000.
238. Ackermann, L. et al., Mast cells in psoriatic skin are strongly positive for interferon-gamma. *Br. J. Dermatol.*, 140, 624–633, 1999.
239. Jiang, W.Y. et al., Mast cell density and IL-8 expression in nonlesional and lesional psoriatic skin. *Int. J. Dermatol.*, 40, 699–703, 2001.
240. Wintroub, B.U. et al., Morphologic and functional evidence for release of mast-cell products in bullous pemphigoid. *N. Engl. J. Med.*, 298, 417–421, 1978.

241. Katayama, I. et al., High histamine level in the blister fluid of bullous pemphigoid. *Arch. Dermatol. Res.*, 276, 126–127, 1984.
242. Rocken, M. and Hultner, L., Heavy functions for light chains. *Nat. Med.*, 8, 668–670, 2002.
243. Chen, R. et al., Mast cells play a key role in neutrophil recruitment in experimental bullous pemphigoid. *J. Clin. Invest.*, 108, 1151–1158, 2001.
244. Ghoreschi, K. et al., Interleukin-4 therapy of psoriasis induces Th2 responses and improves human autoimmune disease. *Nat. Med.*, 9, 40–46, 2003.

# 11 Neutrophils, Eosinophils, and Basophils in the Skin Immune System

*Edward F. Knol, Taco W. Kuijpers, and Dirk Roos*

## CONTENTS



## I. GRANULOCYTE LIFE CYCLE

Granulocytes and macrophages form the nonspecific cellular defense against microorganisms and parasites, and also remove infected host cells, aged cells, and other degraded body constituents. Three types of granulocyte can be distinguished: neutrophilic granulocytes (neutrophils), eosinophilic granulocytes (eosinophils), and basophilic granulocytes (basophils).

Under normal conditions, neutrophils constitute 40 to 70% of the circulating leukocytes, whereas eosinophils and basophils together form at most 5% of the leukocytes. The common morphological feature of these cells is the presence of many granules in the cytoplasm. Neutrophils and eosinophils are capable of phagocytosis of particulate material and use the contents of their granules for killing ingested microorganisms and for extracellular lysis of parasites. Basophils lack this ability; these cells possess histamine-containing granules, which — upon release — cause blood vessel dilatation in local inflammatory reactions. In addition, eosinophils and basophils are involved in the effector phase of allergic inflammations.[1]

0-8493-1959-5/05/$0.00+$1.50

## A. Maturation

Granulocytes develop in the bone marrow from a common primordial stem cell in about 2 weeks. Early in development, granulocyte differentiation diverges. Neutrophil myelocytes share a common precursor with the monocyte/macrophage lineage, whereas basophils and eosinophils develop from a common, separate precursor. During early development of the various granulocytes, differentiation is controlled by many cytokines that lack lineage specificity, such as granulocyte/macrophage colony-stimulating factor (GM-CSF) and interleukin-3 (IL-3). Differentiation of CFU-GM (colony-forming units granulocytes-macrophages) into neutrophils and monocytes is accomplished by granulocyte-CSF (G-CSF) and macrophage-CSF (M-CSF), respectively.[2]

IL-5 is involved in the terminal differentiation of eosinophils, whereas transforming growth factor b (TGF-) selectively induces basophil but not eosinophil differentiation in the presence of IL-3. A close relation between eosinophils and basophils in the myeloid differentiation has further been suggested by their concomitant presence in cultures of myeloid precursor cells from bone marrow or cord blood and by the presence of hybrid eosinophilic/basophilic granulocytes in these cultures. Similar cells with both eosinophilic and basophilic characteristics are found in some leukemic disorders.

Recent insight into the molecular structure and function of many of the adhesion molecules, in particular the integrin receptors, indicates that the adhesion molecules may not only play a role in cell binding (see later), but also in processes such as early gene transcription, cytokine synthesis, and cellular survival. It is intriguing to speculate that adhesion molecules may also modulate granulocyte differentiation, e.g., by binding to specific bone marrow stromal elements.[2]

## B. Morphology

During myeloid differentiation, the cells undergo a series of characteristic changes in morphology. In the promyelocyte stage of neutrophils, azurophil granules are formed. Through cell division, these granules are divided over the daughter cells. In the subsequent neutrophil myelocyte stage, specific granules are formed. Azurophil granules contain cytotoxic proteins; specific granules contain cell surface receptors and enzymes that degrade extracellular matrix proteins (Table 11.1).[1] In fully differentiated neutrophils, the ratio of azurophil to specific granules is about 1:2. Eosinophils possess only one type of granule, in the mature state characterized by a typical crystal core. These eosinophil granules contain a number of negatively charged, cytotoxic proteins that are used for killing parasites, but may also cause tissue damage in allergic reactions (Table 11.1).[3] Basophil granules contain histamine bound to a proteoglycan matrix (Table 11.1). The specific staining of these granules with neutral, acidic, or basic dyes has earned the different granulocytes their names.[4] Recently, it has been described that apart from basophils and eosinophils, also neutrophils can store and release cytokines and chemokines. Via the release of these cytokines the granulocytes have an additional function in modulating the inflammatory immune response. An overview of the cytokines and chemokines stored in granulocytes is given in Table 11.2.

During the second week of differentiation, the granulocytes do not divide anymore, but the nucleus condenses into its final appearance. In neutrophils, the nucleus is strongly lobulated, and these cells are therefore also called polymorphonuclear leukocytes (PMN). Eosinophils are characterized by a typical bilobed nucleus, whereas basophils also contain a lobulated nucleus, which is difficult to discriminate due to many basophilic granules. Figure 11.1 shows an example of each cell type as each appears under the electron microscope.

## C. Tissue Phase

Two days after the granulocytes have reached their mature morphology, they are released from the bone marrow into the blood. The cytokines and adhesion molecules involved in this emigration process are not known, although downregulation of the chemokine receptor CXCR4, to escape

**TABLE 11.1**
**Constituents of Granules**

| Neutrophils | | | Eosinophils | | Basophils |
|---|---|---|---|---|---|
| **Azurophil Granules** | **Specific Granules** | **Secretory Vesicles** | **Specific Granules** | **Secretory Vesicles** | **Granules** |
| *Serine proteases* | | | *Cationic proteins* | | *Cationic proteins* |
| Elastase | | | Major basic protein | | Major basic protein |
| Cathepsin G | | | Eosinophil cationic protein | | |
| Proteinase 3 | | | Eosinophil-derived neurotoxin | | |
| P29b (AGP7) | | | Eosinophil peroxidase | | |
| *Acid hydrolase* | | | | | |
| β-Glucuronidase | | | | | |
| β-Glycerophosphatase | | | | | |
| *N*-Acetyl-β-glucosaminidase | | | | | |
| α-Mannosidase | | | | | |
| Cathepsin B | | | | | |
| Cathepsin D | | | | | |
| *Metalloproteases* | | | | | |
| | Collegenase (MMP-8) | | | | |
| | Gelatinase (MMP-9 | | | | |
| Leukolysin (MMP-25) | Leukolysin (MMP-25) | Leukolysin (MMP-25) | | | |
| *Other proteins* | | | | | |
| Myeloperoxidase | Neutral a-glycosidase | Albumin | Charcol-Leyden crystal protein | Histaminase | Charcol-Leyden crystal protein |
| CRISP3 | CRISP3 | | CRISP3 | | |
| Lysozyme | Lysozyme | Tetranectin | Arylsulfatase B | Albumin | |
| Azurocidin | Histaminase | | Acid phosphatase | CR3 (CD11b/CD18) | Histamine |
| Defensins | Lactoferrin | | BPI | | Proteoglycans |
| BPI | Vitamin $B_{12}$-binding protein | | | | Endopeptidase |
| Protoglycans | γ-Glutamyltransferase | | | | Basogranulin |
| | hCAP-18 | | | | |

**TABLE 11.1 (Continued)**
**Constituents of Granules**

| | Neutrophils | | Eosinophils | | Basophils |
|---|---|---|---|---|---|
| **Azurophil Granules** | **Specific Granules** | **Secretory Vesicles** | **Specific Granules** | **Secretory Vesicles** | **Granules** |
| *In membranes* | | | | | |
| Granulophysin 53 (CD63) | Aminopeptidase N (CD13) | Aminopeptidase N (CD13) | Granulophysin 53 (CD63) | Cytochrome *b*558 | Granulophysin 53 (CD63) |
| CD68 | LFA-1 (CD11a/CD18) | LFA-1 (CD11a/CD18) | | | |
| | CR3 (CD11b/CD18) | CR3 (CD11b/CD18) | CR3 (CD11b/CD18) | | FcεRI subunits |
| | P150, 95 (CD11c/Cd18) | P150, 95 (CD11c/Cd18) | | | CR3 (CD11b/CD18) |
| | Tyrosine phosphatase (CD45) | Tyrosine phosphatase (CD45) | FcεRI subunits | | |
| | CEA-6 (CD66b) | CEA-6 (CD66b) | CEA-6 (CD66b) | CEA-6 (CD66b) | |
| | Cytochrome $b_{558}$ | Cytochrome $b_{558}$ | | | |
| | Flavoproteins | CR1 (CD35) | | | |
| | fMLP receptor | fMLP receptor | | | |
| | | FcγRIIIb | | | |
| | | Alkaline phosphatase | | | |
| | TC-1 | CD14 | | | |

**TABLE 11.2**
**Cytokines and Chemokines Produced by Granulocytes**

| Neutrophils | Eosinophils | Basophils |
|---|---|---|
| IL-1β | IL-1α | IL-1α |
| IL-4 | IL-3 | IL-4 |
| IL-8 | IL-4 | IL-8 |
| IL-10 | IL-5 | IL-13 |
| IL-12 | IL-6 | MIP-1α |
| TGF-β | IL-8 | RANTES |
| VEGF | IL-10 | |
| TNF-α | IL-12 | |
| MIP-1α | IL-16 | |
| MIP-1β | GM-CSF | |
| MIP-3α | TGF-α | |
| IP-10 | TGF-β | |
| | TNF-α | |
| | MIP-1α | |
| | RANTES | |

from the SDF1 generated by the bone marrow stromal cells, has been postulated as an important mechanism. The cells remain in the circulation for only 6 to 10 h, and then move into the tissues to perform their functions (blood-borne infections are eliminated by liver macrophages). In the tissues, granulocytes retain the ability to migrate, which enables fast recruitment of these cells into areas of inflammation. Figure 11.2 shows the presence of neutrophils, eosinophils, and basophils in skin. The molecular details of granulocyte migration are described in the next section of this chapter.

The survival time of granulocytes in the tissues is not exactly known. In healthy individuals, neutrophil survival in the tissues is estimated at 1 to 2 days. During infections and after heavy loss of blood, this period is longer, up to 4 days. Under such conditions, more immature neutrophils with a rodlike nucleus are released in the blood, and the total number can be increased from $10^{11}$ per day in healthy adults to $10^{12}$ per day. In contrast, eosinophils and basophils can have longer tissue survival times (probably up to several weeks). Binding of these cells to extracellular matrix components prolongs their survival. During parasitic infections or manifestations of allergic disease, the production of eosinophils may be dramatically increased, also characterized by the appearance of more immature cells with a less lobulated nucleus.

At the end of their life cycle, granulocytes — if not lost from mucosal tissues — can be disposed in two ways. When the cells have been engaged in phagocytosis and/or degranulation, they will become necrotic due to the toxic properties of their own constituents. When the cells are still intact, apoptosis will end their life. Granulocytes, and especially neutrophils, are programmed for a very limited survival time, which restricts the extent of inflammation. Phagocytosis enhances apoptosis, whereas inflammatory mediators, such as G-CSF, GM-CSF, and chemokines, prolong survival time. Thus, release of G-CSF at an inflammatory site has at least three different effects: it increases the generation of neutrophils in the bone marrow, it enhances the release of these cells from the bone marrow into the circulation, and it increases the survival time of these cells in the tissues. Apoptosis is aimed at protection of the surroundings, because it involves a series of intracellular changes that retards cell lysis. Among these are changes in the plasma membrane, e.g., the exposure of phosphatidyl serine, and fragmentation of the DNA in the nucleus. Necrotic as well as apoptotic cells are then phagocytized and degraded by macrophages. The site of this disposal is not known.

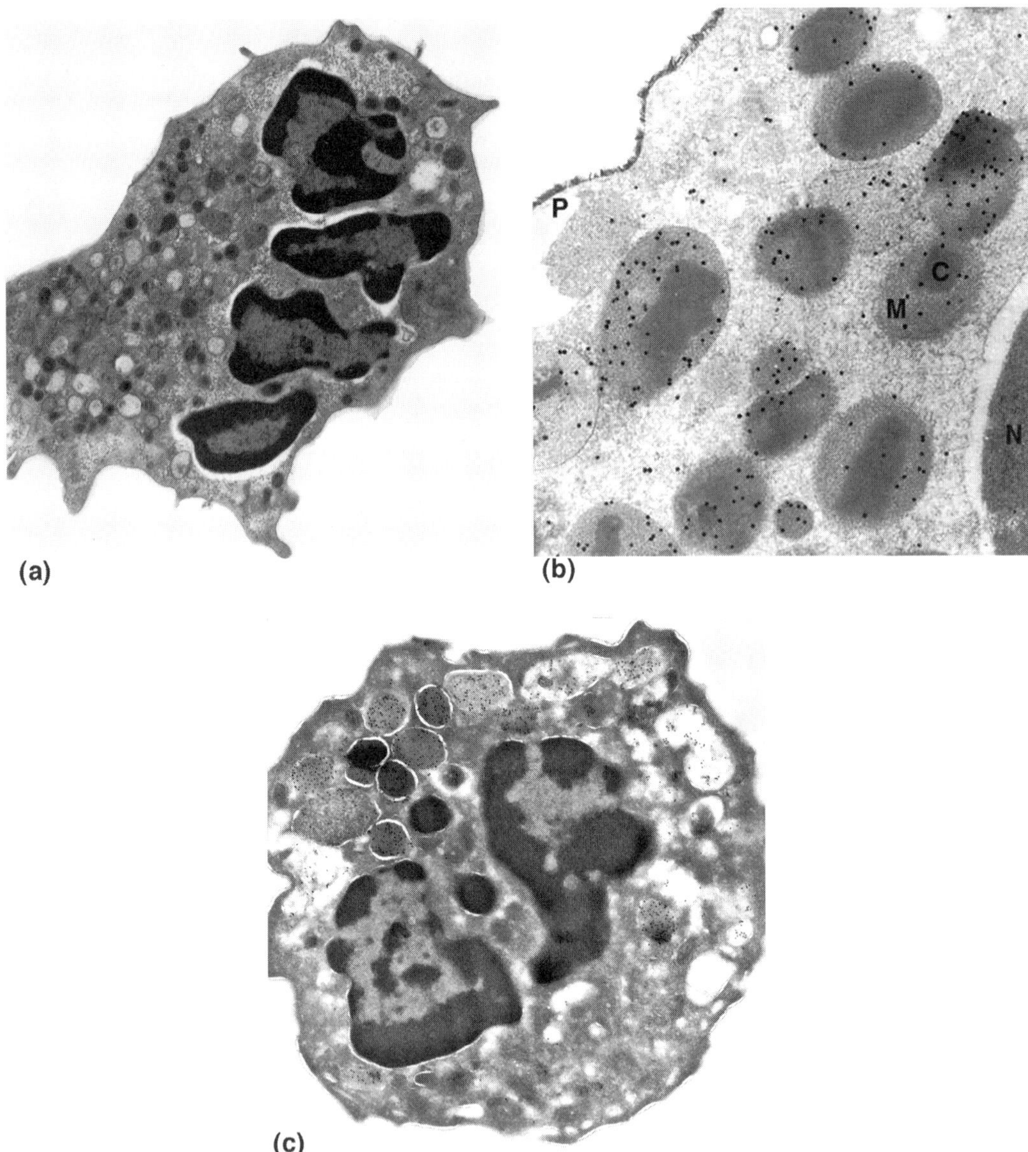


FIGURE 11.1 Morphology of mature neutrophil, eosinophil, and basophil, as depicted by transmission EM. (a) Neutrophil (from human blood). Note the multilobed nucleus, the electron-dense (azurophilic) and electron-lucent (specific) granules and the glycogen-containing storage vesicles (speckled areas). (b) Eosinophil (from human blood). A part of the eosinophil is depicted. The small electron-dense particles depict antibody binding to eosinophil cationic protein. ECP is most prominent in the matrix (M) of the granules and is occasionally found in the core (C) of the granules, the nucleus (N), and cytoplasm. (c) Basophil (from human blood). Note the large number of granules of varying electron density. The small electron-dense particles depict the binding of the BB1 antibody to basogranulin.

## II. GRANULOCYTE MIGRATION

Although a constant movement of granulocytes from the circulation into the tissues exists, not much is known of this process under normal conditions. About half of the total number of granulocytes in the blood is "marginated," i.e., adheres the blood vessel walls. The other half

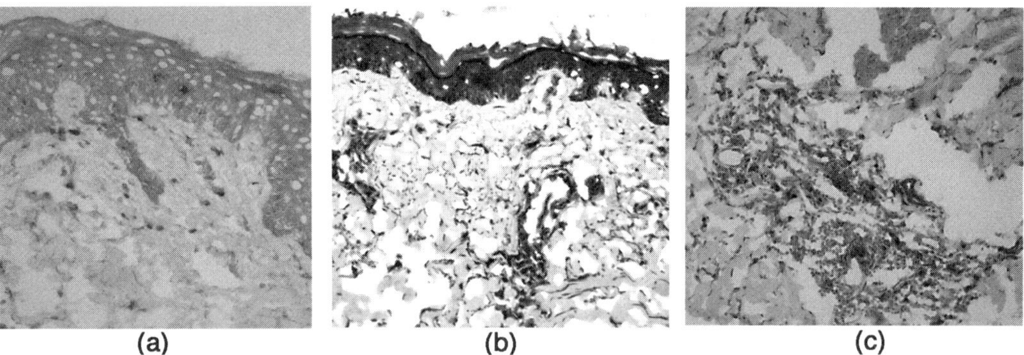


**FIGURE 11.2 (See color insert following page 304.)** Detection of granulocytes in skin by immunohistochemistry. (a) Neutrophil presence in the skin 18 h after UV irradiation of normal healthy skin. Neutrophils (red) are stained for their specific elastase content. Note that apart from neutrophil presence in the dermis, neutrophil infiltration is also found in the epidermis. (b) Eosinophil infiltration in the skin of a patient with AD 24 h after an atopy patch test. Eosinophils (red) are stained with EG2 antibody binding to eosinophil cationic protein. Eosinophil presence is predominantly perivascular. (c) Detail of basophil infiltration in the skin of an allergic patient 18 h after intracutaneous skin testing. Basophils (red) are stained with BB1 antibody binding to basogranulin and are located in the perivascular infiltrate.

circulates with the blood through the body. This marginated pool can be forced to reenter the circulating pool by agents such as adrenalin or exercise.

In inflammatory regions, granulocyte migration into the tissues is strongly increased. Inflammation involves a complex series of events, including vasodilation, increased vascular permeability, and exudation of fluids and plasma proteins. Several chemotactic mediators are generated at the site of the lesion that can bind to specific receptors on the surface of the various leukocytes and induce these cells to move to the inflammatory site. Other inflammatory mediators affect the local vascular endothelial cells by upregulating specific adhesion molecules on these cells. In this way, a coordinated repertoire is started of granulocyte adherence to vascular endothelium, diapedesis out of the bloodstream and subsequent migration into the adjacent tissues toward the site of inflammation.[1]

Most studies on leukocyte adherence and transmigration have been performed with neutrophils. Based on studies *in vitro* with flow chambers and *in vivo* by intravital microscopy, three subsequent processes have been recognized that determine the extravasation of neutrophils to sites of inflammation (Figure 11.3). After initial, weak, and reversible binding to postcapillary endothelial cells, shear force in the circulation will drag the neutrophils over the endothelium, resulting in the first process of so-called "rolling." Rolling decreases the velocity of the neutrophils, and the cells will finally come to a stop or resume circulation in the bloodstream. The rolling phenomenon is mediated by selectin–carbohydrate interactions that are relatively resistant to the shear forces produced by laminar flow. The second process is "adhesion-strengthening" during which the neutrophils also exhibit spreading on the endothelial cells. This occurs through activation of adhesion molecules of the integrin supergene family on the neutrophils. The adhering neutrophils are now able to crawl between the endothelial cells to emigrate in response to locally produced platelet-activating factor (PAF) and IL-8 and to chemotactic factors diffusing from the extravascular site of inflammation. This third process is called endothelial transmigration or diapedesis.[5]

Within the tissues, the neutrophils (and other leukocytes) migrate toward the origin of the chemotactic factor production, i.e., the inflammatory site, by their ability to sense the concentration gradient of these agents. In this process of chemotaxis, reversible integrin activation and deactivation induces crawling of the cells over extracellular matrix components.[6] In the course of these events, transmigration of the leukocytes through mesothelial cell layers (into the peritoneal cavity) and epithelial cell layers (into organ lumen) may also occur.

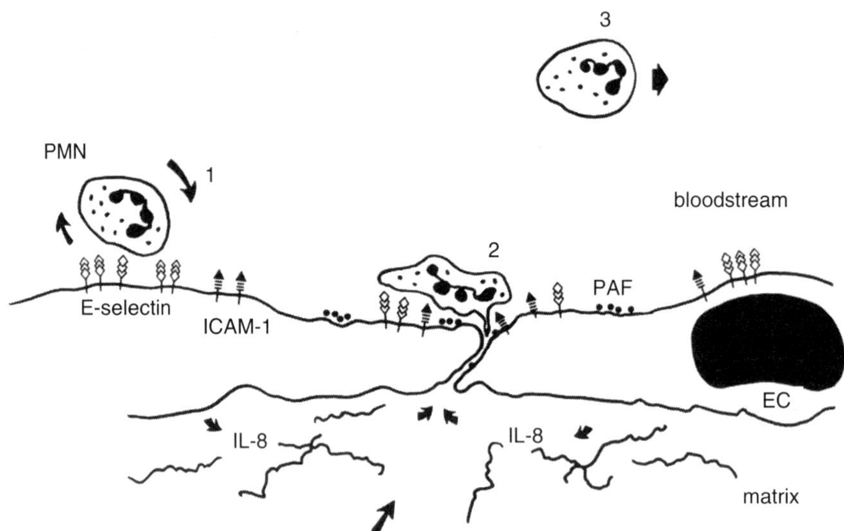


**FIGURE 11.3** Schematic representation of neutrophil rolling, adherence, and diapedesis.1 = Neutrophils in the bloodstream are slowed down by initial, reversible contact of L-selectin on the neutrophils with $Le^x$ sugar ligands on the endothelial cells, and of E-selectin on the endothelial cells with $SLe^x$ sugar ligands on the neutrophils. 2 = This neutrophil rolling changes into stable adhesion by activation of CR3 on the neutrophils, which then binds ICAM-1 on the endothelial cells. PAF and IL-8, produced by activated endothelial cells, form a haptotactic gradient that induces neutrophil diapedesis into the tissues. 3 = Neutrophils without activated CR3 detach from the vessel wall and continue circulation in the bloodstream. (From Kuijpers, T.W. and Roos, D., *Behring Inst. Mitt.*, 92, 10, 1993. With permission,)

## A. Adherence

Selectins are carbohydrate-binding proteins that consist of a lectin domain, an epidermal growth factor domain, a variable number of repetitive short consensus repeats (SCR), an intramembrane domain, and a cytosolic domain. L-selectin (constitutively expressed on leukocytes) contains two SCR domains, E-selectin (on activated endothelial cells) contains six SCR domains, and P-selectin (on degranulated endothelial cells and platelets) contains eight or nine SCR domains (Table 11.3). P-selectin and E-selectin on activated endothelial cells are involved in neutrophil and eosinophil rolling, and this is expected to hold true for the basophils as well. The expression pattern of E-selectin is dependent on *de novo* synthesis and can be induced by the inflammatory cytokines tumor necrosis factor (TNF) and IL-1, or bacterial endotoxins. In activated endothelial cells from umbilical veins, E-selectin expression is maximal at 4 to 6 h, with a decline to near baseline by 24 h. Levels of expression *in vivo* do not seem to follow the same transient time course as is observed *in vitro*.[5]

P-selectin (CD62P) is rapidly and transiently expressed for only 10 to 30 min upon histamine or thrombin treatment of cultured endothelial cells, coinciding with fusion of Weibel–Palade bodies with the plasma membrane. In addition, a role for P-selectin in later phases of leukocyte adherence is predicted by the findings of continued mRNA expression in activated endothelium in mice. This observation is in keeping with the demonstration that CD62P monoclonal antibodies (mAbs) produce prolonged protection against tissue injury following ischemia-reperfusion and lung injury upon massive complement activation. Moreover, P-selectin knockout mice have been demonstrated to be impaired in their leukocyte rolling. To date, such prolonged upregulation has not been established in humans.[7]

The sugar determinants recognized by the three selectin receptors are believed to be related, but not identical oligosaccharide epitopes on glycoproteins and/or glycolipids. All three selectins have in common that they are able to bind to the sialylated Lewis-X antigen ($SLe^x$), which probably

**TABLE 11.3**
**Cell Adhesion Molecules**

| Structure | Antibody Cluster | Ligand |
|---|---|---|
| **Immunoglobulin Superfamily** | | |
| LFA-3 | CD58 | CD2 |
| ICAM-1 | CD54 | LFA-1, CR3, CD43, $\alpha_D\beta_2$ |
| ICAM-2 | CD102 | LFA-1 |
| ICAM-3 | CD50 | $\alpha_D\beta_2$, LFA-1 |
| ICAM-4 | CD242 | LFA-1, CR3, $\alpha_{II}\beta_3$, VLA-4, $\alpha_V\beta_5$ |
| VCAM-1 | CD106 | VLA-4, Fn, $\alpha_4\beta_7$ |
| PECAM-1 | CD31 | PECAM-1 |
| MadCAM-1 | ? | $\alpha_4\beta_7$, L-selectin |

**Integrins**

| Structure | Nomenclature, Antibody Cluster | Ligand |
|---|---|---|
| ***Group I: Very Late Antigens or $\beta_1$ Antigens*** | | |
| $\alpha_1\beta_1$ | VLA-1, CD49a/CD29 | Coll (I,IV), Ln |
| $\alpha_2\beta_1$ | VLA-2, CD49b/CD29 | Coll (I-III), Ln |
| $\alpha_3\beta_1$ | VLA-3, CD49c/CD29 | Coll (I), Ln, Fn |
| $\alpha_4\beta_1$ | VLA-4, CD49d/CD29 | Fn, VCAM, ICAM-4 |
| $\alpha_5\beta_1$ | VLA-5, CD49e/CD29 | Fn |
| $\alpha_6\beta_1$ | VLA-6, CD49f/CD29 | Ln |
| $\alpha_7\beta_1$ | VLA-7, CD49g/CD29 | Ln |
| $\alpha_8\beta_1$ | VLA-8, CD49h/CD29 | Fn |
| $\alpha_9\beta_1$ | VLA-9, CD49i/CD29 | Tenascin |
| $\alpha_v\beta_1$ | alt. FnR, CD51/CD29 | Fn |
| ***Group II:LeuCAM or $\beta_2$ Integrins*** | | |
| $\alpha_L\beta_2$ | LFA-1, CD11a/CD18 | ICAM-1, ICAM-2, ICAM-3, ICAM-4 |
| $\alpha_M\beta_2$ | Mac-1, CD11b/CD18 | ICAM-1, iC3b, Factor X, Fb, Tsp, ICAM-4 |
| $\alpha_X\beta_2$ | p150, 95, CD11c/CD18 | IC3b, Fb |
| $\alpha_D\beta_2$ | ? | ICAM-3, ICAM-1, VCAM-1 |
| ***Group III: Cytoadhesins or $\beta_3$ Integrins*** | | |
| $\alpha_{II}\beta_3$ | GpIIb-IIIa, CD41/CD61 | Fb, Fn, vWF, Vn, Tsp, ICAM-4 |
| $\alpha_V\beta_3$ | VnR, CD51/CD61 | Fb, Fn, vWF, Vn, Tsp |
| $\alpha_R\beta_3$ | LRI, CD-/CD61 | Fb, Fn, vWF, Vn |
| ***Alternative $\beta$ Integrin Groups*** | | |
| $\alpha_6\beta_4$ | $\alpha_E\beta_6$, TSP180, CD49f/CD- | Ln |
| $\alpha_V\beta_5$ | $\alpha_v\beta_5$ | Fn, Vn, ICAM-4 |
| $\alpha_V\beta_6$ | ? | Vn, TGF-β3 |
| $\alpha_e\beta_7$ | M290, i.e., L antigen, βp, $\alpha_{HML}\beta_7$ | E-cadherin |
| $\alpha_4\beta_7$ | LPAM-1, CD49d/CD- | Fn, VCAM-1, MAdCAM-1 |
| $\alpha_V\beta_8$ | ? | Fn, Vn, Ln, Coll (IV), TGF-β |

**Selectins**

| Structure | Nomenclature, Antibody Cluster | Ligand |
|---|---|---|
| E-selectin | ELAM-1, CD62E | $SLe^x$, $SLe^a$, L-selectin, VIM-2, CLA |
| P-selectin | GMP-140, PADGEM, CD62P | $SLe^x$, $SLe^a$, $Le^x$, $Le^a$, L-selectin, PSGL-1, VIM-2 |
| L-selectin | LAM-1, Leu8, CD62L | $SLe^x$, $SLe^a$, CD34, GLYCAM-1, MAdCAM-1, E-selectin, P-selectin, VIM-2, heparin sulfate |

represents a major ligand for E-selectin and P-selectin on granulocytes. The carbohydrate moiety recognized on endothelial cells by granulocyte L-selectin is most probably E-selectin.[8] $SLe^x$ has not been found on the surface of endothelial cells, except for high endothelial venules (HEV) in lymphoid tissues. L- and P-selectin binding may to a certain extent depend on sulfatation of the oligosaccharide(s) involved in cell adhesion. On granulocytes, but not on lymphocytes, L-selectin contains oligosaccharide ligands for both E- and P-selectin, which allows binding of L-selectin to E- or P-selectin under shear stress. The rapid shedding of L-selectin upon granulocyte activation may be one way to regulate this process.[6]

The next phase of granulocyte extravasation involves adhesion strengthening and cell spreading mediated by integrin–ligand binding. Integrins are heterodimeric surface molecules present on many cell types, which bind to extracellular matrix proteins and/or immunoglobulin-like molecules (Table 11.3). Depending on the presence of a common β subunit, the integrins are classified as $\beta_1$, $\beta_2$, $\beta_3$, or alternative β integrins. A specific feature of the integrins is an increase in ligand binding upon cell activation, mediated through a reversible conformation change and cell-surface clustering of the integrins. This cell activation can be induced by binding of chemotactic factors, cytokines, or selectins to granulocyte surface structures.[5]

An important difference between eosinophilic and basophilic granulocytes vs. neutrophils is the expression of $\beta_1$ or very late antigen (VLA) integrin receptors on the first two cell types and only to a very limited extent on neutrophils (Table 11.3). Most attention has been paid to the function of VLA-4 ($\alpha_4\beta_1$) in leukocyte adherence to endothelial cells through binding to vascular cell adhesion molecule-1 (VCAM-1), a member of the immunoglobulin supergene family expressed on endothelial cells following activation by lipopolysaccharide (LPS), TNF, IL-1, IL-4, or IL-13. VLA-4-mediated granulocyte adherence to endothelial VCAM-1 may represent the first stage of an alternative, $\beta_2$-integrin-independent pathway for eosinophils and basophils to emigrate, similar to monocytes and lymphocytes.[9] Human VCAM-1 consists of two different variants, with six or seven Ig-like domains, as a result of alternative splicing. Both the 6- and 7-domain form support VLA-4-dependent cell binding; the 7-domain form predominates on endothelial cells.

VLA-4 also recognizes the extracellular matrix (ECM) protein fibronectin (FN) through binding to an alternatively spliced variant that contains part of the third connective segment (IIICS) domain, the so-called CS-1 domain. Eosinophils do not avidly bind to FN(CS-1) unless stimulated. To date, studies on the regulation of VLA-4 avidity on blood basophils have not been reported. Also, although one may expect the other $\beta_1$ integrin receptors on eosinophils to be regulated in their avidity for ligands as is VLA-4, this remains to be formally proved. Eosinophils and basophils also express $\alpha_4\beta_7$; however, its relevance is as yet obscure.[9]

*In vitro* studies indicate that granulocyte adherence to endothelial cells involves adhesion molecules of the $\beta_2$ integrin (CD11/CD18) subgroup (Table 11.3). These surface proteins are $\alpha_L\beta_2$ (lymphocyte function-associated antigen 1, or LFA-1), $\alpha_M\beta_2$ (macrophage protein 1, or Mac-1, or complement receptor 3, CR3), $\alpha_X\beta_2$ (protein 150, 95, or p150, 95, or CR4), and $\alpha_D\beta_2$. They bind to counterstructures of the immunoglobulin (Ig)-like supergene family — intercellular adhesion molecule (ICAM)-1, ICAM-2, ICAM-4, vascular adhesion molecule (VCAM)-1, and ligand(s) as yet to be identified.

The $\beta_2$ integrin receptors are rapidly upregulated from specific granules and secretory vesicles in neutrophils and eosinophils, and from the histamine-containing granules in basophils, after fusion of these organelles with the plasma membrane. Most likely, upregulation of LFA-1, Mac-1/CR3, and p150, 95 adhesion molecules per se does not contribute as significantly to granulocyte adherence as the aforementioned affinity and avidity changes.[5] Preactivation of eosinophils induces a shift from $\beta_1$ integrin (VLA-4) usage to $\beta_2$ integrin (CR3) usage, as required for extravascular mobility.

The relevance of these *in vitro* observations is found in the leukocyte adhesion deficiency syndromes (LAD)-I and -II. Neutrophils of patients with the LAD-I syndrome (lacking the $\beta_2$ subfamily of integrin receptors) show initial rolling but are unable to emigrate, a response clearly dependent on the expression and function of CD11/CD18 molecules. On the other hand, a few patients are known to suffer from recurrent infections due to lack of $SLe^x$ expression on their leukocytes, coined as the LAD-II syndrome. These patients' neutrophils are unable to show the process of rolling, and only show a reaction of neutrophil emigration when the shear force is reduced (as occurs in the dilated postcapillary venules at sites of inflammation).[5] The integrins on the surface of LAD-II leukocytes can then be activated by chemokines after binding to their respective receptors on the leukocytes.

## B. Diapedesis

After tight adhesion and spreading of granulocytes on vascular endothelium, the granulocytes start to squeeze between the endothelial cells. Several conditions need to be fulfilled for this process. First, the tight junctions between two adjacent endothelial cells have to open up, to allow passage to the granulocytes. Indications exist that this process results from cross-linking of endothelial surface proteins (e.g., ICAM-1 and VCAM-1) by the adhering granulocytes. Second, the connections between endothelial cell ligands and integrin receptors on the granulocytes must be broken, to allow movement of the granulocytes over the endothelial cell surface. Third, to give direction to the granulocyte movement, a concentration gradient of chemotaxins must exist. This gradient may be derived from extravascular origin (infecting microorganisms or activated tissue-dwelling cells) or may originate from activated endothelium. In both situations (often concurrent), the chemotaxins belong to the so-called C-X-C α subgroup or C-C β subgroup of chemokines, depending on the presence or absence of an amino acid between two cysteines at a fixed position in these proteins (Table 11.4). Probably, the endothelium-derived chemokines form a concentration gradient on the endothelial cell surface by attachment to extracellular matrix proteins. Possibly, such a haptotactic gradient activates the granulocytes to form new $\beta_2$-integrin-ligand connections at the

**TABLE 11.4**
**Binding Specificity of Chemotactic Stimuli for Human Leukocytes**

| | Neutrophils | Eosinophils | Basophils |
|---|---|---|---|
| PAF | +++ | +++ | +++ |
| fMLP | +++ | ++ | ++ |
| C3a | – | ++ | ++ |
| C5a | +++ | ++ | ++ |
| C5a(des-Arg) | + | – | ++ |
| $LTB_4$ | + | + | + |
| **C-X-C Family of Chemokines** | | | |
| IL-8 | +++ | ++ | ++ |
| GROα, β, or γ | + | – | + |
| CTAP-III, NAP-2 | + | – | + |
| PF4 | + | – | + |
| **C-X-C Family of Chemokines** | | | |
| RANTES | – | ++ | ++ |
| MIP-1α | – | + | + |
| MIP-1β | – | – | +/– |
| MCP-1 | – | – | +++ |
| MCP-2 | – | + | + |
| MCP-3 | – | + | + |
| MCP-4 | – | + | + |
| Eotaxin, -2, -3 | – | +++ | ++ |

front of the moving granulocytes, and to disrupt such connections at the tail end of these cells.[6] In addition, homologous platelet-endothelial cell adhesion molecule-1 (PECAM-1; CD31) connections between endothelial cells and granulocytes also promote diapedesis.[5]

For neutrophils, endothelium-derived PAF and IL-8 have been shown to be essential agents for diapedesis in case extravascular chemotaxins are lacking.[10] IL-8 acts in a strictly neutrophil-specific fashion, but PAF and β-subgroup chemokines such as monocyte chemoattractant protein-3 (MCP-3) and RANTES (regulated upon activation, normal T-cell expressed and secreted) are candidate chemoattractants involved in eosinophil and basophil diapedesis through endothelium.[11]

Neutrophils are initially the predominant leukocytes at sites of acute inflammation, with the peak of emigration generally occurring in the first few hours. Subsequently, mononuclear phagocytes derived from blood monocytes become the most abundant cell type.[4] Eosinophils and basophils are found especially at sites of allergic inflammation.[9] These differences in kinetics of emigration and accumulation, as well as the site specificity, are probably due to multiple cellular mechanisms, including production of local cytokines and chemoattractants in the inflamed tissues, up- or down-regulation of both leukocytic and endothelial adhesion molecules, and alterations in the avidity of leukocyte integrins. For example, during the process of leukocyte rolling, an eosinophil-specific epitope on L-selectin (recognized by the LAM1-11 mAb), and during the static adhesion, the more abundant expression of VLA-4 on eosinophils and basophils can selectively regulate the adhesion of these cells to the vessel wall. The latter process is also favored by the specific expression of VCAM-1 and the production of MCP-3 and RANTES by IL-4-activated endothelium. By the use of specific mAbs, we have demonstrated that, during diapedesis through a monolayer of cultured human umbilical vein endothelial cells, eosinophils utilize FN(CS-1), and not VCAM-1, as the ligand for VLA-4. IL-5, predominantly produced by T lymphocytes at sites of allergic inflammation, is a specific activator of eosinophils and basophils. Whether adhesion molecules found only at sites of allergic inflammation, as has been demonstrated in murine lung microvasculature, or eosinophil-specific chemokines, as has been demonstrated in guinea pigs, play a role in selective accumulation, is not yet known.[11]

## C. Chemotaxis

Directed cell movement is called chemotaxis. Leukocytes are able to recognize concentration differences in a gradient of inflammatory agents and to direct their movement toward the source of these agents, i.e., toward the inflammatory site. Details of this complicated process are largely unknown. Probably, occupation of a threshold difference in the number of chemotaxin receptors on one side of a leukocyte induces the cytoskeletal rearrangements needed for movement. It is also possible that leukocytes keep crawling in the direction of chemokines exposed on a surface. As in diapedesis, $\beta_2$ integrin connections with the tissue cell proteins or extracellular matrix proteins must be formed at the front of the moving leukocytes and broken at the rear end. Moreover, for continued sensing of the chemotaxin gradient, the chemotaxin receptors on the leukocytes must be freed from their ligand for repeated usage. This occurs through internalization of the receptor–ligand complex, intracellular disruption of the connection, and reappearance of the free receptor on the leukocyte surface.[1]

The chemotaxins involved in granulocyte movement are those of the chemokine α and β subgroup, with different specificities for the various cell types (Table 11.4). These agents are produced by host cells in response to inflammation. In addition, chemotactic peptides are released by infecting microorganisms (e.g., formyl-methionyl-leucyl-phenylalamine, fMLP) and by the host complement system (C5a). Lipid mediators such as leukotriene $B_4$ ($LTB_4$) and PAF are also strong chemotattractants. For each of these agents, specific receptors on the granulocyte surface exist. These receptors belong to the rhodopsin superfamily of integral membrane proteins with seven transmembrane domains. Ligand specificity is created by differences in the extracellular domains. The intracellular domains interact with various trimeric guanidine triphosphate (GTP)-binding proteins, thus establishing a link with signal transduction pathways leading to functional responses.

As described in the previous paragraphs, the effects of chemotaxin binding to granulocytes are manifold: upregulation of adhesion receptors, shedding of L-selectin, activation of integrins, and induction of diapedesis and chemotaxis. At higher concentrations of the chemotaxins, as found in inflammatory foci, the granulocytes may also be activated to degranulate and release reactive oxygen species and inflammatory mediators (see next section of this chapter). This response is strongly affected by the priming (preactivation) state of the granulocytes, induced by various cytokines, and by adhesion of these cells to matrix proteins.[1] For example, TNF-α induces generation of reactive oxygen species by neutrophils bound to a matrix protein, but has no such effect on neutrophils in suspension. Binding of eosinophils to fibronectin primes these cells for enhanced responses to subsequent stimuli, but also prolongs their survival, due to IL-3 and GM-CSF production by these cells.[11]

In conclusion, we may state that the final outcome of an inflammatory reaction in the skin or other organs is defined by a large number of factors, present at different stages of the development or resolution of an inflammatory response. Our increasingly detailed knowledge of adhesion molecules and the mechanisms that control leukocyte traffic suggests that drugs aimed at inhibiting their function may be useful in ameliorating this response. Caution is warranted with integrin blockade, because this goal may not be reached unless a complete immune depression is enforced, which would leave the host severely compromised. On the other hand, inhibiting the relevant sugar determinants that function as ligands for the selectin members may be less harmful, yet less potent as well. The option of selective inhibition at the level of chemokines is obviously a station too far, since ample redundancy has been found in chemokines and chemokine receptors and also we hardly know which chemotactic specificity is hidden in all the different organ-related inflammatory reactions.

## III. CYTOTOXIC POTENTIAL OF GRANULOCYTES

### A. Phagocytosis

Neutrophils, and to a lesser extent eosinophils, are capable of phagocytosis of a large variety of microorganisms, including bacteria, yeasts, fungi, and mycoplasmata, but also nonliving particulate material, such as inorganic crystals and denatured organic matter. This process involves a carefully organized series of events that include adherence of ingestable material to surface receptors on the phagocytes, cytoskeletal rearrangements leading to pseudopod formation, folding of the pseudopods around the material and formation of a closed vesicle (phagosome) that contains the ingested material (Figure 11.4).[1]

The recognition of microorganisms by phagocytic cells depends on a number of systems. One is the direct binding of pattern recognition receptors (PRRs) to pathogen-associated molecular patterns (PAMPs). PRRs exist as secreted proteins and as surface proteins on phagocytes. Examples of secreted PRRs are mannan-binding lectin (MBL) and ficolins, both collectin-like C-type lectins that bind to repeating carbohydrate residues on microorganisms and that able to induce complement activation, leading to opsonization of the microbes. Other examples of secreted PRRs are C-reactive protein (CRP) and serum amyloid protein (SAP), pentraxins that bind to phosphorylcholine on microbial membranes and apoptotic cells, and also induce complement activation. LPS-binding protein (LBP) is a plasma protein that mediates the binding of LPS on microbes to the CD14 molecule on macrophages and neutrophils. Cell-surface PRRs are CD14, which cooperates with Toll-like receptors (TLRs) to activate the phagocytes, and the glycan-recognizing receptors CR3 (complement receptor type 3) and human dectin-1, although as yet not formally proved. In general, opsonization, i.e., covering of microbes with antibodies and/or complement fragments, is needed for efficient uptake by phagocytes. Thus, the soluble PRRs help in the process of opsonization, and the cell-surface PRRs act by turning the bactericidal potential and activity of the phagocytes toward bound or ingested microorganisms.

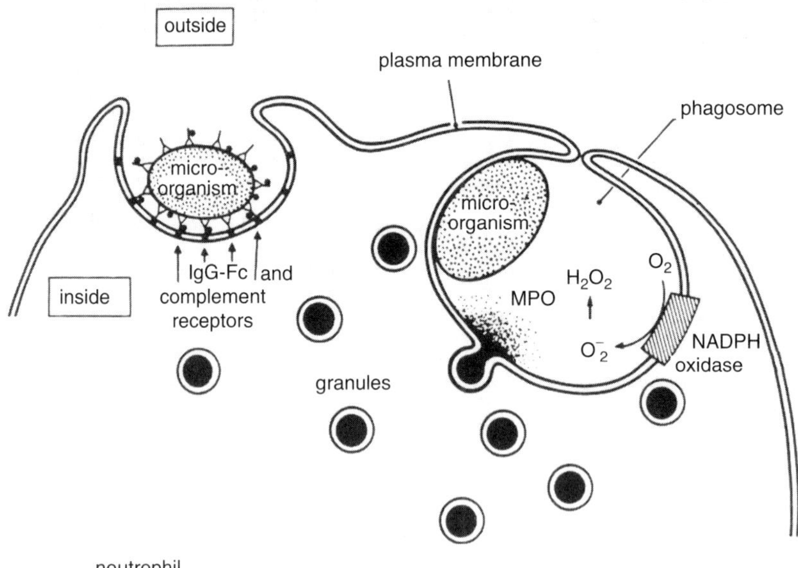


**FIGURE 11.4** Schematic representation of phagocytosis, degranulation, and NADPH oxidase activation. Microorganisms covered with IgG antibodies and C3 fragments are bound to Fcγ and complement receptors on the granulocyte surface. Subsequently, pseudopods from the granulocytes fold around the microorganism and fuse into a phagosome. Within the phagosome, contents of cytoplasmic granules and reactive oxygen compounds are released, which then kill the ingested microorganism. (From Roos, D., *Drug Investigation,* 3(Suppl. 2), 48, 1991. With permission.)

Antibodies bind with their Fab regions to microbial antigens, resulting in close spatial packing of the Fc regions of these antibodies. This configuration induces C1q binding and complement activation via the classical pathway, resulting in deposition of complement components C3b and C3bi to the antibodies or on the microbial surface. Alternatively, MBL or ficolins bind to repeating carbohydrate structures on the microorganisms, followed by binding and activation of certain serine proteases (MBL-binding serine protease 1 and 2, or MASP-1 and -2). These MASPs then activate complement factors 2 and 4, leading — as in the classical pathway — to C3 fragment deposition on the microbes. Some microorganisms also induce direct complement activation via the alternative pathway. Subsequent binding of the microbe-bound complement fragments to complement receptors CR1 (for C3b) and CR3 (for C3bi) then couples the opsonized microorganisms to the phagocytes. Moreover, the spatial arrangement of the antibody Fc regions also induces direct binding of the opsonized microorganisms to Fc receptors on the phagocytes.[1] Most important for this last process are antibodies of the IgG class, for which neutrophils carry two distinct types of receptor: FcγRIIa and FcγRIIIb (Table 11.5). Both receptors have a low affinity for monomeric IgG, but bind immune complexes with several IgG molecules quite well. Eosinophils can bind IgG molecules only to FcγIIa receptors. Neutrophils and eosinophils also contain receptors for IgA molecules, but the opsonizing capacity of these antibodies remains to be proved. Antibodies of the IgM class accelerate complement activation but do not bind directly to phagocytes. Table 11.5 summarizes the known complement and immunoglobulin receptors on granulocytes.

Binding of opsonized microorganisms or other material to phagocyte receptors triggers three distinct processes in these cells: phagocytosis of the opsonized material, fusion of the intracellular granules with the phagosomal membrane (degranulation), and generation of reactive oxygen species. Phagocytosis is induced by local changes in the actin network adjacent to the plasma membrane, i.e., breakdown of this network close to occupied receptors and increased actin connections at some distance. As a result, the cell will form pseudopods around the bound particle. Through subsequent

**TABLE 11.5**
**Function of Fc- and Complement-Receptors on Granulocytes**

| Nomenclature | Cell Type[a] | Ligand | Effect | | |
|---|---|---|---|---|---|
| | | | Phagocytosis | Release Mediators | Cytoxicity |
| FcγR-I (CD64) | N | IgG | + | + | + |
| FcγR-IIa (CD32) | N/E/B | IgG | + | + | + |
| FcγR-IIIb (CD16-I)[b] | N | IgG | ? | +/– | +/– |
| FcαR | N/E | IgA | + | + | + |
| FcεR-I | B/E | IgE | – | + | +/– |
| FcεR-II | B/E | IgE | ? | + | ? |
| CR1 (CD35) | N/E/B | C4b/C3b | + | + | + |
| CR3 (CD11b/CD18) | N/E/B | iC3b[c] | + | + | + |
| CR4 (CD11c/CD18) | N/E/B | iC3b/C3dg[c] | + | + | + |
| C3a receptor | E/B | C3a | – | + | – |
| C5a receptor | N/E/B | C5a | – | + | – |

[a] N, Neutrophils; E, eosinophils; B, basophils.
[b] Linked to the cell membrane by a glycosyl-phosphatidyl-inositol (GPI) anchor.
[c] $\beta_2$ integrin ligands; see Table 11.3.

binding of opsonin receptors on these pseudopods to the antibodies and complement fragments on the particle, the pseudopods are tightly bound to the particle, the whole process increases and the particle will be completely engulfed. Finally, the pseudopods fuse with each other and form a phagosome composed of a piece of the original plasma membrane that tightly fits outside-in around the particle (Figure 11.4). Several particles may be ingested in this way by one single phagocyte, and the phagosomes may fuse with each other into one or more intracellular vesicles.[1]

## B. Degranulation

As a result of membrane fusion, the contents of the granules are released into the phagosome and start to act upon the ingested material. As mentioned before, neutrophils contain at least two types of granule: azurophilic and specific (see Table 11.1). Azurophilic granules resemble lysosomes in other cell types in that they contain acid hydrolases, i.e., with a low pH optimum. These granules also contain myeloperoxiydase, an enzyme that catalyzes the production of hypochlorous acid (HOCl) from hydrogen peroxide ($H_2O_2$) and chloride ions. HOCl is very toxic for many microorganisms, but is rather instable. However, it can react with primary and secondary amines to *N*-chloramines, of which several are stable and strongly microbiocidal. Azurophilic granules further contain a number of serine proteinases, a large amount of defensins (small cationic peptides with a broad spectrum of bactericidal activities) and bactericidal permeability-increasing protein (BPI), a potent antibiotic against Gram-negative bacteria.[1]

In the specific granules of neutrophils we find lactoferrin, an iron-binding and therefore bacteriostatic protein, and vitamin $B_{12}$-binding protein, which probably has a similar function. The metalloproteinases collagenase and gelatinase are also located in the specific granules. These proteins have an important function in inflammatory reactions because they degrade extracellular matrix components and thus enable the neutrophils to reach microorganisms located deep in the tissues. Lysozyme, which hydrolyzes certain peptidoglycans of Gram-positive bacteria, is present in azurophilic as well as in specific granules.[1]

Neutrophils contain also secretory vesicles, small organelles with a large number of receptor molecules in their membrane, such as CR1, CR3, and FcγRIIIb. These secretory vesicles fuse very easily with the plasma membrane and are therefore thought to be involved in rapid upregulation of these receptors on the cell surface. Similar vesicles have been observed in eosinophils. Their existence in basophils remains to be investigated. Separate gelatinase-containing tertiary granules have been suggested to exist in neutrophils, but this issue has not yet been resolved.

As mentioned earlier, eosinophils act, like macrophages, against parasites. These pathogens are far too large to be ingested, however, and hence are killed through an extracellular cytotoxic process. The eosinophils adhere to the parasite wall, a process involving opsonins and complement and Fc receptors, and degranulate into the small space between the eosinophil and the parasite.[3] In a similar fashion, neutrophils are involved in tissue degradation when adhering to immune complexes deposited in the tissues, as in many immune complex diseases. This process is sometimes referred to as frustrated phagocytosis.[1]

The majority of granules found in eosinophils are crystalloid-containing, specific (secondary) granules. Immature eosinophils are characterized by the abundant presence of primary granules. These primary granules lack the typical crystalloid core. Recent results indicate that primary granules develop into specific granules during eosinophil maturation. Both primary and specific granules contain the cationic proteins major basic protein (MBP), eosinophil cationic protein (ECP), eosinophil-derived neurotoxin (EDN) and eosinophil peroxidase (EPO) (see Table 11.1). These cationic proteins are most likely responsible for the tissue damage in allergic inflammations and for the helminthotoxic effects of the eosinophils.

Eosinophil degranulation (quantitated by the amounts of released EDN or ECP) can be induced by exposure of eosinophils to serum-coated surfaces, such as beads or plates. Moreover, surfaces coated with $IgG_1$, IgA, or sIgA are also potent stimuli of eosinophil degranulation. This degranulation can be increased by preincubation of the eosinophils with IL-3, IL-5, or GM-CSF. Surprisingly, soluble stimuli, such as fMLP, PMA (phorbol-myristate acetate), or C5a, activate eosinophils for superoxide release but only induce degranulation when the cortical cytoskeleton is disturbed by cytochalasin B. Recent results indicate that signals from integrins are necessary for eosinophil degranulation.[3]

Basophils contain round cytoplasmic granules with diameters up to 1.2 μm. A subtype of smaller granules has been located between the nuclear lobes. Within these granules histamine is stored, at about 1 to 2 pg/cell. The characteristic metachromatic staining of basophils is due to the presence of proteoglycans in the granule (see Table 11.1). Histamine and a kallikrein-like endopeptidase are bound to this proteoglycan matrix. Basophils share with eosinophils the presence of Charcot–Leyden crystal protein and major basic protein in their granules.[4]

Activation of basophilic granulocytes results in release of inflammatory mediators, such as histamine. The release reaction can be induced via cross-linking of IgE bound to FcεRI on the basophil membrane (Table 11.5). Of all Fc receptors, FcεRI has the highest affinity for its ligand ($\sim 10^{-10}$ *M*). FcεRI is a tetrameric complex composed of one transmembrane α subunit that binds IgE with its extracellular part, one β subunit containing four transmembrane-spanning domains, and two disulfide-linked γ subunits each spanning the plasma membrane once. Both cytoplasmic tails of the β- and γ-chains contain the so-called ITAM (immune-recognition receptor tyrosine-based activation motif) sequences relevant for signaling. Other stimuli of the histamine release reaction are the anaphylatoxins C3a and C5a, leukocyte products such as the so-called histamine-releasing factors, and the chemotactic tripeptide fMLP. Several members of the family of chemokines (see Table 11.4) have been demonstrated to activate basophils to release histamine.[4] MCP-1, 2, and 3 as well as RANTES are potent stimuli of basophil degranulation. Macrophage inflammatory protein (MIP)-1α and platelet factor 4 (PF4) can also induce basophil histamine release but only to a relatively low extent. IL-8 has been found to induce degranulation after preincubation of basophils with IL-3. Although IL-3, IL-5, GM-CSF, NGF (nerve growth factor), and PAF do not induce histamine release from human basophils, they are potent primers of basophil responses to other stimuli.

## C. Production of Oxygen Radicals

Generation of reactive oxygen species is catalyzed by the enzyme NADPH oxidase. This enzyme is present in neutrophils and in eosinophils, but not in basophils, and consists of a membrane-bound component called cytochrome $b_{558}$ and a number of cytosolic regulating proteins. The cytochrome contains not only heme moieties but also a flavin group. It binds NADPH at the cytosolic side of the membrane and transports electrons to oxygen on the other side of the membrane (in the phagosome or on the cell surface). In this way, superoxide ($O_2^-$) is produced, which may subsequently be converted into hydrogen peroxide and other reactive oxygen species (see above). Direct formation of hydroxyl radicals by phagocytes has never been conclusively proved, but may take place within phagocyte targets.

The activity of the NADPH oxidase is well regulated: superoxide formation takes place only during a restricted period after phagocytosis, adherence or encounter of high concentrations of chemotaxins. This activity regulation is accomplished by translocation of the cytosolic regulator proteins to the cytochrome, which allow enzymatic activity by inducing a conformational change in the cytochrome that is needed for NADPH binding.[1] The extent of oxidase activation is also regulated. At the receptor level this is accomplished by integrins and TLRs. Binding of β2 integrins on the phagocyte surface to immobilized ligands leads to the phenomenon of cell "priming," a kind of preactivation that leads to increased reaction to subsequent activation signals (Fc receptor ligands, chemokines, complement fragments). Molecular details of this process are not yet known. TLRs on the cell surface or in the phagosome membrane can "sense" the microbes and regulate the extent of cell activation needed for effective but not excessive defense reactions.

Generation of superoxide and related oxygen products in the phagosome is essential for killing of many different types of organisms, as illustrated by the pathology of patients with an inherited defect in the NADPH oxidase. Recently, it has become clear that oxidase activity not only generates reactive oxygen-derived compounds, but also induces a flux of potassium ions into the phagosome that is essential for liberating the microbiocidal proteases from their proteoglycan matrix in the azurophil granules. Thus, the NADPH oxidase is a two-edged sword with direct and indirect effects against pathogens. Release of reactive oxygen compounds into the extracellular surroundings is also functional: they activate metalloproteinases released by the phagocytes and they inactivate serine proteinase inhibitors in body fluids. As a result, these proteinases can act on tissue components and help destroy unwanted material. However, in chronic inflammations, these reactions may lead to irreversible damage to the tissues and then need to be suppressed by treatment.

### D. Release of Inflammatory Mediators

Apart from the release of prestored mediators, granulocytes also synthesize and release other potent inflammatory mediators. These inflammatory mediators are derived from the phospholipid pool in the plasma membrane. Following the action of phospholipase $A_2$, arachidonic acid is formed. Arachidonic acid in its turn can be converted by lipoxygenases into leukotrienes and other hydroperoxy fatty acids, or it can be converted by cyclo-oxygenases into prostaglandins. Products of the cyclo-oxygenase pathway are not synthesized in large amounts in granulocytes, but 5-lipoxygenase products are abundant after stimulation of granulocytes. Stimulated neutrophils produce and release predominantly leukotriene $B_4$, whereas basophils and eosinophils release leukotriene $C_4$.[12]

The action of phospholipase $A_2$ on membrane phospholipids also results in lyso-phospholipid formation. Acetylation of lyso-phospholids leads to the formation of PAF.[12] The respiratory burst of eosinophils induced by serum-treated zymosan is dependent on autologously produced PAF, which primes these cells in an autocrine fashion.

## IV. GRANULOCYTES AND SKIN DISEASES

Healthy skin contains few, if any, extravasated granulocytes. However, in a broad variety of skin diseases, the presence of subtypes of granulocytes has been described as a characteristic feature.

## A. Presence of Granules in Skin Diseases

Neutrophils are believed to play an important role in the pathophysiology of various infectious skin diseases, such as superficial or deep pyodermal reactions. In vasculitis, characterized by deposition of immune complexes, neutrophils are prominent in the perivascular region in, e.g., Behçet's syndrome and erythema elevatum et diutinum. In skin diseases characterized by local depositions of autoantibodies and complement, neutrophils have been demonstrated in, e.g., bullous pemphigoid, linear IgA dermatosis, IgA pemphigus, and dermatitis herpetiformis. In psoriasis, Sweet's syndrome, and subcorneal pustulosis, neutrophil presence in the skin is thought to be mediated by T-cell activation. It has been hypothesized that pyoderma gangrenosum and neutrophilic hydradenitis belong to this T-cell-mediated group of neutrophil dermatoses.[13] The presence of neutrophils in skin in allergic disorders is not always seen. After allergen skin prick tests, mast cell degranulation is found, as well as a marked neutrophil infiltration. However, in a more appropriate model for atopic dermatitis, the so-called atopy patch test, and in lesional skin of patients with atopic dermatitis (AD), neutrophils are apparently absent, which argues against the role and presence of neutrophils in AD.[14] Mast cell degranulation in skin is more pronounced in urticaria, where prominent neutrophil skin influx has been demonstrated.

Eosinophil and basophil infiltrates in skin are typical of atopic dermatitis and delayed-type hypersensitivity reactions (see Figure 11.2b and c). In intracutaneous allergen skin tests and in atopy patch tests, both cell types are demonstrated after approximately 6 and 24 h, respectively. The presence of basophils has been controversial, due to lack of selective markers, but the availability of the basophil-specific monoclonal antibodies BB1 (see Figures 11.1c and 11.2c) and 2D7, binding within the secretory granules, has recently been helpful in determining the presence of basophils in tissues. Interestingly, in chronically inflamed AD skin, basophils can no longer be found, and intact eosinophils are rare; mostly eosinophil-derived proteins are still found, however. This can be explained by the complete degranulation of eosinophils and basophils once these cells have arrived in the skin. Recently, it has been postulated that eosinophils are able to emigrate from tissue and activate, e.g., lymph node cells, which might be an alternative explanation for the small numbers of intact eosinophils and basophils in chronically inflamed skin.

The role of eosinophils in atopic dermatitis skin is currently under debate. Eosinophil infiltration is one of the hallmarks in allergic inflammatory disorders, such as allergic asthma and atopic dermatitis. However, several novel findings indicate that eosinophil presence is not related to disease outcome or severity. For example, intradermal injection of RANTES induced a marked eosinophil influx and degranulation, but no signs of inflamed skin were noted.[15] Recently, blocking humanized monoclonal antibodies to the eosinophil-specific growth factor IL-5 has been applied in allergic asthma. Despite a drastic reduction in eosinophil numbers in blood and lung, no changes in clinical symptoms were found, which questions the role of eosinophils in allergic asthma.[16] Currently, an international multicenter trial is evaluating the effect of humanized anti-IL-5 in patients with AD. A potent beneficial effect of anti-IL-5 on hypereosinophil syndrome-related dermatitis has been described.[17]

Patients with the LAD-I syndrome (lacking the $\beta_2$ subfamily of integrins) suffer from early omphalitis and necrotic nonsuppurative skin lesions, of which they may succumb if their syndrome concerns the severe LAD-I type (without any $\beta_2$ integrin expression). On the other hand, the few patients with the LAD-II syndrome, lacking $SLe^x$ expression on their leukocytes, do not suffer from major skin problems.[18]

## B. Models to Study Granulocyte Migration in Skin

Granulocyte infiltration in the skin does not only depend on the expression of adhesion molecules, but also on the presence of a chemotactic gradient. Skin blisters provide a convenient model to study the inflammatory response *in vivo* in humans.[19] Migration of leukocytes (90 to 95% neutrophils) into the blister fluid was detectable within 3 h, and appeared to level off at 16 to 24 h. Accompanying the cellular immune response was the accumulation of inflammatory mediators in the fluid. The accumulation of Interferon-γ (IFN-γ) reached a plateau within 3 h. The accumulation of C5a did not peak until 5 h, whereas leukotriene B4 continued to accumulate through 24 h. IL-6 and IL-8 concentrations were minimal at 3 to 8 h, but dramatic by 24 h, while IL-1β, TNF-α, and G-CSF were undetectable within 3 to 8 h, but markedly elevated by 24 h. Upon functional testing of the exudative neutrophils, a significant desensitization of the exudated cells to IL-8 and C5a (in contrast to fMLP) was found, reflecting a previous exposure to these attractants *in vivo*.

Another way to study the skin infiltration of granulocytes is by direct injection of chemokines. Injection of up to 4 μg of RANTES intradermally induced eosinophil, but not neutrophil, influx in the skin of both allergic and non-allergic subjects. Although the final number of infiltrating eosinophils was comparable in both subject groups, allergic subjects demonstrated a more rapid influx, indicative of a preactivated state of the peripheral blood eosinophils and/or skin endothelium.[15] Injection of up to 1000 pmol of the chemokine MIP-1α resulted in the infiltration of eosinophils and neutrophils, as well as increased expression of the adhesion molecule E-selectin on skin endothelium. Infiltration of neutrophils already 2 h after MIP-1α injection is remarkable since expression of its receptor CCR1 has not been demonstrated on purified neutrophils *in vitro*.[20]

## C. Selectivity in Skin Recruitment of Granulocyte Subsets

The steps of recruitment and subsequent activation may be different for the granulocytic subsets among the various diseases, as indicated, e.g., by the extracellular deposition of eosinophil granule major basic protein (MBP) in lesional atopic dermatitis skin, whereas deposition of neutrophil but not eosinophil granule proteins occurs in erythema elevatum et diutinum. This difference in granulocytic subset predominance or reactivity can be explained in several ways, such as chemotaxin receptor expression and receptor affinity regulation (see also Table 11.4), total number of cells attracted, or local survival factors.

Each environment may have its own repertoire in granulocyte recruitment, in part defined by local blood supply and capillary flow physiology as well as by the adhesion molecules involved in the leukocyte/postcapillary endothelial cell interactions. Thus, neutrophils migrate to delayed-type hypersensitivity induced in *joints* but not in *skin*, and this migration is CD18-independent, but migration to intra-articular IL-1 and TNF-α is largely CD18 dependent in both joints and skin.[21] The reaction of neutrophils to C5a may differ as well, as evidenced by the different reactions on neutrophil recruitment in *lung* as compared to *skin*. Eosinophil (or basophil) influx in skin, as occurs in allergic late-phase or delayed-type hypersensitivity (DTH) reactions, is presumed to be dependent on both CD18 and VLA-4/VCAM-1 interactions, but to date the contribution of each of these integrins, or the involvement of alternative molecules such as $\alpha_4\beta_7$ or extraintestinal expression of mucosal addressin cell adhesion molecule (MAdCAM)-1(-like) material, is unknown.

## D. Modulating Skin Immune Response by Granulocytes

Recently, some novel insights in the role of granulocytes in skin have been obtained. With regard to neutrophils, it was demonstrated that, apart from the release of inflammatory mediators and killing of pathogens, neutrophils release multiple cytokines (see Table 11.2). By releasing cytokines neutrophils can modulate the local immune response. An intriguing finding came from the observation that neutrophils enter the skin after ultraviolet (UV) exposure. For a long time, neutrophils that infiltrated UV-exposed skin were thought to be mainly involved in the repair processes of UV-damaged skin.[22] Only recently, it was found that neutrophils can produce immune suppressive cytokines, such as IL-4 and IL-10, once they have arrived in the skin. In the treatment of psoriasis by UV it has been demonstrated that the typical Th2 switch is due to IL-4 release by infiltrating neutrophils.[23] On the other hand, a decreased influx of neutrophils after UV appears to be related to inflammation in polymorphous light eruption.[24] Both findings indicate that, after a specific trigger, neutrophils are able to inhibit local skin inflammation.

## V. CONCLUSION

In conclusion, granulocyte recruitment is a well-regulated process, defined by several adhesion molecules and inflammatory factors, of which IL-8 seems to form the basis for low-level turnover in the skin. On the other hand, little is known about the precise substances that specifically invoke neutrophilic, eosinophilic, or basophilic granulocytes to react in the way they do under certain pathologic conditions. Functional assays *in vivo* are required to (dis)prove the ideas obtained from *in situ* immunohistochemistry and *in vitro* cultures. Transgenic animals in which local production of inflammatory agents have been modulated, as well as application of humanized antibodies and small-molecular-weight inhibiting peptides in human subjects, may be valuable tools for such research. We regard this as the most important goal for future skin research during the next decade.

## REFERENCES


1. Densen, P., Clark, R.A., and Nauseef, W.M., Granulocytic phagocytes, in *Principles on Practice of Infectious Diseases*, Mandell, G.L., Bennett, J.E., and Dolin, R., Eds., Churchill Livingstone, New York, 1994, 221.
2. Delves, P.J. and Lydyard, P.M., Leukocyte development, in *Cellular Immunology,* Delves, P.J., Ed., Blackwell Scientific, Oxford, U.K., 1994, 33.
3. Rosenberg, H.F., Eosinophils, in *Inflammation: Basic Principles and Clinical Correlates*, 3rd ed., Gallin, J.I. and Snyderman, R., Eds., Lippincott, Williams & Wilkins, Philadelphia, 1999, 61.
4. Nilsson, G., Costa, J.J., and Metcalfe, D.D., Mast cells and basophils, in *Inflammation: Basic Principles and Clinical Correlates*, 3rd ed., Gallin, J.I. and Snyderman, R., Eds., Lippincott, Williams & Wilkins, Philadelphia, 1999, 97.
5. Carlos, T.M. and Harlan, J.M., Leukocyte-endothelial adhesion molecules, *Blood,* 84, 2068, 1994.
6. Springer, T.A., Traffic signals for lymphocyte recirculation and leukocyte emigration: the multistep paradigm, *Cell,* 76, 301, 1994.
7. Ley, K. and Tedder, T.F., Leukocyte interactions with vascular endothelium. New insights into selectin-mediated attachment and rolling, *J. Immunol.,* 155, 525, 1995.
8. Zölnner, O. et al., L-selectin from human, but not from mouse neutrophils binds directly to E-selectin, *J. Cell Biol.*, 136,707, 1997.
9. Bochner, B.S. and Schleimer, R.P., The role of adhesion molecules in human eosinophil and basophil recruitment, *J. Allergy. Clin. Immunol.,* 94, 427, 1994.
10. Kuijpers, T.W. et al., Neutrophil migration across monolayers of cytokine-prestimulated endothelial cells: a role of platelet-activating factor and IL-8. *J. Cell Biol.,* 117, 565, 1992.
11. Wardlaw, A.J., Walsh, G.M., and Symon, F.A., Mechanisms of eosinophil and basophil migration, *Allergy,* 49, 797, 1994.
12. Henderson, W.R., Jr., Eicosanoids and platelet-activating factor in allergic respiratory diseases, *Am. Rev. Respir. Dis.,* 143(Suppl.), S86, 1991.
13. Von Den Driesch, D.P., Polymorphonuclears: structure, function, and mechanisms of involvement in skin diseases. *Clin. Dermatol.,* 18, 233, 2000.
14. Langeveld-Wildschut, E.G., et al. Evaluation of the atopy patch test and the cutaneous late- phase reaction as relevant models for the study of allergic inflammation in patients with atopic eczema, *J. Allergy Clin. Immunol.,* 98, 1019, 1996.
15. Beck, L.A. et al., Cutaneous injection of RANTES causes eosinophil recruitment — comparison of nonallergic and allergic human subjects, *J. Immunol.,* 159, 2962, 1997.
16. Bochner, B.S., Verdict in the case of therapies versus eosinophils: the jury is still out, *J. Allergy Clin. Immunol.,* 113, 3, 2004.
17. Plotz, S.G. et al., Use of an anti-interleukin-5 antibody in the hypereosinophilic syndrome with eosinophilic dermatitis, *N. Engl. J. Med.,* 349, 2334, 2003.

18. Von Andrian, U.H. et al., *In vivo* behavior of neutrophils from two patients with distinct inherited leukocyte adhesion deficiency syndromes, *J. Clin. Invest.,* 91, 2893, 1993.
19. Kuhns, D.B. et al., Dynamics of the cellular and humoral components of the inflammatory response elicited in skin blisters in humans, *J. Clin. Invest.,* 89, 1734, 1992.
20. Lee, S.C. et al., Cutaneous injection of human subjects with macrophage inflammatory protein-1 alpha induces significant recruitment of neutrophils and monocytes, *J. Immunol.,* 164, 3392, 2000.
21. Gao, J.X., Issekutz, A.C., and Issekutz, T.B., Neutrophils migrate to delayed-type hypersensitivity reactions in joints, but not in skin. Mechanism is leukocyte function-associated antigen-1-/Mac-1-independent, *J. Immunol.,* 153, 5689, 1994.
22. Hawk, J.L., Murphy, G.M., and Holden, C.A., The presence of neutrophils in human cutaneous ultraviolet-B inflammation, *Br. J. Dermatol.,* 118, 27, 1988.
23. Piskin, G. et al., IL-4 expression by neutrophils in psoriasis lesional skin upon high-dose UVB exposure, *Dermatology,* 207, 51, 2003.
24. Schornagel, I.J. et al., Decreased neutrophil skin infiltration after UVB exposure in patients with polymorphous light eruption, *J. Invest. Dermatol.,* 123, 202, 2004.

# Part III

## Humoral Constituents of the Skin Immune System

# 12 Free Radicals

*Maria Lucia Dell'Anna, Emanuela Camera, and Mauro Picardo*

## CONTENTS



0-8493-1959-5/05/$0.00+$1.50

*If a molecule is reactive enough to be lethal, how can it be specific and reversible enough to participate in signaling?*[1]

# I. INTRODUCTION

The aim of this chapter is to provide a review of the chemical and biological aspects of the most known reactive species, with particular attention to the interaction with the immune system. After a rapid estimation of the chemical characteristics of the most representative free radicals and reactive oxygen species (ROS) and reactive nitrogen species (RNS) generated in biological environment, we focus on the cellular aspects of redox status and on the sites and the modality of ROS production inside the cell. In particular, the role of a correct redox balance in the intracellular signal transduction will be discussed including the link between ROS and transcription factors and/or kinase pathways, and the complex network of the antioxidants. Finally, we illustrate the role of the ROS-mediated pathways in the regulation of the function of the different immune-competent cells in physiological, aged, and pathological conditions. A brief view of a possible therapeutic approach based on antioxidant supplementation closes the chapter.

Free radicals are elements or compounds that possess unpaired electrons in the outer atomic or molecular orbital, respectively. This is the essential feature that provides free radicals with high chemical reactivity and rapid, and sometimes uncontrolled, transfer of signal associated with oxidative stress. Other compounds, even possessing a complete octet, are associated with a high reactivity. In biological systems, the most representative free radicals and reactive species are those derived from the activation of molecular oxygen at the ground state ($^3O_2$). In Table 12.1, the sources of free radicals and ROS are represented. ROS, including RNS, are generated during some physiological activities of the cell, such as the mitochondrial respiration and the synthesis of the melanin by epidermal cells. Moreover, external agents, as in the case of ultraviolet A/B (UVA/B) ray or transition metals, can stimulate their production. Either positive or deleterious actions of the free radicals depend on the chemical reactivity and the relative abundance of the different species, the chemical structure of the target, and the presence of scavenger compounds.

# II. FREE RADICALS AND REACTIVE SPECIES OF OXYGEN AND NITROGEN

## A. Singlet Oxygen

Singlet oxygen ($^1O_2$), an electronically excited state of molecular oxygen, is generated through several cellular, enzymatic, and non-enzymatic reactions and may account for the oxidant species produced during UV exposure in the presence of photosensitizers, causing peroxidation of epidermal lipids.[2,3] Singlet oxygen represents the effector of the lipid hydroperoxide-mediated cytotoxicity, since it is released during the decomposition of lipid peroxides into peroxyl radicals through the Russel mechanism.[4] Even the reaction between peroxynitrite, an RNS, and linoleic acid hydroperoxide can produce $^1O_2$.[5] Nonetheless, the biological generation of $^1O_2$ via chemiexcitation processes is still debated, whereas the production of $^1O_2$ in the extracellular space, through spontaneous anion superoxide dismutation or by the eosinophil peroxidase-$H_2O_2$-bromide system, seems to be physiologically relevant. In both cases, the microenvironment plays a critical role.[6] Proteins are also accounted among the potential targets of $^1O_2$ due to their elevated concentration in cell microenvironment and to the high constant rate of the reaction.[4,7] A peculiar characteristic of $^1O_2$ consists of the ability to transfer excess energy to quenching molecules, like carotenes and carotenoids, thus returning to the ground state. On the other hand, the energy-accepting molecules remain stable even in the excited state or alternatively can dissipate the accumulated energy in the form of heat, thus neutralizing the oxidative potential of $^1O_2$.[8] However, $^1O_2$ itself possesses a relatively long lifetime, which can be even increased in polar environments. $^1O_2$ is able to diffuse through cellular

**TABLE 12.1**
**Reactive Species and Their Generators**

| Species | $^{\bullet}OH$ | $^1O_2$ | $O_2^{\bullet-}$ | $H_2O_2$ | NO |
|---|---|---|---|---|---|
| Sources | Fenton-like reaction | Peroxidase | NADH dehydrogenase | SOD | NOS |
| | Mitochondrial ETC | SOD | Ubiquinone/cytochrome *c* intersection | NOS | $NO_2^-$ ($Fe^{2+}$-mediated) |
| | Peroxynitrite decomposition | UV | Xanthine oxidase | Xanthine oxidase | |
| | | | Aldehyde oxidase | $6BH_4$ recycling | |
| | | | NADPH oxidase | NADPH oxidase | |
| | | | | Pteridine oxidation | |
| | | | | MAO-A | |
| | | | | CoQ oxidation | |
| | | | | TNF-α signal | |

membranes and to cause damage in sites distant from its original sources,[9] such as the modifications of redox sensitive molecules in the blood following UV irradiation of the skin.[10,11]

Singlet oxygen impairs cellular signaling and induces stress response at the cellular level, as in the case of the activation of mitogen-activated protein kinase (MAPK).[3] $^1O_2$ is further implicated even in the survival signaling cascade through the downregulation of the epidermal growth factor receptor (EGFR) in keratinocytes, therefore affecting the protein-level of EGFR and its phosphorilation.[12]

## B. Superoxide Anion

Superoxide anion radical ($O_2^{\bullet-}$) is formed through the net acquisition of an electron by $O_2$, along with its negative charge. The progressive reduction of $O_2$ to $H_2O$ is depicted in the scheme of Reaction 12.1. Inside the cells, the $O_2^{\bullet-}$ can be produced either non-enzymatically, by oxidation of semireduced ubiquinone, catecholamine, and flavins, or by means of enzymatic catalysis of NADPH oxidase and xanthine oxidase.

$$O_2 \rightarrow O_2^{\bullet-} \rightarrow H_2O_2 \rightarrow {}^{\bullet}OH \rightarrow H_2O \qquad (12.1)$$

$O_2^{\bullet-}$ presents an ample spectrum of reactivity. In fact, it interacts with lipids proteins, saccharides, and nucleic acids. As a result of the electric charge, in most cases $O_2^{\bullet-}$ cannot penetrate through cellular membranes and tends to exert its detrimental effects at the site of generation. Diverse biological effects of $O_2^{\bullet-}$ may be attributed to the products of its dismutation or to the formation of thyl radicals by reaction with endogenous thiol groups, frequently found in proteins and enzymes.[13–15] $O_2^{\bullet-}$ dismutates to $H_2O_2$ and $O_2$ either spontaneously or through the catalysis of diverse superoxide dismutase (SOD) isoenzymes. Additionally, $O_2^{\bullet-}$ can react with $H_2O_2$, its own by-product, in a reaction (Haber–Weiss reaction, Reaction 12.2) catalyzed by divalent metals ($Me^{2+}$) and this finally leads to the generation of the highly reactive hydroxyl radical ($^{\bullet}OH$).[16] Moreover, in aqueous environments $O_2^{\bullet-}$ behaves as a strong reducing agent leading transition metal ion ($Cu^{2+}$, $Fe^{2+}$, etc.) to a lower oxidation state associated with higher reactivity and, in turn, promotion of $^{\bullet}OH$ formation.[17]

$$O_2^{\bullet-} + H_2O_2 \rightarrow O_2 + OH^- + {}^{\bullet}OH \qquad (12.2)$$

## C. Hydrogen Peroxide

Hydrogen peroxide ($H_2O_2$) is a small molecule with a high rate of diffusion, capable of crossing the cell membrane, and is easily generated and removed. It is more stable than other ROS, including superoxide anion, even if its half-life depends on cellular pH and redox potential. $H_2O_2$ is an uncharged compound generated by the univalent reduction of oxygen followed by the dismutation of $O_2^{\bullet -}$ as described above and in the schematic sequence (Reaction 12.1). It is formed as a by-product of the basal cellular metabolism and following exposure to pro-oxidant agents.[18] $H_2O_2$ has a moderate oxidant capacity, as compared with other ROS. However, it possesses a broad reactivity toward thyl group proteins, enzymes, and polyunsaturated fatty acids (PUFA), when it can reach relatively high concentrations, as in the skin.[19] $H_2O_2$ acts via specific reversible protein oxidation, targeting cysteine residues and generating sulfenic acid (–SOH) which, in turn, must be reduced by glutathione (GSH) and thioredoxin. However, only the deprotonated and thiolate anion cysteine can be oxidized by $H_2O_2$. Consequently, only a small set of cysteine residues, located near to a positively charged amino acid able to produce a $pK_a$ below 5.0, can be a target for $H_2O_2$ whereas the most part of cysteine residues, with a $pK_a$ of 8.5, are protected from the oxidative insult.[18] $H_2O_2$ is required for the formation of more potent and dangerous oxidants, such as hydroxyl radicals ($^{\bullet}OH$). The latter is induced in the presence of divalent transition metals, in particular iron ($Fe^{2+}$), through Fenton or Fenton-like reactions.[20] In fact, $H_2O_2$ may act in lowering the threshold response for antibodies with low affinity for their corresponding antigens and for antigens present at low concentrations.[18]

## D. Hydroxyl Radical

Among the ROS, hydroxyl radical ($^{\bullet}OH$) is one of the most reactive intermediate with a very short lifespan. $^{\bullet}OH$ is a neutral compound having an unpaired electron, which, due to the high reactivity state, immediately oxidizes susceptible target compounds located in the immediate proximity of its site of generation. Primary targets of $^{\bullet}OH$ are lipids, from which it abstracts hydrogen atoms starting the development of the lipoperoxidation process. Additionally, $^{\bullet}OH$ causes a range of DNA damage, such as structural modifications of the component bases, DNA strand breakage, and inhibition of the repair system.[21]

## E. Hypochlorous Acid

Hypochlorous acid (HClO) is formed from $H_2O_2$ and chloride upon enzymatic catalysis by myeloperoxidase, which plays an important role in the bactericidal activity of phagosomes. HClO is one of the most powerful oxidants released by activated neutrophils and phagocytes at the sites of inflammation. The same mechanism that underlies the bactericidal property of HClO may result in the oxidation of host targets, mainly sulfidril and amine groups of enzymes and proteins.[22] Proofs of an oxidative process implicated in the negative interaction between free radicals and the host defense system are given by the antiproliferative effect exerted by HClO on lymphocytes *in vivo* and by the prevention by ascorbic acid treatment *in vitro*.[23]

## F. Lipoperoxides

Lipoperoxides are the most unstable and reactive compounds originating from the reaction of radicalized unsaturated lipids with oxygen or, alternatively, of unsaturated lipids with excited forms of molecular oxygen. The abstraction of a hydrogen radical is particularly favored for those unsaturated lipids bearing a bis-allilic methylene group or in presence of free radicals as alkyl, alkossi, or hydroxyl radicals. The lipoperoxide compound can decompose and initiate a chain reaction leading to the propagation of damage even to nonlipidic cell structures. The lipoperoxidative process consists of two phases (initiation, Reaction 12.3, and propagation Reactions 12.4 and 12.5) that amplify the progression of the reaction until termination reaction takes place. By-products of lipoperoxidation, such as 4-hydroxy-2-nonenal (4-HNE) and malondialdehyde (MDA), have been implicated in the oxidative stress-mediated cell signaling.[24,25]

$$LH + {}^{\bullet}OH \rightarrow {}^{\bullet}L + H_2O \quad (12.3)$$

$${}^{\bullet}L + O_2 \rightarrow LOO^{\bullet} \quad (12.4)$$

$$LOO^{\bullet} + LH \rightarrow LOOH + {}^{\bullet}L \quad (12.5)$$

### G. Reactive Nitrogen Species

RNS are activated derivatives of nitrogen, even though they contain oxygen and could be regarded also as ROS. The progenitor of the RNS is nitric oxide (${}^{\bullet}NO$). It is generated enzymatically from L-arginine via NO synthase (NOS) in a reaction dependent on the $O_2$ tension.[26] In the absence of $O_2$, as during ischemia, an alternative pathway may be activated based on the $Fe^{2+}$-mediated non-enzymatic generation of NO from $NO_2^-$.[27]

Different isoforms of NOS have been described. The endothelial (eNOS) and the neuronal (nNOS) isoforms are constitutively expressed and are regulated through the calcium/calmodulin couple and phosphorylation, whereas the inducible form of NOS (iNOS) is upregulated during inflammation, and is able to produce NO at higher levels and for a longer period of time than the other two isoenzymes.[18]

In addition to direct activity, NO can react with molecular oxygen, generating nitrosonium ion ($NO^+$), nitrous acid anhydride ($N_2O_3$), and radical $NO^{\bullet}_2$, all able to nitrosylate cysteine residues in proteins. $NO_2$ and $N_2O_3$, through different chemical pathways, are involved in processes of nitration or nitrosilation of tyrosine, amines, and thiols and may be implicated in the loss of function of some proteins. Peroxynitrite ($ONOO^-$) is a potent oxidant formed by interaction of ${}^{\bullet}NO$ with $O_2^{\bullet-}$ according to Reaction 12.6. In turn, $ONOO^-$ may oxidize or nitrate other molecules, or spontaneously decay, giving rise to the highly damaging molecules as ${}^{\bullet}OH$ and ${}^{\bullet}NO_2$.

$$O_2^{\bullet-} + {}^{\bullet}NO \rightarrow ONOO^- \quad (12.6)$$

## III. INTRACELLULAR GENERATION OF ROS

Principal sites of ROS generation are the plasma membrane, the mitochondria, and the peroxisomes. ROS are generated inside the cell by the reduction of oxygen by less than four electrons and its production can be enhanced by several factors, such as hormones, cytokines, drugs, and UV and ionizing radiation.[20,28–30] The main source of the electrons needed for the oxygen reduction is the mitochondrial electron transport chain.[18,28] ROS are produced during the arachidonic acid cascade, triggered by many factors, such as TNF-$\alpha$ or PDGF (platelet-derived growth factor), able to activate phospholipase $A_2$ ($PLA_2$).[18,20] The cytokine-induced ROS synthesis is mediated by the activation of sphingomyelinase — with a subsequent release of ceramide acting on mitochondria.[20] Other sources are the membrane-associated NAD(P)H oxidase, mainly expressed in phagocytes, cytochrome P450 system — located in the endoplasmic reticulum and involved in the unsaturated fatty acids oxidation, xanthine oxidase, COX (cyclooxygenase), LOX (lipooxygenase) — mainly expressed in lymphocytes and astrocytes and $\gamma$-glutamyl transpeptidase ($\gamma$-GT). NADPH oxidase is associated with the membrane and exerts its action within a few minutes after the activation. The enzyme catalyzes the one-electron reduction of $O_2$ to $O_2^{\bullet-}$ using NADPH as electron donor.[12] NADPH oxidase is composed of four subunits: two membrane-spanning, gp91-phox and p22-phox (forming cytb558), and two cytosolic, p47-phox and p67-phox. The subunits assembly is mediated by the G protein rac2 (or rac1), which, upon activation, facilitates the p47/p67 assembly via cytoskeletal reorganization.[18,20,28,31,32] The NADPH oxidase complex has also been found in nonphagocytic cells, such as B lymphocytes, even if not all components appear expressed uniformly by the different cell types. In nonphagocytic cells, rac1 can mediate signals between $PI_3$kinase — activated by platelet-derived growth factor (PDGF), transforming growth factor (TGF-β1) — and NADPH oxidase. In these nonphagocytic cells NADPH oxidase regulates oxygen burst against microorganisms when activated by cytokines — tumor necrosis factor-alpha (TNF-α), interleukin-1beta (IL-1β), IL-3, IL-6 — or growth factors (PDGF, nerve growth factor [NGF], TGF-β, granulocyte-macrophage colony-stimulating factor [GM-CSF], fibroblast growth factor [FGF-2]). Considering that the product ($O_2^{\bullet -}$) of NADPH oxidase, formed outside the cell, is not membrane permeable, the enzyme can modulate the intracellular pathways only after the generation of the diffusible $H_2O_2$, generated from superoxide anion.[18,20,28,29]

## IV. CELL PROTECTIVE SYSTEM AGAINST OXIDATIVE STRESS

The skin immune system is equipped to respond rapidly and effectively to a variety of insults occurring at the interface between the organism and the environment, through the coordinate activities of multiple epidermal and dermal cell populations. Depending on their concentrations, ROS may activate adaptive response or irreversibly damage skin constituents. To regulate the flow of ROS and to reduce the effects of oxidative stimuli, the skin possesses a wide array of related antioxidant defense mechanisms (Table 12.2).[33] Moreover, the higher percentage of PUFA in the membrane of the immunocompetent cells, with respect to other cell types, must be preserved by a high level of intracellular antioxidants, like ascorbic acid, vitamin E, and GSH, confirming the crucial role of a correct balance between oxidants and antioxidants for an appropriate immune surveillance. Many studies *in vitro* and *in vivo* have indicated that antioxidants improve the immune functions, leading to low levels of ROS and pro-inflammatory cytokines.[34,35] Moreover, ROS,

**TABLE 12.2**
**Cellular Antioxidant Pattern**

| Antioxidant | Property | Activity | Localization |
|---|---|---|---|
| SOD | MnSOD (tetrameric 80 kDa)<br>CuZnSOD (dimeric 32 kDa constitutive) | $2H^+ + 2O_2^{\bullet -} \rightarrow H_2O_2 + O_2$ | Mitochondria<br>Cytosol and mitochondria |
| Cat | Contains heme group (constitutive). | $2H_2O_2 \rightarrow 2H_2O + O_2$ | Peroxisomes |
| Lipoic acid system | Lipoic acid + lipoamide deydrogenase | GSH, Vit E, ascorbate, and CoQ regeneration | Cell membrane mitochondria |
| GSH | γ-L-Glutamil-L-cysteinyl-glycine tripeptide (constitutive) | Free radicals direct scavenger; substrate for GPx | Mitochondria and cytosol |
| Vit E | Lipid soluble; lowered by UV (inducible) | Lipoperoxides reduction | Membranes |
| GPx | Se-dependent; GPx1 to GPx4 | $2H_2O_2 \rightarrow 2H_2O + O_2$<br>Lipoperoxide reduction | Mitochondria and cytosol |
| GSH reductase | | GSH regeneration | Mitochondria and cytosol |
| GSH-*s*-transferase | | Lipoperoxide and pirimidine dimers reduction | Mitochondria and cytosol |
| TrxR | NADPH-dependent homodimer | $2H^+ + 2O_2^{\bullet -} \rightarrow H_2O_2 + O_2$<br>Ascorbate reduction | Mitochondria and cytosol |
| Ascorbate | Water soluble (inducible) | Vit E reduction | Cytosol |
| CoQ | Component of electron chain flow; lowered by UV (constitutive) | Lipoperoxide reduction and Vit E regeneration | Inner mitochondrial membrane |

physiologically produced in the skin, are compartmentalized according to the cellular localization of the principal antioxidants, such as SODs, catalase, glutathione, glutathione peroxidases, etc., in order to establish coordinated intracellular steady-state levels of ROS.[21] Within the antioxidant defense system, the cell is able to modulate the expression of redox-sensitive genes codifying for glutathione peroxidase, quinone reductase, catalase, SOD2, heme oxygenase, ferritin, thioredoxin, metallothionein, COX-2, and of genes not directly involved in oxidative stress such as those codifying for chemokines (IL-8 and MIP-1$\alpha$), stromelysin, and collagenase-3. The promoter of the ROS-inducible genes contains binding sites for the transcription factors AP-1, ATF/CREB, NF-$\kappa$B.[12] In the next part of the chapter, only the endogenous constituents of the skin antioxidant system are taken in consideration, even though several exogenously supplied antioxidants are known for their modulating effects on the skin immune system.

## A. Low-Molecular-Weight Antioxidants

Low-molecular-weight antioxidants (LMWA) form a heterogeneous class of compounds sharing the capacity to donate electrons and neutralize the highly reactive species illustrated above. Moreover, LMWA may contribute to the regeneration of oxidized form of each antioxidant. According to a general subdivision, LMWA can be classified in lipophilic and hydrophilic compounds. Vitamin E, $\alpha$-lipoic acid (LA), carotenoids, and ubiquinone belong to the former type, whereas the second class includes vitamin C (L-ascorbate) and reduced glutathione (GSH). Vitamin E ($\alpha$-tocopherol) is introduced in the organism with the diet or with micronutrient supplementation. Because of its lipophilicity, after absorption, it preferentially accumulates in lipid phases and cell membranes. Vitamin E plays a key role in protecting biological membranes from peroxidative damage, mainly for its capacity to neutralize peroxyl radicals and other free radicals and to arrest the initiation and propagation phases of lipoperoxidation.[36] However, the antioxidant activity of vitamin E can be highly affected by the physical state of different lipid systems and by the concentration and distribution of neighboring antioxidants. LA is a liposoluble acid containing a disulfur bridge. In cells, LA forms covalent bonds with the $\varepsilon$-amino group of lysine in cytoplasmic proteins by means of a dihydrolipoamide dehydrogenase, which reduces lipoate to dihydrolipoic acid (DHLA).[37] Enzymes involved in the GSSG reduction, such as glutathione and thioredoxine reductase, can also transform LA in DHLA.[38] DHLA can participate to the scavenging of $^{\bullet}OH$, preventing the promotion of lipoperoxidative reactions. Moreover, LA mimics the antioxidant properties of vitamin E and C and it is highly effective in contrasting the symptoms of their deficit.[39] L-Ascorbate is an important water-soluble antioxidant distributed in both extracellular and intracellular fluids.[40] Within the cells, vitamin C is present in a reduced form whereas in the intercellular space, the oxidative process generates the highly unstable dehydroascorbic acid, which, in turn, is regulated by means of a membrane-mediated reduction before entry into the cells. Intracellular L-ascorbate works as direct antioxidant and may participate in the reduction of the vitamin E radical, restoring its antioxidant capacity.[41] Vitamin C interferes with the antiproliferative effect exerted by HClO on lymphocytes *in vitro*.[42] Several reports have shown the ability of LMWA to act synergistically in preventing oxidative damage. Vitamin A and ascorbic acid help $\alpha$-tocopherol in the reduction of lipid peroxidation.[12,43] The lipoate–DHLA complex can recycle oxidized vitamin C and E.[44] Finally, it is worth taking into account that LMWA, in given conditions, may act as a pro-oxidant agent. Vitamin E at high doses favors lipid peroxidation;[45] ascorbate in association with $Fe^{2+}$ ions and carotenoids, in particular conditions, provides potent oxidant systems and increases lipid peroxidation.[46]

## B. Glutathione System

GSH is a tripeptide ($\gamma$L-gluatmyl-L-cysteinyl-L-glycine) representing the most relevant intracellular low-molecular-weight thiol present in the skin. In most cells, GSH concentration ranges between 1 and 10 m*M* and is regulated by oxidation/reduction balance and by *de novo* synthesis and breakdown. The biosynthesis of GSH is a two-step process in which the first part is the formation of γ-glutamylcysteine from glutamate and cysteine catalyzed by γ-glutamylcysteine synthetase (GCS), the second part gives GSH after the addition of glycine to γ-glutamylcysteine by glutathione synthetase. The cysteine required for the synthesis of GSH is taken from the circulating GSH that is degraded by the membrane-associated enzyme γ-glutamyl transpeptidase (γ-GT).[47] A sufficient supply of GSH is essential for the regulation of the effects caused by ROS. It acts as a free radical scavenger in non-enzymatic reactions and as the substrate of the enzyme glutathione peroxidase (GPx). In both types of reactions, GSH is oxidized to GSSG, which is rapidly recycled back to GSH by NADPH through the action of the enzyme glutathione reductase (GR). GR activity in the skin is fairly high and is warranted by an adequate supply of NADPH by glucose-6-phosphate dehydrogenase. In normal conditions, GSSG accounts for only the 1% of total glutathione. Except for conditions characterized by extended oxidative stress, the concentration of GSSG is only transiently elevated since the reduction to GSH by GR is fairly efficient. Importantly, GSH oxidation may also involve thiol groups of protein and enzymes producing PrSSG disulfides. The enzymes that use and regenerate GSH represent one of the fundamental defense systems against oxidative stress and play a central role in the survival of many cell types, even those of the immune system.[48]

### C. Catalase and Glutathione Peroxidase

The enzyme responsible for the removal of $H_2O_2$ is catalase, a homotetrameric enzyme with an active site containing heme iron.[49] Catalase is primarily placed in peroxysome, the site of major $H_2O_2$ production. However, the capacity of cells to remove $H_2O_2$ is affected by the high sensitivity of catalase to pro-oxidant agents.[50] The antioxidant activity of catalase is complemented by the seleno-enzyme glutathione peroxidase (GPx), even though the latter is located in a different cellular site and has different chemical features and substrate specificities. For example, while catalase is active only toward $H_2O_2$, GPx reduces many different peroxide compounds, including organic hydroperoxides.[12,51,52] Moreover, GPx shows high affinity for its substrates scavenging $H_2O_2$ at concentration lower than 100 μ*M*, whereas catalase acts as second line of defense, when $H_2O_2$ concentration exceeds 100 μ*M*. The reducing activity of GPx is exerted, in most cases, at the expense of the reducing equivalents of GSH-generating GSSG. Two different enzymes belong to GPx family, the classical GPx (cGPx1-3) and the phospholipid hydroperoxide GPx (PHGPx) with nuclear, cytosolic, and mitochondrial distribution. All the GPx are characterized by an active site containing cysteine. On the other hand, whereas the three cGPx forms are tetrameric and use GSH only as a reducing agent, the PHGPx is monomeric and can also utilize other reducing substrates. PHGPx is produced as short (S-PHGPx) and long (L-PHGPx) forms, with an extramitochondrial and a mitochondrial localization, respectively. Even though PHGPx is able to reduce $H_2O_2$, its main function is to protect the cellular membrane from the oxidative stress.[50] As suggested by *in vitro* overexpressing models, L-PHGPx prevents mitochondrial impairment, affecting also ATP production and the cell survival through hydroperoxide reduction. In particular, PHGPx prevents the reaction between hydrogen peroxide and mitochondrial $Fe^{2+}$, which generates hydroxyl radical and lipid hydroperoxide and leads to the "cardiolipin cascade" involved in the cytochrome *c* release. Moreover, PHGPx is able to inhibit several lipoxygenase activities (5-LOX, 12-LOX, and 15-LOX) lowering the level of prostaglandin and leukotriene formation thus directly participating in the modulation of inflammation.[53]

### D. Superoxide Dismutases

Superoxide dismutases (SODs) catalyze the dismutation of $O_2^{\bullet-}$ to $H_2O_2$ and $O_2$. The various SOD isoenzymes are crucial for the $H_2O_2$ formation in both intracellular and extracellular spaces. Schematically, the distribution of SOD isoenzymes in biological compartments includes the following localization. Inside the cells, SOD is present in two forms, one with a prevalent cytosolic

(Cu/ZnSOD, SOD1, molecular weight 32,000) localization and the second principally abundant in the mitochondrial matrix (MnSOD, SOD2, molecular weight 88,000). In the extracellular fluids an additional isoenzyme containing Cu and Zn (EC-SOD, molecular weight 135,000, SOD3) is present.[54] The enzymes work very efficiently and even if NO could react with $O_2^{-\bullet}$ more powerfully than SOD, at low NO intracellular level, SOD is the main $O_2^{\bullet-}$-degrading agent. SODs, principally MnSOD, are induced by inflammatory mediators, such as ROS, endotoxin, and pro-inflammatory cytokines, in different cell types.[55–57]

## V. ROS AS MEDIATORS OF THE SIGNAL

For several years ROS have been considered only because of their known dangerous effect. Recently, this "bad reputation" has been changed. Reactive species, including nitric oxide, are now recognized as essential molecules for a number of physiological activities,[18] by acting as second messengers.[28,58–60]

### ROS as Intracellular Messengers

ROS and RNS can act as intracellular mediators because of their ability to adapt to the environmental modifications, to modulate pathways not contiguous to the generation site, to act as a switch factor or continuous modulator, and finally to be specific mediators for multiple targets. Usually, the specificity features are classified in three types. ROS or RNS, due to their chemistry, correspond to a type III specificity, as they interact covalently with multiple targets, modulating the response to specific ligands. However, the second messenger function of ROS is still debated because the reactive species are easily diffusible and short lived but they are also specific, whereas the second messengers do not possess spatial resolution and target specificity. In addition, it is difficult to accept that potentially dangerous molecules can also take part in signaling pathways. A way to discriminate between cytotoxicity and intracellular signaling is based on the time and extent of ROS production. An example is given by NO, which when produced by NOS at low activity (eNOS and nNOS) triggers $Ca^{2+}$-mediated signals, whereas the NO generated by iNOS acts independently of $Ca^{2+}$ level and causes cell death. An intriguing explanation of these phenomena, which takes into account the non-univocal activity of the different enzyme isoforms, could be that even the death represents a component of the signaling pathway. Additional examples of second messenger activities of the reactive species are provided by SoxR nitrosylation by NO. This leads to a conformational change of SoxR and to a subsequent transactivation of the SoxS gene, thus establishing a positive feedback that controls the antioxidant enzymes synthesis. This situation represents a clear example of a type I specific interaction that requires colocalization of multiple molecular components along a specific pathway, which gives rise to a linear flow of the information, via noncovalent interactions. On the other hand, it is known that hydrogen peroxide can transiently inactivate tyrosine phosphatases, through a type III specificity mechanism, thus acting not as a second messenger but as a secondary messenger, which interferes with the extent of the reactions initiated by other mediators. Initially, guanylyl cyclase and NF-κB were indicated as the main target molecules modulated by reactive species. Indeed, the spectrum of cellular targets appears broader than previously estimated including ion channels, G protein–coupled receptors, small GTPases, phosphatases, kinases, cytoskeletal components, cell-cycle regulators, transcription factors, hystone (de)acetylases, and DNA methylases.[1]

Regarding the specific activities of the cells involved in the immune network, ROS may affect, positively and negatively, multiple cellular functions. An example can be provided directly or indirectly, by means of cytokines release, increase of the cell-to-cell contact and adhesion to the extracellular matrix. Both these events represent a crucial process in the setting of natural and adaptive immune responses.[61]

### 1. From Membrane to Nucleus

Several activities of the immune cells are explicated through a ligand–receptor interaction. The correct exposure and clustering of the receptors represent the early steps in intracellular signal transduction. The polyunsaturated fatty acid configuration confers fluidity to the cell membrane, allowing receptor recruitment, and represents the substrate for the synthesis of some regulatory eicosanoids (prostaglandins and leukotrienes) released by the cells involved in the inflammatory process. The relevance of membrane composition is proved by the evidence that the clustering of the receptor for TNF-α requires raft regions rich in sphingolipids and cholesterol. Rafts represent the liquid-ordered phase of the lipid bilayer. The receptor engagement in raft domain triggers the recruitment of the downstream kinases, whose activation leads to the mitochondrial and nuclear modifications associated with the cell answer.[62] An early event in lymphocyte proliferation is the enrichment of plasma membrane with arachidonic acid (C20:4, n6) subsequent to the activation of lysolecithin acyltransferase, located in proximity of the TCR/CD3 complex. During blastic transformation of the T cells there is an increment of fluidity of the membrane, which is due to the accumulation of oleic (C18:1, n9), docosapentaenoic (C20:5, n3), and docosahexaenoic (C22:6, n3) acids and to a reduction of linoleic (C18:2, n6) and arachidonic acids.[63] Signals depending on the redox status can be transduced from the membrane to the nucleus through a phosphorylation/dephosphorylation process of the tyrosine and serine/threonine residues of cellular proteins. Moreover, changes in the intracellular $Ca^{2+}$ level, depending on the redox status of the thiols, influence the extent of redox-dependent phosphorylation.[61] An example of membrane protein phosphorylation is provided by the UVB-induced activation of the receptors for the growth factors KGF and EGF. The UVB-dependent phosphorylation and internalization of KGFR on fibroblasts is mediated by the time-limited production of ROS within a few minutes, as confirmed by antioxidant-mediated inhibition of the process. The relevance of the membrane modification in the redox signal transmission is further marked by the diminishment of the membrane PUFA after UVB radiation.[64–66]

### 2. From Mitochondria to Nucleus

Mitochondria play a part in the ROS-governed processes, as they are involved in the transduction of the signal to the nucleus, even through a restrained ROS release (Figure 12.1). When ROS

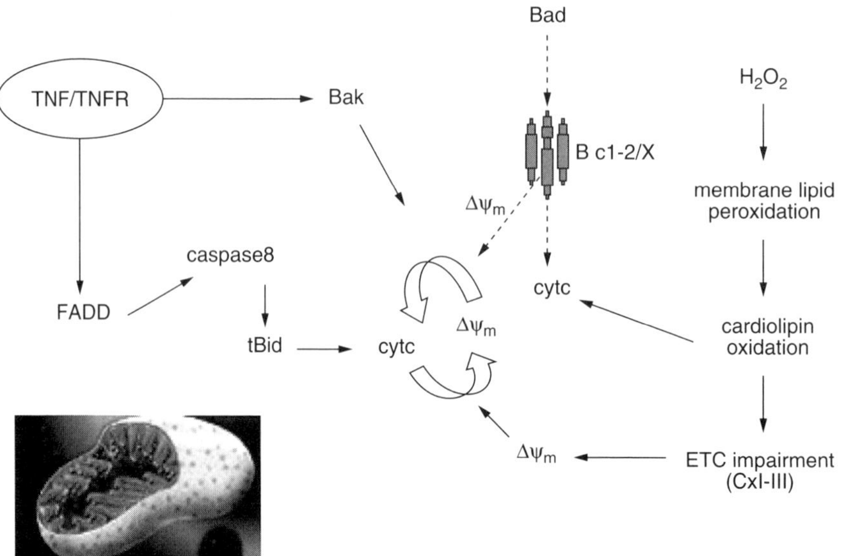


**FIGURE 12.1** Some intramitochondrial events and cell death.

generation is low, nuclear genes that upregulate the metabolic rate, as well as the cell rescue machinery, are activated. In contrast, when ROS exceed a threshold level, they act in reducing the transmembrane potential and in releasing cytochrome *c*, thus triggering an apoptotic process.[67] Mitochondrial function, undoubtedly, represents a crucial link between cellular redox status and apoptotic events, controlled through caspase activation. The relevance of ROS-mediated release of cytochrome *c*, activation of caspases, ASK-1, and p38 are further supported by the effects of antioxidants, such as thioredoxin and thioredoxin peroxidase, that effectively counteract all these events.[68] PHGPx inhibits the generation of cardiolipin hydroperoxide, which represents the first step in cytochrome *c* release. Cardiolipin, located in the inner mitochondrial membrane, binds also to NADH-ubiquinone oxidoreductase, cytochrome *c* oxidase, and adenine nucleotide translocator (ANT), which is known to be implicated in apoptotic-associated membrane remodeling and pro-apoptotic factors release. The link between the levels of mitochondrial membrane lipoperoxides and cytochrome *c* release is illustrated by the following cascade of events. An excessive intracellular ROS generation triggers peroxidation of lipids, including cardiolipin, with a subsequent conformational change of cytochrome *c* and dissociation from cardiolipin; the next step takes place by the release of cytochrome *c* in the extramitochondrial environment with induction and/or amplification of multiple apoptotic pathways. In addition, ANT bears several thiol groups and can be completely inhibited by the cardiolipin hydroperoxide and by the cytochrome *c* itself. Thus, PHGPx, lowering the mitochondrial level of lipid hydroperoxides, directly regulates multiple mitochondrial apoptotic pathways.[69,-70] As in the case of the cell membrane, the mitochondrial membrane composition plays a relevant role in ROS generation. Unsaturated phospholipids, which represent a main constituent of the membrane structure, have two key functions: to properly assemble and maintain the functional state of the protein complexes involved in the electron transport chain and to couple oxidation with phosphorylation. A deficiency of polyunsaturated fatty acids determines an increase of ROS generation and has been associated with some impaired activities of the immune system.

## 3. Redox Signals and $Ca^{2+}$

ROS can elicit $Ca^{2+}$ responses, and calcium channels are known ROS targets. In fact, exogenous $H_2O_2$ reduces the threshold sensitivity of endothelial cells to $IP_3$ (inositol 3 phosphate) at levels able to induce $Ca^{2+}$ release. $Ca^{2+}$-ATPase, $Na^+/Ca^{2+}$ exchanger, and calmodulin activities appear to be under redox control. An additional example is provided by nerve tissue in which agonist stimulation and ROS-mediated oxidation act together to enhance the $Ca^{2+}$ signaling. The effect of ROS on $Ca^{2+}$-driven signal appears to be dose dependent, as a low ROS level exerts mitogenic action on lymphocytes whereas high ROS intracellular concentrations shift the cells toward an apoptotic phenotype. This appears related to the duration of $Ca^{2+}$ flux because nanomolar $H_2O_2$ concentration causes a short, transient release of $Ca^{2+}$ from intracellular stores, followed by ERK1/2 activation and growth response, whereas micromolar $H_2O_2$ concentrations elicit a prolonged $Ca^{2+}$ flux (release from intracellular stores plus influx) associated with cell cycle arrest and upregulation of $p27^{Kip1}$.[28,29,71]

## 4. Cysteine as Redox Sensor and Signal Transducer

The oxidation/reduction of cysteine is crucial in the regulation of intracellular redox homeostasis and appears to be involved in some essential functions of the APC (antigen-presenting cells). The ability of APCs to professionally present the antigens depends on their ability to take protein and enzymatically and chemically modify it, and show the product on the membrane surface in association with MHC II molecules. The oxidation status of cysteine residues present in some enzymes involved in these processes affects their activity and the entire antigen processing.[60] Cysteine ($pK_a$ 4.7 to 5.4) is a thiolate anion at neutral pH and forms a thiol-phosphate intermediate in the protein tyrosine phosphatase pathway. The oxidation of cysteine inhibits the phosphatase activity, leading to phosphorylation and cell proliferation. In addition, the Cys-X-X-Cys motif in redoxins (thioredoxin, glutaredoxin) represents a target for ROS that are able to activate downstream pathways. Thioredoxin is associated with ASK1. In response to cytokines, such as TNF-α, the oxidation of the cysteine motif by ROS leads to its dissociation from ASK1 allowing active kinase. Protein tyrosine phosphatase (PTP) is a cysteine-dependent enzyme characterized by the presence of the PTP signature motif Cys-$(Xaa)_5$-Arg at the catalytic site. The catalytic site containing cysteine has a low $pK_a$ and thus is susceptible to inactivation by ROS.[72] The cysteine redox status appears to be relevant also for the activity of protein tyrosine phosphatase 1B (PTP1B), which acts by attacking its $Cys_{215}$ to phosphotyrosine substrate (pTyr) with the production of a covalent phosphocysteine intermediate. In fact, the peculiar motif of PTP forms a cradle-like conformation where $Cys_{215}$ is stabilized, and represents the functional support for the active site. On the other hand, $Tyr_{46}$ confers the specificity for pTyr substrate. The oxidation of $Cys_{215}$ to sulfenic acid by $H_2O_2$ determines the formation of a sulfenyl-amide bond and an intense modification of the active site. PTP1B can be reactivated by GSH, suggesting the formation of mixed disulfides with $Cys_{215}$. The sulfenyl-amide intermediate prevents the irreversible oxidation of $Cys_{215}$.[70,71]

## 5. Nitric Oxide

Monocytes/macrophages are the main producers of NO, indicating that NO plays a crucial role in antimicrobial defense.[73] In the phagocytic cells, NOS and NAD(P)H oxidase are simultaneously overexpressed after stimulation with cytokines, peptide hormones, and bacterial endotoxins.[20] NO is released by infiltrating macrophages in the presence of $CD4^+$ T cells. It acts as an effector molecule of the cytotoxic machinery and as a modulator of cytokine production, providing the shift toward a Th2 response.[74] The molecular mechanism involved in the NO pathway includes the induction of iNOS in skin dendritic cells, which is positively regulated by JAK2 (janus kinase 2) and NF-κB,[75] which, in turn, act on an iNOS enhancer that contains elements responsive to NF-κB and IFN-γ (Stat1a and IFN-regulatory factors, IRF-1/2).[76] NO, in turn, regulates the activity of NF-κB and AP-1,[74] through a pathway that induces Ras activation and $PI_3$ release. Low concentration of NO activates NF-κB, whereas high levels of NO cause nitrosylation of cysteine in a p50 subunit, therefore preventing its binding to DNA. In the presence of other ROS, NO induces G protein $p21^{Ras}$, heme-oxygenase-1, and COX through the activation of MAPK.[20] Moreover, NO activates PPAR-γ in macrophages with a subsequent decrease of the oxidative burst via downregulation of p47 phagocyte oxidase ($p47^{phox}$), a component of NADPH oxidase. In monocyte/macrophage, NO is able to induce both the interaction between PPAR-γ and DNA and the transactivation of a PPAR-responsive gene within 1 to 2 h. The rapid activation of the PPAR response is consistent with recruitment of a preformed factor and is less likely consistent with enhanced mRNA expression. This process probably accounts for a negative feedback mechanism, which allows containment of free radical release by the cells. Recently, PPAR-γ has been reported to antagonize co-activators such as CREB-protein (cAMP-responsive element-binding protein) leading to a block of TNF-α formation.[73] The effect of NO on transcription factors is bimodal: when the concentrations of ROS and NO are elevated, GSH and proteins, including thioredoxin reductase, can be nitrosylated. The accumulation of oxidized thioredoxin activates ASK1 and JNK. The reaction of NO with high concentration of superoxide anion produces $ONOO^-$ and its accumulation stimulates the apoptotic process via the JNK, p53, Bax, cytochrome *c*, and caspase pathways. On the contrary, at low $O_2^{\bullet -}$ level a cGMP-dependent activation of HSP32 and Bcl-2 takes place, suppressing the apoptotic process. The production of cGMP is the result of the activation of guanylate cyclase, an enzyme highly sensitive to NO because of its prosthetic heme group.[20] The involvement of NO in the apoptotic process of T cells is supported by the finding that its release is induced by pro-apoptotic stimuli, such as TNF-α and IL-1β. However, the relationship between NO and Fas remains unclear. Fas engagement leads to the release of NO with a consequent membrane hyperpolarization, depending on the proton force associated with F1-FoATPase activity. This process plays a protective role

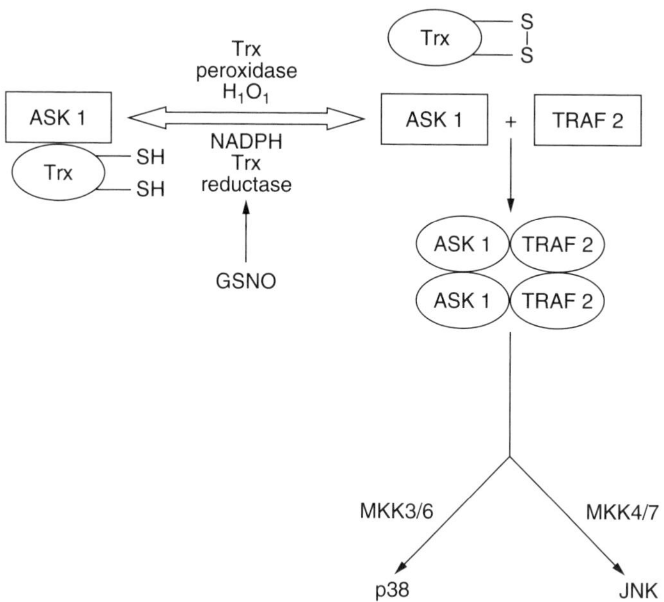


**FIGURE 12.2** Redox regulation of ASK1. (Modified from Turpaev.[20])

against T-lymphocyte apoptosis at least until the pro-apoptotic signals overcome it. A continuous NO overload inhibits mitochondrial respiration, whereas the effect is partially countered by a reversal of F1-FoATPase and ATP production through the glycolitic pathway, which allows extrusion of protons from the matrix and the establishment of a correct transmembrane potential.[28] Finally, NO can act as antioxidant both limiting lipid peroxidation chain reaction and subtracting iron ions. This process represents a mechanism of control against excessive production and release of ROS by infiltrating lymphocytes.[20]

## 6. Intracellular Pathways

Molecular targets of ROS are represented by ERK1/2, JNK (the most sensitive), and p38 MAPK pathways. Schematically, ERK1/2 is involved in lymphocyte proliferation and activation. In addition to the early phases of antigen-dependent activation, the duration of ERK activation represents the threshold for either negative (transient activation) or positive (sustained activation) thymocyte selection.[76,77] The different kinases induced by the $H_2O_2$ level modification within MAPK family regulate specifically the apoptotic pathways (JNK) or cell activation and ICAM-1 expression (p38), thus affecting cellular functions differentially. Among the upstream mediators involved in the MAPK pathways, Fyn and Jak2 activities are required for $H_2O_2$ activation of Ras and ERK1/2. The JNK activation requires Src and Cas but not Fyn, suggesting that c-Src and Fyn act separately in ROS-mediated signal transduction. Finally, ROS stimulation is associated with a tyrosine phosphatase downregulation with a subsequent burst of the opposite kinases.[32,33] The activity of ERK, p38, and JNK is regulated by threonine-tyrosine protein kinases, named kinases of MAP protein kinases (MEK, MKK, MAPKK). The phosphorylation and the activity of these kinases are controlled by specific double-protein phosphatases (MKP1/2, PP2A). In addition, the protein kinase ASK1 (apoptosis signal-regulating kinase 1) (Figure 12.2), a member of MAP3K family, is also involved in the mechanism of the redox-regulation of the MAPK. Interestingly, reduced thioredoxin binds to the ASK1 N-terminal region and inactivates it by blocking the binding site for TRAF2 (TNF receptor-associated factor 2). Consequently, the thioredoxin oxidation, induced by $H_2O_2$ or other ROS, provides for the release of ASK1, which can thus phosphorylate and activate MKK3/6/7 and SEK1. These, in turn, activate p38 and JNK. Thus, the activation of ASK1 by stress inducers,

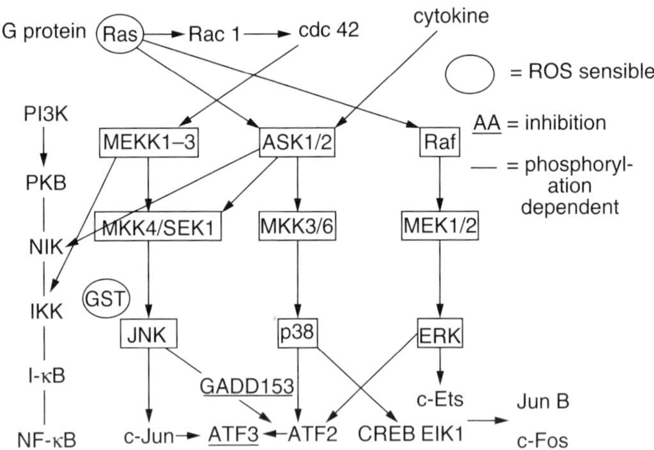


**FIGURE 12.3** MAPK pathways and ROS. (Modified from Turpaev.[20])

such as TNF, UV, or growth factor withdrawal, initiates the apoptotic pathway. ASK1 is controlled by the PP5 (protein serine/threonine phosphatase), which, by dephosphorylating the active ASK1, determines its downregulation. Therefore, the accumulation of unfolded protein in the endoplasmic reticulum activates ASK1, thus delivering an apoptotic signal.[20,78,79] ROS can activate ERK through some membrane-associated proteins, such as G protein $p21^{Ras}$, Rac, tyrosine protein kinase Fyn (Src family), factor $p66^{Shc}$, and the double serine-serine protein kinase Raf. ERK, which is controlled by several growth factors, activates transcription factors Elk-1 and c-Ets, which, in turn, regulate c-Fos, a subunit of AP-1.[20,78] An excessive activation of the MAPK pathway could elicit a negative loop. In T lymphocytes, the engagement of the T-cell receptor (TCR) leads to rapid production of hydrogen peroxide and other ROS, via a MEK1-dependent mechanism, establishing a negative feedback on MEK-ERK activation and the subsequent phosphorylation of regulatory proteins. Probably the ability of ROS to activate or inhibit ERK depends on its oxidative modification of the protein tyrosine phosphatases (PTP1B and SHP-2) (Figure 12.3).[76,77]

## 7. Transcription Factors

The intracellular redox potential affects the activity of several transcription factors (Hif-1α, Ref-1, AP-1, Nrf, STAT, AIF, NF-κB, Sp-1, c-Myb, p53), thus regulating the expression of multiple genes involved in cell survival, functional activation, and death.[80] Moreover, the cellular redox status is conditioned even by the oxidation of NAD cofactors ($NAD^+$, NADH, $NADP^+$, NADPH), acting as redox sensors.[64,81,82]

Exposure of hypoxic cells to $H_2O_2$ helps to establish normoxic conditions through down-modulation of the Hif-1 (hypoxia-induced factor 1). Under normal $pO_2$, Hif-1 is degraded, whereas during hypoxia the ubiquitin pathway of Hif-1α is inhibited leading to an overexpression.[32] To avoid an excessive activation of Hif-1, this factor is hydroxylated to be bound to the von Hippel–Lindau protein and then to the E3 ubiquitin protein ligase.[64] The Hif-1α subunit permits the binding to DNA and is characterized by helix-loop-helix loop (HLH family), in which the Hif-1β subunit promotes the nuclear translocation. The presence of an iron-sulfur cluster in Hif-1α plays a ROS receptor-like role. The hypoxia-induced hyperproduction of ROS by mitochondria causes the oxidation of iron ions and then inhibits Hif-1 degradation allowing its nuclear translocation. Decreased oxygen pressure can indirectly determine (through the production of semiquinones and reduced flavins) the generation of ROS by the mitochondria.[20] Hif-1α, which controls the expression of at least 30 $O_2$-sensitive genes, is directly involved in the leukocyte response to hypoxia and inflammation. In response to an injury, neutrophils arrest the blood flow in the small vessels, allowing migration into the tissue in inflammation areas. The blood flow reduction also determines a low $O_2$ pressure and the migration of macrophage precursors at the site of inflammation. When the pressure of $O_2$ is lowered or the superoxide anion is overproduced by the mitochondrial electron transport chain, the two Hif-1 subunits can associate and activate several genes. In addition, Hif-1α is involved in ATP production via glycolitic enzymes, and this is essential for leukocyte migration in peripheral tissues.[83]

The 37-kDa Ref-1 induces the DNA binding of AP-1 by means of a redox-dependent reduction of cysteines at DNA-binding of c-*fos* and c-*jun*. By this modality Ref-1 also regulates other transcription factors, such as NF-κB, p53, Egr-1, c-Myb, Pax-8. In addition, it exhibits an apurinic/apyrimidinic endonuclease activity, therefore participating in the base excision repair pathway. In different cell types, Ref-1 exerts a protective role against cell death as induced by oxidative stimuli. It prevents nuclear translocation and then activation of NF-κB induced by hypoxia, via the inhibition of the $H_2O_2$-regulated Rac-1. Noteworthy is that Ref-1 does not affect the $H_2O_2$ rate of elimination; rather it acts in containing its intracellular production as induced by hypoxia or TNF-α. Ref-1 activity is located both at nuclear and cytoplasmic levels. The nuclear activity is due to the N-terminus cysteine-mediated reduction of the transcription factors and to C-terminus endonuclease function. The cytoplasmic activity of Ref-1 affects the regulation of $H_2O_2$ production, the activation of IκB kinases, or the IκB affinity. The link between Ref-1 activities and oxidative stress is also supported by evidence of its binding to thioredoxin, which, in turn, is able to bind to NADPH oxidase $p40^{phox}$, thus suggesting an involvement of Ref-1 in the NADPH oxidase control. However, NF-κB regulation by Ref-1 appears more complex, as cytoplasmic Ref-1 inhibits the Rac-1-dependent NF-κB nuclear translocation by lowering ROS production, whereas the nuclear Ref-1 form maintains the NF-κB reduced form and promotes NF-κB-mediated gene transcription.[32,80]

Among the stress-induced transcription factors, the Nrf (nuclear respiratory factor) family should be mentioned. Nrf1 and 2 are involved in the upregulation of NAD(P)H:quinone oxidoreductase, glutathione-*S*-transferase, epoxide hydrolase. The specific DNA-binding sites for Nrf are named antioxidant responsive element (ARE) where the cooperative binding between Nrf and AP-1 transcription factors takes place.[20]

STAT (signal transducers activators transcription) represent well-characterized mediators of cytokines and hormone-induced signals. STAT is activated by intracellular and exogenous ROS. Phosphorylated STAT is then able to translocate into the nucleus where it induces the expression of target genes. The 70- and 90-kDa HSP (heat shock proteins), transactivated by STAT, prevent protein aggregation under stress condition, and may antagonize multiple signals leading to apoptosis. It is likely that the $H_2O_2$-mediated activation of HSP70 may play a part in the mechanism of adaptation to oxidative stress.[84]

Interestingly, proteins involved as transducers of redox signaling are multifunctional proteins. An example is provided by AIF (apoptosis-inducing factor), which can act as NADH oxidase in mitochondria and as scaffolding protein for a caspase-independent nuclear cell death. Moreover, it can work in the electron transport chain, as indicated by the evidence that a genetic deletion of AIF causes an uncoupling of mitochondrial electron flow, an increase of ROS, membrane disruption, and nuclear translocation of AIF.[64,85]

NF-κB induces several genes involved in both natural and adaptive immune responses, in the cellular protection from stress stimuli, and in the apoptotic process. The transcription factor is sequestered in the cytosol until the inhibitor protein IκBα is removed by phosphorylation and targeted to ubiquitin-mediated degradation (IκB kinase, IKK). The catalytic subunit IKKα appears to be involved in B-cell maturation, independently on the general NF-κB activation, and some functions previously assigned to NF-κB were recognized as peculiar to IKKα, such as NF-κB transcriptional activation and p100 and IκBα phosphorylation.[86] ROS trigger NF-κB through several pathways: activation of G protein $p21^{Ras}$, of membrane phosphatidylinositol-3-kinase (PIP3K), and of phosphatidylinositol-3,4,5-triphosphate-dependent protein kinases PKB, $PKC_{\zeta}$, and $PKC_{\theta}$; activation of MEKK1, TAK1, MKK6 members of MAPK cascades JNK and p38; modulation of thioredoxin peroxidase activity.[20,87] Endotoxins, such as LPS, induce an increase of ROS generation, TNF-α release, lipoperoxidation, altered GSSG/GSH ratio, and reduction of Cat and SOD activities in both phagocytes and lymphocytes. All these modifications are associated with the activation of NF-κB.[88] It is well known that the release of ROS induces several cytokines (IL-1β, IL-6, TNF-α) in a dose-dependent-manner. Studies of the molecular pathways connecting redox status, NF-κB activation, and cytokine release indicate that GSH depletion causes an IκBα stabilization with subsequent downregulation of NF-κB translocation.[89,90] The activity of the γ-glutamyltranspeptidase, which hydrolyzes GSH, favors ROS elevation, and finally triggers the transactivation of NF-κB. The ROS-mediated activation of NF-κB appears to be different from those promoted by cytokine-mediated responses, and involves a particular tyrosine residue in IκBα instead of two N-terminal serines.[92]

The presence of cysteine residues in DNA-binding domains of c-Jun, c-Fos, and p50 makes these factors highly sensitive to ROS-mediated oxidation, a process that inactivates the AP-1 and NF-κB transcription factors. The subsequent reduction is possible by means of Redox Factor 1 (Ref-1), a protein containing active thiol groups, which is involved in DNA repair (DNAse activity) and in p53 activation. The inactivation of the transcription factors takes place only at high ROS concentration and this simultaneously causes an increased rate of apoptosis.[20]

## VI. ROS AS MEDIATORS OF THE IMMUNE RESPONSE

### A. Lymphocytes

The extent of ROS generation affects cell functions both directly, by interfering with the activity of some enzymes involved in the signal transduction, and indirectly, by affecting the membrane integrity. Indeed, proper lipid composition of the plasma membrane allows the correct plugging, within the membrane, of the different components of the signal transduction machinery. Consequently, the lipoperoxidative processes, which lead to a loss of membrane fluidity, can substantially impair correct exposure of the receptors, recruitment of the different components of the receptor complexes, and downstream transmembrane protein modifications. All these alterations can then affect the development of the immune response. Regarding the direct effect of the redox status on some specific steps necessary for signal transduction in immunocompetent cells, the involvement of ROS in lymphocyte activation takes place at several levels, such as receptor activation by antigens, kinase induction, and induction of phosphatase-mediated inhibition. The classical B-lymphocyte products, the immunoglobulins, have been recently identified as a possible catalytic center for the $^1O_2$ reduction. Probably, the site is provided by the point of contact between immunoglobulin heavy and light chain variable domains ($V_H$ and $V_L$, respectively), where $H_2O_2$ is ensnared in a hydrophobic pocket. Obviously, the colocalization of NADPH oxidase and immunoglobulins can increase ROS generation. BCR (B-cell receptor) or TCR (T-cell receptor) activation and CD2/LFA3 recruitment[93] are associated with $H_2O_2$ generation, which is implicated in the amplification of the signal transduction (Figure 12.4). Moreover, $H_2O_2$ can mimic the function of the ligand by activating the specific lymphocyte receptor, through the oxidation of the protein, with the subsequent aggregation and activation. Alternatively, the direct downstream PTK activation, or the inhibition of PTP activity, may take place. It is known that the transduction of the signal from the receptor depends on the relative extent of the activation along the pathways of the kinases and phosphatases. Considering that the two enzymes are characterized by different kinetic orders (second-order reaction for PTK and first-order reaction for PTP) and by a significantly different turnover rate (1000-fold higher in PTP than in PTK), ROS, by acting on both kinases and phosphatases, can modulate fine regulation of their activity.[18,94]

A crucial role for B-cell survival is played by the BCR, which is able to rapidly activate NF-κB and the genes under its control, such as Bcl-2 and Bcl-$X_L$. In the BCR-mediated signal the complex produced by Btk (Bruton tyrosine kinase), adapter BLNK (B-cell linker), and PLCγ2 plays

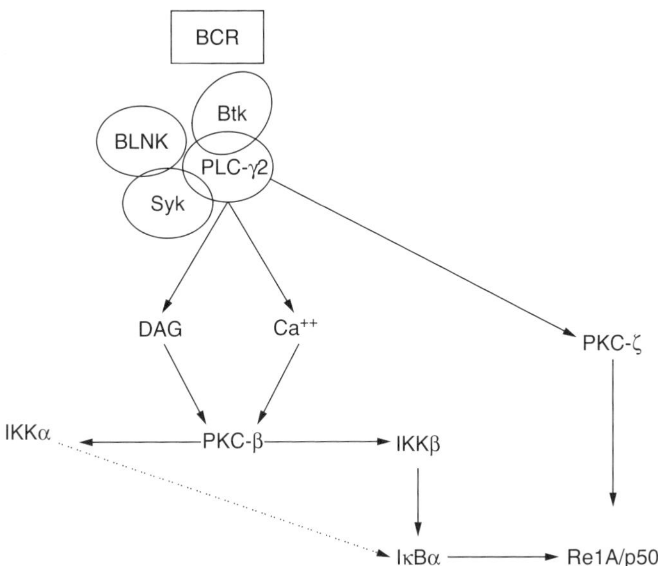


**FIGURE 12.4** Lymphocyte-receptor-mediated pathway. (Modified from Moscat et al.[86])

a central role.[86] In addition, Btk and Akt can interact with each other following $H_2O_2$ generation.[95] The specific ligand engagement of BCR causes a rapid translocation of the receptor to a $H_2O_2$ source, such as NADPH oxidase, confirming a physical and functional association between the two complexes.[18] The proliferation and activation of the lymphocytes are also mediated by the ROS-dependent stimulation of MAPK, $Ca^{2+}_i$ increase, and p56*lck* and p72*syk* activation.[96,97] Even the functional activity of other membrane receptors appears dependent on ROS. The binding and activation of VCAM-1, physiologically expressed by endothelial cells, induces the release of ROS by the specific stimulation of NADPH oxidase and ROS, therefore acting as an intracellular messenger. This induces a change in the endothelial cell cytoskeleton and cellular shape, which allows lymphocyte migration through the blood vessels.[98]

The antioxidants ascorbic acid and *N*-acetylcysteine can counteract the increased adhesion as well as TNF-α release by lymphocytes, as during endotoxic shock experimentally induced in an animal model, confirming the involvement of ROS in the adhesion process.[99,100] Antioxidants, and GSH in particular, are capable of modulating several lymphocyte functions, even by small variations of intracellular GSH concentration or of the GSH/GSSG ratio, since the redox-sensitive site of T-cell activation corresponds to very early components (p56*lck*, p59*fyn*) of the MAPK cascade.[101] In resting naive T cells, the activity of γ-GT is very low, whereas resting memory T cells show a significantly higher expression of this enzymatic activity. GSH synthase also may differentially affect naive and memory cell activities, by altering the NF-κB response and the threshold sensitivity to Fas-induced apoptosis. Memory T lymphocyte seems to be able to administer oxidative stress induced by CD28 engagement or exogenous $H_2O_2$ through the modulation of NF-κB activation. IL-2 production triggered by CD28 engagement depends on the activation of 5-LOX and is associated with a decrease of intracellular GSH.[96] *In vitro* experimental models showed a tight relationship among GSH production, the status of T-cell activation, and the response to NO. Low-GSH-producing T-cell subsets are characterized by a "non-activated" phenotype and by an exacerbated apoptotic response to NO. In addition, the cross-communication between NO and GSH interferes with the amount of IFN-γ produced by T cells in response to activation signals.[102–104] The tight link between antioxidant/pro-oxidant balance and the cell death process in lymphocytes is further supported by evidence of an improvement of cell viability coupled with a reduction of the mitochondrial ROS production after oral intake of a pool of antioxidants.[105,106]

## B. Monocytes

Monocytes, after physical or chemical stimulation, are able to produce and release in the extracellular environment ROS to a higher extent than lymphocytes. ROS production appears to be related to the process of monocyte-to-macrophage differentiation through COX-2 activation.[107] M-CSF (monocyte-colony stimulating factor) is involved in monocyte/macrophage homeostasis and survival by activating Akt and ERK. M-CSF induces ERK activation via PI3K and ROS production. The PI3K products are targets for Vav, a protein acting as exchange factor for the NADPH oxidase and Rac. Rac, when activated, stabilizes the NADPH oxidase complex and promotes ROS production. Akt and ERK work synergistically to activate NF-κB and thus to permit cell viability.[108] ROS production interferes with the ceramide pathway involved in cell death process. Synthetic analogues of ceramides (C2/C6 ceramides) cause an increase of ROS with a subsequent growth arrest, depending on the extent of the GSH depletion.[109,110]

## C. Eosinophils

Eosinophils are involved in inflammatory and allergic diseases and their function appears to be controlled by specific chemokines, such as those of eotaxin family. These chemokines enhance the effector function, by inducing $O_2^{\bullet-}$ production and degranulation. ROS production is associated with the release of granules determining tissue destruction. The eosiniphil peroxidase catalyzed the oxidation of several targets by $H_2O_2$ in the presence of halides, such as bromide.[111]

## D. Neutrophils

Neutrophils represent the first defense against microorganisms, which are phagocytated and destroyed mainly via an oxygen-dependent pathway. The activation of the neutrophils induces the respiratory burst, an accelerated cyanide-insensitive oxygen uptake, which leads to univalent and divalent $O_2$ reduction. In the respiratory burst the crucial events are the receptor–ligand interaction, protein kinase C activation, membrane translocation of NADPH, and finally the oxygen burst. Following stimulation, the different components of the NADPH oxidase complex are assembled and translocate to the membrane,[112] through different mechanisms probably involving the GTP-associated Rac and the redox-sensitive p40 proteins.[12,20,21,35,36] The protein p29 participates to the NADPH oxidase complex and exhibits $Ca^{2+}$-independent $PLA_2$ activity at phosphatidylcholine substrates, protects glutathione synthetase, inactivates $H_2O_2$, and can be considered a peroxiredoxin. Probably, p29 associates with p67 in the cytosol, and in this form it protects NADPH oxidase from $O_2^{\bullet-}$ and the consequent oxidative damage by inactivating $H_2O_2$ and by interfering with $H_2O_2$-mediated signal.[112] The neutrophils involved in the inflammatory process are not responsive to apoptotic signals mediated by Fas. This peculiar behavior appears to be associated with increased levels of GSH and a modified expression of caspases. The effect of the antioxidant could be mediated by mitochondrial membrane stabilization and by a direct inhibition of the caspase activity.[113,114] On the other hand, the pro-inflammatory activity of neutrophils is balanced by some negative feedback circuits involving arachidonic acid metabolism. Arachidonate is a substrate for the neutrophil 5-LOX, which produces the inflammatory leukotriene B4 ($LTB_4$). However, arachidonate also activates 15-LOX, which generates, even from the intermediate leukotriene A4 ($LTA_4$), lipoxin, with anti-inflammatory properties. Through this mechanism, the cell can autoregulate the passage from a pro-inflammatory to an anti-inflammatory phenotype. In addition, COX-2, induced by microbial derivatives, uses arachidonate as substrate to generate PGE2, which is able, in turn, to exert a negative control on 5-LOX but not on 15-LOX.[115] Lipoxin can cut the inflammatory response through different mechanisms: by reducing the recruitment and the activation of the neutrophils and by lowering $O_2^{\bullet-}$ formation, also responsible for the $ONOO^-$ production. Peroxynitrite is able to activate ERK and to act as intracellular second messenger for the IL-8 mRNA expression, via NF-κB and AP-1 nuclear accumulation, whereas lipoxin inhibits both these processes. In particular,

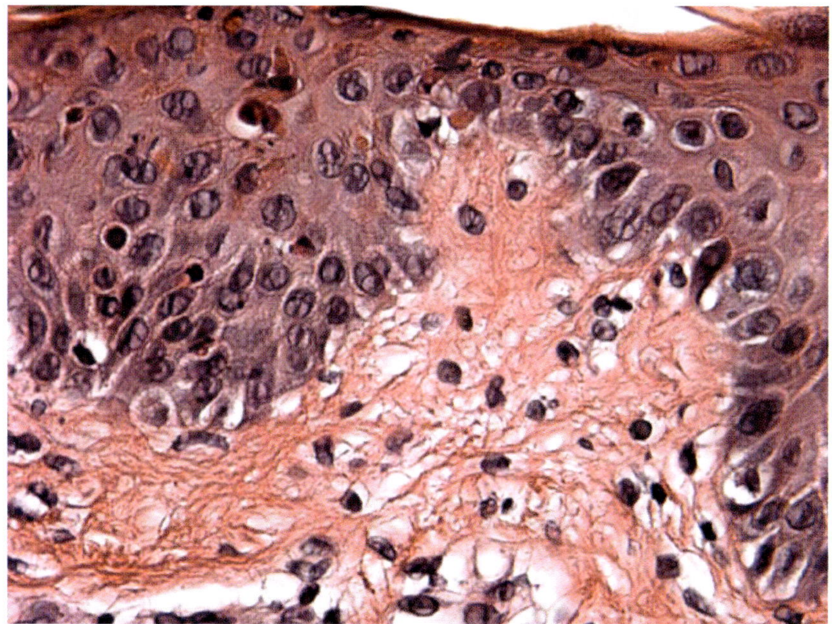

**FIGURE 8.6** UV-light-induced macrophages infiltration into skin after 4 MED UV irradiation, macrophages in papillary dermis and epidermis.

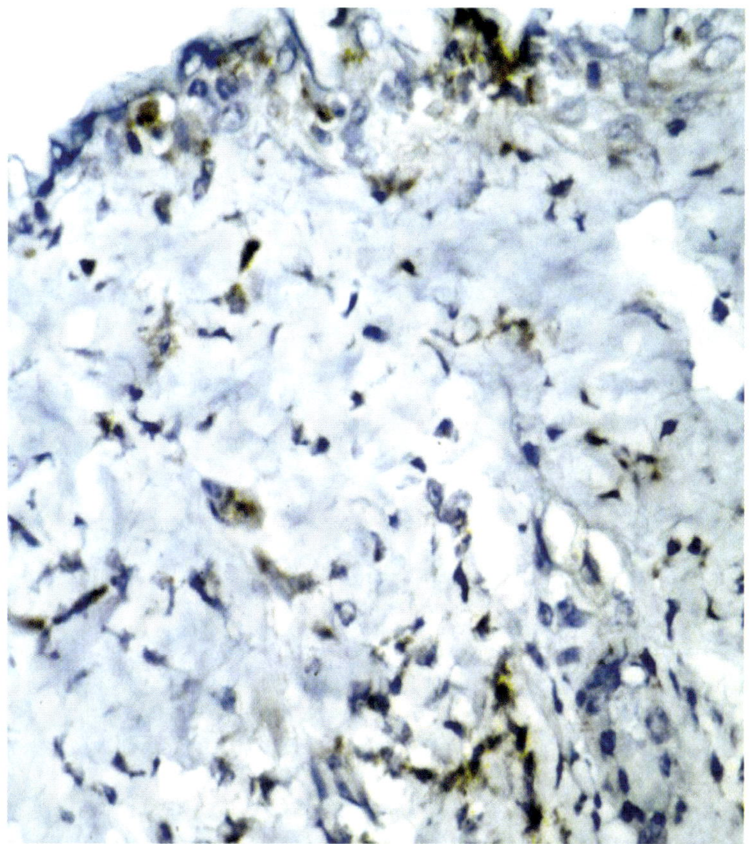

**FIGURE 8.8** Highly significant staining for $H_2O_2$ was observed in UVB-exposed sample. Numerous cells in the dermis and the epidermis exhibit positive staining. Intense staining was observed in cells with large cytoplasm, most likely representing macrophages in the perivascular and epidermal compartments.

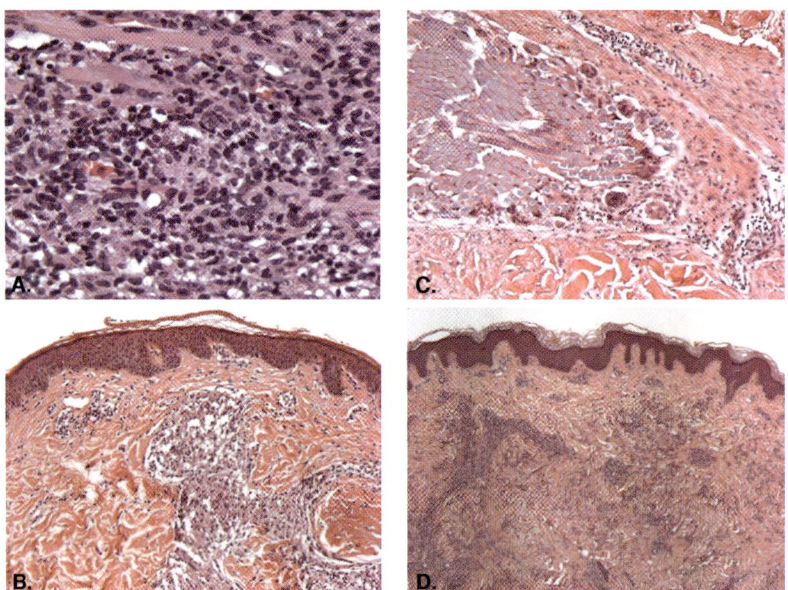


**FIGURE 8.9** Different patterns of macrophage infiltration in skin. (a) Infectious granuloma. Dense infiltrates of histiocytes, some of which contain *Leishmania* organisms. (b) Foreign body granuloma. Collections of macrophages and foreign body giant cells around suture fragments. (c) Sarcoidosis. An epitheloid cell granuloma. (d) Granuloma annulare. A palisaded granuloma with collections of histiocytes around central area of clearing.

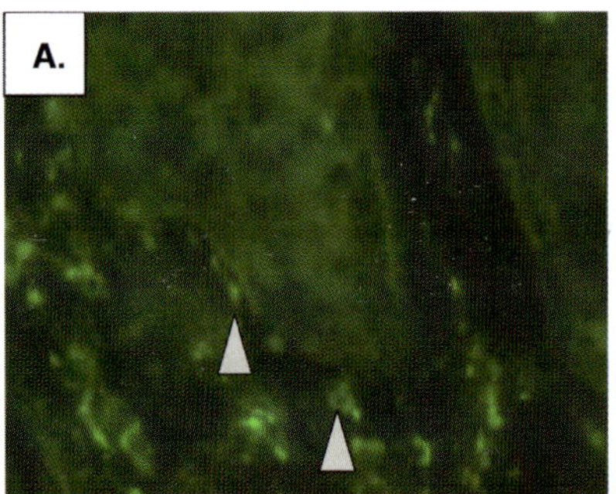


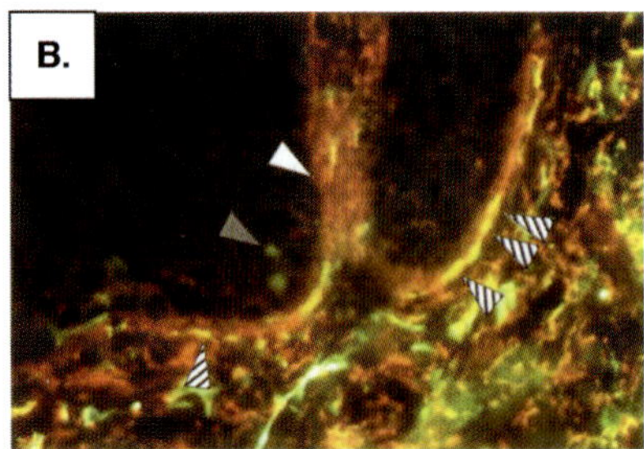


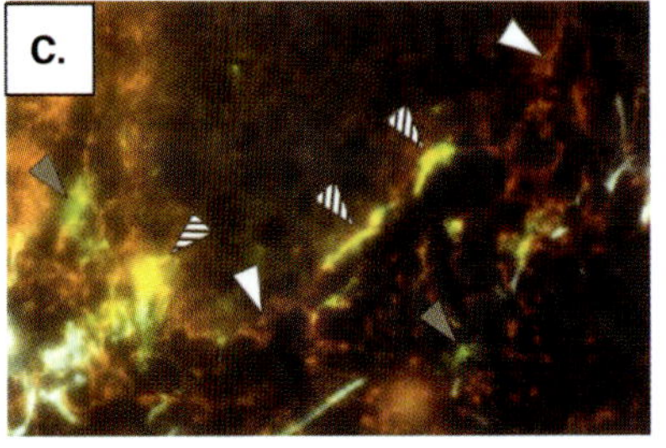


**FIGURE 8.10** CD68$^+$ cells along the DEJ of involved psoriasis tissue are also CD45$^+$ and colocalize with extradomain A (EDA) fibronectin. (a) CD68 expression was detected using a FITC-conjugated anti-CD68-specific antibody. CD68$^+$ cells can be seen lining the DEJ, as well as in the papillary dermis (gray arrows). Double immunohistochemistry staining was performed on involved skin sections. CD45RO (b) or RB (c) and EDA fibronectin antibodies were detected by a FITC-conjugated antibody and a biotinylated antibody, respectively, plus Streptavidin-Rhodamine. Double staining resulted in yellow fluorescence (striped arrows) was present in elongate cells along the DEJ (BandC). EDA fibronectin deposition along the DEJ without CD45$^+$ cell association is noted in red (white arrow). CD45RO$^+$ cells and CD45RB$^+$ cells without EDA fibronectin co-expression is noted in b and c, respectively (gray arrows).

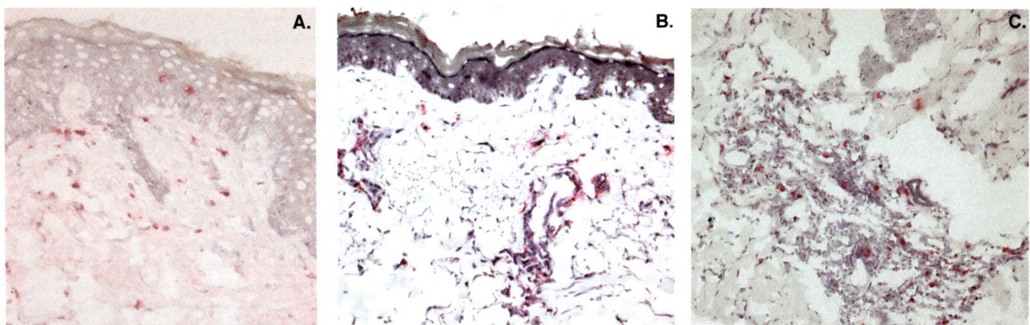


**FIGURE 11.2** Detection of granulocytes in skin by immunohistochemistry. (a) Neutrophil presence in the skin 18 h after UV irradiation of normal healthy skin. Neutrophils (red) are stained for their specific elastase content. Note that apart from neutrophil presence in the dermis, neutrophil infiltration is also found in the epidermis. (b) Eosinophil infiltration in the skin of a patient with AD 24 h after an atopy patch test. Eosinophils (red) are stained with EG2 antibody binding to eosinophil cationic protein. Eosinophil presence is predominantly perivascular. (c) Detail of basophil infiltration in the skin of an allergic patient 18 h after intracutaneous skin testing. Basophils (red) are stained with BB1 antibody binding to basogranulin and are located in the perivascular infiltrate.

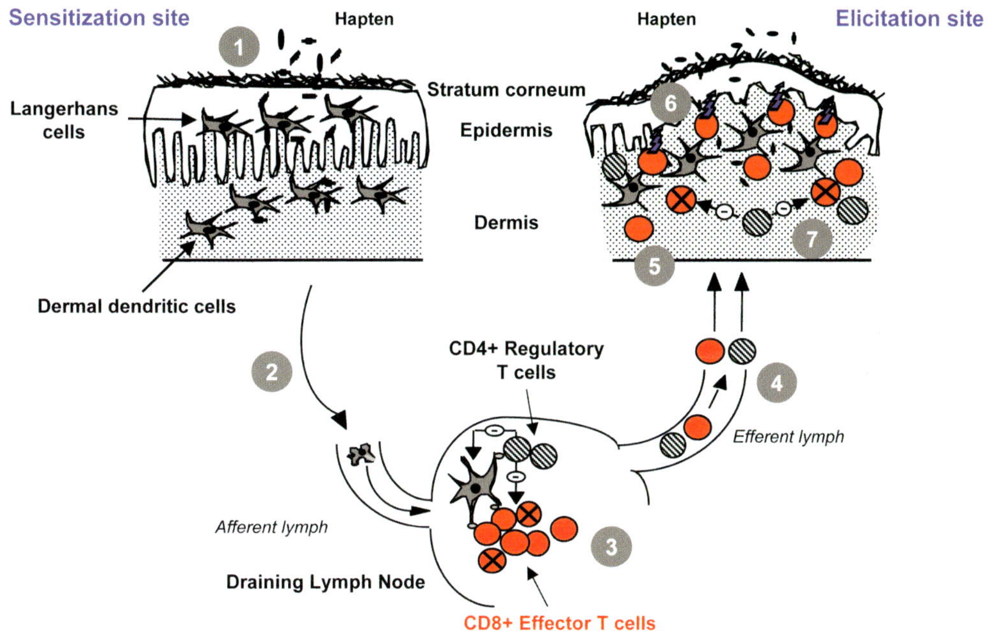


**FIGURE 31.1** Pathophysiology of CHS. *Sensitization step:* Haptens penetrate the stratum corneum. Hapten loading by skin DC (step 1) parallels activation and migration of DC through the afferent lymphatic vessels to the draining lymph nodes (step 2). Migrating DC are located in the paracortical area of the draining LN where they can present haptenated peptides on MHC class I and II molecules to $CD8^+$ and $CD4^+$ T cells, respectively (step 3). Specific T-cell precursors expand clonally in the draining LN and diffuse to the bloodstream through the efferent lymphatic vessels and the thoracic duct (step 4). During this process they acquire skin-specific homing antigens (CLA and CCR4) and become memory T cells. Primed T cells preferentially diffuse in the skin after transendothelial migration. At the end of the sensitization step everything is ready for the development of a CS reaction upon challenge with the relevant hapten. *Elicitation phase:* When the hapten is painted for a second (and subsequent) time, it diffuses through the epidermis and could be loaded by LC or other skin cells expressing MHC molecules, such as keratinocytes and dermal DC, which are then able to activate trafficking specific T cells (step 5). $CD8^+$ cytotoxic T-cell activation initiates the inflammatory process through keratinocyte apoptosis and cytokine/chemokine production (step 6). This is responsible for the recruitment of leukocytes (including regulatory T cells) from the blood to the skin leading to the development of skin lesions (step 7).

the inhibition of NF-κB can be due to the ability of lipoxin to protect IκBα from nitration by peroxynitrite. It is conceivable that lipoxin also interferes with assembly of the NADPH oxidase with cytoskeleton.[116]

## E. Macrophages

Macrophages are involved in the innate immune response, as they can recognize pathogens through unmethylated CpG nucleotides (common in bacteria). This leads to activation of macrophages through induction of NF-κB activation and increased GSSG/GSH ratio, which appears to be the first signal for the activation of the transcription factor.[117] Macrophages, activated by lymphocytes and pathogen by-products, are induced to release proteases, cytokines (mainly TNF-α), ROS, and RNS.[115,118] Bacterial lipopolysaccaride (LPS) quickly induces NADPH-mediated ROS production leading to MAPK activation and then to IL-1 production and release. Indeed, LPS could act at transcriptional (on the p38 kinase and the transcription factor ATF-2), translational, and post-translational levels.[119] However, endogenous mechanisms, including the antioxidant apparatus, operate fine control of the extent of macrophage activation to prevent excessive inflammatory reaction.[81] The cellular redox protection/detoxification systems can be upregulated by ROS production, mainly via an increase of CuZnSOD, MnSOD, and catalase activities. Contextually, a boost of the GSH level takes place ensuring intensification of the redox buffering potential. The administration of the antioxidant *N*-acetylcysteine *in vivo* is able to reduce ROS production and cytokine release, counteracting chemotaxis, adhesion, ROS production, and cytokine release. This takes place mainly by modulation of the NF-κB release from the cytosolic inactive store, thus confirming the importance of a proper redox balance in regulating monocyte functional activities.[120,121]

## F. TNF and TNFR family

The broad spectrum of action of TNF-α is initiated by the engagement of specific receptors (TNFR). After TNFR cross-linking an elevation of intracellular ROS takes place leading to activation of the downstream effectors, including JNK and NF-κB. All the TNFR family members contain as many as six cysteine residues, which renders them highly sensitive to redox status. Stimulation of TNFR1 gives rise to ROS production in mitochondria, via the association between ASK1 and TRAF2 through a redox-sensitive and thioredoxin-dependent mechanism. Among the different intracellular targets of the ROS release induced by the TNF-α, there is also PARP-1 (poly-ADP ribose polymerase 1), which could both directly activate NF-κB and support its activity. Moreover, ROS can activate the caspases, amplifying the apoptotic process. The involvement of the ROS-dependent signal in intracellular signaling is suggested by evidence from *in vitro* models ($\rho^0$ cells), which lack the mitochondrial electron transport chain, are incapable of increasing the ROS level, are inefficient at activating NF-κB following TNF-α stimulation, and are resistant to the apoptotic process induced by the ETC inhibitors.[122,123]

## G. Soluble Factors: Cytokines

ROS can be considered either mediators of various biological actions of cytokines or inducers of their production and release. Cytokines can activate the phagocytic cells during inflammation, leading to ROS hyperproduction, and can promote the intracellular formation of pro-oxidant species. Some activities of cytokines, such as the TNF-α– and IL-1-dependent vascular permeability, are due to the release of ROS by activated polymorphonucleates, i.e., through the oxygen burst. Cytokines induce ROS release, through the activation of xanthine oxidase, $PLA_2$, NADPH oxidase, MnSOD, and leukotriene synthesis. IFN-γ, IL-3, and C5a complement fraction thus can stimulate the oxygen burst. In addition, IL-8, GM-CSF, and GROα prime neutrophils to produce $O_2^{\bullet-}$, upregulating receptor expression for strong stimuli. After contact with microbial agents, the intracellular ROS generation mediated by the respiratory burst leads, in addition to the killing of the trapped microorganisms, to activation of the redox-responsive genes, including those of cytokines and chemokines. CC-chemokines recruit mononuclear cells and, to a lesser extent, eosinophils, basophils, and macrophages, whereas CXC chemokines recruit mainly neutrophils. IL-12, which plays a pivotal role in innate immunity, triggers the release of PAF, thus amplifying ROS function.[124]

## VII. ROS AS MEDIATORS OF THE ALTERED IMMUNE RESPONSE

A complete evaluation of the immune-mediated diseases that involve free radical generation exceeds the scope of this chapter. Herein, our aim is simply to talk about those ROS that play a pivotal role in most skin diseases characterized by the presence of immune cell infiltrates and/or the release of cytokines or diseases caused by environmental agents, such as UV radiation, chemical compounds, or viruses, able to trigger oxidative stress. The tissue damage induced by free radicals is generally ascribed to their role in the induction of cell death through both apoptotic and necrotic processes. UV is able to induce the peroxidation of the skin lipids, mainly of the squalene, in an energy-dependent manner. The extent of squalene peroxidation correlates with the erythemal manifestations. Moreover, by-products of squalene oxidation can downregulate the induction of the contact sensitization and a general immune deregulation involving the expression of adhesion molecules (i.e., ICAM-1), as well as the release of some cytokines (IL-1α, TNF-α). Some of the UV effects depend on modification of the membrane composition and fluidity, generation of $^1O_2$, and *trans/cis*-isomerization of urocanic acid. The modified pattern of saturated and unsaturated fatty acids induced by UV also affects the quantity and the activity of the antioxidants with a consequence impairment of their balance. The photosensitization process requires the generation of free radicals. During the type I photosensitization, the ground state photosensitizer takes up energy entering the unstable triplet state via the short-lived singlet state. In type II photosensitization, the compound reacts with $O_2$ and generates ROS, which is able to modify proteins, lipids, and nucleic acids. As proteins and other cell components are modified, they could be new antigens and escape the normal self-tolerance. UV-mediated ROS overproduction and ICAM-1 expression are also involved in the relapses of photosensitive lupus erythematosus and polymorphous light eruption. UVA irradiation is able to induce locally immunosuppression, characterized by a low number of Langerhans cells in epidermis, due in part to the increased production of NO.[125] During inflammatory skin diseases, $H_2O_2$, released by infiltrating neutrophils, determines increased expression of ICAM-1 on keratinocytes through a post-transcriptional modification (intracellular transport and/or membrane rearrangement). Contact chemical sensitizers, such as dinitrohalobenzene, induce the decrease of GSH level, favoring the generation of reactive species able to amplify the inflammatory reaction (production of TNF-α and IL-8, expression of ICAM-1). Interestingly, the loss of GSH appears to correlate with the extent of allergic manifestations.

Lipid metabolism changes, which affect the lymphocyte membrane and the eicosanoids levels, could play a role in the pathogenesis of the atopic dermatitis. Mechanical or thermal stress can induce urticaria through the generation of ROS able to promote the activation of the transcription factors and then the production of cytokines and eicosanoids. The increased related fraction of membrane PUFA and the reduced catalase activity could render the lymphocytes more susceptible to different peroxidative stimuli.[126] The cellular redox status affects the cellular capability to respond correctly to external insults, such as chemical toxic compounds. Indeed, the threshold sensitivity to the chemical irritants (i.e., sodium dodecyl sulfate) is correlated with the activity of the enzymatic antioxidants in epidermis and in peripheral lymphocytes.[127]

Allergic contact dermatitis to nickel represents the most frequent metal allergy, probably because of the wide nickel diffusion. The ability of nickel to elicit a biological response depends on the redox status in the skin environment, which determines the oxidation status of the metal and the interactions with cellular components. The release of ROS represents an event common to several inflammatory conditions and can contribute to the nickel redox status change, which renders it more active (from Ni(II) to Ni(III) or Ni(IV)). Moreover, in nickel allergy the T-cell-specific immune response, characterized by the expression of activation molecules and by cytokine release, is mediated by intracellular production of ROS. The clinical manifestations and the metabolic pathways elicited by nickel can be counteracted by the presence of zinc, probably due to the different pattern of cytokine (IL-10 and TGF-β).[128,129] The amplification and the persistence of the allergic response could be due also to the ability of nickel to inhibit the NOS, by means of a conversion of the $Ca^{2+}$/calmodulin system into a form unable to activate the enzyme, thus leading to suppression of the NO-dependent regulatory mechanism.[130]

A deficiency of polyunsaturated fatty acids, vitamin E, ubiquinone, and GPx activity has been found also in patients with seropositive HIV, due to an impairment of the desaturase system rather than to an increased lipoperoxidative process. In such patients a hypereosinophilic syndrome with cutaneous pruritus, related to an increased release of IL-4 and IL-5 and of chemokines from $CD4^-CD8^-$ or $CD4^-CD8^{dim}$ T cells, has been reported.[131] In HIV seropositive subjects, the free radical–mediated apoptosis of the lymphocytes participates in the immunodeficiency by means of the loss of $CD4^+$ T cells. The p24 and gp120 structural HIV-1 proteins are able to induce ROS generation by neutrophils and NO release by macrophages. Moreover, the viral regulatory protein Tat can increase the lymphocytic production of ROS. However, the observed oxidative stress in HIV infection is not due exclusively to the viral protein–mediated ROS generation but also to the derangement in antioxidants and oxidant equilibrium.[132]

The involvement of a hyperproduction of free radicals has been suggested in the pathogenesis of vitiligo. Although the vitiligo pathogenetic process is still unclear, an intriguing explanation may involve the intracellular hyperproduction of ROS by mitochondria, primary or secondary to a deficiency of antioxidants, which then leads to the cell damage. As a consequence, melanocytes might express cryptic antigens that support an immune response able to maintain and amplify the damage and the disappearance of the melanocytes.[133–136] A vitamin E deficiency is frequently associated with immune abnormalities involving the NK activity and the antibody-dependent cytotoxicity. The immune response to skin allograft is mediated by infiltrating macrophages producing NO in presence of $CD4^+$ T cells. NO acts by inducing the production of IL-4 and IL-10. The role of NO is confirmed by prolonged graft survival in the presence of iNOS inhibitors.[30]

## VIII. SENESCENCE OF THE IMMUNE SYSTEM

Oxygen-derived free radicals are responsible for the age-associated damage both at cellular and tissue levels. Increased oxidative stress in aging could be the consequence of the imbalance between free radical generation and the antioxidant defense system, which leads to a decline in normal cellular functions, and affects several systems, including the immune system. The concept of immune senescence has been suggested on the basis of the increased incidence of cancer and infectious diseases in aged subjects. The main age-related modification involves cellular immunity. In fact, lymphocytes present impaired adhesion, migration, proliferation, and cytokine production, whereas phagocytes exhibit altered adhesion, migration, phagocytosis, oxygen burst, and cytokine release (TNF-α and IL-1).[38,39] In granulocytes the age-related increase of ROS production is related to the deregulation of protein kinase C activity.[137]

## IX. ANTIOXIDANT SUPPLEMENTATION

Therapeutic strategies to improve the cellular redox balance may represent a powerful tool in the future for the treatment of diseases associated with oxidative stress. The physiological senescence of the immune system and the skin manifestations of excessive exposure to free radicals have been neutralized *in vitro* or in experimental animal models by the addition of SOD/catalase mimetics or by caloric restriction, respectively. In humans, rigorous caloric restriction obviously cannot be proposed. However, topical use of an antioxidant enzyme mimetic has been proposed in the treatment of pigmentary disorders and a dietary intake of a balanced pool of antioxidants can ameliorate the detrimental effects of UV irradiation and of some immunological abnormalities observed in these forms of skin diseases.[133,138] However, mechanisms of adaptation to oxidative stress or modulation of receptor activities may be altered in the presence of elevated reducing equivalents, establishing a condition of "reductive stress." Thus, even though treatment of many disorders with antioxidants is advantageous, the doses and the composition need to be formulated with caution.

## X. CONCLUSIONS

In the immune network, ROS act at both the extracellular level and the intracellular level. By these modalities, ROS provide an efficient and rapid mechanism for intercellular communication and allow fine regulation of the cellular metabolic state in response to external environment. A schematic illustration of this concept is provided by the link between innate and specific immune responses. The release of ROS by activated neutrophils and macrophages, in fact, enhances the lymphocytic kinase pathways and contributes to the activation and amplification of the adaptive (antigen-specific) immune response.

However, at the present time, many open questions lack a definitive answer. What is the identity of some reactive species producing enzymes? Why are they redundant? What is the source for the species generated after PDGF, EGF, NGF activation? Although we know that reactive oxygen and nitrogen species act differently, we still do not know how this is so.[1]

## REFERENCES

1. Nathan, C., Specificity of a third kind: reactive oxygen and nitrogen intermediates in cell signaling, *J. Clin. Invest.,* 111, 769, 2003.
2. Muller, A. et al., Characterization of specific leukotriene C4 binding sites on cultured human keratinocytes, *Br. J. Dermatol.,* 119, 275, 1988.
3. Klotz, L.O. et al., Singlet oxygen-induced signaling effects in mammalian cells, *Photochem. Photobiol. Sci.,* 2, 88, 2003.
4. Davies, M.J., Singlet oxygen-mediated damage to proteins and its consequences, *Biochem. Biophys. Res. Commun.*, 305, 761, 2003.
5. Miyamoto, S. et al., Direct evidence of singlet molecular oxygen [$O_2(^1$DeltaG)] production in the reaction of linoleic acid hydroperoxide with peroxynitrite, *J. Am. Chem. Soc.*, 125, 45, 2003.
6. Tarr, M. and Valenzeno, D.P., Singlet oxygen: the relevance of extracellular production mechanisms to oxidative stress *in vivo*, *Photochem. Photobiol. Sci.*, 2, 355, 2003.
7. Wright, A. et al., Photo-oxidation of cells generates long-lived protein peroxides, *Free Radical Biol. Med.*, 34, 637, 2003.
8. Cantrell, A., McGarvey, D.J., Truscott, T.G., Rancan, F., Bohm, F., Singlet oxygen quenching by dietary carotenoids in a model membrane environment, *Arch. Biochem. Biophys.,* 412, 47, 2003.
9. Ito, T., Cellular and subcellular mechanisms of photodynamic action: the $^1O_2$ hypothesis as a driving force in recent research, *Photochem. Photobiol.*, 28, 493, 1978.
10. Lledias, F. and Hansberg, W., Catalase modification as a marker for singlet oxygen. *Methods Enzymol.*, 319, 110, 2000.
11. Krutmann, J. and Morita, A., Mechanisms of ultraviolet (UV)B and UVA phototherapy, *J. Invest. Dermatol. Symp. Proc.*, 4, 70, 1999.
12. Zhuang, S., Ouedraogo, G.D., and Kochevar, I.E., Downregulation of epidermal growth factor receptor signalling by singlet oxygen through activation of caspase-3 and protein phosphatase, *Oncogene*, 22, 4413, 2003.
13. Borg, D.C. et al., Cytotoxic reactions of free radical species of oxygen, *Photochem. Photobiol.*, 28, 887, 1978.

14. Asada, K. et al., Superoxide dismutases in photosynthetic organisms, *Adv. Exp. Med. Biol.,* 74, 551, 1976.
15. Ross, D., Norbeck, K., and Moldeus, P., The generation and subsequent fate of glutathionyl radicals in biological systems, *J. Biol. Chem.,* 260, 15028, 1985.
16. Rigo, A., Stevanato, R., Finazzi-Agro, A., and Rotilio, G., An attempt to evaluate the rate of Haber Weiss reaction by using OH radical scavengers, *FEBS Lett.,* 80, 130, 1977.
17. Winterbourn, C.C., Superoxide as an intracellular radical sink, *Free Radical Biol. Med.*, 14, 85, 1993.
18. Reth, M., Hydrogen peroxide as second messenger in lymphocyte activation, *Nat. Immunol.,* 3, 1129, 2002.
19. Halliwell, B. and Gutteridge, J.M.C., *Free Radical in Biology and Medicine*, Clarendon Press/Oxford University Press, Oxford, 1989, 160–165.
20. Turpaev, K.T., Reactive oxygen species and regulation of gene expression, *Biochemistry,* 67, 339, 2002.
21. Beckman, K.B. and Ames, B.N., Oxidative decay of DNA, *J. Biol. Chem.,* 272, 19633, 1997.
22. Lapenna, D. and Cuccurullo, F., Hypochlorous acid and its pharmacological antagonism: an update picture, *Gen. Pharmacol.,* 27, 1145, 1996.
23. Smit, M.J. and Anderson, R., Inhibition of mitogen-activated proliferation of human lymphocytes by hypochlorous acid *in vitro*: protection and reversal by acsorbate and cysteine, *Agents Actions,* 3, 338, 1990.
24. Yang, Y., et al., Cells preconditioned with mild, transient UVA irradiation acquire resistance to oxidative stress and UVA-induced apoptosis: role of 4-hydroxynonenal in UVA-mediated signaling for apoptosis, *J. Biol. Chem.,* 278, 41380, 2003.
25. Dissemond, J. et al., Protective and determining factors for the overall lipid peroxidation in ultraviolet A1-irradiated fibroblasts: *in vitro* and *in vivo* investigations, *Br. J. Dermatol.,* 149, 341, 2003.
26. Zwier, J.L., Wang, P., Samouilov, A., and Kuppusamy, P., Enzyme-independent formation of nitric oxide in biological tissues, *Nat. Med,,* 1, 804, 1995.
27. Ignarro, L.J., Ed., *Nitric Oxide: Biology and Pathobiology.* Academic Press, San Diego, 2000.
28. Sauer, H., Wartenberg, M., and Hescheler, J., Reactive oxygen species as intracellular messengers during cell growth and differentiation, *Cell. Physiol. Biochem.,* 11, 173, 2001.
29. Samavati, L. et al., Mitochondrial K(ATP) channel openers activate the ERK kinase by an oxidant-dependent mechanism, *Am. J. Physiol. Cell. Physiol.,* 283, C273, 2002.
30. Shackelford, R.E., Kaufmann, W.K., and Paules, R.S., Oxidative stress and cell cycle checkpoint function, *Free Radical Biol. Med.,* 28, 1387, 2000.
31. Kuribayashi, F. et al., The adaptor protein $p40^{phox}$ as a positive regulator of the superoxide-producing phagocyte oxidase, *EMBO J.,* 21, 6312, 2002.
32. Vignais, P.V., The superoxide-generating NADPH oxidase: structural aspects and activation mechanism, *Cell. Mol. Life Sci.,* 59, 1428, 2002.
33. Salh, B. et al., Dissociated ROS production and ceramide generation in sulfosalazine-induced cell death in Raw 264.7 cells, *J. Leukocyte Biol.,* 72, 790, 2002.
34. De la Fuente, M., Effects of antioxidants on immune system ageing, *Eur. J. Clin. Nutr.,* 56, S5, 2002.
35. Schindowski, K. et al., Age-related increase of oxidative stress-induced apoptosis in mice prevention by *Ginkgo biloba* extract (Egb761), *J. Neural Transm.,* 108, 969, 2001.
36. Frei, B.B. and Ames, B.N., Relative importance of vitamin E in antiperoxidative defences in human blood and low density lipoproteins (LDL), in *Vitamin E in Health and Diseases*. Packer, L. and Fuchs, J., Eds., Marcel Dekker, New York, 1998, 191.
37. Benedetti, M.S. et al., Effects of aging on the content of sulfur-containing amino acids in rat brain, *J. Neural Transm. Gen. Sect.*, 3, 191, 1991.
38. Matsugo, S. et al., Alpha-lipoic acid as a biological antioxidant, *Free Radical Biol. Med.,* 19, 277, 1995.
39. Podda, M. et al., Alpha-lipoic acid supplementation prevents symptoms of vitamin E deficiency, *Biochim. Biophys. Res. Commun.,* 204, 98, 1994.
40. Frei, B. et al., Ascorbate: the most effective antioxidant in human blood plasma, *Adv. Exp. Med. Biol.,* 264, 155, 1990.
41. Goldenberg, H., Landertshamer, H., and Laggner, H., Functions of vitamin C as a transmembrane electron transport in blood cells and related cell culture models, *Antioxidant Redox Signal.,* 2, 189, 2000.

42. Smit, M.J. and Anderson, R., Inhibition of mitogen-activated proliferation of human lymphocytes by hypochlorous acid *in vitro*: protection and reversal by ascorbate and cysteine, *Agent Action,* 3, 338, 1990.
43. Tesoriere, L. et al., Synergistic interactions between vitamin A and vitamin E against lipid peroxidation in phosphatidylcholine liposomes, *Arch. Biochem. Biophys.,* 1, 57, 1996.
44. Matsugo, S. et al., Elucidation of antioxidant activity of dihydrolipoic acid toward hydroxyl radical using a novel hydroxyl generator NP-III, *Biochem. Mol. Biol. Int.,* 37, 375, 1995.
45. Witting, P.K. et al., Assessment of prooxidant activity of vitamin E in low-density lipoprotein in plasma. in *Methods in Enzymology,* Packer, L., Ed., Academic Press, New York, 1999, 362.
46. Palozza, P., Prooxidant actions of carotenoids in biological systems, *Nutr. Rev.,* 9, 257, 1999.
47. Meister, A., Glutathione, ascorbate, and cellular protection, *Cancer Res.,* 54, 1969s, 1994.
48. Pietarinen-Runtti, P. et al., Expression of antioxidant enzymes in human inflammatory cells, *Am. J. Physiol. Cell. Physiol.,* 278, C118, 2000.
49. Schonbaum, G. and Chance, B., Catalase, in *The Enzymes,* Vol. 13, Boyer, P.D., Ed., Academic Press, New York, 1976, 363.
50. Gilchrest, B.A. et al., Glutathione peroxidase, superoxide dismutase and catalase inactivation by peroxide and oxygen derived free radicals, *Mech. Ageing Dev.,* 51, 283, 1990.
51. Jones, D.P. et al., Metabolism of hydrogen peroxide in isolated hepatocytes: relative contribution of catalase and glutathione peroxidase in decomposition of endogenously generated $H_2O_2$, *Arch. Biochem. Biophys.,* 210, 505, 1981.
52. Maiorino, M., et al., Reactivity of phospholipids hydroperoxide glutathione peroxidase with membrane and lipoprotein lipid hydroperoxides, *Free Radical Res. Commun.,* 12–13, 131, 1991.
53. Imai, H. and Nakagawa, Y., Biological significance of phospholipid hydroperoxide glutathione peroxidase (PHGPx, GPx4) in mammalian cells, *Free Radical Biol. Med.,* 34, 145, 2003.
54. Zelko, I.N., Mariani, T., and Folz, R.J., Superoxide dismutase multigene family: a comparison of the CuZn-SOD (SOD1), Mn-SOD (SOD2), and EC-SOD (SOD3) gene structures, evolution, and expression, *Free Radical Biol. Med.,* 33, 337, 2002.
55. Rogers, R.J., Cytokine-inducible enhancer with promoter activity in both the rat and human manganese-superoxide dismutase genes, *Biochem. J.,* 347, 233, 2000.
56. Kifle, Y. et al., Regulation of the manganese superoxide dismutase and inducible nitric oxide synthase gene in rat neuronal and glial cells, *J. Neurochem.,* 66, 2128, 1996.
57. Chang, D.J. et al., Cell killing and induction of manganese superoxide dismutase by tumor necrosis factor-alpha is mediated by lipoxygenase metabolites of arachidonic acid, *Biochem. Biophys. Res. Commun.,* 188, 538, 1992.
58. Finkel, T., Redox-dependent signal transduction, *FEBS Lett.,* 476, 52, 2000.
59. Finkel, T., Reactive oxygen species and signal transduction, *IUBMB Life,* 52, 3, 2001.
60. Soberman, R.J., The expanding network of redox signaling: new observations, complexities, and perspectives, *J. Clin. Invest.,* 111, 571, 2003.
61. Sen, C.H. and Roy, S., Antioxidant regulation of cell adhesion, *Med. Sci. Sports Exerc.,* 33, 377, 2001.
62. Hueber, A.O., Role of membrane microdomain in rafts in TNFR-mediated signal transduction, *Cell Death Dif.,* 10, 7, 2003.
63. Anel, A. et al., Fatty acids metabolism in human lymphocytes. II. Activation of fatty acid desaturase-elongase systems during blastic transformation, *Biochem. Biophys. Acta,* 1044, 332, 1990.
64. Peus, D. et al., $H_2O_2$ is required for UVB-induced EGF receptor and downstream signaling pathway activation, *Free Radical Biol. Med.,* 27, 1197, 1999.
65. Belleudi, F. et al., The endocytic pathway followed by the keratinocyte growth factor receptor, *Histochem. Cell. Biol.,* 118, 1, 2002.
66. Marchese, C. et al., UVB-induced activation and internalization of keratinocyte growth factor receptor, *Oncogene,* 22, 2422, 2003.
67. Lee, H.C. and YH Wei, Y.H., Mitochondrial role in life and death of the cell, *J. Biomed. Sci.,* 7, 2, 2000.
68. Ueda, S. et al., Redox control of cell death, *Antioxidant Redox Signal.,* 4, 405, 2002.
69. Kamata, H. and H Hirata, H., Redox regulation of cellular signaling, *Cell. Signal.,* 11, 1, 1999.
70. Salmeen, A. et al., Redox regulation of protein tyrosine phosphatase 1B involves a sulphenyl-amide intermediate, *Nature,* 423, 769, 2003.

71. van Montfort, R.L.M. et al., Oxidation state of the active-site cysteine in protein tyrosine phosphatase 1B, *Nature,* 423, 773, 2003.
72. Kwon, J., Devadas, S. and Williams, M.S., T cell receptor-stimulated generation of hydrogen peroxide inhibits MEK-ERK activation and lck serine phosphorylation, *Free Radical Biol. Med.,* 35, 406, 2003.
73. von Knethen, A. and Brüne, B., Activation of peroxisome proliferator-activated receptor $\gamma$ by nitric oxide in monocytes/macrophages down-regulates p47$^{phox}$ and attenuates the respiratory burst, *J. Immunol.,* 169, 2619, 2002.
74. Holan, V. et al., Nitric oxide as a regulatory and effector molecule in the immune system. *Mol. Immunol.,* 38, 989, 2002.
75. Cruz, M.T. et al., LPS induction of I kappa B-alpha degradation and iNOS expression in a skin dendritic cell line is prevented by the janus kinase 2 inhibitor, tyrphostin b42, *Nitric Oxide,* 5, 53, 2001.
76. Beltràn, B. et al., Inhibition of mitochondrial respiration by endogenous nitric oxide: a critical step in Fas signaling, *PNAS,* 99, 8892, 2002.
77. Pani, G. et al., Endogenous oxygen radicals modulate protein tyrosine phosphorylation and JNK-1 activation in lectin-stimulated thymocytes, *Biochem. J.,* 347, 173, 2000.
78. Seo, S.R. et al., $Zn^{2+}$-induced ERK activation mediated by reactive oxygen species causes cell death in differentiated PC12 cells, *J. Neurochem.,* 78, 600, 2001.
79. Takeda, K. et al., Roles of MAPKKK ASK1 in stress-induced cell death, *Cell Struct. Function,* 28, 23, 2003.
80. Angkeow, P., Redox factor-1: an extra-nuclear role in the regulation of endothelial oxidative stress and apoptosis, *Cell Death Diff.,* 9, 717, 2002.
81. Rutter, J. et al., Regulation of clock and NPAS2 DNA binding by the redox state of NAD cofactors, *Science,* 293, 510, 2001.
82. Zhang, Q., Piston, D.W., and Goodman, R.H., Regulation of corepressor function by nuclear NADH, *Science,* 295, 1895, 2001.
83. Nathan, C., Oxygen and the inflammatory cell, *Nature,* 422, 675, 2003.
84. Madamanchi, N.R. et al., Reactive oxygen species regulate heat-shock protein 70 via the JAK/STAT pathway, *Arterioscler. Thromb. Vasc. Biol.,* 21, 321, 2001.
85. Lipton, S.A. and Bossy-Wetzel, E., Dueling activities of AIF in cell death versus survival: DNA binding and redox activity, *Cell,* 111, 147, 2002.
86. Moscat, J., Diaz-Meco, M.T., and Rennert, P., NF-kB activation by protein kinase C isoforms and B-cell function, *EMBO Rep.,* 4, 31, 2003.
87. Wang, H. et al., Nicotinic acetylcholine receptor $\alpha 7$ subunit is an essential regulator of inflammation, *Nature* advance online publication, 22 December 2002 (doi:10.1038/nature01339).
88. Victor, V.M. and De la Fuente, M., Immune cells redox state from mice with endotoxin-induced oxidative stress. Involvement of NF-kappaB, *Free Radical Res.,* 37, 19, 2003.
89. Haddad, J.J., Glutathione depletion is associated with augmenting a proinflammatory signal: evidence for an antioxidant/pro-oxidant mechanism regulating cytokines in the alveolar epithelium, *Cytokines Cell Mol. Ther.,* 6, 177, 2000.
90. Haddad, J.J., Redox regulation of pro-inflammatory cytokines and IkappaB-alpha/NF-kappaB nuclear translocation and activation, *Biochem. Biophys. Res. Commun.,* 296, 847, 2002.
91. Accaoui, M.J. et al., Gamma-glutamyltranspeptidase-dependent glutathione catabolism results in activation of NF-kB, *Biochem. Biophys. Res. Commun.,* 276, 1062, 2000.
92. Schoonbroodt, S. and Piette, J., Oxidative stress interference with the nuclear factor-kappa B activation pathway, *Biochem. Pharmacol.,* 60, 1075, 2000.
93. Frossi, B. et al., H(2)O(2) induces translocation of APE/Ref-1 to mitochondria in the Raji B-cell line, *J. Cell. Physiol.,* 193, 180, 2002.
94. Lindvall, J. and Islam, T.C., Interaction of Btk and Akt in B cell signaling, *Biochem. Biophys. Res. Commun.,* 293, 1319, 2002.
95. Carlisle, M.L., King, M.R., and Karp, D.R., $\gamma$-Glutamyl transpeptidase activity alters the T cell response to oxidative stress and Fas-induced apoptosis, *Int. Immunol.,* 15, 17, 2003.
96. Chiaradia, E. et al., Antioxidant systems and lymphocyte proliferation in the horse, sheep and dog, *Vet. Res.,* 33, 661, 2002.

97. Matheny, H.E., Deem, T.L., and Cook-Mills, J.M., Lymphocyte migration through monolayers of endothelial cell lines involves VCAM-1 signaling via endothelial cell NADPH oxidase, *J. Immunol.,* 164, 6550, 2000.
98. Tudor, K.S., Hess, K.L., and Cook-Mills, J.M., Cytokines modulate endothelial cell intracellular signal transduction required for VCAM-1-dependent lymphocyte transendothelial migration, *Cytokine,* 15, 196, 2001.
99. De la Fuente, M. and Victor, V.M., Ascorbic acid and N-acetylcysteine improve *in vitro* the function of lymphocytes from mice with endotoxin-induced oxidative stress, *Free Radical Res.,* 35, 73, 2001.
100. Tatla, S. et al., The role of reactive oxygen species in triggering proliferation and IL-2 secretion in T cells, *Free Radical Biol. Med.,* 26, 14, 1999.
101. Hehner, S.P. et al., Enhancement of T cell receptor signaling by a mild oxidative shift in the intracellular thiol pool, *J. Immunol.,* 165, 4319, 2000.
102. Roozendaal, R. et al., Interaction between nitric oxide and subsets of human T lymphocytes with differences in glutathione metabolism, *Immunology,* 107, 334, 2002.
103. Shenker, B.J. et al., Mercury-induced apoptosis in human lymphocytes: caspase activation is linked to redox status, *Antioxidant Redox Signal.,* 4, 379, 2002.
104. Balamurugan, K. et al., Chromium(III)-induced apoptosis of lymphocytes: death decision by ROS and Src-family tyrosine kinases, *Free Radical Biol. Med.,* 33, 1622, 2002.
105. Mosca, L. et al., Modulation of apoptosis and improved redox metabolism with the use of a new antioxidant formula, *Biochem. Pharmacol.,* 63, 1305, 2002.
106. Hildeman, D.A. et al., Reactive oxygen species regulate activation-induced T cell apoptosis, *Immunity,* 10, 735, 1999.
107. Barbieri, S.S. et al., Reactive oxygen species mediate cyclooxygenase-2 induction during monocyte to macrophage differentiation: critical role of NADPH oxidase, *Cardiovasc. Res.,* 60, 187, 2003.
108. Bhatt, N.Y. et al., Macrophage-colony-stimulating factors-induced activation of extracellular-regulated kinases involves phosphatidylinositol 3-kinase and reactive oxygen species in human monocytes, *J. Immunol.,* 169, 6427, 2002.
109. Hampton, M.B. and S Orrenius, S., Redox regulation of apoptotic death in the immune system, *Toxicol. Lett.,* 102, 355, 1998.
110. Phillips, D.C., Allen, K., and Griffiths, H.R., Synthetic ceramides induce growth arrest or apoptosis by altering cellular redox status, *Arch. Biochem. Biophys.,* 407, 15, 2002.
111. Badewa, A.P., Hudson, C.E., and Heiman, A.S., Regulatory effects of eotaxin, eotaxin-2, and eotaxin-3 on eosinophil degranulation and superoxide anion generation, *Exp. Biol. Med.,* 227, 645, 2002.
112. Leavey, P.J. et al., A 29-kDa protein associated with $p67^{phox}$ expresses both peroxiredoxin and phospholipase $A_2$ activity and enhances superoxide anion production by a cell-free system of NADPH oxidase activity, *J. Biol. Chem.,* 277, 45181, 2002.
113. Watson, R.W.G. et al., Regulation of Fas antibody induced neutrophil apoptosis is both caspase and mitochondrial dependent, *FEBS Lett.,* 453, 67, 1999.
114. Maianski, N.A., Roos, D., and Kuijpers, T.W., Tumor necrosis factor $\alpha$ induces a caspase-independent death pathway in human neutrophils, *Blood,* 101, 1987, 2003.
115. Nathan, C., Points of control in inflammation, *Nature,* 420, 846, 2002.
116. Jòzsef, L. et al., Lipoxin $A_4$ and aspirin-triggered 15-epi-lipoxin $A_4$ inhibit peroxynitrite formation, NF-κB and AP-1 activation, and IL-8 gene expression in human leukocytes, *PNAS,* 99, 13266, 2002.
117. Kirsch, J.D. et al., Accumulation of glutathione disulfide mediates NF-kappaB activation during immune stimulation with CpG DNA, *Antisense Nucleic Acid Drug Dev.,* 12, 327, 2002.
118. Nathan, C. and Shiloh, M.U., Reactive oxygen and nitrogen intermediates in the relationship between mammalian hosts and microbial pathogens, *PNAS,* 97, 8841, 2000.
119. Hsu, H.Y. and Wen, M.H., Lipopolysaccaride-mediated reactive oxygen species and signal transduction in the regulation of interleukin-1 gene expression, *J. Biol. Chem.,* 277, 22131, 2002.
120. Victor, V.M. and De la Fuente, M., *N*-Acetylcysteine improves *in vitro* the function of macrophages from mice with endotoxin-induced oxidative stress, *Free Radical Res.,* 36, 33, 2002.
121. Victor, V.M., Rocha, M., and De la Fuente, M., Regulation of macrophage function by the antioxidant *N*-acetylcysteine in mouse-oxidative stress by endotoxin, *Int. Immunopharmacol.,* 3, 97, 2003.
122. Chandel, N.S., Schumacker, P.T., and Arch, R.H., Reactive oxygen species are downstream products of TRAF-mediated signal transduction, *J. Biol. Chem.,* 276, 42728, 2001.

123. Wajant, H., Pfizenmaier, K., and Scheurich, P., Tumor necrosis factor signaling, *Cell Death Diff.*, 10, 45, 2003.
124. Bussolati, B. et al., Platelet-activating factor synthesized by IL-12-stimulated polymorphonuclear neutrophils and NK cells mediates chemotaxis, *J. Immunol.*, 161, 1493, 1998.
125. Yuen, K.S., Nearn, M.R., and Halliday, G.M., Nitric oxide-mediated depletion of Langerhans cells from the epidermis may be involved in UVA radiation-induced immunosuppression, *Nitric Oxide*, 6, 313, 2002.
126. Briganti, S. et al., Oxidative stress in physical urticarias, *Clin. Exp. Dermatol.*, 26, 284, 2001.
127. Camera, E. et al., Levels of enzymatic antioxidants activities in mononuclear cells and skin reactivity to sodium dodecyl sulphate, *Int. J. Immunopathol. Pharmacol.*, 16, 49, 2003.
128. Santucci, B., Camera, E., and Picardo, M., Biochemical aspects of nickel hypersensitivity: factors determining allergenic action, in *Nickel and the Skin, Absorption, Immunology, Epidemiology, and Metallurgy*, Hostynek, J.J. and Maibach, H.I., Eds., CRC Press, Boca Raton, FL, 2002, 201.
129. Paganelli, R. et al., *In vitro* effects of nickel-sulphate on immune functions of normal and nickel-allergic subjects: a regulatory role for zinc, *J. Trace Elem. Med. Biol.*, 17, 00, 2003.
130. Palumbo, A. et al., $Ni^{2+}$, a double-acting inhibitor of neuronal nitric oxide synthase interfering with L-arginine binding and $Ca^{2+}$/calmodulin-dependent enzyme activation, *Biochem. Biophys. Res. Commun.*, 285, 142, 2001.
131. Paganelli, R. et al., Th2-type cytokines, hypereosinophilia, and interleukin-5 in HIV disease, *Allergy*, 52, 110, 1997.
132. Bautista, A.P., Free radicals, chemokines, and cell injury in HIV-1 and SIV infections and alcoholic hepatitis, *Free Radical Biol. Med.*, 31, 1527, 2001.
133. Schallreuter, K.U. et al., *In vivo* and *in vitro* evidence for hydrogen peroxide (H2O2) accumulation in the epidermis of patients with vitiligo and its successful removal by a UVB-activated pseudocatalase, *J. Invest. Dermatol. Symp. Proc.*, 4, 91, 1999.
134. Maresca, V. et al., Increased sensitivity to peroxidative agents as a possible pathogenic factor of melanocyte damage in vitiligo, *J. Invest. Dermatol.*, 109, 310, 1997.
135. Dell'Anna, M.L. et al., Mitochondrial impairment in peripheral blood mononuclear cells during the active phase of vitiligo, *J. Invest. Dermatol.*, 117, 908, 2001.
136. Dell'Anna, M.L. et al., Alterations of mitochondria in peripheral blood mononuclear cells of vitiligo patients, *Pigment Cell Res.*, 16, 553, 2003.
137. Martins Chaves, M. et al., Correlation between NADPH oxidase and protein kinase C in the ROS production by human granulocytes related to age, *Gerontology*, 48, 354, 2002.
138. Leone, G., Combined phototherapy in vitiligo, presented at 10th Meeting of the European Society for Pigment Cell Research, 26–29 September 2001, Rome, Italy, *Abstr. Book Pigment Cell Res.*, 14, 380, 2001.

# 13 Defensins and Cathelicidins

*Kevin O. Kisich and Donald Y.M. Leung*

## CONTENTS



## I. INTRODUCTION

Among the innate immune defenses of the skin are several families of small peptides, which possess direct antimicrobial activity, or both antimicrobial and immunomodulatory activity. These peptides are essential to defenses against microbial colonization and invasion through the skin. Many of these peptides were first discovered based on their antimicrobial properties, and therefore designated antimicrobial peptides (AMP). However, some peptides originally described as chemokines, such as macrophage inflammatory protein 3$\alpha$ and 3$\beta$ (MIP3$\alpha$/MIB3$\beta$), also have potent antimicrobial activity. Therefore, for the purposes of this discussion we use the abbreviation AMP to signify the antimicrobial properties of the peptides in question, regardless of other activities they may possess. Immunoregulatory activities of classically antimicrobial peptides are discussed as needed.

## II. MAJOR CATEGORIES OF HUMAN ANTIMICROBIAL PEPTIDES

Classical human AMP found in the skin as of 2003 include cathelicidin, dermcidin, and defensins. Dermcidin and cathelicidin are both linear peptides, and are each the only member of their respective

0-8493-1959-5/05/$0.00+$1.50

**TABLE 13.1**
**Summary of Human AMP, Cellular Sources, Antimicrobial, and Immunomodulatory Activities**

| Peptide | Cellular Source(s) | Most Active Against: | Immunomodulatory Activity For: |
|---|---|---|---|
| HD1 | Neutrophils | Gram-negative, enveloped virus, yeast | Cytokine secretion by epithelial cells[5] naive T cell, immature dendritic cell chemotaxis[6] |
| HD2 | Neutrophils | Gram-negative, enveloped virus, yeast | Cytokine secretion by epithelial cells,[5] naive T cell, immature dendritic cell chemotaxis[6] |
| HD3 | Neutrophils | Gram-negative, enveloped virus, yeast | Cytokine secretion by epithelial cells,[5] naive T cell, immature dendritic cell chemotaxis[6] |
| HD4 | Neutrophils | Gram-negative, Gram-positive, yeast | Not reported |
| HD5 | Paneth cells | Gram-negative, yeast | Not reported |
| HD6 | Paneth cells | Gram-negative, yeast | Not reported |
| HBD1 | Epithelial cells | Gram-negative, yeast | Memory T cells, monocytes, dendritic cells via CCR6 |
| HBD2 | Epithelial cells | Gram-negative, yeast | Memory T cells, monocytes, dendritic cells via CCR6,[7] mast cells[79] |
| HBD3 | Epithelial cells | Gram-negative, Gram-positive, yeast | Monocytes |
| HBD4 | Epithelial cells, epididymis, gastric antrum | Staphylococcus carnosus, Pseudomonas aeruginosa | Not reported |
| Dermcidin | Eccrine sweat glands, neural cells (pons) | Gram-negative, Gram-positive, *Candida albicans.* | Not reported |
| LL37 | Epithelial/neutrophils | Gram-negative, Gram-positive, enveloped virus, yeast | Neutrophils, monocytes, T cells, mast cells via FPRL-1 receptor[77] |

gene families in humans.[1,2] Defensins constitute a large family of genes, and differ from dermcidin and cathelicidin both in their primary sequences and characteristic disulfide bonding patterns.[3]

Chemokines constitute an emerging and increasingly recognized group of AMP, and are abundantly expressed in human skin. Keratinocytes have been shown to express at least six chemokines that have also been shown to have antimicrobial activity, including CXCL1, CCL17, CCL20, IP-9, IP-10, and Mig.[4] While the chemokines have no apparent sequence similarity with known AMP, Yang and colleagues have shown that they share similar topological organization with defensins, which may help to explain their antimicrobial activity.[4] The essentials of the human defensins LL37 and dermcidin are summarized in Table 13.1.

## A. Defensins

Tomas Ganz and colleagues initially isolated and characterized three small, cationic peptides from the azurophilic granules of human neutrophils, and named them "defensins."[8] These peptides were subsequently found to be the first members of a large family of peptides sharing homologous primary and secondary structures, which have been evolutionarily conserved throughout vertebrate evolution, and share structural similarities with host defense molecules in insects,[9] mollusks,[10] and plants.[11]

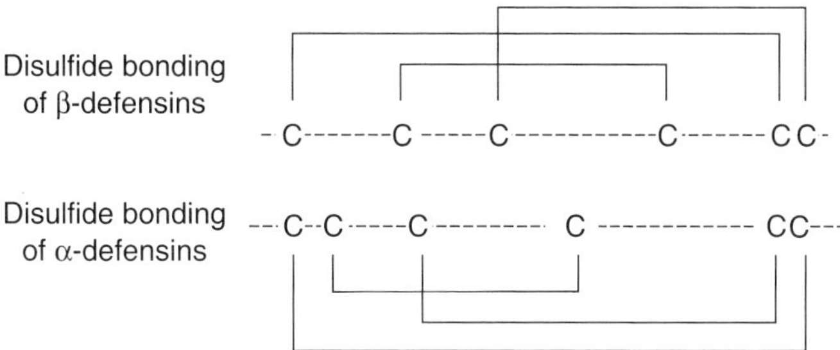


**FIGURE 13.1** Characteristic disulfide binding patterns of α- and β-defensins. Conserved cysteine residues are cross-linked in different orders between the two defensin families, resulting in different topologies.

## B. Alpha and Beta Defensins Have Different Patterns of Disulfide Bonding

The defensin family of peptides has three main branches, which have so far been identified, the α-, β-, and θ-defensins.[8,12,13] The α- and β-defensins each have three disulfide bonds stabilizing their short primary sequences, but the connectivity pattern of the cysteine residues distinguishes these to branches of the defensin family as shown in Figure 13.1. The θ-defensins are unique among defensins in two important ways. First, they are circular molecules, and only have a single disulfide bond stabilizing their structures.[13] Second, they are not genomically encoded, but are instead created post-translationally from proteolytic fragments of two unexpressed α-defensins, which have been designated "demidefensins."[14] The genes for α, β, and the demidefensin constituents of θ-defensins are expressed in most vertebrate classes examined.[3] However, the mRNAs required for translation of the precursor peptides for human θ-defensins have acquired premature stop codons, which prevents expression of the peptides in human cells.

*Humans express six α-defensins, but up to 28 β-defensins.* Human α-defensins are represented by human neutrophil proteins 1, 2, 3, and 4, (HD1–4) along with the intestinal defensins HD5 and 6. HD1–4 are synthesized by immature neutrophils, and stored in azurophilic granules in the cytoplasm.[15] HD5 and 6 are expressed by Paneth cells of the intestinal crypts, where they are important for preventing bacterial invasion of the intestinal mucosa.[16–19] HDs constitute approximately one third of the total protein of the azurophilic granules of human neutrophils.[15] However, defensins have not yet been detected in PMN of mice. Upon phagocytosis of microorganisms, the granule-containing vacuoles fuse with the phagosomes, thus exposing the microorganism to high concentrations of both defensins and other antibiotic proteins such as lysozyme and myeloperoxidase.[14] Rabbit alveolar macrophages and murine macrophages also express defensins, but defensin expression has not yet been demonstrated in human macrophages.

β-Defensins are the other family of human defensins, and are abundantly expressed in the kidney, urinary epithelium, and epithelia of several other organs including skin, trachea, and major conducting airways.[4,19] β-Defensin-1 synthesis does not appear to be inducible, and it has been hypothesized that the major function of hBD1 is in microbial defense of the genitourinary system.[20] A second member of the human β-defensin family, hBD2, is induced upon inflammation of the skin[21] and respiratory tract.[22] HBD-3 has recently been described[23] to have a similar antimicrobial spectrum as hBD-2, with the addition of potent activity against *Staphylococcus aureus*, and is expressed in the adult heart, skeletal muscle, fetal thymus, and is inducible in epidermal cells and tissues. There has been one report of a fourth member of the human β-defensin family, hBD-4, recently reported, unfortunately without information regarding the cellular or tissue sources.[24] Presumably, there will be additional information forthcoming about hBD3 and hBD4 in the near future. An additional 16 to 28 hBD genes have been identified in the human genome. Several of these are expressed in the epididymis, and three in the lung.[25,26] The number of hBD genes expressed in epididymis may indicate that the function of these peptides may extend beyond antimicrobial activity. β-Defensins 1 to 4 are salt sensitive, and it has been hypothesized that inactivation of defensins in the salty epithelial secretions of patients with cystic fibrosis may play a role in susceptibility to bacterial infections.[27]

Both the α- and β-defensin gene clusters are situated near each other on 8p22-p23, suggesting common ancestry for both groups of defensins.[28] However, the defensins have undergone rapid duplication and sequence divergence in primates.[29] Even among humans it has been found that there is extensive variation in the numbers of β-defensin gene copies,[30] and that there are allelic differences that affect antimicrobial activity.[41]

### C. Cathelicidin

The human antimicrobial peptide LL37/hCAP18 (human cationic antimicrobial peptide, 18 kDa) was discovered based on homology to rabbit CAP18.[31,32] This peptide was initially isolated from rabbit leukocytes based on its ability to bind and inhibit various activities of LPS. The mature human LL37 peptide shares the ability to bind LPS with high affinity,[32] and is able to kill both Gram-positive and Gram-negative bacteria, fungi, and some enveloped virus.

*LL37 is generated by proteolytic processing of human cathelicidin.* Human LL37 as well as rabbit CAP-18 are the C-terminal proteolytic fragments of larger proteins.[32] The parent protein contains a 30-aa signal peptide, a 103-aa N-terminal domain of unknown function, the cathelin-like domain, for which they are included in a large family of proteins called cathelicidins, which include porcine protegrins.[33] The LPS-binding and antimicrobial peptide is derived from the 37-aa C-terminal peptide homologous to rabbit cap18. Human cathelicidin is the first and only human member of this protein family identified so far.

*The structure is not stabilized by disulfide bonds, and is distinct from that of defensins.* While the secondary structure of LL37 is not stabilized by disulfide bonds, the primary sequence is rich in proline.[34] The crystal structure of LL37 has yet to be published, but that of a related peptide, porcine protegrin 1 (PG-1), has been extensively studied. The prolines cause the secondary structure in protegrins to adopt a fold, placing two β-sheet domains next to each other in antiparallel orientation.[35] In protegrin 1, this conformation is stabilized by two disulfide bonds, which are absent in human LL37.

### D. Dermcidin

Dermcidin is a recently discovered antimicrobial peptide produced in eccrine sweat glands.[1] Like LL37, it is produced from a larger precursor peptide via proteolytic processing, and does not contain disulfide bonds.[1] However, dermcidin does not share any sequence homology with either LL37 or the defensins. It shares broad-spectrum antimicrobial activity against bacteria and fungi,[1] but there have not yet been any reports of antiviral activity. Dermcidin has independently been identified as a neural survival factor, and is thought to regulate immune function via interactions with IgG.[36,37]

## III. ANTIMICROBIAL ACTIVITIES OF HUMAN AMP

As noted above, human AMP are toxic to bacteria, fungi, and viruses. However, the antimicrobial activity spectrum of each peptide appears to be unique even though there has not yet been a comprehensive study comparing the activities of AMP under a uniform set of assay conditions. Typical assay conditions include a 1- to 4-h exposure of a log-phase culture of the microbe in question at 37°C to the AMP in 10 m*M* phosphate buffer, pH 7.4, containing 0.01× tryptic soy broth.[38] It should be noted, however, that such conditions of low osmotic strength are chosen to optimize the activity of the AMP in question, rather than to mimic the conditions under which they might function *in vivo*. The activities of many human AMP, particularly defensins, are strongly attenuated at salt concentrations approaching physiological.[3] However, it is likely that under the particular conditions that each AMP functions *in vivo*, certain microbes will still be sensitive to their effects, for example, hBD-2 in saliva, and hBD-1 in urine. Discerning which AMP are important for defense against which microbes *in vivo* remains a topic of intense inquiry.

## A. Sensitivities of Different Classes of Microbes

*Bacteria.* All bacteria examined to date, including Gram-positive, Gram-negative, and mycobacteria were killed by one or more human AMP under low salt conditions *in vitro*. The activities of hBD-1, 2, and 3, LL37, and dermcidin are the most pertinent for this review, because they are produced by cells of the skin either constitutively or before induction of local inflammation in response to microbial challenge. A rigorous comparison of their activities against any particular microbe has not been conducted, and different laboratories have used different assay conditions to determine activity against various bacteria. Therefore, it is very difficult to compare their various potencies for any given bacterial species. However, it is important to bear in mind that microbes typically face multiple antimicrobial peptides when encountering human epithelia, including skin. Some pairs of antimicrobial peptides, such as defensin and LL37, have been shown to synergize in killing of more-resistant bacteria, such as *S. aureus*.[39]

*Fungi. Candida albicans* has been the most widely studied fungus for susceptibility to human AMP. Different investigators have found this organism to be sensitive to killing by defensins under low salt conditions, but at slightly higher concentrations than for *Escherichia coli*.[8] Turner et al.[40] have noted that *C. albicans* is sensitive to LL37, but that the activity is inhibited by salt. In the initial description of dermcidin, *C. albicans* was also found to be sensitive to killing by that AMP.[1] *Cryptococcus neoformans* has also been studied, and it has been found to be sensitive to both α– and β-defensins.[8,41] However, its sensitivity to LL37 does not appear to have been documented. Therefore, while there are numerous fungal pathogens of the skin, there has thus far been limited work done on characterizing the sensitivity of many fungi to human AMP.

*Viruses.* AMP of the skin are also likely to play important roles in defense against viral infection. The antiviral activity of defensins was first tested by Daher et al.[42] who demonstrated inactivation of the enveloped viruses herpes simplex virus types 1 and 2 (HSV1/2), cytomegalovirus, vesicular stomatitis virus, and influenza A/WSN by HD1-3. However, two non-enveloped viruses, echovirus type 11 and reovirus type 3, were not affected by defensin exposure.[42] Inactivation of human immunodeficiency virus (HIV) by α-defensins and θ-defensins has been reported, but there have not yet been reports of direct inactivation by β-defensins.[43,44] LL37 also has potent antiviral activity against vaccinia virus, which occurs by destruction of the viral envelope via an unknown mechanism.[45] However, in the same series of experiments, vaccinia virus was insensitive to the effects of defensins.

## B. Mechanism of Action of Human AMP

The detailed mechanisms by which each AMP impairs microbial viability have been the subject of intense inquiry, and are not yet fully understood. Lehrer et al.[46] were able to demonstrate that the ability of rabbit defensins to kill *Candida albicans* correlated well with the ability of the defensins to bind to the fungi. In fact, all of the known AMP present in the skin are rich in lysine and arginine residues, which impart cationic character to the peptides. The cell walls or outer membranes of bacteria tend to bear a net negative charge, which partially explains the high affinity that most AMP have for microbial surfaces under low salt conditions. In addition to binding modes based on ionic interactions, defensins have high affinity for carbohydrate residues,[47] while LL37 binds LPS with high affinity.[40] Therefore, the first step in the process by which AMP kill microbes is necessarily by binding to the microbial surface.

The next step in the microbicidal mechanism appears to involve perturbation of essential microbial membranes. Using the example of *E. coli* and HD-1, Lehrer et al.[48] demonstrated that interaction of the bacteria with HD-1 under conditions that supported killing resulted in permeablization of the outer membrane, followed by permeablization of the inner membrane, and cessation of bacterial RNA, DNA, and protein synthesis. This is explained via results of studies by Kagan et al.,[49] which demonstrated that HD1 forms voltage-dependent, ion-permeable channels in model lipid bilayer membranes. The precise structure of the defensin-mediated pore has not been published, although it has been the subject of intense scrutiny.[50–52]

LL37 has also been found to cause ionic leakage by bacterial membranes,[53] and the mode by which it binds to membranes has recently been studied by Henzler-Wildman et al.[54] Through differential scanning calorimetry and solid state nuclear magnetic resonance (NMR) it was determined that LL37 lies among the phospholipid head groups of the membrane, with the hydrophobic plane of its amphipathic helix oriented into the membrane, and the hydrophilic/cationic surface interacting with the phospholipid head groups and the solvent. This mode is consistent with the "toroidal pore" model of pore formation, rather than the barrel stave or micellar models.[54] Comparable studies have not yet been reported for dermcidin.

Inactivation of enveloped virus by AMP implies that creation of lesions in membranes does not necessarily require a membrane potential, as is the case for bacteria. The specificity of which peptides can inactivate virus also implies a structural basis to binding of the peptides to virus, which is independent of charge, as β-defensins have equivalent levels of charge as LL37 and α-defensins, yet have no direct effect on enveloped viruses.[45]

The debate over the precise conditions under which human AMP function *in vivo* will certainly continue for some time. However, it is clear that although the range of microbes that are killed by individual AMP may be restricted upon introduction of physiological ionic conditions, or media, the summed effects of all the AMP with which microbes must contend remain formidable. This point is illustrated by some strains of *S. aureus* that have developed resistance to defensins,[39] which is mediated by incorporation of lysine residues into the structure of the cell wall under the influence of the MprF gene.[55] However, even resistant *S. aureus* are effectively killed under physiological ionic conditions by the combination of LL37 and defensin, which are highly synergistic.[56] Synergistic killing of microbes by pairs of AMP under physiological salt conditions has been reported for *C. albicans,*[57] *S. aureus,*[56] and *Mycobacterium tuberculosis*.[58] In the case of *M. tuberculosis*, binding of defensins to the cell membrane is inhibited by the poorly permeable mycobacterial cell wall. LL37 binds to the cell wall with high affinity, and causes an increase in permeability. This then allows defensins access to the membrane, which they bind and permeablize.[58] Such cooperative activity among AMP is reflected in the organization of the innate AMP defense of the skin.

## IV. CELLULAR SOURCES AND SYNTHESIS, LAYERS OF DEFENSE

### A. Sweat as a Vehicle for AMP

The organization of AMP in the skin actually begins beyond the limits of keratinized layers, in the sweat. Eccrine sweat glands constitutively secrete both dermcidin and LL37 into the sweat, which are deposited on the skin surface by bulk flow.[1,59] Therefore, microbes contacting the skin from the environment first encounter both dermcidin and LL37. HBD1 is also present during the first encounter of the skin with environmental microbes, as hBD1 is constitutively expressed by keratinocytes, and remains intact during involution and keratinization of the cells.[60] The presence of these three potent AMP on the surface of normal, non-inflamed skin helps explain why most humans support the growth of relatively few microbes on the skin, despite almost continual exposure from the environment.

### B. Epithelial Cells, Including Keratinocytes Produce b-Defensins and Cathelicidin

Potential pathogens that are not killed quickly by the combination of dermcidin, LL37, and hBD1 present at the surface may provoke inflammatory activation of keratinocytes through interaction with surface pattern recognition molecules, such as Toll-like receptors.[61,62] Activation of keratinocytes by microbial products results in initiation of gene expression for additional LL37, hBD2, and hBD3.[63,64] The products of translation of β-defensin mRNAs are pre-propeptides.[65] Proteolytic processing of these precursors to their mature forms is a multistep process that occurs in the endoplasmic reticulum and the Golgi prior to secretion.[66] Secretion of hBD2 has been shown to occur via incorporation into lamellar bodies, which are secreted from the spinous layer of keratinocytes in the epidermis.[67] LL37 is initially translated into the cathelicidin protein, from which the N-terminal signal sequence and 103-aa cathelin-like domains are cleaved, leaving the 37-aa C-terminal peptide.[2] Sorensen et al.[68] have demonstrated that in neutrophils this processing occurs after secretion of cathelicidin into the extracellular space and is dependent on protease-3. The protease responsible for cleavage of LL37 from the cathelicidin precursor following secretion from keratinocytes has not yet been described. However, inhibition of neutrophil elastase activity has been shown to impair maturation of LL37 and clearance of bacteria from wounds.[69]

### C. Immunomodulatory Roles of AMP

The consequences of activating keratinocytes via pattern recognition molecules such as Toll-like receptors include initiation of local inflammation due to secretion of cytokines and chemokines in addition to AMP. Secretion of ILα, TNF-α, IFN-α/β, and IL-8[70–72] result in activation of local postcapillary endothelial venules to release their tight junctions and express cell adhesion molecules.[73] This in turn allows leakage of serum proteins, including immunoglobulins and complement, into the tissue. Neutrophils and other inflammatory cells migrate into the tissue due to chemoattraction by IL-8, and the AMP themselves.[74,75]

LL37 and β-defensins have been shown to play important immunomodulatory roles in recruiting and activating neutrophils, monocytes, immature dendritic cells, and T cells.[75,76] LL37 has been shown to mediate chemoattraction of these cells via formyl-peptide receptor-like 1 (FPRL-1).[77] While immature dendritic cells and memory T cells are attracted via β-defensins binding to CCR-6.[78] In addition, defensins and LL37 have potent chemotactic and activating activities on mast cells, which are transduced via a G protein–coupled phospholipase C pathway.[79,80] These chemotactic and activating activities of AMP may also provide an essential set of signals to initiate an adaptive immune response in cases where the innate microbicidal capacity of the skin is overwhelmed. This subject has recently been reviewed by Yang et al.[81]

### D. Antimicrobial Activities of Chemokines

The observations that the peptides that we know as AMP also have important immunomodulatory activities illustrate that the name "antimicrobial peptide" may fail to capture the spectrum of contributions these molecules make toward host defense. In fact, there have been reports that molecules initially described as chemokines, and which are known to mediate their chemotactic activities through specific chemokine receptors, possess potent, broad-spectrum antimicrobial activities *in vitro*.[4,82] Indeed, Yang and colleagues[4] have surveyed 30 known human chemokines, and found 17 of them to possess antimicrobial activity *in vitro*. Because human keratinocytes are known to produce numerous chemokines upon activation,[83–86] it may be reasonable to view this cell type as functioning not only as a contributor to the epithelial barrier, but also as an active effector cell of the innate immune system. This view is further supported by long-standing recognition that keratinocytes are capable of phagocytosing an array of different particles, including apoptotic cells, melanosomes, liposomes, and starch particles.[87–90]

### E. Skin Diseases Associated with Deficient AMP Production Are Associated with Increased Microbial Burden

The importance of proper coordination of the innate immune functions of skin cells is illustrated in diseases in which inducible antimicrobial responses are affected. Two common skin diseases can be used as examples. In the case of psoriasis, the barrier function of the epidermis is impaired, and there is an overabundance of several Th1 cytokines including TNF and IFN-γ.[91] Elevated levels of these cytokines in psoriatic skin stimulate production of LL37, hBD2, and hBD3.[21,63,92] However, psoriasis is remarkable in that, even though the barrier function is compromised, microbial infections are very rare.

The barrier function of the skin is also compromised in atopic dermatitis (AD);[93] however, the cytokine milieu in the skin of patients with AD is dominated by Th2-derived cytokines, including IL-4, IL-10, and IL-13.[94] Nomura and colleagues[63] have shown that exposure of keratinocytes to IL-4 or IL-13 inhibits stimulation of defensin gene expression in response to IFN-γ and TNF. Indeed, patients with AD are impaired in their ability to induce expression of LL37 and defensins in the skin relative to patients with psoriasis.[95] Patients with AD are prone to microbial infections of the skin, including bacteria, fungi, and enveloped viruses.[96] Thus, properly regulated expression of AMP in the skin is essential for defense against microbial colonization and infection.

## V. SUMMARY AND CONCLUSIONS

The skin is exposed to countless microbial challenges every day. The vast majority of these microbes are never able to colonize the skin, even though it is a nutrient rich environment for many microorganisms. Sweat glands produce at least two potent peptide antibiotics, dermcidin and LL37, which are deposited in large amounts on the skin surface when we sweat. The keratinocytes themselves constitutively express another peptide antibiotic, hBD1, which permeates the keratinized layers of the skin, and can kill many environmental microbes in cooperation with LL37 and dermcidin. The metabolic products of microbes that are not as easily killed by this most superficial line of defense provoke keratinocytes in deeper layers to produce additional LL37, hBD2, hBD3, and several chemokines, which also possess direct antimicrobial activity, as well as cytokines that initiate the inflammatory response. Inflammatory cells including neutrophils, monocytes, immature dendritic cells, and memory T cells are recruited by the chemotactic activities of the AMP, and chemokines produced by the keratinocytes. Once at the site of infection, neutrophils utilize an array of antimicrobial mechanisms, including large amounts of α-defensins, to kill the microbes, while immature dendritic cells and memory T cells activate an adaptive immune response. Failure to produce sufficient levels of AMP in the skin during Th2-cytokine-dominated chronic inflammation, such as AD, is associated with increased microbial burden in the skin.

## REFERENCES


1. Schittek, B., Hipfel, R., Sauer, B. et al., Dermcidin: a novel human antibiotic peptide secreted by sweat glands, *Nat. Immunol.,* 2, 1133, 2001.
2. Larrick, J.W., Lee, J., Ma, S. et al., Structural, functional analysis and localization of the human CAP18 gene, *FEBS Lett.,* 398, 74, 1996.
3. Lehrer, R.I. and Ganz, T., Defensins of vertebrate animals, *Curr. Opin. Immunol.,* 14, 96, 2002.
4. Yang, D., Chen, Q., Hoover, D.M. et al., Many chemokines including CCL20/MIP-3alpha display antimicrobial activity, *J. Leukocyte Biol.,* 74, 448, 2003.
5. van Wetering, S., Mannesse-Lazeroms, S.P., van Sterkenburg, M.A. et al., Neutrophil defensins stimulate the release of cytokines by airway epithelial cells: modulation by dexamethasone, *Inflamm. Res.,* 51, 8, 2002.

6. Yang, D., Chertov, O., Bykovskaia, S.N. et al., Beta-defensins: linking innate and adaptive immunity through dendritic and T cell CCR6, *Science,* 286, 525, 1999.
7. Yang, D., Chen, Q., Chertov, O. et al., Human neutrophil defensins selectively chemoattract naive T and immature dendritic cells, *J. Leukocyte Biol.,* 68, 9, 2000.
8. Ganz, T., Selsted, M.E., Szklarek, D. et al., Defensins. Natural peptide antibiotics of human neutrophils, *J. Clin. Invest.,* 76, 1427, 1985.
9. Bulet, P., Hetru, C., Dimarcq, J.L. et al., Antimicrobial peptides in insects; structure and function, *Dev. Comp. Immunol.,* 23, 329, 1999.
10. Charlet, M., Chernysh, S., Philippe, H. et al., Innate immunity. Isolation of several cysteine-rich antimicrobial peptides from the blood of a mollusk, *Mytilus edulis, J. Biol. Chem.,* 271, 21808, 1996.
11. Thomma, B.P., Cammue, B.P. and Thevissen, K., Plant defensins, *Planta,* 216, 193, 2002.
12. Selsted, M.E., Tang, Y.Q., Morris, W.L. et al., Purification, primary structures, and antibacterial activities of beta-defensins, a new family of antimicrobial peptides from bovine neutrophils, *J. Biol. Chem.,* 268, 6641, 1993.
13. Tran, D., Tran, P.A., Tang, Y.Q. et al., Homodimeric theta-defensins from rhesus macaque leukocytes: isolation, synthesis, antimicrobial activities, and bacterial binding properties of the cyclic peptides, *J. Biol. Chem.,* 277, 3079, 2002.
14. Wang, W., Cole, A.M., Hong, T. et al., Retrocyclin, an antiretroviral theta-defensin, is a lectin, *J. Immunol.,* 170, 4708, 2003.
15. Valore, E.V. and Ganz, T., Posttranslational processing of defensins in immature human myeloid cells, *Blood,* 79, 1538, 1992.
16. Jones, D.E. and Bevins, C.L., Paneth cells of the human small intestine express an antimicrobial peptide gene, *J. Biol. Chem.,* 267, 23216, 1992.
17. Jones, D.E. and Bevins, C.L., Defensin-6 mRNA in human Paneth cells: implications for antimicrobial peptides in host defense of the human bowel, *FEBS. Lett.,* 315, 187, 1993.
18. Ouellette, A.J. and Bevins, C.L., Paneth cell defensins and innate immunity of the small bowel, *Inflamm. Bowel. Dis.,* 7, 43, 2001.
19. Zhao, C., Wang, I. and Lehrer, R.I., Widespread expression of beta-defensin hBD-1 in human secretory glands and epithelial cells, *FEBS. Lett.,* 396, 319, 1996.
20. Valore, E.V., Park, C.H., Quayle, A.J. et al., Human beta-defensin-1: an antimicrobial peptide of urogenital tissues, *J. Clin. Invest.,* 101, 1633, 1998.
21. Harder, J., Bartels, J., Christophers, E. et al., A peptide antibiotic from human skin, *Nature,* 387, 861, 1997.
22. Hiratsuka, T., Nakazato, M., Date, Y. et al., Identification of human beta-defensin-2 in respiratory tract and plasma and its increase in bacterial pneumonia, *Biochem. Biophys. Res. Commun.,* 249, 943, 1998.
23. Harder, J., Bartels, J., Christophers, E. et al., Isolation and characterization of human beta-defensin-3, a novel human inducible peptide antibiotic, *J. Biol. Chem.,* 276, 5707, 2001.
24. Garcia, J.R., Krause, A., Schulz, S. et al., Human beta-defensin 4: a novel inducible peptide with a specific salt-sensitive spectrum of antimicrobial activity, *FASEB. J.,* 15, 1819, 2001.
25. Scheetz, T., Bartlett, J.A., Walters, J.D. et al., Genomics-based approaches to gene discovery in innate immunity, *Immunol. Rev.,* 190, 137, 2002.
26. Kao, C.Y., Chen, Y., Zhao, Y.H. et al., ORFeome-based search of airway epithelial cell-specific novel human [beta]-defensin genes, *Am. J. Respir. Cell. Mol. Biol.,* 29, 71, 2003.
27. Bals, R., Wang, X., Wu, Z. et al., Human beta-defensin 2 is a salt-sensitive peptide antibiotic expressed in human lung, *J. Clin. Invest.,* 102, 874, 1998.
28. Sparkes, R.S., Kronenberg, M., Heinzmann, C. et al., Assignment of defensin gene(s) to human chromosome 8p23, *Genomics,* 5, 240, 1989.
29. Maxwell, A.I., Morrison, G.M. and Dorin, J.R., Rapid sequence divergence in mammalian beta-defensins by adaptive evolution, *Mol. Immunol.,* 40, 413, 2003.
30. Hollox, E.J., Armour, J.A. and Barber, J.C., Extensive normal copy number variation of a beta-defensin antimicrobial-gene cluster, *Am. J. Hum. Genet.,* 73, 591, 2003.
31. Larrick, J.W., Morgan, J.G., Palings, I. et al., Complementary DNA sequence of rabbit CAP18 — a unique lipopolysaccharide binding protein, *Biochem. Biophys. Res. Commun.,* 179, 170, 1991.

32. Larrick, J.W., Hirata, M., Balint, R.F. et al., Human CAP18: a novel antimicrobial lipopolysaccharide-binding protein, *Infect. Immun.*, 63, 1291, 1995.
33. Storici, P. and Zanetti, M., A novel cDNA sequence encoding a pig leukocyte antimicrobial peptide with a cathelin-like pro-sequence, *Biochem. Biophys. Res. Commun,* 196, 1363, 1993.
34. Oren, Z., Lerman, J.C., Gudmundsson, G.H. et al., Structure and organization of the human antimicrobial peptide LL-37 in phospholipid membranes: relevance to the molecular basis for its non-cell-selective activity, *Biochem. J.,* 341 (Pt 3), 501, 1999.
35. Aumelas, A., Mangoni, M., Roumestand, C. et al., Synthesis and solution structure of the antimicrobial peptide protegrin-1, *Eur. J. Biochem.,* 237, 575, 1996.
36. Cunningham, T.J., Hodge, L., Speicher, D. et al., Identification of a survival-promoting peptide in medium conditioned by oxidatively stressed cell lines of nervous system origin, *J. Neurosci.,* 18, 7047, 1998.
37. Cunningham, T.J., Jing, H., Akerblom, I. et al., Identification of the human cDNA for new survival/evasion peptide (DSEP): studies *in vitro* and *in vivo* of overexpression by neural cells, *Exp. Neurol.,* 177, 32, 2002.
38. Valore, E.V. and Ganz, T., Laboratory production of antimicrobial peptides in native conformation., in *Methods in Molecular Biology: Antibacterial Peptide Protocol,* Shafer, W.M., Humana Press, Totowa, NJ, 1999.
39. Midorikawa, K., Ouhara, K., Komatsuzawa, H. et al., *Staphylococcus aureus* susceptibility to innate antimicrobial peptides, beta-defensins and CAP18, expressed by human keratinocytes, *Infect. Immun.,* 71, 3730, 2003.
40. Turner, J., Cho, Y., Dinh, N.N. et al., Activities of LL-37, a cathelin-associated antimicrobial peptide of human neutrophils, *Antimicrob. Agents Chemother.,* 42, 2206, 1998.
41. Circo, R., Skerlavaj, B., Gennaro, R. et al., Structural and functional characterization of hBD-1(Ser35), a peptide deduced from a DEFB1 polymorphism, *Biochem. Biophys. Res. Commun.,* 293, 586, 2002.
42. Daher, K.A., Selsted, M.E. and Lehrer, R.I., Direct inactivation of viruses by human granulocyte defensins, *J. Virol.,* 60, 1068, 1986.
43. Nakashima, H., Yamamoto, N., Masuda, M. et al., Defensins inhibit HIV replication *in vitro*, *AIDS,* 7, 1129, 1993.
44. Cole, A.M., Hong, T., Boo, L.M. et al., Retrocyclin: a primate peptide that protects cells from infection by T- and M-tropic strains of HIV-1, *Proc. Natl. Acad. Sci. U.S.A.,* 99, 1813, 2002.
45. Howell, M.D., Jones, J.F., Kisich, K.O., Streib, J.E., Gallo, R.L., and Leung, D.Y.M., Selective killing of vaccinia virus by LL-37: implications for eczema vaccinatum, *J. Immunol.,* 172, 1763–1767, 2004.
46. Lehrer, R.I., Szklarek, D., Ganz, T. et al., Correlation of binding of rabbit granulocyte peptides to *Candida albicans* with candidacidal activity, *Infect. Immun.,* 49, 207, 1985.
47. Yenugu, S., Hamil, K.G., Birse, C.E. et al., Antibacterial properties of the sperm-binding proteins and peptides of human epididymis 2 (HE2) family; salt sensitivity, structural dependence and their interaction with outer and cytoplasmic membranes of *Escherichia coli*, *Biochem. J.,* 372, 473, 2003.
48. Lehrer, R.I., Barton, A., Daher, K.A. et al., Interaction of human defensins with *Escherichia coli.* Mechanism of bactericidal activity, *J. Clin. Invest.,* 84, 553, 1989.
49. Kagan, B.L., Selsted, M.E., Ganz, T. et al., Antimicrobial defensin peptides form voltage-dependent ion-permeable channels in planar lipid bilayer membranes, *Proc. Natl. Acad. Sci. U.S.A.,* 87, 210, 1990.
50. Cociancich, S., Ghazi, A., Hetru, C. et al., Insect defensin, an inducible antibacterial peptide, forms voltage-dependent channels in *Micrococcus luteus*, *J. Biol. Chem.,* 268, 19239, 1993.
51. Plakhova, V.B., Shchegolev, B.F., Rogachevskii, I.V. et al., A possible molecular mechanism for the interaction of defensin with the sensory neuron membrane, *Neurosci. Behav. Physiol.,* 32, 409, 2002.
52. Yue, G., Merlin, D., Selsted, M.E. et al., Cryptdin 3 forms anion selective channels in cytoplasmic membranes of human embryonic kidney cells, *Am. J. Physiol. Gastrointest. Liver Physiol.,* 282, G757, 2002.
53. Saiman, L., Tabibi, S., Starner, T.D. et al., Cathelicidin peptides inhibit multiply antibiotic-resistant pathogens from patients with cystic fibrosis, *Antimicrob. Agents Chemother.,* 45, 2838, 2001.
54. Henzler Wildman, K.A., Lee, D.K. and Ramamoorthy, A., Mechanism of lipid bilayer disruption by the human antimicrobial peptide, LL-37, *Biochemistry,* 42, 6545, 2003.

55. Peschel, A., Jack, R.W., Otto, M. et al., *Staphylococcus aureus* resistance to human defensins and evasion of neutrophil killing via the novel virulence factor MprF is based on modification of membrane lipids with l-lysine, *J. Exp. Med.,* 193, 1067, 2001.
56. Nagaoka, I., Hirota, S., Yomogida, S. et al., Synergistic actions of antibacterial neutrophil defensins and cathelicidins, *Inflamm. Res.,* 49, 73, 2000.
57. Lehrer, R.I., Szklarek, D., Ganz, T. et al., Synergistic activity of rabbit granulocyte peptides against Candida albicans, *Infect. Immun.,* 52, 902, 1986.
58. Higgins, M.P., Heuizer, H., Heifets, L. et al., Synergistic mechanisms of antimicrobial peptide activity against *Mycobacterium tuberculosis* (submitted).
59. Murakami, M., Ohtake, T., Dorschner, R.A. et al., Cathelicidin anti-microbial peptide expression in sweat, an innate defense system for the skin, *J. Invest. Dermatol.,* 119, 1090, 2002.
60. Marchini, G., Lindow, S., Brismar, H. et al., The newborn infant is protected by an innate antimicrobial barrier: peptide antibiotics are present in the skin and vernix caseosa, *Br. J. Dermatol.,* 147, 1127, 2002.
61. Kawai, K., Shimura, H., Minagawa, M. et al., Expression of functional Toll-like receptor 2 on human epidermal keratinocytes, *J. Dermatol. Sci.,* 30, 185, 2002.
62. Liu, A.Y., Destoumieux, D., Wong, A.V. et al., Human beta-defensin-2 production in keratinocytes is regulated by interleukin-1, bacteria, and the state of differentiation, *J. Invest. Dermatol.,* 118, 275, 2002.
63. Nomura, I., Goleva, E., Howell, M.D. et al., Cytokine milieu of atopic dermatitis, as compared to psoriasis, skin prevents induction of innate immune response genes, *J. Immunol.,* 171, 3262, 2003.
64. Di Nardo, A., Vitiello, A. and Gallo, R.L., Cutting edge: mast cell antimicrobial activity is mediated by expression of cathelicidin antimicrobial peptide, *J. Immunol.,* 170, 2274, 2003.
65. Semple, C.A., Rolfe, M., and Dorin, J.R., Duplication and selection in the evolution of primate beta-defensin genes, *Genome Biol.,* 4, R31, 2003.
66. Ganz, T., Liu, L., Valore, E.V. et al., Posttranslational processing and targeting of transgenic human defensin in murine granulocyte, macrophage, fibroblast, and pituitary adenoma cell lines, *Blood,* 82, 641, 1993.
67. Oren, A., Ganz, T., Liu, L. et al., In human epidermis, beta-defensin 2 is packaged in lamellar bodies, *Exp. Mol. Pathol.,* 74, 180, 2003.
68. Sorensen, O.E., Follin, P., Johnsen, A.H. et al., Human cathelicidin, hCAP-18, is processed to the antimicrobial peptide LL-37 by extracellular cleavage with proteinase 3, *Blood,* 97, 3951, 2001.
69. Cole, A.M., Shi, J., Ceccarelli, A. et al., Inhibition of neutrophil elastase prevents cathelicidin activation and impairs clearance of bacteria from wounds, *Blood,* 97, 297, 2001.
70. Zhang, J.Z., Maruyama, K., Ono, I. et al., Regulatory effects of 1,25-dihydroxyvitamin D3 and a novel vitamin D3 analogue MC903 on secretion of interleukin-1 alpha (IL-1 alpha) and IL-8 by normal human keratinocytes and a human squamous cell carcinoma cell line (HSC-1), *J. Dermatol. Sci.,* 7, 24, 1994.
71. Fujisawa, H., Kondo, S., Wang, B. et al., The expression and modulation of IFN-alpha and IFN-beta in human keratinocytes, *J. Interferon Cytokine Res.,* 17, 721, 1997.
72. Kock, A., Schwarz, T., Kirnbauer, R. et al., Human keratinocytes are a source for tumor necrosis factor alpha: evidence for synthesis and release upon stimulation with endotoxin or ultraviolet light, *J. Exp. Med.,* 172, 1609, 1990.
73. Pober, J.S., Effects of tumour necrosis factor and related cytokines on vascular endothelial cells, *Ciba Found. Symp.,* 131, 170, 1987.
74. Smith, G.S. and Lumsden, J.H., Review of neutrophil adherence, chemotaxis, phagocytosis and killing, *Vet. Immunol. Immunopathol.,* 4, 177, 1983.
75. Yang, D., Biragyn, A., Kwak, L.W. et al., Mammalian defensins in immunity: more than just microbicidal, *Trends Immunol.,* 23, 291, 2002.
76. Lehrer, R.I. and Ganz, T., Cathelicidins: a family of endogenous antimicrobial peptides, *Curr. Opin. Hematol.,* 9, 18, 2002.
77. De, Y., Chen, Q., Schmidt, A.P. et al., LL-37, the neutrophil granule- and epithelial cell-derived cathelicidin, utilizes formyl peptide receptor-like 1 (FPRL1) as a receptor to chemoattract human peripheral blood neutrophils, monocytes, and T cells, *J. Exp. Med.,* 192, 1069, 2000.

78. Hoover, D.M., Boulegue, C., Yang, D. et al., The structure of human macrophage inflammatory protein-3alpha/CCL20. Linking antimicrobial and CC chemokine receptor-6-binding activities with human beta-defensins, *J. Biol. Chem.,* 277, 37647, 2002.
79. Niyonsaba, F., Iwabuchi, K., Matsuda, H. et al., Epithelial cell-derived human beta-defensin-2 acts as a chemotaxin for mast cells through a pertussis toxin-sensitive and phospholipase C-dependent pathway, *Int. Immunol.,* 14, 421, 2002.
80. Niyonsaba, F., Iwabuchi, K., Someya, A. et al., A cathelicidin family of human antibacterial peptide LL-37 induces mast cell chemotaxis, *Immunology,* 106, 20, 2002.
81. Yang, D., Chertov, O., and Oppenheim, J.J., Participation of mammalian defensins and cathelicidins in anti-microbial immunity: receptors and activities of human defensins and cathelicidin (LL-37), *J. Leukocyte Biol.,* 69, 691, 2001.
82. Starner, T.D., Barker, C.K., Jia, H.P. et al., CCL20 Is an inducible product of human airway epithelia with innate immune properties, *Am. J. Respir. Cell. Mol. Biol.,* 29, 627, 2003.
83. Boorsma, D.M., de Haan, P., Willemze, R. et al., Human growth factor (huGRO), interleukin-8 (IL-8) and interferon-gamma-inducible protein (gamma-IP-10) gene expression in cultured normal human keratinocytes, *Arch. Dermatol Res.,* 286, 471, 1994.
84. Albanesi, C., Scarponi, C., Sebastiani, S. et al., A cytokine-to-chemokine axis between T lymphocytes and keratinocytes can favor Th1 cell accumulation in chronic inflammatory skin diseases, *J. Leukocyte Biol.,* 70, 617, 2001.
85. Tohyama, M., Shirakara, Y., Yamasaki, K. et al., Differentiated keratinocytes are responsible for TNF-alpha regulated production of macrophage inflammatory protein 3alpha/CCL20, a potent chemokine for Langerhans cells, *J. Dermatol. Sci.,* 27, 130, 2001.
86. Flier, J., Boorsma, D.M., Bruynzeel, D.P. et al., The CXCR3 activating chemokines IP-10, Mig, and IP-9 are expressed in allergic but not in irritant patch test reactions, *J. Invest. Dermatol.,* 113, 574, 1999.
87. Takashima, A. and Grinnell, F., Human keratinocyte adhesion and phagocytosis promoted by fibronectin, *J. Invest. Dermatol.,* 83, 352, 1984.
88. Okazaki, K., Uzuka, M., Morikawa, F. et al., Transfer mechanism of melanosomes in epidermal cell culture, *J. Invest. Dermatol.,* 67, 541, 1976.
89. Mottaz, J.H. and Zelickson, A.S., The phagocytic nature of the keratinocyte in human epidermis after tape stripping, *J. Invest. Dermatol.,* 54, 272, 1970.
90. Szepfalusi, Z., Parth, E., Jurecka, W. et al., Human monocytes and keratinocytes in culture ingest hydroxyethylstarch, *Arch. Dermatol. Res.,* 285, 144, 1993.
91. Barker, J.N., Psoriasis as a T cell-mediated autoimmune disease, *Hosp. Med.,* 59, 530, 1998.
92. Frohm, M., Agerberth, B., Ahangari, G. et al., The expression of the gene coding for the antibacterial peptide LL-37 is induced in human keratinocytes during inflammatory disorders, *J. Biol. Chem.,* 272, 15258, 1997.
93. Abe, T., Ohkido, M. and Yamamoto, K., Studies on skin surface barrier functions: skin surface lipids and transepidermal water loss in atopic skin during childhood, *J. Dermatol.,* 5, 223, 1978.
94. Reinhold, U., Kukel, S., Goeden, B. et al., Functional characterization of skin-infiltrating lymphocytes in atopic dermatitis, *Clin. Exp. Immunol.,* 86, 444, 1991.
95. Ong, P.Y., Ohtake, T., Brandt, C. et al., Endogenous antimicrobial peptides and skin infections in atopic dermatitis, *N. Engl. J. Med.,* 347, 1151, 2002.
96. Leung, D.Y., Infection in atopic dermatitis, *Curr. Opin. Pediatr.,* 15, 399, 2003.

# 14 Complement as a Part of the Skin Immune System

*Syed Shafi Asghar, Krisztina Klára Timár, and Marcel Christian Pasch*

## CONTENTS



## I. INTRODUCTION

Complement is one of the most powerful affecter systems involved in the body's defense and inflammation. It consists of some 40 proteins, which include soluble as well as membrane-embedded proteins. Among the soluble complement proteins are components of the classical pathway, which kill pathogens in the presence of antibodies. There are components of the lectin pathway that recognize invading pathogens through their surface carbohydrates and kill them in the absence of antibodies. There are components of the alternative pathway that kill pathogens in the absence of antibodies. And, there are soluble regulators of complement activation that regulate different steps of classical, lectin, and alternative pathways in fluid phase. Soluble regulators inhibit complement activation in the fluid phase much more strongly than on the surface of pathogens. In this way they protect self-cell from bystander lysis while allowing efficient killing of the pathogen by the complement system. Among the cell membrane complement proteins are cell surface regulators

0-8493-1959-5/05/$0.00+$1.50

**TABLE 14.1**
**Some Newly Assigned Functions of the Complement System**

| Functions | Ref. |
|---|---|
| 1. Enhancement of immunogenecity of antigens | 2 |
| 2. Regulation of IgE synthesis | 3,4 |
| 3. Regulation of cell survival, proliferation, and apoptosis | 5–7 |
| 4. Development of central nervous system | 8 |
| 5. Cartilage and bone development | |
| Differentiation of mesenchymal cells into early chondriocytes | 9 |
| Differentiation of macrophage like mononuclear cell progenitors into osteoclasts | 10 |
| Cartilage-bone transformation and bone remodeling and vascularization | 11 |
| 6. Reproduction processes | |
| Complement receptors mediated gamete maturation, follicular development and ovulation | 12, 13 |
| Cell surface complement regulator-mediated protection of entire reproduction tract, sperm, and oocytes, maintenance of feto-maternal tolerance, and sperm oocyte fusion | 14–16 |
| 7. Liver regeneration | 17 |
| 8. Early hematopoietic development | 18 |
| 9. Angiogenesis and blood vessel remodeling | 18 |

that inhibit different steps of complement activation on body cells to prevent their killing by autologous complement. Among the membrane complement proteins are also complement receptors that mediate a variety of functions of the cell on which they are expressed. They have long been known to mediate chemotaxis, phagocytosis, mast cell degranulation, and B- and T-cell activation. All these proteins together provide a system capable of destroying a large variety of pathogens either directly by causing their lysis without damaging self-cells or indirectly by recruiting phagocytes cells. Recent studies have assigned many new striking functions[1] to the complement system; some of them have direct or indirect effects on skin under physiopathological conditions. These are listed in Table 14.1.

This chapter briefly describes the three pathways of the complement system, mechanisms of protection of self-cells from detrimental effects of activation of autologous complement, and the ability of skin cells to synthesize complement proteins. It also describes dermatological diseases associated with genetic deficiencies or aberrant expression of proteins of this system.

## II. COMPLEMENT PATHWAYS

Several reviews on the complement system have recently been published;[19–22] therefore, only passing reference to the three pathways of complement is presented here (Figure 14.1). In general, complement activation on foreign target cells via the classical pathway is initiated after antibody molecules bind to a cell surface antigen(s). One of the subunits of C1, C1q, recognizes the bound antibody and interacts with its Fc portion. This results in the activation of other subunits, C1r and C1s, within C1. Activated C1s then splits the fourth component of complement (C4) into a smaller fragment, C4a, and a larger one, C4b. In freshly formed C4b, a thioester bond becomes exposed, which reacts rapidly with any nearby electron-donating group. Thus, some of the freshly formed C4b can react covalently with the amino or hydroxyl group present on the surface of sensitized target cells. C4b also has a binding site for the second component of complement (C2), which leads to the generation of C4b2 complex on the target cell. In this complex, if C2 is appropriately oriented toward activated C1s, activated C1s cleaves C2 into C2a and C2b. C2a remains in the complex but C2b leaves it. The C4b2a complex, thus formed, is a protease with its active site in C2a. This enzyme, known as the C3-convertase of the classical pathway, can cleave native C3 to generate C3b.

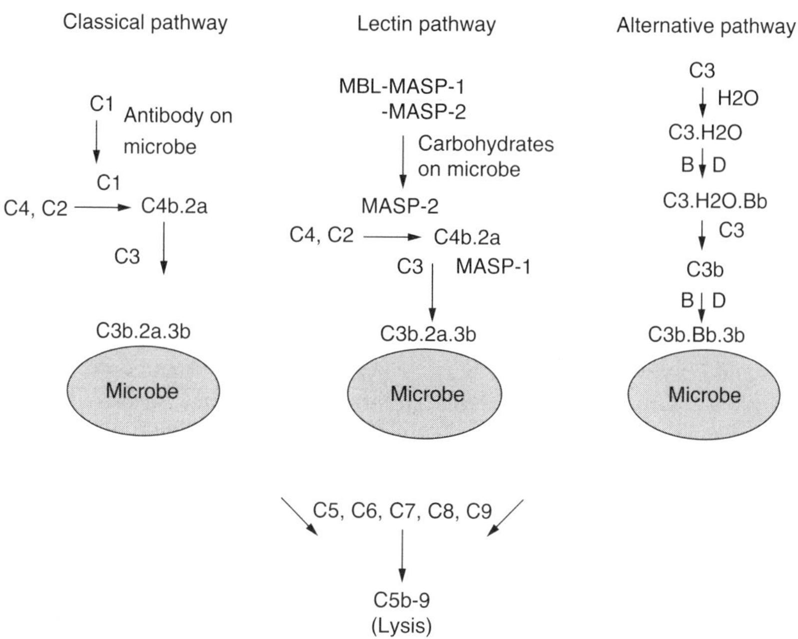


**FIGURE 14.1** Diagrammatic representation of the mechanism of lysis of foreign cell by classical lectin and alternative pathways. (Left) Classical pathway. Binding of antibody to the antigenic determinants on microbe in the presence of components of the classical pathway leads to the formation of activated C1s and generation of C3-convertase (C4b·2a), C5-convertase (C4b.2a.3b), and finally MAC on the microbe. (Middle) Lectin pathway. Binding of MBL and ficolins to an array of carbohydrates on the invading microbe leads to the activation of MASP complex whose MASP-2 serine protease activity splits C4 and C2 resulting in the generation of C3-convertase (C4b·C2a), and MASP-1 activity cleaves C3 into C3b, which results in the assembly of C5-convertase (C4b.2a.3b) and finally MAC on the microbe. (Right) Alternative pathway. C3 through its thioester bond generates C3·$H_2O$, which in the presence of factor B and factor D can form initial C3-convertase (C3·$H_2O$·Bb). This enzyme in the presence of alternative pathway and late components leads to the generation of C3-convertase (C3b·Bb), C5-convertase (C3b.Bb.3b) and finally MAC. MAC formed by any of the three pathways causes lysis of microbe. To keep the diagram simple, smaller complement products have not been depicted and the role of properdin in stabilizing C3/C5-convertases of the alternative pathway has not been illustrated. For details of both pathways, see the text. Factor B and factor D have been abbreviated to B and D, respectively.* Lectin = MBL, H-ficolin, and L-ficolin.

The lectin pathway of complement activation is initiated when recognition units of this pathway bind to specific carbohydrate moieties present on the surface of the invading pathogen. In the lectin pathway three serum proteins, mannan-binding lectin (MBL),[22] L-ficolin[23,24] (elastin-binding protein 37, or EPB-37, ficolin/P35; hucolin), and H-ficolin (hekata antigen)[25] have been identified as recognition units. MBL belongs to the collectin group of proteins. It contains a collagen-like domain and a carbohydrate recognition domain (CRD).[22] Three 32-kDa polypeptides fold together to form a subunit, and three to six subunits constitute MBL molecules of approximately 300 to 650 kDa. Their overall structure resembles that of C1q, the recognition unit of the classical pathway. MBL binds to carbohydrates with three and four hydroxyl groups in pyranose ring in a $Ca^{2+}$-dependent manner. The prominent ligands of MBL are mannose and *N*-acetyl-glucosamine (GlcNAc). Ficolins are a group of proteins that contain a collagen-like and a fibrinogen-like domain. The carbohydrate recognition site of ficolins resides within the fibrinogen-like domain. Ficolins have carbohydrate specificities different from that of MBL. L-ficolin binds to GlcNAc residues next to galactose of complex-type oligosaccharides but not to mannose.[26] H-ficolin binds to Glc.NAc and *N*-acetyl-galactosamine (GalNAc), but not to mannose and lactose.[25] Because of these steric specificities,

MBL, L-ficolin, and H-ficolin bind to carbohydrates present on pathogenic microorganisms but not on self-cells. MBL, L-ficolin, and H-ficolin exist in serum in association with MBL-associated serine proteases (MASPs) through their collagen-like domains. MASP complex consists of several subunits — MASP-1, MASP-2, MASP-3 and a truncated form of MASP-2 known as MAP-19 or sMAP.[27,28] These subunits are held together by $Ca^{2+}$ ions and electrostatic interactions. There are similarities in modular structures of subunits within the complex and between these subunits and C1r and C1s.[29,30] When a pathogenic microbe such as bacteria, fungus, parasite, or virus enters the body, MBL and L- and H-ficolins bind to their respective surface carbohydrate ligands. This binding results in the activation of serine protease subunits of the MASP complex that are associated with MBL and ficolins. Detailed molecular events related to the activation of serine proteases of this complex remain unknown. MASP-1 and MASP-2 are converted from single polypeptide proenzymes to activated enzymes consisting of two polypeptides, heavy A and light B chain, linked by a disulfide bond.[29,30] B-chains contain serine protease active centers. Activated MASP-2 cleaves C4 and C2, and activated MASP-1 cleaves C3 and C2.[31] MASP-3 regulates the C4 and C2 cleaving activity of MASP-2. The function of sMAP in this activated complex remains unknown. The net result of the activation of MASP-2 is the generation of C3 convertase (C4b.2a), the enzyme generated during the activation of classical pathway described above. C3-convertase and activated MASP-1 can cleave native C3 to generate C3b.

The activation of the alternative pathway is initially dependent on the continuous but slow exposure of a thioester bond otherwise buried inside the C3 molecule.[32] This exposure takes place likely as a result of normal thermal unfolding of the C3 molecule. The exposed thioester bond is highly reactive and reacts with nucleophilic groups such as amino and hydroxyl groups. Until recently this reaction was considered nonspecific, but now the thioester bond is known to react preferentially to C3b, C4b, and IgG and this specificity may be an important factor in further complement activation. In human $IgG_1$ and C4b, $Thr^{144}$ and $Ser^{1213}$, respectively, are the major sites of the thioester bond attachment.[33] In the fluid phase, most of the C3 with an exposed thioester bond reacts with water to form $C3{\cdot}H_2O$. This intermediate can combine with factor B present in body fluids to generate $C3{\cdot}H_2O{\cdot}B$ complex, which in the presence of an enzyme factor D is converted to $C3{\cdot}H_2O{\cdot}Bb$ complex. This complex is an enzyme known as the initial C3-convertase of the alternative pathway. It can cleave C3 to generate C3b fragments. At this point, freshly formed C3b molecules can combine with factor B through their mutual binding sites in the fluid phase or bind covalently to hydroxyl or amino groups of molecules present in the membranes of foreign target cells or self-cells present in the immediate vicinity. Binding of C3b to factor B in the fluid phase generates C3b·B, which in the presence of factor D is converted to fluid-phase C3b·Bb complex known as C3-convertase of the alternative pathway. Binding of C3b to membranes of foreign or self-cell results in membrane-bound C3b that combines with factor B to generate membrane bound C3b.B. This complex in the presence of factor D is converted to membrane-bound C3b·Bb complex, the C3-convertase of the alternative pathway. A complement protein, properdin, combines with fluid-phase as well as membrane-bound C3-convertase to generate C3b.Bb.P, a comparatively more stable C3-convertase of the alternative pathway. Fluid-phase as well as membrane-bound C3-convertase generates large amounts of C3b and thus cause amplification of C3b generation and C3-convertase formation in the fluid phase and on cell surfaces. On foreign target cells, this enzyme continues to perform its function of cleaving C3 to C3b, whereas on self-cells, it is destroyed, as discussed below in Section III.B.

C3b generated by the classical, lectin, or alternative pathway C3-convertases combines with the respective bimolecular C3-convertases (C4b.2a and C3b.Bb, respectively). This results in generation of C5-convertases of the classical and lectin ($C4b.2a.3b_n$) and alternative (C3b.Bb.3b) pathways. Alternative pathway C5-convertase is stabilized by properdin. C5-convertases are formed mainly on the cell surface but not significantly in the fluid phase because of the low degree of quick availability of an appropriate orientation for attachment of C3b to soluble C3b.Bb. C5 then combines with C4b and C3b subunits of C5-convertase of the classical/lectin pathway or C3b and Bb subunits of C5-convertase of the alternative pathway in an orientation suitable for cleavage by

C2a or Bb subunit, respectively, within these C5-convertases. C5-convertases cleave C5 to C5a and C5b. Metastable C5b remains loosely bound to C5-convertases; C6 then combines with it. The binding of C7 to C5b6 complex causes the formation of C5b-7 complex, which is released from the C5-convertases. This release exposes the metastable membrane-binding site of C5b-7. At this point, the C5b-7 complex can bind to a foreign invading target cell or to a host cell present in the immediate vicinity. C8 and C9 then join C5b-7 complex resulting in the assembly of the membrane attack complex (C5b-9; MAC). MAC generated on the surface of a foreign cell can form pores in its membrane that results in its lysis. On self-cell the self-assembly of late components generates noncytolytic MAC as described in the following section.

## III. MECHANISMS THAT PROTECT BODY CELLS FROM AUTOLOGOUS COMPLEMENT

As described above, C3b generated by C3-convertases of classical, lectin, and alternative pathway can bind covalently to the surface of invading pathogen as well as self-cell and cause subsequent activation of complement and lyse them. While elimination of invading pathogen by the complement system is highly desirable, damage to self-cells must be prevented. Damage to self-cells is prevented by the following fluid phase and cell surface mechanisms.

### A. Control of Complement Activation in Fluid Phase by Soluble Regulators

The mechanisms that protect self-cells from classical-, lectin-, or alternative pathway-mediated lysis by keeping complement dormant in the fluid phase involve several plasma inhibitors and inactivators that act at virtually every step of the complement cascade. These regulators minimize the formation and maximize the inactivation of complement fragments, such as C4b and C3b, and complement complexes, such as C5b-7, so that a minimum of them in active form collide with self-cells and a minimum of complement activation on self-cells occurs. These include C1-inhibitor (C1-INH), MASP-3, factor H, C4-binding protein (C4BP), factor I, vitronectin, and clusterin (Table 14.2).

The primary and tertiary structure of C1-INH and its functions have recently been reviewed.[34] C1-INH keeps the activation of C1 checked in circulation and body fluids. It efficiently interacts with activated C1r and activated C1s to form C1r–C1s–$(C1\text{-}INH)_2$ complex and dissociates C1q subunit from C1 complex. Inhibition of activated C1 results in the inhibition of cleavage of C4 as well as C2 and thereby in the inhibition of formation of active fragments C4b and C2a. C1-INH inhibits C1 approximately 100 times more strongly in the fluid phase than on the cell surface.[35] C1-INH also appears to regulate lectin pathway at an early stage. It forms stable complexes with both MASP-1 and MASP-2 and inhibits their proteolytic activities.[27] In addition, C1-INH in combination with $\alpha_2$-macroglobulin renders the lectin pathway unable to activate complement on *Neisseria gonorrhoeae*;[36] $\alpha_2$-macroglobulin binds to MASP-1 covalently and to MBL noncovalently in a $Ca^{2+}$-dependent manner to inhibit complement activation by the lectin pathway.

Although a very limited number of studies have been carried out on the functions of MASP-3, its ability to inhibit C4 cleaving activity of MBL-MASP-2 complex[28] may be held as a hypothesis that MASP-3 may be a soluble regulator of the lectin pathway.

The structures and functions of C4BP,[37,38] both molecular species of factor H, FH (155 kDa) and FHL-1 (factor H-like protein-1) (45 kDa),[39] and factor I[40] have recently been reviewed. They prevent the assembly of C3/C5-convertases of the classical and alternative pathways in fluid phase. C4BP and factor H combine with freshly formed C4b and C3b, respectively. They then develop cofactor activities for the enzyme factor I, which cleaves the α-chains of C4b and C3b, respectively, to inactivate them before they collide with self-cells. In this way, they protect self-cells. MBL appears to regulate classical and alternative pathways exquisitely by enhancing the binding of C4BP to C4b and binding of factor H to C3b.[41]

**TABLE 14.2**
**Fluid-Phase and Cell Surface Regulators of Complement Activation**

| Regulator | Ligand Specificity | Functional Activity |
|---|---|---|
| | **Fluid Phase Regulators** | |
| **C1 stage** | | |
| C1-INH | C1r/C1s | Inhibits C1r and C1s mainly in fluid phase |
| **MASP stage** | | |
| MASP-3 | MASP-2 | Inhibits cleavage of C4 and C2 by MASP-2 |
| **C3/C5 convertase formation stage** | | |
| C4BP | C4b | Cofactor for factor I in cleavage of C4b |
| Factor H | C3b | Cofactor for factor I in cleavage of C3b |
| Factor I | Factor H/C4BP MCP/CR1 | Cleaves C3b and C4b using cofactors |
| **MAC formation stage** | | |
| Vitronectin | C5b-8/C9 | Prevents the assembly of cytolytic MAC |
| Clusterin | C5b-8/C9 | Prevents the assembly of cytolytic MAC |
| | **Membrane-Embedded Regulators** | |
| **C3/C5-convertase formation stage** | | |
| DAF | C4b/C3b | Dissociates C2a and Bb from C4b and C3b |
| MCP | C4b/C3b | Cofactor for factor I in cleaving C4b and C3b |
| CR1 | C4b/C3b | Cofactor for factor I in cleaving C4b and C3b |
| **MAC formation stage** | | |
| CD59 | C5b-8/C9 | Prevents assembly of cytolytic MAC on self-cell |

*Abbreviations:* INH, C1-inhibitor; MASP, MBL-associated serine proteases; C4BP, C4b-binding protein; CR1, complement receptor-1; DAF, decay-accelerating factor; MAC, membrane attack complex; MCP, membrane cofactor protein.

*Source:* Adapted from Asghar, S.S. and Pasch, M.C., *Frontiers Biosci.*, 5, 63–81, 2000; and Bos, J.D. et al., *Clin. Dermatol.*, 19, 563–572, 2001. With permission.

Two structurally distinct serum proteins, vitronectin[42] and clusterin,[43] which exhibit a variety of functions, have recently been reviewed. Both these proteins also inhibit MAC formation by identical mechanisms. Both bind to C5b-7 as it is assembled in fluid phase. C5b-7 complex in which vitronectin or clusterin has been incorporated is unable to fix on cell membranes but can take up C8 and C9 molecules to form nonlytic C5b-9 complexes. Thus, vitronectin and clusterin, by rendering the MAC nonlytic, offer protection to the self-cell.

## B. Control of Complement Activation on Self-Cell by Cell Surface Regulators

Despite the efficient control of activation of the classical, lectin, and alternative pathways by soluble regulators, some complement fragments and complement complexes can escape regulation, become deposited on self-cells, and activate the rest of the complement cascade on their surfaces.[19,20,44,45] Activation of complement by any of the three pathways can potentially damage self-cells. Activation of complement on self-cells is, however, inhibited by multiple membrane-embedded regulators of complement. These include decay-accelerating factor (DAF), membrane cofactor protein (MCP), complement receptor-1 (CR1), and CD59. The ligand specificities and functional activities of these regulators are summarized in Table 14.2.

DAF, MCP, and CR1 have recently been reviewed.[20] They restrict complement activation on self-cells at the C3/C5-convertase formation stage. When C4b and C3b are fixed on a self-cell, DAF present in the membrane of the same cell binds to the deposited C4b and C3b and inhibits the interaction of C2 with C4b and of factor B with C3b. It also dissociates C2a and Bb from preformed C4b2a and C3bBb, respectively. Thus, DAF inhibits activation of complement on the surface of a self-cell at the C3-convertase formation stage and protects the cell from all the three pathways of autologous complement. MCP is also expressed on a wide variety of cell types. When C4b and C3b formed during complement activation are fixed on the membrane of a self-cell, MCP present in the membrane of the same cell combines with these fragments and develops cofactor activity for factor I. Factor I then proteolytically degrades C4b and C3b to inactive products iC4b and iC3b, respectively. Thus, MCP interferes with ongoing classical, lectin, and alternative pathways on a self-cell by intercepting the formation of C3/C5-convertases and mediating their inactivation. CR1 is present on a limited number of cell types. When C4b and C3b formed during complement activation are fixed on the membrane of a CR1 bearing self-cell, CR1 combines with these fragments and acts as a cofactor for the enzyme factor I, which cleaves C3b to iC3b, iC3b to C3c and C3dg, C4b to iC4b, and iC4b to C4c and C4d. Thus, CR1 can regulate the formation and activities of C3/C5-convertases of complement on CR1 bearing cells.

CD59 has recently been reviewed.[20] It controls complement activation on the surface of a self-cell at the MAC formation stage. It accomplishes this by binding to an epitope on α-chain of C8 that is exposed when C8 interacts with the C5b-7 complex on the cell membrane, on the one hand, and by binding to an exposed site of C9, on the other.

DAF, MCP, and CD59 (and CR1 on CR1-bearing cells) act synergistically to control different steps of complement activation on self-cells and protect them from all three pathways of the complement system.

### C. Control of Lysis of Self-Cell by Elimination of Membrane Attack Complex

The above-described humoral and membrane-associated mechanisms, in most instances, do not allow formation of cytolytic MAC on self-cells. However, if activation of complement is so excessive that a limited number of cytolytic MAC complexes have been formed on the body cells, these complexes are eliminated by vesicular shedding and endocytosis.[7,46]

## IV. MEDIATION OF CELL FUNCTIONS BY COMPLEMENT RECEPTORS

Complement receptors mediate a variety of functions of a cell on which they are expressed; using complement fragments as signaling molecules.[5] The key players are CR1, CR2, CR3, CR4, C3aR, C5aR, and C1qR. CR1 is a receptor for C3b present on phagocytic cells. CR1 in conjunction with CR3 mediates phagocytosis. CR1 also acts as a regulator of activation of complement on body cells as described above. CR2 is the receptor for iC3b, C3dg, and C3d. On B cells it mediates C3d-dependent enhancement of immunogenicity of antigens[2] and regulates IgE production through CD23 ligation.[3,4] CR3 is a receptor for iC3b and iC4b. CR3 is involved in several monocyte and macrophage functions including phagocytosis, which as described above requires CR1. CR4 is a receptor for iC3b. It has multiple functions including mediation in iC3b-mediated phagocytosis, elimination of opsonized apoptotic cells by phagocytes, and involvement in adherence of cells such as monocytes and neutrophils to endothelium and other substrates. Several C1q receptors (C1qRs) have been described.[47] The most characterized of these are cC1qR (60kd)[48] and C1qRp (126 kDa).[49] cC1qR seems to be involved in C1q-mediated enhancement of phagocytosis and C1qRp in C1q-mediated cell functions during complement activation in inflammatory conditions. Both bind to C1q and other molecules having collagen-like regions such as MBL, conglutinin, and lung surfactant protein-A. C3aR and C5aR bind small chemotactic complement fragments C3a and C5a, respectively.

MAC formed during local activation of complement can also have profound nonlethal effects on self-cells without involving any receptor. These effects include cell activation and release of inflammatory and non-inflammatory mediators.[5]

## V. SYNTHESIS OF COMPLEMENT IN THE SKIN

The primary site of the synthesis of almost all plasma complement proteins is the liver. Among the few exceptions are factor D synthesized in adipose tissue, C1 in gut epithelium, and H-ficolin in bile duct epithelial cells.[50] The primary sites of synthesis of several components of the lectin pathway and properdin remain unknown. Many cell types of other tissues produce complement components although they may not be the primary sites of synthesis of plasma complement. These include monocytes/macrophages, fibroblasts, astrocytes, endothelial cells, leukocytes, cells of renal glomerulus, and synovial lining cells.[51–53] Some cell types such as astrocytes produce almost all complement components, whereas others such as adipocytes produce a limited number of complement proteins. Locally produced complement is believed to be involved in inflammation at local tissue level when recruitment of plasma complement does not occur. Brain,[51] kidney,[53] and heart[54] have been shown to synthesize all the components of complement. In this part of the chapter we focus on the synthesis of complement in the skin.

In the skin, the epidermal compartment is avascular. In the dermal compartment, the passage of large plasma proteins of molecular weight more than 40 kDa from blood into the tissues is effectively restricted by endothelial cells and underlying basement membrane.[55] Thus, under normal circumstances little or no plasma complement will reach the dermis (and the epidermis). The absence of plasma complement in dermis and epidermis in extravascular areas is perhaps an advantage in that a potential source of damage to self-cells is not there. It is a disadvantage in that one of the systems of immune defense is missing in these compartments. The ideal situation would be that under normal circumstances there is no or a very low level of complement in these compartments but complement is produced when it is needed, e.g., during microbial infection or inflammation. This seems to be the case in the skin. In the epidermal compartment, the major cell type is keratinocyte, which constitutionally synthesizes very low, perhaps negligible, amounts of complement. During microbial invasion or other inflammatory conditions, keratinocytes are believed to release a number of cytokines.[56,57] Under these conditions, infiltrated cells can also release cytokines. Cytokines released from keratinocytes and inflammatory cells can differentially upregulate the synthesis of complement by keratinocytes that can presumably kill a pathogen. Thus, complement becomes available when needed. The same appears to be true for the dermis where the major cell type is the fibroblast. The cytokines produced by fibroblasts and infiltrated inflammatory cells can induce fibroblasts to synthesize complement when it is needed. We and others have examined the cytokines that can induce these epidermal and dermal cells to produce complement proteins.

### A. Synthesis of Complement in the Epidermis

Of the three major resident cell types in the epidermis — keratinocytes, melanocytes, and Langerhans cells — keratinocyte is by far the best-studied cell type (Table 14.3).

#### 1. Expression of Complement Proteins by Keratinocytes

##### a. *Complement Components*

The possibility that keratinocytes may be capable of synthesizing C3 was first raised by Basset-Seguin and co-workers,[58,59] who showed that C3dg, a 41-kDa fragment of α-chain of C3, is an

**TABLE 14.3**
**Expression of Complement Proteins by Resident Skin Cells**

| Fluid Phase Proteins | Source | Membrane Proteins | Source |
|---|---|---|---|
| **Classical pathway** | | Regulators | |
| C1q | F | DAF (CD55) | K, Me, Ma |
| C1r | F | MCP (CD46) | K, Me, Ma |
| C1s | F | CD59 | K, Me, Ma |
| C4 | F, K* | | |
| C2 | F | Complement receptors | |
| **Lectin pathway** | | CR1 (CD35) | K |
| MBL | ND | CR2 (CD21) | K |
| L-Ficolin | ND | CR3 (CD11b/CD18) | L, Ma** |
| H-Ficolin | ND | CR4 (CD11c/CD18) | Ma |
| M-Ficolin | ND | C5aR (CD88) | L, Ma, K** |
| MASP-1 | ND | C3aR | Ma |
| MASP-2 | ND | cC1qR | K |
| MASP-3 | ND | C1qRp | K NExp* |
| sMAP | ND | | |
| **Alternative pathway** | | | |
| Factor B | K, F | | |
| Factor D | ND | | |
| Properdin | ND | | |
| **Terminal components** | | | |
| C3 | K, F | | |
| C5 | K* | | |
| C6 | F | | |
| C7 | F | | |
| C8 | F | | |
| C9 | F | | |
| **Regulators** | | | |
| C1-INH | F | | |
| MASP-3 | ND | | |
| C4BP | ND | | |
| Factor H | K, F | | |
| Factor I | K* | | |
| Clusterin | ND | | |
| Vitronectin | ND | | |

*Note:* K = keratinocyte; F = fibroblast; Me = melanocytes; Ma = mast cell; L= Langerhans cells; ND = not yet studied in any of the resident skin cell.

* Preliminary results; see the text.

** Expression only in inflammatory skin diseases; see the text. NExp = not expressed.

integral part of the lamina densa and sublamina densa regions of the basement membrane of normal skin. These workers hypothesized that epidermal keratinocytes synthesize C3 whose breakdown product, C3dg, is passively incorporated into the adjacent epidermal basement membrane and becomes its integral part. Dovezenski et al.[60] showed the *in situ* expression of C3 and factor B by epidermal keratinocytes and the release of C3 by cultured keratinocytes. Basset-Seguin et al.[61] and

Yancey et al.[62] confirmed the synthesis of C3 and factor B in human keratinocytes and A431 cells at the protein and mRNA level.

Demonstration of constitutive synthesis of C3 and factor B led to the question of what regulates the synthesis of these components in keratinocytes. We have shown that the constitutive secretion of C3 by keratinocytes in culture was low but synthesis of C3 was greatly enhanced by interleukin-1α (IL-1α), interferon-γ (IFN-γ), and tumor necrosis factor-α (TNF-α) in increasing order.[63] Terui et al.[64] who studied a large number of cytokines and growth factors obtained similar results and showed that TNF-α and IFN- are the main cytokines that regulate the synthesis of C3 in human keratinocytes and that IL-1α and IL-1β also regulate it to some extent. The increase in C3 protein synthesis by these cytokines was shown in our laboratory to be associated with the increase in C3 mRNA.[63] We also showed that the constitutive secretion of factor B by keratinocytes was very low but the synthesis and secretion of factor B were enhanced significantly by IL-1α and interleukin-6 (IL-6) and greatly by IFN-γ and that this increase in factor B protein synthesis was associated with the increase in factor B message.[63]

Synthesis of components of lectin (MBL, H-ficolin, L-ficolin, MASP-1, MASP-2, MASP-3, and sMAP), classical (C1q, C1r, C1s, C2), and alternative (factor D, properdin) pathways is yet to be investigated. There is some preliminary evidence that C4 is synthesized by keratinocytes and its synthesis is regulated by IFN-γ (unpublished observations). Are keratinocytes able to synthesize other components of complement? Preliminary experiments in our laboratory using an ELISA whose minimum detection limit was 10 pg/ml showed that C5 was not released into the culture medium but was present in cell lysates. C5 mRNA could be detected by reverse transcriptase–polymerase chain reaction (RT-PCR). C5 protein release could not be induced by supernatant of activated mononuclear cells, which by virtue of having a large number of cytokines induces the synthesis of many complement proteins in many cell types. C5 release could also not be induced by activators of protein kinase C (phorbol 12-myristate, or PMA, and $Ca^{2+}$ ionophore A23187) and protein kinase A (dibutyryl cAMP). These results, although preliminary, indicate that perhaps keratinocytes are capable of synthesizing C5 but its synthesis and release are tightly regulated. Tight regulation of C5 synthesis could perhaps be yet another mechanism by which keratinocytes protect themselves from damage by their own complement. Nevertheless, the factors that regulate the synthesis and release of C5 need to be investigated. Synthesis of other late components of complement by keratinocytes also needs to be studied.

### b. *Fluid-Phase Regulators of Complement Activation*

Keratinocyte-derived complement can provide immune defense against pathogens, but it may also damage cells in the epidermis. As part of the mechanism of prevention of this damage, keratinocytes may also be expected to produce soluble regulators of complement activation, namely, C1-INH, MASP-3, C4BP, factor H, factor I, clusterin, and vitronectin. Of these, only the synthesis of factor H has been studied in some detail. Both molecular species of factor H, FH (155 kDa) and factor H-like protein-1 (FHL-1; 45 kDa), are produced by keratinocytes, and synthesis of both is upregulated by IFN-γ.[65] Keratinocytes also constitutively synthesize functionally active factor I whose synthesis is upregulated by IFN-γ (unpublished observations).

### c. *Cell Surface Regulators of Complement Activation*

Membrane-embedded regulators of complement, DAF, MCP, and CD59, are expected to be expressed by keratinocytes for prevention of complement-mediated damage. Indeed, human keratinocytes have been shown to express DAF, MCP, and CD59.[66] Owing to the high level of expression of membrane regulators, human keratinocytes[67] and human keratinocyte cell line SCC-12F[68] are extremely resistant to complement lysis. In a recent study in our laboratory,[66] recombinant transforming growth factors-1, 2 and 3 (TGF-1, TGF-2, and TGF-3) were found to upregulate MCP and CD59 but not DAF. An additional factor present among the mediators released from activated mononuclear cells also appears to upregulate MCP and CD59. So far, this factor has not been identified.

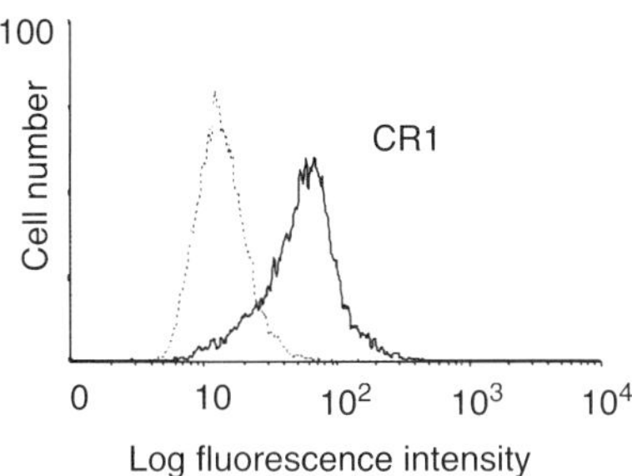


**FIGURE 14.2** Expression of CR1 by cultured human keratinocytes. Cultured human keratinocytes were washed and $10^4$ cells were analyzed for the expression of CR1 by flow cytometry. The continuous line shows keratinocyte staining of CR1; broken line shows staining with isotype control.

### *d. Complement Receptors*

Dovezenski et al.[60] have shown the expression of CR1 and CR2 *in situ* on epidermal as well as cultured keratinocytes. They have also shown expression of these receptors on epidermal keratinocytes by *in situ* hybridization. Figure 14.2 shows the expression of CR1 on cultured keratinocytes as detected by flow cytometry in our laboratory. CR2 expression in cultured keratinocytes and keratinocyte cell lines RHEK-1 and HeLa has been shown at the protein and mRNA level.[69] There are no reports, as yet, on the expression of CR3 and CR4 on keratinocytes.

C5aR does not appear to be expressed on normal keratinocytes. This is suggested by the fact that C5a did not cause transient $Ca^{2+}$ fluxes in keratinocytes and C5aR mRNA could not be detected in keratinocytes or in HaCat.[70] *In situ* hybridization studies[71] have shown that normal epidermal keratinocytes do not express detectable levels of C5aR transcripts, but those in lesional skin of patients with pyogenic granuloma and lichen planus do express C5aR message. A tight coexpression of C5aR and IL-6 mRNAs was observed in keratinocytes from lesions of these patients. Thus, C5aR appears to play an as-yet-unknown role in the pathogenesis of some skin diseases. C3aR on keratinocytes remains to be studied.

Expression of cC1qR and C1qRp on human keratinocytes was tested in our laboratory by flow cytometry (Figure 14.3). Antibodies directed against cC1qR[48] but not against C1qRp[49] recognized the receptor on keratinocytes. This does not necessarily mean that keratinocytes are not capable of expressing C1qRp because expression of C1qRp has not yet been studied (1) in normal keratinocytes at mRNA level, (2) in keratinocytes stimulated with cytokines and other potential inducers, and (3) in inflammatory diseases of the skin. The expression of complement receptors on keratinocytes is summarized in Table 14.3. The regulation of expression of complement receptors on keratinocytes has not yet been studied.

The results of the studies carried out so far on the regulation of synthesis of other complement proteins in keratinocytes are summarized in Table 14.4.

## 2. Synthesis of Complement Proteins by Melanocytes and Langerhans Cells

The contribution of melanocytes and Langerhans cells in the production of soluble complement proteins in epidermis remains unknown. So far, melanocytes have been shown to express only complement regulatory molecules[72] and Langerhans cells only C5aR[73] and CR3[74] (Table 14.3). The fact that Langerhans cells belong to the monocyte/macrophage lineage of cells may be held as a hypothesis that these cells may be capable of synthesizing several if not all soluble complement proteins. They will undoubtedly be shown to express most, if not all, membrane-embedded complement regulatory molecules. Definitive studies on synthesis of complement by Langerhans cells are restricted by the fact that they are difficult to purify in sufficient yield. It is likely that melanocytes and Langerhans cells may also contribute to local synthesis of complement significantly and that

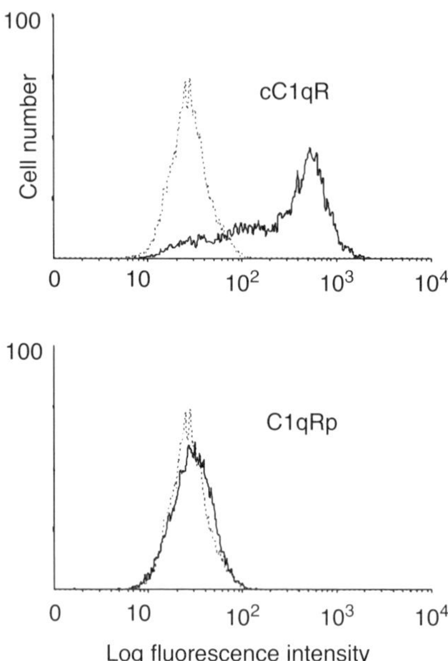


**FIGURE 14.3** Expression of cC1qR on human keratinocytes. Cultured human keratinocytes were washed and $10^4$ cells were analyzed for the expression of cC1qR and C1qRp. The continuous line in upper panel represents staining of keratinocytes by monoclonal anti-cC1qR. (Courtesy of Prof. Daha, Leiden, the Netherlands.) The continuous line in the lower panel represents staining by monoclonal anti-C1qRp (R139). (Courtesy of Dr. Tenner; see Neopmuceno et al.[49]) Broken lines in both panels represent staining by respective isotype control. Note strong expression of cC1qR but no expression of C1qRp on keratinocytes. U937 cell line showed strong expression of cC1qR as well as C1qRp (data not shown).

**TABLE 14.4**
**Cytokine Regulation of Synthesis of Complement Proteins by Keratinocytes**

| C Protein | Cytokines That Regulate the Synthesis |
|---|---|
| C3 | IL-1α, TNF-α, IFN-γ |
| Factor B | IL-1α, IL-6, IFN-γ |
| C5 | ND |
| Factor I | IFNγ |
| Factor H (45 and 155 kDa) | IFN-γ |
| MCP | TGF-1, TGF-2, TGF-3 |
| CD59 | TGF-1, TGF-2, TGF-3 |

ND = Regulators not known; see the text.

some components found not to be synthesized by keratinocytes may possibly be synthesized by these cells.

### B. Synthesis of Complement in the Dermis

Because of the property of endothelium to act as a molecular sieve,[55] complement produced by endothelial cells will enter the lumen side rather than the dermal side. Thus, there is likely to be virtually no or little contribution of cutaneous endothelial cells in the production of complement in the skin.

**TABLE 14.5**
**Cytokine Regulation of Complement Synthesis in Skin Fibroblasts**

| C Protein | Regulatory Cytokines | Ref. |
|---|---|---|
| C1r | TNF-α | 84 |
| C1s | TNF-α | 84 |
| C2* | IFN-γ, TNF-α, IL-1 | 74, 84 |
| C4 | IFN-γ (TNF-α shows synergistic effect) | 74 |
| C3 | TNF-α (IL-4 shows synergistic effect), IL-1, IL-6 | 79, 84 |
| | IL-13 (in TNF-α stimulated cells) | 85 |
| | IL-17 | 86 |
| Factor B | TNF-α, IL-1, IL-6 (IL-4 inhibits TNF-α, IL-1, and LPS induced synthesis) | 79 |
| | IFN-γ (synergism with LPS) | 80 |
| | IL-13 (in TNF-α-stimulated cells) | 85 |
| | IL-17 | 86 |
| C1-INH | TNF-α | 82 |
| Factor H (45 and 155 kDa) | IFN-γ | 81 |

Skin fibroblasts have been shown to synthesize several components of classical (C1q, C1r, C1s, C4, and C2)[75–77] and alternative (C3 and factor B)[78–80] pathways, late components (C5 to C9),[78] and two fluid-phase regulators of complement (C1-INH and factor H)[81–83] (Table 14.3 and Table 14.5). Cytokine regulation of the synthesis of these components is summarized in Table 14.5.

In spite of the propensity of stimulated mast cells to release a large number of preformed as well as *de novo* synthesized mediators and their involvement in several skin diseases such as atopic dermatitis,[87] their ability to produce soluble complement proteins has not yet been investigated. However, expression of several cell surface complement proteins in mast cells has been studied (see Table 14.3). Human skin mast cells and human mast cell line HMC-1 express C3aR as well as C5aR and undergo chemotaxis in response to C3a and C5a[88] but not in response to their des-Arg forms.[89,90] This may perhaps explain rapid accumulation of mast cells at sites of inflammation. Two types of C3aR have been identified on HMC-1 cell line — a high-affinity (C3aR1) and a low-affinity (C3aR2) receptor.[91] C5aR was detectable on mast cells in normal human skin and in psoriatic plaque but not in wheal and flare reactions or in urticaria pigmentosa.[92] HMC-1 cell line also expresses low levels of CR3 and CR4, which were upregulated by a protein kinase C activator, PMA, both at the protein and mRNA level.[93] CR4 was present on a low number of normal mast cells. A higher number of mast cells bearing the common chain of CR3 and CR4 were seen in inflammatory diseases such as psoriasis vulgaris, atopic dermatitis, and lichen planus. These observations led to the speculation that these complement receptors play an important role in homing of immature mast cells as well as in interaction of activated mast cells with other inflammatory cells. Mast cells isolated from juvenile foreskin and mammary skin have been shown to express complement regulatory molecules, DAF, MCP, and CD59.[94]

### C. Contribution of Migrating Cells to Complement Biosynthesis in the Skin

Cytokines and growth factors produced by inflammatory cells recruited during inflammatory conditions may induce complement synthesis by inflammatory cells as well as by resident cells of the skin. Mononuclear cells are known to produce all the components of classical and alternative pathways[52] and polymorphonuclear cells synthesize and store at least some late components.[95] The ability of these cells to synthesize components of lectin pathway remains obscure. Because cells of bone marrow origin contribute to more than 5% of plasma complement, the amount of complement produced locally by infiltrated cells should be functionally significant. As cytokines can cross the dermal-epidermal basement membrane,[96] they may induce the synthesis of complement in both compartments.

## VI. COMPLEMENT DEFICIENCIES AND SKIN DISEASES

### A. Complement Components

O'Neil,[97] Frank,[98] and Walport[99] have published excellent reviews on complement deficiencies. Pickering et al.[100] have described the details of age, gender, race, ethnic group, and clinical abnormalities (including skin aberrations) in individual complement-deficient patients. Discussion on these deficiencies will, therefore, be avoided except to make a passing comment that, in cases of homozygous deficiencies of C3, factor H, and factor I, C3dg is not formed and therefore lamina densa and sublamina densa regions are likely to be devoid of this integral structural protein. It is not known whether absence of C3dg in these regions contributes to any of the skin abnormalities seen in these deficiencies. In the last decade the deficiency of a component of the lectin pathway, MBL, has also been described. This is the only known deficiency of this pathway.[101] Patients have low levels of MBL in their serum. The defect is surprisingly common; approximately 5% of individuals in the general population have this deficiency. They suffer from severe infections in early life before their adaptive immunity is developed. MBL deficiency can also increase the severity of infectious diseases in adults. For example, patients with acquired deficiency syndrome who have MBL deficiency show shorter survival time than patients without this deficiency.[102] A link between MBL deficiency and disease severity of rheumatoid arthritis, cystic fibrosis, and systemic lupus erythematosus (SLE) has been suggested. MBL deficiency is caused by promoter polymorphism and three mutations in the collagen-like domain. Alterations in the structure of the collagen-like domain caused by these mutations render MBL susceptible to cleavage by matrix metalloproteinases.[103] MBL from normal individuals shows high-molecular-weight oligomeric structure that is required for complement activation, whereas MBL from patients consists of low-molecular-weight forms.

### B. Soluble Regulators

The genetic deficiency of C1-INH leads to the disease hereditary angioneurotic edema (HANE). The clinical, genetic, and mechanistic aspects of HANE have recently been reviewed.[104] In this disease, recurrent attacks of acute edema of extremities, gastrointestinal tract, and orificial areas occur. Edema of the larynx can be fatal. Approximately 85% of the patients have type I HANE in which C1-INH antigenic levels are low (5 to 30% of normal) and about 15% have type II HANE in which normal levels of dysfunctional C1-INH protein occur. There is also an acquired form of HANE with identical symptoms. This often is associated with other diseases, mainly B-cell disorders, and with antibodies to C1-INH. Because C1-INH also inhibits contact activation[34] (activation of factor XII, pre-kallikrein, high-molecular-weight kininogen, and factor XIa), any event that can cause its local consumption can cause activation of C1, serine protease subunits of MASP complex, and contact activation system. This results in the generation of C2-kinin and bradykinin. Both these vasoactive substances were thought to induce the attack of edema in HANE but now it is becoming clear that angioedema in HANE is most likely mediated by bradykinin.[105]

Several patients with factor I deficiency are known.[40,106–109] In this deficiency regulation of C3/C5-convertases of complement pathways is abrogated. Patients have very low circulating levels of native C3 and very high levels of C3b, which is not inactivated in absence of factor I. The levels of C3bi or C3d are not increased. These patients have very low levels of factor B, most of which is consumed to generate C3b·Bb, which does not easily decay in absence of factor I. In factor I deficiency, C profiles are very consistent from patient to patient but clinical manifestations are variable. Recurrent infections or sepsis is quite common. Arthritis has been recorded in two kindreds, and skin abscesses in one and osteomyelitis in another. The deficiency has been observed in association with Klinefelter's syndrome, hemolytic anemia, and polyarteritis nodosa.

In homozygous factor H deficiency,[40,110–112] the pattern of derailment of the complement system was very much similar to that seen in factor I deficiency.[40,106] Classical and alternative pathway activities were undetectable. C3 and factor B levels were very low. C5 to C9 levels were greatly depressed. C profiles were consistent from patient to patient but clinical manifestations were different: collagen vascular disease (mostly SLE-like), glomerulonephritis, recurrent lung infections, hemolytic uremic syndrome, meningitis, and sepsis.

C4BP deficiency has been reported in a family in which C4BP levels in the patient and in a healthy sister and the father were 15 to 25% of normal.[113] Another sister had normal C4BP concentration. Immunochemical levels of C1 to C9, factor B, factor I, factor H, properdin, and C1-INH and functional levels of C1-INH were normal. *In vitro* activation of the classical pathway in patient serum, by aggregated IgG, resulted in greater C3 consumption than in normal sera due to diminished inactivation of C4b·2a. The proband was presented with intermittent facial angioedema and features of Behçet's disease: cutaneous vasculitis, genital and oral ulceration, arthralgia, and joint effusion.

Homozygous or heterozygous deficiencies of vitronectin and clusterin have not yet been described.

### C. Cell Surface Regulators

Genetic deficiency of DAF has been described in six patients.[114–117] Erythrocytes in this disorder become slightly more susceptible to lysis than normal, *in vitro*. The deficiency does not cause proxysmal nocturnal hemoglobulinuria (PNH)-like syndrome. Most of the patients develop gastrointestinal problems including protein-losing enteropathy and Crohn's disease. Patients with dermatological diseases have not yet been described. Crohn's disease is often associated with pyoderma gangrenosum but genetic deficiency of DAF in this dermatological condition has also not yet been reported.

Two patients with genetic deficiency of CD59 on all cells have been described.[118,119] One presented with PNH-like disease, the other with cerebral infarction.[118] None presented with any dermatological condition.

Genetic deficiencies of MCP and CR1 have not yet been described.

## VII. ABERRANCY IN THE EXPRESSION OF COMPLEMENT PROTEINS AND SKIN DISEASES

Aberrant expression of membrane-bound complement regulators has been seen in several human diseases.[44] Here, discussion is confined to dermatological diseases only.

Absence or very low expression of MCP and DAF was seen in cutaneous vascular endothelium of lesional and nonlesional skin of patients with limited and diffuse systemic sclerosis.[120] CD59 expression was also low in some patients with both subsets of the disease. Aberrant expression of MCP and DAF was endothelial cell-specific and was postulated to render endothelial cells susceptible to slow damage by physiologically activated autologous complement and accelerated damage by occasional pathologically activated complement. Time to time systemic activation of complement is known to be associated with extensive visceral involvement in systemic sclerosis.[121] The mechanism of decreased expression of these molecules on endothelial cells remains obscure.

Greatly decreased expression of MCP and DAF was seen in the endothelium of lesional but not in nonlesional skin of patients with morphea.[122] Expression of CD59 was normal. Aberrant expression of MCP and DAF, the mechanism of which remains unknown could be the part of the mechanism of endothelial cell damage in lesional skin of these patients. UVA-1 phototherapy has been successfully tried for the treatment of dermal sclerosis in systemic sclerosis and morphea, but it is not known whether this treatment upregulates the expression of MCP and DAF on endothelial cells in these patients.

Expression of MCP and DAF was found to be lower in lesional and perilesional epidermis in comparison to lesional epidermis of patients with vitiligo.[72] Low expression was seen in whole epidermis. It was hypothesized that in lesional skin, the overall number of MCP and DAF molecules may be so low that they may not be able to protect melanocytes from lysis by antimelanocyte membrane antibodies, present in patients with vitiligo,[123–125] and complement. Thus, aberrant expression of MCP and DAF in lesional epidermis including melanocytes could be the part of the mechanism of loss of melanocytes in vitiligo lesion.[126]

In SLE, immune complex elimination is impaired.[19,127] This impairment was thought to be due to the low levels of CR1 on erythrocytes; erythrocyte CR1 takes up C3b-bearing immune complexes and transports them to spleen and liver for eventual elimination. The clinical significance of this reduction is in question, as approximately 65% patients with SLE have low CR1 levels on erythrocytes but 20 to 30% of normal controls also have a similar decrease. Whether the decrease in CR1 on erythrocytes in this disease is genetic or acquired is also controversial. Most of the evidence suggests that reduction in erythrocyte CR1 levels is acquired. Recently, decreased expression of CR1 has been observed on neutrophils in atopic dermatitis, and the decrease has been correlated with disease activity.[128] Decreased expression was also found on eosinophils in this disease, but this decrease was not correlated with the disease activity.

## VIII. CONCLUDING REMARKS

The feeling of many immunologists that all that had to be discovered about the complement system has been discovered is proving to be unjust. The work on complement is still progressing in several directions. Several components of the lectin pathway have recently been discovered and the functions of some are under investigation. New findings related to complement in the physiology of skin and pathology of skin diseases are being reported. Local synthesis of complement in the skin and its regulation are under investigation. Many crucial questions related to the physiopathological importance of the synthesis of complement in the skin have yet to be addressed. Do skin cells synthesize components of the lectin pathway? Can complement synthesized in skin by itself eliminate skin invasive organisms? Can it contribute to solubilization and elimination of immune complexes in the skin, outside the vascular compartment? What physiological and pathological role do complement receptors play on skin cells? Do complement activation products in the lesions of skin diseases such as psoriasis and pemphigus arise from locally synthesized complement? Therapeutic agents are being developed to treat complement-mediated diseases (see Chapter 38 of this volume).

## REFERENCES

1. Mastellos, D. and Lambris, J.D., Complement: more than a "guard" against invading pathogens? *Trends Immunol.* 23, 485, 2002
2. Demsey, P.W., Allison, M.E.D., Akkaraju, S., Goodnow, C.C., and Fearon, D.T., C3d of complement as a molecular adjuvant: bridging innate and acquired immunity. *Science* 271, 348, 1996.
3. Reljic, R., Cosentinc, G., and Gould, H.J., Function of CD23 in the response of human B cells to antigen. *Eur. J. Immunol.* 27, 572, 1997
4. Bonnefoy, J.-Y., Pochon, S., Aubry, J.P., Garber, P., Gauchat, J.F., Jansen, K., and Flores-Romo, L., A pair of surface molecules involved in human IgE regulation. *Immunol. Today* 14, 1, 1993.
5. Asghar, S.S. and Pasch, M.C, Complement as a promiscuous signal transduction device. *Lab. Invest.* 78, 1203, 1998.
6. Farkas, I., Takahashi, M., Fukud, A., Yamamoto, N., Akatsu, H., Baranyi, L., Tateyama, H., Yamamoto, T., Okada, N., and Okada, H., Complement C5a receptor-mediated signaling may be involved in neurodegradation in Alzheimer's disease. *J. Immunol.* 170, 5764, 2003.

7. Rus, H.G., Niculescu, F.I., and Shin, M.L., Role of the C5b-9 complement complex in cell cycle and apoptosis. *Immunol. Rev.* 180, 49, 2001.
8. O'Barr, S.A., Caguioa, J., Gruol, D., Perkins, G., Ember, J.A., Hugli, T., and Cooper, N.R., Neuronal expression of a functional receptor for the C5a complement activation fragment. *J. Immunol.* 166, 4154, 2001.
9. Maeda, T., Abe, M., Kurisu, K., Jikko, A., and Furukawa, S., Molecular cloning and characterization of a novel gene, CORS26, encoding a putative secretary protein and its possible involvement in skeletal development. *J. Biol. Chem.* 276, 3628, 2001.
10. Sato, T., Abe, E., Jin, C.H., Hong, M.H., Katagiri, T., Kinoshita, T., Amizuka, N., Ozawa, H., and Suda, T., The biological roles of the third component of complement in osteoclast formation. *Endocrinology* 133, 397, 1993.
11. Andrades, J.A., Nimni, M.E., Becerra, J., Eisenstein, R., Davis, M., and Sorgente, N., Complement proteins are present in developing endochondral bone and may mediate cartilage cell death and vascularization. *Exp. Cell Res.* 227, 208, 1996.
12. Hasty, L.A., Lambris, J.D., Lessey, B.A., Pruksananoda, K., and Lytte, C.R., Hormonal regulation of complement components and receptors throughout the menstrual cycle. *Am. J. Obstet. Gynecol.* 170, 169, 1994.
13. Vacquier, V.D., Evolution of gamete recognition proteins. *Science* 291, 1995, 1998.
14. Rooney, I.A., Oglesby, T.J. and Atkinson, J.P., Complement in human reproduction — activation and control. *Immunol. Res.* 12, 276, 1993.
15. Xu, C., Mao, D., Holers, V.M., Palanca, B., Cheng, A.M., and Molina H, A critical role for murine complement regulator crry in fetomaternal tolerance. *Science* 287, 498, 2000.
16. Anderson, D.J., The role of complement component C3b and its receptors in sperm-oocyte interaction. *Proc. Natl. Acad. Sci. U.S.A.* 90, 10051, 1993.
17. Mastellos, D., Papadimitriou, J.C., Franchini, S., Tsonis, P.A., and Lambris, J.D., A novel role of complement: mice deficient in the fifth component of complement (C5) exhibit impaired liver regeneration. *J. Immunol.* 166, 2479, 2001.
18. Petrenko, O., Beavis, A., Klaine, M., Kittapa, R., Godin, I., and Memiseka, I.R., The molecular characterization of the fetal stem cell marker RR4. *Immunity,* 10, 691, 1999.
19. Asghar, S.S., Complement and complement regulatory proteins, in *Skin Immune System,* 2nd ed., Bos, J.D., Ed., CRC Press, Boca Raton, FL, 1997, 239–254.
20. Liszewski, M.K., Farries, T.C., Lubin, D.M., Rooney, I.A., and Atkinson, J.P., Control of the complement system. *Adv. Immunol.* 61, 201, 1996.
21. Morgan, B.P., The complement system: an overview. *Methods Mol. Biol.* 150, 1–13, 2000.
22. Holmskov, U., Thiel, S., and Jensenius, J.C., Collectins and ficolins: humoral lectins of the innate immune defense. *Annu. Rev. Immunol.* 21, 547, 2003.
23. Matsushita, M., Endo, Y., Taira, S., Sato, Y., Fujita T, Ichikawa N, Nakata, M., and Mizuochi, T., A novel human serum lectin with collagen- and fibrinogen-like domains that functions as an opsonin. *J. Biol. Chem.* 271, 2448, 1996.
24. Harumiya, S., Takeda, K., Sugiura, T., Fukumoto, Y., Tachikawa, H., Miyazono K, Fujimoto, D., and Ichijo, H., Characterization of ficolins as novel elastin-binding protein and molecular cloning of human ficolin-1. *J. Biochem.* 120, 745, 1996.
25. Sugimoto, R., Yae, Y., Akaiwa, M., Kitajima, S., Shibata, Y., Sato, H., Hirata, J., Okochi, K., Izuhara, K., and Hamasaki, N., Cloning and characterization of the Hakata antigen, a member of the ficolin/opsonin p35 lectin family. *J. Biol. Chem.* 273, 20721, 1998.
26. Le, Y., Lee, S.H., Kon, O.L., and Lu, J, Human L-filicin: plasma levels, sugar specificity, and assignment of its lectin activity to the fibrinogen-like (FBG) domain. *FEBS Lett.* 425, 367, 1998.
27. Matsushita, M., Endo, Y., and Fujita, T., Complement activating complex of ficolin and mannose-binding lectin associated serine protease. *J. Immunol.* 164, 2281, 2000.
28. Dahl, M.R., Thiel, S., Matsushita, M., Fujita, T., Willis, A.C., Christiansen, T., Vorup-Jensen, T., and Jensenius, J.C., MASP-3 and its association with distinct complexes of the mannose-binding lectin complement activation pathway. *Immunity* 15, 127, 2001.
29. Sato, T., Endo, Y., Matsushita, M., and Fujita, T., Molecular characterization of a novel serine protease involved in activation of the complement system by mannose binding protein. *Int. Immunol.* 6, 665, 1994.

30. Thiel, S., Vorup-Jensen, T., Stover, C.M., Schwaeble, W., Laursen, S.B., Poulsen, K., Willis, A.C., Eggleton, P., Hansen, S., Holmskov, U., Kenneth, B., Reid, M., and Jensenius, J.C., A second serine protease associated with mannan-binding lectin that activates complement. *Nature* 386, 506, 1997.
31. Matsushita, M., Takahashi, M., Thiel, S., Jensenius, J.C., and Fujita T., Distinct proteolytic activities of MASP-1 and MASP-2. *Mol. Immunol.* 35, 349, 1998.
32. Law, S.K.A. and Dodds, A.W., The internal thioester and the covalent binding properties of the complement proteins C3 and C4. *Protein Sci.* 6, 263, 1997.
33. Sahu, A. and Lambris, J.D., Structure and biology of complement protein C3, a connecting link between innate and acquired immunity. *Immunol. Rev.* 180, 35, 2001.
34. Calieze, C., Wuillemin, W.A., Zeerleder, S., Redondo, M., Eisele, B., and Hack, C.E., C1-estersae inhibitor: an anti-inflammatory agent and its potential use in the treatment of diseases other than hereditary angioedema. *Pharm. Rev.* 52, 91, 2000.
35. Tenner, A.J. and Frank, M.M., Activator bound C1 is less susceptible to inactivation by C1-inhibitor than is fluid phase C1. *J. Immunol.* 137, 625, 1986.
36. Gulati, S., Sastry, K., Jensenius, J.C., Rice, P.A., and Ram, S., Regulation of the mannan-binding lectin pathway of complement on *Neisseria gonorrhoeae* by C1-inhibitor and $\alpha_2$-macroglobulin. *J. Immunol.* 168, 4078, 2002.
37. Hessing, M., The interaction between complement component C4b-binding protein and the vitamin K-dependent protein S forms a link between blood coagulation and the complement system. *Biochem. J.* 277, 581, 1991.
38. Villoutreix, B.O., Blom, A.M., Webb, J., and Dahlback, B., The complement regulator C4b-binding protein analyzed by molecular modeling, bioinformatics and computer-aided experimental design. *Immunopharmacology* 42, 121, 1999.
39. Zipfel, P.F., Jokiranta, T.S., Hellwage, J., Koistinen, V., and Meri, S., The factor H protein family. *Immunopharmacology* 42, 53, 1999.
40. Sim, R.B., Kolble, K., McAleer, M.A., Dominguez, O., and Dee, V.M., Genetics and deficiencies of soluble regulatory proteins of the complement system. *Int. Rev. Immunol.* 10, 65, 1993.
41. Suankratay, C., Mold, C., Zhang, Y., Lint, T.F., and Gewurz, H., Mechanism of complement-dependent hemolysis via the lectin pathway: role of the complement regulatory proteins. *Clin. Exp. Immunol.* 117, 442, 1999.
42. Schvartz, I., Seger, D., and Shaltiel, S., Vitronectin. *Int. J. Biochem. Cell Biol.* 31, 539, 1999.
43. Trougakos, I.P. and Gonos, E.S., Clusterin/apolipoprotein J in human aging and cancer. *Int. J. Biochem. Cell Biol.* 34, 1430, 2002.
44. Asghar, S.S., Membrane regulators of complement activation and their aberrant expression in disease. *Lab. Invest.* 72, 254, 1995.
45. Meri, S. and Jarva, H., Complement regulation. *Vox Sang* 74(Suppl. 2), 291, 1998.
46. Morgan, B.P., Effects of membrane attack complex of complement on nucleated cells. *Curr. Top. Microbiol. Immunol.* 178, 115, 1992.
47. Eggleton, P., Tenner, A.J., and Reid, K.B., C1q receptors. *Clin. Exp. Immunol.* 120, 406, 2000.
48. van den Berg, R.H., Faber-Krol, M., van Es, L.A., and Daha, M.R., Regulation of the function of the first components of C by human C1q-receptor. *Eur. J. Immunol.* 25, 2206, 1995.
49. Nepomuceno, R.R., Henschen-Edman, A.H., Burgess, W.H., and Tenner, A.J., cDNA cloning and primary structure analysis of C1qRp, the human C1q/MBL/SPA receptor that mediates enhanced phagocytosis *in vitro*. *Immunity* 6, 119, 1997.
50. Akaiwa, M., Yae, Y., Sugimoto, R., Suzuki, S.O., Iwaki, T., Izuhara, K., and Hamasaki, N., Hakata antigen, a new member of the ficolin/opsonin p35 family is a novel human lectin secreted into bronchus/alveolus and bile. *J. Histochem. Cytochem.* 47, 777, 1999.
51. Morgan, B.P. and Gasque, P., Expression of complement in the brain: role in health and disease. *Immunol. Today* 17, 461, 1996.
52. Morgan, B.P. and Gasque, P., Extra hepatic complement biosynthesis. Where, when and why? *Clin. Exp. Immunol.* 107, 1, 1997.
53. Andrews, P.A., Zhou, W., and Sacks, S.H., Tissue synthesis of complement as immune regulator. *Mol. Med. Today* 1, 202, 1995.
54. Yasojima, K., Schwab, C., McGeer, E.G., and McGeer, P.L., Human heart generates complement proteins that are up regulated and activated after myocardial infarction. *Circ. Res.* 83, 860, 1998.

55. Malik, A.B., Lynch, J.J., and Cooper, J.A., Endothelial barrier function. *J. Invest. Dermatol.* 93: 62s, 1989.
56. Luger, T.A., Beissert, S., and Schwarz, T., The epidermal cytokine network, in *Skin Immune System,* 2nd ed., Bos, J.D., Ed., CRC Press, Boca Raton, FL, 1997, 271–310.
57. Barker, J.N.W.N., Epidermis as a pro-inflammatory organ, in *Skin Immune System,* 2nd ed., Bos, J.D., Ed., CRC Press, Boca Raton, FL, 1997, 339–345.
58. Basset-Seguin, N., Dersookian, M., Cehrs, K., and Yancey, K.B., C3d,g is present in normal human epidermal basement membrane. *J. Immunol.* 141, 1273, 1988.
59. Basset-Seguin, N., Porneuf, M., Dereure, O., Mils, V., Tesnieres, A., Yancey, K., and Guilhou, J.-J., C3d,g deposits in inflammatory skin diseases: use of psoriatic skin as a model of cutaneous inflammation. *J. Invest. Dermatol.* 101, 827, 1993.
60. Dovezenski, N., Billetta, R., and Gigli, I., Expression and localization of proteins of the complement system in human skin. *J. Clin. Invest.* 90, 2000, 1992.
61. Basset-Seguin, N., Wright Caughman, S., and Yancey, K., A-431 cells and human keratinocytes synthesize and secrete the third component of complement. *J. Invest. Dermatol.* 95, 621, 1990.
62. Yancey, K., Overholster, O., Domloge-Hultsch, N., Li, L.-J., Wright Caughman, S., and Bisalbtra, P., Human keratinocytes and A-431 cells synthesize and secrete factor B, the major zymogen protease of the alternative complement pathway. *J. Invest. Dermatol.* 98, 379, 1992.
63. Pasch, M.C., van den Bosch, N.H.A., Daha, M.R., Bos, J.D., and Asghar, S.S., Synthesis of complement components C3 and factor B in human keratinocytes is differentially regulated by cytokines. *J. Invest. Dermatol.* 114, 78, 2000.
64. Terui, T., Ishii, K., Ozawa, M., Tabata, N., Kato, T., and Tagami, H., C3 production of cultured human epidermal keratinocytes is enhanced by IFN-$\gamma$ and TNF-$\alpha$ through different pathways. *J. Invest. Dermatol.* 108, 62, 1997.
65. Timár, K.K., Pasch, M.C., van den Bosch, N.H.A., Jarva, H., Meri, S., Bos, J.D., and Asghar, S. S., Human keratinocytes synthesize factor H: synthesis is regulated by interferon-. Submitted.
66. Pasch, M.C., Bos, J.D., Daha, M.R., and Asghar, S.S., Transforming growth factor:$\beta$ isoforms regulate the surface expression of membrane cofactor protein (CD46) and CD59 on human keratinocytes. *Eur. J. Immunol.* 29, 100, 1999.
67. Norris, D.A., Ryan, S.B., Kissinger, R.M., Fritz, K.A., and Boyce, S.T., Systemic comparison of antibody mediated mechanisms of keratinocyte lysis *in vitro*. *J. Immunol.* 135, 1073, 1985.
68. Whitlow, M.B. and Klein, L.M., Response of SSC-12F, a human squamous cell carcinoma cell line, to complement attack. *J. Invest. Dermatol.* 109, 39, 1997.
69. Birkenbach, M., Tong, X., Bradbury, L.E., Tedder, T.F., and Kieff. E., Characterization of an Epstein-Barr virus receptor on human epithelial cells. *J. Exp. Med.* 176, 1405, 1992.
70. Werfel, T., Zwirner, J., Oppermann, M., Sieber, A., Begemann, G., Drommer, W., Kapp, A., and Gotze, O., CD88 antibodies specifically bind to C5aR on dermal CD117$^+$ and CD14$^+$ cells and react with a desmosomal antigen in human skin. *J. Immunol.* 157, 1729, 1996.
71. Fayyazi, A., Sandau, R., Duong, L.Q., Gotze, O., Radzun, H.J., Schweyer, S., Soruri, A., and Zwirner, J., C5a receptor and interleukin-6 are expressed in tissue macrophages and stimulated keratinocytes but not in pulmonary and intestinal epithelial cells. *Am. J. Pathol.* 154, 495, 1999.
72. van den Wijngaard, R.M.J.G.J., Asghar, S.S., Pijnenborg, Y., Tigges, B.J., Westerhof, W., and Das, P.K., Aberrant expression of complement regulatory proteins, membrane cofactor protein (MCP) and decay accelerating factor (DAF), in the lesional epidermis of patients with vitiligo. *Br. J. Dermatol.* 146, 80, 2000.
73. Morelli, A., Larregina, A., Chuluyan, E., Kolkowski, E., and Fainboim, L., Functional expression and modulation of C5a receptor (CD88) on skin dendritic cells. Chemotactic effect of C5a on skin dendritic cells. *Adv. Exp. Med. Biol.* 417, 133, 1997.
74. De Panfilis, G., Soligo, D., Manara, G.C., Ferrari, C., Torresani, C., and Zucchi, A., Human normal-resting epidermal Langerhans cells do express the type 3 complement receptor. *Br. J. Dermatol.* 122, 127, 1990.
75. Al-Adnani, M.S. and McGee, J.O., C1q production and secretion by fibroblasts. *Nature* 263, 145, 1976.
76. Morris, K.M., Colten, H.R., and Bing, D.H., The first component of complement: a quantitative comparison of its biosynthesis in culture by human epithelial and mesenchymal cells. *J. Exp. Med.* 148, 1007, 1978.

77. Kulics, J., Circolo, A., Strunk, R.C., and Colten, H.R., Regulation of synthesis of complement protein C4 in human fibroblasts: cell- and gene-specific effects of cytokines and lipopolysaccharide. *Immunology* 82: 509, 1994.
78. Gerred, P., Hetland, G., Mollnes, T.E., and Stoervold, G., Synthesis of C3, C5, C6, C7, C8, and C9 by human fibroblasts. *Scand. J. Immunol.* 32, 555, 1990.
79. Katz, Y. and Strunk, R.C., Enhanced synthesis of factor B induced by tumor necrosis factor in human skin fibroblasts is decreased by IL-4. *J. Immunol.* 144, 4675, 1990.
80. Katz, Y., Cole, F.S., and Strunk, R.C., Synergism between gamma interferon and lipopolysaccharide for synthesis of factor B, but not C2, in human fibroblasts. *J. Exp. Med.* 167, 1, 1988.
81. Katz, Y. and Strunk, R.C., Synthesis and regulation of factor H in human skin fibroblasts. *J. Immunol.* 141, 559, 1988.
82. Katz, Y. and Strunk, R.C., Synthesis and regulation of C1-inhibitor in human skin fibroblasts. *J. Immunol.* 142, 2041, 1989.
83. Adult, B.H., Schmidt, B.Z., Fowler, N.L., Kashtan, C.E., Ahmed, A.E., Vogt, B.A., and Colten, H.R., Human factor H deficiency. Mutations in framework cysteine residues and block in H protein secretion and intracellular catabolism. *J. Biol. Chem.* 272, 25168, 1997.
84. Katz, Y. and Strunk, R.C., IL-1 and tumour necrosis factor. Similarities and differences in stimulation of expression of complement and IFN-beta/IL-6 genes in human fibroblasts. *J. Immunol.* 142, 3862, 1988.
85. Katz, Y., Stav, D., Barr, J., and Passwell, J.H., IL13 results in differential regulation of the complement protein C3 and factor B in tumor necrosis factor (TNF)-stimulated fibroblasts. *Clin. Exp. Immunol.* 101, 150, 1995.
86. Katz, Y., Nadiv, O., Rapoport, M.J., and Loos, M., IL-17 regulates gene expression and protein synthesis of the complement system, C3 and factor B, in skin fibroblasts. *Clin. Exp. Immunol.* 120, 22, 2000.
87. van Loveren, H., Redegeld, F., Matsuda, H., Buckley, T., Teppema, J.S., and Garssen, J., Mast cells, in *Skin Immune System,* 2nd ed., Bos, J.D., Ed., CRC Press, Boca Raton, FL, 1997, 159–184.
88. Hartmann, K., Henz, B.M., Kruger-Krasagakes, S., Kohl, J., Burger, R., Guhl, S., Haase, I., Lippert, U., and Zuberbier, T., C3a and C5a stimulate chemotaxis of human mast cells. *Blood* 89, 2863, 1997.
89. Zwirner, J., Gotze, O., Sieber, A., Kapp, A., Begemann, G., Zuberbier, T., and Werfel, T., The human mast cell line HMC-1 binds and responds to C3a but not C3a (desArg). *Scand. J. Immunol.* 47, 19, 1998.
90. Werfel, T., Oppermann, M., Butterfield, J.H., Begemann, G., Elsner, J., Gotze, O., and Zwirner, J., The human mast cell line MHC-1 expresses C5a receptors and responds to C5a but not C5a (desArg). *Scand. J. Immunol.* 44, 30, 1996.
91. Legler, D.F., Loetscher, M., Jones, S.A., Dahinden, C.A., Arock, M., and Moser, B., Expression of high and low affinity receptors for C3a on the human mast cell line, HMC-1. *Eur. J. Immunol.* 26, 753, 1996.
92. Werfel, T., Oppermann, M., Begemann, G., Gotze, O., and Zwirner, J., C5a receptors are detectable on mast cells in normal human skin and in psoriatic plaques but not in wheal and flare reactions or in urticaria pigmentosa by immunohistochemistry. *Arch. Dermatol. Res.* 289, 83, 1997.
93. Weber, S., Babina, M., Feller, G., and Henz, B.M., Human leukemic (HMC-1) and normal skin mast cells express beta 2-integrins: characterization of beta 2-integrins and ICAM-1 on MHC-1 cells. *Scand. J. Immunol.* 45, 471, 1997.
94. Ghannadan, M., Baghestanian, M., Wimazal, F., Eisenmenger, M., Latal, D., Karrgul, G., Walchshofer, S., Sillaber, C., Lechner, K., and Valent, P., Phenotypic characterization of human skin mast cells by combined staining with toluidine blue and CD antibodies. *J. Invest. Dermatol.* 111, 689, 1998.
95. Hogasen, A.K., Wurzner, R., Abrahamsen, T.G., and Dierich, M.P., Human polymorphonuclear leukocytes store large amounts of terminal complement components C7 and C6, which may be released on stimulation. *J. Immunol.* 154, 4734, 1995.
96. Kondo, S., Kooshesh, F., and Saunder, D.N., Penetration of keratinocyte-derived cytokines into basement membrane. *J. Cell. Physiol.* 171, 190, 1997.
97. O'Neil, K.M., Complement deficiency. *Clin. Rev. Allergy Immunol.* 19, 83, 2000.
98. Frank, M.M., Complement deficiencies. *Pediatr. Clin. North Am.* 47, 1339, 2000.
99. Walport, M.J., Complement. *N. Engl. J. Med.* 344, 1058, 2001.

100. Pickering, M.C., Botto, M., Taylor, P.R., Lachmann, J., and Walport, M.J., Systemic lupus erythematosus, complement deficiency and apoptosis. *Adv. Immunol.* 76, 227, 2000.
101. Turner, M.W., Mannose-binding lectin (MBL) in health and disease. *Immunobiology* 199, 327, 1999.
102. Gerred, P., Madsen, H.O., Balslev, U., Hofman, B., Pedersen, C., Gerstoft, J., and Svejgaard, A., Susceptibility to HIV infection and progression of AIDS in relation to variant alleles of mannose-binding lectin. *Lancet* 349, 236, 1997.
103. Butler, G.S., Sim, D., Tam, E., Devine, D., and Overall, C.M., Mannose-binding lectin (MBL) mutants are susceptible to matrix metalloproteinase proteolysis: potential role in human MBL deficiency. *J. Biol. Chem.* 277, 17511, 2002.
104. Carugati, A., Pappalardo, E., Zinagle, L.C., and Cicardi, M., C1-inhibitor deficiency and angioedema. *Mol. Immunol.* 38, 161, 2001.
105. Nussberger, J., Cugno, M., and Cicardi, M., Bradykinin-mediated angioedema. *N. Engl. J. Med.* 347, 621, 2002.
106. Bonnin, A.J., Zeitz, H.J., and Gewurz, A., Complement factor I deficiency with recurrent aseptic meningitis. *Arch. Intern. Med.* 153, 1380, 1993.
107. Naked, G.M., Florido, M.P., Ferreira d Paula, P., Vinet, A.M., and Inostroza, J.S., Deficiency of human complement factor I associated with lowered factor H. *Clin. Immunol.* 96, 162, 2000.
108. Sadallah, S., Gudat, F., Laissue, J.A., Spath, P.J., and Schifferli, J.A., Glomerulonephritis in a patient with complement factor I deficiency. *Am. J. Kidney Dis.* 33, 1153, 1999.
109. Amadei, N., Baracho, G.V., Nudelman, V., Bastos, W., Florido, M.P., and Issac, L., Inherited factor I deficiency associated with systemic lupus erythematosus, higher susceptibility to infection and low levels of factor H. *Scand. J. Immunol.* 53, 615, 2001.
110. Zipfel, P.F., Complement factor H: physiology and physiopathology. *Semin. Thromb. Hemost.* 27, 191, 2001.
111. Sanchez-Corral, P., Bellavia, D., Amico, L., Brai, M., and Rodriguez de Cordoba, S., Molecular basis of factor H, FHL-1 deficiency in an Italian Family. *Immunogenetics* 51, 366, 2000.
112. Schmidt, B.Z., Fowler, N.L., Hidvegi, T., Perlmutter, D.H., and Colten, H.R., Disruption of disulfide bond is responsible for impaired secretion in human complement factor H deficiency. *J. Biol. Chem.* 274, 11782, 1999.
113. Trapp, R.G., Fletcher, M., Forristall, J., and West, C. D., C4 binding protein deficiency in a patient with atypical Behcet's disease. *J. Rheumatol.* 14, 135, 1987.
114. Merry, A.H., Rawlinson, V.I., Uchikawa, M., Daha, M.R., and Sim, R.B., Studies on the sensitivity to complement-mediated lysis of erythrocytes (Inab phenotype) with a deficiency of DAF (decay accelerating factor). *Br. J. Haematol.* 73, 248, 1989.
115. Tate, C.G., Uchikawa, M., Tanner, M.J.A., Judson, P.A., Parsons, S.F., Mallinson, G., and Antee, D.J., Studies on the defect which causes absence of decay accelerating factor (DAF) from the peripheral blood cells of an individual with the Inab phenotype. *Biochem. J.* 261, 489, 1989.
116. Morgan, B.P., Clinical complementology: recent progress and future trends. *Eur. J. Clin. Invest.* 24, 219, 1994.
117. Shichishima, T., Saitoh, Y., Terasawa, T., Noji, H., Kai, T., and Maruyama, Y., Complement sensitivity of erythrocytes in a patient with inherited complete deficiency of CD59 or with the Inab phenotype. *Br. J. Haematol.* 104, 303, 1999.
118. Yamashima, M., Ueda, E., Kinoshita, T., Takami, T., Ojima, A., Ono, H., Tanaka, H., Kondo, N., Norii, T., Okada, N., Okada, H., Inoue, K., and Kitani, T., Inherited complete deficiency of 20 kilodalton homologous restriction factor (CD59) as a cause of paroxysmal nocturnal hemoglobulinuria. *N. Engl. J. Med.* 323, 1184, 1990.
119. Taguchi, R., Fanahashi, Y., Ikezawa, H., and Nikashima I. Analysis of PI (phosphatidylinositol)-anchoring antigens in a patient of paroxysmal nocturnal hemoglobulin4uria (PNH) reveals deficiency of IF-5 antigen (CD59), a new complement regulatory factor. *FEBS Lett.* 261, 142, 1990.
120. Venneker, G.T., van den Hoogen F.H.J., Boerbooms, A.M.T., Bos, J.D., and Asghar, S.S., Aberrant expression of membrane cofactor protein (MCP) and decay accelerating factor (DAF) in the endothelium of patients with systemic sclerosis: A possible mechanism of vascular damage. *Lab. Invest.* 70, 830, 1994.
121. Senaldi, G., Lupoli, S., Vergani, D., and Black, C. M., Activation of the complement system in systemic sclerosis — relationship to clinical severity. *Arthritis Rheum.* 32, 1262, 1989.

122. Venneker, G.T., Das, P.K., Naafs, B., Tiggers, A.J., Bos, J.D., and Asghar, S.S., Morphia lesions are associated with aberrant expression of membrane cofactor protein (MCP) and decay accelerating factor (DAF) in vascular endothelium. *Br. J. Dermatol.* 131, 237, 1994.
123. Yu, H.S., Kao, C.H., and Yu, C.L., Coexistence and relationship of anti-keratinocyte and anti-melanocyte antibodies in patients with non-segmental type vitiligo. *J. Invest. Dermatol.* 100, 823, 1993.
124. Cui, J., Arita, Y., and Bystryn, J.C., Cytolytic antibodies to melanocytes in vitiligo. *J. Invest. Dermatol.* 100, 812, 1993.
125. Harning, R., Cui, J., and Bystryn, J. C., Relationship between the incidence and level of pigment cell antibodies and disease activity in vitiligo. *J. Invest. Dermatol.* 97, 1078, 1991.
126. Le Poole, I.C., van den Wijngaard, R.M.J.G.J., Westerhof, W., Dutrieux, R.P., and Das, P.K., Presence or absence of melanocytes in vitiligo lesions. An immunohistochemical investigation. *J. Invest. Dermatol.* 100, 816, 1993.
127. Davies, K.A., Peters, A.M., Beynon, H.L., and Walport, M.J., Immune complex processing in patients with systemic lupus erythematosus. *In vivo* imaging and clearance studies. *J. Clin. Invest.* 90, 2075, 1992.
128. Yoshida, T., Kubota, Y., Nishimoto, M., Okada, H., and Hirashima, M., CD35 expression on peripheral blood granulocytes of patients with atopic dermatitis. *J. Dermatol. Sci.* 28, 42, 2002.

# 15 The Skin Cytokine Network

*Martin Steinhoff and Thomas A. Luger*

## CONTENTS



0-8493-1959-5/05/$0.00+$1.50

## I. INTRODUCTION

Cytokines are an essential part of the body's defense mechanism against microbiological agents, allergens, toxins, tumor cells, and ultraviolet (UV) light. In addition to chemokines, radical oxygen species, prostanoids, neuropeptides, and amines, for example, cytokines exert important immunoregulatory capacities in an autocrine, paracrine, juxtacrine, or even endocrine fashion.

Cytokines are structurally related polypeptides or glycoproteins that mediate their effects at concentrations within the pico- or nanomolar range. Originally, they were regarded as immunocompetent cell-derived immunomodulators. However, recent knowledge demonstrates that a clear-cut differentiation between cytokines, growth factors, neurotransmitters, and hormones is not possible (Table 15.1). However, the predominant role of cytokines is to control inflammation, host defense, and tissue injury. Cytokines determine the direction as well as the outcome of an immune response and control tissue integrity following injury. Thus, the quality and quantity of cytokine production within the injured tissue determines whether the immune system is directed into a humoral, cytotoxic, cell-mediated, or allergic response. Moreover, cytokines (among other mediators) determine the switch of the immune system from a pro-inflammatory to an anti-inflammatory state.

During the last decades enormous knowledge has been accumulated on the role of cytokines in cutaneous inflammation. They are ultimately involved in all phases of inflammation. While pro-inflammatory cytokines induce the body's response to external or internal danger, anti-inflammatory cytokines are capable of restoring tissue homeostasis by suppressing inflammatory processes. Various molecular biological and modern immunological techniques were applied to cytokine research, and the genes for the currently known factors have been cloned and characterized in the skin. These studies clearly demonstrate that many cytokines exert pleiotropic functions. For example, interleukin 1 (IL-1) was originally described as a leukocytic pyrogen, endogenous pyrogen, B-cell-activating factor, and lymphocyte-activating factor. Today, it is well known that various skin cells including keratinocytes use IL-1 to communicate with neighboring cells in the skin during inflammation.[1] Thus, the IL nomenclature was introduced to avoid the older descriptive and often misleading names.

To gain a better understanding of the role of cytokines in skin inflammation, one has to differentiate between human and animal studies as well as between *in vitro* and *in vivo* data. The availability of recombinant cytokines and cytokine antagonists helped tremendously to verify specific effects of cytokines *in vivo*. Modern techniques such as genomic and proteomic approaches gave new insight into the regulatory mechanisms underlying the effects of cytokines. Moreover, the use of cytokine and cytokine receptor gene–deficient mice helps to understand the specific role of these molecules during cutaneous inflammation. However, it has to be considered that during the *in vivo* situation a cocktail of several cytokines simultaneously or sequentially acts upon the inflammatory microenvironment. Thus, the biological activities of cytokines during inflammation are the sum of well-tuned synergistic and antagonistic processes.

Cytokines utilize different cell biological mechanisms to modulate inflammation. Some cytokines such as IL-1, IL-2, or IL-4, for example, exert their effects by exclusively binding to cell surface receptors. Others, such as transforming growth factor-beta (TGF-β) or IL-6 may additionally interact with components of the extracellular matrix to modulate skin function during inflammation. They influence different components of the cell such as phagocytosis, receptor internalization, expression of major histocompatibility complex (MHC) antigens, production of radical oxygen species, other cytokines a.o.

In the skin, cytokines are released by keratinocytes, Langerhans cells (LC), melanocytes, fibroblasts, endothelial cells, monocytes, dendritic cells (DC), T cells, B cells, mast cells, granu-

**TABLE 15.1**
**Cytokines**

| | |
|---|---|
| Interleukins (IL) | IL-1 to IL-29, IL-1 RA, IL-18 RA, MIF |
| Tumor necrosis factors (TNF) | TNF-α, TNF-β |
| Chemokines | C-X-C type: IL-8, Gro-α, ENA-78, IP-10 |
| | MIG, GCP-2 |
| | C-C type: MCP-1N–3, RANTES, I-309 |
| | MIP-1α, MIP-1β, C10, CCL27 |
| | C type: lymphotactin |
| | Fractelkine |
| Hematopoietic growth factors | Erythropoietin, stem cell factor |
| | Colony-stimulating factors (IL-3, GM-CSF, G-CSF, M-CSF), Flt3 ligand |
| Interferons (IFN) | IFN-α, -β, -γ, -ω |
| Growth factors | EGF, TGF, TGF-β, FGF, PDGF, NGF, IGF, KGF, LIF, VEGF, Oncostatin M |

*Abbreviations:* APC, antigen-presenting cell; CSF, colony stimulating factor; DC, dendritic cell; EGF, epidermal growth factor; ENA-78, epithelial neutrophil-activating protein-78; FGF, fibroblast growth factor; GCP-2, granulocyte chemotactic protein-2; Gro, growth-regulated oncogene; ICAM, intercellular cell adhesion molecule; IGF, insulin-like growth factor; IFN, interferon; IL, interleukin; IP-10, interferon-inducible protein-10; KGF, keratinocyte growth factor; LC, Langerhans cell; MCP-1, microbial cationic protein-1; MIF, macrophage migration-inhibitory factor; MIG, macrophage interferon-inducible gene; MIP, macrophage inflammatory protein; NGF, nerve growth factor; PDGF, platelet-derived growth factor; RANTES, regulated upon activation, normal T expressed, and presumably secreted; TGF, transforming growth factor; TNF, tumor necrosis factor; VCAM, vascular cell adhesion molecule; VEGF, vascular endothelial growth factor.

locytes, and platelets. Importantly, cytokines have pleiotropic effects in the various cell types depending on the microenvironment and the activation state of the different cell types; i.e., they exert different functions. This is — at least in part — due to the different intracellular signaling mechanisms, which may be activated by cytokine receptor activation and vary among the cell types and states of activation. Nuclear transcription factor-κB (NF-κB), for example, mediates pro-inflammatory effects when the maximum of activation occurs after 1 h. When the maximal stimulation of this transcription factor takes place at 4 h, NF-κB mediates anti-inflammatory properties.[2]

## II. PRIMARY PRO-INFLAMMATORY CYTOKINES

Interleukins are polypeptides participating in all normal and reactive cell functions. So far 29 interleukins have been described and characterized. Some of them are prime cells, making them responsive to other agents, and most act in synergistic ways.

### A. Interleukin-1

The first cytokine being detected in the skin was IL-1, which originally was named epidermal thymocyte activating factor (ETAF).[1] Cytokines of the IL-1 family are key players of immunity and inflammation in virtually every organ of the body. So far the members of the IL-1 family that have been discovered include IL-1α, IL-1β, IL-1RA, IL-1H, IL-1F7b, IL-18, and IL-18BP. They may function as agonistic or antagonistic ligands for the members of the IL-1 receptor family. IL-1α and IL-18 are structurally very closely related and both are synthesized as biologically inactive precursor molecules lacking a signal peptide. Upon stimulation, almost any cell of the body including keratinocytes was found to synthesize many of the IL-1 family members. In some cells such as macrophages, fibroblasts, endothelial cells, and DC, IL-1 may also exist as a membrane-bound form.

The currently known ten members of the IL-1R family are defined as membrane-spanning molecules that consist of at least one Ig-like domain exterior to the cell and, except for IL-1RII, a Toll/IL-1R (TIR) domain in the cytoplasm. The type I IL-1R (IL-1R) binds both IL-1α and IL-1β. In addition, a homologue of the IL-1R, known as IL-1R accessory protein (AcP), which has no affinity on its own for either of the IL-1 forms, is required for IL-1 signaling. The second natural IL-1 binding protein is the IL-1RII, which has a high affinity for IL-1α, but a much lower affinity for IL-1β or IL-1RA.

IL-1RI is expressed on keratinocytes, fibroblasts, endothelial cells, lymphocytes, and other cells. IL-1RII can be detected on B lymphocytes and neutrophils. An endogenous soluble IL-1 receptor antagonist (IL-1RA type I) was found to act as a competitive IL-1R inhibitor. There is evidence of differences in responses mediated via each receptor. Cultured keratinocytes predominantly express mRNA for IL-1, but *in vivo* in normal epidermis IL-1α is also detectable. Accordingly, IL-1 was found in the stratum granulosum, and considerable amounts have also been detected in psoriatic scales.[3] However, this is confined to IL-1, which is functionally inactive, while active IL-1α is reduced.[4]

IL-1 is a pro-inflammatory cytokine, stimulates repair and differentiation, and is an important mediator of immune regulation. It is mitogenic for thymocytes and T cells and induces IL-2 synthesis and IL-2 receptor expression. Furthermore, IL-1 is a growth factor for B cells, by inducing proliferation and enhancing antibody formation, and it also increases natural killer (NK) cell activity. IL-1 also activates macrophages and neutrophils as well as the release of their enzymes, and induces prostaglandin synthesis.

It has been contended that, despite the large amounts of IL-1 detected in epidermis, it is largely inactive and contributes little to the inflammatory response. Nevertheless, injection of keratinocyte IL-1 and recombinant IL-1 (rIL-1) into mice[5,6] and rabbits induces edema, erythema, and neutrophil infiltration. There is also evidence that during wound healing, human keratinocyte IL-1 stimulates the synthesis of prostaglandin $E_2$ ($PGE_2$) by subpopulations of human fibroblasts, which subsequently results in the stimulation of keratinocyte proliferation and differentiation.[7]

IL-1 is increased in the early phase of numerous skin diseases and induces the release of further cytokines, growth factors, and the recruitment of T lymphocytes in the inflammatory tissue. IL-1 participates in the regulation of microvascular dermal endothelial cells by the upregulation of cell adhesion molecules like ICAM-1 or E-selectin, for example. On keratinocytes IL-1 also regulates the expression of ICAM-1 participating in the recruiting of lymphocytes in the epidermis. An even more far-reaching relevance at inflammatory dermatoses can be suspected via activation of IL-6 or NF-κB.[4]

IL-1 is also considered as a key cytokine in the pathogenesis of autoimmune diseases such as pemphigus vulgaris. Accordingly, increased levels of IL-1α and tumor necrosis factor-alpha (TNF-α) have been detected in lesional skin of patients with pemphigus. Acantholysis of keratinocytes was found to be inhibited by antibodies directed against IL-1α and TNF-α. Furthermore, in IL-1α and TNF-α receptor-deficient mice a decreased susceptibility for pemphigus was observed.

## B. Interleukin-6

IL-6 is mainly generated by monocytes, but also by bone marrow cells, fibroblasts, endothelial cells, certain T cells, B cells, and keratinocytes.[8] IL-6 is involved in the regulation of the function of T, B, and NK cells that express both of the IL-6 receptor chains. It plays an essential role in the maturation of B cells and antibody production, and also participates in inflammation by inducing the formation of acute-phase proteins by hepatocytes. In T cells, IL-6 mediates activation, growth, and differentiation. Thus, IL-6 is an "early" pro-inflammatory cytokine and induces acute-phase protein production, and increased formation of IL-6 by fibroblasts, endothelial cells, and keratinocytes stimulated by IL-1 and TNF-α may represent a significant amplifying process in inflammation.[9,10] Despite the finding of increased IL-6 serum levels in autoimmune diseases such as systemic lupus erythematosus (SLE), systemic scleroderma, and pemphigus vulgaris, a specific role of IL-6 in any skin disease is not established.[11,12] Recently, an essential role of IL-6 during wound healing has been described.[13]

## C. Tumor Necrosis Factor

TNF, also defined as *cachectin* and *endogenous pyrogen*, is a protein of 17 kDa, which exists in a secreted and transmembrane form and builds dimers or trimers after being released.[14] It is secreted by monocytes and macrophages, mast cells, fibroblasts, smooth muscle cells, endothelial cells, keratinocytes, T cells, and certain NK cells. It has multiple pro-inflammatory as well as anti-inflammatory activities, and is also a growth factor in normal physiological regeneration and wound healing.[15] Upon stimulation by exogenous factors such as bacterial lipopolysaccharide (LPS), staphylococcal toxin, viruses, and other organisms, or by endogenous mediators like C5a, IL-1, IL-2, granulocyte-macrophage colony-stimulating factor (GM-CSF), substance P, bradykinin, and TNF itself, large amounts are released within minutes, and the synthesis is rapidly increased. The rate of synthesis is controlled by interferon-gamma (IFN-γ),[16] but several other cytokines may antagonize and influence further release, e.g., TGF-β, IL-6, $PGE_2$, or vitamin $D_3$, for example. TNF-α is activated after processing at the cell membrane by a transmembrane enzyme (TNF-α-converting enzyme) (TACE).

Three types of TNF receptors have been identified: TNF-R1 (CD 120a, p55) and TNF-R2 (CD 120b, p75), which are expressed by almost all cells and bind both TNF-α and TNF-β, and TNF-R3, which is generated only by human hepatocytes and binds TNF-α. Each receptor appears to mediate different cellular responses.[17] TNF receptors also belong to the superfamily of death receptors, which are able to induce apoptosis in keratinocytes and leukocytes during cutaneous inflammation.

The soluble forms of the receptors, released from cell membranes, neutralize both forms of TNF, thereby preventing systemic effects resulting from local inflammation.[18] The soluble receptors occur in the blood and urine of normal persons, and were found to be markedly increased during various inflammatory disorders and sepsis.[18–20] Besides receptors, TNF-binding proteins (TBPs) are capable of regulating TNF function after release into the extracellular space.

TNF has many biological properties, similar to those of IL-1, which synergistically may enhance TNF activity. It induces septic shock and fever,[21] cachexia,[22] and is a potent mediator of inflammation, increasing macrophage and neutrophil chemotaxis, phagocytosis, cytotoxicity, and the respiratory burst activity.[23–28] The protective role of TNF is supported by the observation that mice lacking the gene for TNF do not develop sepsis but otherwise are lacking an efficient defense against systemic infection. Thus, an important role of TNF is to protect the tissue by limiting the inflammation to a local response. On the other hand, once the infection has come to a systemic stage, TNF may have deleterious effects leading to sepsis and shock reaction.[29] Some of these effects may be aggravated by the ability of TNF to stimulate synthesis of many other cytokines and mediators, including IL-1, GM-CSF, platelet-derived growth factor (PDGF), TGF-β, prostaglandins, and leukotrienes.

In the skin, TNF-α has been found to exert numerous effects. Toxins, haptens, as well as UV light, are potent inducers of TNF-α release from keratinocytes. TNF receptors are ultimately involved in the regulation of keratinocyte apoptosis.[30] TNF-α also induces the intensive expression of ICAM-1 in keratinocytes. Via activation of NF-κB and C/EBPβ, TNF-α regulates the synthesis of cytoskeletal proteins participating in epidermal responses to inflammation or wound healing. In contrast to its tissue-damaging properties, TNF is also a growth factor, stimulating fibroblast proliferation and synthesis, and exhibits synergy with epidermal growth factor (EGF), by increasing the EGF receptor, PDGF, and insulin.[14]

In endothelial cells, TNF promotes leukocyte adherence by increasing the expression of E-selectin, ICAM-1, and VCAM, probably via activation of the transcription factor NF-kB. TNF-α is also a potent activator of neutrophils, leading to the regulation of cell recruitment, chemotaxis, degranulation, and release of cytokines and oxidative burst mediators. TNF-α has been identified as one of the cytokines required for the maturation of DC and therefore also plays a role in the initiation of an immunoresponse. The pathophysiological relevance of TNF-α was demonstrated in various models for infection, inflammation, and autoimmune disease.[31,32] This is further supported by the successful use of biologics targeting TNF-α for the treatment of T-cell-mediated skin diseases such as psoriasis.[33,34] Moreover, diseases associated with mutations within the TNF-receptor type I have been described. Accordingly, the TNF-receptor-associated periodic syndrome (TRAPS) is a rare hereditary disease characterized by prolonged periodic fever attacks and severe localized inflammatory reactions.[35]

## III. LYMPHOCYTE-ACTIVATING CYTOKINES

### A. Interleukin-2

IL-2, or T-cell growth factor, is an essential mediator for developing an immune response. Activated T lymphocytes secrete IL-2, and express IL-2 receptors resulting in their proliferation and clonal expansion. IL-2 is also an important mediator for the proliferation of B lymphocytes and the activation of NK cells. Furthermore, IL-2 most importantly participates in the regulation of T-cell functions in Th1-mediated skin diseases such as psoriasis, cutaneous T-cell lymphoma, and melanoma. The important role of IL-2 in these diseases recently has been proved by the successful therapeutic use of specific anti-IL-2 strategies.[36–38]

### B. Interleukin-4

Originally named B-cell growth factor, IL-4 acts mainly on immunocompetent cells, and induces proliferation of activated mature T cells, enhances T-cell cytotoxic properties, but suppresses cytokine formation by Th1 cells, and thereby reduces delayed-type hypersensitivity (DTH) responses. On B cells, IL-4 stimulates MHC class II expression, and the expression of the low-affinity IgE receptor (CD23). IgE synthesis is regulated by IL-4 together with IL-13, and is inhibited by IFN-γ and TGF-β. Cytokines such as IL-2, IL-5, IL-6, and IL-9 synergize with IL-4 and IL-13 to enhance IgE production. On macrophages, however, IL-4 decreases CD23 expression. Mast cell growth is stimulated by IL-4, as is the growth of precursor hematopoietic cells, both directly and indirectly, by stimulating granulocyte colony-stimulating factor (G-CSF) and macrophage CSF (M-CSF) production in monocytes. IL-4 is important for the differentiation toward a Th2 T-cell subtype. In contrast, cytokines such as IL-12, IL-18, and IL-23 inhibit the differentiation of IL-4-producing T cells. Although IL-4 is generated in high amounts by T cells, there is also evidence that IL-4 is released in the skin by keratinocytes or mast cells. The IL-4 receptor was detected on T and B cells, macrophages, dendritic cells, mast cells, fibroblasts, and keratinocytes. Accordingly, IL-4 turned out to be an essential mediator for the differentiation of dendritic cells.[39] *In vivo* IL-4 was found to mediate immunodeviation toward Th2 and therefore in preliminary studies successfully has been used for the treatment of Th1-mediated skin diseases such as psoriasis, and antibodies to IL-4 have been tested as therapeutics for the treatment of atopic dermatitis.[40]

### C. Interleukin-5

IL-5, a helper T-cell lymphokine, induces growth and differentiation of activated B cells, and is a key mediator of switching immunoglobulin class synthesis. It is the most important promoter of eosinophil formation and differentiation. Mature eosinophils are activated, and their survival is prolonged in parasitic infestations. IL-5 works synergistically with IL-3 and GM-CSF on eosinophils.

### D. Interleukin-7

IL-7, synthesized by monocytes and T cells, is a hematopoietic growth factor, stimulating T-cell and B-cell proliferation. Moreover, immune functions like the proliferation of cytotoxic T cells and

NK cells as well as the activation of monocytes and macrophages can be triggered by IL-7. Therefore, administration or neutralization of IL-7 may allow the modulation of immune functions in patients with lymphocyte depletion, tumors, or autoimmune diseases.[41]

Two different IL-7R have been characterized mainly on lymphoid and myeloid cells. There is evidence that primarily IL-7Rα but not IL-7Rβ expression is required for T-lymphocyte proliferation. Recently, an IL-7-like cytokine thymic stromal lymphopoietin (TSLP) was described that binds to heterodimers consisting of the IL-7Rα chain and a common γ-like receptor chain also named TSLP receptor. TSLP was found to be highly expressed in keratinocytes from patients with inflammatory skin diseases such as atopic dermatitis (AD). TSLP activates $CD11^+$ dendritic cells to migrate and to initiate a Th2 immune response.[42]

### E. Interleukin-9

IL-9 is produced by $CD4^+$ T lymphocytes and was originally described in the murine system as P40, TCGF III and mast cell growth-enhancing activity (MEA). IL-9 is a growth factor for Th lymphocytes, mast cells, and megakaryoblastic leukemic cells and stimulates the development of erythropoietic colonies as well as the IL-4-induced IgE production by B lymphocytes. IL-9 transcripts also were detected in Hodgkin lymphomas and large cell anaplastic lymphomas, suggesting a role of IL-9 in the pathogenesis of these tumors.

### F. Interleukin-11

IL-11 stimulates precursor/progenitor hematopoietic blast cell mitosis, and synergizes with GM-CSF, IL-3, and IL-4. It also promotes an immunodeviation toward Th2, induces the formation of acute-phase proteins by the liver, stimulates fibroblast functions, supports differentiation of lymphocytes, but depresses differentiation of adipocytes and inhibits abnormal keratinocyte differentiation. Accordingly, first clinical trials have shown that IL-11 appears to be effective in the treatment of psoriasis. Moreover, a role for IL-11 in tissue remodeling during severe asthma has been suggested.[43]

### G. Interleukin-12

IL-12 is generated by monocytes/macrophages, dendritic cells, B cells, neutrophils, mast cells, and keratinocytes. The active form is a heterodimer consisting of a p40 and a p35 subunit. Interestingly, homodimers and monomers of p40 serve as competitive antagonists by binding to the IL-12 receptor without activating the signal transduction cascade. There is now evidence for an IL-12 family of heterodimeric cytokines, which share similar functions in innate as well as adaptive immunity but also have differentiated effects. Currently, the IL-12 family consists of five members including IL-23, Il-27, cardiotrophin-like cytokine/soluble cyliary neutrotrophic factor receptor (CLC/sCNTFR), and CLC/cytokine-like factor 1 (CLC/CLF-1).[44] IL-12 is an important activator of NK cells. It further increases IFN-γ production, modulates T-cell functions, and inhibits tumor angiogenesis.[45] In the skin, the production of IL-12 is induced by bacterial products or UV light, for example. Recently, a protective effect of IL-12 on UV-induced DNA damage was described in keratinocytes.[46]

### H. Interleukin-13

IL-13 shares many effects with IL-4 and was found to be released by T cells, mast cells, or keratinocytes. It affects the function of B cells as well as monocytes and decreases the production of pro-inflammatory cytokines in keratinocytes and endothelial cells. IL-13 also reduces the chemokine-induced chemotaxis of T cells, which altogether is evidence for an inflammatory role of IL-13.[47] Finally, IL-6 expression on monocytes is inhibited by both IL-4 and IL-13.

## I. Interleukin-14

IL-14 (high-molecular-weight, HMW, B-cell growth factor, BCGF) is a cytokine implicated in the generation and maintenance of normal memory B cells. It is produced by malignant B cells and normal as well as malignant T cells.[48]

## J. Interleukin-15

IL-15 shares many of the activities of IL-2 but is characterized by the use of a unique α-chain of its receptor. Both receptors use a common β- and γ-chain. The major sources of IL-15 are macrophages, epithelial cells including keratinocytes and fibroblasts, whereas T cells do not express IL-15. A major stimulus for IL-15 production are by IFN-α, and -β. Like IL-2, IL-15 functions as a T-cell growth factor, is chemotactic for T cells, activates NK cells, stimulates B-cell growth as well as differentiation and plays a role in the maturation of dendritic cells.[49] In human keratinocytes, IL-15 inhibits the anti-Fas and methylcellulose-induced apoptosis.[50] Because of its IFN-γ- and IgE-synthesis-modulating function, a relevance in the pathophysiology of the atopic dermatitis is attributed to IL-15.

## K. Interleukin-16

IL-16 is secreted from keratinocytes and Langerhans cells and is an important chemokine for the recruitment of $CD4^+$ T cells, monocytes, eosinophils, and Langerhans cells into the inflamed skin. Serum and RNA expression of this cytokine seems to correlate positively with the acuity of atopic dermatitis.[51]

## L. Interleukin-17

IL-17 is expressed by activated T cells of the memory phenotype ($CD4^+CD45R0^+$) and also eosinophils. IL-17 activates macrophages, fibroblasts, keratinocytes, and endothelial cells.[48,49] In keratinocytes, IL-17 initiates the release of growth-regulated oncogene-alpha (GRO-α), GM-CSF, IL-6, and the IFN-γ-induced expression of ICAM-1. In dermal endothelial cells, IL-17 induces the IL-1 secretion as well as the upregulation of cell adhesion molecules. Fibroblasts are stimulated by IL-17 to an increased IL-6 secretion and collagen synthesis, suggesting role of IL-17 in the pathophysiology of the systemic scleroderma.[52–54]

## M. Interleukin-18

The production of IL-18 has been described in dendritic cells, macrophages, keratinocytes, osteoblasts, microglia cells, and fibroblasts, and IL-18 mRNA expression can be stimulated by LPS, GM-CSF, and Fas ligand. IL-18 is also synthesized by human keratinocytes and was found be significantly upregulated in inflammatory skin diseases. The receptor for IL-18 is expressed by keratinocytes, which refers to an autocrine regulation by IL-18.[55] Functional IL-18 requires activation by an IL-18 converting enzyme (ICE or caspase-1) or proteinase-3.[56]

Together with IL-12, IL-18 significantly stimulates the production of IFN-γ. IL-18 also induces the maturation of T cells and NK cells, and stimulates the release of cytokines and chemokines. It increases Fas-mediated NK-cell cytotoxicity, induces IgE production by B cells, and synergizes with IL-2 to enhance IL-4 production. However, the effects of IL-18 on T cells seem to vary dependent on endogenous and exogenous factors such as the maturation state and the micromilieu. In basophils, IL-18 contributes to IL-4 and IL-13 production and in macrophages IL-18 induces the production of cytokines such as IL-6 and IFN-γ, TNF-α, and IL-1β. Moreover, IL-18 stimulates the synthesis of IL-6, IL-8, ICAM-1, and matrix metalloproteinases by endothelial cells.

IL-18 binds to a unique heterodimer receptor, which is upregulated by IL-12. IL-18-binding protein (IL-18BP) is a secreted protein able to bind IL-18 with high affinity, leading to inhibition of IL-18-induced IFN-γ and IL-8 production and NF-κB activation. Recently, another secreted protein, IL-1H, was observed to have also IL-18R antagonist activity (see also IL-1).[57]

In the skin, IL-18 modulates the migration of LC cells, the activity of T-helper cells, and wound healing.[58] IL-18 also regulates ICAM-1 expression on microvascular endothelial cells, indicating a role in leukocyte/endothelial interactions during inflammation. The pathophysiological relevance of IL-18 at present is discussed in connection with some diseases such as atopic dermatitis.[59] Enhanced expression of IL-18 was found in patients with lupus erythematodes and psoriasis. Finally, IL-18 also seems to be an important regulator during host defense in viruses, bacteria, fungi, and protozoa.

### N. Interleukin-21

IL-21 is a new member of the type I cytokine superfamily, which is mainly produced by activated T cells and has close structural similarities with IL-15, IL-2, and IL-4. It has a unique receptor chain, IL-21R, that pairs with the common γ-chain. The multiple biological functions of IL-21 include activation of NK cells, T cells, and B cells, and recently it also was found to inhibit the activation and maturation of DCs.[60]

### O. Interleukin-23

IL-23 is an only recently discovered cytokine belonging to the IL-12 cytokine family. Transgenic mice overexpressing the IL-23 show an intensive inflammatory infiltrate of lymphocytes and macrophages, among others, in numerous organs including the skin.[61] There is also recent evidence that in the skin IL-23, via increasing the number of LC with a more mature phenotype, enhances cutaneous immunity[62] (see also IL-12).

### P. Interleukin-25

Two new members of the IL-17 cytokine family, IL-17F and IL-25, have been described recently. IL-25 is produced by Th2 cells as well as mast cells, and via inducing the production of IL-4, IL-5, and IL-13 it is capable of amplifying allergic type inflammatory responses.[63]

### Q. Interleukin-27

Recently, a new member of the IL-12 family of heterodimeric cytokines was described, and defined as IL-27.[64] As an early product of activated antigen-presenting cells (APC), IL-27 is able to induce the clonal expansion of naive $CD4^+$ T cells. Synergistically with IL-12 it induces the production of IFN-γ by Th1- and NK cells. IL-27 probably binds on the orphan-receptor WSX-1/TCCR belonging to the IL-6/IL-12 receptor family, identified as the IL-27R.[65] These results commonly point at an important relevance of IL-27 for the proliferation and activation of naive T cells.[66]

### R. Interleuken-31

In a very recent paper, IL-31 was cloned. The authors demonstrated IL-31 to be an important cytokine preferentially produced by T helper type 2 cells. It may be involved in inflammation, keratinocyte function and pruritus.[66a]

## IV. IMMUNOSUPPRESSIVE CYTOKINES

In addition to pro-inflammatory cytokines, certain cytokines exert potent anti-inflammatory effects including IL-1 RA, TGF-β, and members of the IL-10 family. The physical state of cytokines in body fluids has been rarely investigated. Detection of a cytokine by immunological techniques allows only conclusions concerning its presence, but not about its potential activity. The cytokine may be coupled to another molecule that prevents binding to the specific receptor. Coupling may occur as (1) dissociable complexes with a protective lipoprotein that releases the cytokine to react with its receptor; (2) firmly bound complexes of cytokine and a carrier protein that interferes with receptor linkage;[67,68] or (3) complexes of cytokine with its specific soluble receptor that blocks interaction with cell receptors.[69] Anti-inflammatory cytokines exert their effects by (1) regulation of cytokine secretion, and differences of the agonists to stimulate secretion; (2) regulation of cytokine receptor expression; (3) receptor competition of different cytokines; (4) soluble binding factors and/or inhibitors; (5) regulation of proteases that activate the cytokine proform (converting enzymes), such as TRACE (TNF-receptor-activating co-enzyme), for example.[70]

## A. IL-10 Family of Cytokines

Because of their similarity to IL-10 function, IL-10, -19, -20, -22, -24, and -26 have been grouped to the IL-10 family. IL-28 and IL-29 share similarities to both type I IFNs and IL-10 cytokines.

### 1. Interleukin-10

Originally, IL-10 was described as a cytokine secreted by Th2 cells that inhibits the release of cytokines from Th1 cells.[71] Later it was found that IL-10 can be synthesized by Th1 as well as Th2 lymphocytes, cytotoxic T cells, mast cells, B cells, and monocytes; the last is the major source for IL-10 in humans. Today there is evidence for an IL-10 family of related cytokines, comprising different members of viral or cellular origin, including IL-19, IL-20, IL-22 (IL-10-related T-cell-derived inducible factor), IL–24 (melanoma differentiation-associated antigen 7), and IL-26 (AK155).[72] The different receptors for the IL-10 family belong to the cytokine receptor family type 2 resulting in diverse biological effects by activating signal transducer and activator of transcription (STAT) factors[73] (see cytokine suppressors and inhibitors).

IL-10 diminishes IFN-γ and IL-2 production by Th1 cells, as well as IL-4 and IL-5 generation by Th2 cells. IL-10 inhibits release of IL-1β, IL-6, IL-8, IL-12, and TNF-α in monocytes, as well an IFN-γ and TNF-α in NK cells. In monocytes or DCs, IL-10 also downregulates the expression and the release of MHC class II molecules, CD23, ICAM-I, and the accessory B7 molecule. Thus, IL-10 is an important cytokine for the regulation of antigen presentation and suppression of Th1 as well as Th2 cytokine production.

The anti-inflammatory effect of IL-10 is due to the inhibition of pro-inflammatory cytokines like IL-1, IL-2, IL-6, TNF-α or IFN-γ, further due to the inhibition of chemokines (IL-8) and chemokine receptors like (CXC-2 R). In eosinophils, IL-10 inhibits eosinophil survival and IL-4-induced IgE synthesis indicating an important role of this cytokine in allergic responses. In contrast, IL-10 activates the proliferation and Ig production of B cells. Thus, IL-10 is also a survival and differentiation factor for B cells. In conclusion, IL-10 contributes to inhibition of cellular and allergic immune responses while stimulating humoral and cytotoxic immune mechanisms.[74]

Increased expression of IL-10 was proved in patients with allergic contact dermatitis.[75] Accordingly, IL-10-deficient mice show a delayed immune response (CHS, $TH_1$ reaction).[76] Stimulators of the IL-10 synthesis in keratinocytes are contact allergens or the UVB light, for example. The effect of IL-10 is mediated via a specific IL-10 receptor expressed on numerous cells of the skin.[77] IL-10 also has been proposed as a therapeutic target for the treatment of inflammatory diseases such as psoriasis, atopic diseases such as AD and asthma, as well as other autoimmune diseases.[78]

### 2. Interleukin-19

IL-19 is a member of the IL-10 family that is released by monocytes and macrophages upon stimulation by LPS and GM-CSF. It also can be released by B cells. IL-19 exerts its effects by stimulating the receptors of IL-20 or IL-22.[79]

### 3. Interleukin-20

IL-20 exhibits a distinctive homology with IL-10 and was also found to be expressed in the skin and trachea. Overexpression of IL-20 in transgenic mice causes skin lesions similar to that of psoriasis. Two putative receptors for IL-20 were identified on keratinocytes. Moreover, IL-20 receptors are highly expressed in psoriatic skin further providing evidence for a role of this cytokine in the pathophysiology of psoriasis[80] (see also IL-10).

### 4. Interleukin-22

IL-22 (IL-10-related T-cell-derived inducible factor) is generated in $CD4^+$ T cells and mast cells, for example, and its production can be stimulated by IL-9 and LPS. The IL-22 receptor has also been detected in the skin.[81] Opponents of this receptor–ligand interaction are two soluble IL-22-receptor antagonists (IL-22RA1 and -RA2).[82] The IL-22RA2 is expressed by immunocompetent cells as well as epithelial cells. In contrast to other members of the IL-10 family of cytokines, IL-22 mediates acute-phase responses in the inflamed tissue and hepatocytes (see also IL-10).

### 5. Interleukin-24

IL-24 (melanoma differentiation-associated antigen 7) is a member of the IL-10 cytokine family, which is generated by Th2 cells in an IL-4-inducible manner. It was also found to be produced by differentiated melanoma cells and LPS-stimulated monocytes. IL-24 was shown to inhibit the proliferation of tumor cells including melanoma by inducing specific apoptotic pathways.[83]

### 6. Interleukin-26

IL-26 (AK155), generated by monocytes and various T-cell types, is involved in the transformed phenotype of human T cells after infection by herpes virus.[84,85]

### 7. Interleukin-28 and -29

Very recently, three novel cytokines designated IL-28A, IL-28B, and IL-29 have been identified.[86] They are induced by viral infection and are distantly related to type I IFNs and the IL-10 family because of their antiviral activity. IL-28 and IL-29 bind to a heterodimeric class II cytokine receptor, consisting of IL-10R$\beta$, and an orphan class II receptor chain IL-28R$\alpha$.

## B. IL-1RA and IL-18 RA

Two types of specific blocking agents for IL-1 activity have been identified. The first is a soluble receptor without a transmembrane structure that binds to free IL-1 thereby inactivating its binding site. The second, IL-1 receptor antagonist (IL-1RA), is an inactive IL-1 homologue that blocks specific IL-1 receptor sites on cells. IL-1RA is normally secreted during inflammatory reactions. Its production and release are modulated by many cytokines such as IL-4, IL-6, IL-13, or TGF-$\beta$, for example. The important function of IL-1RA is to potentially inhibit the deleterious effects of IL-1 during inflammation. Keratinocytes, fibroblasts, and monocytes are also capable of generating an intracellular form of IL-1RA. Its function and regulation, however, are not fully understood.[87]

IL-1$\alpha$ or IL-1$\beta$ activity normally follows binding of the cytokine to the IL-1R type I receptor on all responding cells.[88] Other cells, such as B cells and neutrophils, express another IL-1R, the IL-1R type II. It has been suggested that the IL-1RII can be shed from the cell surface and bind with free IL-1, thus ultimately blocking its ability to couple to cell-bound IL-R1. An alternative inhibitory molecule is an inactive homologue of IL-1, IL-1RA, which binds to cellular receptors without inducing a signal. The inert homologue therefore blocks the receptor, and subsequently prevents later binding of active IL-1.[89–92] This type of antagonist is peculiar to IL-1. It is secreted mainly by monocytes and macrophages, but also by neutrophils and fibroblasts. It has been designated secreted interleukin-1 receptor antagonist (sIL-1RA).

Both the IL-1α- and the IL-18 precursor require cleavage into an active mature molecule by an intracellular cysteine protease called IL-1α-converting enzyme (ICE), which is also known as capsase-1. Thus ICE inhibitors may limit the activity of IL-1α as well as IL-18. IL-1RA is a physiological antagonist that has similar structure with IL-1α as well as IL-β and thus competes with the binding of the natural ligand to the receptor. IL-18BP is a naturally occurring antagonist that is able to bind IL-18 with high affinity and to neutralize its activity, but not that of IL-1. Recently, another IL-18 antagonist IL-1H was discovered that has sequence homology with IL-1RA and binds the IL-18R but is not able to bind the IL-1R. IL-1F7b shares sequence homology with IL-18 and binds the IL-18Rα but has no IL-18-like agonistic or antagonistic activity. IL-F7b binds to IL-18BP and subsequently may block the IL-18Rα, which ultimately results in the inhibition of IL-18 activity.

A nonreceptor-soluble protein that may function as a protective carrier protein or inhibitory substance is $\alpha_2$M; it is a carrier for IL-1, IL-6, and PDGF, but inactivates IL-2 and FGF.[93–95] Other soluble inhibitors, mainly against IL-1, have been found in the medium of UV-exposed keratinocyte cultures, and in the sera of UV-exposed mice and humans. The identity of this substance, which blocks the activity of IL-1, however, is still unknown.[96]

### C. Transforming Growth Factor

TGF-β belongs to a family of peptides involved in growth and differentiation in almost all cells generated. It is ultimately involved in the regulation of extracellular matrix proteins and pathophysiological processes such as fibrosis, wound healing, and scar formation. Within the immune system, TGF-β downregulates the function of T cells, B cells, monocytes, and NK cells. T cells, undergoing apoptosis, release TGF-β leading to immunosuppressive effects in the inflammatory micromilieu.[97] TGF-β also diminishes mast cell function by inhibiting mast cell proliferation and IgE synthesis. TGF-β reduces the synthesis of IL-1 and IL-2. TGF-β, secreted in an inactive form, after exposure to acid pH in wound fluid, can bind weakly to EGFR on keratinocytes and endothelium, and compete with the stimulating molecules EGF and TGF-β, thereby reducing keratinocyte and endothelial proliferation.

## V. INTERFERONS

Interferons were originally described as factors that "interfere" with the replication of viruses. They comprise a family of cytokines to which a great significance is attributed, especially as defense against cancer cells and viral infections. Moreover, IFNs are key regulatory agents with many activities in normal tissue physiology, inflammation, and the immune responses.

IFN-α and IFN-β are rapidly released after viral infections upon stimulation via double-stranded RNA. In contrast, IFN-γ is induced indirectly during the inflammatory response against pathogens but also contributes to host defense. The major cellular source of IFN-α are macrophages and B cells, whereas IFN-β is produced by fibroblasts, and IFN-γ is synthesized by activated T cells. Very recently, a novel member of the type I IFN family was cloned, and defined as IFN-κ. It induces the release of several cytokines from monocytes and DCs, and inhibits IL-12 release from monocytes. The synthesis of IFN-κ is induced by IFN-γ in monocytes as well as DCs. It also can be detected in these cells in lesional skin of AD and psoriasis.[98]

The three IFNs have specific receptors and different properties, which may act in a synergistic or antagonistic fashion. IFN-α and IFN-β exert their effects by inhibiting the virus replication in host cells. Additionally, both molecules not only affect infected cells but also activate defense mechanisms in neighboring "healthy" cells in a paracrine manner. Activation of the receptor by IFN-α and IFN-β leads to the induction of intracellular signaling pathways involved in inflammation and host defense such as signal transducers of transcription (STATs), P1-kinase, and Mx-protein, all of which increase the resistance of cells to viral replication.[99]

IFN-γ induces the formation of MHC class II molecules on monocytes and keratinocytes,[100–102] while IFN-α and IFN-β upregulate expression of the MHC class I antigens on many cell types leading to an optimized presentation to cells of the adaptive immune system such as T cells. Interferons activate NK-cell activity leading to the successful killing of infected cells. In contrast, interferons save non-infected cells from destruction by NK cells by inducing MHC-I molecules on these cells. In addition, IFN-γ stimulates the activity of a proteinase, cathepsin S.[103] The release of vascular growth factors (VEGF) is induced in keratinocytes and suppressed in fibroblasts by IFN-γ, indicating that this cytokine is involved in the regulation of angiogenesis.[104]

IFN-γ also augments monocyte secretion of TNF-α and TNF-, which contribute to the antiviral and antiproliferative properties of IFNs,[105] and increases the expression of IL-2R and ligand binding on human leukemic and normal lymphocytes.[106] All three IFNs augment the activity of NK lymphocytes and macrophages,[107] and stimulate macrophage synthesis of arachidonic acid products.[108] IFN-α may also stimulate the formation of IgG and IgM by B cells.[109] Thus, interferons directly function as important mediators of both the innate as well as the adaptive immune response.

In inflammatory skin diseases like the AD, a beneficial effect of IFN-γ treatment has been reported. Moreover, in mice mast cells appear to contribute to the regulation of IFN-γ in the inflamed skin.[110] A role for IFN-γ has also been implicated in autoimmune diseases such as lupus erythematosus. Accordingly, the overexpression of IFN-γ in the epidermis leads to SLE-similar skin alterations. Interestingly, humans and mice deficient in Fas, TNF-receptor family member, cannot induce apoptosis of autoreactive cells, and consequently develop progressive lymphoproliferative disorders and lupus-like autoimmune diseases. CD137, another TNF-receptor family member, activates T cells and induces rejection of allografts and established tumors. Monoclonal antibodies to CD137 (2A) blocks lymphadenopathy and spontaneous autoimmune diseases in Fas-deficient mice leading to prolonged survival. Notably, 2A treatment rapidly augments IFN-γ production, and induces the depletion of autoreactive B cells and abnormal double-negative T cells, possibly by increasing their apoptosis through Fas- and TNF receptor-independent mechanisms. These results demonstrate that antibodies specific for co-stimulatory molecules can be used as novel therapeutic agents to delete autoreactive lymphocytes and block autoimmune disease progression.[111] Together, IFNs not only “interfere” as antiviral agents but are also important mediators of inflammatory and immune responses within the skin.

## VI. HEMATOPOIETIC GROWTH FACTORS

Hematopoietic growth factors (HGF) or hematopoietins are produced by many different cell types and act on cells of the hematopoietic system. They include the CSFs, erythropoietin (Epo), stem cell factor (SCF), and several other cytokines,[112] thereby regulating differentiation as well as proliferation of hematopoietic stem cells. They can be either expressed as transmembrane molecules or released into the environment where they mediate their effects in an autocrine, paracrine, or endocrine fashion. Multilineage CSFs such as IL-3, GM-CSF, and IL-4 regulate early stages of development of multipotential progenitors, whereas already committed progenitors are controlled by late-acting, lineage-specific factors such as Epo, IL-5, and M-CSF. Other early-acting cytokines are G-CSF, IL-6, IL-11, IL-12, IL-13, leukemia inhibitory factor (LIF), and SCF, which are strictly regulated after activation.[113] Upon stimulation, for example, during ontogenesis or after infection, CSFs are rapidly upregulated up to 1000×. CSF also induce the production of other growth factors and peptides resulting in the regulation of mitogenesis or cell-cycle regulation. In addition to CSF, Epo, and SCF, other factors have been demonstrated to be involved in the regulation of hematopoiesis such as TGF-β,[114] IL-6,[115] or even neuropeptides such as substance P,[116] for example. Thus, HGFs comprise many factors of different families orchestrating the regulation of hematopoiesis and cell differentiation in the bone marrow and the periphery.

## A. Colony-Stimulating Factors

Originally, CSFs were described as molecules released by feeder cells *in vitro* to promote colony growth. Most of them are *N*- or *O*-glycosylated cytokines, which prevents them from proteolysis. CSFs are produced by most cutaneous and immune cells such as keratinocytes, endothelial cells, smooth muscle cells, fibroblasts, neutrophils, mast cells, and T cells, for example. They show significant effects in the picomolar range making them powerful mediators of growth and differentiation. The classical CSFs comprise of G-CSF, GM-CSF, MEG-(megacaryocytic)-CSA, and IL-3. While G-CSF and GM-CSF are lineage-specific agents, IL-3 and MEG-CSA are multifunctional hematopoietic factors. The biological functions of CSFs are mediated by specific transmembrane receptors. Receptor–ligand interactions are mostly terminated by receptor internalization.

The use of CSF can be therapeutically used for patients suffering from various hematopoietic diseases or during chemotherapy, when the quantity of certain blood cells is dramatically diminished. Interestingly, some CSF also show tumoricidal and cytotoxic capacity making them prospective beneficial tools for tumor therapy.

GM-CSF is a multilineage CSF, which stimulates the function of neutrophils, eosinophils, and macrophages and is a growth factor for myeloleukemic cells. Moreover, GM-CSF inhibits the migration of neutrophils, induces phagocytosis, eicosanoid production, and antibody-dependent cytotoxicity (ADCC) and stimulates the tumoricidal and antimicrobial activity as well as cytokine production of macrophages.[117,118] The GM-CSF receptor, which is expressed on several myeloid and nonmyeloid cells, shares a common signal-transducing β-chain with the IL-3 and IL-5 receptor.[119] Interestingly, GM-CSF-deficient mice show normal numbers of peripheral blood cells, bone marrow progenitors, and tissue hematopoietic cells. Even mutant bone marrow cells were able to reconstitute lethally irradiated mutant mice.[120] Therefore, the common belief that GM-CSF plays a central role in myelopoiesis must now be modified.

GM-CSF-production within the skin has been demonstrated both at the mRNA as well as at the protein level in keratinocytes, fibroblasts, mast cells, macrophages, and endothelial cells[121] (Table 15.2). Upon various stimuli such as antigen or irritant application, IL-1, UV irradiation, or during inflammatory skin diseases, keratinocytes respond with enhanced GM-CSF release.[122,123] GM-CSF receptors have been found on epidermal LCs, macrophages, and DCs.[124] GM-CSF appears to play an important role in cutaneous immunity, and it maintains LC viability during short-term *in vitro* culture, but also induces profound alterations of LC function when investigated *in vitro*. It is essential for the ability of epidermal APCs to sensitize naive, unprimed T cells, although upregulation of MHC class II molecules on LC during *in vitro* culture appears to be independent of GM-CSF.[124,125] Moreover, GM-CSF also was found to be an essential factor triggering the migration of LC.[126] The

**TABLE 15.2**
**Keratinocyte-Derived Cytokines and Chemokines**

| | |
|---|---|
| Resting keratinocytes | IL-1, IL-6, IL-7, IL-11, IL-15, TNF, GM-CSF, G-CSF, TGF-β |
| Activated keratinocytes (UV, endotoxin, phorbol ester, cytokines) | IL-1/β, IL-6, IL-7, IL-10, IL-11, IL-12, IL-13, IL-15, IL-1RA, TNF,IL-8, Gro-α,-β, ENA-78, IP-10, MIP-2, MCP-1, RANTES, IL-3, G-CSF, M-CSF, GM-CSF, SCF, IFN-α, IFN-β, TGF, TGF-β, PDGF, bFGF |

*Abbreviations:* IL, interleukin; TNF, tumor necrosis factor; GM-CSF, granulocyte-macrophage colony-stimulating factor; G-CSF, granulocyte colony-stimulating factor; TGF, transforming growth factor; Gro, growth regulated oncogene; ENA-78, epithelial neutrophil-activating protein-78; IP-10, interferon-inducible protein-10; MIP-2, macrophage inflammatory protein-2; MCP-1, microbial cationic protein-1; RANTES, regulated upon activation, normal T expressed, and presumably secreted; M-CSF, macrophage colony-stimulating factor; SCF, stem cell factor; IFN, interferon; PDGF, platelet-derived growth factor; bFGF, basic fibroblast growth factor.

**TABLE 15.3**
**Cytokine Production by Langerhans Cells**

| | Cytokine |
|---|---|
| In situ | IL-1β |
| | TNF |
| | IFN |
| | MIP-1 |
| | MIP-2 |
| Fresh LC | IL-1β, IL-12, IL-15 |
| | MIP-1 |
| | MIP-2 |
| | SCF |
| Cultured LC | IL-1β, IL-6 |
| | MIP2 |

*Abbreviations:* IL, interleukin; TNF, tumor necrosis factor; IFN, interferon; MIP-1, macrophage inflammatory protein-1; SCF, stem cell factor.

functional changes of LC induced by GM-CSF can be antagonized by TNF-α.[127] GM-CSF also appears to be involved in immunosurveillance toward neoplastic growth, since effective sensitization against tumor antigens was found to be greatly upregulated by GM-CSF.[128] In addition to its effects on LC, GM-CSF may also be a growth-promoting factor for other resident or recruited cells within the skin.[129] Interestingly, the hematopoietic effects of GM-CSF (as well as G-CSF and IL-3) can be antagonized by serine proteases such as neutrophil-derived elastase.[130] Many signal transduction pathways including phosphatidyl-inositol-3-kinase ($PI_3K$) and c-myc may be involved in the transduction of the GM-CSF-mediated hematopoietic proliferatory effects.[131]

IL-3 is a nonspecific hematopoietic growth factor, which in the murine system is identical with mast cell growth factor (MCGF). In addition to affecting stem cell differentiation, IL-3 is a growth factor for some myeloid cell lines and induces phagocytosis of macrophages.[132] The IL-3 receptor was identified on stem cells, monocytes, and T cells. Like the IL-5R and the GM-CSFR, the IL-3R consists of two distinct chains of which the β-chain is identical for all three cytokine receptors.[133] IL-3 is mainly produced by T lymphocytes; however, it recently was shown that keratinocytes and melanocytes also can produce IL-3[134] (Table 15.2). In cooperation with TGF-β, IL-3 mediates a GM-CSF independent differentiation of human $CD34^+$ hematopoietic progenitor cells into DCs with an LC phenotype.[135] However, the ability of TGF-β to polarize the differentiation of hematopoietic progenitor cells to LCs was weaker in cooperation with IL-3 as compared to M-CSF since LC did not express Birbeck granula in the latter case (Table 15.3).

G-CSF is the principal cytokine regulating granuolopoiesis and induces the formation of granulocyte colonies. In addition to its effect on stem cells, G-CSF also activates mature neutrophils, induces phagocytosis, chemotaxis, enzyme release, and ADCC. G-CSF is produced by many different cells including keratinocytes[136] (Table 15.2). The receptor for G-CSF recently was characterized on neutrophils.[137] Recent studies using G-CSF receptor knockout mice are neutropenic but show only a modest reduction of committed myeloid precursors. This is in favor of compensatory mechanisms that are not clear as of yet. It is suggested that G-CSF-receptor-mediated signaling pathways play a pivotal role in directing the commitment of hematopoietic precursors to the various myeloic lineages.[138]

In contrast to the other CSFs, M-CSF is a disulfide bridge linked homodimer. The M-CSF receptor was found to be expressed on monocytes and to be identical with the product of the c-fms oncogene. M-CSF induces the proliferation and differentiation of macrophage progenitor cells.

In addition, M-CSF stimulates the production of cytokines, tumor cytotoxicity, and enzyme release in macrophages. M-CSF also was found to be produced by many different cells, including keratinocytes[139,140] (Table 15.2). Moreover, M-CSF, in cooperation with TGF-β, induces LC development from hematopoietic progenitor cells independent of GM-CSF.[141]

### B. Stem Cell Factor

SCF (CD 117) or mast cell growth factor (MGF) is a highly conserved hematopoietic growth factor that was identified as a ligand of the c-kit gene product and therefore also was named c-kit ligand. In mice, SCF is the product of the SI (steel) locus, whereas the W locus codes for the c-kit tyrosinase receptor, and thus SCF, was also named steel factor.[142,143] SCF gene mutations or deletions result in embryonic lethality due to marked anemia and severe impairment of the hematopoietic system including mast cell deficiency. Both a soluble and a transmembrane form can be achieved by alternative splicing. Many cells have been identified as a source of SCF, and in the skin keratinocytes, LC, mast cells, fibroblasts, and endothelial cells are able to produce SCF[144–146] (Table 15.2 and Table 15.3). *In vitro*, SCF stimulates the proliferation of IL-3-dependent and mature murine mast cells and therefore was described as "mast cell growth factor."[143,146]

Recent data indicate a close interaction between mast cells and T cells. For example, MCs proliferate in response to TH2 cytokine release such as IL-4, Il-5, and IL-9.[147] For example, SCF along with IL-4 stimulates the proliferation and differentiation of CD3$^+$ cells, and IL-4 induces the expression of the Fcε receptor on mast cells suggesting that SCF together with IL-4 can induce T-cell proliferation, differentiation, and maturation from cord blood precursor cells.[148,149] In many tissues, SCF synergizes with other growth factors, such as G-CSF, GM-CSF, IL-7, Epo, and TGF-β, for example. *In vivo* application of SCF results in enhanced blood counts of megakaryocytes and platelets. Thus, SCF may be an important stimulator of platelet generation.

A recent observation demonstrates that CSF seems to play a role in the pathogenesis of mastocytosis. Mast cells express the CSF receptor, defined as c-kit. By activating this receptor, SCF not only induces histamine, tryptase, and leukotriene C4 in mast cells, but is also chemotactic for these cells.[150] Finally, CSF prevents mast cells from apoptosis. In the skin of patients with cutaneous mastocytosis, an altered distribution and an abnormal production of MGF were demonstrated in comparison to normal skin. This appears to be due to increased proteolytic processing. Moreover, mast cell tumor lines may also express CSF suggesting that CSF/c-kit interactions may be responsible for growth-promoting events in mast cell tumors. Therefore, soluble MGF may be responsible for the accumulation of mast cells and hyperpigmentation found in cutaneous mastocytosis.[150]

SCF is essential for the development of hematopoietic, germ, and pigment cell lineages. It synergizes with other hematopoietic cytokines such as GM-CSF, G-CSF, IL-3, and Epo to stimulate progenitor cells of myeloid and erythroid lineages.[142] There is recent evidence indicating that SCF also functions as a growth-promoting signal for human DC in culture. Whereas the differentiation of human CD34$^+$ bone marrow cells requires TNF-α and GM-CSF, they can be expanded for several weeks in culture with SCF.[151,152] An important function of SCF is its melanocyte-stimulating capacity. Accordingly, in patients with piebaldism, which is an autosomal dominant defect in melanocyte development characterized by patches of hypopigmented skin and hair, a mutant of the c-kit gene was detected.[153] Similarly, a mutation of the mouse c-kit gene is associated with depigmentation, a defective proliferation and differentiation of stem cells and germ cells.[154]

## VII. CONCLUSION

There is no doubt that a fine-tuned network of mediators including cytokines, chemokines, and growth factors are crucially involved in the regulation of skin function both under physiological and pathophysiological conditions. Many studies have proved that — upon appropriate stimulation

— every cell within the epidermis and dermis is capable of releasing these factors and of expressing their respective high-affinity receptors. Cytokines exert many effects in the skin during inflammation, immune responses, infection, cell growth, and differentiation. They can act synergistically or antagonize each other, thereby maintaining homeostasis and limited inflammation. There is some redundancy among different cytokines and other mediators as they have overlapping activities and may use similar signal-transducing pathways. Therefore, it is of major importance to further elucidate the cytokine cascade, which will allow new insight into the pathomechanisms of inflammatory and immune reactions. It will be important to further explore the receptor–ligand interactions of cytokine receptors and further delineate the subsequent intracellular signal transduction pathways to understand the molecular mechanisms by which cytokines regulate gene transcription in the various cell types. This will help to develop new strategies for the treatment of inflammatory, infectious, autoimmune, and tumorigenic diseases in the skin.

## ACKNOWLEDGMENTS

This work has been supported by grants from the Federal Ministry of Education and Research (IZKF, Fö.01KS9604/0), Deutsche Forschungsgemeinschaft (STE 1014/1-1; SFB 293; SFB 492 to M.S.), C.E.R.I.E.S., Paris, Noratis Foundation, and Boltzmann-Institute, Münster, Germany (to T.L. and M.S.).

## REFERENCES

1. Luger, T.A., Stadler, B.M., Luger, B.M., Mathieson, B.J., Mage, M., Schmidt, J.A., and Oppenheim, J.J., Murine epidermal cell-derived thymocyte-activating factor resembles murine interleukin 1, *J. Immunol.*, 128, 2147, 1982.
2. Lawrence, T., Gilroy, D.W., Colville-Nash, P.R., and Willoughby, D.A., Possible new role for NF-κB in the resolution of inflammation, *Nat. Med.*, 7, 1291, 2001.
3. Camp, R.D.R., Fincham, N., Cunningham, F.M. et al., Psoriatic skin lesions contain biologically active amounts of an interleukin 1-like compound, *J. Immunol.*, 137, 3469, 1986.
4. Abeyama, K., Eng, W., Jester, J.V., Vink, A.A., Edelbaum, D., Cockerell, C.J., Bergstresser, P.R., and Takashima, A., A role for NF-kappaB-dependent gene transactivation in sunburn, *J. Clin. Invest.*, 105, 1751, 2000.
5. Nakae, S., Komiyama, Y., Narumi, S., Sudo, K., Horai, R., Tagawa, Y., Sekikawa, K., Matsushima, K., Asano, M., and Iwakura, Y., IL-1-induced tumor necrosis factor-alpha elicits inflammatory cell infiltration in the skin by inducing IFN-gamma-inducible protein 10 in the elicitation phase of the contact hypersensitivity response, *Int. Immunol.*, 15, 251, 2003.
6. Lee, W.Y., Lockniskar, M.F., and Fischer, S.M., Interleukin-1 alpha mediates phorbol ester-induced inflammation and epidermal hyperplasia, *FASEB J.*, 8, 1081, 1994.
7. Rauschmayr, T., Groves, R.W., and Kupper, T.S., Keratinocyte expression of the type 2 interleukin 1 receptor mediates local and specific inhibition of interleukin 1-mediated inflammation, *Proc. Natl. Acad. Sci. U.S.A.*, 94, 5814, 1997.
8. Neuner, P., Urbanski, A., Trautinger, F., Möller, A., Kirnbauer, R., Kapp, A., Schopf, E., Schwarz, T., and Luger, T.A., Increased IL-6 production by monocytes and keratinocytes in patients with psoriasis, *Proc. Natl. Acad. Sci. U.S.A.*, 86, 6367, 1991.
9. Grossman, R.M., Krueger, J., Yourish, D., Granelli Piperno, A., Murphy, D.P., May, L.T., Kupper, T.S., Sehgal, P.B., and Gottlieb, A.B., Interleukin 6 is expressed in high levels in psoriatic skin and stimulates proliferation of cultured human keratinocytes, *Proc. Natl. Acad. Sci. U.S.A.*, 86, 6367, 1989.
10. Neuner, P., Urbanski, A., Trautinger, F., Möller, A., Kirnbauer, R., Kapp, A., Schopf, E., Schwarz, T., and Luger, T.A., Increased IL-6 production by monocytes and keratinocytes in patients with psoriasis, *J. Invest. Dermatol.*, 97, 27, 1991.
11. Turksen, K., Kupper, T., Degenstein, L., Williams, I., and Fuchs, E., Interleukin 6: insights to its function in skin by overexpression in transgenic mice, *Proc. Natl. Acad. Sci. U.S.A.*, 89, 5068, 1992.

12. Lopez-Robles, E., Avalos-Diaz, E., Vega-Memije, E., Hojyo-Tomoka, T., Villalobos, R., Fraire, S., Domiguez-Soto, L., and Herrera-Esparza, R., TNFalpha and IL-6 are mediators in the blistering process of pemphigus, *Int. J. Dermatol.,* 40, 185, 2001.
13. Gallucci, R.M., Sloan, D.K., Heck, J.M., Murray, A.R., and O'Dell, S.J., Interleukin-6 indirectly induces keratinocyte migration, *J. Invest. Dermatol.,* 122, 764, 2004.
14. Balkwill, FR., Tumour necrosis factor, *Br. Med. Bull.*, 45, 389–400, 1989.
15. Tracey, K.J., Vlassara, H., and Cerami, A., Cachetin/tumour necrosis factor, *Lancet,* 1122, 1989.
16. Beutler, B., Tkacenko, V., Milsark, I. et al., Effect of gamma interferon on cachetin expression by mononuclear phagocytes. Reversal of lpsd (endotoxin resistance) phenotype, *J. Exp. Med.,* 164, 1791, 1986.
17. Vilcek, J. and Lee, T.H., Tumour necrosis factor. New insights into the molecular mechanisms of its multiple actions, *J. Biol. Chem.,* 266, 7313, 1991.
18. Van Zee, K.J., Kohno, T., Fischer, E., et al., Tumour necrosis factor soluble receptors circulate during experimental and clinical inflammation and can protect against excessive tumour necrosis factor *in vitro* and *in vivo*, *Proc. Natl. Acad. Sci. U.S.A.*, 89, 4845, 1992.
19. Digel, W., Porzsolt, F., Schmid, M., et al., High levels of circulating soluble receptors for tumour-necrosis factor in hairy-cell leukemia and type-B chronic lymphatic leukemia, *J. Clin. Invest.*, 89, 1690, 1992.
20. Aderka, D., Wysenbeek, A., Engelmann, H., et al., Correlation between serum levels of soluble tumour necrosis factor receptor and disease activity in systemic lupus erythematosus, *Arth. Rheum.,* 36, 1111, 1993.
21. Tracey, K.J., Beutler, B., Lowry, S.F., et al., Shock and tissue injury induced by recombinant human cachetin, *Science,* 234, 470, 1986.
22. Tracey, K.J., Wei, H., Manogue, K.R., et al., Cachetin tumour necrosis factor induces cachexia, anemia, and inflammation, *J. Exp. Med.,* 167, 1211, 1988.
23. Djeu, J.Y., Blanchard, D.K., and Richards, A.L., Tumour necrosis factor induction by *Candida albicans* from human natural killer cells and monocytes, *J. Immunol.,* 141, 4047, 1988.
24. Shalaby, M.R., Aggarwal, B.B., Rinderknect, E., et al., Activation of human polymorphonuclear functions by interferon gamma and tumour necrosis factor, *J. Immunol.,* 135, 2069, 1985.
25. Beutler, B. and Cerami, A., The biology of cachectin/TNF – a primary mediator of the host response, *Annu. Rev. Immunol.,* 7, 625, 1989.
26. Perez, C., Albert, I., DeFay, K., Zachariades, N., Gooding, L., and Kriegler, M., A nonsecretable cell surface mutant of tumor necrosis factor (TNF) kills by cell-to-cell contact, *Cell,* 63, 251, 1990.
27. Tartaglia, L.A. and Goeddel, D.V., Two TNF receptors, *Immunol. Today,* 13, 151, 1992.
28. Tracey, K.J., Fong, Y., Hesse, D.G., Manogue, K.R., Lee, A.T., Kuo, G.C., Lowry, S.F., and Cerami, A., Anti-cachectin/TNF monoclonal antibodies prevent septic shock during lethal bacteraemia, *Nature,* 330, 662, 1987.
29. Hultgren, O., Eugster, H.P., Sedgwick, J.D., Korner, H., and Tarkowski, A., TNF/lymphotoxin-alpha double-mutant mice resist septic arthritis but display increased mortality in response to *Staphylococcus aureus*, *J. Immunol.,* 161, 5937, 1998.
30. Wakugawa, M., Nakamura, K., Akatsuka, M., Nakagawa, H., and Tamaki, K., Interferon-gamma-induced rantes production by human keratinocytes is enhanced by IL-1beta, TNF-alpha, IL-4 and IL-13 and is inhibited by dexamethasone and tacrolimus, *Dermatology,* 202, 239, 2001.
31. Nakayama, T., Fujisawa, R., Yamada, H., Horikawa, T., Kawasaki, H., Hieshima, K., Izawa, D., Fujiie, S., Tezuka, T., and Yoshie, O., Inducible expression of a CC chemokine liver- and activation-regulated chemokine (LARC)/macrophage inflammatory protein (MIP)-3 alpha/CCL20 by epidermal keratinocytes and its role in atopic dermatitis, *Int. Immunol.,* 13, 95, 2001.
32. Vestergaard, C., Bang, K., Gesser, B., Yoneyama, H., Matsushima, K., and Larsen, C.G., A Th2 chemokine, TARC, produced by keratinocytes may recruit CLA+CCR4+ lymphocytes into lesional atopic dermatitis skin, *J. Invest. Dermatol.,* 115, 640, 2000.
33. Gottlieb, A.B., Infliximab for psoriasis, *J. Am. Acad. Dermatol.*, 49, S112, 2003.
34. Leonardi, C.L., Powers, J.L., Matheson, R.T., Goffe, B.S., Zitnik, R., Wang, A., and Gottlieb, A.B., Etanercept Psoriasis Study Group. Etanercept as monotherapy in patients with psoriasis, *N. Engl. J. Med.,* 349, 2014, 2003.
35. Hentgen, V. and Reinert, P., TNF receptor-associated periodic syndrome (TRAPS): clinical aspects and physiopathology of a rare familial disease, *Arch. Pediatr.,* 10, 45, 2003.

36. Atzpodien, J., Neuber, K., Kamanabrou, D., Fluck, M., Brocker, E.B., Neumann, C., Runger, T.M., Schuler, G., von den Driesch, P., Muller, I., Paul, E., Patzelt, T., and Reitz, M., Combination chemotherapy with or without s.c. IL-2 and IFN-alpha results for a prospectively randomized trial of the Cooperative Advanced Malignant Melanoma Chemoimmunotherapy Group (ACIMM), *Br. J. Cancer*, 86, 179, 2002.
37. Arienti, F., Sule-Suso, J., Belli, F., Mascheroni, L., Rivoltini, L., Melani, C., Maio, M., Cascinelli, N., Colombo, M.P., and Parmiani, G., Limited antitumor T cell response in melanoma patients vaccinated with interleukin-2 gene-transduced allogenic melanoma cells, *Human Gene Ther.*, 7, 1955, 1996.
38. Takada, T., Kato, K., Yagita, H., Hamada, H., and Okumura, K., Effects of immunization with tumor cells double transfected with interleukin-2 (IL-2) and interleukin-12 (IL-12) genes on artificial metastasis of colon 26 cells in BALB/c mice, *Clin. Exp. Metastasis*, 17, 125, 1999.
39. Romani, N., Gruner, S., Brang, D., Kampgen, E., Lenz, A., Trockenbacher, B., Konwalinka, G., Fritsch, P.O., Steinman, R.M., and Schuler, G., Proliferating dendritic cell progenitors in human blood, *J. Exp. Med.,* 180, 83, 1994
40. Biedermann, T., Kneilling, M., Mailhammer, R., Maier, K., Sander, C.A., Kolias, G., Kunkel, S.L., Hultner, L., and Rocken, M., Mast cells control neutrophil recruitment during T cell-mediated delayed-type hypersensitivity reactions through tumor necrosis factor and macrophage inflammatory protein 2, *J. Exp. Med.*, 192, 1441, 2000.
41. Fry, T.J. and Mackall, C.L., Interleukin-7: from bench to clinic, *Blood*, 99, 3892, 2002.
42. Soumelis, V., Reche, P.A., Kanzler, H., Yuan, W., Edward, G., Homey, B., Gilliet, M., Ho, S., Antonenko, S., Lauerma, A., Smith, K., Gorman, D., Zurawski, S., Abrams, J., Menon, S., McClanahan, T., de Waal-Malefyt, Rd. R., Bazan, F., Kastelein, R.A., and Liu, Y.J., Human epithelial cells trigger dendritic cell mediated allergic inflammation by producing TSLP, *Nat. Immunol.,* 3, 673, 2002.
43. Zheng, T., Zhu, Z., Wang, J., Homer, R.J., and Elias, J.A., 11: insights in asthma from overexpression transgenic modeling, *J. Allergy Clin. Immunol.,* 108, 489, 2001.
44. Trinchieri, G., Pflanz, S., and Kastelein, R.A., The IL-12 family of heterodimeric cytokines: new players in the regulation of T cell responses, *Immunity*, 19, 641, 2003.
45. Lamont, A. and Adorini, L., IL-12: a key cytokine in immune regulation, *Immunol. Today*, 17, 214, 1996.
46. Schwarz, A., Ständer, S., Berneburg, M., Böhm, M., Kulms, D., van Steeg, H., Grosse-Heitmeyer, K., Krutmann, J., and Schwarz, T., Interleukin-12 suppresses ultraviolet radiation-induced apoptosis by inducing DNA repair, *Nat. Cell. Biol.*, 4, 26, 2002.
47. Obara, W., Kawa, Y., Ra, C., Nishioka, K., Soma, Y., and Mizoguchi, M. T., Cells and mast cells as a major source of interleukin-13 in atopic dermatitis, *Dermatology*, 205, 11, 2002.
48. Ford, R., Tamayo, A., Martin, B., Niu, K., Claypool, K., Cabanillas, F., and Ambrus, J. Jr., Identification of B-cell growth factors (interleukin-14; high molecular weight-B-cell growth factors) in effusion fluids from patients with aggressive B-cell lymphomas, *Blood*, 86, 283, 1995.
49. Lodolce, J., Burkett, P., Koka, R., Boone, D., Chien, M., Chan, F., Madonia, M., Chai, S., and Ma, A., Interleukin-15 and the regulation of lymphoid homeostasis, *Mol. Immunol.,* 39, 537, 2002.
50. Ruckert, R., Asadullah, K., Seifert, M., Budagian, V.M., Arnold, R., Trombotto, C., Paus, R., and Bulfone-Paus, S., Inhibition of keratinocyte apoptosis by IL-15: a new parameter in the pathogenesis of psoriasis? *J. Immunol.,* 165, 2240, 2002.
51. Frezzolini, A., Paradisi, M., Zaffiro, A., Provini, A., Cadoni, S., Ruffelli, M., and De Pita, O., Circulating interleukin 16 (IL-16) in children with atopic/eczema dermatitis syndrome (AEDS): a novel serological marker of disease activity, *Allergy,* 57, 815, 2002.
52. Moseley, T.A., Haudenschild, D.R., Rose, L., and Reddi, A.H., Interleukin-17 family and IL-17 receptors, *Cytokine Growth Factor Rev.,* 14, 155, 2003.
53. Katz, Y., Nadiv, O., Rapoport, M.J., and Loos, M., IL-17 regulates gene expression and protein synthesis of the complement system, C3 and factor B, in skin fibroblasts, *Clin. Exp. Immunol.,* 120, 22. 2000.
54. Kurasawa, K., Hirose, K., Sano, H., Endo, H., Shinkai, H., Nawata, Y., Takabayashi K., and Iwamoto, I., Increased interleukin-17 production in patients with systemic sclerosis, *Arthritis Rheum.*, 43, 2455, 2000.
55. Gracie, J.A., Robertson, S.E., and McInnes, I.B., Interleukin-18, *J. Leukoc. Biol.,* 73, 213, 2003.
56. Koizumi, H., Sato-Matsumura, K.C., Nakamura, H., Shida, K., Kikkawa, S., Matsumoto, M., Toyoshima, K., and Seya, T., Distribution of IL-18 and IL-18 receptor in human skin: various forms of IL-18 are produced in keratinocytes, *Arch. Dermatol. Res.*, 293, 325, 2001.

57. Steinhoff, M., Brzoska, T., and Luger, T.A., Role of keratinocytes in epidermal immune response, *Trends All. Clin. Immunol.*, 1, 27, 2001.
58. Kampfer, H., Paulukat, J., Muhl, H., Wetzler, C., Pfeilschifter, J., and Frank, S., Lack of interferon-gamma production despite the presence of interleukin-18 during cutaneous wound healing, *Mol. Med.*, 6, 1016, 2000.
59. Lametschwandtner, G., Biedermann, T., Schwarzler, C., Gunther, C., Kund, J., Fassl, S., Hinteregger, S., Carballido-Perrig, N., Szabo, S.J., Glimcher, L.H., and Carballido, J.M., Sustained T-bet expression confers polarized human TH2 cells with TH1-like cytokine production and migratory capacities, *J. Allergy Clin. Immunol.*, 113, 987, 2004.
60. Parrish-Novak, J., Foster, D.C., Holly, R.D., and Clegg, C.H., Interleukin-21 and the IL-21 receptor: novel effectors of NK and T cell responses, *J. Leukoc. Biol.*, 72, 856, 2002.
61. Wiekowski, M.T., Leach, M.W., Evans, E.W., Sullivan, L., Chen, S.C., Vassileva, G., Bazan, J.F., Gorman, D.M., Kastelein, R.A., Narula, S., and Lira, S.A., Ubiquitous transgenic expression of the IL-23 subunit p19 induces multiorgan inflammation, runting, infertility, and premature death, *J. Immunol.*, 166, 7563, 2001.
62. Kopp, T., Lenz, P., Bello-Fernandez, C., Kastelein, R.A., Kupper, T.S., and Stingl, G., IL-23 production by cosecretion of endogenous p19 and transgenic p40 in keratin 14/p40 transgenic mice: evidence for enhanced cutaneous immunity, *J. Immunol.*, 170, 5438, 2003.
63. Hurst, S.D., Muchamuel, T., Gorman, D.M., Gilbert, J.M., Clifford, T., Kwan, S., Menon, S., Seymour, B., Jackson, C., Kung, T.T., Brieland, J.K., Zurawski, S.M., Chapman, R.W., Zurawski, G., and Coffman, R.L., New IL-17 family members promote Th1 or Th2 responses in the lung: *in vivo* function of the novel cytokine IL-25, *J. Immunol.*, 169, 443, 2002
64. Pflanz, S., Timans, J., Cheung, J., Rosales, R., Kanzler, H., Gilbert, J., Hibbert, L., Churakowa, T., Travis, M., Vaisberg, E., Blumenschein, W., Mattson, J., Wagner, J., To, W., Zurawski, S., McClanahan, T.K., Gorman, D., Bazan, J., de Waal Malefyt, R., Rennik, D., and Kastelein, R., IL-27, a heterodimeric cytokine composed of EBI3 and p28 protein, induces proliferation of naive CD4+ T cells, *Immunity*, 16, 779, 2002.
65. Trinchieri, G., Interleukin-12 and the regulation of innate resistance and adaptive immunity, *Nat. Rev. Immunol.*, 3, 133, 2003.
66. Lucas, S., Ghilardi, N., Li, J., and de Sauvage, F.J., IL-27 regulates IL-12 responsiveness of naive CD4+ T cells through Stat1-dependent and -independent mechanisms, *Proc. Natl. Acad. Sci. U. S. A.*, 100, 15047, 2003.
66a. Dillon, S.R., Sprecher, C., Hammond, A., Bilsborough, J., Rosenfeld-Franklin, M., Presnell, S.R., Haugen, H.S., Maurer, M., Harder, B., Johnston, J., Bort, S., Mudri, S., Kiujper, J.L., Bukowski, T., Shea, P., Dong, D.L., Dasovich, M., Grant, F.J., Lockwood, L., Levin, S.D., LeCiel, C., Waggie, K., Day, H., Topouzis, S., Kramer, J., Kuesner, R., Chen, Z., Foster, D., Parrish-Novak, J., and Gross, J.A., Interleukin 31, a cytokine produced by activated T cells, induces dermatitis in mice, *Nat. Immunol.*, 5(7), 752–760, 2004.
67. Fernandez-Botran, R., Soluble cytokine receptors: their role in immuno-regulation, *FASEB J.*, 5, 2567, 1991.
68. Sims, J.E., Gayle, M.A., Slack, J.L., et al., Interleukin 1 signalling occurs exclusively via the type I receptor, *Proc. Natl. Acad. Sci. U.S.A.*, 90, 6155, 1993.
69. Dinarello, C.A., Interleukin-1 and interleukin-1 antagonism, *Blood*, 77, 1627, 1991.
70. Dripps, D.J., Brandhuber, B.J., Thompson, R.C., and Eisenberg, S.P., Interleukin-1 (IL-1) receptor antagonist binds to the 80-kDa IL-1 receptor but does not initiate IL-1 signal transduction, *J. Biol. Chem.*, 266, 10331, 1991.
71. Fickenscher, H., Hor, S., Kupers, H., Knappe, A., Wittmann, S., and Sticht, H., The interleukin-10 family of cytokines, *Trends Immunol.*, 23, 89, 2002.
72. Knappe, A., Hor, S., Wittmann, S., and Fickenscher, H., Induction of a novel cellular homolog of interleukin-10, AK155, by transformation of T lymphocytes with herpesvirus saimiri, *J. Virol.*, 74, 3881, 2000.
73. Conti, P., Kempuraj, D., Frydas, S., Kandere, K., Boucher, W., Letourneau, R., Madhappan, B., Sagimoto, K., Christodoulou, S., and Theoharides, T.C., IL-10 subfamily members: IL-19, IL-20, IL-22, IL-24 and IL-26, *Immunol. Lett.*, 88, 171, 2003.
74. Berg, D.J., Leach, M.W., Kuhn, R., Rajewsky, K., Muller, W., Davidson, N.J., and Rennick, D., Interleukin 10 but not interleukin 4 is a natural suppressant of cutaneous inflammatory responses, *J. Exp. Med.*, 182, 99, 1995.

75. Enk, A.H., Saloga, J., Becker, D., Mohamadzadeh, M., and Knop, J., Induction of hapten-specific tolerance by interleukin 10 *in vivo*, *J. Exp. Med.*, 182, 99, 1994.
76. Nickoloff, B.J., Fivenson, D.P., Kunkel, S.L., Strieter, R.M., and Turka, L.A., Keratinocytes interleukin-10 expression is upregulated in tape-stripped skin, poison ivy dermatitis and Sezary syndrome, but not in psoriatic plaques, *Clin. Immunol. Immunopathol.*, 73, 63, 1994.
77. Asadullah, K., Docke, W.D., Sabat, R.V., Volk, H.D., and Sterry, W., The treatment of psoriasis with IL-10: rationale and review of the first clinical trials, *Expert. Opin. Investig. Drugs*, 9, 95, 2000.
78. Asadullah, K., Sterry, W., and Volk, H.D., Interleukin-10 therapy—review of a new approach, *Pharmacol. Rev.*, 55, 241, 2003.
79. Chen, Q., Ghilardi, N., Wang, H., Baker, T., Xie, M.H., Gurney, A., Grewal, I.S., and de Sauvage, F.J., Development of Th1-type immune responses requires the type I cytokine receptor TCCR, *Nature*, 407, 916, 2000.
80. Romer, J., Hasselager, E., Norby, P.L., Steiniche, T., Thorn Clausen, J., and Kragballe, K., Epidermal overexpression of interleukin-19 and -20 mRNA in psoriatic skin disappears after short-term treatment with cyclosporine a or calcipotriol, *J. Invest. Dermatol.*, 121, 1306, 2003.
81. Xie, M.H., Aggarwal, S., Ho, W.H., Foster, J., Zhang, Z., Stinson, J., Wood, W.I., Goddard, A.D., and Gurney, A.L., Interleukin (IL)-22, a novel human cytokine that signals through the interferon receptor-related proteins CRF2-4 and IL-22R, *J. Biol. Chem.*, 275, 31335, 2000.
82. Pestka, S., Krause, C.D., Sarkar, D., Walter, M.R., Shi, Y., and Fisher, P.B., Interleukin-10 and related cytokines and receptors, *Annu. Rev. Immunol.*, 22, 929, 2004.
83. Chada, S., Sutton, R.B., Ekmekcioglu, S., Ellerhorst, J., Mumm, J.B., Leitner, W.W., Yang, H.Y., Sahin, A.A., Hunt, K.K., Fuson, K.L., Poindexter, N., Roth, J.A., Ramesh, R., Grimm, E.A., and Mhashilkar, A.M., MDA-7/IL-24 is a unique cytokine–tumor suppressor in the IL-10 family, *Int. Immunopharmacol.*, 4, 649, 2004.
84. Langer, J.A., Cutrone, E.C., and Kotenko, S., The Class II cytokine receptor (CRF2) family: overview and patterns of receptor-ligand interactions, *Cytokine Growth Factor Rev.*, 15 33, 2004.
85. Hor, S., Pirzer, H., Dumoutier, L., Bauer, F., Wittmann, S., Sticht, H., Renauld, J.C., de waal Malefyt, R., and Fickenscher, H., The T-cell lymphokine interleukin-26 targets epithelial cells through the interleukin-20 receptor 1 and interleukin-10 receptor 2 chains, *J. Biol. Chem.*, 2004.
86. Sheppard, P., Kindsvogel, W., Xu, W., Henderson, K., Schlutsmeyer, S., Whitmore, T.E., Kuestner, R., Garrigues, U., Birks, C., Roraback, J., Ostrander, C., Dong, D., Shin, J., Presnell, S., Fox, B., Haldeman, B., Cooper, E., Taft, D., Gilbert, T., Grant, F.J., Tackett, M., Krivan, W., McKnight, G., Clegg, C., Foster, D., and Klucher, K.M., IL-28, IL-29 and their class II cytokine receptor IL-28R, *Nat. Immunol.*, 4, 63, 2003.
87. Companjen, A.R., van der Wel, L.I., Boon, L., Prens, E.P.,and Laman, J.D., CD40 ligation-induced cytokine production in human skin explants is partly mediated via IL-1, *Int. Immunol.*, 14, 669, 2002.
88. Arend, W.P., Malyak, M., Guthridge, C.J., and Gabay, C., Interleukin-1 receptor antagonist: role in biology, *Annu. Rev. Immunol.*, 16, 27, 1998.
89. Kupper, T.S. and Groves, R.W., The interleukin-1 axis and cutaneous inflammation, *J. Invest. Dermatol.*, 105, 62, 1995.
90. Dickinson, A.M., Cavet, J., Cullup, H., Wang, X.N., Jarvis, M., Sviland, L.,and Middleton, P.G., Predicting outcome in hematological stem cell transplantation, *Arch. Immunol. Ther. Exp. (Warsz.)*, 50, 371, 2002.
91. Granowitz, E.V., Clark, B.D., Mancilla, J., and Dinarello, C.A., Interleukin-1 receptor antagonist competitively inhibits the binding of interleukin-1 to the type II interleukin-1 receptor, *J. Biol. Chem.*, 266, 14147, 1991.
92. Kupper, T.S. and Groves, R.W., The interleukin-1 axis and cutaneous inflammation, *J. Invest. Dermatol.*, 105, 625, 1995.
93. Hannum, C.H., Wilcox, C.J., Arend, W.P. et al., Interleukin-1 receptor antagonist activity of a human interleukin-1 inhibitor, *Nature*, 343, 336, 1990.
94. James, K., Interactions between cytokines and α2-macroglobulin, *Immunol. Today*, 11, 163, 1990.
95. Borth, W. and Luger, T.A., Identification of α2-macroglobulin as a cytokine binding plasma protein, *J. Biol. Chem.*, 264, 5818, 1989.
96. Krutmann, J., Schwarz, T., Kirnbauer, R., Urbanski, A., and Luger, T.A., Epidermal cell-contra-interleukin 1 inhibits human accessory cell function by specifically blocking interleukin 1 activity, *Photochem. Photobiol.*, 52, 783, 1990.

97. Chen, W.J., Frank, M. E., Jin, W. et al., TGF-b released by apoptotic T cell contributive to an imunosuppressive milieu, *Immunity*, 14, 715, 2001.
98. Nardelli, B., Zaritskaya, L., Semenuk, M., Cho, Y.H., LaFleur, D.W., Shah, D., Ullrich, S., Girolomoni, G., Albanesi, C., and Moore, P.A., Regulatory effect of IFN-kappa, a novel type I IFN, on cytokine production by cells of the innate immune system, *J. Immunol.*, 169, 4822, 2002.
99. Chang, Y.E. and Laimins, L.A., Microarray analysis identifies interferon-inducible genes and Stat-1 as major transcriptional targets of human papillomavirus type 31, *J. Virol.*, 74, 4174, 2000.
100. Bashman, T.Y., Nickoloff, B.J., Merigan, T.C., et al., Recombinant gamma interferon induces HLA-DR expression on cultured human keratinocytes, *J. Invest. Dermatol.*, 83, 88, 1984.
101. Kaplan, G., Witmer, M.D., Nath, I. et al., Influence of delayed immune reactions on human epidermal keratinocytes, *Proc. Natl. Acad. Sci. U.S.A.*, 3, 3469, 1986.
102. Kelly, V.E., Fiers, W., and Strom, T.B., Cloned human interferon-g but not interferon-b or -a induces expression of HLA-DR determinants by fetal monocytes and myeloid leukaemic cell lines, *J. Immunol.*, 132, 240, 1984.
103. Schwarz, G., Boehncke, W.H., Braun, M., Schroter, C.J., Burster, T., Flad, T., Dressel, D., Weber, E., Schmid, H., and Kalbacher, H., Cathepsin S activity is detectable in human keratinocytes and is selectively upregulated upon stimulation with interferon-gamma, *J. Invest. Dermatol.*, 119, 44, 2002.
104. Trompezinski, S., Denis, A., Schmitt, D., and Viac, J., IL-10 is unable to downregulate VEGF expression in human activated keratinocytes, *Arch. Dermatol. Res.*, 294, 377, 2002.
105. Nedwin, G.E., Svedersky, L.P., Bringham, T.S. et al., Effect of interleukin 2, interferon gamma and mitogens on the production of tumour necrosis factor alpha and beta, *J. Immunol.* 135, 2492, 1985.
106. Herrmann, F., Cannistra, S.A., Levine, H. et al., Expression of interleukin 2 receptors and binding of interleukin 2 by gamma-interferon-induced human leukaemic and normal monocytic cells, *J. Exp. Med.*, 162, 1111, 1985.
107. Herberman, R.B., Ortaldo, J.R., Djeu, J.Y. et al., Role of interferon in regulation of cytotoxicity by natural killer cells and macrophages, *Ann. N.Y. Acad. Sci.*, 350, 63, 1980.
108. Boraschi, D., Censini, S., Bartalini, M. et al., Regulation of arachidonic acid metabolism in macrophages by immune and non-immune interferons, *J. Immunol.*, 135, 502, 1985.
109. Rodriguez, M.A., Prinz, W.A., Sibbitt, W.L. et al., $\alpha$-Interferon increases immunoglobulin production in cultured human mononuclear leukocytes, *J. Immunol.* 130, 1215, 1983.
110. Alenius, H., La, Mast cells regulate IFN-gamma expression in the skin and circulating IgE levels in allergen-induced skin inflammation, *J. Allergy Clin. Immunol.*, 109, 106–113, 2002.
111. Sasseville, D., Ghamdi, W.A., and Khenaizan, S.A., Interferon-induced cutaneous necrosis, *J. Cutan. Med. Surg.*, 35, 917, 1999.
112. Schrader, J.W., Colony stimulating factors and the skin, in *Epidermal Growth Factors and Cytokines.*, Luger, T.A. and Schwarz, T., Eds., Marcel Dekker, Inc., New York, 1993, 147.
113. Langer, J.C., Henckaerts, E., Orenstein, J., and Snoeck, H.W., Quantitative trait analysis reveals transforming growth-factor-{beta}$\Sigma$ as a positive regulator of early hematopoietic progenitor and stem cell Function, *J. Exp. Med.*, 199, 5, 2004.
114. Sun, Y., Chen, H.M., Subudhi, S.K., Chen, J., Koka, R., Chen, L., and Fu, Y.X., Costimulatory molecule-targeted antibody therapy of a spontaneous autoimmune disease, *Nat. Med.*, 8, 1405, 2002.
115. Vollmer, P., Peters, M., Ehlers, M., Yagame, H., Matsuba, T., Kondo, M., Yasukawa, K., Buschenfelde, K.H., and Rose-John, S., Yeast expression of the cytokine receptor domain of the soluble interleukin-6 receptor, *J. Immunol. Meth.*, 199, 47, 1996.
116. Rameshwar, P., Zhu, G., Donnelly, R.J., Qian, J., Ge, H., Goldstein, K.R., Denny, T.N., and Gascon, P., The dynamics of bone marrow stromal cells in the proliferation of multipotent hematopoietic progenitors by substance P: an understanding of the effects of a neurotransmitter of the differentiating hematopoietic stem cell, *J. Neuroimmunol.*, 121, 22, 2001.
117. Lieschke, G.J. and Burgess, A.W., Granulocyte colony-stimulating factor and granulocyte-macrophage colony-stimulating fator, *N. Engl. J. Med.*, 327, 28, 1992.
118. Husain, B., Lendemans, S., Ackermann, M., Wendel, A., Schade, F.U., and Flohe, S., GM-CSF counteracts hemorrhage-induced suppression of cytokine-producing capacity, *Inflamm. Res.*, 53, 13, 2004.
119. Tavernier, J., Devos, R., Cornelis, S., Tuypens, T., Van der Heyden, J., Fiers, W., and Plaetinck, G., A human high affinity interleukin-5 receptor (IL5R) is composed of an IL5-specific alpha chain and a beta chain shared with the receptor for GM-CSF, *Cell*, 66, 1175, 1991.

120. Dranoff, G., Crawford, A.D., Sadelain, M., Ream, B., Rashid, A., Bronson, R.T., Dickersin, G.R., Bachurski, C.J., Mark, E.L., Whitsett, J.A. et al., Involvement of granulocyte-macrophage colony-stimulating factor in pulmonary homeostasis, *Science*, 264, 713, 1994.
121. Schwarz, T. and Luger, T.A., Pharmacology of cytokines in the skin, in *Pharmacology of the Skin*, Muhktar, H., Ed., CRC Press, Boca Raton, FL, 1992, 283.
122. Nozaki, S., Abrams, J.S., Pearce, M.K., and Sauder, D.N., Augmentation of granulocyte/macrophage colony-stimulating factor expression by ultraviolet irradiation is mediated by interleukin 1 in Pam 212 keratinocytes, *J. Invest. Dermatol.,* 97, 10, 1991.
123. Becker, D. and Knop, J., Epidermal cell-derived cytokines and delayed-type hypersensitivity., in *Epidermal Growth Factors and Cytokines.*, Luger, T.A. and Schwarz, T., Eds., Marcel Dekker, Inc., New York, 1993, 365.
124. Romani, N., Heufler, C., Koch, F., Topar, G., Kämpgen, E., and Schuler, G., Cytokines and Langerhans cells, in *Epidermal Growth Factors and Cytokines.*, Luger, T.A. and T. Schwarz, Eds., Marcel Dekker, Inc., New York, 1993, 345.
125. Denfeld, R.W., Hara, H., Tesmann, J.P., Martin, S., and Simon, J.C., UVB-irradiated dendritic cells are impaired in their APC function and tolerize primed Th1 cells but not naive CD4+ T cells, *J. Leukoc. Biol.*, 69, 548, 2001.
126. Rupec, R., Magerstaedt, R., Schirren, C.G., Sander, E., and Bieber, T., Granulocyte/macrophage-colony stimulating factor induces the migration of human epidermal langerhans cells *in vitro*, *Exp. Dermatol.*, 5, 115, 1996.
127. Noirey, N., Staquet, M.J., Gariazzo, M.J., Serres, M., Dezutter-Dambuyant, C., Andre, C., Schmitt, D., and Vincent, C., Withdrawal of TNF-alpha after the fifth day of differentiation of CD34+ cord blood progenitors generates a homogeneous population of Langerhans cells and delays their maturation, *Exp. Dermatol.*, 12, 96, 2003.
128. Grabbe, S. and Granstein, R. D., Mechanisms of ultraviolet radiation carcinogenesis, in *Mechanisms of Immune Regulation.*, Granstein, R.D., Ed., Karger, Basel, 1994, 291.
129. Kaplan, G., Walsh, G., Guido, L.S., Meyn, P., Burkhardt, R.A., Abalos, R.M., Barker, J., Frindt, P.A., Fajardo, T.T., Celona, R., and Cohn, Z.A., Novel responses of human skin to intradermal granulocyte/macrophage-colony-stimulating factor: Langerhans cell recruitment, keratinocyte growth, and enhanced wound healing, *J. Exp. Med.*, 175, 1717, 1992.
130. El Ouriaghli, F., Fujiwara, H., Melenhorst, J.J., Sconocchia, G., Hensel, N., and Barrett, A.J., Neutrophil elastase enzymatically antagonizes the *in vitro* action of G-CSF: implications for the regulation of granulopoiesis, *Blood,* 101, 1752, 2003.
131. Kobayashi, N., Saeki, K., and Yuo, A., Granulocyte-macrophage colony-stimulating factor and interleukin-3 induce cell cycle progression through the synthesis of c-Myc protein by internal ribosome entry site-mediated translation via phosphatidylinositol 3-kinase pathway in human factor-dependent leukemic cells, *Blood,* 102, 3186, 2003.
132. Moore, M.A.S. Interleukin-3, an overview, in *Lymphokines, Vol. 15*, Schrader, J.W., Ed., Academic Press, San Diego, 1988, 219.
133. Luger, T.A., Köck, A., Kirnbauer, R., Schwarz, T., and Ansel, J.C., Keratinocyte-derived interleukin 3, *Ann. N.Y. Acad. Sci.*, 548, 253, 1988.
134. Köck, A., Schwarz, T., Micksche, M., and Luger, T.A., Cytokines and human malignant melanoma. Immuno- and growth regulatory peptides in melanoma biology, in *Cancer Treatment and Research, Vol. 5*, Nathanson, L., Ed., Kluwer Academic, Norwell, MA, 1991, 41.
135. Mollah, Z.U., Aiba, S., Nakagawa, S., Mizuashi, M., Ohtani, T., Yoshino, Y., and Tagami, H., Interleukin-3 in cooperation with transforming growth factor beta induces granulocyte macrophage colony stimulating factor independent differentiation of human CD34+ hematopoietic progenitor cells into dendritic cells with features of Langerhans cells, *J. Invest. Dermatol.,* 121, 1397, 2003.
136. Dalloul, A.H., Arock, M., Fourcade, C., Beranger, J.Y., Jaffray, P., Debre, P., and Mossalayi, M.D., Epidermal keratinocyte-derived basophil promoting activity. Role of interleukin-3 and soluble CD23., *J. Clin. Invest.*, 90, 1242, 1992.
137. Cosman, D., Colony-stimulating factors *in vivo* and *in vitro*, *Immunol. Today*, 9, 97, 1988.
138. Nicola, N.A. and Metcalf, D., Subunit promiscuity among hemopoietic growth factor receptors, *Cell*, 67, 1, 1991.

139. Richards, M.K., Liu, F., Iwasaki, H., Akashi, K., and Link, D.C., Pivotal role of granulocyte colony-stimulating factor in the development of progenitors in the common myeloid pathway, *Blood*, 102, 3562, 2003.
140. Chodakewitz, J.A., Lacy, J., Edwards, S.E., Birchall, N., and Coleman, D.L., Macrophage colony-stimulating factor production by murine and human keratinocytes. Enhancement by bacterial lipopolysaccharide, *J. Immunol.*, 144, 2190, 1990.
141. Mollah, Z.U., Aiba, S., Nakagawa, S., Mizuashi, M., Ohtani, T., Yoshino, Y., and Tagami, H., Interleukin-3 in cooperation with transforming growth factor beta induces granulocyte macrophage colony stimulating factor independent differentiation of human CD34+ hematopoietic progenitor cells into dendritic cells with features of Langerhans cells, *J. Invest. Dermatol.,* 121, 1397, 2003.
142. Geissler, E.N., Liao, M., Brook, J.D., Martin, F.H., Zsebo, K.M., Housman, D.E., and Galli, S.J., Stem cell factor (SCF), a novel hematopoietic growth factor and ligand for c-kit tyrosine kinase receptor, maps on human chromosome 12 between 12q14.3 and 12qter, *Somat. Cell Mol. Genet.*, 17, 207, 1991.
143. Williams, D.E., Eisenman, J., Baird, A., Rauch, C., Van Ness, K., March, C.J., Park, L.S., Martin, U., Mochizuki, D.Y., Boswell, H.S. et al., Identification of a ligand for the c-kit proto-oncogene, *Cell*, 63, 167, 1990.
144. Grabbe, J., Welker, P., Dippel, E., and Czarnetzki, B.M., Stem cell factor, a novel cutaneous growth factor for mast cells and melanocytes, *Arch. Dermatol. Res.*, 287, 78, 1994.
145. Nakamura, K., Tanaka, T., Morita, E., Kameyoshi, Y., and Yamamoto, S., Enhancement of fibroblast-dependent mast cell growth in mice by a conditioned medium of keratinocyte-derived squamous cell carcinoma cells, *Arch. Dermatol. Res.*, 287, 91, 1994.
146. Weiss, R.R., Whitaker Menezes, D., Longley, J., Bender, J., and Murphy, G.F., Human dermal endothelial cells express membrane-associated mast cell growth factor, *J. Invest. Dermatol.*, 104, 101, 1995.
147. Tsuji, K., Zsebo, K.M., and Ogawa, M., Murine mast cell colony formation supported by IL-3, IL-4, and recombinant rat stem cell factor, ligand for c-kit, *J. Cell Physiol.*, 148, 362, 1991.
148. Lora, J.M., Al-Garawi, A., Pickard, M.D., Price, K.S., Bagga, S., Sicoli, J., Hodge, M.R., Gutierrez-Ramos, J.C., Briskin, M.J., and Boyce, J.A., FcepsilonRI-dependent gene expression in human mast cells in differentially controlled by T helper type 2 cytokines, *J. Allergy Clin. Immunol.*, 112, 1119, 2003.
149. Lee, E., Min, H.K., Oskeritzian, C.A., Kambe, N., Schwartz, L.B., and Wook Chang, H., Recombinant human (rh) stem cell factor and rhIL-4 stimulate differentiation and proliferation of CD3(+) cells from umbilical cord blood and CD3(+) cells enhance FcepsilonR1 expression on fetal liver-derived mast cells in the presence of rhIL-4, *Cell Immunol.,* 226, 30, 2003.
150. Longley, B.J., Jr., Morganroth, G.S., Tyrrell, L., Ding, T.G., Anderson, D.M., Williams, D.E., and Halaban, R., Altered metabolism of mast-cell growth factor (c-kit ligand) in cutaneous mastocytosis, *N. Engl. J. Med.*, 328, 1302, 1993.
151. Young, J.W., Szabolcs, P., and Moore, M.A., Identification of dendritic cell colony-forming units among normal human CD34+ bone marrow progenitors that are expanded by c-kit-ligand and yield pure dendritic cell colonies in the presence of granulocyte/macrophage colony-stimulating factor and tumor necrosis factor alpha, *J. Exp. Med.*, 182, 1111, 1995.
152. Szabolcs, P., Moore, M.A., and Young, J.W., Expansion of immunostimulatory dendritic cells among the myeloid progeny of human CD34+ bone marrow precursors cultured with c-kit ligand, granulocyte-macrophage colony-stimulating factor, and TNF-alpha, *J. Immunol.*, 154, 5851, 1995.
153. Giebel, L.B. and Spritz, R.A., Mutation of the KIT (mast/stem cell growth factor receptor) protooncogene in human piebaldism, *Proc. Natl. Acad. Sci. U.S.A.*, 88, 8696, 1991.
154. Tsujimura, T., Hirota, S., Nomura, S., Niwa, Y., Yamazaki, M., Tono, T., Morii, E., Kim, H.M., Kondo, K., Nishimune, Y. et al., Characterization of Ws mutant allele of rats: a 12-base deletion in tyrosine kinase domain of c-kit gene, *Blood*, 78, 1942, 1991.

# 16 Chemokines of Human Skin

*Saveria Pastore, Andrea Cavani, Cristina Albanesi, and Giampiero Girolomoni*

## CONTENTS



## I. INTRODUCTION

The skin provides a major boundary between the host and the external environment, and consequently it is adequately equipped to mount effective immune responses against microorganisms and other environmental threats. The skin is also a frequent site of hypersensitivity reactions against apparently harmless antigens, such as the haptens causing allergic contact dermatitis (ACD), and of complex immunopathological reactions with a strong genetic component, such as atopic dermatitis (AD) and psoriasis. Dendritic cells (DCs), including epidermal Langerhans cells (LCs) and dermal DCs, are specialized in the recognition and capture of foreign antigens as well as in the activation of naive T cells, all essential steps in the induction of immune responses. Finally, T lymphocytes transduce antigen recognition into effector mechanisms to eliminate pathogens. The recruitment of T cells and other leukocytes at the site of skin inflammation is therefore the critical step for an efficient response to potentially dangerous signals. Keratinocytes, mast cells, and endothelial cells, which constitute the static component of the skin immune system, as well as DCs, attract discrete T-cell subsets in the skin via the release of a variety of chemoattractants, including lipid metabolites and proteins. This chapter specifically focuses on the role of chemokines in skin inflammation. We discuss the vast body of experimental evidence that documents the unique potential of chemokines to selectively attract distinct leukocyte subtypes to the restricted site of a skin lesion, and their implication not only in the perpetuation of inflammation, but also in complete tissue repair.

0-8493-1959-5/05/$0.00+$1.50

## II. CHEMOKINES AND THEIR RECEPTORS

### A. Redundancy of the Chemokine–Chemokine Receptor System

Chemokines are a superfamily of structurally related, small (6 to 14 kDa) proteins that regulate the traffic of various types of leukocytes, including lymphocytes, DCs, monocytes, neutrophils, and eosinophils.[1–6] Advances in molecular cloning techniques as well as the development of expressed sequence tag databases allowed the rapid identification of a vast array of chemokine-related genes, and, to date, more than 50 human chemokines have been characterized (see http://cytokine.medic.kumamoto-u.ac.jp/). Chemokines are classified in four subfamilies according to the position of two highly conserved cysteine residues at the N-terminus of the molecule (Table 16.1). Upon secretion, chemokines bind to extracellular matrix and cell membrane proteoglycans forming stable gradients from the site of their production. CX3CL1/Fractalkine is an exception, as it is expressed as a membrane integral protein that can be shed from the membrane.[7] Although their main function is to regulate cell trafficking, chemokines also play important roles in governing leukocyte activation and differentiation.[8,9] The specific effects of chemokines on target cells are mediated by seven transmembrane-spanning, G –protein–coupled receptors.[10,11] To date, about 20 chemokine receptor-encoding genes have been identified, mostly located in clusters on chromosomes 2 and 3 (Table 16.1). Of note, the chemokine–chemokine receptor axis is often highly promiscuous, allowing a single chemokine to bind different receptors and a chemokine receptor to be activated by distinct chemokines. In contrast to this notion, some recently identified chemokines show a very high receptor and tissue specificity, and are thought to contribute to tissue-restricted leukocyte trafficking.[12,13] In particular, CCL27/CTACK is predominantly expressed in the skin and binds specifically CCR10.[14,15] Also the CCL17/TARC-CCR4 system has been proposed to be determinant for the selective homing of CCR4-bearing T lymphocytes to inflamed skin.[12] Moreover, the same chemokine may initiate different signals according to the bound receptor: for example, CXCL9/Mig, CXCL10/IP-10, and CXCL11/I-TAC are agonists to CXCR3, but they also bind CCR3, antagonizing receptor activation by CCR3 ligands.[16] Similarly, CCL11/eotaxin is a natural agonist for CCR3 and CCR5 and an antagonist for CCR2 and CXCR3.[17–19] These data support the concept of the opposing roles of CCR3 and CXCR3 in Th1/Th2 polarization.

Depending on their function, regulation, and site of production, chemokines can be classified as "inflammatory" and "lymphoid," these last known also as "homeostatic." Inflammatory chemokines are expressed in inflamed tissues by resident or infiltrating cells, and recruit effector cells. Homeostatic chemokines, such as CCL19/ELC/MIP3-β and CXCL13/BCA1, are primarily produced within lymphoid tissues and are involved in the maintenance of the constitutive lymphocyte traffic and cell compartmentalization within these organs.[1,4,6] Also the CCL21(SLC)/CCR7 axis was conceived as being essentially involved in a pure homeostatic function, exclusively controlling the appropriate naive T-cell migration to secondary lymphoid organs.[1] Quite recently, however, this axis has been found prominently upregulated in skin sites affected by distinct T-cell-mediated skin diseases, including AD, graft-vs.-host-disease, and lichen planus, with CCL21 over-induced in endothelial cells and CCR7 highly expressed on infiltrating cells, including memory T cells and DCs.[20]

### B. Chemokine Receptors on T-Cell Subsets

T-lymphocyte circulation in peripheral tissues encompasses a series of complex events including adhesion to endothelial cells mediated by selectins, integrins, and adhesion molecules and by the local expression of chemotactic stimuli.[21] Chemokines are physiological activators of rapid lymphocyte arrest along high endothelial venules (HEV) in secondary lymphoid organs, and play a central role in selective tissue homing. Transient tethering and rolling precede firm adhesion of circulating leukocytes and are essential to slow leukocyte motion, thus facilitating microenvironmental sampling and subsequent interaction with pro-adhesive chemokines presented by the

**TABLE 16.1**
**Principal Human Chemokines and Chemokine Receptors**

| Systematic Name | Current Name | Receptor(s) |
|---|---|---|
| | **CXC Family** | |
| CXCL1 | Growth-related oncogene (GRO)-α, MGSA-α, NAP-3 | CXCR2 |
| CXCL2 | GRO-β, MGSA-β, MIP-2α | CXCR2 |
| CXCL3 | GRO-γ, MGSA-γ, MIP-2β | CXCR2 |
| CXCL4 | PF4 | Unknown |
| CXCL5 | ENA-78 | CXCR1, CXCR2 |
| CXCL6 | GCP-2, CKA-3 | CXCR1 |
| CXCL7 | NAP-2 | CXCR2 |
| CXCL8 | IL-8 | CXCR1, CXCR2 |
| CXCL9 | Monokine-induced by IFN-γ (Mig) | CXCR3, *CCR3** |
| CXCL10 | IFN-induced protein of 10 kDa (IP-10), C7 | CXCR3, *CCR3** |
| CXCL11 | IFN-induced T-cell α-chemoattractant (I-TAC), IP-9 | CXCR3, *CCR3** |
| CXCL12 | Stromal-derived factor (SDF)-1α/β | CXCR4 |
| CXCL13 | B-cell-activating chemokine (BCA)-1, BLC | CXCR5 |
| CXCL14 | Breast and kidney chemokine (BRAK), bolekine, MIP-2γ | Unknown |
| CXCL15 | Lungkine | Unknown |
| CXCL16 | SR-PSOX | CXCR6 |
| | **CC Family** | |
| CCL1 | I-309 | CCR8 |
| CCL2 | Monocyte chemotactic protein (MCP)-1, MCAF, SMC-CF. | CCR1, 2 |
| CCL3L1 | LD78β | CCR1, CCR5 |
| CCL3 | Macrophage inflammatory protein (MIP)-1α, LD78α, SISα | CCR1, CCR5 |
| CCL4 | MIP-1β, LAG-1 | CCR1, CCR5 |
| CCL5 | Regulation and activated normal T cell expressed and secreted (RANTES) | CCR1, CCR3, CCR5 |
| CCL7 | MCP-3 | CCR1, 2, 3, *CCR5** |
| CCL8 | MCP-2 | CCR1, 2, 3, 4, 5 |
| CCL11 | Eotaxin-1 | CCR3, CCR5, *CXCR3,** *CCR2** |
| CCL13 | MCP-4, NCC-1 | CCR1, 2, 3, CCR5 |
| CCL14 | HCC-1, HCC-3, NCC-2 | CCR1, 3, 5 |
| CCL15 | HCC-2, Lkn-1, MIP-1δ, NCC-3 | CCR1, 3 |
| CCL16 | HCC-4, LEC, NCC-4 | CCR1 |
| CCL17 | Thymus- and activation-regulated chemokine (TARC) | CCR4 |
| CCL18 | Dendritic cell chemokine 1 (DC-CK1), PARC, AMAC-1, MIP-4 | Unknown |
| CCL19 | MIP-3β, ELC, exodus-3 | CCR7, 11 |
| CCL20 | MIP-3α, LARC, exodus-1, ST-38 | CCR6 |
| CCL21 | Secondary lymphoid tissue chemokine (SLC), 6Ckine, exodus-2 | CXCR3, CCR7, CCR11 |
| CCL22 | Macrophage-derived chemokine (MDC), STCP-1 | CCR4 |
| CCL23 | MPIF-1 | CCR1 |
| CCL24 | Eotaxin-2, MPIF-2 | CCR3 |
| CCL25 | Thymus-expressed chemokine (TECK) | CCR9, 11 |
| CCL26 | Eotaxin-3, MIP-4α | CCR3 |
| CCL27 | Cutaneous T-cell-attracting chemokine (CTACK), ILC | CCR10 |
| CCL28 | Mucosae-associated epithelial chemokine (MEC) | CCR10 |
| | **C Family** | |
| XCL1 | Lymphotactin, SCM-1α, ATAC | XCR1 |
| XCL2 | SCM-1β | XCR1 |
| | **CXXXC Family** | |
| CX3CL1 | Fractalkine | $CX_3CR1$ |

*Note:* Chemokine binding to the receptors in italics (*) antagonizes natural agonistic chemokines.

**TABLE 16.2**
**Chemokine Receptors Expressed by Resting/Activated CD4⁺ T-Cell Subsets**

| | CD4+ T Cells | | |
|---|---|---|---|
| | **Th1** | **Th2** | **Tr1** |
| CCR1 | ++/+ | ++/+ | ++/+ |
| CCR2 | ++/+ | ++/+ | ++/+ |
| CCR3 | –/– | +++/+ | +/+ |
| CCR4 | ±/+ | +++/+++ | ++/++ |
| CCR5 | +++/+ | +/± | ++/+ |
| CCR8 | –/– | ++/+ | +++/++ |
| CXCR1 | +/– | +/– | +/– |
| CXCR2 | –/– | –/– | –/– |
| CXCR3 | +++/+ | ±/– | ++/+ |
| CXCR4 | +/+ | +/+ | ++/+ |
| $CX_3CR1$ | +++/nd | ±/nd | nd |

*Note:* nd, not determined.

endothelial cells. Tethering and rolling of leukocytes on vessel walls are primarily mediated by specialized selectins and mucins. These relatively loose adhesive interactions are rapidly converted into integrin-dependent firm adhesion upon chemokine receptor engagement, and generation of intracellular signals. The functions of adhesion molecules and chemokine receptors are reciprocally regulated. Quantitative variations in chemokine receptor expression level and ligand engagement may alter the selectivity of integrin-dependent lymphocyte adhesive responses, suggesting a mechanism by which chemokine networks may either generate or break the specificity of lymphocyte subset recruitment.[22] On the other hand, adhesion molecule triggering changes chemokine receptor expression.

Chemokine receptor asset on T lymphocytes varies depending on their activation stage, differentiation pattern, and tissue targeting. Naive T lymphocytes are mostly home to lymph nodes, where they are experienced by antigen-loaded DCs that migrated from peripheral tissues. Physiologically, lymph node entry of naive T cells is regulated by the expression of CCR7, which is bound by SLC produced by the endothelial cells of the HEV.[23] CCR7–SLC interaction increases $\alpha_L\beta_2$ integrin adhesiveness for ICAM-1/2 on endothelial cells, thus promoting the processes of firm adhesion and transmigration of T cells. Once T cells have crossed the HEV, their interaction with DCs is favored by MIP-3β and CCL18/DC-CK1/PARC, which are secreted by DCs and which attract naive T lymphocytes via recognition of the MIP-3β cognate receptor CCR7. In addition, DCs are the most abundant source of CCL22/MDC and TARC, which bind CCR4 expressed on the surface of recently activated T cells.[1,24] Once experienced, T lymphocytes completely rearrange their chemokine receptor profile, and acquire new migratory capacity to allow their homing in peripheral tissues. Importantly, acquisition of discrete chemokine receptors parallels the differentiation and cytokine polarization of T cells (Table 16.2). T helper (Th) 1 lymphocytes are rich in CXCR3 and CCR5, whereas Th2 cells express CCR3, CCR4, and CCR8.[1,25,26] The recently identified T-regulatory (Tr) cells, producing high amounts of IL-10, co-express both Th1- and Th2-associated receptors, with high levels of CCR8 and moderate amounts of CCR7.[27,28] CCR8, together with CCR4, is also highly expressed on the recently identified CD4⁺CD25⁺ regulatory T cells.[29] These findings suggest that the CCR8/I-309 axis may have a central role in the recruitment of multiple T-cell populations involved in the control of peripheral immune responses. In contrast to the large body of information regarding the migratory behavior of CD4⁺ T cells, chemokine responsiveness of CD8⁺ T lymphocytes has been less investigated. Recent data indicate that skin-homing CD8+ T cytotoxic cells type 1 (Tc1) and type 2 (Tc2) cells both express high amount of CXCR3, whose expression in CD4+ cells is mainly limited to the Th1 subset, and promptly respond to IP-10 in chemotaxis assays. Conversely, Tc1 and Tc2 cells show lower expression of CCR4, when compared to Th1 and Th2 lymphocytes.[30] Thus, the local expression of chemokines during an inflammatory process may contribute to the selective accumulation of different T-cell subsets. Importantly, T-cell activation strongly affects chemokine receptor expression, with most receptors for inflammatory chemokines downregulated, except for CCR4 and CCR8, which are transiently upregulated.[26,31] Receptor down-regulation promotes a switch from a migratory to a stationary behavior, so that T lymphocytes can better exert their effector activities. Besides naive T cells, a pool of central memory T cells express CCR7.[32] Once activated, these lymphocytes upregulate CCR7 and migrate to lymph nodes, where they can provide strong help for DC maturation and differentiate into effector cells.

The existence of subsets of memory T cells that preferentially migrate to the skin is well documented. Most of the skin-homing T lymphocytes express the cutaneous lymphocyte-associated antigen (CLA), the ligand for E-selectin expressed by activated endothelial cells of the skin microvasculature.[33] It has been recently described that skin-seeking CD4+ T lymphocytes express CCR4 independent from their cytokine releasing profile. CCR4 permits T-lymphocyte adhesion to TARC, which is exposed on the surface of activated endothelium at the site of skin inflammation.[12] CCR4 triggering by TARC induces T-lymphocyte integrin activation and promotes the firm adhesion of circulating lymphocytes to the endothelium. CCR6, albeit also expressed in gut migrating lymphocytes, has been described as an important chemokine receptor that favors T-cell migration into the skin.[34] In particular, TNF-α-activated dermal microvascular endothelial cells produce large amounts of CCL20/MIP-3α, which is critical for the arrest of CCR6+ memory T cells.[35] Finally, CTACK is a newly identified tissue-specific chemokine predominantly produced by epidermal keratinocytes, which recruits CCR10+ skin-homing T lymphocytes into the inflamed skin.[14,15,36]

## C. Chemokine Production by Resident Skin Cells

Resident skin cells greatly contribute to T-lymphocyte recruitment during inflammation.[37] A limited amount of specific chemokines is expressed in unperturbed skin, and is probably involved in the basal trafficking of memory T cells and DCs, although no conclusive data are available so far. Keratinocytes are a relevant source of chemokines, with resting cells releasing low levels of CXCL8/IL-8 and expressing CTACK and CXCL12/SDF-1 mRNA.[14,38] Constitutive keratinocyte production of MIP-3α has been implicated in the basal recruitment of LCs in the epidermis,[39] although other groups have failed to show significant production by unstimulated keratinocytes or expression in normal epidermis.[15,40,41] Following activation, keratinocytes rapidly upregulate IL-8 and CTACK, and synthesize CXCL1/Gro-α, IP-10, Mig, I-TAC, CCL5/RANTES, CCL2/MCP-1, MIP-3α, MDC, and CCL1/I-309. TARC is constitutively expressed at very low levels by primary keratinocyte cultures, and its induction in response to cytokines has been shown by Vestergaard et al.,[42] but we were not able to confirm this finding.[22,43] IP-10, MCP-1, and IL-8 are the most abundant chemokines released by activated keratinocytes. *In vitro* investigations have indicated that inflammatory and T-cell-derived cytokines are the most potent stimuli for keratinocyte activation. In particular, IL-1 and TNF-α strongly induce MIP-3α, RANTES, and IL-8.[40,41,44] Type 1 cytokine IFN-γ, alone or together with TNF-α, rapidly promotes the secretion of very high levels of CXCR3 agonists and MCP-1, and low amounts of I-309 and MDC.[43,44] IL-17, a cytokine produced by part of Th1 and Th2 lymphocytes, modulates the effects of IFN-γ on keratinocytes by augmenting IL-8, and decreasing RANTES release.[44,45] Notably, IL-4, a type 2 cytokine, enhances IFN-γ-induced release of IP-10, Mig, and I-TAC by cultured keratinocytes,[46] indicating that the Th2 to Th1 switch observed in some chronic inflammatory skin diseases (e.g., AD) could partly depend on the predilection of keratinocytes to release Th1-active chemokines.[43]

Keratinocytes from genetically determined inflammatory skin disorders may have intrinsic abnormalities in their capacity to produce chemokines. For example, keratinocytes cultured from patients with AD show an exaggerated production of RANTES, whereas psoriatic keratinocytes overproduce IL-8, MCP-1, and IP-10.[47,48] These defects may help to explain the accumulation of distinct leukocyte types in these two diseases. Recent findings from our group have demonstrated that the expression of the chemokines IP-10, Mig, and MCP-1 induced by IFN-γ in human keratinocytes can be abrogated by overexpression of the negative regulators of IFN-γ signaling: suppressor of cytokine signaling (SOCS)1 and SOCS3.[49] SOCS molecules are strongly expressed by keratinocytes in lesional skin of psoriasis and ACD patients, and to a lesser extent in AD lesions. These observations identify SOCS1 and SOCS3 molecules as new potential molecular targets for those IFN-γ-dependent skin diseases where chemokines are aberrantly expressed by keratinocytes. Finally, we recently identified a feedback mechanism through which the epidermis physiologically controls its own chemokine expression in response to pro-inflammatory cytokines. Central to these events is keratinocyte autocrine activation of epidermal growth factor receptor (EGFR), which not only drives an effective promotion of tissue repair mechanisms, but also downregulates the expression of potent chemokines, including IP-10, RANTES, and MCP-1. In the mouse model of ACD to 2,4-dinitro-fluorobenzene, pharmacological abrogation of EGFR signaling induces deranged expression of these chemokines and consequently an amplification of both irritant and immune-specific inflammation in response to hapten painting.[50]

Other resident cells can contribute to chemokine production during skin inflammation. Dermal fibroblasts produce IL-8, RANTES, MIP-3α, and Gro-α when stimulated with IL-1 and TNF-α.[40,51] Moreover, these cells constitutively express the mRNA for CCL11/eotaxin, CCL24/eotaxin-2, and CCL26/eotaxin-3, which are upregulated in response to TNF-α and IL-4.[52,53] Dermal fibroblasts also express CCL13/MCP-4 mRNA in response to pro-inflammatory cytokines.[54] All these chemokines are strong attractants of eosinophils and Th2 cells, and may play a relevant role in AD and other diseases in which eosinophils are involved.[51] Apart from acting as major effector cells in the elicitation of allergic inflammation, mast cells may promote T-cell recruitment by release of chemotactic stimuli such as IL-8, XCL1/lymphotactin, and IL-16.[55] DCs represent another relevant source of chemokines, whose production follows a precise sequential order during maturation.[32] After an initial burst of inflammatory chemokines (MIP-1α, MIP-1β, RANTES, MCP-1, and IL-8), maturing DCs produce lymphoid chemokines such as TARC, MDC, PARC, and ELC, the last two active on naive T cells. Interestingly, different DC subsets appear to express a similar pattern of chemokines attracting T cells.[56] Extracellular nucleotides (e.g., ATP) may represent constitutive signals that can alert the immune system of abnormal cell death. Relatively high doses of nucleotides induce rapid release of pro-inflammatory mediators and favor pathogen killing. However, recent findings on antigen-presenting cells (APCs), particularly DCs, revealed a more complex role for these molecules. ATP affects the pattern of chemokine release from DCs by upregulating the constitutive production of MDC and inhibiting the LPS-induced secretion of IP-10 and RANTES. This results in a selectively impaired capacity of DCs to recruit type 1 but not type 2 lymphocytes.[57] In contrast, IFN-γ-treated DCs markedly upregulate the release of IP-10 while significantly reducing the secretion of TARC; hence, they improve the attraction of Th1 rather than Th2 cells, and consequently induce a more effective Th1 polarization of the immune response.[58] DCs are the largest source of MDC, and *in situ* MDC staining is most evident in mature CD83$^+$ DCs, with the number of MDC$^+$ DCs much higher in AD lesional skin than in skin affected with psoriasis or ACD.[24] In the complex process of leukocyte recruitment, some chemokines have been shown to induce firm arrest via integrins, both *in vitro* and *in vivo*. Upon exposure to inflammatory signals, endothelial cells express MIP-3α, SDF-1, SLC, TARC, MCP-1, IL-8, RANTES, Gro-α, and MIP-1β, some of which are involved in the arrest of lymphocytes under physiologic flow conditions.[21] In particular, TARC has been detected in venules of inflamed human skin and determines adhesion of skin memory T cells to ICAM-1 *in vitro*.[12] Moreover, Fitzhugh et al.[35] demonstrated that MIP-3α produced by endothelial cells may be critical for the arrest of CCR6$^+$ T lymphocytes on activated dermal endothelium, suggesting a role for this chemokine in T-cell recruitment in psoriatic skin where infiltrating CCR6$^+$ leukocytes are numerous. Finally, CX3CL1/fractalkine is expressed on the membrane of endothelial cells and modulated by inflammatory signals and cytokines. The fractalkine/CX3CR1 axis can be part of an amplification circuit of polarized type 1 responses, as suggested by the higher expression of this chemokine in psoriatic as compared to AD lesions.[59]

## III. THE ROLE OF CHEMOKINES IN INFLAMMATORY SKIN DISEASES

Chemokines appear to be crucial regulators of both the induction and expression of chronic inflammatory skin diseases. ACD serves as a valuable model for understanding the specific contribution of different T-cell subsets as well as the mechanisms underlying the generation and regulation of T-cell responses. The kinetics and pattern of chemokine expression during ACD resemble those observed during wound healing, with IL-8 and MCP-1 expressed first, followed by RANTES, and finally by CXCR3 receptor agonists,[60,61] suggesting that the skin sets up a standard sequential pattern of chemokine expression in response to different types of injuries.[62] Most of the studies on the role of chemokines in the mouse model of ACD have looked at the induction phase and few, if any, have addressed the expression phase. However, work in other models of Th1-mediated inflammation has provided further comprehension of the molecular mechanisms implicated in this type of disease.[63,64] By contrast, psoriasis and AD differ substantially in the pattern of chemokines expressed in the skin (Table 16.3). In the following subsections, we overview the whole experimental evidence that currently establishes the chemokine–chemokine receptor axis as the most relevant — and complex — network involved in the expression of chronic inflammatory skin diseases.

### A. Allergic Contact Dermatitis

ACD is a T-cell-mediated inflammatory reaction occurring in sensitized individuals at the site of hapten challenge. Valuable animal models of ACD are available and the disease can be easily induced in humans, allowing detailed analysis of the cell types and molecules involved in its induction, expression, and regulation. Thus, ACD represents a prototype for T-cell-mediated skin immune responses, and many of the cellular and molecular mechanisms described in this reaction have been applied to the understanding of other lymphocyte-driven disorders. In the sensitization phase, hapten penetrated into the skin is picked up by skin DCs, which then migrate to the draining lymph nodes and present the hapten-peptide-MHC complexes to naive antigen-specific T lymphocytes. This process leads to the clonal expansion of specific T cells, which can then be recruited to the skin. The migration of skin DCs to the lymph nodes is regulated by various factors, including a profound rearrangement in the pattern of chemokine receptors, that allow DCs to encounter naive T cells.[65,66] In mice deficient in CCR7 or its ligand, SLC, skin DCs do not migrate to the lymph nodes and contact hypersensitivity (CH) does not develop.[67,68] In sensitized subjects, a reexposure to the antigen determines the activation and expansion of specific memory T cells. The inflammatory infiltrate in ACD is mainly composed of CD4$^+$ and CD8$^+$ T cells, monocytes, and DCs, with an early and transient presence of neutrophils. The expression of both murine CH and human ACD correlates with the activity of hapten-specific CD8$^+$ T cells, which exert their effector function through direct cytotoxic activity as well as the release of cytokines.[69–73] On the other hand, CD4$^+$ T cells play a more complex role, with Th1 and Th2 subsets contributing to disease expression, and Tr cells primarily involved in its modulation and/or termination.[27,74] In addition, Th2 cells may also exert a regulatory role as IL-4 administration or passive transfer of hapten-specific Th2 lymphocytes can reverse established murine CH.[75] However, CH is reduced or unmodified in IL-4$^{-/-}$ mice and decreased in STAT-6 deficient mice, in which Th2 responses are impaired.[76]

During ACD, leukocyte recruitment is under the control of the sequential and coordinated release of chemokines from resident and immigrating cells. In a recent work, Goebeler et al.[61]

**TABLE 16.3**
**Chemokine Expression in Inflammatory Skin Diseases**

| | Major Cell Sources | Allergic Contact Dermatitis | Psoriasis | Atopic Dermatitis |
|---|---|---|---|---|
| IL-8 | Keratinocytes | | | |
| | Mast cells | ++ | ++ | + |
| IP-10 | Keratinocytes | | | |
| | T cells | +++ | ++ | + |
| | Monocytes, DCs | | | |
| I-309 | Keratinocytes | | | |
| | T cells | + | nd | nd |
| | Monocytes | | | |
| Eotaxin | Fibroblasts | | | |
| | T cells | nd | nd | ++ |
| | Mast cells | | | |
| MCP-1 | Keratinocytes | | | |
| | T cells, mast cells | ++ | ++ | ++ |
| | Monocytes, DCs | | | |
| MCP-3, MCP-4 | Fibroblasts | + | + | +++ |
| RANTES | Keratinocytes | | | |
| | T cells | ++ | ++ | ++ |
| | Monocytes, DCs | | | |
| MDC | DCs | + | + | +++ |
| TARC | Dendritic cells | | + | + |
| | Endothelial cells | + | | |
| CTACK | Keratinocytes | ++ | ++ | ++ |
| MIP-3α | Keratinocytes | | | |
| | Endothelial cells | ++ | +++ | nd |
| Fractalkine | Keratinocytes | | | |
| | Endothelial cells | ++ | ++ | + |

*Note*: nd, not determined.

analyzed the expression pattern of chemokines in the skin at different time points after hapten application. By using *in situ* hybridization, they showed that MCP-1 is already detectable at 6 h after hapten challenge, whereas RANTES and MDC appear at 12 h concomitantly with the infiltration of mononuclear cells in the dermis and epidermis. The expression of IP-10, Mig, TARC, and CCL18/PARC begins at 12 h and peaks at 72 h, paralleling the strong infiltration of lymphocytes. The variety of chemokines expressed during ACD determines a robust and rapid recruitment of leukocytes into the skin. MCP-1 seems to play a relevant role in ACD. In fact, transgenic mice overexpressing MCP-1 in basal keratinocytes showed enhanced CH responses together with an increased number of infiltrating DCs.[77] It is still unclear which chemokine(s) drives the initial influx of T cells, the cellular source(s), as well as the nature of the induction stimulus. Keratinocytes may represent important contributors to this phase, although a TNF-α-mediated induction by haptens has been demonstrated only for IL-8.[78] Activated endothelial cells can conceivably contribute to early leukocyte arrival in the skin, by expressing both adhesion molecules and chemokines.[12,21,35] During the elicitation of ACD, upregulated expression of epidermal CTACK is already observed after 6 h. After 24 h, CTACK immunoreactivity is also detectable free in the papillary dermis and on dermal microvessels, most likely as the consequences of secretion from keratinocytes followed by absorption on extracellular matrix proteins and endothelial cells, respectively. At 24 to 48 h, the number of $CCR10^{+}$ T cells increases dramatically first in the perivascular and subepidermal areas and then in the epidermis.[36] Also, mast cells and platelets might be indirectly involved in this early T-cell recruitment through the release of serotonin, which together with TNF-α activates the endothelium and facilitates cell entrance. This phenomenon seems to be C5a dependent, as C5a knockout mice do not show T-cell infiltration at the sites of hapten challenge.[79] Moreover, mast cells can be importantly involved in neutrophil recruitment through the release of TNF-α and MIP-2, the functional analogue of human IL-8 in murine CH.[80] Infiltrating monocytes and DCs are themselves a source of chemokines for successive boosts of lymphocyte arrival. The activation of some hapten-specific T lymphocytes into the skin leads to the production of cytokines like IFN-γ, TNF-α, and IL-4, which in turn stimulate keratinocytes and other cells to produce IP-10, Mig, and I-TAC, the ligands for CXCR3.[43,44,46] These chemokines selectively attract T lymphocytes, which then rapidly accumulate in the epidermis. Indeed, keratinocytes, continuously stimulated by T-cell-derived cytokines, produce large amounts of CXCR3 ligands, thus contributing to further accumulation of CXCR3-bearing T cells. The result is that more than 70% of ACD infiltrating T lymphocytes are $CXCR3^+$.[46,62] The higher expression of CXCR3 and CCR4 on skin-homing nickel-specific $CD8^+$ and $CD4^+$ T cells suggests that trafficking of these two populations at the site of skin inflammation differs, with $CD4^+$ and $CD8^+$ cell recruitment primarily directed by the CCR4/TARC and CXCR3/IP-10 axis, respectively.[30] Once recruited into the skin, activated T lymphocytes represent a relevant source of chemokines. Upon T-cell receptor triggering, Th1 and Th2 cells produce similar sets of chemokines, including RANTES, I-309, IL-8, and MDC.[8] Some differences seem to exist in terms of chemokine production between $CD4^+$ and $CD8^+$ T lymphocytes. In a mouse model it has been shown that IP-10 expression is primarily mediated by $CD8^+$ and inhibited by $CD4^+$ T lymphocytes during the elicitation phase of CH.[81]

Resolution of ACD is likely due to multiple mechanisms, including induction of T-cell anergy and active suppression, and may involve several cell types. In this process, IL-10-producing T cells (Tr lymphocytes) might play a central role.[27,82,83] We recently demonstrated that Tr cells migrate *in vitro* in response to various chemokines including MCP-1, MIPs, and TARC. More interestingly, I-309, which is not active on Th1 cells, attracts more vigorously Tr lymphocytes than Th2 cells. Consistent with these results, Tr lymphocytes express higher levels of CCR8 compared to Th2 cells. I-309 is produced by both keratinocytes and activated T cells, and is expressed in ACD skin with an earlier kinetics compared to IL-4 and IL-10.[28] These data indicate that I-309/CCR8 may contribute relevantly to the termination of ACD through the recruitment of Tr lymphocytes. Also CCR6, the receptor of MIP-3α, seems to be involved in the modulation of CH, as CCR6-deficient mice show increased and persistent CH responses probably in relation to an impaired recruitment of $CD4^+$ regulatory cells.[84]

## B. Psoriasis

Psoriasis is a genetically determined skin disease characterized by aberrant proliferation and differentiation of keratinocytes as well as cutaneous inflammation. T-cell-mediated immune mechanisms have a primary role in the pathogenesis of psoriasis.[85–87] In particular, activated Th1 cells releasing IFN-γ and TNF-α stimulate keratinocytes to produce cytokines, chemokines, and adhesion molecules, which further amplify the inflammatory response. Various studies have documented a strong chemokine expression in psoriatic keratinocytes in lesional skin, and keratinocyte production of chemokines may contribute relevantly to the establishment of the inflammatory infiltrate.[88] Specifically, IL-8 and related chemokines are responsible for the intraepidermal collection of neutrophils.[38,89] MCP-1, RANTES, IP-10, and other CXCR3 ligands attract predominantly monocytes and Th1 cells,[90,91] whereas MIP-3α recruits immature LCs and DCs, and $CLA^+$ T cells.[40,92] In line with these observations, T cells bearing CCR4, CXCR3, and CCR6 receptors are well represented in psoriatic skin lesions.[92,93] In particular, $CXCR3^+CD8^+$ T cells are increased tenfold in psoriatic epidermis compared with the frequency of these cells in peripheral blood of patients with psoriasis.[93] MCP-4 is also strongly expressed in the basal layers of the psoriatic epidermis and together with MIP-3α can direct the traffic of immature DCs.[94] CTACK is abundantly present in basal and suprabasal keratinocytes of psoriatic lesions as well as in the dermis, together with a high number of CCR10+ T cells.[36] Consistent with the Th1-dominated immunity underlying psoriasis, CCR10 is preferentially expressed by skin-homing CLA+ memory T cells secreting TNF-α and IFN-γ, but minimal IL-10 and IL-4 upon activation.[95] Activation of endothelial cells may represent an early event in the pathogenesis of psoriatic lesions, and allow the initial accumulation of T cells, which in turn can amplify the inflammatory response by releasing cytokines. Expression of MIP-3α on dermal endothelial cells may thus play an important role in the arrest of CCR6+ immature DCs and memory T cells,[35,92] whereas expression of TARC is important for the arrest of CCR4+ T cells.[22] Dermal endothelial cells of psoriasis lesions, but not those of AD, are strongly positive for fractalkine, a membrane-bound chemokine that is induced by IFN-γ and whose receptor (CXCR1) is preferentially expressed by Th1 cells and natural killer (NK) cells.[59]

The genetic predisposition to psoriasis may include an altered control of inflammatory gene expression in the skin. In particular, psoriatic keratinocytes may have intrinsic defects leading to exaggerated synthesis of certain chemokines such as IL-8, MCP-1, and IP-10,[48,89,96] and also display increased expression of IL-8R, which can mediate an increased proliferative response of keratinocytes to the chemokine.[88,97] Moreover, psoriatic keratinocytes activated *in vitro* with IFN-γ and TNF-α showed a ICAM-1 induction higher than normal keratinocytes. The signal transduction initiated by IFN-γ and TNF-α principally involves cooperation between STAT-1 and NF-κB transcription factors. In contrast, AP-1 is known to be less important in the signaling elicited by these cytokines. We have shown that in transiently transfected keratinocytes, IFN-γ and TNF-α induced a strong NF-κB and STAT-1 binding activity, whereas the induction of AP-1 function was less evident. Interestingly enough, psoriatic keratinocytes exhibited a more prominent NF-κB and STAT-1, but not AP-1 activity compared to control keratinocytes.[96] Indeed, perturbation in signal transduction pathways and in the activation of transcription factors has been implicated in the dysregulated functions of psoriatic keratinocytes.[98,99]

Increasing evidence indicates that nitric oxide (NO) is involved in the maintenance of skin homeostasis as well as in the modulation of inflammatory reactions. NO is a short-lived radical produced from the L-arginine pathway by different isoforms of NO synthase (NOS), which are expressed by various cell types residing in the skin. High levels of NO have been measured in the skin affected with psoriasis, AD, or ACD.[100,101] In these conditions, pro-inflammatory cytokines stimulate keratinocytes to express inducible NOS (iNOS), which in turn catalyzes NO production. Fibroblasts and DCs also become iNOS-positive after exposure to bacterial endotoxin and IFN-γ, and endothelial cells express iNOS after activation with IL-1β. The role of NO in the regulation of inflammatory responses has been extensively investigated. Depending on the concentration, the cell type, and its state of activation, as well as the presence of other inflammatory mediators, NO can either block or stimulate inflammatory responses.[102] A novel function of NO is its ability to modulate chemokine expression. Recently, we tested whether synthetic NO donors could modulate the expression of chemokines and ICAM-1 in keratinocyte primary cultures established from healthy subjects and patients with psoriasis. NO donors (*S*-nitrosoglutathione and NOR-1) diminished in a dose-dependent manner and at both mRNA and protein levels IP-10, RANTES, and MCP-1 expression in keratinocytes cultured from healthy subjects and patients with psoriasis. In contrast, constitutive and induced IL-8 production was unchanged. *In vivo,* NO-treated psoriatic skin showed reduction of IP-10, RANTES, and MCP-1, but not IL-8 expression by keratinocytes. Moreover, the number of CD14+ and CD3+ cells infiltrating the epidermis and papillary dermis diminished significantly. NO donors also downregulated ICAM-1 protein expression without affecting mRNA accumulation *in vitro*, and suppressed keratinocyte ICAM-1 *in vivo*. These results define NO donors as negative regulators of chemokine production by keratinocytes, both *in vitro* and *in vivo*.[96] The clinical efficacy of novel targeted immunomodulatory therapies of psoriasis, such as IL-10 and dimethylfumarate, is associated with a downregulation of chemokine production and signaling pathway. In particular, administration of IL-10 to patients with chronic plaque psoriasis inhibited the epidermal IL-8 pathway by reducing the expression of IL-8, its receptor CXCR2, and its inducer IL-17.[103,104] Consistently, dimethylfumarate suppresses the IFN-γ-induced production of Gro-α, IL-8, Mig, IP-10, and I-TAC in keratinocytes and peripheral blood mononuclear cells.[105]

## C. Atopic Dermatitis

AD is a chronic inflammatory disease that results from complex interactions between genetic and environmental factors.[106] An altered lipid composition of the stratum corneum is responsible for the xerotic aspect of the skin, and may determine a higher permeability to allergens and irritants. Indeed, specific immune responses against a variety of environmental allergens are implicated in AD pathogenesis with a bias toward Th2 immune responses. In particular, DCs expressing membrane IgE receptors play a critical role in the amplification of allergen-specific T-cell responses.[107,108] Cross-linkage of specific IgE receptors on dermal mast cells provokes release and synthesis of a vast series of mediators. Following their recruitment and activation into the skin, eosinophils are also thought to contribute to tissue damage. Keratinocytes of patients with AD exhibit a propensity to an exaggerated production of cytokines and chemokines, a phenomenon that can be relevant in promoting and maintaining inflammation, and may play a major role in localizing the atopic diathesis to the skin.[109] Thus, a complex network of cytokines and chemokines contributes to establish a local milieu that favors the permanence of inflammation in AD skin. Patients with AD exhibit exaggerated Th2 responses, and initiation of AD lesions is thought to be mediated by early skin infiltration of Th2 lymphocytes releasing high levels of IL-4, IL-5, and IL-13. Subsequently, the accumulation of activated monocytes, mature DCs, and eosinophils determines a rise in IL-12 expression and the appearance of a mixed Th2/Th1 cytokine pattern, with reduced IL-4 and IL-13 and the presence of IFN-γ.

The proportion of $CD4^+$ T lymphocytes expressing CCR4 in the peripheral blood of patients with AD is higher compared to $CD4^+$ T cells of healthy controls. In contrast, patients with AD bear a lower percentage of circulating $CXCR3^+CD4^+$ T cells.[42,110–112] Moreover, the percentage of blood $CCR4^+CD4^+$ cells correlates positively with disease severity and IL-4 and IL-13 secretion by $CD4^+$ T cells.[112,113] $CCR4^+CD4^+$ T cells are also positive for the skin-homing receptor, CLA, and infiltrate in a high number AD lesions,[111,112] indicating not only increased generation of $CCR4^+$ T cells, but also enhanced recruitment into AD skin. The ligands for CCR4 are TARC and MDC, two chemokines present in high amounts in the plasma of patients with AD and whose levels correlate with disease activity.[114–116] Both TARC and MDC are produced abundantly by immature DCs and even more by mature DCs *in vitro*. TARC is expressed by microvascular endothelial cells in AD lesions, thus possibly playing a role in the recruitment of $CCR4^+$ T cells from the circulation,[22] but also by epidermal keratinocytes, as recently evidenced by *in situ* RT-PCR.[117] *In situ* studies have also shown that MDC immunoreactivity in AD skin is mostly confined to $CD1a^+CD83^+$ mature DCs, and identified this cell type as the major source of MDC *in vivo*.[22,24] In aggregate, these data point to a relevant role for $CCR4^+$ T cells in the pathogenesis of AD, and suggest that DCs may guide not only their activation but also their preferential accumulation in this disease.

Other chemokines that participate in the accumulation of T cells in AD include RANTES, MCP-1, eotaxin, MIP-3α, CTACK, and IL-16. RANTES and MCP-1, which attract both Th1 and Th2 cells, are expressed by infiltrating leukocytes but especially by keratinocytes in diseased skin,[48] although only RANTES has been found elevated in the serum of patients.[118] Together with its receptor CCR3, eotaxin is expressed in the dermis of AD lesions in particular by mononuclear cells and fibroblasts.[119,120] Also MIP-3α mRNA is found expressed in AD skin, although less abundantly than in psoriasis,[121] with specific immunostaining localized in the basal epidermis and $CCR6^+$ cells, with these last identified mainly as DCs and T cells.[41] Interestingly, disruption of the epidermal permeability barrier has been shown to upregulate the expression of epidermal MIP-3α mRNA in the epidermis.[121] This molecular mechanism is reasonably implicated in the initial influx of DCs and T cells in AD skin, which is characterized by an intrinsic permeability barrier dysfunction. Similarly to psoriasis, acute and chronic AD lesions exhibit strong CTACK expression in the epidermis and numerous CCR10$^+$ T cells.[36] Recently, an elevation of circulating IL-16 has been associated to active AD in children.[122] Increased expression of IL-16 has already been detected in the epidermis of AD lesions,[123] and LCs have been recognized as the most relevant source of this chemokine in this disease.[124] IL-16 is a strong inducer of migratory responses in CD4$^+$ T cells, monocytes, and eosinophils.[125] *In vitro* experiments indicate that IL-16 is a major chemotactic signal from DCs toward themselves and CD4$^+$ T cells.[126] It is thus possible to speculate that LC-derived IL-16 may critically contribute to T-cell recruitment in AD. Indeed, lesional skin of patients with AD exhibits an increased number of cells belonging to the DC lineage, including epidermal LCs, dermal DCs, and a unique population of epidermal CD1a$^+$ DCs expressing CD1b and/or CD36, which closely resemble DCs generated *in vitro* by culturing monocytes in the presence of GM-CSF and IL-4. Such DCs can efficiently present IgE-bound allergens to T lymphocytes, since they display an upregulated expression of both the high-affinity (FcεRI) as well as the low-affinity (FcεRII/CD23) IgE receptors.[127] Furthermore, FcεRI engagement has been shown to upregulate IL-16 production in LCs derived from atopic donors.[128]

Eventually, the selective uptake of allergens and the subsequent induction of specific T-cell responses may further provide a mechanism to perpetuate skin inflammation. LC-derived IL-16 can also attract eosinophils into the skin. Although eosinophils are not prominent in AD infiltrate, they are potent effector cells, and contribute to inflammation by the release of a variety of cytotoxic species such as eosinophil cationic protein, eosinophil peroxidase major basic protein, and eosinophil-derived neurotoxin/eosinophil protein X. In the context of acute and chronic AD lesions, eosinophils are attracted by resident skin populations through the increased expression of CCR3 binding molecules, including RANTES, MCP-4, and eotaxin.[119,120] *In situ* hybridization experiments performed on skin biopsies soon after challenge with a proper provocation factor have demonstrated a prominent neosynthesis of RANTES and MCP-3 by dermal fibroblasts. In acute AD, eosinophil attraction could be predominantly performed by these cells, whose eotaxin and MCP-4 secretion is potently increased in response to T-cell-derived IL-4.[52,54]

In contrast to psoriasis, IL-8 and IP-10 are only weakly expressed in some limited areas of the epidermis in AD lesions. *In vitro* studies have shown that keratinocytes from patients with AD produced increased amounts of RANTES, but reduced levels of IP-10, in response to IFN-γ or TNF-α when compared to keratinocytes from normal controls or patients with psoriasis.[48] RANTES is not the only pro-inflammatory factor whose expression has been found upregulated in keratinocytes cultured from patients with AD, as they displayed overproduction of spontaneous as well as IL-1α- and IFN-γ-induced GM-CSF release, when compared to healthy control keratinocytes.[129]

Numerous functional polymorphisms in the regulatory/coding regions of clusters of cytokine/chemokine genes, including RANTES, have been found in patients with AD,[130,131] which could be implicated in an overproduction by keratinocytes. However, apart from genes coding for Th2 cytokines, polymorphisms for other inflammatory genes were not confirmed in other studies.[132] Indeed, the genes that contribute to complex diseases are difficult to identify, because they typically exert small effects on disease risk. In addition, the magnitude of their effects is likely to be modified by other unrelated genes as well as environmental factors. Thus, susceptibility loci for complex diseases identified in one study may not be replicated in other populations.

In the search for a molecular mechanism underlying abnormal GM-CSF production, we have found that AD keratinocytes express higher constitutive and/or induced levels of members of the AP-1 family of transcription factors, including c-Jun, JunB, and c-Fos, compared to keratinocytes from normal controls.[47] AP-1 is prominently activated by various cytokines, including IL-4, IFN-γ, and TNF-α, and AP-1 binding sites are strategically located in the promoters of a vast array of cytokines and chemokines, including RANTES. Our data support the concept that keratinocytes from patients with AD or psoriasis bear intrinsic alterations in their response to pro-inflammatory stimuli, and that these abnormalities contribute to establish a pro-inflammatory environment in these diseases. In particular, epithelial/DC interactions may be very important in the initiation and persistence of inflammation in AD. The distinct propensity of keratinocytes to produce higher than normal levels of growth factors (GM-CSF), chemokines (RANTES), and cytokines (TNF-$\alpha$, thymic stromal lymphopoietin/TSLP) may greatly stimulate DC differentiation from precursors, and recruit as well as activate DCs in AD skin. This activation includes high production of chemokines attracting CCR4$^+$ Th2 lymphocytes and increased stimulation of T-cell responses.[133] The triggers that activate keratinocytes in the very early phases may include the altered epidermal permeability barrier functions,[121,134] as previously mentioned. In contrast to what has been described with bronchial epithelial cells, environmental allergens such as those of the house dust mite do not seem to stimulate keratinocyte production of chemokines or cytokines.[135]

## IV. CHEMOKINES AND CHEMOKINE RECEPTORS AS POTENTIAL THERAPEUTIC TARGETS IN INFLAMMATORY SKIN DISORDERS

The growing knowledge on the mechanisms controlling the recruitment of T cells in the skin during inflammatory and immune responses suggests that targeting chemokines or their receptors could be an effective approach for the therapy of inflammatory diseases. Given the redundancy of the chemokine network, it is crucial to establish the validity of targeting the system for therapeutic intervention. Intense investigation in this field is currently applied not only to prevent HIV infection, but also for the possible cure of a variety of disorders, including cancer, autoimmune diseases such as multiple sclerosis and rheumatoid arthritis, and asthma, and to prevent transplant rejection.[136] Nonetheless, this therapeutic strategy has received a limited amount of attention by investigative dermatologists so far. Antibodies directed to MCP-1 administered to rats undergoing cutaneous delayed-type hypersensitivity were reported to abolish T cell migration and inflammatory sequelae almost completely.[137] These initial observations led to the conclusion that MCP-1 could be a useful therapeutic target for skin diseases driven by T cells, although experiments on MCP-1$^{-/-}$ mice did not sustain this hypothesis. These mice displayed inability to recruit specifically monocytes into the lesions of both delayed-type and contact sensitivity, but the swelling response was normal.[138]

The simultaneous expression of multiple chemokines and receptors in the course of an inflammatory disease and the low number of chemokine receptors as compared to the number of their soluble ligands suggest that any strategy that is aimed at antagonizing multiple chemokine receptor interactions is likely to be more effective than therapies that target a single chemokine. Recently, anti-CXCR3 antibodies were shown effective in inhibiting a delayed-type hypersensitivity in the mouse via blockade of activated T-cell transmigration to the peripheral inflammatory sites.[139] CXCR3 is also a dominant factor directing T cells into mouse skin allografts to induce acute rejection, and the blockade of CXCR3 expression by means of systemic administration of peptide nucleic acid CXCR3 antisense significantly prolonged skin allograft survival.[140] Previously, a significant attenuation of allograft rejection in heart-transplanted mice could be found in CXCR3$^{-/-}$ mice, but also in mice treated with a neutralizing antibody to CXCR3, thus confirming the critical role of this receptor in this disease.[141] Also, the observation that CCR7$^{-/-}$ mice lack both CH and delayed-type hypersensitivity reactions assumes a particular relevance to encourage the validation of chemokine receptor targeting for the cure of inflammatory diseases of the skin.[67]

Several companies are now deeply involved in the development of selective small-molecule chemokine receptor antagonists, and some of these compounds have entered phase I clinical trials.[142] Among the possible clinical applications of this new class of drugs, special attention is currently devoted to the therapy of allergic diseases, in particular asthma.[143] Promising indication has been obtained with dual-receptor antagonists, such as Met-RANTES, which antagonizes the actions of RANTES on both CCR1 and CCR5, and dramatically reduces eosinophilia in a pulmonary Th2-mediated inflammation model,[144] but also tissue damage in a colitis model and disease symptoms in collagen-induced arthritis, these last conceived as typical Th1-mediated disease models.[145] CCR1 antagonism has also shown potential indications in a variety of inflammatory disorders.[136,146] Positive results in phase I clinical trials in patients with multiple sclerosis have been reported with BX471, a small compound belonging to the piperazine class, with selective CCR1 antagonism. However, the finding that CCR1$^{-/-}$ mice have a decreased resistance to *Toxoplasma gondii* infection suggests that potential negative consequences of these types of therapies should be seriously evaluated.[147]

As it is specifically involved in the recruitment of eosinophils and Th2 cells, impairment of CCR3 function is considered an interesting approach especially against allergic inflammation.[143] Indeed, work on CCR3$^{-/-}$ mice has demonstrated that CCR3 plays an essential role in eosinophil recruitment to the skin at sites of antigen sensitization, as well as during airway hyperresponsiveness following inhaled antigen challenge of epicutaneously sensitized mice.[148] Chemical modification of the N-terminal residue of the T-cell chemoattractant CCL18/MIP-4 provides an extremely potent and selective peptidic CCR3 antagonist, called Met-chemokine β7, which has been shown to efficiently oppose eosinophil chemotaxis at very low concentrations (in the order of 1 n*M*).[149] Finally, numerous small-molecule CCR3 antagonists have been described recently, and are now under intense preclinical investigation.[142,150–152] Given that CCR1 has high homology (62.5%) to CCR3, a major concern is to increase their binding selectivity toward CCR3, hence reducing the possibility of undesired CCR1-linked side effects. A further complexity factor in the validation of effective CCR3 antagonists arises because their proven efficacy in the blockade of CCR3 on human cells (e.g., eosinophils) cannot be easily transferred to animal models for further functional characterization, due to high species selectivity in their binding to human CCR3.[136]

## V. CONCLUSION

Since the quite recent discovery of the superfamily of chemokines and their receptors, there has been an intense effort to define their role in the complex orchestration of the leukocyte trafficking. Using a variety of experimental approaches, recent studies have provided irrefutable evidence that chemokines are essential mediators in the pathophysiology of inflammatory skin diseases. The correct, controlled trafficking of leukocytes is a fundamental feature of the immune response to infection. By contrast, a characteristic feature of all inflammatory processes is the excessive recruitment of leukocytes to the site of inflammation. In chronic, recurrent inflammatory disorders of the skin, such as psoriasis and AD, resident populations of the skin appear to facilitate this process via intense production of diverse chemokines, while no efficient tissue repair seems to take place concomitantly. In this context, the strategy of selectively blocking leukocyte recruitment to the skin should be extensively investigated. In the last few years, significant progress has been made in the design of a number of inhibitors that can be used to limit chemokine activity in *in vivo* disease models. However, the search for proper drug targets will critically depend on the availability of animal models to mirror human dermatological diseases.

## REFERENCES


1. Sallusto, F., Mackay, C.F., and Lanzavecchia, A., The role of chemokine receptors in primary, effector, and memory immune responses, *Annu. Rev. Immunol.*, 18, 59, 2000.
2. Zlotnik, A. and Yoshie, O., Chemokines: a new classification system and their role in immunity, *Immunity*, 12, 121, 2000.
3. Mackay, C.R., Chemokines: immunology's high impact factors, *Nat. Immunol.*, 2, 95, 2001.
4. Moser, B. and Loetscher, P., Lymphocyte traffic control by chemokines, *Nat. Immunol.*, 2, 123, 2001.
5. Kunkel, E.J. and Butcher, E.C., Chemokines and the tissue-specific migration of lymphocytes, *Immunity*, 16, 1–4, 2002.
6. Luster, A.D., The role of chemokines in linking innate and adaptive immunity, *Curr. Opin. Immunol.*, 14, 129, 2002.
7. Bazan, J.F. et al., A new class of membrane-bound chemokine with a CX3C motif, *Nature*, 385:640–644, 1997.

8. Sallusto, F. et al., Switch in chemokine receptor expression upon TCR stimulation reveals novel homing potential for recently activated T cells, *Eur. J. Immunol.*, 29, 2037, 1999.
9. Luther, S.A. and Cyster, J.G., Chemokines as regulators of T cell differentiation, *Nat. Immunol.*, 2, 102, 2001.
10. Rossi, D. and Zlotnik, A., The biology of chemokines and their receptors, *Annu. Rev. Immunol.*, 18, 217, 2000.
11. Mellado, M. et al., Chemokine signaling and functional responses: the role of receptor dimerization and TK pathway activation, *Annu. Rev. Immunol.*, 19, 397, 2001.
12. Campbell, J.J. et al., The chemokine receptor CCR4 in vascular recognition by cutaneous but not intestinal memory T cells, *Nature*, 400, 776, 1999.
13. Zabel, B.A. et al., Human G protein-coupled receptor GPR9-6/CC chemokine receptor 9 is selectively expressed on intestinal homing T lymphocytes, mucosal lymphocytes, and thymocytes and is required for thymus-expressed chemokine-mediated chemotaxis, *J. Exp. Med.*, 190, 1241, 1999.
14. Morales, J. et al., CTACK, a skin-associated chemokine that preferentially attracts skin-homing memory T cells, *Proc. Natl. Acad. Sci. U.S.A.*, 96, 14470, 1999.
15. Homey, B. et al., The orphan chemokine receptor G protein-coupled receptor-2 (GPR-2, CCR10) binds the skin associated chemokine CCL27 (CTACK/ALP/ILC), *J. Immunol.*, 164, 3465, 2000.
16. Loetscher, P. et al., The ligands of CXC receptor 3, I-TAC, Mig, and IP-10 are natural antagonists for CCR3, *J. Biol. Chem.*, 276, 2986, 2001.
17. Uguccioni, M. et al., High expression of the chemokine receptor CCR3 in human blood basophils. Role in activation by eotaxin, MCP-4, and other chemokines, *J. Clin. Invest.*, 100, 1137, 1997.
18. Weng, Y. et al., Binding and functional properties of recombinant and endogenous CXCR3 chemokine receptors. *J. Biol. Chem.*, 273, 18288, 1998.
19. Ogilvie, P. et al., Eotaxin is a natural antagonist for CCR2 and an agonist for CCR5, *Blood*, 97, 1920, 2001.
20. Christopherson, K.W. et al., Endothelial induction of the T-cell chemokine CCL21 in T-cell autoimmune diseases, *Blood*, 101, 801, 2003.
21. Von Andrian, U.H., and Mackay, C.R., T-cell function and migration. Two sides of the same coin, *N. Engl. J. Med.*, 343, 1020, 2000.
22. D'Ambrosio, D. et al., Quantitative differences in chemokine receptor engagement generate diversity in integrin-dependent lymphocyte adhesion, *J. Immunol.*, 169, 2303, 2002.
23. Gunn, M.D. et al., A chemokine expressed in lymphoid high endothelial venules promotes the adhesion and chemotaxis of naive T lymphocytes, *Proc. Natl. Acad. Sci. U.S.A.*, 95, 258, 1998.
24. Vulcano M. et al., Dendritic cells as a major source of macrophage-derived chemokine/CCL22 *in vitro* and *in vivo*, *Eur. J. Immunol.*, 31, 812, 2001.
25. Bonecchi, R. et al., Differential expression of chemokine receptors and chemotactic responsiveness of type 1 T helper cells (Th1s) and Th2s, *J. Exp. Med.*, 187, 129, 1998.
26. D'Ambrosio, D. et al., Selective up-regulation of chemokine receptors CCR4 and CCR8 upon activation of polarized human type 2 Th cells, *J. Immunol.*, 161, 5111, 1998.
27. Cavani, A. et al., Effector and regulatory T cells in allergic contact dermatitis, *Trends Immunol.*, 22, 118, 2001.
28. Sebastiani, S. et al., Chemokine receptor expression and function in $CD4^+$ T lymphocytes with regulatory activity, *J. Immunol.*, 116, 996, 2001.
29. Iellem, A. et al., Unique chemotactic response profile and specific expression of chemokine receptors CCR4 and CCR8 by $CD4^+CD25^+$ regulatory T cells, *J. Exp. Med.*, 194, 847, 2001.
30. Sebastiani, S. et al., Nickel-specific $CD8^+$ and $CD4^+$ T cells display distinct migratory response to chemokines produced during allergic contact dermatitis, *J. Invest. Dermatol.*, 118, 1052, 2002.
31. Sallusto, F. et al., Two subsets of memory T lymphocytes with distinct homing potential and effector function, *Nature*, 401, 708, 1999.
32. Sallusto, F. et al., Distinct patterns and kinetics of chemokine production regulate dendritic cell function, *Eur. J. Immunol.*, 29, 1617, 1999.
33. Robert, C. and Kupper, T.S., Inflammatory skin diseases, T cells, and immune surveillance, *N. Engl. J. Med.*, 341, 1817, 1999.
34. Liao, F. et al., CC-chemokine receptor 6 is expressed in diverse memory subsets of T cells and determines responsiveness to macrophage inflammatory protein 3$\alpha$, *J. Immunol.*, 162, 186, 1999.

35. Fitzhugh, D.J. et al., C-C chemokine receptor 6 is essential for arrest of a subset of memory T cells on activated dermal microvascular endothelial cells under physiologic flow conditions *in vitro*, *J. Immunol.*, 165, 6677, 2000.
36. Homey, B. et al., CCL27-CCR10 interactions regulate T cell-mediated skin inflammation, *Nat. Med.*, 8, 157, 2002.
37. Garcia-Ramallo, E. et al., Resident cell chemokine expression serves as the major mechanism for leukocyte recruitment during local inflammation, *J. Immunol.*, 169, 6467, 2002.
38. Anttila, H.S. et al., Interleukin-8 immunoreactivity in the skin of healthy subjects and patients with palmoplantar pustulosis and psoriasis, *J. Invest. Dermatol.*, 98, 96, 1992.
39. Charbonnier, A.-S. et al., Macrophage inflammatory protein 3α is involved in the constitutive trafficking of epidermal Langerhans cells, *J. Exp. Med.*, 190, 1755, 1999.
40. Dieu-Nosejan, M.-C. et al., Macrophage inflammatory protein 3α is expressed at inflamed epithelial cell surfaces and is the most potent chemokine known in attracting Langerhans cell precursor, *J. Exp. Med.*, 192, 705, 2000.
41. Nakayama, N. et al., Inducible expression of a CC chemokine liver- and activation-regulated chemokine (LARC)/macrophage inflammatory protein (MIP)-3α/CCL20 by epidermal keratinocytes and its role in atopic dermatitis, *Int. Immunol.*, 13, 95, 2000.
42. Vestergaard, C. et al., TARC, produced by keratinocytes may recruit $CLA^+CCR4^+$ lymphocytes into lesional atopic dermatitis skin, *J. Invest. Dermatol.*, 115, 640, 2000.
43. Albanesi, C. et al., A cytokine-to-chemokine axis between T lymphocytes and keratinocytes can favor Th1 cell accumulation in chronic inflammatory skin diseases, *J. Leukocyte Biol.*, 70, 617, 2001.
44. Albanesi, C., Cavani, A., and Girolomoni, G., Interleukin-17 is produced by nickel-specific T lymphocytes and regulates ICAM-1 expression and chemokine production in human keratinocytes. Synergistic or antagonist effects with interferon-γ and tumor necrosis factor-α, *J. Immunol.*, 162, 494, 1999.
45. Albanesi, C. et al., Interleukin 17 is produced by both Th1 and Th2 lymphocytes, and modulates interferon-γ- and interleukin 4-induced activation of human keratinocytes, *J. Invest. Dermatol.*, 115, 81, 2000.
46. Albanesi, C. et al., IL-4 enhances keratinocyte expression of CXCR3 agonistic chemokine, *J. Immunol.*, 165, 1395, 2000.
47. Pastore, S. et al., Dysregulated activation of activator protein 1 in keratinocytes of atopic dermatitis patients with enhanced expression of granulocyte/macrophage-colony stimulating factor, *J. Invest. Dermatol.*, 115, 1134, 2000.
48. Giustizieri, M.L. et al., Keratinocytes from patients with atopic dermatitis and psoriasis show a different chemokine production profile in response to T cell-derived cytokines, *J. Allergy Clin. Immunol.*, 107, 871, 2001.
49. Federici, M et al., Impaired IFN-γ-dependent inflammatory responses in human keratinocytes overexpressing the suppressor of cytokine signaling 1, *J. Immunol.*, 169, 434, 2002.
50. Mascia, F. et al., Blockade of the EGF receptor induces a deranged chemokine expression in keratinocytes leading to enhanced skin inflammation, *Am. J. Pathol.*, 163, 303, 2003.
51. Schröder, J.M. and Mochizuki, M., The role of chemokines in cutaneous allergic inflammation, *Biol. Chem.*, 389, 889, 1999.
52. Mochizuki, M. et al., IL-4 induces eotaxin: a possible mechanism of selective eosinophils recruitment in helminth infection and atopy, *J. Immunol.*, 160, 60, 1998.
53. Dulkys, Y. et al., Detection of mRNA for eotaxin-2 and eotaxin-3 in human dermal fibroblasts and their distinct activation profile on human eosinophils, *J. Invest. Dermatol.*, 116, 498, 2001.
54. Petering, H. et al., Detection of MCP-4 in dermal fibroblast and its activation of the respiratory burst in human eosinophils, *J. Immunol.*, 160, 555, 1998.
55. Mekory, Y.A. and Metcalfe, D.D., Mast cell-T cell interactions, *J. Allergy Clin. Immunol.*, 104, 517, 1999.
56. Vissers, J.L.M. et al., Quantitative analysis of chemokine expression by dendritic cell subsets *in vitro* and *in vivo*, *J. Leukocyte Biol.*, 69, 785, 2001.
57. la Sala, A. et al., Dendritic cells exposed to extracellular adenosine triphosphate acquire the migratory properties of mature cells and show a reduced capacity to attract type 1 T lymphocytes, *Blood*, 99, 1715, 2002.

58. Corinti, S. et al., Erythrocytes deliver Tat to interferon-γ-treated human dendritic cells for efficient initiation of specific type 1 immune responses *in vitro*, *J. Leukocyte Biol.*, 71, 652, 2002.
59. Fraticelli, P. et al., Fractalkine (CX3CL1) as an amplification circuit of polarized Th1 responses, *J. Clin. Invest.*, 107, 1173, 2001.
60. Engelhardt, E. et al., Chemokines IL-8, Gro-α, MCP-1, IP-10, and MIG are sequentially and differentially expressed during phase-specific infiltration of leukocyte subset in human wound healing, *Am. J. Pathol.*, 153, 1849, 1998.
61. Goebeler, M. et al., Differential and sequential expression of multiple chemokines during elicitation of allergic contact hypersensitivity, *Am. J. Pathol.*, 158, 431, 2001.
62. Flier, J. et al., The CXCR3 activating chemokines IP-10, Mig, and IP-9 are expressed in allergic but non in irritant patch test reactions, *J. Invest. Dermatol.*, 113, 574, 1999.
63. Fife, B.T. et al., CXCL10 (IFN-γ-inducible protein-10) control of encephalitogenic $CD4^+$ T cell accumulation in the central nervous system during experimental autoimmune encephalomyelitis, *J. Immunol.*, 166, 7617, 2001.
64. Salomon, I. et al., Targeting the function of IFN-γ-inducible Protein 10 suppresses ongoing adjuvant arthritis, *J. Immunol.*, 169, 2685, 2002.
65. Sozzani, S. et al., Differential regulation of chemokine receptors during dendritic cell maturation: a model for their trafficking properties, *J. Clin. Immunol.*, 20, 151, 2000.
66. Rennert, P.D. et al., Essential role of lymph nodes in contact hypersensitivity revealed in lymphotoxin-α-deficient mice, *J. Exp. Med.*, 193, 1227, 2001.
67. Förster, R. et al., CCR7 coordinates the primary immune response by establishing functional microenvironments in secondary lymphoid organs, *Cell*, 99, 23, 1999.
68. Gunn, M.D. et al., Mice lacking expression of secondary lymphoid organ chemokine have defects in lymphocyte homing and dendritic cell localization, *J. Exp. Med.*, 189, 451, 1999.
69. Bouloc, A., Cavani, A., and Katz, S.I., Contact hypersensitivity in MHC class II-deficient mice depends on $CD8^+$ T lymphocytes primed by immunostimulating Langerhans cells, *J. Invest. Dermatol.*, 111, 44, 1998.
70. Kehren, J. et al., Cytotoxicity is mandatory for $CD8^+$ T cell-mediated contact hypersensitivity, *J. Exp. Med.*, 189, 779, 1999.
71. Traidl, C. et al., Disparate cytotoxic activity of nickel-specific $CD8^+$ and $CD4^+$ T cell subsets against keratinocytes, *J. Immunol.*, 165, 3058, 2000.
72. Trautmann, A. et al., T-cell-mediated Fas-induced keratinocyte apoptosis plays a key pathogenetic role in eczematous dermatitis, *J. Clin. Invest.*, 106, 25, 2000.
73. Wang, B. et al., $CD4^+$ Th1 and $CD8^+$ type 1 cytotoxic T cells both play a crucial role in the full development of contact hypersensitivity, *J. Immunol.*, 165, 6783, 2000.
74. Girolomoni, G. et al., T-cell subpopulations in the development of atopic and contact allergy, *Curr. Opin. Immunol.*, 13, 733, 2001.
75. Biedermann, T. et al., Reversal of established delayed type hypersensitivity reactions following therapy with IL-4 or antigen-specific Th2 cells, *Eur. J. Immunol.*, 31, 1582, 2001.
76. Yokozeki, H. et al., Signal transducer and activator of transcription 6 is essential in the induction of contact hypersensitivity, *J. Exp. Med.*, 191, 995, 2000.
77. Nakamura, K., Williams, I.R., and Kupper, T.S., Keratinocyte-derived monocyte chemoattractant protein 1 (MCP-1): analysis in a transgenic model demonstrates MCP-1 can recruit dendritic and Langerhans cells to skin, *J. Invest. Dermatol.*, 105, 635, 1995.
78. Griffiths, C.E.M. et al., Modulation of leukocyte adhesion molecule, a T-cell chemotaxin (IL-8) and a regulatory cytokine (TNF-α) in allergic contact dermatitis (rhus dermatitis), *Br. J. Dermatol.*, 124, 519, 1991.
79. Tsuji, R.I. et al., Early local generation of C5a initiates the elicitation of contact sensitivity by leading to early T cell recruitment, *J. Immunol.*, 165, 1588, 2000.
80. Biedermann, T. et al., Mast cells control neutrophil recruitment during T cell-mediated delayed-type hypersensitivity reactions through tumor necrosis factor and macrophage inflammatory protein 2, *J. Exp. Med.*, 192, 1441, 2000.
81. Abe, M. et al., Interferon-γ inducible protein (IP-10) expression is mediated by $CD8^+$ T cells and is regulated by $CD4^+$ T cells during the elicitation phase of contact hypersensitivity, *J. Invest. Dermatol.*, 107, 360, 1996.

82. Cavani, A. et al., Human CD4+ T lymphocytes with remarkable regulatory functions on dendritic cells and nickel-specific Th1 immune responses, *J. Invest. Dermatol.*, 114, 295, 2000.
83. Schwarz, A. et al., Evidence for functional relevance of CTLA-4 in ultraviolet-radiation-induced tolerance, *J. Immunol.*, 165, 1824, 2000.
84. Varona, R. et al., CCR6-deficient mice have impaired leukocyte homeostasis and altered contact hypersensitivity and delayed-type hypersensitivity responses. *J. Clin. Invest.*, 107, R37, 2001.
85. Nickoloff, B.J. et al., Is psoriasis a T-cell disease? *Exp. Dermatol.*, 9:359, 2000.
86. Asadullah, K., Volk, H.-D., and Sterry, W., Novel immunotherapies for psoriasis, *Trends Immunol.*, 23, 47, 2002.
87. Krueger, J.G., The immunologic basis for the treatment of psoriasis with new biological agents, *J. Am. Acad. Dermatol.*, 46, 1, 2002.
88. Schön, M.P. and Ruzicka, T., Psoriasis: the plot thickens ..., *Nat. Immunol.*, 2, 91, 2001.
89. Nickoloff, B.J. et al., Aberrant production of interleukin-8 and thrombospondin-1 by psoriatic keratinocytes mediates angiogenesis, *Am. J. Pathol.*, 144, 820, 1994.
90. Gillitzer, R. et al., MCP-1 mRNA expression in basal keratinocytes of psoriatic lesions, *J. Invest. Dermatol.*, 101, 127, 1993.
91. Gottlieb, A.B. et al., Detection of a $\gamma$ interferon-induced protein IP-10 in psoriatic plaques, *J. Exp. Med.*, 168, 941, 1988.
92. Homey, B. et al., Up-regulation of macrophage inflammatory protein 3$\alpha$/CCL20 and CC chemokine receptor 6 in psoriasis, *J. Immunol.*, 164,6621, 2000.
93. Rottman, J.B. et al., Potential role of the chemokine receptors CXCR3, CCR4, and the integrin $\alpha E\beta 7$ in the pathogenesis of psoriasis vulgaris, *Lab. Invest.*, 8, 335, 2001.
94. Vanbervliet, B. et al., Sequential involvement of CCR2 and CCR6 ligands for immature dendritic cell recruitment: possible role at inflamed epithelial surfaces, *Eur. J. Immunol.*, 32, 231, 2002.
95. Hudak, S. et al., Immune surveillance and effector functions of CCR10+ skin homing T cells, *J. Immunol.*, 169, 1189, 2002.
96. Giustizieri, M.L. et al., Nitric oxide donors suppress chemokine production by keratinocytes *in vitro* and *in vivo*, *Am. J. Pathol.*, 161, 1409, 2002.
97. Kulke, R. et al., The CXC receptor 2 is over-expressed in psoriatic epidermis, *J. Invest. Dermatol.*, 110, 90, 1998.
98. Karvonen, S.L. et al., Psoriasis and altered calcium metabolism: downregulated capacitative calcium influx and defective calcium-mediated cell signaling in cultured psoriatic keratinocytes, *J. Invest. Dermatol.*, 114, 693, 2000.
99. Haase, I. et al., A role for mitogen-activated protein-kinase activation by integrins in the pathogenesis of psoriasis, *J. Clin. Invest.*, 108, 527, 2001.
100. Sirsjo, A. et al., Increased expression of inducible nitric oxide synthase in psoriatic skin and cytokine-stimulated cultured keratinocytes, *Br. J. Dermatol.*, 134, 643, 1996.
101. Ormerod, A.D. et al., Detection of nitric oxide and nitric oxide synthases in psoriasis, *Arch. Dermatol. Res.*, 290, 3, 1998.
102. Bodgan, C., Nitric oxide and the immune response, *Nat. Immunol.*, 2, 907, 2001.
103. Asadullah, K. et al., Effects of systemic interleukin-10 therapy on psoriatic skin lesions: histologic, immunohistologic, and molecular biology findings, *J. Invest. Dermatol.*, 116, 721, 2001.
104. Reich, K. et al., Response of psoriasis to interleukin-10 is associated with suppression of cutaneous type 1 inflammation, down-regulation of the epidermal interleukin-8/CXCR2 pathway and normalization of keratinocyte maturation, *J. Invest. Dermatol.*, 116, 319, 2001.
105. Stoof, T.J. et al., The antipsoriatic drug dimethylfumarate strongly suppresses chemokine production in human keratinocytes and peripheral blood mononuclear cells, *Br. J. Dermatol.*, 144, 1114, 2001.
106. Leung, D.Y., and Soter, N.A., Cellular and immunologic mechanisms in atopic dermatitis, *J. Am. Acad. Dermatol.*, 44, S1, 2001.
107. von Bubnoff, D., Geiger, E., and Bieber, T., Antigen-presenting cells in allergy, *J. Allergy Clin. Immunol.*, 108, 329, 2001.
108. Kraft, S. et al., Aggregation of the high-affinity IgE receptor Fc$\varepsilon$RI on human monocytes and dendritic cells induces NF-$\kappa$B activation, *J. Invest. Dermatol.*, 118, 830, 2002.
109. Girolomoni, G. and Pastore, S., Epithelial cells and atopic diseases, *Curr. Allergy Asthma Rep.*, 1, 481, 2001.

110. Yamamoto, J. et al., Differential expression of the chemokine receptors by the Th1- and Th2-type effector populations within circulating CD4+ T cells, *J. Leukocyte Biol.*, 68, 568, 2000.
111. Nakatani, T. et al., CCR4+ memory CD4+ T lymphocytes are increased in peripheral blood and lesional skin from patients with atopic dermatitis, *J. Allergy Clin. Immunol.*, 107, 353, 2001.
112. Wakugawa, M. et al., CC chemokine receptor 4 expression on peripheral blood CD4+ T cells reflects disease activity of atopic dermatitis, *J. Invest. Dermatol.*, 117, 188, 2001.
113. Okazaki, H. et al., Characterization of chemokine receptor expression and cytokine production in circulating CD4+ T cells from patients with atopic dermatitis: up-regulation of C-C chemokine receptor 4 in atopic dermatitis, *Clin. Exp. Allergy*, 32, 1236, 2002.
114. Fujisawa, T. et al., Presence of high contents of thymus and activation-regulated chemokine in platelets and elevated plasma levels of thymus and activation-regulated chemokine and macrophage-derived chemokine in patients with atopic dermatitis, *J. Allergy Clin. Immunol.*, 110, 139, 2002.
115. Horikawa, T. et al., IFN-γ-inducible expression of thymus and activation-regulated chemokine/CCL17 and macrophage-derived chemokine/CCL22 in epidermal keratinocytes and their roles in atopic dermatitis, *Int. Immunol.*, 14, 767, 2002.
116. Kakinuma, T. et al., Serum macrophage-derived chemokine (MDC) levels are closely related with the disease activity of atopic dermatitis, *Clin. Exp. Immunol.*, 27, 270, 2002.
117. Zheng, X. et al., Demonstration of TARC and CCR4 mRNA expression and distribution using *in situ* RT-PCR in the lesional skin of atopic dermatitis, *J. Dermatol.*, 30, 26, 2003.
118. Kaburagi, Y. et al., Enhanced production of CC-chemokines (RANTES, MCP-1, MIP-1α, MIP-1β, and eotaxin) in patients with atopic dermatitis, *Arch. Dermatol. Res.*, 293, 350, 2001.
119. Yawalkar, N. et al., Enhanced expression of eotaxin and CCR3 in atopic dermatitis, *J. Invest. Dermatol.*, 113, 43, 1999.
120. Taha, R.A. et al., Evidence for increased expression of eotaxin and monocyte chemotactic protein-4 in atopic dermatitis, *J. Allergy Clin. Immunol.*, 105, 1002, 2000.
121. Schmuth, M. et al., Expression of the C-C chemokine MIP-3α/CCL20 in human epidermis with impaired permeability barrier function, *Exp. Dermatol.*, 11, 135, 2002.
122. Frezzolini, A. et al., Circulating interleukin 16 (IL-16) in children with atopic/eczema dermatitis syndrome (AEDS): a novel serological marker of disease activity, *Allergy*, 57, 815, 2002.
123. Laberge, S. et al., Association of increased CD4+ T-cell infiltration with increased IL-16 expression in atopic dermatitis, *J. Allergy Clin. Immunol.*, 102, 645, 1998.
124. Reich, K. et al., Evidence for a role of Langerhans cell-derived IL-16 in atopic dermatitis, *J. Allergy Clin. Immunol.*, 109, 681, 2002.
125. Cruikshank, W.W., Kornfeld, H., and Center, D.M., Interleukin-16, *J. Leukocyte Biol.*, 67, 757, 2000.
126. Kaser, A. et al., A role for IL-16 in the cross-talk between dendritic cells and T cells, *J. Immunol.*, 163, 3232, 1999.
127. Stingl, G. and Maurer, D., IgE-mediated allergen presentation via Fc epsilon RI on antigen-presenting cells, *Int. Arch. Allergy Immunol.*, 113, 24, 1997.
128. Reich, K. et al., Engagement of FcεRI stimulates the production of IL-16 in Langerhans cell-like dendritic cells, *J. Immunol.*, 167, 6321, 2001.
129. Pastore, S. et al., Granulocyte macrophage colony-stimulating factor is overproduced by keratinocytes in atopic dermatitis. Implications for sustained dendritic cell activation in the skin, *J. Clin. Invest.*, 99, 3009, 1997.
130. Nickel, R.G. et al., Atopic dermatitis is associated with a functional mutation in the promoter of the C-C chemokine RANTES, *J. Immunol.*, 164, 1612, 2000.
131. Elliot, K., and Forrest, S., Genetics of atopic dermatitis, in *Atopic Dermatitis*, Bieber, T. and Leung, D.Y.M., Eds., Marcel Dekker, New York, 2002, 81.
132. Kozma, G.T. et al., Lack of association between atopic eczema/dermatitis syndrome and polymorphisms in the promoter region of RANTES and regulatory region of MCP-1, *Allergy*, 57, 160, 2002.
133. Soumelis, V. et al., Human epithelial cells trigger dendritic cell mediated allergic inflammation by producing TSLP, *Nat. Immunol.*, 3, 673, 2002.
134. Elias, P.M., Wood, L.C., and Feingold, K.R., Epidermal pathogenesis of inflammatory dermatoses, *Am. J. Contact Dermatitis*, 10, 119, 1999.
135. Mascia, F. et al., House dust mite allergen exerts no direct proinflammatory effects on human keratinocytes, *J. Allergy Clin. Immunol.*, 109, 532, 2002.

136. Proudfoot, A.E.I., Chemokine receptors: multifaceted therapeutic targets, *Nat. Rev. Immunol.*, 2, 106, 2002.
137. Rand, M.L. et al., Inhibition of T cell recruitment and cutaneous delayed-type hypersensitivity-induced inflammation with antibodies to monocyte chemoattractant protein-1, *Am. J. Pathol.*, 158, 855, 1996.
138. Lu, B. et al., Abnormalities in monocyte recruitment and cytokine expression in monocyte chemoattractant protein 1-deficient mice, *J. Exp. Med.*, 16, 601, 1998.
139. Xie, J.H. et al., Antibody-mediated blockade of the CXCR3 chemokine receptor results in diminished recruitment of T helper 1 cells into sites of inflammation, *J. Leukocyte Biol.*, 73, 771, 2003.
140. Jiankuo, M. et al., Peptide nucleic acid antisense prolongs skin allograft survival by means of blockade of CXCR3 expression directing T cells into graft, *J. Immunol.*, 170, 1556, 2003.
141. Hancock, W.W. et al., Requirement of the chemokine receptor CXCR3 for acute allograft rejection, *J. Exp. Med.*, 192, 1515, 2000.
142. Carter, P.H., Chemokine receptor antagonism as a approach to anti-inflammatory therapy: "just right" or plain wrong? *Curr. Opin. Chem. Biol.*, 6, 510, 2002.
143. Ono, S.J. et al., Chemokines: roles in leukocyte development, trafficking, and effector function, *J. Allergy Clin. Immunol.*, 111, 1185, 2003.
144. Gonzalo, J.A. et al., The coordinated action of CC chemokines in the lung orchestrates allergic inflammation and airway hyperresponsiveness, *J. Exp. Med.*, 188, 157, 1998.
145. Ajuebor, M.N. et al., The chemokine RANTES is a crucial mediator of the progression from acute to chronic colitis in the rat, *J. Immunol.*, 166, 552, 2001.
146. Saeki, T. and Naya, A., CCR1 chemokine receptor antagonist, *Curr. Pharm. Design*, 9, 1201, 2002.
147. Khan, I.A. et al., Mice lacking the chemokine receptor CCR1 show increased susceptibility to *Toxoplasma gondii* infection, *J. Immunol.*, 166, 1930, 2001.
148. Ma, W. et al., CCR3 is essential for skin eosinophilia and airway hyperresponsiveness in a murine model of allergic skin inflammation, *J. Clin. Invest.*, 109, 621, 2002.
149. Nibbs R.J. et al., C-C chemokine receptor 3 antagonism by the beta-chemokine macrophage inflammatory protein 4, a property strongly enhanced by an amino-terminal alanine-methionine swap, *J. Immunol.*, 164, 1488, 2000.
150. Sabroe, I. et al., A small molecule antagonist of chemokine receptors CCR1 and CCR3, *J. Biol. Chem.*, 275, 25985, 2000.
151. Saeki, T. et al., Identification of a potent and nonpeptidyl CCR3 antagonist, *Biochem. Biophys. Res. Commun.*, 281, 779, 2001.
152. White, J.R. et al., Identification of potent, selective non-peptide CC chemokine receptor-3 antagonist that inhibits eotaxin, eotaxin-2, and monocyte chemotactic protein-4-induced eosinophil migration, *J. Biol. Chem.*, 275, 36626, 2000.

# 17 Neuropeptides in the Skin

*James N. Baraniuk*

## CONTENTS



## I. INTRODUCTION

The cutaneous nervous system responds immediately to many stimuli including skin irritation, injury, and ambient temperature changes. These nerves include large-diameter, myelinated fine touch, proprioception, and specialized sensory organ neurons, minimally myelinated Type Aδ fibers that sense cold and high heat sensation, and a family of novel and sensation-selective unmyelinated Type C nociceptive neurons. Activation of these systems can lead to local, spinal cord, and central nervous system (CNS) (Table 17.1) responses in proportion to the perceived threat of the stimulus. Because these neural mechanisms are highly species dependent, studies in rodents should not be extrapolated to humans.[1] This chapter focuses on the roles of human Type C sensory neurons.

Type C neurons act as sentinels to detect and transmit specific sensations such as itch and pain nociceptive messages to the CNS. Different subpopulations of C fibers are responsible for different sensory modalities. Type C neurons are also unique because they mediate immediate cutaneous responses to these potentially injurious stimuli. The prototypic local, neurally mediated skin response to injury is the triple response of Lewis.[2] Firm, blunt injury such as strong stroking of the skin is followed by development of a "white line," "red line," "flare," local edema ("wheal") if the injury is severe enough, and local hyperalgesia. To understand this fundamental cutaneous defense mechanism, we must appreciate the complex innervation of the skin, the central spinal cord connections

0-8493-1959-5/05/$0.00+$1.50

**TABLE 17.1**
**Effects of Capsaicin, CGPR, SP, and Their Antagonists on Vasodilation[118]**

| | Capsaicin | CGRP | SP |
|---|---|---|---|
| Duration of vasodilation | Long | Long | Short |
| hCGRP8-37 (CGRP antagonist) | Inhibited | Inhibited | No effect |
| SR-140.333 (NK1-antagonist) | No effect | No effect | Inhibited |

*Note:* Capsaicin → C fibers → CGRP → Vasodilation = Flare.

*Source:* Rinder, J. and Lundberg, J.M., *Allergologie*, 1, 48, 1996. With permission.

of sensory nerves, the identities of the neurotransmitters, and the intricate coordination of nerves, blood vessels, and other elements that are involved in the skin inflammatory response.

Parasympathetic and sympathetic systems play critical homeostatic roles by regulating vascular and other processes. They regulate body temperature by conserving heat during cold exposure (vasoconstriction, contraction of erector pili muscles to create an insulating layer of air beneath elevated hairs), and promote heat loss by vasodilation, sweating, and evaporative cooling during exercise and heat exposure.

Although specific neuropeptides are generally associated with each of the three peripheral nervous systems, there are wide variations in the combinations of neuropeptides and other neurotransmitters that are expressed in neurons in different tissues and species. Neuroregulators released by end organ target cells can regulate the nature of the neurotransmitters required for their proper functioning. This would explain the release of acetylcholine by sympathetic nerves to activate sweat gland muscarinic receptor-mediated functions (sweating during physiological stressors). Neurons are also highly plastic in their neuropeptide expression, and may change these patterns during active inflammatory states. These complex signaling processes permit "customization" of neurotransmitter content to fit the specific tasks of the nerve in its central and peripheral sites.

## II. NEUROGENIC INFLAMMATION, CAPSAICIN, AND TRP PROTEINS

Early scientific evidence for the involvement of the nervous system in the development of inflammatory responses came from the experiments of Bayliss[3] in 1901 and others who used chemical stimuli, such as capsaicin, mustard oil, xylene, and electrical stimulation to demonstrate that wheal and flare reactions were dependent on intact polymodal, small, nonmyelinated C fibers. The wheal and flare were considered sufficient for the reaction to be termed "neurogenic inflammation." Their hypothesis has been supported by several observations. Sensory neuropeptides such as substance P (SP) are released in the skin from nerve endings by noxious or electrical stimulation.

Neuropeptides induce vasodilation and vascular permeability when injected intradermally. SP antagonists can inhibit heat-induced or electrically induced edema in rat skin (but are less effective in humans). Flare (vasodilation) reactions do not occur in skin areas affected by congenital analgesia, analgesia induced by herpes zoster, local anesthetics, or diabetic neuropathy, and do not spread beyond the dermatome of the initially stimulated neurons. Cutaneous neurogenic responses can be prevented by local pretreatment with the sensory nerve toxin capsaicin.

Capsaicin, trans-8-methyl-*n*-vanillyl-6-nonenamide, the hot, spicy essence of red peppers, depolarizes a population of nociceptive Type C (and potentially some Aδ) sensory nerves by activating a nonselective cation channel (Figure 17.1).[4] This channel was cloned and named the vanilloid

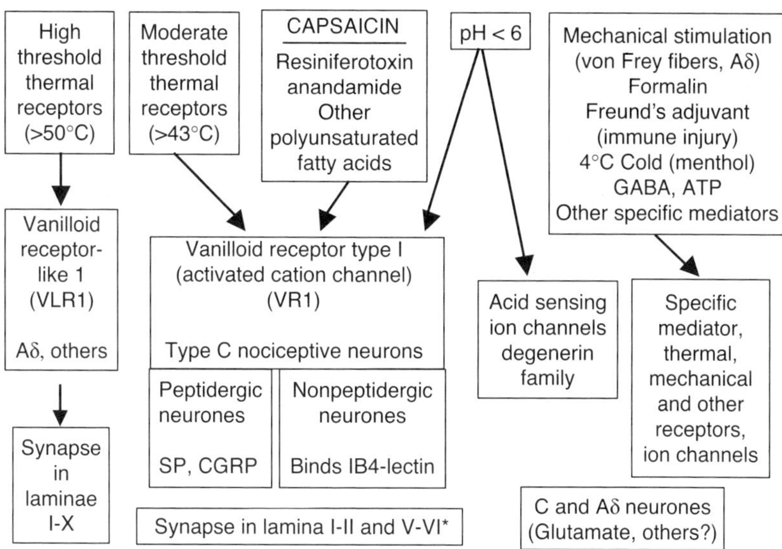


**FIGURE 17.1** Multiple nociceptive stimuli (nocifers, alogens) act upon VR1 (TRPV1) and other receptors to depolarize discrete populations of Type C and Aδ peripheral nerves. The Type C neurons may be divided into peptidergic, and nonpeptidergic, isolectinB4$^+$ subsets.

receptor 1 (VR1).[5] Low threshold heat (>43°C), pH < 5, arachidonic acid metabolites that form endogenous cannibinoids such as the CB1 agonist *N*-arachadonoyl-dopamine (NADA),[6] and other cationic lipids may also be endogenous agonists of VR1.

Acute capsaicin administration to rats and guinea pigs causes an influx of $Na^+$ and $Ca^{2+}$ that depolarizes neurons and causes the release of SP, calcitonin gene-related peptide (CGRP), somatostatin (SOM), neurokinin A (NKA), eledoisin, prostaglandins, and acetylcholine. Intradermal and topical capsaicin induces dose-dependent flare and hyperalgesia responses.[7] Thermography identified reproducible punctuate regions that likely represented dilated arterioles that supplied blood to the superficial dermal plexus for the flare response.[8] Capsaicin treatment induced mechanical and heat hyperalgesia (accentuated pain responses induced by lower levels of stimulation by each modality). The sharply defined regions of hyperalgesia corresponded to the thermographic flare. The flare, temperature changes, and hyperalgesia were blocked by local anesthetics. A limitation is that 10 µl of 1% capsaicin was injected. This dose may activate "silent" C and Aδ nociceptors that are hypothesized to be activated by skin injury.[9]

Repeated topical use desensitizes the skin to noxious chemical, mechanical, and heat stimuli without affecting touch, pressure, vibration, cold, or Aδ-fiber-mediated sensations in humans, guinea pigs, and rats.[10] Local capsaicin treatment in humans reduced the flare response to chemical irritants, intradermally injected histamine, anti-IgE, and antigen, but did not affect wheal responses. High doses administered to neonatal rats induced mitochondrial swelling and a reduction in cytoplasmic vesicles in small dorsal root ganglion cells that contain SP and SOM, and degeneration of various types of neuropeptide-containing sensory C fibers.[4] By contrast, ingestion of up to 30 to 60 g of capsaicin per day is considered a culinary delight in some chronically capsaicin-desensitized societies.

The capsaicin receptor VR1 is a member of the transient receptor potential channel (TRP) hexahelical transmembrane protein superfamily. At least 26 TRP proteins have been identified. They are classified into vanilloid (TRPV), canonical channel (TRPC), melastatin (TRPM), and PKD (TRPP) subfamilies. The proteins organize as heterotetrameric structures with preferred partners such as TRPC3/6/7, TRPC4/5, and possibly TRPC1/4/5 forming the functional complexes.[11] The loop between the fifth and sixth transmembrane region forms the ion pore. Each tetramer has specific agonists and antagonists, stoichiometry, and pore capacities. Sensor diversity is enhanced by splice variants of these proteins that may also alter their sensitivities and functions. Their major function is to sense specific stimuli and induce a rapid inward flux of $Ca^{2+}$ and other cations that depolarizes the neuron.

The vanilloid subfamily contains TRPV1 (VR1), the TRPV2 vanilloid-like receptor 1 (VRL-1, high heat sensitivity, Aδ nerve fibers), TRPV3 (another heat sensitive receptor), and TRPV4, an osmotic and mechanicosensitive receptor.[12] The sensory modality detected by each protein depends upon co-expressed subfamily members, other associated proteins, and potentially the local lipid membrane microenvironment. In *Caenorhabditis elegans*, for example, TRPV4 alone responds to hypotonic stimuli. When coupled with other proteins including a specific G protein α subunit, TRPV4 responds to hyperosmolar and mechanical stimuli. Other proteins can modulate the temperature sensitivity of TRPV4 function. Combinations of these sensory cation channels, other ion channels (e.g., proton channels), G protein–coupled receptors (GPCR), and other receptor proteins may account for the different sensations conveyed by nociceptors. There may be plasticity in their expression during inflammation, which could explain apparent changes in the sensitivity to certain stimuli ("peripheral hyperalgesia").

The TRPV proteins are not limited to nerves. TRPV1 is expressed in keratinocytes.[13] These epidermal receptors could respond to noxious stimuli such as topical capsaicin or intradermally injected neuropeptides with the release of interleukin (IL)-1 and other mediators that in turn activate mast cells, Langerhans cells, and populations of C fibers. The acute toxic effect of capsaicin supports this hypothesis. Exposures in industrial chili pepper workers or victims of high doses of "pepper spray" self-defense products can develop damage to keratinocytes and fibroblasts,[14] extremely severe erythema, edema, desquamation analogous to third-degree burns, mucosal irritation including lacrimation, rhinorrhea, cough, and potentially bronchoconstriction. These data would indicate that intradermal injections of peptides or other TRP agonists could be sufficient to cause toxicity reactions. If so, then many years of investigations using intradermal injections of micromolar concentrations to various neuropeptides may have to be reinterpreted or considered artifacts to epidermal toxicity.

## III. SENSORY NERVES

Sensory nerves convey the entire spectrum of cutaneous sensations from the skin to specific layers of the substantia gelatinosa of the spinal cord.[15,16] Large Aβ and Aδ myelinated fibers, and fine, nonmyelinated C fibers are found in the deep dermis as bundles and fibers near blood vessels, sweat glands, and hair follicles. The larger neurons innervate various specialized mechanical and temperature-sensitive end organs in the upper dermis near the epidermal–dermal junction zone. C fibers are found as fine, nonmyelinated free endings in the dermis and epidermis, and form cage- or basket-like arborizations around vessels, glands, and the upper portions of hair follicles.

Mechanical, chemical, and thermal stimuli activate polymodal nociceptive C fibers, which conduct electrical impulses centrally to the spinal cord. It appears that the chemosensory neurons may also depolarize locally in retrograde fashion throughout the extensively branched dermal ramifications of these neurons (Figure 17.1). Neurosecretory swellings, or varicosities, are strung like beads on a string, and release neurotransmitters as waves of depolarization pass along the branches. Neuropeptides diffuse to specific receptors on local vessels, glands, epidermis, resident connective tissue cells, and immune cells such as lymphocytes and mast cells. This "efferent" neurosecretory response stimulated by "afferent" sensory nerves has been termed the "axon-reflex"[2] and is implicated in flare generation. Separate "pain" and "itch" chemosensory C fibers are present in the "nociceptive" neuron pool, a finding that must be kept in mind when extrapolating neurogenic responses of painful stimuli to other sensations.

Various combinations of neurotransmitters are present in these neurons. The list of candidate sensory neurotransmitters is ever-increasing and includes SP, CGRP, NKA (substance K), neurokinin B (NKB, neuromedin K), SOM, vasoactive intestinal peptide (VIP), cholecystokinin (CCK), dynorphin (DYN), neurotensin (NT), galanin (GAL), secretoneurin, and potentially endothelins and excitatory amino acids (Table 17.1). Not all have been examined in human skin.

## IV. TACHYKININS

Tachykinins, or NKs, share a common C-terminal pentapeptide sequence (Phe-X-Gly-Leu-Met where X is Phe in SP) and an aminidated C-terminal.[17] A series of tachykinin genes produces a family of preprotachykinin mRNAs and tachykinin peptides.[18] Three tachykinin receptors have been cloned. NK-1 receptors are most sensitive to SP, and likely mediate SP-induced arterial vasodilation and venous dilation with increased venular permeability and plasma extravasation. NK-2 receptors prefer NKA. Their most important function is mediation of tachykinin-induced bronchial contraction. NK-3 receptors bind NKB, and are likely important only in the CNS. NK-1 receptors activate mitogen-activated protein kinase (MAPK), nuclear factor of activated T cells (NF-AT), nuclear factor for kappa chains in B cells (NFκB).[19,20]

SP binding sites are found in endothelial cells, dermal papillae, adnexal structures, and epidermis.[21] Endothelial and vascular smooth muscle effects include vasodilation that may be mediated by nitric oxide.[22] Activation of endothelium leads to plasma extravasation in rodents. Rapid upregulation of adhesion molecules may occur in concert with extravasation. Injection of SP and NKA cause perivascular cuffing by neutrophils in normal humans and by neutrophils and eosinophils in atopic subjects.[23] SP and NKA may have trophic or modulatory effects on endothelium, keratinocytes, and other dermal cells.[24]

Many of the effects of SP and other peptides have been attributed to their ability to degranulate mast cells. Functional connections between SP-releasing neurons and mast cells have been proposed. Indeed, SP, NKA, NKB, SOM, and VIP produce triple responses after intradermal injection.[25] The reactions last about 1 h. SP can cause degranulation of bovine skin mast cells.[26] However, the SP analogue $NH_2$-Arg-Pro-Lys-Pro-$C_{12}H_{25}$ is an equally effective histamine-releasing agent.[27] Its structure suggests a nonselective biophysical membrane interaction. The ability of SP, SP analogues, bradykinin, VIP, and other basically charged peptides to release rat peritoneal mast cell histamine was correlated with their ability to release mast cell histamine and produce a flare, but not the wheal response.[27] However, electrical depolarization of nociceptive neurons can induce vascular permeability without mast cell degranulation.[28] These data suggest that the SP–mast cell concept is an attractive hypothesis that may be applicable in rodents, but that it is more difficult to embrace in humans.

## V. CALCITONIN GENE-RELATED PEPTIDE

CGRP-α and -β are potent vasodilators (Table 17.2). Intermittent and transient release may mediate "hot flashes."[29] The CGRP/adrenomedullin family of seven-transmembrane receptors is coupled to adenylate cyclase. The cAMP production induces arteriolar smooth muscle relaxation and long-lasting erythema. CGRP potentiates the arterial vasodilation induced by other agents and SP release, and promotes the transmission of nociceptive information induced by mechanical stimulation.[30,31] Intradermal injection of 15 pmol of CGRP produces erythema within 1 min, which peaks in intensity at 1 h and lasts for 5 to 6 h. This flare response resembles the erythema seen near burned and injured skin. CGRP does not produce an appreciable wheal. However, it does accentuate the edema caused by SP, NKA, NKB, histamine, bradykinin, platelet-activating factor (PAF), C5a des-Arg, $LTB_4$, and f-Met-Leu-Phe. This is probably a direct consequence of the CGRP vasodilatory effect,

**TABLE 17.2**
**Histologic Localization of Neuropeptides in Human Skin**

| Location | CGRP | SP | NKA | SOM | VIP | PHM | NPY | NT |
|---|---|---|---|---|---|---|---|---|
| Epidermis | | | | | | | | |
| Basal cells | – | – | – | – | – | – | + | – |
| Free endings | + | + | + | – | + | – | – | – |
| Merkel cells | – | – | – | – | + | – | – | – |
| Merkel cell axons | – | – | – | – | – | – | – | – |
| Dermis | | | | | | | | |
| Subepidermal zone | ++ | + | + | + | + | + | – | – |
| Free endings | ++ | + | + | + | + | – | – | – |
| Bundles | ++ | + | + | – | ++ | + | – | – |
| Dermal folds | ++ | + | + | – | – | – | – | – |
| Meissner's corpuscles | + | + | – | – | – | – | – | – |
| Smooth muscle bundles | – | – | – | – | + | – | – | – |
| Vessels | | | | | | | | |
| Temporal artery | ++ | ± | – | – | – | – | ++ | – |
| Dermal arteries | + | ± | – | + | ++ | + | + | – |
| Arterioles | + | + | + | + | + | + | + | – |
| AV Anastamosis | | | | | | | | |
| Arterial | + | + | + | – | ++ | + | ++ | ++ |
| Venous | + | + | + | – | + | + | + | + |
| Capillaries | ++ | + | + | – | – | – | – | – |
| Venules | + | + | + | – | + | + | + | – |
| Veins | + | – | – | – | + | + | + | – |
| In glands | + | + | + | – | + | + | + | – |
| Glands | | | | | | | | |
| Eccrine | + | – | – | ± | ++ | + | ++ | + |
| Apocrine | – | – | – | ± | ++ | + | ++ | – |
| Sebaceous | – | – | – | – | – | ± | ± | – |
| Ducts | – | ± | ± | – | + | + | + | + |
| Myoepithelial cells | – | – | – | – | + | – | – | + |
| Meibomian gland | – | + | – | – | ++ | – | – | + |
| Hair Follicles | | | | | | | | |
| Upper follicles | + | + | – | ± | ++ | ± | + | + |
| Erector pili muscle | – | – | – | – | + | – | – | – |

*Note:* ++ present with intense staining; + present; ± occasionally reported in given location; – not identified in studies to date.

which increases local blood flow.[31] Significantly, coadministration of the sympathetic nerve vasoconstrictor neuropeptide tyrosine (NPY) reduces this edema.[32]

## VI. REGULATION BY PEPTIDASES

Tachykinins, VIP, opioids, endothelins, bradykinin, and many other peptides are metabolized by membrane-bound neutral endopeptidase (EC 3.4.24.11; "enkephalinase"; neutral endopeptidase [NEP]).[33] Degradation limits the duration of peptide action. Dipeptidyl peptidase, angiotensin-converting enzyme (ACE), carboxypeptidase, and aminopeptidase activities are also active *in vivo*. Dysfunction or inhibition of NEP or ACE leads to exaggerated peptide effects (e.g., ACE inhibitor-induced cough).

## VII. PARASYMPATHETIC NERVES

Large-diameter parasympathetic fibers release acetylcholine. A smaller-diameter population appears to contain combinations of VIP, PHM (polypeptide with histidine at the N-terminal and methionine at the C-terminal, originally described as PHI in porcine tissues), PACAP (pituitary adenyl cyclase–activating peptide), and neuronal nitric oxide. VIP and PHM are derived from a single gene, which explains their colocalization. They have similar vasodilatory, bronchodilatory, and secretomotor effects, although VIP is consistently more potent.[34] The combinations of neurotransmitters in postganglionic parasympathetic neurons depend upon the structure innervated, and presumed function of that nerve. Guinea pig sphenopalatine neurons that innervate facial hair follicles and glands are innervated by neurons containing VIP, NPY, enkephalin, and SP, indicating that there is a high degree of target specificity of these nerves, with "customized" combinations of neurotransmitters released as dictated by the required functions of those nerves, and the innervated structure.[35] Neuronal NOS is colocalized with VIP in small-diameter peribronchial ganglia in ferrets and humans suggesting a vasodilator role for these neurons. Their presence and function in the skin is less well understood. At least five muscarinic receptors have been cloned, and it is likely that M3 receptor activation is important for gland cell exocytosis, while M2 receptors act as inhibitory autoreceptors that inhibit or "turn off" neural depolarization.

## VIII. SYMPATHETIC NERVES

Adrenergic sympathetic fibers release either norepinephrine or norepinephrine plus NPY,[34] while cholinergic sympathetic neurons innervate sweat glands. Postsynaptic α-adrenergic and NPY receptors stimulate vasoconstriction, and counter the vasodilatory effects of SP, CGRP, VIP, bradykinin, and histamine.[34,36] While NPY Y1 receptors are likely responsible, it is unclear which of the cloned $\alpha 1_{A/D}$, $\alpha 1_B$, $\alpha 1_C$, $\alpha 2_{c10}$, $\alpha 2_{c2}$, or $\alpha 2_{c4}$ gene products are responsible for vasoconstriction *in vivo*.[37] Atrial natiuretic peptide (ANP) is found in sympathetic cholinergic fibers near sweat glands in human axillary skin.[38]

## IX. NERVE DISTRIBUTIONS AND NEUROPEPTIDE LOCALIZATION

Highly innervated skin areas such as the fingertips contain large amounts of CGRP (5.1 pmol/g), SP (2.4 pmol/g), SOM (0.23 pmol/g), VIP (2.3 pmol/g), and NPY (4.0 pmol/g), while less sensitive areas such as the thigh contain less CGRP (0.5 pmol/g), SP (0.07 pmol/g), SOM (0.05 pmol/g), VIP (0.2 pmol/g), and NPY (0.5 pmol/g).[32]

Histologic localization of CGRP, SP, NKA, SOM, VIP, PHM, NPY, neurotensin (NT), GAL, and ANP in human skin is summarized below and in Table 17.2.[15,32] The epidermis contains free nerve endings that stain for CGRP, SP, NKA, and VIP. VIP is also present in granules in Merkel cells, basal epidermal neural crest-derived secretory cells that are in intimate contact with bare axons. The neurotransmitters of these axons are not yet known. The dermis contains large numbers of CGRP, SP, NKA, SOM, VIP, and PHM nerve bundles and free endings in the interstitial connective tissue and alongside arterial vessels. Some Meissner's corpuscles are innervated by CGRP or SP.[39] Smooth muscle bundles in the prepuce and scrotum are innervated by VIP.

Dermal vessels are extensively innervated (Table 17.2). Individual varicose fibers and dense plexuses are present adjacent to or in the adventitial-medial area. The most intensely innervated regions are the precapillary sphincters of metarterioles and the arterial portions of ateriovenous anastomoses. Capillaries also receive numerous CGRP fibers. In larger vessels, such as temporal and occipital arteries, CGRP and NPY are present. The distributions of these neuropeptides define the potential targets of sensory neuron-mediated dilation (CGRP, SP, and NKA in arterioles, capillaries, postcapillary venules, and other vessels), parasympathetic vasodilation (VIP and PHM in dermal arteries, arterial portion of arteriovenous anastomoses, veins, glands), and sympathetic vasoconstriction (NPY in muscular arteries, arterial portion of arteriovenous anastomoses, and veins). Glands are heavily innervated by VIP and NPY fibers. Glandular myoepithelial cells appear to be innervated by VIP- and NT- containing neurons. Meibomian glands of the upper eyelid are also heavily innervated by VIP.

Hair follicles contain VIP fibers at erector pili muscles, and dense plexuses of VIP, SP, CGRP, NT, and NPY fibers are present in the upper follicle region. These may participate in propioception and other sensory functions. NPY immunoreactivity of unknown significance is located in the basal epidermal layer and outer root sheath of hair follicles.

Some epidermal bare nerve endings contain VIP. In humans, VIP does not appear to colocalize with other sensory neuropeptides. The locations of most VIP and PHM fibers are consistent with their functions as secretomotor and vasodilatory parasympathetic fibers. VIP has two receptors that activate adenylate cyclase activity in sweat gland acinar and myoepithelial cells.

Specific combinations of sensory neuropeptides are found in different species and organs. In human skin, CGRP + SOM, and CGRP + SP fibers are found. NKA is colocalized with SP, as they are derived from the same genes. SP and SOM are rarely found together. GAL appears to colocalize with CGRP. In the guinea pig, nerves containing dynorphin (DYN) + cholecystokinin (CCK) + CGRP + SP or SP alone are found as free endings in epidermis, dermis, and near capillaries; CGRP + SP are found in the airways, systemic vessels, and vessels of the thoracic and abdominal viscera; CGRP + SP + DYN are found in the airways and pelvic viscera; and CGRP + SP + CCK are found in the small vessels of striated muscle.[40] Specific combinations are also found in rat visceral, splanchnic, and peripheral nerves that project to different layers of the substantia gelatinosa.[16]

## X. THE TRIPLE RESPONSE OF LEWIS REVISITED

The triple response of Lewis[2] can now be reexamined (Figure 17.2). A light injury does not lead to the triple response. Instead, a "white line" is produced by the emptying of capillaries under the contact site. Endothelial cell swelling has been reported. The reaction begins within seconds and may last 15 min. The response has not been systematically studied because it is difficult to induce reproducibly. The white line response is reminiscent of white dermographism and $\alpha$-adrenoceptor-mediated blanching.

After a firm, blunt stroke, epidermal cell disruption is seen.[41] These cells release factors that produce transient, local vasodilation with the formation of the "red line."[42] Although largely undefined, these factors could include ATP, $K^+$, or IL-1. They could lead to nociceptor activation, mast cell degranulation, or granulocyte and endothelial cell activation. The red line effect is likely to be fundamentally different from the axon reflex mechanism of flare development, as vascular permeability and edema can occur along the red line, but not in the region of the flare. In subjects who display dermographism,[41] blunt stroking generates itchy, erythematous, elevated wheals that develop as urticarial wheals rather than macular flare responses. These dramatic responses can last an hour or more. The mechanism is not understood.

Contraction of endothelial cells within the vascular basement membrane of postcapillary venules causes them to pull away from each other. This forms gaps. Hydrostatic pressure drives albumin, IgG, IgM, complement, fibrinogen, high-molecular-weight kininogen, and other plasma proteins flood into the interstitial space. The plasma flux exceeds the capacity of lymphatics to remove the fluid leading to local edema. The presence of exogenous chemicals, bacteria, foreign bodies, or endogenously released enzymes could activate complement, coagulation, plasmin, or other cascades, and escalate inflammatory responses. The generation of chemotactic factors such as C5a, $LTB_4$, PAF, and others could lead to the extravasation of granulocytes, macrophages, and lymphocytes, which could in turn augment the response. Edema fluid containing exogenous chem-

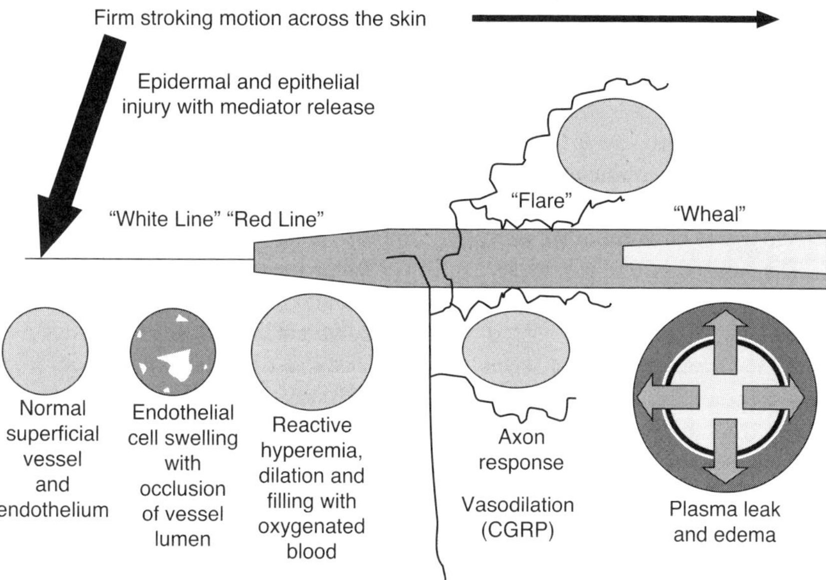


**FIGURE 17.2** The triple response of Lewis revisited. Firm stroking of the skin generates a stereotyped response. The stroking injures the epidermis and endothelium of superficial vessels, leading to mediator release. The endothelial cells respond by swelling and transiently occluding the vessels. The relative lack of oxygenated blood causes the "white line" under the stroked region. Reactive hyperemia follows with dilation of the superficial vessels and maintenance of the thin "red line." The mediators cause endothelial contraction, which pulls them away from each other and allows plasma extravasation. The edema over the red line causes the minimal "wheal" associated with this response. The epidermal injury, mediator release, or direct stimulation of neural mechanoreceptors depolarizes a population of Type C neurons. These are highly branched and innervate superficial vessels and the helical arterioles. Dilation of these vessels allows hot ("calor"), highly oxygenated ("rubor") blood flush into the superficial vessels to cause the "flare." CGRP is the probable neurotransmitter mediator of this widespread vasodilation event. The axon carries news of the scratch or stroking to the spinal cord, where it may be conveyed to cortical centers and reach the level of consciousness.

icals, antigens, activated antigen-presenting cells, leukocytes, and cellular and other debris flow via lymphatic vessels to lymph nodes where they are available for immune processing and presentation.

## XI. ACTIVATION OF SENSORY RECEPTORS, NERVE DEPOLARIZATION, AND THE AXON RESPONSE

Depolarization of nociceptive nerves is regulated by several groups of receptors. Excitatory autoreceptors cause depolarization. Agonists such as histamine, bradykinin, and acetylcholine probably act via GPCR. Other depolarizing agents may be released by degranulating mast cells (histamine), platelets (serotonin), IL-1 (keratinocytes), or Merkel cells; proteolytically cleaved plasma protein products such as bradykinin (generated from kininogen) or anaphylatoxins C3a and C5a; and products of injured or hypoxic cells such as $H^+$, $K^+$, ATP, prostaglandin $E_2$ ($PGE_2$), and other arachidonic acid metabolites. These excitatory, depolarizing GPCRs act in concert with the previously described TPR cation channels and other as yet poorly understood sensor systems.

Inhibitory autoreceptors include NPY Y2, $GABA_B$, 5-HT3, histamine H3, μ-opioid, α2c2- and β2-adrenergic receptors.[43,44] Activation of these receptors hyperpolarizes the neurons so that more intense stimuli are required to cause depolarization and pain.

Prostaglandins and leukotrienes, especially $LTB_4$, reduce polarization and so make it easier for other stimuli to fully depolarize and activate the neurons. Activation of the peripheral ends of nociceptive neurons by IL-1, IL-6, IL-8, tumor necrosis factor-alpha (TNF-$\alpha$), and nerve growth factor (NGF) may also contribute to hyperalgesia (increased pain with innocuous stimulation).[45] Similar effects on itch neurons are postulated but less well studied.

The wave of depolarization is transmitted to the axon and into the spinal cord. However, depolarization can also proceed through each neural branching point in the peripheral nerve.[8,15,16,45] These branches generally follow arteriolar vessels to the capillaries, postcapillary venules, and into the epidermis. Depolarization of these branches and their varicosities releases combinations of CGRP, SP, NKA, and possibly other neurotransmitters. These act on their respective receptors on end organs. The most important effect in the skin is probably the arteriolar vasodilation that increases the flux of internal body temperature ("hot," calor), highly oxygenated ("red," rubror) blood to the superficial vascular plexus. As discussed above, the "tumor," or edema, does not appear to be neurogenically medicated in human skin.

This issue has been examined by inserting microdialysis catheters into the dermis, and perfusing them with micromolar concentrations of SP or CGRP.[46] This may mimic the effects of dermal, interstitial, axon response-mediated neuropeptide release. SP- and CGRP-induced vasodilation. SP, but not CGRP, caused plasma extravasation. Inhibition of NOS activities reduced baseline vasodilation by 30%, SP-induced vasodilation by a maximum of 40%, but had no effect on CGRP effects.[47] As mentioned already, caution must be used in interpreting these and intradermal injection experiments, as the amounts of peptide injected were five to six orders of magnitude larger than tissue interstitial fluid neuropeptide concentrations. Other microdialysis studies indicate baseline concentrations of about 20 pg/ml for CGRP and 15 to 35 pg/ml for SP (nanomolar ranges).[1] Cutaneous electrical stimulation (4 Hz) doubled CGRP concentrations in humans, but had less dramatic effects on SP and no effects on total protein (a measure of vascular permeability).[1] This again demonstrates that the axon response in humans is limited to a flare without plasma extravasation.

Influences that determine the extent of the flare are not known. The size of the flare is proportional to the stimulus intensity.[7] Dose-dependent flare responses have been demonstrated for both histamine and capsaicin. The axon reflex theory suggests that the extent of the flare is determined by the area of distribution of the stimulated neuron's network of branches and the arterioles that they innervate and can dilate after depolarization and neuropeptide release. Dose dependence suggests that the original stimulus intensity may determine the extent of depolarization of the branched neural network. Such an arrangement also implies that there should be an upper limit to the area of flare that can be produced by increasing doses of agonist. Such a theoretical upper limit to the flare response has been suggested.[48] This limitation would apply if one or a series of neurons is initially depolarized, and requires that no additional neurons be recruited. Alternative theories suggest that there may not be any upper limit to the flare because sufficiently intense release of neuropeptides may lead to secondary depolarization of adjacent neuron branches with development of their own secondary axon response flares. In particular, release of SP has been hypothesized to cause mast cell degranulation with release of mediators that depolarize a secondary ring of histamine-sensitive and other neurons. Evidence for the latter is based predominantly on animal experiments and intradermal experiments using supraphysiological doses of SP. Finally, spinal cord activation may lead to retrograde depolarization of additional primary afferent C fibers that release their neuropeptides in the skin and increase the size of the flare.

Nerve impulses are carried from epidermal and dermal free endings to layers I and II of the spinal cord substantia gelatinosa where combinations of CGRP, SOM, SP, NKA, and perhaps other neurotransmitters are released by these different populations of fibers. Messages of mechanicosensitive, chemosensitive, and itch neurons synapse on different sets of dorsal horn neurons. Itch and pain are conveyed by distinct lateral spinothalamic pathways to separate thalamic nuclei.[49] Pain can be appreciated at the thalamic level. Interactions with sympathetic afferent nerves, autonomic and motor reflexes, and other pathways are in need of further investigation. They may play roles in chronic pain, sympathetic reflex dystrophy, complex regional pain syndromes, and related conditions.[50]

## XII. SUBTYPES OF TYPE C NEURONS: ITCH, PAIN, AND MECHANICAL SENSITIVITY

Populations of nonmyelinated neuropeptide-containing sensory C fibers may be differentially depolarized by the application of a wide variety of molecules. Distinct patterns of these mediators have been associated with separate itch and pain sensations. This suggests distinct neural receptor expression patterns on each subtype of nerve.

Separate populations of Type C neurons mediate itch and pain.[51] Electrical stimulation of "itch" neurons generates itch that does not change into a painful sensation. Changes in stimulation intensity (voltage and frequency) had no effect. The specificity of itch and pain neurons was assessed by applying neuroactive substances through intradermal microdialysis membranes.[51] Capsaicin always caused pain but never itching. Histamine always provoked itching and rarely pain. Overall, pain severity was ranked capsaicin > acetylcholine > bradykinin > serotonin > histamine. Itch was ranked histamine >> $PGE_2$ = serotonin = acetylcholine > bradykinin > capsaicin. $PGE_2$ led to moderate itching. Serotonin, acetylcholine, and bradykinin induced more pain than itching.

Microneurography of the human lateral peroneal nerve identified distinct patterns of sensory modalities within Type C neurons.[51] Neurons responsive to mechanical stimulation ($n = 89$, "polymodal nociceptors") had weak responses to histamine, $PGE_2$, and acetylcholine. Mechanosensitive neurons had electrical thresholds of 1 to 14 mA compared to 34 to 82 for mechanoinsensitive neurons. $PGE_2$ and serotonin did not induce mechanical hyperalgesia (lower thresholds for pain). These two populations also differed in their responses to heat stimulation. Mechanosensitive units had lower temperature thresholds (40.8 ± 3.1°C; mean ± SD; temperature inducing pain responses) than mechanoinsensitive units (49.0 ± 2.8°C; $p < 0.001$). This defined these units as low-electrical-threshold mechanosensitive neurons. Iontopheresis of $PGE_2$ into the skin significantly decreased the temperature threshold of the mechanoinsensitive subset to 45.1 ± 2.8°C ($p < 0.0001$). $PGE_2$ had no effect on temperature thresholds in the mechanothermal sensitive subset.

The mechanoinsensitive Type C neurons could be further divided into two subsets. The larger subset ($n = 52$) responded to capsaicin with intense pain like the mechanosensitive group, and had weak responses to histamine, $PGE_2$, and acetylcholine.

The second mechanoinsensitive subset ($n = 24$) conveyed itch. These nerves were most responsive to histamine and $PGE_2$, and less sensitive to serotonin, acetylcholine, bradykinin, and capsaicin. This histamine-sensitive subset had the slowest neural conduction rates ever recorded (0.70 ± 0.17 m/s; $p < 0.01$ compared to the mechanoinsensitive subset that was not responsive to histamine).

Paradoxically, capsaicin and bradykinin stimulated depolarization of these "itch" neurons, but pain was not induced. The paradox can be explained by the yin–yang relationship between itch and pain. Scratching, capsaicin, and electrical stimulation activate mechanosensitive neural endings that convey painful sensations.[52,53] The pain overcomes and inhibits any itch response that may also have been induced via the histamine-sensitive subset. Pain suppression of itch sensations appears to be based in the dorsal horn of the spinal cord. This is supported by the effects of opioids. They reduce pain but are accompanied by increased spinal cord–mediated itch.[54] The itching that follows the reduction of pain by opioids can be blocked by the opioid antagonists (and antipruritic drugs) naloxone and naltrexone.[55] Itch is also increased by giving local anesthetics that block peripheral sources of pain.[56] This pain–itch cross-regulation must occur at the dorsal horn level, as the two sensations are conveyed by distinct secondary ascending neurons in separate spinothalamic pathways.[49]

The itch and pain nerves have different-sized flare reactions. Laser-induced heating of the epidermis generates smaller flares compared to histamine and capsaicin when assessed at roughly comparable levels of discomfort.[57] Histamine-activated nerves generate significantly larger flares suggesting extensive areas of cutaneous innervation by highly branched superficial neural processes. This indicates a functional link between itch and the flare response. These findings are consistent with the activation of these histamine-responsive itch neurons during allergic reactions with mast cell degranulation. In anaphylaxis, there is an increase in blood CGRP. This may mediate the long-lasting arteriolar vasodilation and refractory hypotension of severe anaphylaxis.[58]

## XIII. ISOLECTIN B4 IMMUNOREACTIVE TYPE C NERVES

In addition to the peptide-containing Type C neurons, there is a separate set of ganglion cells that do not generally express peptides. Instead, they are identified by expression of isolectin B4.[59] This α-D-galactose-binding protein from *Griffonia simplicifolia* labels CNS microglia, nearly all peripheral gustatory axons, and about half of small-diameter dorsal root ganglion cells (Type C neurons) and postganglionic efferent and visceral afferent sensory sympathetic nerves. A sensory function is suggested by the observation that most isolectin-B4-positive dorsal root ganglion cells express the P2X3 receptor subunit of the P2X ATP-gated ion channel family. This suggests a role in responses to tissue injury with cellular purine release.[60] The neurotransmitters may be excitatory amino acids, although there is some overlap with peptidergic nerves in some dorsal root ganglion systems. However, some of the peptidergic cells may be transiently activated by peripheral inflammation or nerve injury and have temporary expression of SP and other neuropeptides as an indication of their plasticity.[61]

Isolectin B4 immunoreactive cells in rat skin included the epidermal plasma membranes, glands, hair follicles, endothelium, and single nonmyelinated neurons that traversed the dermis and extended to the epidermal junction.[62] Only 2% of hairs were innervated. Sweat glands were more densely innervated than sebaceous glands. These may represent cholinergic sympathetic neurons. Smooth muscles of arterioles and potentially some capillaries were innervated. These were considered to be of sympathetic origin, although some may have been sensory. No specialized skin sensory organs were innervated. The distributions, sensations conveyed, and functions of these nerves in skin are largely unknown. Glial cell line–derived neurotrophic factor is a survival factor for isolectin-B4-positive, but not VR-1-positive murine neurons.[63] It is anticipated that this subset of nociceptive nerves will have novel sensory and regulatory effects in skin physiology.

## XIV. NEUROPEPTIDES AND IMMUNITY

Neuropeptides from SP to corticotropin-releasing hormone (CRH) have potent effects on many types of immune cells.[64] They can be synthesized by lymphocytes, mast cells, and eosinophils, and express their receptors in a functional fashion. Modulation of SP and other neuropeptide receptors on lymphocytes may be of prognostic importance in cutaneous tumor infiltration.[62] SP nerves were identified in Peyer's patches and the spleen.[65] Culture of human nasal mucosal explants *in vitro* with SP causes an increase in IL-1β and IL-6 mRNA production in tissue from normal subjects, but increases in a wide range of cytokine mRNAs in atopic subjects.[66] The mRNAs may originate from immune cells, or resident cells such as epithelium or endothelium. SP antagonists reduce cutaneous inflammation induced by tuberculin (delayed-type hypersensitivity) and benzoic acid–induced contact urticaria, but not inflammation induced by benzalkonium chloride (irritant delayed reaction) or UVB irradiation.[67]

Neurogenic stimulation may cause granulocyte chemoattraction after 24 h. Intradermal CGRP injection leads to perivascular neutrophil accumulation.[23] SP was a chemotactic agent for neutrophils and macrophages, increased their adhesion to endothelium, and caused lysosomal enzyme release. The C-terminal end of SP (SP[5-11]) was the chemotactic principle. This portion also induced a wheal without a flare. The N-terminal region promoted phagocytosis by macrophages and neutrophils.

Intradermal injection of SP and CGRP stimulated endothelial cells to transport preformed adhesion markers P- and E-selectin from intracellular Weibel–Palade bodies to the endothelial surface.[23] ICAM-1 and VCAM were not altered. VCAM-1 had been upregulated by SP *in vitro*,[69] demonstrating the importance of human *in vivo* models for determining relevance to human pathophysiology. The SP- and CGRP-induced upregulation of endothelial E-selectin was followed by modest tissue infiltration by neutrophils in this model. In addition, SP caused a significant eosinophilic infiltration in atopic subjects. These data suggest that E-selectin adhesion marker expression and modest neutrophilic and eosinophilic granulocyte infiltration were components of neurogenic inflammation. The "nonspecific," mild granulocytic infiltrate may be deceptive, since neutrophils and eosinophils become activated as they diapedese, and may release their granule contents such as neutrophil elastase, eosinophil major basic protein (EG-2) or eosinophilic cationic protein (ECP). As a result, very little cellular "infiltrate" may be apparent by hematoxylin and eosin staining alone. Instead, neutrophil elastase, EG-2 or ECP, may be detected in tissue by immunohistochemistry as has been shown for atopic dermatitis.[70]

## XV. WOUND HEALING

In healing wounds, there appears to be a complex interplay between neuropeptides from regenerating axons and the surrounding, regenerating skin.[71] Sensory nerves sprout extensively in the first 3 weeks after a wound, and then return to their normal fiber density. These nerves may have a trophic influence as seen in amphibians where leg regeneration does not occur in denervated limbs. Autonomic nerves sprout into regenerating tissue after sensory nerves.[72] In humans, SP and NKA stimulate connective tissue cell and skin fibroblast growth that is blocked by the SP antagonist spantide. SOM, VIP, and CGRP had no effect. However, the SP, CGRP, and SOM content of newly synthesized skin is decreased from normal. Gastrin-releasing peptide, a member of the bombesin family of peptides, promotes wound healing.[73]

Nerve growth factor (NGF) likely plays an essential role in neural regeneration and homeostasis. SP and NKA may stimulate NGF release from fibroblasts.[24] Keratinocytes, endothelial cells, Langerhans cells, and T lymphocytes are other sources in psoriasis,[74] wound healing,[75] and diverse inflammatory conditions.[76] NGF receptors have been identified in rat innervated keratinocytes, Merkel cells, the outer root sheaths of hair follicles, hair follicle receptors, Schwann cells, and neurons.[77]

## XVI. NEUROPEPTIDES IN DERMATOLOGIC DISEASE

Atopic dermatitis has increased densities of SP-immunoreactive nerves with expression of NPY in epidermal cells.[78] SOM-immunoreactive neurons were found only in normal skin. CGRP- and VIP-immunoreactive fibers were not altered. However, VIP receptor expression was decreased.[79] Galanin immunoreactivity was diffusely present in epidermal cells, while neurotensin- and NKA-immunoreactive materials were absent. Smaller wheal and flare responses to SP, NKA, NT, and histamine, and smaller flare responses to CGRP may be due to tachyphylaxis of skin structures as a result of excessive endogenous neuropeptide release.[80] Peripheral levels of these neuropeptides and NGF may serve as markers of disease severity in atopic dermatitis.[81] Disruption of these sensory systems at the peripheral and dorsal horn levels is likely to contribute to the pruritus of this disorder.[82] CNS regulation of peripheral neural responses and interactions with the cutaneous immune system may also be dysfunctional in atopic dermatitis since computerized testing provides a systemic stressor that enhances responses such as allergic wheal responses.[83,84] Such stressors may affect skin barrier functions even in healthy subjects.[85]

SP-immunoreactive nerve density may be increased in lesions of psoriasis.[86] NGF may play a role as well.[78] In patients with nickel sensitivity, SOM, SP, and VIP induce peripheral blood T-cell proliferation *in vitro*.[87] Neuropeptide-based drugs, such as a CGRP antagonist, are in development for allergic contact dermatitis.[88] Plasma and skin NPY levels may be useful for monitoring vitiligo.[89] Acne and alopecia areata may be associated with neural dysfunction due to altered glandular neutral endopeptidase and other peptidase expression.[90–93] As would be expected, SP, CGRP, VIP, SOM, and NPY are present in the painful, spontaneous blisters of inflammatory bullous diseases such as bullous pemphigoid, eczema, and burns.[93]

Sensory nerves have been implicated in acquired cold- and heat-induced urticaria,[94] but their precise roles as causes or secondarily activated systems are still under investigation. In idiopathic urticaria, secondary release of histamine from mast cells is most likely responsible for the itch and the vascular leak that causes the edema. The dose–response curve for histamine-induced vascular leak is shifted to the left of the dose–response curve for the perception of itch.

SP was absent in the dorsal horns of victims of familial dysautonomia.[95] Patients with multiple system atrophy (Shy–Drager syndrome) have significantly reduced SP, NKA, CGRP, SOM, and GAL concentrations in the dorsal spinal cord, yet have intact cutaneous wheal and flare responses to histamine.[96] Other hereditary neuropathies and notalgia paresthetica have distinct patterns of neural dysfunction and altered neuropeptides.[97,98]

The SP content of human skin and nerves decreases with age, suggesting reduced axon response activity in older populations.[99] Whether neuropeptides activate common mechanisms of skin aging requires further investigation.[100]

Decreases in CGRP neuron density are reported in diabetes,[101,102] Raynaud's phenomenon, and systemic sclerosis (scleroderma).[103,104] Peripheral blood CGRP, other neuropeptides, and NGF may be useful markers of disease activity in scleroderma.[104] Imbalances between vasoconstrictors such as endothelin and angiotensin II and the vasodilators nitric oxide and CGRP may contribute to these neurovascular diseases.[103] A decrease in CGRP neurons may contribute to HIV-associated xerosis.[105] CGRP has been implicated in the flushing associated with medullary carcinoma of the thyroid.[106] CGRP may play a valuable role as a potent, long-lasting vasodilator in the treatment of congestive heart failure,[107] cardiac arrhythmias,[108] Raynaud's disease,[109] erectile dysfunction,[110] and salvage of traumatic tissue flaps with compromised blood supply.[110]

SOM immunoreactivity has been found in diabetic lipodystrophy and in the Golgi and cytoplasm of epidermal and dermal dendritic cells of patients with urticaria pigmentosa.[111] SOM has been used to treat the necrolytic migratory erythema of glucagonoma.[112]

VIP staining cells are present in lichen sclerosis and atrophicus and mast cells in cutaneous mastocytosis.[113] VIP nerves are reported absent near sweat glands and ducts in patients with cystic fibrosis. Plasma VIP levels are reduced in patients with Raynaud's disease.[114] Transient cutaneous nerve stimulation produces vasodilation and increased plasma VIP levels.

Capsaicin has been used to treat post-herpetic neuralgia, psoriasis, and prurigo nodularis.[115] However, capsaicin intensified the reactions to UV irradiation, nonimmune contact dermatitis (benzoic acid), irritant contact reactions (benzalkonium chloride), tuberculin reactions, and allergic contact dermatitis.[116] Roles for pain- but not itch-conveying nociceptive nerves and axon responses are anticipated in sunburn and UV light-induced immunosuppression.[117]

## XVII. CONCLUSIONS

The identification of multiple subsets of Type C neurons with different triggers, markers, physical characteristics, anatomical connections, peripheral and central functions is the most exciting development in the study of peripheral nerves in recent years. Cloning of the capsaicin receptor, and other members of the transient receptor potential (TRP) channel superfamily of cation channels, discovery of their roles as osmo- and mechanosensors, identification of distinct isolectin B4 neurons, and new functional studies have clarified the mechanisms of itch and pain. New-found correlations between other sensations, neurotransmitter combinations, and peripheral actions of these and potentially other novel neural subsets will dramatically shift our views of nociceptive nerves and redefine "neurogenic inflammation."

## ACKNOWLEDGMENTS

Support was provided by U.S. Public Health Service Award RO1 AI 42403.

## ABBREVIATIONS

| | |
|---|---|
| ANP | atrial natruietic peptide |
| BOMB | bombesin (other family members: gastrin-releasing peptide, neuromedin B) |
| CCK | cholecystekinin |
| CGRP | calcitonin gene-related peptide |
| CNS | central nervous system |
| DYN | dynorphin |
| GAL | galanin |
| GPCR | G protein–coupled receptor |
| IL | interleukin |
| met-ENK | met-enkephalin |
| NKA | neurokinin A |
| NKB | neurokinin B |
| NPY | neuropeptide Y |
| NT | neurotensin |
| PAF | platelet-activating factor |
| $PGE_2$ | prostaglandin $E_2$ |
| PHI | peptide histidine isoleucine |
| PHM | peptide histidine methionine |
| SOM | somatostatin |
| SP | substance P |
| TPR | transient receptor potential |
| TPRC | transient receptor potential canonical |
| TRPM | transient receptor potential melastatin |
| TRPP | transient receptor potential phosphokinase D |
| TPRV | transient receptor potential vanilloid |
| VIP | vasoactive intestinal peptide |
| VLR1 | vanilloid-like receptor 1 |
| VR1 | vanilloid receptor 1 |

## REFERENCES


1. Sauerstein, K., Klede, M., Hilliges, M., and Schmelz, M., Electrically evoked neuropeptide release and neurogenic inflammation differ between rat and human skin. *J. Physiol.,* 529, 803–810, 2000.
2. Lewis, T., *The Blood Vessels of the Human Skin and Their Responses,* Shaw & Sons, London, 1927.
3. Bayliss, W.M., On the origin from the spinal cord of the vasodilator fibres of the hind limb and on the nature of these fibers, *J. Physiol.,* 26, 173, 1901.
4. Holzer, P., Capsaicin: cellular targets, mechanisms of action, and selectivity for thin sensory neurons. *Pharmacol. Rev.,* 43, 143–201, 1991
5. Caterina, M.J., Vanilloid receptors take a TRP beyond the sensory afferent, *Pain,* 105, 5–9, 2003.
6. Huang, S., Bisogno, T., Trevisani, M., Al-Hayani, A., De Petrocellis, L., Fezza, F., Tognetto, M., Petros, T.J., Krey, J.F., Chu, C.J., Miller, J.D., Davies, S.N., Geppetti, P., Walker, J.M., and Di Marzo, V., An endogenous capsaicin-like substance with high potency at recombinant and native vanilloid VR1 receptors, *PNAS,* 99, 8400–8405, 2002.
7. Iadarola. M.J., Berman, K.F., Zeffiro, T.A., Byas-Smith, M.G., Gracely, R.H., Max, M.B., and Bennett, G.J., Neural activation during acute capsaicin-evoked pain and allodynia assessed with PET, *Brain,* 121, 931–947, 1998.
8. Serra, J., Campero, M., and Ochoa, J., Flare and hyperalgesia after intradermal capsaicin injection in human skin, *J. Neurophysiol.,* 80, 2801–2810, 1998.
9. Serra, J., Campero, M., and Ochoa, J., Sensitization of "silent" C-nociceptors in areas of secondary hyperalgesia (SH) in humans, *Neurology,* 45, A365, 1995.

10. Simone, D.A., Nolano, M., Johnson, T., Wendelschafer-Crabb, G., and Kennedy, W.R., Intradermal injection of capsaicin in humans produces degeneration and subsequent reinnervation of epidermal nerve fibers: correlation with sensory function, *J. Neurosci.*, 18, 8947–8959, 1998.
11. Birnbaumer, L., Yidirim, E., and Abramowitz, J., A comparison of the genes coding for canonical TRP channels and their M, V and P relatives, *Cell Calcium,* 33, 419–432, 2003.
12. Liedtke, W., Tobin, D.M., Bargmann, C.L., and Friedman, J.M., Mammalian TRPV4 (VR-OAC) directs behavioral responses to osmotic and mechanical stimuli in *Caenorhabditis elegans, PNAS*, 100, 14531–14536, 2003.
13. Southall, M.D., Li, T., Gharibova, L.S., Pei, Y., Nicol, G.D., and Travers, J.B., Activation of epidermal vanilloid receptor-1 induces release of proinflammatory mediators in human keratinocytes, *J. Pharmacol. Exp. Ther.*, 304, 217–222, 2003.
14. Ko, F., Diaz, M., Smith, P., Emerson, E., Kim, Y.J., Krizek, T.J., and Robson, M.C., Toxic effects of capsaicin on keratinocytes and fibroblasts, *J. Burn Care Rehabil.,* 19, 409–413, 1998.
15. Hua, X.Y., Tachykinins and calcitonin gene-related peptide in relation to peripheral functions at capsaicin-sensitive sensory neurons, *Acta Physiol. Scand.,* 127, 1, 1986.
16. Gibbins, I.L., Waltchow, D., and Coventry, B., Two immunohistochemically identified populations of calcitonin gene related peptide (CGRP) immunoreactive axons in human skin, *Brain Res.,* 414, 143, 1987.
17. Severini, C., Improta, G., Falconieri-Erspamer, G., Salvadori, S., and Erspamer, V., The tachykinin peptide family, *Pharmacol. Rev.,* 54, 285–322, 2002.
18. Kurtz, M.M., Wang, R., Clements, M.K., Cascieri, M.A., Austin, C.P., Cunningham, B.R., Chicchi, G.G., and Liu, Q., Identification, localization and receptor characterization of novel mammalian substance P-like peptides, *Gene*, 21, 205–212, 2002.
19. Quinlan, K.L., Naik, S.M., Cannon, G., Armstrong, C.A., Bunnett, N.W., Ansel, J.C., and Caughman, S.W., Substance P activates coincident NF-AT- and NF-kappa B-dependent adhesion molecule gene expression in microvascular endothelial cells through intracellular calcium mobilization, *J. Immunol.,* 163, 5656–5665, 1999.
20. Okabe, T., Hide, M., Koro, O., and Yamamoto, S., Substance P induces tumor necrosis factor-alpha release from human skin via mitogen-activated protein kinase, *Eur. J. Pharmacol.,* 398, 309–315, 2000.
21. Pincelli, C., Fantini, F., Giardino, L., Zanni, M., Calza, L., Sevignani, C., and Giannetti, A., Autoradiographic detection of substance P receptors in normal and psoriatic skin, *J. Invest. Dermatol.,* 101, 301–304, 1993.
22. Busija, D.W. and Chen, J., Effects of trigeminal neurotransmitters on piglet pial arterioles, *J. Dev. Physiol.*, 18, 67–72, 1992.
23. Smith, C.H., Barker, J.N.W.N., Morris, R.W., MacDonald, D.M., and Lee, T.H., Neuropeptides induce rapid expression of endothelial cell adhesion molecules and elicit granulocytic infiltration in human skin, *J. Immunol.*, 151, 3274–3282, 1993.
24. Burbach, G.J., Kim, K.H., Zivony, A.S., Kim, A., Aranda, J., Wright, S., Naik, S.M., Caughman, S.W., Ansel, J.C., and Armstrong, C.A., The neurosensory tachykinins substance P and neurokinin A directly induce keratinocyte nerve growth factor, *J. Invest. Dermatol.,* 117, 1075–1082, 2001.
25. Wallengren, J. and Hakanson, R., Effects of substance P, neurokinin A, and calcitonin gene related peptide in human skin and their involvement in sensory nerve-mediated responses, *Eur. J. Pharmacol.,* 143, 267, 1987.
26. Hunt, T.C., Cambell, A.M., Robinson, C., and Holgate, S.T., Structural and secretory characteristics of bovine lung and skin mast cells: evidence for the existence of heterogeneity, *Clin. Exp. Allergy,* 21, 73–82, 1991.
27. Repke, H. and Beinert, M., Mast cell activation — a receptor independent mode of substance P action? *FEBS Lett.,* 221, 236, 1987.
28. Baraniuk, J.N., Kowalski, M.L., and Kaliner, M.A., Relationships between permeable vessels, nerve fibers and mast cells in rat cutaneous neurogenic inflammation, *J. Appl. Physiol.,* 68, 2305–2311, 1990.
29. Spetz, A.C., Pettersson, B., Varenhorst, E., Theodorsson, E., Thorell, L.H., and Hammar, M., Momentary increase in plasma calcitonin gene-related peptide is involved in hot flashes in men treated with castration for carcinoma of the prostate, *J. Urol.,* 166, 1720–1723, 2001.
30. Brain, S.D. and Williams, T.J., Inflammatory oedema induced by synergism between calictonin gene-related peptide (CGRP) and mediators of increased vascular permeability, *Br. J. Pharmacol.,* 86, 855, 1985.

31. Steenbergh, P.H., Hoppener, J.W.M., Zandberg, J., Lips, C.J.M., and Jansz, J.S., A second human calcitonin/CGRP gene, *FEBS Lett.,* 183, 403, 1985.
32. Wallengren, J., Ekman, R., and Sundler, F., Occurrence and distribution of neuropeptides in the human skin, *Acta Derm. Venereol.* (Stockholm), 67, 185, 1987.
33. Roques, B.P., Noble, F., Dauge, V., Fournie-Zaluski, M.C., and Beaumont, A., Neutral endopeptidase 24.11: structure, inhibition, and experimental and clinical pharmacology, *Pharmacol. Rev.*, 45, 87–146, 1993.
34. Polak, J.M. and Bloom, S.R., Regulatory peptides in autonomic and sensory neuron systems, *Exp. Brain Res.,* 16, 11, 1987.
35. Gibbins, I.L., Target-related patterns of co-existence of neuropeptide Y, vasoactive intestinal peptide, enkephalin, and substance P in cranial parasympathetic neurons innervating the facial skin and exocrine glands of guinea-pigs, *Neuroscience*, 38, 541–560, 1990.
36. Daly, R.N. and Heible, J.P., Neuropeptide Y modulates adrenergic nerve transmission by an endothelium dependant mechanism, *Eur. J. Pharmacol.,* 138, 445, 1987.
37. Bylund, D.B., Subtypes of $\alpha$1- and $\alpha$2-adrenergic receptors, *FASEB J.*, 7, 832–839, 1992.
38. Tainio, H., Vaalasti, A., and Rechardt, L., The distribution of substance P-, CGRP-, galanin-, and ANP-like immunoreactive nerves in human sweat glands, *Histochem. J.,* 19, 375, 1987.
39. Johansson, O., Fantini, F., and Hu, H., Neuronal structural proteins, transmitters, transmitter enzymes and neuropeptides in human Meissner's corpuscles: a reappraisal using immunohistochemistry, *Arch. Dermatol. Res.,* 291, 419–424, 1999.
40. Gibbins, I.L., Furness, J.B., and Costa, M., Pathway specific patterns of co-existence of substance P, calcitonin gene related peptide, cholecystekinin, and dynorphin in neurons of the dorsal root ganglion of the guinea pig, *Cell Tissue Res.,* 248, 417, 1987.
41. Cauna, N. and Levine, M.I., The fine morphology of the human skin in dermographism, *J. Allergy,* 45, 266, 1970.
42. Morhenn, V.B., Firm stroking of human skin leads to vasodilatation possibly due to the release of substance P, *J. Dermatol. Sci.,* 22, 138–144, 2000.
43. Stein, C., The control of pain in peripheral tissue by opioids, *N. Engl. J. Med.,* 332, 1685–1690, 1995.
44. Stander, S., Gunzer, M., Metze, D., Luger, T., and Steinhoff, M., Localization of $\mu$-opioid receptor 1A on sensory nerve fibers in human skin, *Regul. Pept.*, 110, 75–83, 2002.
45. Dray, A., Urban, L., and Dickenson, A., Pharmacology of chronic pain, *TiPS,* 15, 190–197, 1994.
46. Weidner, C., Klede, M., Rukwied, R., Lischetzki, G., Neisius, U., Skov, P.S., Petersen, L.J., and Schmelz, M., Acute effects of substance P and calcitonin gene-related peptide in human skin: a microdialysis study, *J. Invest. Dermatol.,* 115:1015–20, 2000
47. Klede, M., Clough, G., Lischetzki, G., and Schmelz, M., The effect of the nitric oxide synthase inhibitor *N*-nitro-L-arginine-methyl ester on neuropeptide-induced vasodilation and protein extravasation in human skin, *J. Vasc. Res.*, 40, 105–114, 2003.
48. Buckely, C.E., III, Lee, K.L., and Burdick, D.S., Methacholine-induced cutaneous flare response: bivariate analysis of responsiveness and sensitivity, *J. Allergy Clin. Immunol.,* 69, 25, 1983.
49. Andrew, D. and Craig, A.D., Spinothalamic lamina 1 neurons selectively sensitive to histamine: a central neural pathway for itch, *Nat. Neurosci*., 4, 72–77, 2001.
50. Weber, M., Birklein, F., Neundorfer, B., and Schmelz, M., Facilitated neurogenic inflammation in complex regional pain syndrome, *Pain*, 91, 251–257, 2001.
51. Schmelz, M., Schmidt, R., Weidner, C., Hilliges, M., Torebjork, H.E., and Handwerker, H.O., Chemical response pattern of different classes of C-nociceptors to pruritogens and algogens, *J. Neurophysiol.*, 89, 2441–2448, 2003.
52. Brull, S.J., Atasassoff, P.G., Silverman, D.G., Zhang, J., and LaMotte, R.H., Attenuation of experimental pruritus and mechanically evoked dysesthesiae in an area of cutaneous allodynia, *Somatosens. Mot. Res.,* 16, 299–303, 1999.
53. Nilsson, H.J., Levinsson, A., and Schouenborg, J., Cutaneous field stimulation (CFS): a powerful method to combat itch, *Pain*, 71, 49–55, 1997.
54. Schmeltz, M., A neural pathway for itch, *Nat. Neurosci.,* 4, 9–10, 2001.
55. Odou, P., Azar, R., Luyckx, M., Brunet, C., and Dine, T., A hypothesis for endogenous opioid peptides in uraemic pruritis: role of enkephalin, *Nephrol. Dial. Transpl.,* 16, 1953–1954, 2001.

56. Atanassoff, P.G., Brull, S.J., Zhang, J., Greenquist, K., Silverman, D.G., and LaMotte, R.H., Enhancement of experimental pruritus and mechanically evoked dysesthesiae with local anesthetic, *Somatosens. Mot. Res.,* 16, 291–298, 1999.
57. Algermissen, B., Hermes, B., Henz, B.M., Muller, U., and Berlien, H.P., Laser-induced weal and flare reactions: clinical aspects and pharmacological modulation, *Br. J. Dermatol.,* 146, 863–868, 2002.
58. Volcheck, G.W., Butterfield, J.H., Yunginger, J.W., and Klee, G.G., Elevated serum levels of calcitonin gene-related peptide in Hymenoptera sting-induced anaphylaxis, *J. Allergy Clin. Immunol.,* 102, 149–151, 1998.
59. Wang, H., Rivero-Melian, C., Robertson, B., and Grant, G., Transganglionic transport and binding of the isolectin B4 from *Griffonia simplicifolia* I in rat primary sensory neurons, *Neuroscience,* 62, 539–551, 1994.
60. Vulchanova, L., Reidl, M., Shuster, S., Wang, J., Buell, G., Surprenant, A., North, R.A., and Elde, R., Immunohistochemical localization of the P2X3 receptor subunit in rat dorsal root ganglion (DRG) neurons, *Soc. Neurosci. Abstr.,* 22, 1810, 1996.
61. Hunter, D.D., Myers, A.C., and Undem, B.J., Nerve growth factor-induced phenotypic switch in guinea pig airway sensory neurons, *Am. J. Respir. Crit. Care Med.*, 161, 1985–1990, 2000.
62. Petruska, J.C., Streit, W.J., and Johnson, R.D., Localization of unmyelinated axons in rat skin and mucocutaneous tissue utilizing the isolectin GS-I-B4, *Somatosens. Mot. Res.*, 14, 17–26, 1997.
63. Zwick, M., Davis, B.M., Woodbury, C.J., Burkett, J.N., Koerber, H.R., Simpson, J.F., and Albers, K.M., Glial cell line-derived neurotrophic factor is a survival factor for isolectin B4-positive, but not vanilloid receptor 1-positive, neurons in the mouse, *J. Neurosci.,* 22, 4057–4065, 2002.
64. Luger, T.A., Neuromediators: a crucial component of the skin immune system, *J. Dermatol. Sci.*, 30, 87–93, 2002.
65. Misery, L., Bourchanny, D., Kanitakis, J., Schmitt, D., and Claudy, A., Modulation of substance P and somatostatin receptors in cutaneous lymphocytic inflammatory and tumoral infiltrates, *J. Eur. Acad. Dermatol. Venereol.,* 15, 238–241, 2001.
66. Stanisz, A.M., Scicchitano, R., Dazin, P., Bienenstock, J., and Payan, D.G., Distribution of substance P receptors on murine spleen and Peyer's patch T and B cells, *J. Immunol.,* 139, 749, 1987.
67. Okayama, Y., Shirotori, K., Kudo, K., Ishikawa, K., Ito, E., Togawa, K., and Saito, I., Cytokine expression after the topical administration of substance P to human nasal mucosa, *J. Immunol.*, 151, 4391–4398, 1993.
68. Wallengren, J., Substance P antagonist inhibits immediate and delayed type cutaneous hypersensitivity reactions, *Br. J. Dermatol.*, 124, 324–328, 1991.
69. Quinlan, K.L., Song, I.S., Naik, S.M., Letran, E.L., Olerud, J.E., Bunnett, N.W., Armstrong, C.A., Caughman, S.W., and Ansel, J.C., VCAM-1 expression on human dermal microvascular endothelial cells is directly and specifically up-regulated by substance P, *J. Immunol.,* 162, 1656–1661, 1999.
70. Leiferman, K.M.S., Acherman, J., Sampson, H.A., Haugen, H.S., Venecie, P.Y., and Gleich, G.J., Dermal deposition of eosinophil granule major basic protein in atopic dermatitis: comparison with onchocerciasis. *N. Engl. J. Med.,* 313, 282–285, 1985.
71. Altun, V., Hakvoort, T.E., van Zuijlen, P.P., van der Kwast, T.H., and Prens, E.P., Nerve outgrowth and neuropeptide expression during the remodeling of human burn wound scars. A 7-month follow-up study of 22 patients, *Burns*, 27, 717–722, 2001.
72. Karanth, S.S., Dhital, S., Springall, D.R., and Polak, J.M., Reinnervation and neuropeptides in mouse skin flaps, *J. Autonom. Nerv. Syst.,* 31, 127–134, 1990.
73. Yamaguchi, Y., Hosokawa, K., Nakatani, Y., Sano, S., Yoshikawa, K., and Itami, S., Gastrin-releasing peptide, a bombesin-like neuropeptide, promotes cutaneous wound healing, *Dermatol. Surg.*, 28, 314–319, 2002.
74. Pincelli, C., Nerve growth factor and keratinocytes: a role in psoriasis, *Eur. J. Dermatol.*, 10, 85–90, 2000.
75. Gibran, N.S., Tamura, R., Tsou, R., and Isik, F.F., Human dermal microvascular endothelial cells produce nerve growth factor: implications for wound repair, *Shock*, 19, 127–130, 2003.
76. Ansel, J.C., Neuromediators and inflammation, *Exp. Dermatol.*, 10, 352–353, 2001.
77. Riberio-da-Silva, A., Kenigsberg, R.L., and Cuello, A.C., Light and electron microscopic distribution of nerve growth factor receptor-like immunoreactivity in the skin of the rat lower lip, *Neuroscience*, 43, 631–646, 1991.

78. Pincelli, C., Fantini, F., Massimi, P., Girolomoni, G., Seidenari, S., and Giannetti, A., Neuropeptides in the skin from patients with atopic dermatitis: an immunohistochemical study, *Br. J. Dermatol.*, 122, 745–750, 1990.
79. Groneberg, D.A., Welker, P., Fischer, T.C., Dinh, Q.T., Grutzkau, A., Peiser, C., Wahn, U., Henz, B.M., and Fischer, A., Down-regulation of vasoactive intestinal polypeptide receptor expression in atopic dermatitis, *J. Allergy Clin. Immunol.*, 111, 1099–1105, 2003.
80. Giannetti, A. and Girolomi, G., Skin reactivity to neuropeptides in atopic dermatitis, *Br. J. Dermatol.*, 121, 681–688, 1989.
81. Toyoda, M., Nakamura, M., Makino, T., Hino, T., Kagoura, M., and Morohashi, M., Nerve growth factor and substance P are useful plasma markers of disease activity in atopic dermatitis, *Br. J. Dermatol.*, 147, 71–79, 2002.
82. Stander, S. and Steinhoff, M., Pathophysiology of pruritus in atopic dermatitis: an overview, *Exp. Dermatol.*, 11, 12–24, 2002.
83. Kimata, H., Enhancement of allergic skin wheal responses and *in vitro* allergen-specific IgE production by computer-induced stress in patients with atopic dermatitis, *Brain Behav. Immun.*, 17, 134–8, 2003.
84. Katayama, I., Bae, S.J., Hamasaki, Y., Igawa, K., Miyazaki, Y., Yokozeki, H., and Nishioka, K., Stress response, tachykinin, and cutaneous inflammation, *J. Invest. Dermatol. Symp. Proc.*, 6, 81–86, 2001.
85. Altemus, M., Rao, B., Dhabhar, F.S., Ding, W., and Granstein, R.D., Stress-induced changes in skin barrier function in healthy women, *J. Invest. Dermatol.*, 117, 309–317, 2001.
86. Naukkarinen, A., Harvima, I.T., Aalto, M.L., and Horsmanheimo, M., Mast cell tryptase and chymase are potential regulators of neurogenic inflammation in psoriatic skin, *Int. J. Dermatol.*, 33, 361–366, 1994.
87. Nordlind, K. and Mutt, V., Modulating effect of beta-endorphin, somatostatin, substance P and vasoactive intestinal peptide on the proliferative response of peripheral blood T lymphocytes of nickel-allergic patients to nickel sulphate, *Int. Arch. Allergy Appl. Immunol.*, 81, 368, 1986.
88. Wallengren, J., Dual effects of CGRP-antagonist on allergic contact dermatitis in human skin. *Contact Dermatitis*, 43, 137–143, 2000.
89. Tu, C., Zhao, D., and Lin, X., Levels of neuropeptide-Y in the plasma and skin tissue fluids of patients with vitiligo, *J. Dermatol. Sci.*, 27, 178–182, 2001.
90. Toyoda, M., Nakamura, M., Makino, T., Kagoura, M., and Morohashi, M., Sebaceous glands in acne patients express high levels of neutral endopeptidase, *Exp. Dermatol.*, 11, 241–247, 2002.
91. Toyoda, M. and Morohashi, M., New aspects in acne inflammation, *Dermatology*, 206, 17–23, 2003.
92. Toyoda, M., Makino, T., Kagoura, M., and Morohashi, M., Expression of neuropeptide-degrading enzymes in alopecia areata: an immunohistochemical study, *Br. J. Dermatol.*, 144(1), 46–54, 2001.
93. Wallengren, J., Ekman, R., and Moller, H., Substance P and vasoactive intestinal peptide in bullous and inflammatory skin disease, *Acta Derm. Venereol.* (Stockholm), 66, 23, 1986.
94. Wallengren, J., Moller, H., Ekman, R., Occurrence of substance P, vasoactive intestinal peptide, and calcitonin gene-related peptide in dermographism and cold urticaria, *Arch. Dermatol. Res.*, 279, 512, 1987
95. Pearson, J., Brandeis, L., and Cuello, A.C., Depletion of substance P-containing axons in substantia gelantinosa of patients with diminished pain sensitivity, *Nature*, 295, 61, 1982.
96. Anand, P., Bannister, R., McGregor, G.P., Ghatei, M.A., Mulderry, P.K., and Bloom, S.R., Marked depletion of dorsal spinal cord substance P and calcitonin gene-related peptide with intact skin flare responses in multiple system atrophy, *J. Neurol. Neurosurg. Psychiatr.*, 51:192, 1988.
97. Verze, L., Viglietti-Panzica, C., Plumari, L., Calcagni, M., Stella, M., Schrama, L.H., and Panzica, G.C., Cutaneous innervation in hereditary sensory and autonomic neuropathy type IV, *Neurology*, 55, 126–128, 2000.
98. Savk, E., Dikicioglu, E., Culhaci, N., Karaman, G., and Sendur, N., Immunohistochemical findings in notalgia paresthetica, *Dermatology*, 204, 88–93, 2002.
99. Helme, R.D. and McKernan, S., Effects of age on the axon reflex response to noxious chemical stimulation, *Clin. Exp. Neurol.*, 22, 57, 1985.
100. Giacomoni, P.U. and Rein, G., Factors of skin ageing share common mechanisms, *Biogerontology*, 2, 219–229, 2001.
101. Levy, D.M., Terenghi, G., Gu, X.H., Abraham, R.R., Springall, D.R., and Polak, J.M., Immunohistochemical measurements of nerves and neuropeptides in diabetic skin: relationship to tests of neurological function, *Diabetologia*, 35, 889–897, 1992.

102. Vinik, A.I., Erbas, T., Park, T.S., Stansberry, K.B., Scanelli, J.A., and Pittenger, G.L., Dermal neurovascular dysfunction in type 2 diabetes, *Diabetes Care,* 24, 1468–1475, 2001.
103. Terenghi, G., Bunker, C.B., Lui, Y.F., Springall, D.R., Cowen, T., Dowd, P.M., Polak, J.M., Image analysis quantification of peptide-immunoreactive nerves in the skin of patients with Raynaud's phenomenon and systemic sclerosis, *J. Pathol.*, 164, 245–252, 1991.
104. Matucci-Cerinic, M., Giacomelli, R., Pignone, A., Cagnoni, M.L., Generini, S., Casale, R., Cipriani, P., Del Rosso, A., Tirassa, P., Konttinen, Y.T., Kahaleh, B.M., Fan, P.S., Paoletti, M., Marchesi, C., Cagnoni, M., and Aloe, L., Nerve growth factor and neuropeptides circulating levels in systemic sclerosis (scleroderma), *Ann. Rheum. Dis.*, 60, 487–494, 2001.
105. Rowe, A., Mallon, E., Rosenberger, P., Barrett, M., Walsh, J., and Bunker, C.B., Depletion of cutaneous peptidergic innervation in HIV-associated xerosis, *J. Invest. Dermatol.,* 12, 284–289, 1999.
106. Brain, S.D., Tippins, J.R., Morris, H.R., MacIntyre, I., and Williams, T.J., Potent vasodilator activity of calcitonin gene related peptide in human skin, *J. Invest. Dermatol.,* 87, 533, 1986.
107. Stevenson, R.N., Roberts, R.H., and Timmins, A.D., Calcitonin gene related peptide: a hemodynamic study of a novel vasodilator in patients with severe chronic heart failure, *Int. J. Cardiol.,* 37, 407–414, 1992.
108. Zhang, J.F., Lui, J., and Lui X.Z. Stabilization of cardiac rhythm in subsequently life-threatening ventricular tachycardia and fibrillation by calcitonin gene related peptide, *Int. J. Cardiol.*, 34, 101–103, 1992.
109. Shawket, S., Dickerson, C., Hazleman, B., and Brown, M.J., Prolonged effect of CGRP in Raynaud's patients: a double-blind randomized comparison with prostacyclin, *Br. J. Clin. Pharmacol.,* 32, 209–213, 1991.
110. Djamilian, M., Stief, C.G., Kuczyk, M., Jonas, U., Follow-up results of a combination of calcitonin gene related peptide and prostaglandin E1 in the treatment of erectile dysfunction, *J. Urol.*, 149:1296–1298, 1993.
111. Johansson, O., Morphologic characterization of the somatostatin-immunoreactive dendritic skin cells in urticaria pigmentosa by patients in computerized image analysis, *Scand. J. Immunol.,* 21, 431, 1985.
112. Elsborg, L. and Glenthoj, A., Effect of somatostatin in necrolytic migratory erythema of glucagonoma, *Acta Med. Scand.*, 218, 245, 1985.
113. Wesley, J.R., Vinik, A.I., O'Dorisio, T.M., Glaser, B., and Fink, A., A new syndrome of symptomatic cutaneous mastocytoma producing vasoactive intestinal peptide, *Gastroenterology*, 82, 963, 1982.
114. Daada, B., Olsen, E., and Eielson, O.P., In search of mediators of skin vasodilation induced by transcutaneous nerve stimulation. III. Increase in VIP in normal subjects and in Raynaud's disease, *Gen. Pharmacol.*, 15:107, 1984.
115. Stander, S., Luger, T., and Metze, D., Treatment of prurigo nodularis with topical capsaicin, *J. Am. Acad. Dermatol.*, 44, 471–478, 2001.
116. Wallengren, A. and Moller, H., The effect of capsaicin on some experimental inflammations in human skin, *Acta Derm. Venereol.* (Stockholm), 66, 373, 1986.
117. Seiffert, K. and Granstein, R.D., Neuropeptides and neuroendocrine hormones in ultraviolet radiation-induced immunosuppression, *Methods,* 28, 97–103, 2002.
118. Rinder, J. and Lundberg, J.M., Effects of hCGRP8-37 and the NK1-receptor antagonist SR140.333 on capsaicin-evoked vasodilation in the pig nasal mucosa *in vivo, Allergologie*, 1, 48, 1996.

# Part IV

## Response Patterns of the Skin Immune System

# 18 Signal Transduction Pathways in the Skin

*Lars Iversen and Knud Kragballe*

## CONTENTS



## I. INTRODUCTION

Signal transduction at the cellular level refers to the movement of signals from outside the cell to inside. It is a way by which the cell can communicate with the environment. Signal transduction pathways control a number of cellular processes including cell cycle, proliferation, differentiation, and apoptosis. Signal transduction pathways are cascades of chemical interactions that ultimately lead to the activation or deactivation of certain cellular processes mostly by initiating or repressing the transcription of specific genes. Aberrant signaling leads to altered homeostasis and is part of the pathogenesis and pathophysiology of many skin diseases including inflammatory skin diseases and neoplasms. This chapter describes the fundamental concepts of signaling in the cell and discusses more thoroughly selected signaling pathways important in the skin.

Fundamentally, cellular signaling can be mediated through two different signaling mechanisms: (1) through binding to a receptor at the outer surface of the cellular membrane and a subsequent

0-8493-1959-5/05/$0.00+$1.50

**TABLE 18.1**
**Cytokine Receptors**

| Receptor Family | Example of Receptor | Dominant Signal Transduction Pathway |
|---|---|---|
| IL-1 receptor family | IL-1R, type 1 | Activation of NF-κB |
| TNF receptor family | TNF-R1 | Activation of NF-κB |
| Hematopoietin receptor family (class I receptors) | IL-2R | Activation of Jak-Stat pathway |
| Interferon/IL-10 receptor family (class II receptors) | IFN-γR and IL-20R | Activation of Jak-Stat pathway |
| Immunoglobulin superfamily | M-CSFR | Activation of intrinsic tyrosine kinase |
| TGF-β receptor family | TGF-βR | Activation of intrinsic serine/threonine kinase |
| Chemokine receptor family | CCR1 | Seven-transmembrane receptors coupled to G-proteins |

*Source:* Modified from Freedberg, I.M. et al., Eds., *Fitzpatrick's Dermatology in General Medicine*, 6th ed., McGraw-Hill, New York, 2003, 286.

activation of a signal transduction cascade; (2) through binding to nuclear receptors and subsequent regulation of gene transcription.

## II. MEMBRANE RECEPTORS

Cell signaling by cytokines and peptide hormones is in general mediated through external and membrane-bound receptors, whereas smaller and more lipophilic signaling molecules such as steroid hormones and some vitamins signal through nuclear receptors.

General features of cytokines are their pleiotropism and redundancy. Pleiotropism refers to the ability of one cytokine to act on different cell types, which reflects that different cell types may have the same type of receptors on their membrane surface. Redundancy refers to the property of multiple cytokines having the same functional effect, which can be explained by the fact that the same receptor or receptor type can bind different cytokines.

Cell surface receptors have three general domains in common: the extracellular domain responsible for ligand binding, the middle hydrophobic segment, and the intracellular portion responsible for initiating intracellular signaling pathways. Receptors for cytokines often have a very high affinity for their ligand and as a consequence only small quantities of the ligand are needed to elicit biological responses. The intracellular signaling pathways are typically activated by ligand-induced clustering of the receptors. Typically, the cytoplasmic portions of two or more receptors are brought together after ligand binding.

Different ways of classifying cytokine membrane receptors have been applied. In this chapter cytokine receptors have been classified into seven major families (Table 18.1).

### A. IL-1 Receptor Family

Two forms (the α and β form) of interleukin (IL)-1 are present with less than 30% homology at the amino acid level. The main biological function of IL-1α and IL-1β is as mediator of the host inflammatory response to infections and other inflammatory stimuli. Both IL-1α and β bind to the cell surface receptor, IL-1R1, and mediate the same biologic activities. IL-1R1 is expressed on almost all cell types and is the major receptor for IL-1-mediated responses. Signal transduction is mediated through its cytoplasmic domain, which bears only little homology to other cytokine receptors. After IL-1α or β binding to IL-1R1 the receptor associates with another protein called IL-1R-associated protein (IL-1RAcP) that is homologous to IL-1R1. Both IL-1R1 and IL-1RAcP are essential to for IL-1 signaling, as demonstrated in mice deficient in either of these molecules.[1] Binding of IL-1 to IL-1R1 and complex formation with IL-1RAcP leads to changes of the cytoplasmic domain of the IL-1R1, recruitment of an adaptor protein called MyD88, and a serine-threonine kinase called IL-1 receptor–associated kinase (IRAK) followed by association with TRAF-6. This complex formation finally leads to activation of the NF-κB and AP-1 transcription factors (see below).[2] An IL-1R antagonist (IL-1Ra) is also known. It binds to the IL-1R but does not recruit the IL-1RAcP and does not induce signal transduction.[3] In keratinocytes, different isoforms of IL-1Ra have been shown.[4] Another way of antagonizing IL-1 responses is through expression of IL-1R2. IL-1R2 does not induce responses to IL-1. It acts predominantly as a decoy receptor that competitively inhibits IL-1 binding to the IL-1R1 receptor. Its expression can be induced by a number of different stimuli such as glucocorticoids as well as inflammatory cytokines like interferon-gamma (IFN-γ) and IL-1, and this has been demonstrated in keratinocytes.[5] The biological role of IL-1Ra and IL-1R2 is probably to limit the inflammatory response.

IL-18 is another cytokine that signals through a similar mechanism as IL-1. The cytoplasmic part of the IL-1R1 and IL-18R are homologues and it is now becoming evident that there is a large family of receptor homologues to IL-1R1 and IL-18R.[6]

## B. TNF Receptor Family

TNF is a key player in acute inflammatory responses and responsible for many of the systemic complications of severe infections. TNF-α is also an important mediator of cutaneous inflammation and has been shown to be synthesized in human keratinocytes.[7] TNF-α is the prototype cytokine in a family of TNF-related signaling molecules that also include TNF-β, lymphotoxin α and β, Fas ligand (FASL), TNF-related apoptosis-inducing ligand (TRAIL), TNF-related activation-induced cytokine (TRANCE), and CD40 ligand (CD154).

The soluble form of TNF-α is homotrimers, and trimerization of the TNF receptor family members is also required for induction of signal transduction.[8] There are two distinct TNF receptors, TNF-RI with a molecular mass of 55 kDa and TNF-RII with a molecular mass 75 kDa. Most biological effects of TNF-α are mediated through TNF-RI although TNF-RII is also capable of inducing signal transduction. Cytokine binding to TNF receptor family members leads to the recruitment of proteins called TNF receptor-associated factors (TRAFs) to the cytoplasmic domain of the receptor and activation of transcription factors, especially NF-κB and AP-1.

Signal transduction through the TNF receptor family seems important in a number of inflammatory skin diseases, and targeting TNF-α is very effective in the treatment of inflammatory diseases like psoriasis and rheumatoid arthritis.

## C. Hematopoietin Receptor Family (Class I Receptors)

The hematopoietin receptor superfamily is the largest of the cytokine receptor families. It is a group of structurally related type I membrane-bound glycoproteins characterized by one or more copies of a domain with two conserved pairs of cysteine residues. Each receptor subtype contains a ligand-binding domain with a characteristic amino acid composition expressing the specificity for the individual cytokines of the receptors. The cytoplasmic domain contains one or more signal-transducing chains, which are often shared by receptors for different cytokines. After ligand binding the receptors oligomerize and phosphorylate intracellular substrates, which results in signal transduction.[9] The main signal transduction pathway for this class of cytokine receptors is the Jak/Stat pathway, although the class I receptors are less specific than the class II receptors and as a consequence therefore also activate a number of other signal transductions pathways beside the Jak/Stat pathway.

A number of cytokines, including IL-2, IL-3, IL-4, IL-5, IL-6, IL-7, IL-9, IL-11, IL-12, IL-13, IL-15, GM-CSF, G-CSF, and growth hormone, signal through the hematopoietin receptor family[9] and several of these cytokines are present in the skin.

## D. Interferon/IL-10 Receptor Family (Class II Receptors)

The class II cytokine receptors are a second major class of cytokine receptors. The extracellular domains of the receptors are composed of tandem fibronectin type III domains with a characteristic pattern of proline and cysteine residues. There is no homology within the intracellular and transmembrane domain of this group of receptors, and only low homology in their extracellular domain.[10] Today there are 12 known members of this class II cytokine receptor family: four receptor subunits (IFN-αR1, IFN-αR2, IFN-γR1, and IFN-γR2) for the type I (IFN-α and IFN-β) and type II (IFN-γ) IFNs, two IL-10 receptor subunits (IL-10R1 and IL-10R2), four receptors utilized by IL-10-related cytokines (IL-20R1, IL-20R2, IL-22R1, and IL-22BP), the tissue factor (TF) that binds FVIIa and one currently orphan receptor.[11,12]

Class II receptors are composed of two distinct receptor chains denoted R1 and R2, e.g., IL-10R1 and IL-10R2. The R1 type subunit binds ligands with high affinity, whereas the R2 type subunit does not bind ligands on its own. Therefore, the R1 type subunit determines the specificity of the receptor. The R1 type subunit has a long intracellular domain that is associated with Jak1 tyrosine kinase whereas the R2 type subunit has a short intracellular domain associated with Jak2 or Tyk2 tyrosine kinase (see below). Ligand binding to the R1 type subunit induces oligomerization of the receptor subunits, recruitment of particularly Stat transcription factors, followed by Jak- or Tyk-mediated tyrosine phosphorylation and activation of the Stat transcription factor. The role of the R2 type subunit is to initiate the signal transduction events.[12]

IFN-αR1, IFN-αR2, IFN-γR1, and IFN-γR2 are the receptors for the IFNs (α, β, γ) that possess antitumor, antiviral, and immunomodulatory properties. Because these receptors are expressed on many cell types of the skin, IFN-α has either been tested in clinical trials or suggested for the treatment in melanoma, cutaneous T-cell lymphoma, Kaposi's sarcoma, basal cell carcinoma, human papillomavirus-associated lesions, and atopic dermatitis.[13]

IL-10 is another cytokine that signals through receptors belonging to the class II receptors. The predominant role of IL-10 is immunomodulation.[14] Although the expression of IL-10Rs in keratinocytes is still controversial, only IL-10R2 has been demonstrated.[15] However, treatment of psoriasis with IL-10 has led to improvement.[13]

IL-19, IL-20, and IL-24 are recently discovered members of the IL-10 family.[16] All three cytokines signal through the IL-20R1/IL-20R2 heterodimer, whereas IL-20 and IL-24 also signal through the IL-20R2/IL-22R heterodimer.[17] All three receptors are expressed in the epidermis.[16] Overexpression of IL-20 in transgenic mice led to severe cutaneous inflammation and altered epidermal proliferation and differentiation, and therefore IL-20 has been suggested to play an important role in the pathogenesis of psoriasis.[16] In keeping with this hypothesis, increased IL-19 and IL-20 mRNA expression has been found in psoriatic skin, whereas no regulation of the IL-20R1, IL-20R2, and IL-22R was found.[18]

## E. Immunoglobulin Superfamily

Some cytokine receptors contain extracellular immunoglobulin (Ig) domains and are classified as members of the immunoglobulin superfamily. They represent a novel family of inhibitory and stimulatory receptors expressed both in myeloid and lymphoid cells.[19] Their role in the skin is unknown, although lymphocytes expressing members of this receptor superfamily have been isolated from the skin and the blood in patients with transformed mycosis fungoides, Sezary's syndrome, and lymphomatoid papulosis.[20]

## F. TGF-β Receptor Family

More than 30 members of the TGF-β family have been identified. The TGF-β family members are made as precursors that are biologically inactive. Once activated by cleavage of a large prodomain,

TGF-β binds to the ligand-binding type II receptor, which then associates with a type I receptor. The type I/type II receptor complex possesses serine/threonine kinase activity resulting in downstream signal transduction primarily through a family of cytoplasmic Smad transcription factors that translocate to the nucleus and regulate gene transcription.[21] In the skin, treatment of fibroblasts with TGF-β results in increased synthesis of collagen and other extracellular matrix proteins, which may be important in wound healing.[22] Furthermore, TGF-β-induced signal transduction has also been suggested to be important in such diseases as scleroderma.[23]

### G. Chemokine Receptor Family

Chemokines represent a large family of structurally related small (8 to 14 kDa) polypeptide signaling molecules.[24] They bind to the chemokine receptor family, which are seven-transmembrane G protein–coupled receptors.[25] The long list of chemokines and chemokine receptors has been extensively reviewed by Zlotnik et al.[24] Originally chemokines were characterized by their ability to induce leukocyte chemotaxis in response to inflammatory stimuli. However, more recently groups of chemokines have been shown also to play a role in homeostatic migration pathways and to act on other cell types including keratinocytes, dendritic cells (Langerhans cells), endothelial cells, and tumor cells eliciting cell proliferation and angiogenesis.[24,26]

The chemokines and their respective receptors are grouped into four subfamilies, the CXC, CC, C, and $CX_3C$, based on the position of their conserved two N-terminal cysteine residues. There is a considerable redundancy and promiscuity in chemokine signaling because many chemokines share the same receptors. Since chemokines act as chemoattractants to T cells, a differential expression of chemokine receptors may contribute to the homing and activation of specific T-cell subsets. It has been demonstrated that differential tissue expression of specific chemokines recruits corresponding T-cell subtypes.[27]

After ligand binding the chemokine receptors associate with intracellular heterotrimeric G proteins.[24] The G protein family contains a large number of family members and therefore the formation of heterotrimeric G proteins may account for the action specificity of the various chemokine receptors. Chemokine receptor–induced G protein–linked signal transduction results in downstream activation of a number of signaling pathways. Activation of phospholipase C (PLC), diacylglycerol (DAG) formation, hydrolysis of phosphotidylinositol triphosphate, calcium influx into the cell, and PKC, $PI_3K$, Rac, and Rho activation have been demonstrated.[28] G protein signal transduction also activates the MAPK signaling pathway, which was recently demonstrated with the monocyte chemoattractant protein-1 (MCP-1) chemokine to involve parallel signaling pathways.[29]

The role of chemokines and chemokine signaling in human skin is discussed in Chapter 16.

## III. JAK/STAT PATHWAY

To date, seven distinct but homologues members of the mammalian signal transducers and activators of transcription (STAT) family have been identified and designated Stat1, Stat2, Stat3, Stat4, Stat5A, Stat5B (Stat5A and 5B are encoded by different genes), and Stat6.[30] The JAK/STAT pathway is activated by a number of different cytokines (Table 18.2) through cytokine binding and oligomerization of plasma membrane receptors (Figure 18.1). This is followed by cross-phosphorylation and activation of receptor associated Janus (JAK) kinases. The JAKs are a small family of four members (Jak1, Jak2, Jak3, and Tyk2) known as tyrosine kinases, which are associated with many cytokine and growth factor receptors, and JAKs have been shown to be critical for all subsequent downstream signaling.[31] JAK activation is followed by phosphorylation of tyrosine residues on the cytoplasmic part of the receptor. Then latent cytoplasmic STAT proteins are recruited to the phosphorylated tyrosine residues via an Src homology-2 (SH2) domain–phosphotyrosine interaction. Next the STAT proteins become phosphorylated by JAKs on conserved carboxy-terminus tyrosine leading to dimerization (homo- or heterodimers) and translocation to the nucleus where

**TABLE 18.2**
**Activation of Jak and Stat by Cytokines and Growth Factors**

| Cytokine/Growth Factor | Jak Activation | Stat Activation |
|---|---|---|
| IFN-α/IFN-β | Jak1, Tyk2 | Stat1, Stat2 |
| IFN-γ | Jak1, Jak2 | Stat1 |
| IL-2 | Jak1, Jak3 | Stat3, Stat5 |
| IL-3 | Jak1, Jak2 | Stat5 |
| IL-4 | Jak1, Jak3 | Stat6 |
| IL-5 | Jak1, Jak2 | Stat1, Stat3, Stat5 |
| IL-6 | Jak1, Jak2, Tyk2 | Stat1, Stat3 |
| IL-7 | Jak1, Jak3 | Stat1, Stat3, Stat5 |
| IL-9 | Jak1, Jak3 | Stat1, Stat3, Stat5 |
| IL-10 | Jak1, Tyk2 | Stat1, Stat3 |
| IL-11 | Jak1, Jak2, Tyk2 | Stat3 |
| IL-12 | Jak2, Tyk2 | Stat1, Stat3, Stat4 |
| IL-13 | Jak1, Jak2 | Stat6 |
| IL-15 | Jak1, Jak3 | Stat5 |
| IL-17 | | Stat2, Stat3 |
| IL-19 | | Stat3 |
| IL-20 | | Stat3 |
| IL-21 | Jak1, Jak3 | Stat1, Stat3 |
| IL-22 | | Stat1, Stat3, Stat5 |
| IL-24 | | Stat1, Stat3 |
| GM-CSF | Jak1, Jak2 | Stat5 |
| EGF | Jak1 | Stat1, Stat3, Stat5 |

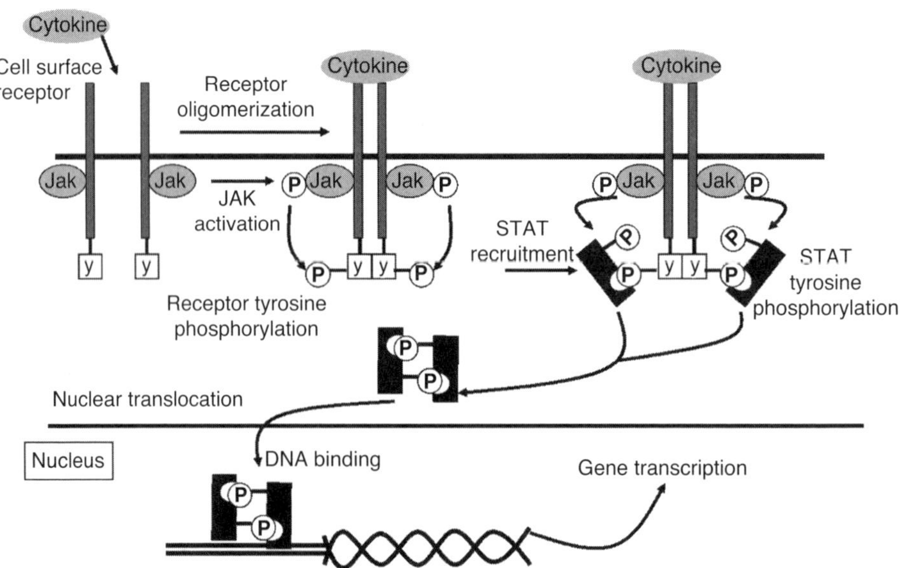


**FIGURE 18.1** Cytokine signaling by JAK and STAT.

STATs, through binding to specific DNA response elements on STAT responsive target genes, induce gene transcription (Figure 18.1).[32]

IFN receptors were the first described activators of JAK/STAT signaling, but afterward the JAK/STAT signaling pathway has been shown to be used by all type I and type II cytokine receptors; therefore, it can be activated by a number of different cytokines and growth factors. As shown in Table 18.2 the same STAT proteins can be involved in signaling by multiple different cytokines. One intriguing question that arises is therefore what determines the specificity of responses to the many different cytokines. The specificity of the response to a certain cytokine may depend on cell-specific receptor expression, modification of STAT responses by coactivators, repressors, and other transcription factors expressed at different levels in different cell types, as well as cross talk with other signaling pathways. Negative regulators of STAT are also known. They include cytoplasmic tyrosine phophatases counteracting JAK, induced suppressor of cytokine signaling (SOCS), which inhibit receptor and JAK function, proteins that inhibit activated STAT (PIAS) by preventing STAT/DNA binding, and nuclear phosphatases that deactivate STAT.

STAT-dependent target genes influence a number of different cellular functions including cellular growth, survival, apoptosis, host defense, and regulation of stress and differentiation as demonstrated in knockout studies of STAT family proteins in mice.[33,34] In normal cells, ligand-dependent activation of the STATs is a transient process lasting for minutes to hours. In contrast, inappropriate persistent STAT activation has been associated with oncogenesis.[35]

The expression of the JAK and STAT family proteins was determined in human epidermis by immunolocalization.[36] JAK1, STAT1, and STAT5 were found to be expressed at almost the same level through the various layers of the epidermis. JAK3, TYK2, STAT2, STAT3, STAT4, and STAT6 were more abundantly expressed in the granular layer than in the lower layers of the epidermis. A striking differential expression was also seen in the granular and the horny keratinized layers of the epidermis where JAK2, JAK3, STAT1, and STAT5 were expressed in much higher amounts than JAK1, TYK2, STAT2, STAT3, STAT4, and STAT6.

The role of STAT3 has been investigated especially in the epidermis. Epidermal cells and keratinocytes that are defective in STAT3 gene expression show impaired growth-factor-dependent *in vitro* migration,[37] and it was also demonstrated that while the development of the epidermis and hair follicles appeared normal, hair cycle and wound healing were severely compromised in STAT3 mutant mice. These results indicate that STAT3 is essential for skin remodeling such as wound healing and hair cycle regulation.

Abnormal signaling in the JAK–STAT signaling pathway has also been suggested in psoriasis. STAT1 activation in response to IFN-$\gamma$ in keratinocytes from psoriasis has been shown to be reduced compared to normal kerationocytes,[38] and an aberrant response to IFN-$\gamma$ may be important for the altered apoptosis and desquamation seen in psoriasis.

## IV. MAPKS

The MAP kinase cascade is one of the most ancient and evolutionarily conserved signaling pathways in the mammalian cell. The kinases control a wide variety of cellular events from very complex cellular programs such as cell differentiation, cell proliferation, apoptosis, and processes involved in immune responses to short-term changes important in maintaining homeostasis.

At least four different and distinctly regulated groups of MAP kinases have been described. These include the extracellular signal-regulated protein kinases (ERK),[39] the c-Jun $NH_2$-terminal kinases (JNK),[40] the p38 MAP kinases,[41,42] and ERK5.[43] The MAPK cascade represents a family of protein kinases that utilizes sequential phosphorylation of specific kinases to regulate the various cellular processes. Each cascade activation includes a MAPKKK, which activates a MAPKK, which again activates a MAPK[44] (Figure 18.2). Each pathway then in turn regulates specific downstream targets including transcription factors as described below.

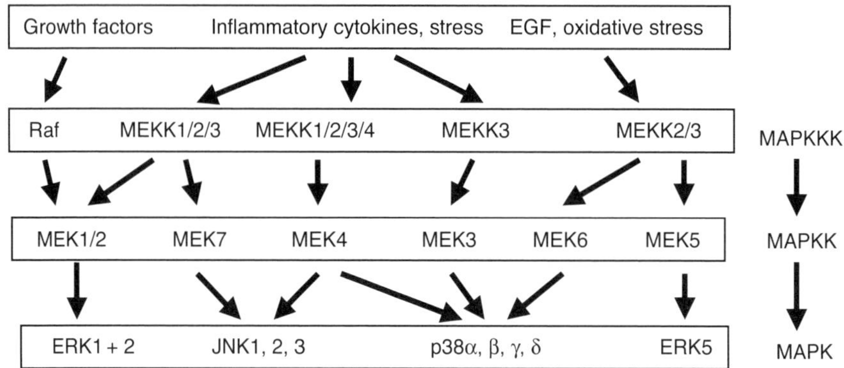


**FIGURE 18.2** The MAP kinase pathway.

MAPKKK regulation represents the entry point to the MAPK pathway and has been shown to involve membrane recruitment, oligomerization, and phosphorylation.[45] The stepwise activation of the various MAPKs through a MAPKKK/MAPKK/MAPK signaling cascade is greatly simplified. As indicated in Figure 18.2, a number of different MAPKKKs and MAPKKs are known and several studies have revealed extensive cross talk between the various cascades.

In the keratinocytes MAPKs play a key role in regulating cell differentiation, apoptosis, and inflammation.[46]

## A. ERK1 and 2

The ERKs were the first MAPK family to be characterized. Two isoforms of ERK, ERK1 and 2, which are sometimes referred to as p44/p42 MAP kinases, have been characterized. They have been shown to be 83% identical, with most differences outside the kinase core.[47] ERK1 and ERK2 are widely expressed and often involved in the regulation of cell growth and differentiation by regulating meiosis, mitosis, and postmitotic functions in different cells. Many different stimuli, including growth factors, cytokines, virus infection, ligands for heterotrimeric guanine nucleotide-binding protein (G protein)–coupled receptors, transforming agents, and carcinogens activate the ERK1 and ERK2 pathway.

Cell surface receptors transmit activating signals to MAP kinases through a variety of mechanisms. One example is the tyrosine kinase receptor activation by growth factors (Figure 18.2), which leads to Ras activation and subsequently activation of Raf kinases.[48] Mammals possess three Raf proteins: Raf-1, A-Raf, and B-Raf.[49] All three Raf isoforms are serine/threonine-specific kinases that integrate upstream input signals. They all three have Ras as a common upstream activator and MEK as the only downstream substrate.[39] Raf activates both MEK1 and MEK2 with similar efficacy *in vitro* and MEK can activate ERK1 and ERK2 via phosphorylation of Thr-Glu-Tyr-motif in the activation loop. Inactivated ERK1 and ERK2 are retained in the cytosol as part of a complex with MEK1, but upon stimulation a substantial portion of the ERK pool translocates to the nucleus. Nuclear translocation is essential for ERK-dependent activation of gene expression and regulation of the cell cycle.

The specificity of ERK signaling depends in part on which isoform of Raf is activated. Mouse knockout studies have shown that each of the three Raf isoforms have distinct roles.[49]

Although the four MAPK modules run in parallel (Figure 18.2), there is a considerable degree of cross talk between them, which creates multiple opportunities for modulating or fine-tuning responses to different signals. As shown in Figure 18.2, ERK1 and ERK2 can also be activated by inflammatory cytokines and cellular stress through a MEKK1/2/3dependent pathway.

Because ERKs like other MAPKs are activated by phosphorylation, the protein phosphatases dephosphorylating MAPKs are key elements in controlling ERK activity. Once ERK1 and 2 have been activated, they can target cytoplasmic proteins, membrane proteins, cytoskeletal proteins, and nuclear proteins. An important role of ERK activation is regulation or modulation of gene expression, which is mediated in two ways. ERK1 and 2 can target a group of protein kinases including Rsk 1 to 3, MAPKAP kinase 2 and 3, and Mnk1 and 2, which enhance gene expression through increasing the accessibility of DNA in the cell.[50] However, ERK1 and ERK2 also phosphorylate transcription factors directly and thereby stimulate their activity. ERK1 and 2 have been demonstrated to phosphorylate a number of transcription factors including c-Fos and c-Jun, which form the AP-1 transcription factor (see below), ELK1, the estrogen receptor, the nuclear factor of activated T cells (NFATc), and family members of the STAT family.[50–52]

ERK1 and ERK2 have both been demonstrated in the epidermis as well as in normal human keratinocytes *in vitro* and have been suggested to play a key role in regulating keratinocyte proliferation, differentiation, and survival.[46,51] Increased ERK activity has also been suggested to play an important role in the pathogenesis of inflammatory and malignant skin diseases. Increased ERK1 and ERK2 expression in the basal and lower suprabasal layer of lesional psoriatic skin has been demonstrated,[53] as well as an increase in the activated form of ERK.[54] Furthermore, an increase in activated ERK was reported in hyperproliferative cultured fibroblasts from psoriatic skin.[55] IL-15, which has been suggested to play an important role in the pathogenesis of psoriasis, has also been demonstrated to induce cellular proliferation and inhibit apoptosis in the human epidermal keratinocyte cell line, HaCaT through an ERK1- and ERK2-dependent mechanism.[56]

ERK activation seems also to be important in a number of human cancers. Numerous solid tumors are known to express constitutive levels of activated ERK1 and ERK2, and ERK activation is critical for a large number of Ras-induced cellular responses. Interestingly, the Ras family of proteins is activated by mutation in approximately 30% of human cancers.[57] Raf kinases are the direct downstream mediators of the Ras proteins, and therefore Raf kinases have also been ascribed a role in the development and maintenance of human malignancies. Raf mutations have been identified in a wide range of human tumors,[58] and especially mutations of the B-Raf gene have been detected in a range of human tumors, e.g., in 66% of malignant melanomas.[59] Recently, increased ERK activation has also been demonstrated in malignant acanthosis nigricans.[60]

Based on this accumulating evidence, indicating a role of ERK activation in epidermal hyperproliferation as well as a role in the development and maintenance of human malignancies, inhibition of ERK activity has now become an important objective in the development of new treatment modalities in a number of hyperproliferative and malignant diseases.

## B. JNK1 TO 3

The c-Jun N-terminal kinase (JNK) was originally identified as the UV-induced factor responsible for phosphorylating and thereby activating the proto-oncogene transcription factor c-Jun.[61] Three highly related but distinct gene products, JNK1, JNK2, and JNK3, can be expressed as a total of ten isoforms as a result of variable mRNA splicing.[62] JNK1 and JNK2 show a broad tissue distribution whereas JNK3 has been considered brain specific. However, recently keratinocytes have been demonstrated to express both JNK1 and JNK3.[63]

JNKs respond to a variety of stress signals including heat shock, osmotic stress, pro-inflammatory cytokines, ischemia, and UV exposure. The JNKs are activated through the MAPKKK/MAPKK cascade (Figure 18.2). Phosphorylation on Thr183 and Tyr185 by the dual-specificity kinases MKK4 and MKK7 results in JNK activation. Although MKK4 and MKK7 can phosphorylate both residues they may exhibit different preference for the phosphate acceptor sites, and the full activation of JNK may need both kinases.

Because JNKs like the other MAPKs are activated by phosphorylation, the protein phosphatases that dephosphorylate MAPKs are key elements in their control. The activity of JNK can be turned off by a number of phosphatases, including MAPK phosphatases,[40] and interestingly JNK activation can also be negatively regulated by NF-κB-mediated inhibition.[64] TNF-α can activate the JNK signaling pathway through binding to TNF receptors, and, conversely, the expression of the TNF gene is regulated by JNK activity. Glucocorticoids have been shown to specifically repress the activity of the JNK signaling pathway. Dexamethasone inhibits TNF-α– and lipopolysaccharide (LPS)-induced activation of JNK whereas no regulation was seen of the ERK and p38 MAPK pathway.[65]

JNKs are active as dimers and translocate across the nuclear membrane. They were originally identified as the major kinases responsible for the phosphorylation of c-Jun, leading to increased activity of the nuclear transcription factor activator protein-1 (AP-1) (see below). Other nuclear transcription factors are now also known to be targets for the JNKs. They include ATF-2, Elk-1, Myc, Smad3, p53, and NFAT4[66]. JNKs exert their effects only on transcription factors in the nucleus. This is in contrast to the other MAPKs, which phosphorylate targets both inside and outside the nucleus.

Activation of the JNK signaling pathway plays an important role in regulating apoptosis as well as tumorigenesis and inflammation. In general, JNK activation is considered to lead to apoptosis although this has been controversial. However, compelling evidence for a pro-apoptotic function of JNK comes from studies with mouse embryonic fibroblasts isolated from JNK1$^{-/-}$ and JNK2$^{-/-}$ mice. These cells were resistant to UV irradiation-induced apoptosis due to failure to activate the mitochondrial-dependent death pathway.[67] This pro-apoptotic effect is most likely mediated through activation of c-Jun transcription since mouse embryonic fibroblasts in which the endogenous c-Jun alleles were replaced with c-Jun resistant to JNK-mediated phosphorylation and activation showed insensitivity to UV-induced cell death.[68]

In the skin, JNK1 and JNK3 have been demonstrated in cultured normal human keratinocytes *in vitro*, and immunohistochemical analyses of normal human skin have revealed that phosphorylated active JNK is expressed in the nuclei in the suprabasal-granular cell layer,[69] indicating that JNK participates in regulation of gene transcription in differentiating normal human keratinocytes. In one study, JNK expression and activation have also been investigated in psoriasis. Here, increased phosphorylated active JNK was found in the nuclei of keratinocytes in involved psoriatic skin compared to uninvolved psoriatic skin.[54] No regulation of the expression of total JNK was found.

UV light often affects the human skin. It acts as an initiator of cellular stress and activates signal transduction resulting in regulation of transcription factors. In keratinocytes only UVB and UVC activate JNK, while in other cell types UVA, UVB, and UVC do.[63] These findings demonstrate that in the epidermis UV light acts as a specific agent regulating highly specialized responses, which may be important for the role of JNK in regulating tumor development. Studies with JNK1-deficient mice have suggested that JNK1 is a crucial suppressor of skin tumor development.[70]

## C. p38 MAPK

The p38 MAPK family has been shown to consist of four different isoforms: p38α,[71] p38β,[72] p38γ,[73] and p38δ.[74] Different expression, activation, and substrate specificity of each specific p38 isoform result in their different physiological functions. While p38α and p38β are ubiquitously expressed, p38γ and p38δ have been shown to be expressed in a more restricted and tissue specific manner. p38γ expression has not been detected in the epidermis, which is in accordance with a recent study where p38γ was shown not to be expressed in keratinocytes.[75] p38δ on the other hand is expressed in the epidermis[75] and plays a key role in regulating epidermal differentiation and apoptosis.[76]

p38 MAPKs are predominantly activated by inflammatory cytokines like TNF-α and IL-1 and they play a key role in regulating the cellular responses to these cytokines. However, p38 MAPKs can also be activated by a number of physical and chemical stresses like oxidative stress[77] and UV irradiation.[78] The signal transduction cascade leading to activation of the various p38 MAPK isoform is rather complex (Figure 18.2). MEK3 and 6 are phosphorylated and activated by a plethora of MEKKs and their relative contribution to the p38 pathway is not fully understood.

MEKK1 to 3 preferentially activate JNKs and ERKs, but they also participate in p38 activation.[79] MEK4 transmits the MEKK1 signal to p38[80] and in a co-transfection study MEK3 was shown to transmit the MEKK3 signal.[79] Reflecting the specificity and selectivity of the MAPK signaling system MEK3 has been shown to activate only p38α, γ, and δ, whereas, for example, MEK6 activates all four isoforms.[72,81,82] In MEK4$^{-/-}$ fibroblasts both JNK and p38 lost their responsiveness to TNF-α and IL-1,[83] whereas p38 activation was selectively inhibited in MEK3$^{-/-}$ mouse embryonic fibroblasts in response to TNF-α but not to IL-1.[84] These results demonstrate the complexity of the MAPK signal transduction cascade.

p38α and β act in many ways similarly and therefore most studies do not distinguish between the two isoforms. p38γ and p38β are both inhibited by pyridinyl imidiazole drugs[85] of which the compound SB203580 is the most extensively characterized, while p38β and p38δ are completely unaffected of these drugs.[85] Similar to other cellular systems, p38α and β MAPK-dependent activity was found in keratinocytes treated with UV light, $H_2O_2$, TNF-α, or IL-1β, suggesting an important role of these two isoforms in mediating keratinocyte responses to cellular stress.[76,86] In HaCaT cells and human keratinocytes p38α and β activation leads to increased COX2 gene expression,[76] increased IL-13Rα2 chain expression in response to IL-4 and IL-13,[87] increased cell proliferation,[88] and in response to TNF-α increased cell toxicity.[89] In other cell types, p38α and β has been shown to induce the expression of IL-1β, IL-5, IL-10, IFN-γ, and TNF-α.[90–94]

p38δ is expressed in epidermis, testis, lung, pancreas, kidney, and small intestine.[74,75] Thus, although p38δ is abundantly expressed in keratinocytes, its physiological role in keratinocytes is only incompletely understood. However, p38δ has been shown to play an important role in inducing keratinocyte differentiation,[76] and in a very recent study data strongly suggested p38δ as the major p38 isoform in driving the expression of the keratinocyte differentiation marker involucrine.[95] p38δ has also been ascribed a key role in the induction of apoptosis in keratinocytes.[76] p38δ expression and/or activity has never been systematically investigated in different skin diseases.

Upon activation p38 was reported to translocate from the cytosol to the nucleus,[96] but the subcellular localization following stimulation is only incomplete.

A number of downstream targets of p38 have been demonstrated. In the nucleus, p38 regulates the activity of a number of transcription factors including ATF-1/2, Elk-1, p53, NF-κB, and AP-1.[50] An inflammatory stimulus has been shown to induce p38α- and/or p38β-dependent phosphorylation of histone H3 in the promoter region of a subset of NF-κB-dependent cytokine and chemokine genes resulting in increased NF-κB recruitment and subsequently increased gene transcription.[97] This demonstrates that p38 plays an important role in regulating inflammatory and immune responses. AP-1 DNA binding activity is indirectly regulated through the induction of c-fos and c-jun expression as well as through a direct phosphorylation of AP-1 components,[50,76] and this may be a way to regulate, e.g., keratinocyte differentiation. A number of keratinocyte differentiation markers have AP-1 binding sites in their promoter region (see below). Other substrates downstream of p38 include different protein kinases, e.g., MAPKAP kinase-2, MAPKAP kinase-3, MAPKAP kinase-5, and MNK1,[98–101] which act both at the transcriptional and the translational level, as well as acting in a feedback mechanism by modulating p38 activity.

The expression and regulation of these downstream targets of p38 MAPK have not been investigated in human skin although it is intriguing to speculate that an imbalance in these protein kinases may be important in the pathogenesis of various skin diseases.

The importance of p38 MAPKs in the regulation of keratinocyte differentiation has been studied *in vitro*, but the role p38 in the pathogenesis of skin diseases characterized by abnormal keratinocyte differentiation has never been investigated. However, p38 MAPK has been suggested as a molecular target for inhibition of pro-inflammatory cytokines.[102] In a mouse model, p38 MAPK has also been demonstrated to play a key role in contact hypersensitivity induced by 2,4-dinitro-1-fluorobenzene (DNFB) and in this study p38 was suggested as an important target for the treatment of contact hypersensitivity.[103] Finally, p38 has been demonstrated to have a pro-apoptotic effect in keratinocytes after UVB irradiation.[46]

### D. ERK5

ERK5 is a relatively recently identified MAPK that is being studied intensely.[43] It is a 90 to 100 kDa protein and one of the largest MAP kinase family members. In the catalytic domain at the N-terminus of ERK5 it is 51% identical to ERK2.

The stimuli that activate ERK5 have not been comprehensively characterized, but ERK5 activation has been demonstrated by such environmental stresses as oxidative stress, as well as by stimuli inducing both cell proliferation and growth such as growth factors and serum[50] (Figure 18.2). In addition, vasoactive peptides or inflammatory cytokines like TNF can activate ERK5.[104]

The signal transduction pathway leading to ERK5 activation involves the MEKK2/3 and MEK5 cascade. MEK5 is the only known MEK that influences ERK5 activity. ERK5 is expressed in many human tissues, but most abundantly in heart and skeletal muscle.[43] It has never been studied in human skin but it has been shown to be expressed in mast cells[105] and in fibroblasts.[106]

Similar to the ERK1 and 2 pathway, ERK5 also activates a distinct set of transcription factors implicated in cell cycle regulation. ERK5 contributes to AP-1 activation by stimulating the expression of genes encoding AP-1 components such as c-jun and c-fos,[107] and AP-1 is involved in keratinocyte proliferation and differentiation as discussed below. NF-κB has also been demonstrated as a downstream target of ERK5 and it has been suggested as an integration point for ERK5 and ERK1 and 2 signaling.[108] Most recently the ERK5 cascade has been shown to induce transcriptional activation of the cyclin D1 gene.[109] The cyclin D1 promoter region contains both AP-1 and NF-κB binding sites among several others and induction of transcriptional activity has been demonstrated to each of these sites. Cyclin D1 is expressed in keratinocytes and has been suggested to mediate the proliferation of stem cells in the epidermis into more differentiated transient amplifying cells in the suprabasal layer.[110] Furthermore, cyclin D1 overexpression is frequently an early step in neoplastic transformation, particularly in mammary epithelium. Because cyclin D1 is a novel target of the ERK5 cascade, it may be interesting to further investigate the role of ERK5 in cancers such as squamous cell carcinomas involving cyclin D1 dysregulation.

## V. TRANSCRIPTION FACTORS

A transcription factor consists of one or more regulatory proteins that bind to specific DNA sequences in a gene. The result of the protein binding to the DNA sequence is usually transcriptional activation resulting in gene transcription and subsequently protein synthesis.

### A. AP-1

The transcription factor AP-1 mediates regulation of gene transcription in response to a variety of extracellular stimuli, and although its physiological functions are still being unraveled it has been demonstrated to regulate inflammatory responses as well as cell proliferation and survival.

AP-1 is not a single protein, but a dimer formed of proteins belonging to the Jun (c-jun, JunB, JunD), Fos (c-fos, FosB, Fra-1, and Fra-2), Maf (c-Maf, MafB, MafA, MafG/F/K, and Nrl) and ATF (ATF2, Lrf1/ATF3, B-ATF, JDP1, JDP2) subfamilies.[111] This discussion focuses mainly on Jun and Fos.

Unlike transcription factors such as NF-κB and STAT, which are constitutively present within the cells, activation of the AP-1 family of transcription factors is regulated predominantly at the transcriptional level with rapid induction of Fos and Jun proteins. Thus, AP-1 DNA binding activity can also be regulated through regulation of Jun and Fos protein turnover and post-translational modification of AP-1 subunit proteins.

The Jun and Fos proteins are known as early responsive genes, which are rapidly but transiently transcribed in response to extracellular stimuli such as growth factors, cytokines, neurotransmitters, bacterial and viral infections, and a variety of physical and chemical stresses.[111]

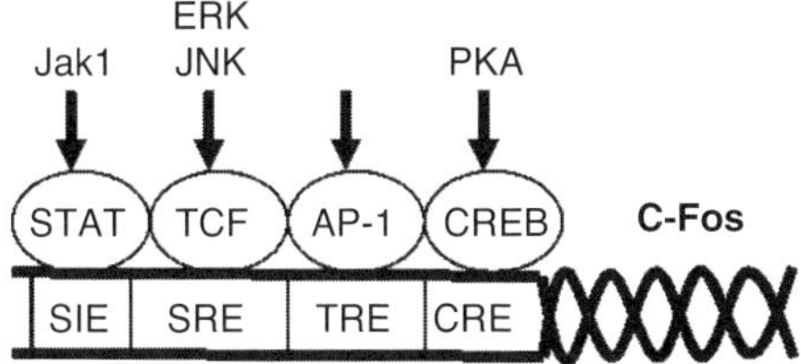


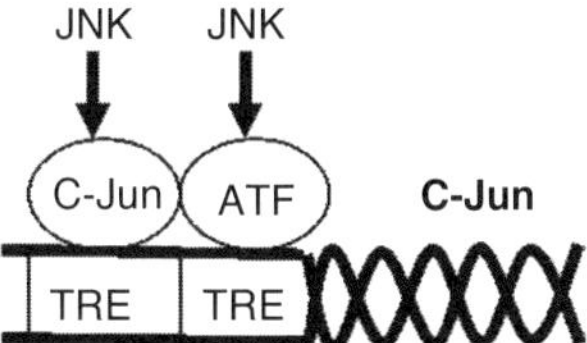


**FIGURE 18.3** Transcriptional activation of AP-1.

The c-fos gene is well characterized and has been shown to contain *cis*-inducible elements (SIE), serum response elements (SRE), TPA response elements (TRE), and cAMP response element (CRE) in its promoter region. These response elements bind various transcription factors such as STAT, ternary complex factor (TCF), AP-1, and cyclic adenosine monophosphate response element–binding protein (CREB) (Figure 18.3).[112–114] The SRE binds TCF, which is activated by growth factors, cytokines, and other stimuli activating the MAPK cascade. The c-jun promoter contains two TREs. In most cell types c-jun is expressed prior to stimulation. Following stimulation that activates especially the JNK signal transduction pathway, c-jun and activating transcription factor (ATF) become phosphorylated resulting in binding to TRE in the c-jun gene promoter region and subsequently gene transcription (Figure 18.3).[112] These newly synthesized AP-1 family proteins then dimerize to form the AP-1 transcription factor either as Jun-Fos heterodimers or Jun-Jun homodimers.

Although Ap-1 DNA binding activity is predominantly regulated at the transcriptional level of the AP-1 family proteins, post-translational regulation can also take place. Both preexisting and newly synthesized Jun and Fos proteins are modulated through their phosphorylation by several kinases including MAPKs, protein kinase A and protein kinase C.[115,116] Phosphorylation of Jun and Fos proteins alters their capacity to dimerize, their DNA-binding capacity, as well as their transcriptional activity.

AP-1 has also been suggested to play a pivotal role in regulating epidermal homeostasis. The expression pattern of Jun and Fos proteins has been studied in both mouse and human epidermis.[117,118] In human epidermis c-jun was found only in the granular layer whereas c-fos was found both in the spinous and granular layer but not in the basal layer. JunB and JunD were ubiquitously expressed in all epidermal layers. This distinct expression pattern of the AP-1 subunits in the epidermis as well as the expression of a number of target genes including keratin 1 and 5, involucrine, and transglutaminase indicate that AP-1 may play a pivotal role in normal and pathological skin physiology, although this could not be confirmed in a knockout mouse model. Mice lacking c-fos, FosB, or JunD did not show any specific skin phenotype.[119] AP-1 regulates a number of genes linked to keratinocyte differentiation and AP-1 activation has also been shown to induce keratinocyte differentiation *in vitro*.[116,118]

Recently, decreased AP-1 DNA binding activity has been found in lesional psoriatic skin compared to nonlesional and normal skin (unpublished results) indicating a role of AP-1 in the pathogenesis of psoriasis. This is further supported by the finding that topical treatment of lesional psoriatic skin with the vitamin D analogue calcipotriol leads to a normalization of the AP-1 DNA binding activity preceding the morphological normalization of the skin.

AP-1 also plays a role in skin carcinogenesis.[111] Inhibition of malignant transformation of the skin is observed in mice expressing a dominant negative c-jun transgene. However, transgenic overexpression of c-jun alone does not increase skin tumor incidence. Skin carcinogenesis requires additional activation of the AP-1 transcription factor.[111]

It also appears that AP-1 is an important transcription factor for controlling cellular responses to injury, as many of the downstream target genes containing the AP-1 binding site in their promoters produce key proteins involved in wound healing and reepithelialization.[112] Furthermore, increased expression of Jun and Fos genes has been demonstrated in response to cellular injury in several models.

## B. NF-κB

Nuclear factor-κB (NF-κB) is a dimeric transcription factor formed by hetero- or homodimerization of the five Rel family proteins: RelA (p65), RelB, cRel, p52, and p50.[120] NF-κB is believed to play a pivotal role in immune and inflammatory responses and in the regulation of cell proliferation and apoptosis. It regulates the transcription of genes encoding pro-inflammatory cytokines (e.g., IL-1, IL-2, TNF-α, and GM-CSF), chemokines (e.g., IL-8 and RANTES), adhesion molecules (e.g., ICAM, VCAM, and E-selectin), inducible enzymes (e.g., COX2 and iNOS), and also the MHC proteins important for the adaptive immune response.[121] Furthermore, the gene coding for the tumor suppressor protein p53 as well as other regulators of apoptosis and cell proliferation (e.g., c-IAP-1, c-IAP-1 Bcl-$X_L$, and c-*myc*) are regulated by NF-κB.[122]

In resting cells, NF-κB is usually retained inactive in the cytoplasm through binding to a member of the NF-κB inhibitor protein family, which contains seven members, IκBα, IκBβ, IκBγ, IκBε, Bcl-3, and the precursor Rel proteins p100 and p105.[123] A wide variety of agonists including the pro-inflammatory cytokines TNF-α and IL-1 have been shown to activate NF-κB. NF-κB activation is mediated through agonist binding to specific cell surface receptors, which then trigger signal transduction pathways that converge on the activation of a specific IκB kinase (IKK) and a subsequent phosphorylation of IκB molecules. Once phosphorylated, IκB is targeted for ubiquitination and degradation by proteosomes allowing translocation of the NF-κB dimer to the nucleus where it binds to specific response elements in the promoter region of the various target genes[124] (Figure 18.4). The IKKs consists of four subunits: α, β, γ, and ε. Activation of IKKβ is considered the classical pathway and it has together with IKKγ been shown to be responsible for NF-κB activation in response to pro-inflammatory stimuli, whereas activation through the IKKα pathway plays a role in mediating cell–cell interaction. IKKε is the most recently discovered IKK.[125] Not much is known about its biological functions but it has been suggested as a key kinase in integrating signals from the NF-κB and C/EBP signaling pathways during inflammatory and immune responses.[126]

NF-κB is ubiquitously expressed in almost all tissues investigated. Although first discovered as a key regulatory factor of immune and inflammatory responses, NF-κB is now recognized as an important player in controlling cellular growth and homeostasis including epidermal proliferation and differentiation.[127–129] Although the precise function of NF-κB in epidermal homeostasis is still

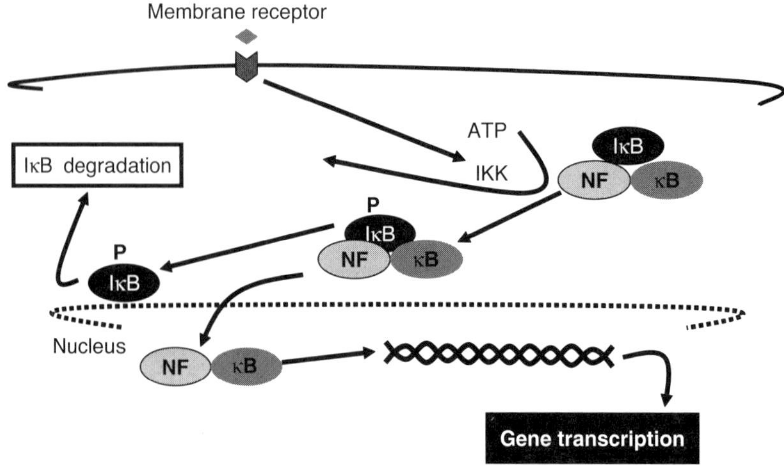


**FIGURE 18.4** Activation of the NF-κB pathway.

mysterious, the NF-κB subunits p50, p65, RelB, and c-Rel have been detected in keratinocytes and normal epidermis.[130] The expression of p52 is not yet fully elucidated. Forced expression of an artificial transactivating form of p50 or p65 in the basal layer of mouse epidermis resulted in cell cycle arrest, hypoplasia, and differentiation,[131,132] whereas epidermis-specific abrogation of NF-κB activation by forced expression of a nondegradable form of IκBα has been shown to lead to hyperplasia and hyperkeratinization.[131] It is unclear whether the observed hyperplasia represents a keratinocyte-cell-autonomous phenomenon or is a secondary effect related to altered immune homeostasis. Mice with an epidermis-specific deletion of IKKβ develop a severe inflammatory skin disease caused by a TNF-mediated, T-cell-independent inflammatory response.[133] These mice were born with a normal epidermis but developed a severe inflammatory dermatitis during the first few weeks. These results demonstrate that IKKβ regulation of NF-κB activity in the epidermis plays an important role in maintaining the immune homeostasis of the skin.

Another IKK family member, IKKα, regulates epidermal differentiation in an NF-κB-independent manner by inducing synthesis of a differentiation-inducing polypeptide.[134]

Besides the effects on differentiation and proliferation, evidence has also been presented demonstrating that NF-κB plays an antiapoptotic role in the epidermis.[135]

Regulation of the transcription of distinct sets of NF-κB target genes is carried out by the activation of specific signal transduction pathways followed by the formation of different NF-κB dimers. Recently, it was shown that NF-κB activation in leukocytes during the onset of inflammation is associated with pro-inflammatory gene expression whereas such activation during the resolution of inflammation was associated with the expression of anti-inflammatory genes and genes important for the induction of apoptosis.[136] Similarly, a change in the predominant NF-κB dimer was seen from 6 to 48 h after the onset of inflammation. A subunit specific function for NF-κB proteins in the regulation of dendritic cell development, survival, and cytokine production has also recently been demonstrated.[137] NF-κB also causes a cell type-dependent divergent gene regulation.[138] This was demonstrated by comparison of the expression of 12,435 genes in keratinocytes and fibroblasts after activation of NF-κB.[138]

An inhibition of NF-κB has been suggested as part of the mechanism of action of several anti-inflammatory drugs. Glucocorticoids have immunomodulatory effects and part of these effects has been ascribed to an inhibitory effect on NF-κB activation.[139–141] Cyclosporine A, which among other indications is used for systemic treatment of inflammatory skin diseases, has also been shown to inhibit NF-κB activation in an animal model with acute hypovolemic shock.[142] Recently, it was demonstrated that dimethylfumarate selectively prevents the nuclear entry of activated NF-κB, and it was suggested that this may be the basis of its beneficial effect in psoriasis.[143] An inhibition of NF-κB activation has also been suggested as the key mechanism for anti-TNF-α antibodies effective in psoriasis.[144]

In keeping with these observations, NF-κB has also been ascribed a key role in the pathogenesis of a number of different skin disorders. Psoriasis is an inflammatory, hyperproliferative skin disease with disturbances in epidermal proliferation. In lesional psoriatic skin several pro-inflammatory cytokines such as IL-1β, TNF-α, IL-6, and IL-8 are upregulated suggesting that they may play a pivotal role in the pathogenesis of psoriasis. These cytokines contain a κB binding site in their promoter region indicating that NF-κB participates in the regulation of their expression. Based on the disturbances in the epidermal proliferation and differentiation and the expression of a number of pro-inflammatory cytokines it is tempting to speculate that disturbances in NF-κB activation may play a pivotal role in the pathogenesis leading to psoriasis. Results from our group have shown that there is an increase in NF-κB binding to the κB motif in the IL-8 promoter region and a decrease in NF-κB binding to the κB motif in the p53 promoter region in lesional psoriatic skin compared to nonlesional psoriatic skin, which is also reflected by an increase in IL-8 expression and decrease in p53 expression. These results demonstrate that NF-κB regulation is very complex, and that there is a high degree of specificity of the genes transactivated by NF-κB in psoriasis. Others have also found disturbances in NF-κB activation in psoriatic keratinocytes,[145,146] whereas the expression levels of p50 and p65 were found not to be altered in lesional psoriatic skin compared to nonlesional psoriatic skin.[147]

Incontinentia pigmenti is a rare X-linked dominantly inherited genodermatosis, which is usually lethal to the male fetus. Recently, deletion mutations of the NEMO/IKKγ gene were shown to account for most cases of incontinentia pigmenti.[148] The mutation in NEMO/IKKγ results in an inhibition of NF-κB signaling and in male NEMO/IKKγ knockout mice NF-κB activation by pro-inflammatory cytokines was completely blocked.[149]

The involvement of NF-κB in sunburn reactions has also been demonstrated. Because most incident solar UV radiation is absorbed in the epidermis and dermis, the effect on the NF-κB pathway is of particular interest. UV irradiation leads to NF-κB activation and in Balb/c mice treatment either topically or systemically with NF-κB decoy oligonucleotides followed by exposure to UVB light significantly reduced UV-induced cutaneous swelling, epidermal hyperplasia, and secretion of the pro-inflammatory cytokines IL-1β, TNF-α, and IL-6.[150]

There is also strong evidence suggesting that NF-κB plays an important role in carcinogenesis. In a malignant melanoma cell line, IKK activity has been shown to be increased compared to normal human epidermal melanocytes and also an enhanced nuclear localization of p50/p65 was seen.[151] NF-κB may also play a role on squamous cell carcinomas. In the SENCAR mouse squamous cell carcinoma model, p50 and p52 were found to be overexpressed in the carcinoma tissue compared to normal epidermis.[152] In another study, blockade of NF-κB predisposes murine skin to squamous cell carcinoma.[153]

NF-κB activation has also been suggested to play a role in some autoimmune diseases[154] as well as being a part of the pathogenesis in the infection with *Borrelia burgdorfei,* also called Lyme disease.[155]

## VI. NUCLEAR RECEPTORS

More than 65 different nuclear receptors form the nuclear receptor superfamily. Nuclear receptors act as transcription factors and are known to be important transcriptional regulators in cellular proliferation, differentiation, and metabolic response to environmental stimuli.[156] In this chapter only selected nuclear receptors are discussed.

### A. PPAR

The peroxisome proliferator-activated receptor (PPAR) family comprises three subtypes PPARα, PPARγ, and PPARδ. All three subtypes are expressed in human keratinocytes.[157,158] PPARs require heterodimerization with retinoid X receptors (RXR) for effective DNA binding and induction of gene transcription[159] (Figure 18.5). The PPARs serve as ligand-activated pleiotropic regulators of cellular proliferation, differentiation, and homeostasis, acting through binding to specific peroxisome proliferator response elements (PPRE) in responsive genes.

PPARα was first identified more than 10 years ago and numerous studies have revealed the importance of PPARα in the control of lipid homeostasis.[160] It is expressed preferentially in the liver and in other tissues with a high fatty acid catabolism. However, PPARα also plays an important role in the regulation of inflammation. PPARα ligands are long-chain polyunsaturated fatty acids including linoleic acid and arachidonic acid, and PPARα activation has been demonstrated to reduce inflammatory responses[161] especially to reduce the duration of leukotriene $B_4$-induced inflammatory responses.[162]

PPARγ is abundantly expressed in adipose tissue and is known as an important regulator of adipocyte differentiation and lipid storage.[163] Although expressed at a much lower level, PPARγ is also found in hepatocytes, fibroblast, myocytes, and breast and colon epithelial cells where activation promotes cell differentiation. In addition to these effects, PPARγ agonists have also been shown to act as potent anti-inflammatory compounds[159] suggesting a role in the treatment of inflammatory

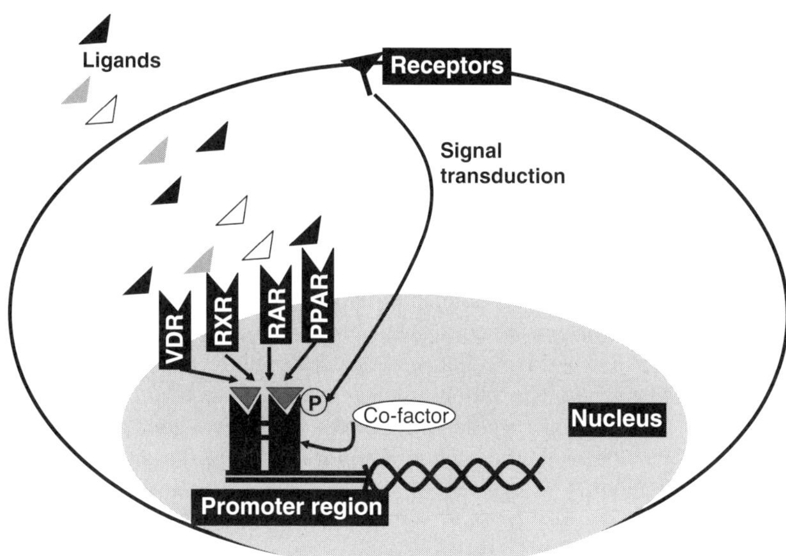


**FIGURE 18.5** Nuclear receptor activation.

diseases. Although a number of different PPARγ ligands have been identified including polyunsaturated fatty acids, some prostaglandins of the J-series, 9- and 13-HODE (hydroxyoctadecadienoic acid), as well as thiazolidinediones, which comprise a novel class of synthetic insulin-sensitizing agent, the true natural ligand may yet have to be discovered.

PPARδ is the most ubiquitously expressed isotype but its biological significance has remained more elusive. PPARδ has been associated with embryo implantation, colonocyte growth, cholesterol metabolism, myelization, and obesity, which was supported by data obtained in PPARδ-deficient mice.[164] PPARδ is activated by ligands such as fatty acids, fibrates, and tetradecylthioacetic acid (TTA).[158]

In the human skin all three different PPAR subtypes are expressed. PPARδ is the predominant subtype in the epidermis whereas PPARα and PPARγ are expressed at much lower levels.[147,158] PPARδ has been suggested to play a role in keratinocyte differentiation and proliferation, and treatment of normal human keratinocytes *in vitro* with a PPARδ selective ligand induces expression of keratinocyte differentiation marker genes, whereas PPARα and PPARγ selective ligands had only negligible effect.[158] Furthermore, targeted disruption of PPARα in a mouse model[165] as well as PPARγ null mice[166] do not exhibit any specific skin phenotype suggesting that these two subtypes do not play a role in epidermal differentiation and proliferation. In contrast, PPARδ knockout mice exhibit a hyperplastic response of the epidermis to TPA application[164] suggesting that this receptor may function as a molecular switch controlling basal cell proliferation and initiation of keratinocyte differentiation.

In the hyperproliferative psoriatic epidermis the expression of PPARδ is significantly upregulated compared to uninvolved psoriatic skin, whereas the expression of PPARα and PPARγ are more controversial.[147,167] Furthermore, several of the hydroxylated eicosanoids that accumulate in psoriatic lesions are potent PPARδ agonists.

Activation of PPARα has also been shown to decrease the inflammatory response in both an irritant and an allergic contact dermatitis animal model.[168] Furthermore, PPARα and PPARδ but not PPARγ have been suggested to play a role in wound healing.[159]

Another interesting finding demonstrating the complexity of signal transduction is that PPARα, PPARγ, and PPARδ have been shown to be involved in the modulation of inflammatory responses via negative cross talk with transcription factors such as NF-κB and AP-1.[147,169]

### B. RXR AND VDR

A ligand for a nuclear receptor is generally referred to as a nuclear hormone. These nuclear hormones all must be small lipophilic compounds because they have to be able to cross the cellular membrane easily. In the skin nuclear hormones like the vitamin A derivative, retinoic acid (RA) and 1α,25-dihydroxyvitamin $D_3$ (vitamin $D_3$) have been shown to play an important role in maintaining homeostasis, and their derivatives are also used in the treatment of various skin diseases such as psoriasis.[170]

RA can modulate the response of keratinocytes to mitogens and is a pleiotropic regulator of epidermal differentiation. RA has both stimulatory and inhibitory effects on keratinocyte differentiation. These diverse effects are mediated through binding to specific subtypes of receptors, the retinoic acid receptors (RARs) and the retinoid X receptors (RXRs), which leads to activation of different sets of responsive genes. The various nuclear receptors can then bind to specific response elements in the promoter region of specific target genes and induce gene transcription. However, in most cases the affinity of a monomeric nuclear receptor for a single binding motif is not sufficient for stable receptor–DNA binding.[171] Most nuclear receptors therefore form homo- or heterodimers with a second nuclear receptor (Figure 18.5) and this is also an elegant way to generate diversity from a limited number of transcription factors.

Vitamin $D_3$ is another important nuclear hormone ligand that regulates keratinocyte homeostasis[172] by decreasing cell proliferation and inducing differentiation. Vitamin $D_3$ binds to its specific nuclear receptor, the vitamin $D_3$ receptor (VDR). The VDR/ligand complex can then dimerize with the thyroid receptor (TR), the RXR, the RAR, or another VDR, but the biologically most important complex is the VDR/RXR heterodimer allowing for cross talk between these two signaling pathways.

After ligand binding and dimerization the nuclear receptor complex binds to specific response elements in the promoter region of the various target genes and induces gene transcription. However, a number of cofactor proteins have also been identified. The cofactor proteins may either act as co-activators of the nuclear receptor complex leading to increased transactivation or act as co-repressors decreasing transactivation (Figure 18.5). Another way of stimulating the transcriptional activity of ligand activated nuclear receptors is through phosphorylation. Signaling molecules reaching the cell surface can bind to membrane receptors and through different signal transduction cascades induce phosphorylation of specific nuclear receptors (Figure 18.5) and thereby modulate the transcriptional activity. This is a way to integrate signals from the cell surface receptors with signals at the nuclear receptor level.

Not all effects of the nuclear receptor ligands can be fully explained by ligand-induced transactivation of the nuclear receptor complex. Nuclear receptors have also been shown to participate in transcriptional cross talk by protein–protein interaction with other transcription factors like AP-1 and NF-κB or kinases involved in other signal transduction cascades.[173]

## REFERENCES

1. Cullinan, E.B. et al., IL-1 receptor accessory protein is an essential component of the IL-1 receptor, *J. Immunol.*, 161, 5614, 1998.
2. Cao, Z. et al., TRAF6 is a signal transducer for interleukin-1, *Nature*, 383, 443, 1996.
3. Hannum, C.H. et al., Interleukin-1 receptor antagonist activity of a human interleukin-1 inhibitor, *Nature*, 343, 336, 1990.
4. Muzio, M. et al., Cloning and characterization of a new isoform of the interleukin receptor antagonist, *J. Exp. Med.*, 182, 336, 1990.
5. Groves, R.W. et al., Inducible expression of type 2 IL-1 receptors by cultured human keratinocytes. Implications for IL-1-mediated processes in epidermis, *J. Immunol.*, 154, 4065, 1995.

6. Sims J.E. et al., IL-1 and IL-18 receptors, and their extended family, *Curr. Opin. Immunol.*, 14, 117, 2002.
7. Kock, A. et al., Human keratinocytes are a source for tumor necrosis factor alpha: evidence for synthesis and release upon stimulation with endotoxin or ultraviolet light, *J. Exp. Med.*, 172, 1609, 1990.
8. Vandevoorde, V. et al., Induced expression of trimerized intracellular domains of the human tumor necrosis factor (TNF) p55 receptor elicits TNF effects, *J. Biol. Chem.*, 137, 1627, 1997.
9. Abbas, A.K., Lichtman, A.H., and Pober, J.S., *Cellular and Molecular Immunology*, 4th ed., W.B. Saunders, Philadelphia, 2000, chap. 11.
10. Thoreau, E. et al., Structural symmetry of the extracellular domain of the cytokine/growth hormone/prolactine receptor family and interferon receptors revealed by hydrophobic cluster analysis, *FEBS Lett.*, 282, 26, 1991.
11. Kotenko, S.V. and Pestka, S., Jak-Stat signal transduction pathway through the eyes of cytokine class II receptor complexes, *Oncogene*, 19, 2557, 2000.
12. Kotenko, S.V., The family of IL-10-related cytokines and their receptors: related, but to what extent? *Cytokine Growth Factor Rev.*, 217, 1, 2002.
13. Asadullah, K., Sterry, W., and Trezer, U., Cytokines: interleukin and interferon therapy in dermatology, *Clin. Exp. Dermatol.*, 27, 578, 2002.
14. Moore, K.W. et al., Interleukin-10 and interleukin-10 receptor, *Annu. Rev. Immunol.*, 19, 683, 2001.
15. Seifert, M. et al., Keratinocyte unresponsiveness towards interleukin-10: lack of specific binding due to deficient IL-10 receptor 1 expression, *Exp. Dermatol.*, 12, 137, 2003.
16. Blumenberg, H. et al., Interleukin 20: discovery, receptor identification, and role in epidermal function, *Cell*, 104, 9, 2001.
17. Parrish-Novak, J. et al., Interleukin 19, 20, and 24 signal through two distinct receptor complexes, *J. Biol. Chem.*, 277, 47517, 2002.
18. Romer, J. et al., Epidermal over expression of interleukin 19, 20 mRNA in psoriatic skin disappears after short term treatment with cyclosporine A or calcipotriol, *J. Invest. Dermatol.*, 121, 1306, 2003.
19. Borges, L. and Cosman, D., LIRs/ILTs/MIRs, inhibitory and stimulatory Ig-superfamily receptors expressed in myeloid and lymphoid cells, *Cytokine Growth Factor Rev.*, 11, 209, 2000.
20. Wechler, J. et al., Killer cell immunoglobulin-like receptor expression delineates *in situ* Sezary syndrome lymphocytes, *J. Pathol.*, 199, 77, 2003.
21. Miyazono, K. et al., TGF-β signalling by Smad proteins, *Adv. Immunol.*, 75, 115, 2000.
22. Takehara, K., Growth regulation of skin fibroblasts, *J. Dermatol. Sci.*, 24, S70, 2000.
23. Trojanowska, M., Molecular aspects of scleroderma, *Front. Biosci.*, 7, d608, 2002.
24. Zlotnik, A. and Yoshei, O., Chemokines a new classification system and their role in immunity, *Immunity*, 12, 121, 2000.
25. Murphy, P.M., Chemokine receptor structure, function and role in microbial pathogenesis, *Cytokine Growth Factor Rev.*, 7, 47, 1996.
26. Petering, H. et al., Characterization of the CC chemokine receptor 3 on human keratinocytes, *J. Invest. Dermatol.*, 116, 549, 2001.
27. Sebastiani, S. et al., Chemokine receptor expression and function in CD4$^+$ T lymphocytes with regulatory activity, *J. Immunol.*, 166, 996, 2001.
28. Mukaida, N., Interleukin 8. An expanding universe beyond neutrophil chemotaxis and activation, *Int. J. Hematol.*, 72, 391, 2000.
29. Jiminez-Sainz, M.C. et al., Signalling pathways for monocyte chemoattractant protein 1- mediated extracellular signal-regulated kinase activation, *Mol. Pharmacol.*, 64, 773, 2003.
30. Leonard, W.J. and O'Shea, J.J., Jaks and STATs: biological implications, *Annu. Rev. Immunol.*, 16, 293, 1998.
31. Ihle, J.N., The Janus protein tyrosine kinase family and its role in cytokine signalling, *Adv. Immunol.*, 60, 1, 1995.
32. Ihle, J.N. et al., Signalling by the cytokine receptor superfamily: Jaks and Stat, *Trends Biochem. Sci.*, 19, 222, 1994.
33. Takeda, K. and Akira, S., STAT family of transcription factors in cytokine-mediated biological responses, *Cytokine Growth Factor Rev.*, 11, 199, 2000.

34. Levy, D.E. and Darnell, J.E., STATs: transcriptional control and biological impact, *Nat. Rev. Mol. Cell Biol.*, 3, 651, 2002.
35. Bromberg, J. and Darnell, J.E., The role of STATs in transcriptional control and their impact on cellular function, *Oncogene*, 19, 2468, 2000.
36. Nishiio, H. et al., Immunolocalisation of the janus kinases (JAK) — signal transducers and activators of transcription (STAT) pathway in human epidermis, *J. Anat.*, 198, 581, 2001.
37. Sano, S. et al., Keratinocyte-specific ablation of Stat3 exhibits impaired skin remodeling, but does not affect skin morphogenesis, *EMBO J.*, 18, 4657, 1999.
38. Jackson, M. et al., Psoriatic keratinocytes show reduced IRF-1 and STAT-1$\alpha$ activation in response to $\gamma$-IFN, *FASEB J.*, 13, 495, 1999.
39. Schaeffe, H.J. and Weber, M.J., Mitogen-activated protein kinases: specific messengers from ubiquitous messengers, *Mol. Cell Biol.*, 19, 2435, 1999.
40. Davis, R.J., Signal transduction by the JNK group of MAP kinases, *Cell*, 103, 239, 2000.
41. Han, J. et al., A MAP kinase targeted by endotoxin and hyperosmolarity in mammalian cells, *Science*, 265, 808, 1994.
42. Han, J. and Ulevitch, R.J., Emerging targets for anti-inflammatory therapy, *Nat. Cell Biol.*, 1, E39, 1999.
43. Zhou, G., Bao, Z.G., and Dixon, J.E., Components of a new human protein kinase signal transduction pathway, *J. Biol. Chem.*, 270, 12665, 1995.
44. Robinson, M.J. and Cobb, M.H., Mitogen-activated protein kinase pathway, *Curr. Opin. Cell. Biol.*, 9, 180, 1997.
45. Kyriakis, J.M. et al., The stress-activated protein kinase subfamily of c-Jun kinases, *Nature*, 369, 160, 1994.
46. Eckert, R.L. et al., Keratinocyte survival, differentiation and death: many roads lead to mitogen-activated protein kinase. *J. Invest. Dermatol. Symp. Proc.*, 7, 36, 2002.
47. Boulton, T.G. et al., ERKs: a family of protein-serine/threonine kinases that are activated and tyrosine phosphorylated in response to insulin and NGF, *Cell*, 65, 663, 1991.
48. Hamad, N.M. et al., Distinct requirements for Ras oncogenesis in human versus mouse cells, *Genes Dev.*, 16, 2045, 2002.
49. Hagemann, C. and Rapp, U.R., Isotype-specific functions of Raf kinases, *Exp. Cell Res.*, 253, 34, 1999.
50. Chen, Z. et al., MAP kinases, *Chem. Rev.*, 101, 2449, 2001.
51. Johansen, C. et al., 1$\alpha$,25(OH)$_2$D$_3$ stimulates AP-1 DNA binding activity by a PI3-kinase/Ras/MEK/ERK1/2 and JNK1 dependent increase in c-Fos, Fra1 and c-Jun expression in human keratinocytes, *J. Invest. Dermatol.*, 120, 561, 2003.
52. Porter, C.M. et al., Identification of amino acid residues and protein kinases involved in the regulation of NFATc subcellular localization, *J. Biol. Chem.*, 275, 3543, 2000.
53. Haase, I. et al., A role for mitogen-activated protein kinase activation by integrins in the pathogenesis of psoriasis, *J. Clin. Invest.*, 108, 527, 2001.
54. Takahashi, H. et al., Extracellular regulated kinase and c-Jun N-terminal kinase are activated in psoriatic involved epidermis, *J. Dermatol. Sci.*, 30, 94, 2002.
55. Dimon-Gadal, S. et al., MAP kinase abnormalities in hyperproliferative cultured fibroblasts from psoriatic skin, *J. Invest. Dermatol.*, 110, 872, 1998.
56. Yano, S. et al., Interleukin 15 induces the signals of epidermal proliferation through ERK and PI 3-kinase in a human epidermal keratinocyte cell line, HaCaT, *Biochem. Biophys. Res. Commun.*, 301, 841, 2003.
57. Bos, J.L., Ras oncogenes in human cancer: a review, *Cancer Res.*, 49, 4682, 1989.
58. Storm, S.M. and Rapp, U.R., Oncogene activation: c-raf-1 gene mutations in experimental and naturally occurring tumors, *Toxicol. Lett.*, 67, 201, 1993.
59. Davies, H. et al., Mutations of the BRAF gene in human cancer, *Nature*, 417, 949, 2002.
60. Haase, I. and Hunzelmann, N., Activation of epidermal growth factor receptor/ERK signalling correlates with suppressed differentiation in malignant acanthosis nigricans, *J. Invest. Dermatol.*, 118, 891, 2002.
61. Hibi, M. et al., Identification of an oncoprotein and UV-responsive protein kinase that binds and potentiates the c-Jun activation domain, *Genes Dev.*, 7, 2135, 1993.
62. Gupta, S. et al., Selective interaction of JNK protein kinase isoforms with transcription factors, *EMBO J.*, 15, 2760, 1996.

63. Adachi, M. et al., Specificity in stress response: epidermal keratinocytes exhibit specialized UV-responsive signal transduction pathways, *DNA Cell Biol.*, 22, 665, 2003.
64. Tang, G. et al., Inhibition of JNK activation through NF-κB target genes, *Nature*, 414, 313, 2001.
65. Gonzales, M. et al., Glucocorticoids antagonize AP-1 by inhibiting the activation/phosphorylation of JNK without affecting its subcellular distribution, *J. Cell Biol.*, 150, 1199, 2000.
66. Cowan, K.J. and Storey, K.B., Mitogen-activated protein kinases: new signalling pathways functioning in cellular responses to environmental stress, *J. Exp. Biol.*, 206, 1107, 2003.
67. Tournier, C. et al., Requirement of JNK for stress-induced activation of the cytochrome c-mediated death pathway, *Science*, 288, 870, 2000.
68. Behrens, A. et al., Amino-terminal phosphorylation of c-Jun regulates stress-induced apoptosis and cellular proliferation, *Nat. Genet.*, 21, 326, 1999.
69. Takahashi, H. et al., Expression of human cystatin A by keratinocytes is positively regulated via the Ras/MEKK1/MKK7/JNK signal transduction pathway but negatively regulated via the Ras/Raf-1/MEK1/ERK pathway, *J. Biol. Chem.*, 276, 36632, 2001.
70. She, Q.B. et al., Deficiency of c-Jun-NH(2)-terminal kinase-1 in mice enhances skin tumor development by 12-*O*-tetradecanoylphorbol-13-acetate, *Cancer Res.*, 62, 1343, 2002.
71. Han, J., Endotoxin induces rapid protein tyrosine phosphorylation in 70Z/3 cells expressing CD14, *J. Biol. Chem.*, 268, 25009, 1993.
72. Jiang, Y. et al., Characterization of the structure and function of a new mitogen-activated protein kinase (p38beta), *J. Biol. Chem.*, 271, 17920, 1996.
73. Lechner, C. et al., ERK6, a mitogen-activated protein kinase involved in C2C12 myoblast differentiation, *Proc. Natl. Acad. Sci. U.S.A.*, 93, 4355, 1996.
74. Kumar, S. et al., Novel homologues of CSBP/p38 MAP kinase: activation, substrate specificity and sensitivity to inhibition by pyridinyl imidazoles, *Biochem. Biophys. Res. Commun.*, 235, 533, 1997.
75. Dashti, S.R., Efimova, T., and Eckert, R.L., MEK7-dependent activation of p38 MAP kinase in keratinocytes, *J. Biol. Chem.*, 276, 8059, 2001.
76. Eckert, R.L. et al., p38 mitogen-activated protein kinases on the body surface — a function for p38δ, *J. Invest. Dermatol.*, 120, 823, 2003.
77. Shiozaki, K. and Russell, P., Cell-cycle control linked to extracellular environment by MAP kinase pathway in fission yeast, *Nature*, 378, 739, 1995.
78. Hazzalin, C.A. et al., p38/RK is essential for stress-induced nuclear responses: JNK/SAPKs and c-Jun/ATF-2 phosphorylation are insufficient, *Curr. Biol.*, 6, 1028, 1996.
79. Deacon, K. and Blank, J.L. MEK kinase 3 directly activates MKK6 and MKK7, specific activators of the p38 and c-Jun NH2-terminal kinases, *J. Biol. Chem.*, 274, 16604, 1999.
80. Guan, Z. et al., Interleukin-1beta-induced cyclooxygenase-2 expression requires activation of both c-Jun NH2-terminal kinase and p38 MAPK signal pathways in rat renal mesangial cells, *J. Biol. Chem.*, 273, 28670, 1998.
81. Wang, X.S. et al., Molecular cloning and characterization of a novel p38 mitogen-activated protein kinase, *J. Biol. Chem.*, 272, 23668, 1997.
82. Enslen, H., Raingeaud, J., and Davis, R.J. Selective activation of p38 mitogen-activated protein (MAP) kinase isoforms by the MAP kinase kinases MKK3 and MKK6, *J. Biol. Chem.*, 273, 1741, 1998.
83. Ganiatsas, S. et al., SEK1 deficiency reveals mitogen-activated protein kinase cascade cross regulation and leads to abnormal hepatogenesis, *Proc. Natl. Acad. Sci. U.S.A.*, 95, 6881, 1998.
84. Wysk, M. et al., Requirement of mitogen-activated protein kinase 3 (MKK3) for tumor necrosis factor-induced cytokine expression, *Proc. Natl. Acad. Sci. U.S.A.*, 96, 3763, 1999.
85. Lee, J.C. et al., p38 mitogen-activated protein kinase inhibitors — mechanisms and therapeutic potentials, *Pharmacol. Ther.*, 82, 389, 1999.
86. Garmyn, M. et al., Human keratinocytes respond to osmotic stress by p38 map kinase regulated induction of HSP70 and HSP27, *J. Invest. Dermatol.*, 117, 1290, 2001.
87. David, M. et al., Induction of the IL-13 receptor alpha2-chain by IL-4 and IL-13 in human keratinocytes: involvement of STAT6, ERK and p38 MAPK pathways, *Oncogene*, 20, 6660, 2001.
88. Zhang, L. et al., Bacterial heat shock protein-60 increases epithelial cell proliferation through the ERK1/2 MAP kinases, *Exp. Cell Res.*, 266, 11, 2001.
89. Ravid, A. et al., Vitamin D inhibits the activation of stress-activated protein kinases by physiological and environmental stresses in keratinocytes, *J. Endocrinol.*, 173, 525, 2002.

90. Foey, A.D. et al., Regulation of monocyte IL-10 synthesis by endogenous IL-1 and TNF-alpha: role of the p38 and p42/44 mitogen-activated protein kinases, *J. Immunol.*, 160, 920, 928, 1998.
91. Rincon, M. et al., Interferon-gamma expression by Th1 effector T cells mediated by the p38 MAP kinase signalling pathway, *EMBO J.*, 17, 2817, 1998.
92. Lu, H.T. et al., Defective IL-12 production in mitogen-activated protein (MAP) kinase kinase 3 (MKK3)-deficient mice, *EMBO J.*, 18, 1845, 1999.
93. Mori, A. et al., p38 mitogen-activated protein kinase regulates human T cell IL-5 synthesis, *J. Immunol.*, 163, 4763, 1999.
94. Brook, M. et al., Regulation of tumour necrosis factor alpha mRNA stability by the mitogen-activated protein kinase p38 signalling cascade, *FEBS Lett.*, 483, 57, 2000.
95. Efimova, T., Broome, A.M., and Eckert, R.L., A regulatory role for p38 delta MAPK in keratinocyte differentiation. Evidence for p38 delta-ERK1/2 complex formation, *J. Biol. Chem.*, 278, 34277, 2003.
96. Ben-Levy, R. et al., Nuclear export of the stress-activated protein kinase p38 mediated by its substrate MAPKAP kinase-2, *Curr. Biol.*, 8, 1049, 1998.
97. Saccani, S., Pantano, S., and Natoli, G., p38-dependent marking of inflammatory genes for increased NF-κB recruitment, *Nat. Immunol.*, 3, 69, 2002.
98. Freshney, N.W., Interleukin-1 activates a novel protein kinase cascade that results in the phosphorylation of Hsp27, *Cell*, 78, 1039, 1994.
99. McLaughlin, M.M., Identification of mitogen-activated protein (MAP) kinase-activated protein kinase-3, a novel substrate of CSBP p38 MAP kinase, *J. Biol. Chem.*, 271, 8488, 1996.
100. Ni, H., MAPKAPK5, a novel mitogen-activated protein kinase (MAPK)-activated protein kinase, is a substrate of the extracellular-regulated kinase (ERK) and p38 kinase, *Biochem. Biophys. Res. Commun.*, 243, 492, 1998.
101. Waskiewicz, A.J., Mitogen-activated protein kinases activate the serine/threonine kinases Mnk1 and Mnk2, *EMBO J.*, 16, 1909, 1997.
102. Adams, J.L. et al., p38 MAP kinase: molecular target for the inhibition of pro-inflammatory cytokines, *Prog. Med. Chem.*, 38, 1, 2001.
103. Takanami-Ohnishi, Y. et al., Essential role of p38 mitogen-activated protein kinase in contact hypersensitivity, *J. Biol. Chem.*, 277, 37896, 2002.
104. Abe, J.I. et al., Big mitogen-activated protein kinase 1 (BMK1) is a redox-sensitive kinase, *J. Biol. Chem.*, 271, 16586, 1996.
105. Wei, W. et al., MEF2C regulates c-Jun but not TNF-alpha gene expression in stimulated mast cells, *Eur. J. Immunol.*, 33, 2903, 2003.
106. Squires, M.S. Nixon, P.M., and Cook, S.J., Cell-cycle arrest by PD184352 requires inhibition of extracellular signal-regulated kinases (ERK) 1/2 but not ERK5/BMK1, *Biochem. J.*, 366, 673, 2002.
107. Karin, M. Liu, Z.G., and Zandt, E., AP-1 function and regulation, *Curr. Opin. Cell Biol.*, 9, 240, 1997.
108. Pearson, G. et al., ERK5 and ERK2 cooperate to regulate NF-kappaB and cell transformation, *J. Biol. Chem.*, 276, 7927, 2001.
109. Mulloy, R. et al., Activation of cyclin D1 expression by the ERK5 cascade, *Oncogene*, 22, 5387, 2003.
110. Xu, X. et al., Differential expression of cyclin D1 in the human hair follicle, *Am. J. Pathol.*, 163, 969, 2003.
111. Shaulian, E. and Karin, M., AP-1 as a regulator of cell life and death, *Nat. Cell Biol.*, 4, E131, 2002.
112. Yates, S. et al., Transcription factor activation in response to cutaneous injury: role of AP-1 in reepithelialization, *Wound Rep. Reg.*, 10, 5, 2002.
113. Karin, M., The regulation of AP-1 activity by mitogen-activated protein kinases, *J. Biol. Chem.*, 270, 16482, 1995.
114. Treisman, R., The serum response element, *Trends Biochem. Sci.*, 17, 423, 1992.
115. Abate, C. et al., Dimerization and DNA binding alter phosphorylation of Fos and Jun, *Proc. Natl. Acad. Sci U.S.A.*, 90, 6766, 1993.
116. Johansen, C. et al., 1α,25-Dihydroxyvitamin $D_3$ induced differentiation of cultured human keratinocytes is accompanied by a PKC-independent regulation of AP-1 DNA binding activity, *J. Invest. Dermatol.*, 114, 1174, 2000.
117. Welter, J.F. et al., Differential expression of the fos and jun family members c-fos, fosB, Fra-1, Fra-2, c-jun, junB and junD during epidermal keratinocyte differentiation, *Oncogene*, 11, 2681, 1995.
118. Rutberg, S.E. et al., Differentiation of mouse keratinocytes is accompanied by PKC-dependent changes in AP-1 proteins, *Oncogene*, 13, 167, 1996.

119. Jochum, W. et al., AP-1 in mouse development and tumourigenesis, *Oncogene*, 20, 2401, 2001.
120. Foo, S.Y. and Nolan G. P., NF-κB to the rescue: RELs, apoptosis and cellular transformation, *Trends Genet.*, 15, 229, 1999.
121. Baldwin, A.S., The transcription factor NF-κB and human disease, *J. Clin. Invest.*, 107, 3, 2001.
122. Baldwin, A.S., Control of oncogenesis and cancer therapy resistance by the transcription factor NF-κB, *J. Clin. Invest.*, 107, 241, 2001.
123. Ghosh, S. May, M.J., and Kopp, E.B., NF-kappa B and Rel proteins: evolutionary conserved mediators of immune responses, *Annu. Rev. Immunol.*, 16, 225, 1998.
124. Rothwarf, D.M. and Karin, M., The NF-kappaB activation pathway: a paradigm in information transfer from membrane to nucleus, *Sci. STKE.*, 1999, RE1, 1999.
125. Shimada, T. et al., IKK-i, a novel lipopolysaccharide-inducible kinase that is related to IkappaB kinases, *Int. Immunol.*, 11, 1357, 1999.
126. Kravchenko, V. et al., IKKi/IKKε plays a key role in integrating signals induced by pro-inflammatory stimuli, *J. Biol. Chem.*, 278, 26612, 2003.
127. Ghosh, S. and Karin, M., Missing pieces in the NF-κB puzzle, *Cell*, 109, S81, 2002.
128. Kaufman, C.K. and Fuchs, E., It's got you covered: NF-κB in the epidermis, *J. Cell Biol.*, 149, 999, 2000.
129. Barnes, P.J. and Karin, M., Nuclear factor-B: a pivotal transcription factor in chronic inflammatory diseases, *N. Engl. J. Med.*, 336, 1066, 1997.
130. Takao, J. et al., Expression of NF-kappaB in epidermis and the relationship between NF-kappaB activation and inhibition of keratinocyte growth, *Br. J. Dermatol.*, 148, 680, 2003.
131. Seitz, C.S. et al., Alteration in NF-κB function in transgenic epithelial tissue demonstrate a growth inhibitory role for NF-κB, *Proc. Natl. Acad. Sci. U.S.A.*, 95, 2307, 1998.
132. Seitz, C. et al., Nuclear factor κB subunits induce epithelial cell growth arrest, *Cancer Res.*, 60, 4085, 2000.
133. Pasparakis, M. et al., TNF-mediated inflammatory skin disease in mice with epidermis-specific deletion of IKK2, *Nature*, 417, 861, 2002.
134. Hu, Y. et al., IKKα controls formation of the epidermis independently of NF-κB, *Nature*, 410, 710, 2001.
135. Qin, J.Z. et al., Role of NF-κB activity in apoptotic response of keratinocytes mediated by interferon-γ, tumor necrosis factor-α, and tumor-necrosis-factor-related apoptosis-inducing ligand, *J. Invest. Dermatol.*, 117, 898, 2001.
136. Lawrence, T. et al., Possible new role of NF-κB in the resolution of inflammation, *Nat. Med.*, 7, 1291, 2001.
137. Ouaaz, F. et al., Dendritic cell development and survival require distinct NF-kappaB subunits, *Immunity*, 16, 257, 2002.
138. Hinata, K. et al., Divergent gene regulation and growth effects by NF-κB in epithelial and mesenchymal cells of human skin, *Oncogene*, 22, 1955, 2003.
139. Scheinman, R.I. et al., Role of transcriptional activation of I kappa B alpha in mediation of immunosuppression by glucocorticoids, *Science*, 270, 283, 1995.
140. Auphan, N. et al., Immunosuppression by glucocorticoids: inhibition of NF-kappa B activity through induction of I kappa B synthesis. *Science*, 270, 286, 1995.
141. Bosscher, K.D. et al., Glucocorticoid-mediated repression of nuclear factor-B-dependent transcription involves direct interference with transactivation, *Proc. Natl. Acad. Sci. U.S.A.*, 94, 13504, 1997.
142. Altavilla, D. et al., Nuclear factor-kappaB as a target of cyclosporin in acute hypovolemic hemorrhagic shock, *Cardiovasc. Res.*, 52, 143, 2001.
143. Loewe, R. et al., Dimethylfumarate inhibits TNF-induced nuclear entry of NF-kappa B/p65 in human endothelial cells, *J Immunol.*, 168, 4781, 2002.
144. Chaudhari, U. et al., Efficacy and safety of infliximab monotherapy for plaque-type psoriasis: a randomised trial, *Lancet*, 357, 1842, 2001.
145. Danning, C.L. et al., Macrophage-derived cytokine and nuclear factor kappaB p65 expression in synovial membrane and skin of patients with psoriatic arthritis, *Arthritis Rheum.*, 43, 1244, 2000.
146. McKenzie, R.C. and Sabin, E., Aberrant signalling and transcription factor activation as an explanation for the defective growth control and differentiation of keratinocytes in psoriasis: a hypothesis, *Exp. Dermatol.*, 12, 337, 2003.
147. Westergaard, M. et al., Expression and localization of peroxisome proliferator-activated receptors and nuclear factor κB in normal and lesional psoriatic skin, *J. Invest. Dermatol.*, 121, 1104, 2003.

148. Smahi, A. et al., Genomic rearrangement in NEMO impairs NF-kappaB activation and is a cause of incontinentia pigmenti. The International Incontinentia Pigmenti (IP) Consortium, *Nature*, 405, 466, 2000.
149. Schmidt-Supprian, M. et al., NEMO/IKK gamma-deficient mice model incontinentia pigmenti, *Mol. Cell*, 5, 981, 2000.
150. Abeyama, K. et al., A role for NF-kappaB-dependent gene transactivation in sunburn, *J. Clin. Invest.*, 105, 1751, 2000.
151. Yang, J. and Richmond, A., Constitutive IkappaB kinase activity correlates with nuclear factor-kappaB activation in human melanoma cells, *Cancer Res.*, 61, 4901, 2001.
152. Pandolfi, F. et al., Expression of cell adhesion molecules in human melanoma cell lines and their role in cytotoxicity mediated by tumor-infiltrating lymphocytes, *Cancer*, 69, 1165, 1992.
153. Dajee, M. et al., NF-κB blockade and oncogenic Ras trigger invasive human epidermal neoplasia, *Nature*, 421, 639, 2003.
154. Bell, S. et al., Involvement of NF-κB signalling in skin physiology and disease, *Cell. Signalling*, 15, 1, 2002.
155. Ebnet, K. et al., *Borrelia burgdorferi* activates nuclear factor-kappa B and is a potent inducer of chemokine and adhesion molecule gene expression in endothelial cells and fibroblasts, *J. Immunol.*, 158, 3285, 1997.
156. Mangelsdorf, D.J. et al., The nuclear receptor superfamily: the second decade, *Cell*, 83, 835, 1995.
157. Rivier, M. et al., Differential expression of peroxisome proliferator-activated receptor subtypes during the differentiation of human keratinocytes, *J. Invest. Dermatol.*, 111, 1116, 1998.
158. Westergaard, M. et al., Modulation of keratinocyte gene expression and differentiation by PPAR-selective ligand tetradecylthioacetic acid, *J. Invest. Dermatol.*, 116, 702, 2001.
159. Kuenzli, S. and Saurat, J.-H., Peroxisome proliferator-activated receptors in cutaneous biology, *Br. J. Dermatol.*, 149, 229, 2003.
160. Willson, T.M. et al., The PPARs: from orphan receptors to drug discovery, *J. Med. Chem.*, 43, 527, 2000.
161. Staels, B. et al., Activation of human aortic smooth-muscle cells is inhibited by PPARalpha but not by PPARgamma activators, *Nature*, 393, 790, 1998.
162. Devchand, P.R. et al., The PPARalpha-leukotriene B4 pathway to inflammation control, *Nature*, 384, 39, 1996.
163. Vamecq, J. and Latruffe, N., Medical significance of peroxisome proliferators-activated receptors, *Lancet*, 354, 141, 1999.
164. Peters, J.M. et al., Growth, adipose, brain, and skin alterations resulting from targeted disruption of the mouse peroxisome proliferator-activated receptor beta (delta), *Mol. Cell Biol.*, 20, 5119, 2000.
165. Lee, S.S. et al., Targeted disruption of the alpha isoform of the peroxisome proliferators-activated receptor gene in mice results in abolishment of the pleiotropic effects of peroxisome proliferators, *Mol. Cell Biol.*, 15, 3012, 1995.
166. Barak, Y. et al., PPAR gamma is required for placental, cardiac, and adipose tissue development, *Mol. Cell*, 4, 585, 1999.
167. Ellis, C.N. et al., Troglitazone improves psoriasis and normalizes models of proliferative skin disease: ligands for peroxisome proliferators-activated receptor-γ inhibit keratinocyte proliferation, *Arch. Dermatol.*, 136, 609, 2000.
168. Sheu, M.Y. et al., Topical peroxisome proliferator activated receptor-alpha activators reduce inflammation in irritant and allergic contact dermatitis model, *J. Invest. Dermatol.*, 118, 94, 2002.
169. Delerive, P.De B. et al., Peroxisome proliferator-activated receptor α negatively regulates the vascular inflammatory gene response by negative cross-talk with transcription factors NF-κB and AP-1, *J. Biol. Chem.*, 274, 32048, 1999.
170. Kragballe, K. et al., Double-blind, right/left comparison of calcipotriol and betamethasone valerate in treatment of psoriasis vulgaris, *Lancet*, 337, 193, 1991.
171. Carlberg, C. et al., The nuclear receptor superfamily, *Retinoids*, 15, 71, 1999.
172. Kang, S. et al., Pharmacology and molecular action of retinoids and vitamin D in skin, *J. Invest. Dermatol. Symp. Proc.*, 1, 15, 1996.
173. Göttlicher, M. Heck, S., and Herrlich, P., Transcriptional cross-talk, the second mode of steroid hormone receptor action, *J. Mol. Med.*, 76, 480, 1998.

# 19 Epidermis as a Pro-Inflammatory Organ

*Jonathan N.W.N. Barker*

## CONTENTS



## I. INTRODUCTION

For many years, it was thought that the skin protected the host from a wide variety of injurious environmental agents such as harmful microbes and physical or chemical trauma, including ultraviolet (UV) radiation simply by acting as an inert physical barrier. This function was subserved through the production of dense connective tissue within the dermis and by the production of the stratum corneum within the epidermis. It was not until the mid-1970s that this view started to change. Before then, it was assumed that if the skin, particularly the epidermis, was injured in any way, immunological responses were initiated elsewhere, with the skin involved purely in a passive way, as a bystander to ongoing immunological and inflammatory processes. The ultrastructural studies of Silberberg et al.[1] demonstrating that epidermal Langerhans cells could be identified in close apposition to T lymphocytes infiltrating the epidermis in allergic contact dermatitis as early as 24 h were the studies to challenge this view. Since then, of course, there has been an explosion of data concerning the pivotal role of Langerhans cells in cutaneous acquired immune responses. Indeed, basic immunological knowledge concerning Langerhans cell function has been turned into potential therapeutic benefit through progress in dendritic cell vaccine technology (see Chapter 39).

Epidermal keratinocytes, which comprise 95% of the mass of human epidermis, are principally responsible for the structural integrity of the epidermis through the production of a corneified cell envelope, and for maintenance of a barrier, through biosynthesis lipids, proteins, and proteoglycans. The view that keratinocytes may also participate actively in epidermal immune responses gained substance when, in 1981, epidermal thymocyte activating factor (ETAF), was identified in supernatants of keratinocyte cultures.[2] ETAF was subsequently shown to be identical to interleukin-1 (IL-1). Thus, keratinocytes had been demonstrated to produce a secretable molecule with multiple effects on immune responses including lymphocyte activation and endothelial/leukocyte adhesion.

0-8493-1959-5/05/$0.00+$1.50

The range of immunomodulatory molecules that keratinocytes produce and either express on their cell surface or secrete has risen inexorably and is reviewed elsewhere in this book (see Chapters 5, 15, and 16).

Since the last edition of this book, major advances have been made in our understanding of innate immune mechanisms.[3] This describes the rapid, nonspecific response by cells to a series of conserved motifs, for example, bacterial lipopolysaccharide (LPS) leading to downstream cellular events in large part orchestrated by the nuclear transcription factor NF-κB. Essential cellular components of the innate immune system include neutrophils, natural killer cells, and mast cells. It is now apparent that the skin, as a primary defense organ, provides a barrier to harmful environmental insults, not only physically but also through the initiation of both innate and acquired immune mechanisms.[4] Innate mechanisms require pattern recognition of molecules such as bacterial LPS by specific cell surface receptors. Keratinocytes possess several of these receptors and further produce peptide antibacterial agents such as defensins.[5] Thus, it has been shown that epidermal keratinocytes play a key role in both acquired and innate cutaneous immune responses.

The remainder of this chapter concentrates on the role of keratinocytes in epidermal immune/inflammatory responses, and in particular their ability to modulate leukocyte recruitment and T-cell effector function in response to epicutaneous stimulation.

## II. ROLE OF KERATINOCYTES IN EPIDERMAL IMMUNE RESPONSES

It is now apparent that keratinocytes exhibit the capacity to produce a wide variety of soluble peptide mediators of inflammation, termed cytokines, which exert their activity through interaction with specific receptors on the surface of target cells. These cytokines include interleukins, chemokines, interferons, growth factors, and angiogenic factors (see Chapters 5, 15, and 16). Once secreted, cytokines may act in an autocrine, juxtacrine, or paracrine fashion to influence multiple different resident cell types within the skin including endothelial cells, macrophage/dendritic cells, neutrophils, lymphocytes, fibroblasts, Langerhans cells, and keratinocytes themselves.

In 1991, it was postulated that a pivotal event in the ability of diverse environmental stimuli responsible for inducing cutaneous inflammation including contact allergens (e.g., $NiSO_4$, urushiol, and DNCB) and irritants (e.g., croton oil, dithranol), UV radiation, particularly UVB, and microbial pathogens, was their ability to directly activate keratinocytes, thus, through the production of specific pro-inflammatory cytokines and leukocyte adhesion molecules, inducing an inflammatory cascade.[6] The consequences of keratinocyte activation are numerous:

1. Modulation of leukocyte accumulation
2. Modulation of antigen presentation within the skin
3. Production of antimicrobial peptides and induction of innate immune mechanisms
4. Promotion of vascular proliferation
5. Modulation of keratinocyte growth, motility, and apoptosis

### A. Cellular Effects of Environmental Challenge

Within minutes to hours after epidermal challenge with stimuli such as allergen, irritant, or UVB, inflammatory changes occur within the skin, including the accumulation of neutrophils and specific subsets of T lymphocytes (skin homing, memory T cells). Immunostaining of skin biopsies taken sequentially after challenge with antigen demonstrates induction of E-selectin and VCAM-1 and upregulation of ICAM-1 on dermal blood vessels.[7] These changes can be observed as early as 8 h after challenge, with staining intensity increasing to a maximum at 24 to 48 h. Concomitant with induction of these vascular adhesion molecules, neutrophils and skin-homing memory T lymphocytes accumulate in the perivascular compartment. Leukocytes then migrate through the dermis toward the epidermis where they may interact with Langerhans cells as observed by Silberberg.

It is of note that these early steps are also observed in "nonantigenic" driven conditions such as irritant dermatitis and UVB-induced inflammation,[8] as well as "antigenic" conditions such as allergic contact dermatitis, suggesting that common mechanisms control these initial events. It has been demonstrated that nonantigen-specific effects of haptens contribute significantly to the elicitation of contact hypersensitivity responses, implying that contact allergens must also possess an "irritant" effect.[9] Urushiol, for example, the allergen responsible for poison ivy dermatitis, causes a rash on primary exposure, a potentially important phenomenon in its allergic capability. There are increasing data that the mechanisms responsible for early events following stimulus involve pathways critical to innate immunity. Although direct measurement of NF-κB in skin *in vivo* is difficult, it seems likely that it is involved. Certainly tumor necrosis factor-alpha (TNF-α) is upregulated early in such events (see below). Further, the alerting of the acquired immune system to environmental events that may be detrimental to the host occurs via the presence of "danger signals."[10] These include molecules such as heat shock proteins and induce, for example, dendritic cell maturation leading to enhanced antigen presentation.

## B. Keratinocyte Responses to Environmental Stimuli

One potential explanation to account for the ability of diverse environmental stimuli to cause inflammation is that they directly induce production and/or secretion of pro-inflammatory cytokines by epidermal cells. *In vitro,* keratinocytes produce multiple cytokines in response to such stimulation including IL-1, TNF-α, IL-6, and IL-8, as assessed by mRNA analysis of cell lysates and protein and bioassay of supernatants. *In vivo,* epicutaneous challenge leads to the detection of multiple cytokines,[11] IL-1, TNF-α, IL-6, and IL-8, as assessed by many techniques such as immunostaining and reverse transcription polymerase chain reaction (RT-PCR). Thus, *in vitro* and *in vivo* evidence exists that keratinocytes are "activated" by environmental stimuli to produce mediators of inflammation.

For keratinocytes to influence inflammatory cell accumulation and subsequent immunological events, it is necessary to postulate that the soluble cytokines detailed above can diffuse from the epidermis into the dermis to effect changes in dermal blood vessels. Anatomically, these events are likely to take place at the tips of dermal papillae, where the potential space between keratinocytes and capillary loops is very small. Furthermore, some studies demonstrate that it is basal keratinocytes in these sites that maximally express molecules such as ICAM-1 and IL-8. The spatial alignment between keratinocytes and endothelial cells within the dermal papilla is analogous to Bowman's capsule in the kidney. Influx of cells at this site is likely to provide the basis for the morphological description of the squirting papilla of Pinkus and Mehregan,[12] observed in psoriasis and seborrheic dermatitis.

Indirect evidence that secreted products of keratinocytes reach the circulation is provided by experiments showing that certain cytokines, namely, IL-1, IL-6, and TNF-α,[13] can be detected within the circulation following whole-body irradiation with UVB. VEGF, thought to be derived from keratinocytes in erythrodermic psoriasis, may account for systemic symptoms such as proteinuria observed in some of these patients.[14] More directly, grafting of genetically manipulated human keratinocytes expressing apolipoprotien-E (apo-E) on to mice, results in detection of apo-E in the mouse peripheral circulation.[15] Keratinocyte-derived cytokines may therefore influence a considerable range of inflammatory events both locally and systemically.

Studies of transgenic mice provide direct evidence that keratinocyte products affect cutaneous immune responses and inflammatory cell accumulation. Mice in which the genes encoding TNF-α[6] and IL-1 are linked to keratin 14 promoter and are overexpressed in the basal layer of the epidermis and produce spontaneous inflammation within the skin. In addition, delayed-type hypersensitivity responses to topically applied antigen are exaggerated in transgenic mice overexpressing a number of other immunomodulatory molecules in the basal epidermis. These include ICAM-1,[17] IL-1 receptor,[18] and MCP-1.[19] Importantly, MCP-1 transgenic mice display an increase in dendritic cells within the dermis, particularly along the dermoepidermal junction in non-inflamed skin, confirming that keratinocyte products possess the capacity to influence leukocyte migration within the dermis, including Langerhans cells and dermal dendrocytes.[20] Interestingly, transgenic mice in which molecules not classically linked to the immune system also provoke an inflammatory response often with features suggestive of human skin diseases. Examples of these include β-integrin (involucrin promoter 21) and VEGF (K14 promoter), both of which lead to psoriasiform inflammation.[22]

### C. Leukocyte Trafficking

Leukocyte infiltration into skin is a multistep process. Interaction between circulating leukocytes and the blood vessel wall, mediated by surface adhesion molecules, is followed by diapedesis of the leukocyte into the perivascular space. Chemotaxins, including a major role for chemokines, then allow directed migration through tissue toward the inflammatory stimulus.[27] Once at the site of inflammation, leukocytes adhere to target cells, including in the case of T helper cells, antigen presenting cells. Two keratinocyte-derived cytokines that are likely to play a pivotal role in the initiation of such reactions in the skin are IL-1 and TNF-α, termed "primary cytokines" by Kupper.[23]

Normal human epidermis contains preformed IL-1. Perturbation of the epidermis leads to release of this cytokine together with gene transcription for both IL-1 and TNF-α. *In vitro,* both are potent inducers of the vascular adhesion molecules E-selectin, ICAM-1, and VCAM-1. In normal human skin *in vivo*, direct intradermal injection of these cytokines leads to a time-dependent increase of the above adhesion molecules on the dermal vasculature, with a concomitant leukocyte dermal infiltrate.[24,25] Following epidermal stimulation, chemotaxins can also be detected in the skin including IL-8 and MCP-1. *In vitro,* keratinocytes produce biologically active amounts of these chemokines and it seems likely that keratinocytes are a major cell type responsible for their production *in vivo*. Given their anatomical site, keratinocytes are uniquely situated to provide the directed migrational stimuli required to attract leukocytes toward the epidermis. A possible mechanism to explain production of the chemokines is that environmental stimuli induce keratinocyte production of IL-1 and TNF-α, which act in both an autocrine and juxtacrine fashion leading to the production of a second "wave" of cytokines.

## III. EPIDERMAL CONTROL OF T-CELL FUNCTION

As stated earlier in this chapter, Langerhans cells are the primary antigen-presenting cell of the epidermis and the mechanisms documented above have, as one of their main aims, delivery of T helper cells to Langerhans cells within the epidermis. Keratinocyte-derived cytokines influence epidermal immune responses not just by modulating leukocyte trafficking but also by directly influencing the antigen-presenting capacity of Langerhans cells. Critical cytokines in this respect are IL-1 and granulocyte-macrophage colony-stimulating factor (GM-CSF). For example, freshly isolated Langerhans cells are poor antigen-presenting cells but after 3 days in culture they potently present antigen. This functional change is attributed to IL-1 and GM-CSF, secreted by contaminating keratinocytes within the culture supernatant.[26]

Langerhans cells have been shown to produce cytokines. These may also be involved in leukocyte recruitment, adhesion, and antigen presentation by Langerhans cells. In addition, evidence exists that keratinocytes may act as antigen-presenting cells. These data are at present conflicting, with some studies showing no effect, others showing resultant T-cell activation, and others revealing induction of tolerogenic signals. An explanation for these conflicting results is that the type of antigen used in the assays, whether nominal or alloantigen, processed or nonprocessed, is varied. The *in vivo* significance remains to be determined.

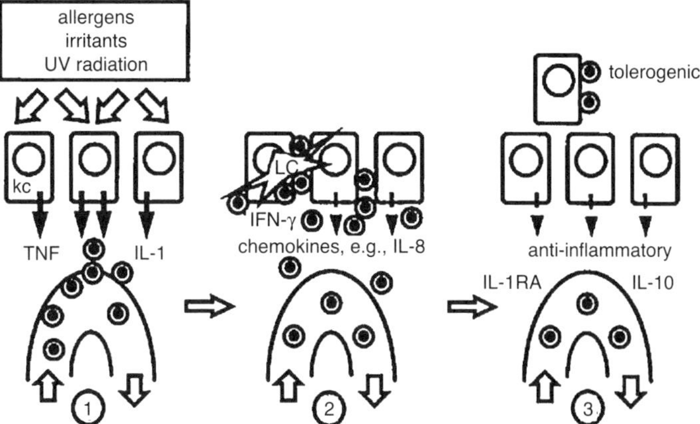


**FIGURE 19.1** Schematic representation of model of keratinocytes as orchestrators of cutaneous inflammation. Step 1: Environmental factors that provoke cutaneous inflammation induce production of "primary cytokines" (TNF-α and IL-1) by keratinocytes (KC). These diffuse into the dermis where the dermal vasculature is activated to express adhesion molecules required for leukocyte recruitment. Step 2: TNF-α and IL-1 produce autocrine and juxtacrine effects including induction of chemokines and other pro-inflammatory cytokines. Lymphocytes become spatially aligned with antigen-presenting cells, particularly Langerhans cells (LC), and produce effector cytokines including IFN-γ. Step 3: Cutaneous inflammation is suppressed by production of anti-inflammatory cytokines and tolerogenic signals provided to lymphocytes by keratinocytes acting as antigen presenting cells.

## IV. MODEL: KERATINOCYTES AS ORCHESTRATORS OF CUTANEOUS INFLAMMATION

### A. Initiation

Epicutaneous contact with environmental stimuli (allergen, irritant, UV radiation, etc.) leads directly to keratinocyte activation and release of the primary cytokines IL-1 and TNF-α. These cytokines diffuse through the dermo-epidermal barrier into the dermis, where they interact with receptors on vascular endothelial cells leading to activation and induction of specific leukocyte adhesion molecules. The result is accumulation of specific subsets of circulating leukocytes (notably neutrophils and/or skin-homing T lymphocytes, depending on the stimulus) in the perivascular compartment.

Autocrine and juxtacrine effects of IL-1 and TNF-α lead to keratinocyte production of chemoattractants including many chemokines, which allow directed migration of leukocytes toward the epidermis. These events occur predominantly within the dermal papillae and are not antigen specific (Figure 19.1).

### B. Amplification

The processes allow close apposition of epidermal cells (Langerhans cells and keratinocytes) and infiltrating leukocytes. Reciprocal interactions between these cells then occur, predominantly mediated by cytokines, to augment the inflammatory response leading to further leukocyte accumulation, activation, proliferation, and cytokine production. Furthermore, certain cytokines likely to be present in such an epidermal environment have synergistic activity with respect to cytokine and adhesion molecule production.

Antigen-driven events may then occur, predominantly through Langerhans cells, but influenced by keratinocyte-derived cytokines.

### C. Resolution

In addition to the production of pro-inflammatory cytokines, keratinocytes produce cytokines that have an anti-inflammatory effect, including IL-1 receptor antagonist. Furthermore, when keratinocytes act as antigen-presenting cells, in many situations the resulting response is an antigen-specific tolerogenic signal. It is therefore possible that sequelae of the events detailed above include activation of these "anti-inflammatory" activities by keratinocytes leading to resolution. Homeostasis, with respect to inflammation, within the epidermis may therefore be critically dependent upon appropriate keratinocyte function. Recently, a subset of T lymphocytes has been identified and named regulatory T cells (Tr). The possibility exists that keratinocytes either directly or through soluble mediators affects the function of these cells.

## REFERENCES


1. Silberberg, I., Baer, R.L., and Rosenthal, S.A., The role of Langerhans cells in allergic contact hypersensitivity. A review of findings in man and guinea pigs [review], *J. Invest. Dermatol.*, 66, 210–217, 1976.
2. Luger, T.A., Stadler, B.M., Katz, S.I., and Oppenheim, J.J., Epidermal cell (keratinocyte)-derived thymocyte-activating factor (ETAF), *J. Immunol.,* 127, 1493–1498, 1981.
3. Medzhitov, R. and Janeway, C., Innate immunity, *N. Engl. J. Med.,* 343, 338–344, 2000.
4. Nickoloff, B.J., Skin innate immune system in psoriasis: friend or foe? *J. Clin. Invest.*, 104(9), 1161–1164, 1999.
5. Ali, R.S., Falconer, A., Ikram, M., Bissett, C.E., Cerio, R., and Quinn, A.G., Expression of the peptide antibiotics human beta defensin-1 and human beta defensin-2 in normal human skin, *J. Invest. Dermatol.*, 117(1), 106–111, 2001.
6. Barker, J.N., Mitra, R.S., Griffiths, C.E., Dixit, V.M., and Nickoloff, B.J., Keratinocytes as initiators of inflammation [see comments] [review], *Lancet*, 337, 211–214, 1991.
7. Griffiths, C.E., Barker, J.N., Kunkel, S., and Nickoloff, B.J., Modulation of leukocyte adhesion molecules, a T-cell chemotaxin (IL-8) and a regulatory cytokine (TNF-alpha) in allergic contact dermatitis (rhus dermatitis), *Br. J. Dermatol.,* 124, 519–526, 1991.
8. Norris, P., Poston, R.N., Thomas, D.S., Thornhill, M., Hawk, J., and Haskard, D.O., The expression of endothelial leukocyte adhesion molecule-1 (ELAM-1), intercellular adhesion molecule-1 (ICAM-1), and vascular cell adhesion molecule-1 (VCAM-1) in experimental cutaneous inflammation: a comparison of ultraviolet B erythema and delayed hypersensitivity, *J. Invest. Dermatol.*, 96, 763–770, 1991.
9. Grabbe, S, and Schwarz, T.. Immunoregulatory mechanisms involved in elicitation of allergic contact hypersensitivity, *Immunol. Today,* 19(1), 37–44, 1998.
10. Raulet, D.H., Roles of the NKG2D immunoreceptor and its ligands, *Nat. Rev. Immunol.*, 3(10), 781–790, 2003.
11. Kondo, S. and Sauder, D.N., Epidermal cytokines in allergic contact dermatitis, *J. Am. Acad. Dermatol.*, 33, 786–800, 1995.
12. Pinkus, H. and Mehregan, A.H., The primary histologic lesion of seborrheic dermatitis and psoriasis, *J. Invest. Dermatol.*, 46, 109–115, 1966.
13. Kock, A., Schwarz, T., Kirnbauer, R., Urbanski, A., Perry, P., Ansel, J.C., and Luger, T.A., Human keratinocytes are a source for tumor necrosis factor alpha: evidence for synthesis and release upon stimulation with endotoxin or ultraviolet light, *J. Exp. Med.,* 172, 1609–1614, 1990.
14. Creamer, D., Allen, M., Jaggar, R., Stevens, R., Bicknell, R., and Barker, J., Mediation of systemic vascular hyperpermeability in severe psoriasis by circulating vascular endothelial growth factor, *Arch. Dermatol.*, 138(6), 791–796, 2002.
15. Fenjves, E.S., Gordon, D.A., Pershing, L.K., Williams, D.L., and Taichman, L.B., Systemic distribution of apolipoprotein E secreted by grafts of epidermal keratinocytes: implications for epidermal function and gene therapy, *Proc. Natl. Acad. Sci. U.S.A.*, 86, 8803–8807, 1989.

16. Williams, I.R and Kupper, T.S., Epidermal expression of intercellular adhesion molecule 1 is not a primary inducer of cutaneous inflammation in transgenic mice, *Proc. Natl. Acad. Sci. U.S.A.*, 91, 9710–9714, 1994.
17. Cheng, J., Turksen, K., Yu, Q.C., Schreiber, H., Teng, M., and Fuchs, E., Cachexia and graft-vs.-host-disease-type skin changes in keratin promoter-driven TNF alpha transgenic mice, *Genes Dev.*, 6, 1444–1456, 1992.
18. Groves, R.W. and Williams, I.R., Overexpression of keratinocyte type1 IL-1 receptor in transgenic mice results in exaggerated IL-1 dependent cutaneous inflammation *in vivo*, *J. Invest. Dermatol.*, 105, 453, 1995 (abstr.).
19. Nakamura, K., Williams, I.R., and Kupper, T.S., Keratinocyte-derived monocyte chemoattractant protein 1 (MCP-1): analysis in a transgenic model demonstrates MCP-1 can recruit dendritic and Langerhans cells into skin, *J. Invest. Dermatol.*, 105, 635–643, 1995.
20. Barker, J.N., Jones, M.L., Swenson, C.L., Sarma, V., Mitra, R.S., Ward, P.A., Johnson, K.J., Fantone, J.C., Dixit, V.M., and Nickoloff, B.J., Monocyte chemotaxis and activating factor production by keratinocytes in response to IFN-gamma, *J. Immunol.*, 146, 1192–1197, 1991.
21. Carroll, J.M., Romero, M.R., and Watt, F.M., Suprabasal integrin expression in the epidermis of transgenic mice results in developmental defects and a phenotype resembling psoriasis, *Cell*, 83(6), 957–968, 1995.
22. Detmar, M., Brown, L.F., Schon, M.P., Elicker, B.M., Velasco, P., Richard, L., Fukumura, D., Monsky, W., Claffey, K.P., and Jain, R.K., Increased microvascular density and enhanced leukocyte rolling and adhesion in the skin of VEGF transgenic mice, *J. Invest. Dermatol.*, 111(1), 1–6, 1998.
23. Kupper, T.S., Immune and inflammatory processes in cutaneous tissues. Mechanisms and speculations [published erratum appears in *J. Clin. Invest.*, 87(2), 753, 1991] [review], *J. Clin. Invest.*, 86, 1783–1789, 1990.
24. Groves, R.W., Ross, E., Barker, J.N., Ross, J.S., Camp, R.D., and MacDonald, D.M., Effect of *in vivo* interleukin-1 on adhesion molecule expression in normal human skin, *J. Invest. Dermatol.*, 98, 384–387, 1992.
25. Groves, R.W., Allen, M.H., Ross, E.L., Barker, J.N., and MacDonald, D.M., Tumour necrosis factor alpha is pro-inflammatory in normal human skin and modulates cutaneous adhesion molecule expression, *Br. J. Dermatol.*, 132, 345–352, 1995.
26. Witmer-Pack, M.D., Olivier, W., Valinsky, J., Schuler, G., and Steinman, R.M., Granulocyte/macrophage colony-stimulating factor is essential for the viability and function of cultured murine epidermal Langerhans cells, *J. Exp. Med.*, 166, 1484–1498, 1987.
27. Schon, M.P., Zollner, T.M., and Boehncke, W.H., The molecular basis of lymphocyte recruitment to the skin: clues for pathogenesis and selective therapies of inflammatory disorders, *J. Invest. Dermatol.*, 121(5), 951–962, 2003.

# 20 Adhesion Molecules and Inflammatory Cell Migration Pathways in the Skin

*Kenneth B. Gordon and Brian J. Nickoloff*

## CONTENTS



## I. INTRODUCTION

The inhibition of inflammatory cell migration in and out of the skin has been recognized as a potentially vital aspect of the immune process in health and disease. The interactions between adhesion molecules on the cutaneous endothelium and keratinocytes with lymphocytes, macrophages, and neutrophils, along with other inflammatory cells of bone marrow origin have become an intriguing target for skin specific targeted immune-modulating therapy for inflammatory disease.

The classic teachings in inflammatory cell migration are based on the rolling, adhesion, and transmigration model.[1] This model predicted that inflammatory cells would migrate into tissues, including the skin, in a nonrandom fashion and would be directed by a specific series of cell–cell interactions between the inflammatory cells in the circulation and the endothelium. The model has been expanded to include migration of cells out of the skin, in a way different from normal recirculation pathways, based on the presence of inflammation in the local environment. What has become increasingly clear in the past few years is that these physical interactions are accompanied by complex signaling events that change the morphology and activity of adhesion molecules that lead to the movement of cells in and out of the circulatory compartment. In this chapter, we discuss the cell surface proteins involved in interactions between inflammatory cells and the endothelium that mediate the physical movement of cells and the interaction between the inflammatory cells and keratinocytes.

0-8493-1959-5/05/$0.00+$1.50

**TABLE 20.1**
**Inflammatory Cell Migration**

| Step in Leukocyte Migration | Lymphocyte Adhesion Molecule | Endothelial Adhesion Molecule |
|---|---|---|
| Rolling | CLA | E-Selectin |
| | PSGL-1 | P-Selectin |
| | sLex | P-Selectin |
| Adherence | LFA-1 | ICAM-1 |
| | LFA-1 | ICAM-2 |
| | VLA-4 | VCAM-1 |
| Transmigration | PECAM-1 | PECAM-1 |
| | ? | JAM |

## II. ADHESION MOLECULE–MEDIATED INFLAMMATORY CELL INTERACTIONS WITH ENDOTHELIUM AND MIGRATION INTO THE SKIN

Although blood-borne lymphocytes migrate in and out of tissues frequently and in great number, it has been recognized for many years that these cells preferentially enter tissues, including the skin, in sites of an active inflammatory process. This process is a stepwise series of events that depends on the physical interaction between adhesion molecules expressed on the surface of both inflammatory cells and endothelium.[1] Moreover, the specific adhesion molecules expressed may have a significant impact on the tissues to which the inflammatory cells migrate. The entire process of an inflammatory cell migrating to the tissue is broken down into three independent movements: rolling, adhesion, and transmigration (Table 20.1).

### A. Rolling

Much of the specificity of inflammatory cell migration into the skin is due to the interactions referred to as rolling.[2] Inflammatory cells in the circulation tend not to bind to resting endothelium due to the shear forces encountered in the bloodstream. To slow the cells for endothelial adherence in sites of inflammation, there are a series of quickly reversible binding interactions between the two cell types causing the circulating cells to alter their linear motion and slow. This movement pattern is called rolling. In many tissues, inflammatory cell migration is not particularly dependent on adhesion molecule–mediated rolling. However, in the skin and the gut, there is a significant requirement for interactions between selectins, a group of carbohydrate-mediated adhesion proteins, and their ligands on inflammatory cells.

In the skin, the selectin expressed on the endothelium of greatest importance is E-selectin (ELAM-1) along with the less-skin-specific P-selectin.[3] These molecules are greatly upregulated in the cutaneous endothelium in areas of acute inflammation, with E-selectin expression more sensitive to an inflammatory environment.[4] In particular, expression of E-selectin is increased in response to exposure to the pro-inflammatory cytokines interferon-gamma (IFN-$\gamma$) and tumor necrosis factor-alpha (TNF-$\alpha$). These selectins may also play differing roles in the rolling process. P-selectin seems to mediate non-inflammation-related cell migration into the skin while E-selectin plays a more central role in inflammation-related migration. P-selectin plays a role in the number of rolling events in an endothelial bed, whereas E-selectin is more important for the amount of slowing of a blood-borne cell.[5,6] The importance of selectins on inflammatory cell migration varies in different vascular beds in animal models as skin is much more sensitive than muscle.[5,7] Moreover, type I helper T cells seem to be recruited into the skin more readily via E-selectin than type II cells.[8]

While the expression of specific selectins on the endothelial surface seems to afford some specificity to inflammatory cell migration, a great deal of research has focused on the expression of the ligands for E-selectin on T cells. Selectin ligands are carbohydrates that can be classified as L-selectin, which binds in the high endothelial venules and mediates migration to the lymph nodes and spleen, and those that bind the endothelial selectins, E-selectin and P-selectin. The most basic ligand is a sialomucin molecule called P-selectin glycoprotein ligand -1 (PSGL-1). PSGL-1 and other functional ligands for P-selectin including sialylated Lewis X ($sLe^x$) are expressed constitutively on neutrophils in the circulation.[9–11] However, naïve T cells express little to no endothelial selectin ligands and, thus, tend to migrate back to the primary lymph organs. In T cells that have undergone primary activation in the draining lymph nodes of the skin, however, there is expression of a modified PSGL-1 called cutaneous lymphocyte antigen (CLA).[12,13] CLA expression is under the control of an enzyme, $\alpha$(1,3)-glucosyltransferase VII (FucT-VII).[13–16] FucT-VII itself is regulated by IL-12 and TGF-$\beta$1 thereby accounting for the increased expression of CLA on T cells of the type I phenotype.[17]

CLA expression affords much of the specificity in migration in cutaneous immune responses involving T cells. While only about 10 to 25% of T cells in the peripheral blood and 5 to 10% in the tonsils or lymph nodes stain positively with HECA-452, a monoclonal antibody that recognizes CLA, 80 to 90% of T cells at sites of cutaneous inflammation stain positively with this antibody.[18,19] This effect seems to be directed by the local environment although the exact mechanism for inducing CLA on T cells is not fully established.[20,21] Thus, potential skin targeted therapy could be developed to block this skin-specific interaction for the treatment of cutaneous inflammatory disease.

### B. Chemokines and Integrin Triggering and Adhesion

After rolling has slowed inflammatory cells from their flow in the vasculature, the integrins that mediate adherence to the endothelium must be altered in their morphology. Like rolling, the mediators that influence this process, primarily chemokines, imbue some level of skin specificity. The integrins on T cells that interact primarily in the adhesive step are lymphocyte function associated antigen-1 (LFA-1) ($\alpha1\beta2$) and VLA-4 ($\alpha4\beta1$).[1,22] These bind to ligands on the endothelium of the immunoglobulin superfamily, ICAM-1,2 and VCAM-1, respectively. All of these adhesion molecules are upregulated by an inflammatory environment.[23–27] In the resting state, these integrins have a low affinity for their ligands and must undergo a morphological change prior to adherence to the endothelium. This triggering of the integrins on the T-cell surface is mediated by a superfamily of small-molecular-weight proteins called chemokines.

Chemokines are bound to the endothelium and interact with both specific and nonspecific receptors on inflammatory cells. These interactions lead to definitive but transitory changes in integrin molecules that greatly increase the affinity and avidity of integrins for their ligands and, thus, allow for the adhesions step. These morphologic changes are related to multiple intracellular signaling steps through protein kinase C and intracellular calcium, depending upon the intergrin.[28,29] In the skin, $CLA^+$ cells tend to migrate and adhere in the presence of the chemokines called CCL17(TARC) and CCL27(CTACK).[30] CCL17 binds to the chemokine receptor CCR4 and is expressed at high levels in active immune responses[31] primarily atopic dermatitis.[32] CCL27, a molecule that binds the chemokine receptor CCR10, is secreted constitutively by keratinocytes but is also increased by pro-inflammatory cytokines.[33] Moreover, this chemokine seems to be expressed selectively in the skin.[34] In mice, either of these chemokines is sufficient for triggering integrins and the blockade of lymphocyte recruitment while the blockade of both molecules is needed to inhibit migration.

### C. Transendothelial Migration

The movement of inflammatory cells through the wall of the blood vessel into the skin is termed transendothelial migration (TEM). The interactions that govern this process are less well understood than those of the preceding steps and do not seem to confer the same level of tissue specificity as rolling and adhesion. In order for the blood-borne cells to migrate into the tissue, they must squeeze between endothelial cells held together with multiple junctions. These junctions include tight junctions, cadherin molecules, and multiple other connections on the lateral walls of endothelial cells. These junctions must separate and then reform to allow for the migration of inflammatory cells but do not show any signs of damage. Electron microscopic evaluation of this process demonstrates T-cell pseudopods pushing through the junctions.[35] Specific adhesion molecules that localize to the lateral aspects of endothelial cells seem to play a crucial role in this process. These adhesion molecules, platelet/endothelial cell adhesion molecule-1 (PECAM-1) and junctional adhesion molecule (JAM), are components of junctions between endothelial cells. PECAM-1 is a member of the immunoglobulin superfamily that has as its primary ligand PECAM-1 on the surface of another cell.[36,37] It is expressed on endothelium as well as platelets and most leukocytes.[38,39] It is not clear if homotypic interactions act as a physical guide for transmigration or signaling events through β-catenin help to initiate the migration of cells through the endothelium.[40,41] Similarly, while antibodies to JAM seem to block monocyte migration into tissue, the mechanism of this interaction remains unknown.[42]

## III. ADHESION MOLECULES, INFLAMMATORY CELL MIGRATION WITHIN THE SKIN AND INTERACTIONS WITH KERATINOCYTES

One of the key insights in the structure of the cutaneous immune system was the recognition that keratinocytes play an active role in many of the responses seen in the skin. Among the central findings was that keratinocytes express adhesion molecules that mediate adherence as well as movement of inflammatory cells within the skin. This binding step was first recognized when it became clear that, in the setting of pro-inflammatory cytokines, lymphocytes would adhere to keratinocytes. With further study, multiple potential interactions have become clear. In this section we discuss the interactions between keratinocytes and immune cells of bone marrow origin with particular emphasis on the role adhesion molecules play during an inflammatory reaction.

### A. Inflammatory Cell Migration in and out of the Epidermis

The best-studied adhesion molecule–mediated interaction between keratinocytes and lymphocytes is that between LFA-1 on lymphocytes and ICAM-1 on T cells. IFN-γ has generally been considered the primary regulatory cytokine for ICAM-1 expression on keratinocytes;[43,44] however, multiple stimuli have been demonstrated to increase the production of this adhesion molecule.[45] Among the identified stimuli are external factors including perturbation of the barrier function of the skin, bacterial superantigens, irritants, and ultraviolet light.[46] Other cytokines including TNF-α may also upregulate ICAM-1 on keratinocytes. This upregulation of ICAM will often precede pathologic T-cell infiltration.[47] Differentiation of keratinocytes will inversely correlate with the ability of these cells to express ICAM-1, accounting for the greater accumulation of T cells in the lower layers of the epidermis.[48,49]

The role of the ICAM-1/LFA-1 interaction in maintaining cell–cell interactions between keratinocytes and lymphocytes is well studied. In a similar fashion to the adherence phase in lymphocyte binding to the endothelium, the ICAM/LFA binding can mediate a keratinocyte/lymphocyte adherence that functionally fixes the T cell to the epidermis for a time.[50] Epidermal T cells are of central importance in many inflammatory diseases of the skin including psoriasis, lichen planus, and cutaneous T-cell lymphoma. In the presence of inflammatory cytokines or an infectious process, a chemokine gradient will attract lymphocytes to the epidermis.[51] However, it is likely that the ICAM/LFA interaction is central to maintaining cells in this compartment.[52] Other integrins on lymphocytes like αEβ7 that can bind to keratinocyte E-cadherin[53] may also play a role in this compartmentalization.[54,55] Some observers believe that the maintenance of T cells in the epidermis is of critical importance and the blockade of this interaction could be a central mechanism of action of drugs that block LFA-1.

Similar compartment-specific responses are seen with other adhesion reactions between keratinocytes and inflammatory cells. Perhaps the best studied of these interactions involves the migration of Langerhans cells out of the epidermis during an active challenge with antigen. One of the primary adhesion molecules in junctions between keratinocytes is E-cadherin.[56] This molecule binds homotypically and is also important for the binding of melanocytes to the epidermis. Langerhans cells also express E-cadherin when they are in their resting state,[57] which mediates attachment to keratinocytes.[58] However, a number of inflammatory mediators, including interleukin (IL)-1β and TNF-α, can downregulate the expression of E-cadherin on Langerhans cells.[58] This allows these dendritic cells to lose their tight binding to the epidermis and migrate to local lymph nodes. This migration is central to their ability to activate naive T cells with the lymph nodes to perpetuate the immune response against a novel antigen or an invading organism.

## B. Adhesion Molecule–Mediated Signaling Reactions

While the binding of inflammatory cells to keratinocytes is likely of great importance in the immune processes of the skin, it has been increasingly clear over the past few years that these adhesion molecule–mediated reactions are not simply passive interactions juxtaposing cells together. Important signaling events take place in the course of these interactions that can lead to physical and chemical changes within the epidermal and the inflammatory cells, which may have significant impact on immune reactions. These signals can be in the form of directed interactions between keratinocytes and lymphocytes as well as keratinocytes acting as an accessory to ongoing immune interactions.

The ICAM-LFA interaction has clearly been demonstrated to have two-way signaling. That is, when this ligation takes place, there are signaling events in both the T cell and the keratinocyte that influence the behavior of both involved cells. Ligation of LFA-1 on the surface of T cells has a profound influence on the behavior pattern of the cell beyond simple adhesion. This interaction can alter cellular functions including the induction of apoptosis, cell proliferation, and the production of effector cytokines along with potentially increasing the activation state during the presentation of antigen.[59,60] Additionally, this interaction may have a significant impact upon keratinocytes. Physical adherence between keratinocytes and T cells through ICAM-LFA binding was necessary for continued upregulation of ICAM-1 on keratinocytes as well as the production of cytokines, especially TNF-α.[60] Thus, not only does ICAM-LFA binding hold keratinocytes and lymphocytes together and influence cell migration in the epidermis, but it also seems to profoundly upregulate the potential for the production of pro-inflammatory mediators, creating an ever-increasing cytokine cascade with T-cell migration into the epidermal compartment.

The final potential role of adhesion molecules in the epidermis is as a potential accessory to the relationship between T cells and professional antigen presenting cells in the skin. Keratinocytes express multiple adhesion molecules along with ICAM-1, which are part of the immunological synapse. Among these are LFA-3 and CD40, ligands for CD2 and CD40 ligand on T cells, respectively.[61,62] While the potential role of keratinocytes acting as antigen presenting cells directly remains controversial, blockade of these interactions in the epidermis has been demonstrated to inhibit many of the normal immune responses in the skin.[63,64] Among these responses is contact sensitivity and immune responses to tumors. It has been theorized that keratinocytes may provide accessory second signaling to T cells through these interactions. In other words, as keratinocytes are adjacent to T cells undergoing immune stimulation with professional antigen presenting cells, keratinocytes may be providing signals through cells surface ligation that increase the activation state of the immune cells.[65–67] Interestingly, activation of CD40 with an agonistic monoclonal antibody can initiate Langerhans cell migration out of the skin.[68] While this relationship is far from definitively demonstrated, the potential for keratinocytes delivering co-stimulatory signals may play a vital role in determining the efficacy of targeted medications directed against the immunological synapse.

## IV. SUMMARY

In the past decade, the role of adhesion molecules in the skin has been clarified at the same time that new adhesion molecule–mediated interactions have been proposed and new questions asked. The vital role of adhesion relationships between endothelial cells and migrating inflammatory cells in the regulation of immune responses has been well defined. What is still being evaluated, however, is how these interactions are regulated on a molecular level. Additionally, the expression of adhesion molecules in the epidermis has opened new avenues of research to evaluate the potential influence these surface proteins may have, not only on cell migration in and out of the epidermis, but also on the activity of the immune response itself.

Of greatest importance, it is central to identify how each of these functions of adhesion molecules in the skin influences the specific immune responses to tumors, invasive organisms, and in immune-mediated diseases, as well as the molecular regulation of these interactions and their signals. This understanding may lead to specific therapeutic approaches to target these interactions and provide new directions in the treatment of immunity of the skin in disease and health. For example, if it were possible to upregulate adhesion molecules in the vascular beds surrounding a skin cancer, a more effective tumor-specific immune response could be developed. Moreover, downward regulation of T-cell migration into lesions of psoriasis, atopic dermatitis, or lichen planus, could lead to effective therapy with a minimum of side effects for the systemic immune response. Thus, the issues discussed in this chapter may hold many of the keys for future therapeutic modalities in treating many diseases of the skin.

## REFERENCES


1. Springer, T.A., Traffic signals for lymphocyte recirculation and leukocyte emigration: the multistep paradigm. *Cell* 76, 301–314, 1994.
2. Lawrence, M.B. and Springer, T.A., Leukocytes roll on a selectin at physiologic flow rates: distinction from and prerequisite for adhesion through integrins. *Cell* 65, 859–873, 1991.
3. Yan, H.C. et al., Leukocyte recruitment into human skin transplanted onto severe combined immunodeficient mice induced by TNF-alpha is dependent on E-selectin. *J. Immunol.* 152, 3053–3063, 1994.
4. Picker, L.J., Kishimoto, T.K., Smith, C.W., Warnock, R.A., and Butcher, E.C., ELAM-1 is an adhesion molecule for skin-homing T cells. *Nature* 349, 796–799, 1991.
5. Hickey, M.J. et al., Varying roles of E-selectin and P-selectin in different microvascular beds in response to antigen. *J. Immunol.* 162, 1137–1143, 1999.
6. Weninger, W. et al., Specialized contributions by alpha(1,3)-fucosyltransferase-IV and FucT-VII during leukocyte rolling in dermal microvessels. *Immunity.* 12, 665–676, 2000.
7. Erdmann, I. et al., Fucosyltransferase VII-deficient mice with defective E-, P-, and L-selectin ligands show impaired $CD4^+$ and $CD8^+$ T cell migration into the skin, but normal extravasation into visceral organs. *J. Immunol.* 168, 2139–2146, 2002.
8. Austrup, F. et al., P- and E-selectin mediate recruitment of T-helper-1 but not T-helper-2 cells into inflamed tissues. *Nature* 385, 81–83, 1997.
9. Phillips, M.L. et al., ELAM-1 mediates cell adhesion by recognition of a carbohydrate ligand, sialyl-Lex. *Science* 250(1), 1130–1132, 1990.
10. Walz, G., Aruffo, A., Kolanus, W., Bevilacqua, M., and Seed, B., Recognition by ELAM-1 of the sialyl-Lex determinant on myeloid and tumor cells. *Science* 250(1), 1132–1135, 1990.

11. Berg, E.L., Magnani, J., Warnock, R.A., Robinson, M.K., and Butcher, E.C., Comparison of L-selectin and E-selectin ligand specificities: the L-selectin can bind the E-selectin ligands sialyl Le(x) and sialyl Le(a. *Biochem. Biophys. Res. Commun.* 184, 1048–1055, 1992.
12. Armerding, D. and Kupper, T.S., Functional cutaneous lymphocyte antigen can be induced in essentially all peripheral blood T lymphocytes. *Int. Arch. Allergy Immunol.* 22, 119, 212–222, 1999.
13. Fuhlbrigge, R.C., Kieffer, J.D., Armerding, D., and Kupper, T.S., Cutaneous lymphocyte antigen is a specialized form of PSGL-1 expressed on skin-homing T cells. *Nature* 389, 978–981, 1997.
14. Homeister, J.W. et al., The alpha(1,3)fucosyltransferases FucT-IV and FucT-VII exert collaborative control over selectin-dependent leukocyte recruitment and lymphocyte homing. *Immunity.* 15(2), 115–126, 2001.
15. Knibbs, R.N. et al., The fucosyltransferase FucT-VII regulates E-selectin ligand synthesis in human T cells. *J. Cell Biol.* 133, 911–920, 1996.
16. Maly, P. et al., The alpha(1,3)fucosyltransferase Fuc-TVII controls leukocyte trafficking through an essential role in L-, E-, and P-selectin ligand biosynthesis. *Cell* 86, 643–653, 1996.
17. Wagers, A.J. and Kansas, G.S., Potent induction of alpha(1,3)-fucosyltransferase VII in activated CD4+ T cells by TGF-beta 1 through a p38 mitogen-activated protein kinase-dependent pathway. *J. Immunol.* 165, 5011–5016, 2000.
18. Berg, E.L. et al., The cutaneous lymphocyte antigen is a skin lymphocyte homing receptor for the vascular lectin endothelial cell-leukocyte adhesion molecule 1. *J. Exp. Med.* 174, 1461–1466, 1991.
19. Picker, L.J., Kishimoto, T.K., Smith, C.W., Warnock, R.A., and Butcher, E.C., ELAM-1 is an adhesion molecule for skin-homing T cells. *Nature* 349, 796–799, 1991.
20. Chu, A., Hong, K., Berg, E.L., and Ehrhardt, R.O., Tissue specificity of E- and P-selectin ligands in Th1-mediated chronic inflammation. *J. Immunol.* 163, 5086–5093, 1999.
21. Kulidjian, A.A., Issekutz, A.C., and Issekutz, T.B., Differential role of E-selectin and P-selectin in T lymphocyte migration to cutaneous inflammatory reactions induced by cytokines. *Int. Immunol.* 14, 751–760, 2002.
22. Santamaria Babi, L.F. et al., Migration of skin-homing T cells across cytokine-activated human endothelial cell layers involves interaction of the cutaneous lymphocyte-associated antigen, CLA), the very late antigen-4, VLA-4), and the lymphocyte function-associated antigen-1, LFA-1. *J. Immunol.* 154, 1543–1550, 1995.
23. Briscoe, D.M., Cotran, R.S., and Pober, J.S., Effects of tumor necrosis factor, lipopolysaccharide, and IL-4 on the expression of vascular cell adhesion molecule-1 *in vivo*. Correlation with CD3+ T cell infiltration. *J. Immunol.* 149, 2954–2960, 1992.
24. Groves, R.W., Ross, E.L., Barker, J.N., and MacDonald, D.M., Vascular cell adhesion molecule-1: expression in normal and diseased skin and regulation *in vivo* by interferon gamma. *J. Am. Acad. Dermatol.* 29, 67–72, 1993.
25. Heckmann, M., Eberlein-Konig, B., Wollenberg, A., Przybilla, B., and Plewig, G., Ultraviolet-A radiation induces adhesion molecule expression on human dermal microvascular endothelial cells. *Br. J. Dermatol.* 131, 311–318, 1994.
26. Gille, J., Swerlick, R.A., Lawley, T.J., and Caughman, S.W., Differential regulation of vascular cell adhesion molecule-1 gene transcription by tumor necrosis factor alpha and interleukin-1 alpha in dermal microvascular endothelial cells. *Blood* 87, 211–217, 1996.
27. Haraldsen, G., Kvale, D., Lien, B., Farstad, I.N., and Brandtzaeg, P., Cytokine-regulated expression of E-selectin, intercellular adhesion molecule-1, ICAM-1), and vascular cell adhesion molecule-1, VCAM-1) in human microvascular endothelial cells. *J. Immunol.* 156, 2558–2565, 1996.
28. Lub, M., van Kooyk, Y., van Vliet, S.J., and Figdor, C.G., Dual role of the actin cytoskeleton in regulating cell adhesion mediated by the integrin lymphocyte function-associated molecule-1. *Mol. Biol. Cell* 8, 341–351, 1997.
29. Stewart, M.P., McDowall, A., and Hogg, N., LFA-1-mediated adhesion is regulated by cytoskeletal restraint and by a $Ca^{2+}$-dependent protease, calpain. *J. Cell Biol.* 140, 699–707, 1998.
30. Reiss, Y., Proudfoot, A.E., Power, C.A., Campbell, J.J., and Butcher, E.C., CC chemokine receptor, CCR)4 and the CCR10 ligand cutaneous T cell-attracting chemokine, CTACK) in lymphocyte trafficking to inflamed skin. *J. Exp. Med.* 194, 1541–1547, 2001.

31. Kakinuma, T. et al., IL-4, but not IL-13, modulates TARC, thymus and activation-regulated chemokine)/CCL17 and IP-10, interferon-induced protein of 10kDA)/CXCL10 release by TNF-alpha and IFN-gamma in HaCaT cell line. *Cytokine* 20, 1–6, 2002.
32. Zheng, X. et al., TGF-beta1-mediated regulation of thymus and activation-regulated chemokine, TARC/CCL17) synthesis and secretion by HaCaT cells co-stimulated with TNF-alpha and IFN-gamma. *J. Dermatol. Sci.* 30, 154–160, 2002.
33. Homey, B. et al., CCL27-CCR10 interactions regulate T cell-mediated skin inflammation. *Nat. Med.* 8, 157–165, 2002.
34. Morales, J. et al., CTACK, a skin-associated chemokine that preferentially attracts skin-homing memory T cells. *Proc. Natl. Acad. Sci. U. S. A.* 96, 14470–14475, 1999.
35. Luscinskas, F.W., Ma, S., Nusrat, A., Parkos, C.A., and Shaw, S.K., Leukocyte transendothelial migration: a junctional affair. *Semin. Immunol.* 14, 105–113, 2002.
36. Sun, Q.H. et al., Individually distinct Ig homology domains in PECAM-1 regulate homophilic binding and modulate receptor affinity. *J. Biol. Chem.* 271, 11090–11098, 1996.
37. Newton, J.P., Buckley, C.D., Jones, E.Y., and Simmons, D.L., Residues on both faces of the first immunoglobulin fold contribute to homophilic binding sites of PECAM-1/CD31. *J. Biol. Chem.* 272, 20555–20563, 1997.
38. Delisser, H.M., Newman, P.J., and Albelda, S.M., Molecular and functional aspects of PECAM-1/CD31. *Immunol. Today* 15, 490–495, 1994.
39. Watt, S.M., Gschmeissner, S.E., and Bates, P.A., PECAM-1: its expression and function as a cell adhesion molecule on hemopoietic and endothelial cells. *Leukocyte Lymphoma* 17, 229–244, 1995.
40. Matsumura, T., Wolff, K., and Petzelbauer, P., Endothelial cell tube formation depends on cadherin 5 and CD31 interactions with filamentous actin. *J. Immunol.* 158, 3408–3416, 1997.
41. Ilan, N., Mahooti, S., Rimm, D.L., and Madri, J.A., PECAM-1, CD31) functions as a reservoir for and a modulator of tyrosine-phosphorylated beta-catenin. *J. Cell Sci.* 112(18), 3005–3014, 1999.
42. Johnson-Leger, C., Aurrand-Lions, M., and Imhof, B.A. The parting of the endothelium: miracle, or simply a junctional affair? *J. Cell Sci.* 113(6), 921–933, 2000.
43. Griffiths, C.E., Voorhees, J.J., and Nickoloff, B.J., Characterization of intercellular adhesion molecule-1 and HLA-DR expression in normal and inflamed skin: modulation by recombinant gamma interferon and tumor necrosis factor. *J. Am. Acad. Dermatol.* 20, 617–629, 1989.
44. Nickoloff, B.J., and Griffiths, C.E., T lymphocytes and monocytes bind to keratinocytes in frozen sections of biopsy specimens of normal skin treated with gamma interferon. *J. Am. Acad. Dermatol.* 20, 736–743, 1989.
45. Griffiths, C.E., Esmann, J., Fisher, G.J., Voorhees, J.J., and Nickoloff, B.J., Differential modulation of keratinocyte intercellular adhesion molecule-I expression by gamma interferon and phorbol ester: evidence for involvement of protein kinase C signal transduction. *Br. J. Dermatol.* 122, 333–342, 1990.
46. Treina, G. et al., Expression of intercellular adhesion molecule-1 in UVA-irradiated human skin cells *in vitro* and *in vivo*. *Br. J. Dermatol.* 135, 241–247, 1996.
47. Griffiths, C.E. and Nickoloff, B.J., Keratinocyte intercellular adhesion molecule-1, ICAM-1) expression precedes dermal T lymphocytic infiltration in allergic contact dermatitis, Rhus dermatitis. *Am. J. Pathol.* 135, 1045–1053, 1989.
48. Kashihara-Sawami, M. and Norris, D.A., The state of differentiation of cultured human keratinocytes determines the level of intercellular adhesion molecule-1, ICAM-1) expression induced by gamma interferon. *J. Invest Dermatol.* 98, 741–747, 1992.
49. Little, M.C., Gawkrodger, D.J., and Mac, N.S., Differentiation of human keratinocytes is associated with a progressive loss of interferon gamma-induced intercellular adhesion molecule-1 expression. *Br. J. Dermatol.* 135, 24–31, 1996.
50. Dustin, M.L., Singer, K.H., Tuck, D.T., and Springer, T.A. Adhesion of T lymphoblasts to epidermal keratinocytes is regulated by interferon gamma and is mediated by intercellular adhesion molecule 1, ICAM-1. *J. Exp. Med.* 167, 1323–1340, 1988.
51. Barker, J.N. et al., Modulation of keratinocyte-derived interleukin-8 which is chemotactic for neutrophils and T lymphocytes. *Am. J. Pathol.* 139, 869–876, 1991.
52. Shiohara, T. et al., Evidence for involvement of lymphocyte function-associated antigen 1 in T cell migration to epidermis. *J. Immunol.* 146, 840–845, 1991.

53. Higgins, J.M. et al., Direct and regulated interaction of integrin alphaEbeta7 with E-cadherin. *J. Cell Biol.* 140, 197–210, 1998.
54. Dietz, S.B., Whitaker-Menezes, D., and Lessin, S.R., The role of alpha E beta 7 integrin, CD103) and E-cadherin in epidermotropism in cutaneous T-cell lymphoma. *J. Cutaneous Pathol.* 23, 312–318, 1996.
55. Pauls, K. et al., Role of integrin alphaE(CD103)beta7 for tissue-specific epidermal localization of CD8+ T lymphocytes. *J. Invest Dermatol.* 117, 569–575, 2001.
56. Jakob, T., Brown, M.J., and Udey, M.C., Characterization of E-cadherin-containing junctions involving skin-derived dendritic cells. *J. Invest Dermatol.* 112, 102–108, 1999.
57. Blauvelt, A., Katz, S.I., and Udey, M.C., Human Langerhans cells express E-cadherin. *J. Invest Dermatol.* 104, 293–296, 1995.
58. Tang, A., Amagai, M., Granger, L.G., Stanley, J.R., and Udey, M.C., Adhesion of epidermal Langerhans cells to keratinocytes mediated by E-cadherin. *Nature* 361, 82–85, 1993.
59. Nickoloff, B.J. et al., Accessory cell function of keratinocytes for superantigens. Dependence on lymphocyte function-associated antigen-1/intercellular adhesion molecule-1 interaction. *J. Immunol.* 150, 2148–2159, 1993.
60. Symington, F.W. and Santos, E.B., Lysis of human keratinocytes by allogeneic HLA class I-specific cytotoxic T cells. Keratinocyte ICAM-1, CD54) and T cell LFA-1, CD11a/CD18) mediate enhanced lysis of IFN-gamma-treated keratinocytes. *J. Immunol.* 146, 2169–2175, 1991.
61. Naderi, S. et al., CD2-mediated CD59 stimulation in keratinocytes results in secretion of IL-1alpha, IL-6, and GM-CSF: implications for the interaction of keratinocytes with intraepidermal T lymphocytes. *Int. J. Mol. Med.* 3, 609–614, 1999.
62. Pasch, M.C., Bos, J.D., Daha, M.R., and Asghar, S.S., Transforming growth factor-beta isoforms regulate the surface expression of membrane cofactor protein, CD46) and CD59 on human keratinocytes [corrected]. *Eur. J. Immunol.* 29, 100–108, 1999.
63. Companjen, A.R., van der Wel, L.I., Boon, L., Prens, E.P., and Laman, J.D., CD40 ligation-induced cytokine production in human skin explants is partly mediated via IL-1. *Int. Immunol.* 14, 669–676, 2002.
64. Denfeld, R.W. et al., CD40 is functionally expressed on human keratinocytes. *Eur. J. Immunol.* 26, 2329–2334, 1996.
65. Fuller, B.W., Nishimura, T., and Noelle, R.J., The selective triggering of CD40 on keratinocytes *in vivo* enhances cell-mediated immunity. *Eur. J. Immunol.* 32, 895–902, 2002.
66. Gaspari, A.A., Sempowski, G.D., Chess, P., Gish, J., and Phipps, R.P., Human epidermal keratinocytes are induced to secrete interleukin-6 and co-stimulate T lymphocyte proliferation by a CD40-dependent mechanism. *Eur. J. Immunol.* 26, 1371–1377, 1996.
67. Grousson, J., Concha, M., Schmitt, D., and Peguet-Navarro, J., Effects of CD40 ligation on human keratinocyte accessory function. *Arch. Dermatol. Res.* 290, 325–330, 1998.
68. Jolles, S., Christensen, J., Holman, M., Klaus, G.B., and Ager, A., Systemic treatment with anti-CD40 antibody stimulates Langerhans cell migration from the skin. *Clin. Exp. Immunol.* 129, 519–526, 2002.

# 21 Physiology and Pathology of Skin Photoimmunology

*Sreedevi Kodali, Stephan Beissert, and Richard D. Granstein*

## CONTENTS



## I. INTRODUCTION

Ultraviolet radiation (UVR) is part of the nonvisible component of the electromagnetic spectrum of sunlight ranging from 200 to 400 nm. It is typically divided into the following three subtypes based on wavelength: UVA (320 to 400 nm), UVB (280 to 320 nm), and UVC (200 to 280). UVR wavelength is directly related to its skin-penetrating ability, but inversely related to energy. For example, UVC radiation has the shortest wavelength, but also carries the most energy and has the most potential for damaging effects.[1] However, most UVC radiation is absorbed by the atmosphere and is not responsible for the deleterious effects of UVR.[2] UVB radiation, which falls in the middle in terms of wavelength and energy, is largely filtered by the ozone layer, but unlike UVC radiation, a substantial portion still reaches the Earth's surface. UVB radiation, although mainly absorbed in the epidermis, has been primarily implicated in the carcinogenic and immunosuppressive properties of UVR. UVB radiation is also largely responsible for UVR-induced erythema and melanogenesis.[3] UVA radiation carries the least energy, but due to its long wavelength penetrates the skin the deepest with as much as 50% reaching the dermis. It is also the most abundant on the Earth's surface, accounting for 95% of UVR that reaches the surface; only 5% is UVB radiation. Due to its low

0-8493-1959-5/05/$0.00+$1.50

energy, it is about 1000 times less biologically active than UVB radiation. However, recent studies have shown that it is a significant contributor to UVR-induced immunosuppression and that it plays a major role in photoaging.[3–5]

The most deleterious effects of UVR are its well-known carcinogenic and immunosuppressive properties, which appear to be linked. Photocarcinogenesis appears to arise from accumulated cellular DNA damage as well as a failure of the immune system to recognize those damaged cells as foreign and eradicate them. Understanding the mechanisms by which UVR exerts its immunosuppressive effects may lead to the development of new methods for combating cutaneous malignancies.[6]

This chapter focuses on the mechanisms of UVR-induced local and systemic immunosuppression and its relation to UVR-induced skin disease and the development of chemopreventative agents.

## II. IMMUNOLOGIC ASPECTS OF PHOTOCARCINOGENESIS

The relationship between UVR and cutaneous malignancy is well established. In humans, there is a direct link between sun exposure and development of sqamous cell carcinoma (SCC), basal cell carcinoma (BCC), and malignant melanoma.[7] In the United States, there is an increased incidence of all three types of cancers with increasing ambient UVR exposure.[8] This evidence is further supported by studies in mice, which have also been shown to develop cutaneous malignancies after long-term UVR exposure.[9, 10]

Part of the carcinogenic potential of UVR is related to its ability to induce DNA mutations. UVC (not relevant at the terrestrial surface), UVB, and UVA radiation, to a lesser extent, induce many types of DNA damage, the most common of which are cyclobutane pyrimidine dimers between neighboring pyrimidine bases and 6-4 photoproduct formation at dipyrimidine sites. This damage is enzymatically excised and replaced by unscheduled DNA synthesis. In most cases the damage is repaired and there are no overt consequences; however, a lifetime of sun exposure can lead to the gradual accumulation of errors in this repair mechanism. These errors can give rise to mutations in tumor suppressor genes leading to unregulated cell proliferation.[11]

Mutations in the tumor suppressor gene *p53* are the most strongly implicated in UV-induced carcinogenesis. Following UVR exposure, there is elevated nuclear *p53* expression, which induces cell cycle arrest and DNA repair or apoptosis. However, mutations in this gene can lead to unregulated cell growth and eventually carcinoma. *p53* mutations have been found in human BCC and SCC and experimentally induced murine carcinomas.[11,12] Since the discovery of *p53*, mutations in other genes have also been implicated in skin cancer. There is a correlation between the tumor suppressor gene *ptc* and BCC, but not the other skin cancers.[6] The *ptc* gene encodes a protein that is part of the sonic hedgehog (*SHH*) signaling pathway and plays an important role in embryonic development.[11] In patients with basal cell nevus syndrome, which is characterized by developmental abnormalities and numerous cutaneous BCC, the genetic defect was localized to chromosome 9 in the human homologue of the *Drosophila ptc* gene.[13] Mutations in *ptc* play an important role in nonfamilial BCC as well. One study looking at sporadic BCC demonstrated that there was a mutation in *ptc* in over one third of the cases.[14] BCC from patients with xerodermal pigmentosum (XP), who have an inherited defect in a DNA repair enzyme, had increased levels of *ptc* mutations.[15] Furthermore, heterozygous *ptc* knockout mice had enhanced BCC formation upon UVR exposure.[16] It is believed that *SHH* binds to *ptc* and inhibits its normal activity similar to mutations in the *ptc* gene. Thus, transgenic mice overexpressing *SHH* in the skin demonstrated many characteristics of basal cell nevus syndrome including cutaneous BCC.[17] In contrast to SCC and BCC, different genes have been linked to melanoma induction. Some familial cutaneous melanomas and melanoma cell lines were shown to have potentially UVR-induced mutations in the *Cdkn2a* locus on chromosome 9, which encodes two proteins *Ink4a* and *Arf*. *Ink4a* is a cyclin-dependent kinase inhibitor (CDK); thus, its loss may lead to unregulated cell growth. *Arf* binds to the protein MDM2 and interferes with the degradation of p53, further protecting the cell from DNA damage and unregulated cell growth.[11] Thus, there is a great deal of evidence demonstrating that UVR-induced DNA damage can lead to the formation of skin cancers.

Several lines of evidence demonstrate that these UVR-induced tumors are highly antigenic and that UVR-induced immunosuppression is a major factor in the development of skin cancers. Landmark experiments done in the 1970s by Kripke et al. showed that when UV-induced tumors were transplanted to normal (non-UVR-exposed) syngeneic mice, these tumors disappeared.[18] However, when these tumors were placed on mice treated with subcarcinogenic levels of UVR, the tumors continued to grow.[18] Furthermore, it was shown that this characteristic was specific to UVR-induced tumors as UV-irradiated mice were able to reject transplantation of syngeneic non-UVR-induced tumors.[19]

In humans, immunosuppression also leads to a higher risk of nonmelanoma skin cancer. Organ transplant patients who are chronically immunosuppressed have higher rates of SCC and BCC as well as a poorer prognosis due to the more aggressive nature of their tumors. In some studies the incidence of developing skin cancers was as high as 66% in the 10 years following organ transplantation.[20]

Numerous studies in both mice and humans employing basic immunologic tests have shown that UVR suppresses the normal immune response and induces tolerance both locally and systemically. In the local murine model, low-dose UVR (~1 J/m$^2$ of UVB radiation) exposure suppresses the induction of contact hypersensitivity (CHS) to haptens painted on UVR-exposed skin. Furthermore, UVR induces hapten-specific tolerance, meaning that the animal cannot be resensitized to the same hapten at a later time. However, there is no immunosuppression or tolerance seen when the haptens are painted on unexposed skin. In the systemic model, when the animal is exposed to high-dose UVR (~2 kJ/m$^2$), immune reactions such as the induction of CHS or delayed-type hypersensitivity (DTH) are inhibited even at non-irradiated sites. For example, CHS induction is suppressed and hapten-specific tolerance results, even when the hapten is painted on unirradiated skin.[2]

There is considerable evidence that human immune reactions can also be suppressed locally and systemically by exposure to UVB radiation.[21] There is also evidence that individuals may be heterogeneous with respect to the development of CHS after application of a sensitizer to UVB-irradiated skin, with 40% of individuals exhibiting a decreased response to application of sensitizer to UVB-exposed skin. It was also found that in patients with a history of nonmelanoma skin cancer, 92% demonstrated inhibition of the induction of CHS. When these susceptible individuals were immunized a second time on unirradiated skin, 45% of those with a history of skin cancer remained unresponsive, demonstrating tolerance, while none of the individuals without a history of cancer showed tolerance.[22] This study suggests that susceptibility to UVB-induced tolerance may be a risk factor for development of skin cancer.

## III. MECHANISMS UNDERLYING UVR-INDUCED IMMUNOSUPPRESSION AND TOLERANCE

### A. Chromophores in the Skin

#### 1. UVR-Mediated DNA Damage and Its Relationship to Immunosuppression

It has been hypothesized that UVR-induced DNA damage and UVR-induced immunosuppression facilitate one another in the development of skin cancers. This hypothesis ultimately raises the question of which event happens first and how the two events are interrelated. Studies by several groups in both mice and humans have demonstrated that DNA damage causes immunosuppression and is the likely initiating event in UVR-induced immunosuppression.

Some of the first conclusive studies made use of the marsupial *Monodelphis domestica,* which has an endogenous enzyme activated by visible light that repairs UVR-induced pyrimidine dimers ("photoreactivating enzyme"). In these animals, UVB radiation suppressed the induction of CHS both locally and systemically. Treatment with visible light following UVB radiation exposure abrogated the inhibition of CHS by activating the endogenous DNA repair enzyme, thus demonstrating that without DNA damage there was no ensuing immune impairment.[23] A similar experiment in mice employed the excision repair enzyme T4 endonuclease 5 (T4N5), which can be applied to the skin via liposomes and is taken up by epidermal cells. When liposomes containing this enzyme were applied to murine skin following UVB radiation exposure, the mice no longer showed the classic UVR-induced suppression of local CHS. Furthermore, application of this enzyme prevented the induction of T suppressor cells, one of the hallmarks of UVR-mediated immunosuppression and tolerance (see below).[24] Several studies demonstrated that DNA damage affects other mediators in UVR-induced immune suppression including cytokines. In murine skin *in vivo* and in murine keratinocytes, application of liposomes containing T4N5 blocked UVB radiation induced production of interleukin-10 (IL-10).[25] Furthermore, in human skin *in vivo* and in a human DNA repair-deficient cell line, treatment with T4N5 following UVB radiation prevented the upregulation of IL-10 and tumor necrosis factor-alpha (TNF-$\alpha$).[26,27]

To demonstrate that DNA damage alone without UVR exposure causes immunosuppression, one group applied the HindIII restriction endonuclease to murine epidermal cells *in vivo* and *in vitro*. As predicted, this impaired induction of CHS both locally and systemically. However, it did not replicate UVR-induced tolerance or transferable suppression. *In vitro,* HindIII-induced DNA damage induced IL-10 and TNF-$\alpha$, cytokines both implicated in UV-induced immunosuppression (see below).[28]

Because there are many cell types in the epidermis, applying repair enzymes to the skin does not provide clues regarding which, if any, cell type is being specifically affected. Attempts to localize the cellular level of this damage resulted in the conclusion that some of the DNA damage responsible for UVR-induced immunosuppression occurs at the level of the antigen-presenting cell (APC). APC from UVB-irradiated mice painted with the hapten FITC were isolated from draining lymph nodes. When these APCs were used to immunize non-irradiated mice, they failed to induce an immune reaction. However, if these APCs were treated *in vitro* with a photo-reactivating pyrimidine dimer repair enzyme, they were subsequently able to induce an immune reaction in naive mice.[29] This clearly demonstrated that DNA damage in APC affected their ability to effectively present antigen and induce an immune response. While likely that DNA damage at the level of the APC may play an important role in UVR-induced immunosuppression, it does not appear to account for some of the other aspects of UVR-induced immunosuppression such as cytokine production.

## 2. *cis*-Urocanic Acid

In addition to DNA, urocanic acid (UCA) is another chromophore within the epidermis that has been found to play a role in UVR-induced immune suppression. It has an absorption spectrum very similar to that of DNA. *trans*-UCA accumulates within the stratum corneum of the epidermis after deamination of histidine. Upon UVR exposure, it is converted to *cis*-UCA.[4] In the 1980s, it was first discovered that the action spectrum for UVR-induced suppression of CHS was maximal at 270 nm and that tape stripping the epidermis to remove the stratum corneum blocked UVR-induced immunosuppression. This led to the belief that UCA was the photoreceptor underlying this effect due to its superficial location and closely matched absorption spectrum.[30] Since this first discovery, numerous studies have demonstrated the critical role of *cis*-UCA.

A few hours following UVB radiation exposure of mice, *cis*-UCA was found in the serum and was detectable for about 2 days. Prolonged levels of serum *cis*-UCA could have implications for UVR-induced systemic immunosuppression.[31] Treatment of mice with *cis*-UCA inhibited both the induction of CHS and DTH and induced antigen-specific T-suppressor cells.[32–34] Exposure of Langerhans cells (LC) to *cis*-UCA inhibited their ability to present antigen both for induction and elicitation of DTH in mice. The same effect was not seen with *trans*-UCA.[35] Furthermore, application of topical *cis*-UCA enhanced tumor growth in UV-irradiated mice.[36]

The effects of *cis*-UCA may be a result of its modulation of the critical UVR-related cytokines TNF-α, IL-10, and IL-12. When *cis*-UCA was injected into mice, it inhibited the induction of CHS; however, injection of anti-TNF-α antibodies eliminated this effect.[37] *In vitro,* spleen cells incubated in *cis*-UCA had enhanced CD4+ T-cell IL-10 production, which could account for some of the systemic immunosuppressive effects of UVR.[38] Inhibition of LC antigen presentation was reversed with the addition of IL-12, implying that UCA downregulates IL-12 production.[39] These studies all demonstrate that administration of exogenous *cis*-UCA mimics the effects of UVR.

Somewhat different results were observed using anti-*cis*-UCA antibodies to block endogenous *cis*-UCA. Two groups had very similar results on the role of *cis*-UCA in UVR-mediated immunosuppression. The antibody administered prior to UVR exposure blocked the suppression of DTH, but had no effect on CHS, although in both cases suppressor T-cell formation was blocked. APC function was also restored with the antibody and UVR-induced decrease in LC density in the skin was also abrogated. However, the antibody had no effect on the dendritic cell increase in lymph nodes draining the site of irradiation.[40,41] In a study more relevant to photocarcinogenesis, mice chronically exposed to UVR had a decreased incidence of tumor formation when they were treated with anti-*cis*-UCA antibodies.[39]

Clearly, *cis*-UCA appears to account for part of the immunosuppressive and photocarcinogenic effects of UVR possibly through modulation of cytokine production and LC antigen presentation function, although it is unknown exactly how it mediates these effects.

### 3. UVR-Induced Oxidative Damage

In addition to UVRs, direct damage to DNA, and conversion of *trans*-UCA to *cis*-UCA, UVR induces the formation of reactive oxygen species and free radicals that interact with the cell membrane and cause lipid peroxidation.[4]

This membrane damage was shown to activate Src tyrosine kinases, which subsequently activate a cascade involving Ha-Ras, Raf-1, and JNK leading to the phosphorylation of c-jun and activation of the transcription factors AP-1 and NF-κB. Previously these transcription factors were thought to be activated as a result of DNA damage, but it has been shown that this same pattern of activation can be seen in enucleated cells. Elevation of intracellular glutathione (a free radical scavenger) inhibited this response, indicating that it may be initiated by oxidative stress.[42,43] A similar study showed an increase in NF-κB with increasing doses of UVB radiation. This NF-κB activation was also seen in cytosolic protein extracts treated with UVR, implying that the signal does not originate in the nucleus.[44] Another study demonstrated that UVR induced cell surface changes, such as clustering and internalization of receptors for epidermal growth factor (EGF), TNF, and IL-1, thereby altering normal cell signaling pathways.[45]

This pathway of activating transcription factors via free radical damage at the level of the cell membrane may cause activation of genes that mediate aspects of UVR-induced immunosuppression (Figure 21.1).

## B. The Role of Cytokines and Other Soluble Mediators

Exposure to UVR suppresses the induction of CHS when a hapten is applied at the same site of UVR exposure, but also at higher doses when the hapten is applied at a distant site. This implies that UVR exposure causes systemic release of factors that account for the immunosuppression seen at the non-irradiated site. Based on this hypothesis, it was discovered that UV-irradiated skin cells such as keratinocytes and mast cells release cytokines, which may account for some of UVR's immune effects.[2] The following studies demonstrate how cytokines modulate local and systemic

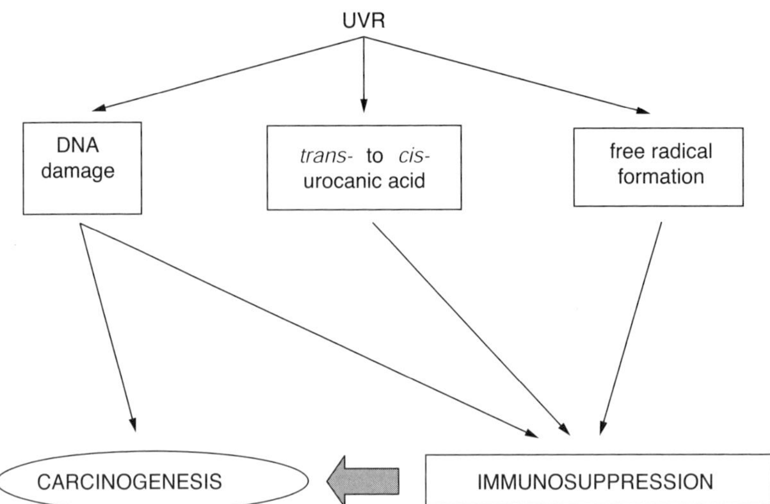


**FIGURE 21.1** Possible mechanisms of UVR-induced carcinogenesis.

immunosuppression and induction of tolerance. Although UVR induces release of many cytokines, IL-10, TNF-α, and IL-12 have assumed more central roles based on their effects.

TNF-α has been implicated in UVR-induced suppression of the induction of CHS, but not DTH or tolerance.[46,47] Injection of TNF-α either locally or systemically prior to application of DNFB inhibits the induction of CHS similar to UVR exposure. In addition, treatment of UV-irradiated mice with anti-TNF-α antibodies abrogates the immunosuppressive effects of UVR on induction of CHS.[47,48] This effect was later shown to be mediated via the TNF-receptor 2 (p75).[46] However, the effect of TNF-α is controversial as one group demonstrated that mice deficient in both TNF-receptor 1 and 2 (p55 and p75) were still susceptible to UVR-induced suppression of CHS in both the local and systemic models.[49]

IL-10 has been implicated in UVR-induced hapten-specific tolerance. Injection of IL-10 prior to sensitization with dinitrofluorobenzene (DNFB) did not affect the induction of CHS when the mice were challenged with DNFB 1 week later. However, when DNFB was reapplied to the same mice 2 weeks later, the mice displayed tolerance to DNFB challenge. Administration of anti-IL-10 antibody prevented UVR-induced tolerance, but had no effect on the UVR-mediated suppression of the induction of CHS.[50]

In multiple experimental models, IL-10 has also been found to play a role in the UVR-induced suppression of DTH. When supernatants from keratinocytes exposed to UVR were administered to mice, it mimicked the suppression of DTH seen with UVR exposure. Treating these supernatants with anti-IL-10 abrogated the suppressive nature of the supernatants. However, administering anti-IL-10 antibody *in vivo* to UV-irradiated mice only partially reversed the suppression of DTH, implying that other factors may also be involved.[51,52] The above studies were further confirmed in IL-10 knockout mice, which were found to be resistant to UVB-induced suppression of DTH. However, these mice were sensitive to UVB-mediated suppression of the induction of CHS. This further shows that the DTH and CHS responses are regulated by different pathways and that IL-10 is involved in DTH suppression, but not CHS suppression.[53]

It is well known that IL-10 suppresses Th1-type immune responses and favors activation of the Th2 subset. Thus, well-documented upregulation of IL-10 by UVR would seem to inhibit Th1 responses and favor Th2 responses. This is further strengthened by the UVR-induced increase in IL-4, which is well known to drive Th2 responses.[54] The role of IL-12 began to be studied as it is one of the crucial Th1 cytokines. It was hypothesized that its downregulation may be involved in UVR-induced immune suppression. Administration of IL-12 either before sensitization or before challenge abrogated the UVR-mediated suppression of local CHS.[55] IL-12 injection also abrogated UVR-induced hapten-specific tolerance. Moreover, IL-12 addition blocked the UVR-induced suppression of DTH and prevented the formation of T suppressor cells.[56] IL-12 was found to exert its affects by reversing the UVR-induced production of IL-10 and TNF-$\alpha$, but did not affect interferon-gamma (IFN-$\gamma$) production.[57]

It was previously believed that these cytokines came only from epidermal keratinocytes. In the past it has been shown that UV-irradiated murine keratinocytes produced cytokines such as IL-10 and TNF-$\alpha$. Furthermore, supernatants from UV-irradiated keratinocytes mimicked some of the immunosuppressive effects of UVR.[51,58] However, in recent years, other sources of cytokines have also come to light. Several studies have shown that mice lacking mast cells are not susceptible to UVB-induced systemic immunosuppression of CHS and DTH. Administering histamine to these mice mimicked the effects of UVB radiation. However, these mice remained susceptible to UVB-induced local CHS suppression, implying that perhaps mast cells are not important for local CHS suppression.[59] Another group reported opposite results regarding the importance of mast cells in local CHS suppression. They showed that mast cell degranulation suppressed CHS locally, and that this suppression could be reversed with administration of anti-TNF-$\alpha$ antibody. Furthermore, local induction of CHS was not impaired in UVB-irradiated mast cell–deficient mice.[60] They also demonstrated that mast cell degranulation induces hapten-specific tolerance, which can be blocked with anti-IL-10 antibodies. In addition, mast cell–deficient mice were not susceptible to UVB-induced hapten-specific tolerance.[61] These studies demonstrate the importance of mast cell–derived factors such as histamine, TNF-$\alpha$, and IL-10 in UVR-mediated immunosuppression. A study in humans has demonstrated another source of cytokines. It was shown that the main source of IL-10 in human skin following UVB radiation exposure is infiltrating $CD11b^+$ macrophages.[62]

Only in the past several years have the molecular events upstream of cytokine production been examined. Although still unclear, there are several current hypotheses. One group demonstrated that IL-10 production upon UVR exposure is linked to IL-4 and prostaglandin $E_2$ ($PGE_2$) production. In mice, UVB radiation induced a dose-dependent increase in serum IL-4 that could be blocked with a COX-2 inhibitor, implying that $PGE_2$ drives IL-4 production. Anti-IL-4 antibodies blocked UVB-induced suppression of DTH. Furthermore, treating irradiated mice with anti-IL-4 suppressed the increase in serum IL-10 production normally seen upon UVB radiation exposure. Injecting normal mice with $PGE_2$ led to an increase in serum IL-4 and IL-10, further implying that $PGE_2$ drives IL-4 and subsequently IL-10 production, eventually leading to systemic immunosuppression. The source of the $PGE_2$ was hypothesized to be keratinocytes as other studies have demonstrated that keratinocytes upregulate $PGE_2$ production following UVR exposure. The source of the serum IL-4 was unknown, but determined not to be keratinocytes in the present study.[63,64]

More recent evidence also implicates factors working upstream of COX, such as platelet-activating factor (PAF). PAF is not expressed in normal skin, but is produced by UV-irradiated keratinocytes, which also upregulate PAF receptor expression following UVR exposure. PAF also upregulates COX-2 expression and $PGE_2$ expression by keratinocytes.[4] Thus, PAF could serve as the upstream mediator of the above-described cytokine cascade. One group demonstrated that both UVR and PAF activated IL-10 gene transcription in a reporter gene construct. Furthermore, administration of PAF suppressed DTH *in vivo* and treating UV-irradiated mice with a PAF receptor antagonist blocked UVR-induced immune suppression.[65]

Another group has demonstrated in a detailed set of experiments that, upon UVB radiation exposure, *cis*-UCA induces neuropeptides such as CGRP and substance P to be released, which subsequently cause mast cell degranulation and histamine release, which then induces prostaglandin production.[66] Although both theories ultimately conclude that it is $PGE_2$ production that drives cytokine production and that mast cells play a crucial role, it is ultimately unclear what the initiating factors may be.

There is also some evidence that iC3b (the bioactive product of C3) and its ligand CD11b are important for UVR-induced immunosuppression in humans. iC3b is generated in the dermis following exposure to UVB radiation and appears to inhibit the differentiation of monocytes into

$CD1c^+$ dendritic cells and induces $CD1c^-CD14^+$ cells.[67] Treatment of mice by *in vivo* anti-CD11b antibody abrogates immunosuppression in the local UVB-induced immunosuppression model. Furthermore, C3-deficient mice cannot be immunosuppressed by local exposure to UVB radiation, and treatment of mice with an agent that inhibits C3 activation and accelerates degradation of iC3b also inhibits UVB radiation–induced immunosuppression.[68] However, it is unclear how iC3b may be related to other aspects of UVR-induced immunosuppression such as cytokine production.

## C. T-Suppressor Cells

The ability of UVR exposure to result in the generation of suppressor T cells that can transfer UVR-induced tolerance to non-UVR-exposed mice was demonstrated more than 20 years ago and has been reproduced by many groups. However, there has been a great deal of controversy regarding the phenotype of these cells and how they develop and function with many questions still unanswered.

UVR-induced tumors are rejected when transplanted onto normal syngeneic mice. However, if these recipients are also exposed to UVR, the transplanted tumor continues to grow.[18] It was then shown that transfer of lymphoid cells from the irradiated host into naive mice permitted tumor growth. Lymphoid cells from UVB-irradiated mice were injected into γ-irradiated donors. These recipients were then challenged with syngeneic UVR-induced tumors. Mice injected with lymphoid cells from UV-irradiated mice were not able to resist challenge with tumor while mice injected with normal lymphoid cells rejected the tumor.[69] The cells responsible for this phenomenon were found to be T cells (i.e., T-suppressor cells).

One group clearly showed the relationship between carcinogenesis and T-suppressor cell development, demonstrating that both UVR-induced carcinogenesis and immune suppression contribute to skin cancer development. Mice were γ-irradiated and repopulated with either normal T cells or T cells from UVB-irradiated mice. These two groups were then grafted with skin from UVB-exposed mice, thus separating the carcinogenic effects of UVR from the immunosuppressive effects. As expected, those mice given T cells from UVB-exposed mice developed significantly more tumors than those mice given normal T cells, which presumably were better at rejecting the tumors. Similarly, mice injected with suppressor T cells and then exposed to UVB radiation had a much shorter latency period for the development of skin cancers than mice injected with normal T cells.[70]

Hapten-specific suppressor T cells were also found to develop in the local model of CHS. Adoptive transfer of spleen and lymph node suspensions from UVB-irradiated hapten-painted mice into γ-irradiated syngeneic recipients induced hapten-specific unresponsiveness. These recipient mice, however, mounted a normal CHS response to other haptens. Furthermore, UVR in the UVB range was necessary to generate these suppressor cells and UVA radiation alone was insufficient. These suppressor cells were also shown to affect the induction of CHS and not the elicitation phase. When these cell suspensions were depleted of $Thy1.2^+$ cells, suppression of CHS in the recipients was blocked, implying that the cells that transfer suppression are in fact T cells. Furthermore, depletion of $CD4^+$ cells also abrogates suppression while depletion of $CD8^+$ cells partially eliminates suppression. This study demonstrates that the cells that transfer suppression are in fact T cells and likely of the $CD4^+$ or $CD4^+CD8^+$ phenotype.[71] Similar studies by another group showed that the phenotype of suppressor cells that allow growth of a syngeneic UVB-induced tumor is $CD4^+CD8^-Ia^-$. Similarly, the suppressor cells generated from UVB-exposed mice from painting hapten on non-irradiated skin were also $CD4^+CD8^-Ia^-$, suggesting that tumor rejection and systemic CHS may operate via the same immunologic pathways. However, the cells generated from UVA-exposed mice from painting hapten on non-irradiated skin was $CD4^+CD8^+$, suggesting that UVA and UVB radiation exert their suppressive effects through different mechanisms.[72]

Antigen-specific suppressor T cells were also found after UVR-induced inhibition of DTH. Further, one group found that injecting supernatants from UV-irradiated keratinocytes into mice led to suppression of DTH. T-suppressor cells were generated of the phenotype $CD3^+CD4^+CD8^-$, implying that a soluble factor may regulate development of these cells.[73,74]

Recently, there has been a more detailed characterization of the somewhat confusing and controversial phenotype of these cells. Using mice congenic at the Thy1 locus, it was demonstrated that suppressor T cells arise from the UVB-irradiated donors and they are $CD4^+CD8^-TCR\alpha/\beta^+$, MHC (major histocompatibility complex) restricted. Clones produced from these cells secreted IL-10, but not IL-4 or IFN-γ. They also blocked APC function and IL-12 production, implying that these cells favor a Th2 phenotype and downregulate Th1-mediated function.[75]

While the above group showed the identity of suppressor cells elicited from the local model of CHS, another group identified another suppressor cell population involved in the elicitation of DTH and tumor immunity. This cell was an NK T cell expressing NK1.1, DX5, Ly49a and secreting high amounts of IL-4. Transferring even small amounts of these cells from UV-irradiated, immunized mice into non-irradiated immunized mice suppressed the elicitation of DTH. When these cells were depleted from the cell suspension prior to injection, there was no suppression of DTH. Furthermore, when these NK T cells from UVR-exposed mice were used to reconstitute γ-irradiated mice, they were unable to reject a transplanted UVR-induced tumor compared with mice injected with conventional $CD4^+$ T cells.[76]

Possible mechanisms by which these cells function have also been elucidated more recently. Two groups have studied the role of Fas/FasL in UVR-induced immune suppression/suppressor cell generation. Hill et al.[77] have shown that FasL deficient mice are not susceptible to UVR-induced suppression of CHS or DTH (except DTH to allogeneic spleen cells) and also lack transferable suppressor cell activity. Schwarz et al.[78] demonstrated similar findings working with two strains of mice deficient in either Fas or FasL. They showed that these mice do not develop UVR-induced tolerance and that, in order to transfer suppression, the recipient mice (but not the donor) need to express both Fas and FasL. Furthermore, they showed *in vitro* that UVR-generated T-suppressor cells enhanced the death rate of dendritic cells and that this was mediated by Fas/FasL and could be prevented by addition of IL-12.[77,78]

Schwarz et al.[78,79] also demonstrated the importance of CTLA-4, a negative T-cell regulatory molecule, in transfer of UVR-induced tolerance. When suppressor cells from UV-irradiated mice were depleted of CTLA-$4^+$ cells there was no longer immune tolerance. In addition, enrichment of CTLA-$4^+$ cells necessitated the use of far fewer cells to transfer suppression. Injection anti-CTLA-4 antibody into mice blocked UVR-induced tolerance and transfer of suppression. Like the cells cloned by Shreedhar et al.,[75] these produced high levels of IL-10, but also made IFN-γ and transforming growth factor-beta (TGF-β), but little IL-2 and no IL-4, similar to T-regulatory type 1 cells.[79,80]

T-suppressor cells clearly play a crucial role in UVR-mediated immune suppression/tolerance and carcinogenesis. There appear to be several different types of suppressor cells that are generated depending on whether there is local vs. systemic suppression. However, their exact mechanism of action remains to be elucidated (Figure 21.2).

## IV. UVR EFFECTS ON CUTANEOUS CELLS

### A. Antigen Presenting Cells

UVR has profound effects on the resident APC (LC) within the epidermis as well as APC in the whole body at higher doses. Not only does it cause a depletion of LC from the skin, but it also significantly impairs their antigen-presenting function. Following UVB radiation exposure, there is a dose-dependent increase in LC migration out of the epidermis as well as morphological changes such as cytoskeletal blebbing and mitochondrial swelling. Collection of these migrating cells further demonstrates that they have a decreased antigen-presenting capacity as assessed by their ability to stimulate T-cell proliferation.[81] *In vivo,* injection of LC conjugated with hapten from UVR-treated mice into normal mice suppressed their ability to induce an immune response to that hapten compared to LC from non-UV-irradiated mice.[82]

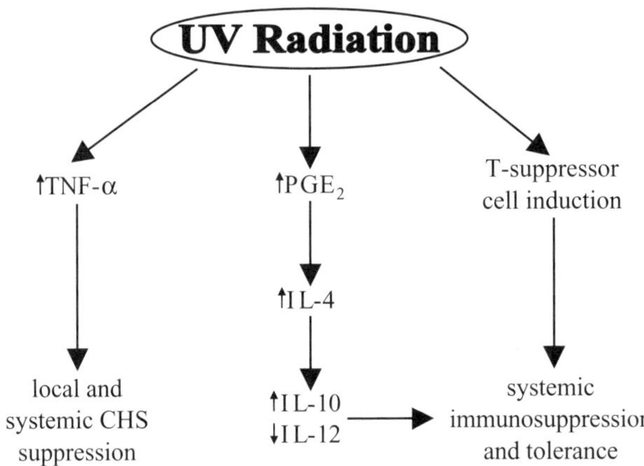


**FIGURE 21.2** Possible mechanisms of UVR-induced immunosuppression and tolerance.

A similar study also demonstrated *in vitro* that UVB radiation–treated LC and other APC were not able to present antigen to a CD4+ Th1 clone. Furthermore, these APC induced anergy in these T cells because the T cells were subsequently unable to be stimulated by non-UVB-radiation-exposed APC. This effect is likely due to a lack of a co-stimulatory signal because supernatants from UVB radiation–exposed cells did not inhibit T-cell proliferation.[83] UVB radiation exposed APC also lose their ability to stimulate Th1 cells, but retain their ability to stimulate cells of the Th2 subset.[84] This was supported by another group that demonstrated that APC isolated from the lymphoid organs of UVR-exposed mice produced insufficient amounts of IL-12 and were incapable of stimulating IFN-γ production by T cells. This defect was mimicked when mice were injected with IL-10 instead of being exposed to UVR.[85] One study using a murine LC-like line showed that exposing dendritic cells to UVB radiation caused subsequent apoptosis of the dendritic cells upon co-culture with T cells, implying that this may be a possible mechanism for UVR-induced immunosuppression and tolerance at the APC level.[86]

## B. Keratinocytes

Keratinocyte damage can be seen several hours after UVR exposure. There is intracellular and intercellular edema and the formation of sunburn cells, which are damaged keratinocytes that will undergo apoptosis.[1] Following UVR exposure, keratinocytes *in vitro* have been shown to secrete a number of cytokines that have been implicated in UVR-induced immunosuppression such as IL-10 and TNF-α.[51] In addition, keratinocytes also make IL-1 and IL-6, whose role in UVR-mediated immune regulation is not as clear or well studied.[87,88] It is believed that keratinocyte DNA damage may be the initiating event in cytokine production because treating UV-irradiated keratinocytes with DNA repair enzymes abrogates IL-10 secretion.[25]

DNA damage and dysregulated growth of keratinocytes lead to skin cancers. As such, UVR-mediated defects in the normal keratinocyte apoptotic pathway have been implicated as an early event in UVR-induced carcinogenesis. It has been shown that keratinocytes upregulate Fas/FasL expression following UVR exposure and treatment with a FasL neutralizing antibody significantly reduced UVR-induced apoptosis.[89] In murine UVR-induced skin tumors, there was no change in Fas expression, but a loss of FasL expression, emphasizing that the Fas/FasL pathway is important for UVR-induced apoptosis and regulation of cell growth.[90] Supporting this hypothesis, another group demonstrated that cultured senescent keratinocytes were more resistant to apoptosis than young keratinocytes, implying a possible mechanism for increased skin cancers with aging.[91]

### C. Mast Cells

Dermal mast cells have been shown to be important in regulating UVR-induced suppression of systemic CHS. One study reports that mast cell–deficient mice are not susceptible to systemic UVB-mediated immune suppression. In these mice, histamine, but not UVB radiation was able to induce systemic immune suppression. Thus dermal mast cells appear to be a key element in UVR-mediated immunosuppression, likely acting via release of histamine. In mice, the prevalence of dermal mast cells was also shown to determine UVR susceptibility. The more sensitive the mouse to UVR-induced immunosuppression, the higher number of dermal mast cells.[59] A similar phenomenon was shown in humans. Patients with previous BCC were demonstrated to have higher prevalence of mast cells in non-sun-exposed buttock tissue.[92] It was also shown that *cis*-UCA could not exert its immunosuppressive effects in mast cell–deficient mice, and it is known that *cis*-UCA can degranulate mast cells *in vitro*.[93] However, recent evidence has shown that *cis*-UCA may mediate its effects by causing release of neuropeptides, which in turn cause degranulation of mast cells. *cis*-UCA did not suppress CHS in mice depleted of neuropeptides with capsaicin.[66] Furthermore, histamine receptor antagonists partially reversed UVB-mediated suppression of CHS. Indomethacin and a histamine receptor antagonist did not cause an additional reversal of the immunosuppression implying that they act through the same pathway.[94]

## V. CLINICAL PHOTOMEDICINE

### A. Wavelengths Implicated in UVR-Induced Immunosuppression and Carcinogenesis

In the past, most studies involving UVR have relied on the use of FS40 sunlamps, which have a high UVB:UVA output (~60 to 65% UVB radiation) in contrast to natural sunlight, which is 95% UVA radiation and 5% UVB radiation. Thus, mainly UVB radiation has been extensively studied and implicated in the immunosuppressive and carcinogenic properties of UVR. The role of UVB radiation in carcinogenesis is clear. In the 1950s, Blum[95] presented some of the first evidence that demonstrated that wavelengths of light from 260 to 300 nm were the most effective at inducing skin cancer. Furthermore, UVR signature DNA mutations such as the pyrimidine dimers and 6,4-photoproducts are primarily the result of UVB radiation and these are often found in *p53* and *ptc* mutations in skin cancers.[6,11]

However, the role of UVA radiation in immune suppression and carcinogenesis has not been clear, with contradicting studies in the past. However, UVA radiation appears to play a crucial role as studies have demonstrated that UVA + UVB radiation was more effective at inducing skin cancers than UVB radiation alone.[96] Several recent studies have helped define the role of UVA radiation more clearly.

To evaluate the UVR wavelengths that were responsible for suppressing the elicitation of DTH, mice were first immunized to *Candida albicans* and then exposed to UVA + UVB radiation (290 to 400 nm), or UVA radiation (320 to 400 nm), or UVA I radiation alone (340 to 400 nm), followed by later challenge with the same antigen. The combination of UVA + UVB radiation and UVA radiation alone suppressed the mice's ability to mount a DTH response. However, UVA I radiation alone did not suppress the immune response. These results imply that UVA II radiation (320 to 340 nm) is primarily responsible for suppressing the elicitation of established immune responses.[97,98] Furthermore, to characterize the mechanism by which UVA radiation exerts its effects, they showed that injection of anti-IL-10 antibody or injection of IL-12 blocked the immunosuppressive effects of UVA radiation. In addition, UVA radiation generated suppressor T cells and application of the DNA repair enzyme T4N5 to mouse skin exposed to UVA radiation also blocked its effects, demonstrating that all UVR may share similar mechanisms of action.[99]

UVA radiation has also been implicated in the induction of malignant melanoma in a fish model. In this model, wavelengths greater than 320 nm were more effective at inducing melanoma.[100] Another study in opossums showed that UVB radiation was more effective than UVA radiation at inducing nonmelanoma skin cancers, but that UVB and UVA radiation were equally effective at inducing melanocytic hyperplasia, a possible melanoma precursor.[101] One group studied the role of UVB radiation in melanoma development using mice transgenic for SV40 coupled to the tyrosinase gene promoter. In these mice, the oncogene SV40 is preferentially expressed in pigmented cells and these mice are more susceptible to melanoma development. UVB radiation of these mice led to the development of melanocytic lesions resembling pigmented macules, nevi, or early melanomas. As these mice have a short lifespan, skin samples containing some of these lesions were grafted after 20 weeks of UVB exposure to longer-lived unirradiated hosts of a different transgenic line. Ten of these lesions subsequently developed into malignant melanoma.[102] In a different experiment, RAG-1 mice were grafted with human newborn foreskin and treated with either the carcinogen 7,12-dimethyl(*a*)benzanthracene (DMBA) alone, UVB radiation alone, or UVB radiation and DMBA. Solar lentigines developed in 23% treated with UVB radiation alone and in 38% of those treated with both UVB radiation and DMBA. Histologic changes resembling lentigo and lentigo maligna were seen in several skin grafts treated with both DMBA and UVB radiation and one animal developed a human malignant melanoma.[103] The above studies indicate that UVA and UVB radiation may play a role in the development of malignant melanoma.

## B. Chemoprevention

The most well known preventative measure aside from sun avoidance is topical sunscreen application. The effectiveness of sunscreens is evaluated on their ability to prevent erythema in human skin, with the higher SPFs (sun protection factor) having the greatest ability to prevent erythema.[4]

One study demonstrated that sunscreens (SPF 15) applied before UV irradiation in mice significantly reduced the incidence of p53 mutations in irradiated skin.[104] Furthermore, a similar study by the same group using a solar simulator (which more accurately mimics the UVA/UVB ratio of natural sunlight) showed that after 16 weeks of UV irradiation 56 to 69% of the control group had p53 mutations, but less than 5% of the mice who had sunscreen (SPF 15 to 22) applied prior to UV irradiation had developed p53 mutations. More importantly, while 100% of control mice developed skin tumors, only 2% of mice treated with sunscreen developed tumors. This demonstrates not only the usefulness of using p53 mutations as a measure of sunscreen efficacy, but also the importance of sunscreens as a whole in possibly reducing the risk of skin cancer.[105]

One study in humans tested the ability of three different sunscreens all with an SPF of 10 to prevent UVR-induced suppression (using a solar simulator) of the CHS response to nickel. They showed that only the two broad-spectrum sunscreens blocking both UVA and UVB radiation were effective in preventing immunosuppression.[106] A similar study in humans looking at elicitation of DTH (to recall antigens) yielded similar results using both a solar simulator as well as natural sunlight. In both cases, use of a sunscreen with greater UVA radiation protection blocked UVR-induced suppression of DTH.[107]

The recent data demonstrating that UVA radiation is responsible for suppressing elicitation of DTH were further proved by testing UVB radiation absorbing sunscreens vs. a sunscreen that absorbs both UVA and UVB radiation in mice. The UVB radiation blocking sunscreen did not block immunosuppression while the UVA + UVB blocking sunscreen did. Both sunscreens had an SPF of 15. Another study in mice by a different group also demonstrated that increased UVA radiation protection in a broad-spectrum sunscreen more effectively blocked UVR-induced systemic suppression of CHS.[108] These results imply that immune suppression or DNA damage may be a better end point to measure a sunscreen's effectiveness. Furthermore, it may be more effective to use sunscreens that offer protection against UVA + UVB radiation.

There is also some evidence that T4N5 may be useful for chemoprevention. In mice, topical application of liposomes containing T4N5 during the period of chronic, repetitive exposure to UVB radiation led to reduction in the number of tumors per mouse compared to controls not treated with T4N5.[109] In patients with xeroderma pigmentosum, a genetic disorder in which there is a defect in DNA repair, topical treatment with a lotion containing T4N5 liposomes for 1 year led to a decreased incidence of new actinic keratoses and BCC compared to controls not treated with T4N5. It is unknown whether these results would apply to normal individuals.[110]

COX-2 inhibitors have also been found to be protective against the carcinogenic effects of UVR as they inhibit $PGE_2$ production, a potential mediator in UVR-induced immunosuppression. In one study, mice were UV-irradiated until they had developed one tumor. They were then administered a COX-2 inhibitor, and it was found that mice given the COX-2 inhibitor developed significantly less tumors than the untreated group.[111] A similar study also showed that mice fed COX-2 inhibitors or general NSAIDS (nonsteroidal anti-inflammatory drugs) before UVR exposure had a dose-dependent decrease in tumor yield.[112] More recently, skin tumors were induced in mice, after which UVR was stopped and the mice were administered a COX-2 inhibitor, an ornithine decarboxylase (ODC) inhibitor, or both. The mice given either drug showed significant tumor regression, which was even greater in the mice administered both drugs. However, when the drugs were stopped, the tumors returned, demonstrating that in order to be effective these drugs may need to be constantly administered.[113]

Another class of agents used to protect against UVR-induced damage are the antioxidants, which can block UVR-induced production of free radicals and cell membrane damage. Among these are the green tea polyphenols, silymarin, curcumin, apigenin, and resveratrol. All of these agents have been shown to inhibit UVR-mediated induction of COX and ODC as well as decrease hydrogen peroxide and free radical content in the skin following UVR treatment. Furthermore, green tea, silymarin, and apigenin were all shown to decrease tumor incidence in mice exposed to UVR. This class of agents represents an additional mechanism for combating the deleterious effects of UVR.[114]

## VI. CONCLUSION

The link between UVR-induced immunosuppression and carcinogenesis is well documented. Numerous studies have demonstrated that preventing immunosuppression by blocking some of the key pathways involved decreased the incidence of skin cancers in UVR-exposed mice. This has direct implications for humans and emphasizes the importance of finding agents to prevent UVR-mediated immune suppression given the rising incidence of sun exposure and skin cancer in many parts of the world. At the current time, the various factors and pathways that have been implicated in UVR-induced immunosuppression cannot be fit together in a coherent and complete system to explain all of the observed effects. In most of the experimental models described, inhibition of any one factor or pathway causes loss of most or all of the immunosuppressive effect. Thus, large gaps remain in our knowledge of how these various pathways interrelate. Nonetheless, it is clear that UVR-induced suppression of immunity has medical and public health consequences.

An interesting question is why the system of UVR-induced suppression exists. It may have been expected that such a deleterious system would be selected against by evolution. One hypothesis is that UVR-induced immunosuppression has evolved to protect against autoimmunity after sunlight exposure. In this hypothesis, cell death or injury following environmental UVR exposure leads to release of immunostimulatory cytokines and hidden antigens with a subsequent increased risk of induction of autoimmunity. If true, selection for mechanisms of immunosuppression would have a survival advantage.

At the current time, it seems prudent to recommend that all individuals use broad-spectrum sunscreens providing both UVA and UVB coverage as a public health measure to afford the best protection against the deleterious effects of environmental UVR exposure.

## REFERENCES


1. Clydesdale, G.J., Dandie, G.W., and Muller, H.K., Ultraviolet light induced injury: immunological and inflammatory effects. *Immunol. Cell. Biol.*, 79, 547, 2001.
2. Schwarz, T., Photoimmunosuppression. *Photodermatol. Photoimmunol. Photomed.*, 18, 141, 2002.
3. Slominski, A. and Pawelek, J., Animals under the sun: effects of ultraviolet radiation on mammalian skin. *Clin. Dermatol.*, 16, 503, 1998.
4. Ullrich, S.E., Photoimmune suppression and photocarcinogenesis. *Front. Biosci.*, 7, d684, 2002.
5. Krutmann, J., Ultraviolet A radiation-induced biological effects in human skin: relevance for photoaging and photodermatosis. *J. Dermatol. Sci.*, 23(Suppl. 1), S22, 2000.
6. Ouhtit, A. and Ananthaswamy, H.N., A model for UV-induction of skin cancer. *J. Biomed. Biotechnol.*, 1, 5, 2001.
7. de Gruijl, F.R., Skin cancer and solar UV radiation. *Eur. J. Cancer*, 35, 2003, 1999.
8. Armstrong, B.K. and Kricker, A., The epidemiology of UV induced skin cancer. *J. Photochem. Photobiol. B*, 63, 8, 2001.
9. Kligman, L.H. and Kligman, A.M., Histogenesis and progression in ultraviolet light-induced tumors in hairless mice. *J. Natl. Cancer Inst.*, 67, 1289, 1981.
10. Hoover, T.L., Morison, W.L., and Kripke, M.L., Ultraviolet carcinogenesis in athymic nude mice. *Transplantation*, 44, 693, 1987.
11. de Gruijl, F.R., van Kranen, H.J., and Mullenders, L.H., UV-induced DNA damage, repair, mutations and oncogenic pathways in skin cancer. *J. Photochem. Photobiol. B*, 63, 19, 2001.
12. Brash, D.E. et al., A role for sunlight in skin cancer: UV-induced p53 mutations in squamous cell carcinoma. *Proc. Natl. Acad. Sci. U.S.A.*, 88, 10124, 1991.
13. Hahn, H. et al., Mutations of the human homolog of *Drosophila* patched in the nevoid basal cell carcinoma syndrome. *Cell*, 85, 841, 1996.
14. Gailani, M.R. et al., The role of the human homologue of *Drosophila* patched in sporadic basal cell carcinomas. *Nat. Genet.*, 14, 78, 1996.
15. Bodak, N. et al., High levels of patched gene mutations in basal-cell carcinomas from patients with xeroderma pigmentosum. *Proc. Natl. Acad. Sci. U.S.A.*, 96, 5117, 1999.
16. Aszterbaum, M. et al., Ultraviolet and ionizing radiation enhance the growth of BCCs and trichoblastomas in patched heterozygous knockout mice. *Nat. Med.*, 5, 1285, 1999.
17. Oro, A.E. et al., Basal cell carcinomas in mice overexpressing sonic hedgehog. *Science*, 276, 817, 1997.
18. Kripke, M.L., Antigenicity of murine skin tumors induced by ultraviolet light. *J. Natl. Cancer Inst.*, 53, 1333, 1974.
19. Kripke, M.L. et al., Further characterization of immunological unresponsiveness induced in mice by ultraviolet radiation. Growth and induction of nonultraviolet-induced tumors in ultraviolet-irradiated mice. *Transplantation*, 28, 212, 1979.
20. Jemec, G.B. and Holm, E.A., Nonmelanoma skin cancer in organ transplant patients. *Transplantation*, 75, 253, 2003.
21. Kelly, D.A. et al., A single exposure of solar simulated radiation suppresses contact hypersensitivity responses both locally and systemically in humans: quantitative studies with high-frequency ultrasound. *J. Photochem. Photobiol. B*, 44, 130, 1998.
22. Yoshikawa, T. et al., Susceptibility to effects of UVB radiation on induction of contact hypersensitivity as a risk factor for skin cancer in humans. *J. Invest. Dermatol.*, 95, 530, 1990.
23. Applegate, L.A. et al., Identification of the molecular target for the suppression of contact hypersensitivity by ultraviolet radiation. *J. Exp. Med.*, 170, 1117, 1989.
24. Kripke, M.L. et al., Role of DNA damage in local suppression of contact hypersensitivity in mice by UV radiation. *Exp. Dermatol.*, 5, 173, 1996.
25. Nishigori, C. et al., Evidence that DNA damage triggers interleukin 10 cytokine production in UV-irradiated murine keratinocytes. *Proc. Natl. Acad. Sci. U.S.A.*, 93, 10354, 1996.
26. Kibitel, J. et al., UV-DNA damage in mouse and human cells induces the expression of tumor necrosis factor alpha. *Photochem. Photobiol.*, 67, 541, 1998.
27. Wolf, P. et al., Topical treatment with liposomes containing T4 endonuclease V protects human skin *in vivo* from ultraviolet-induced upregulation of interleukin-10 and tumor necrosis factor-alpha. *J. Invest. Dermatol.*, 114, 149, 2000.

28. O'Connor, A. et al., DNA double strand breaks in epidermal cells cause immune suppression *in vivo* and cytokine production *in vitro*. *J. Immunol.*, 157, 271, 1996.
29. Vink, A.A. et al., The inhibition of antigen-presenting activity of dendritic cells resulting from UV irradiation of murine skin is restored by *in vitro* photorepair of cyclobutane pyrimidine dimers. *Proc. Natl. Acad. Sci. U.S.A.*, 94, 5255, 1997.
30. De Fabo, E.C. and Noonan, F.P., Mechanism of immune suppression by ultraviolet irradiation *in vivo*. I. Evidence for the existence of a unique photoreceptor in skin and its role in photoimmunology. *J. Exp. Med.*, 158, 84, 1983.
31. Moodycliffe, A.M. et al., Characterization of a monoclonal antibody to *cis*-urocanic acid: detection of *cis*-urocanic acid in the serum of irradiated mice by immunoassay. *Immunology*, 79, 667, 1993.
32. Ross, J.A. et al., Induction of suppression of delayed type hypersensitivity to herpes simplex virus by epidermal cells exposed to UV-irradiated urocanic acid *in vivo*. *Viral Immunol.*, 1, 191, 1987.
33. Kurimoto, I. and Streilein, J.W., Deleterious effects of *cis*-urocanic acid and UVB radiation on Langerhans cells and on induction of contact hypersensitivity are mediated by tumor necrosis factor-alpha. *J. Invest. Dermatol.*, 99, 69S, 1992.
34. Ross, J.A. et al., Ultraviolet-irradiated urocanic acid suppresses delayed-type hypersensitivity to herpes simplex virus in mice. *J. Invest. Dermatol.*, 87, 630, 1986.
35. Beissert, S. et al., Regulation of tumor antigen presentation by urocanic acid. *J. Immunol.*, 159, 92, 1997.
36. Reeve, V.E. et al., Topical urocanic acid enhances UV-induced tumour yield and malignancy in the hairless mouse. *Photochem. Photobiol.*, 49, 459, 1989.
37. Kurimoto, I. and Streilein, J.W., *cis*-urocanic acid suppression of contact hypersensitivity induction is mediated via tumor necrosis factor-alpha. *J. Immunol.*, 148, 3072, 1992.
38. Holan, V. et al., Urocanic acid enhances IL-10 production in activated CD4+ T cells. *J. Immunol.*, 161, 3237, 1998.
39. Beissert, S. et al., IL-12 prevents the inhibitory effects of *cis*-urocanic acid on tumor antigen presentation by Langerhans cells: implications for photocarcinogenesis. *J. Immunol.*, 167, 6232, 2001.
40. el-Ghorr, A.A. and Norval, M., A monoclonal antibody to *cis*-urocanic acid prevents the ultraviolet-induced changes in Langerhans cells and delayed hypersensitivity responses in mice, although not preventing dendritic cell accumulation in lymph nodes draining the site of irradiation and contact hypersensitivity responses. *J. Invest. Dermatol.*, 105, 264, 1995.
41. Moodycliffe, A.M. et al., Differential effects of a monoclonal antibody to *cis*-urocanic acid on the suppression of delayed and contact hypersensitivity following ultraviolet irradiation. *J. Immunol.*, 157, 2891, 1996.
42. Devary, Y. et al., The mammalian ultraviolet response is triggered by activation of Src tyrosine kinases. *Cell*, 71, 1081, 1992.
43. Devary, Y. et al., NF-kappa B activation by ultraviolet light not dependent on a nuclear signal. *Science*, 261, 1442, 1993.
44. Simon, M.M. et al., UVB light induces nuclear factor kappa B (NF kappa B) activity independently from chromosomal DNA damage in cell-free cytosolic extracts. *J. Invest. Dermatol.*, 102, 422, 1994.
45. Rosette, C. and Karin, M., Ultraviolet light and osmotic stress: activation of the JNK cascade through multiple growth factor and cytokine receptors. *Science*, 274, 1194, 1996.
46. Kurimoto, I. and Streilein, J.W., Tumor necrosis factor-alpha impairs contact hypersensitivity induction after ultraviolet B radiation via TNF-receptor 2 (p75). *Exp. Dermatol.*, 8, 495, 1999.
47. Rivas, J.M. and Ullrich, S.E., The role of IL-4, IL-10, and TNF-alpha in the immune suppression induced by ultraviolet radiation. *J. Leukocyte Biol.*, 56, 769, 1994.
48. Yoshikawa, T. and Streilein, J.W., Tumor necrosis factor-alpha and ultraviolet B light have similar effects on contact hypersensitivity in mice. *Reg. Immunol.*, 3, 139, 1990.
49. Amerio, P. et al., Rethinking the role of tumour necrosis factor-alpha in ultraviolet (UV) B-induced immunosuppression: altered immune response in UV-irradiated TNFR1R2 gene-targeted mutant mice. *Br. J. Dermatol.*, 144, 952, 2001.
50. Niizeki, H. and Streilein, J.W., Hapten-specific tolerance induced by acute, low-dose ultraviolet B radiation of skin is mediated via interleukin-10. *J. Invest. Dermatol.*, 109, 25, 1997.
51. Rivas, J.M. and Ullrich, S.E., Systemic suppression of delayed-type hypersensitivity by supernatants from UV-irradiated keratinocytes. An essential role for keratinocyte-derived IL-10. *J. Immunol.*, 149, 3865, 1992.

52. Ullrich, S.E., Mechanism involved in the systemic suppression of antigen-presenting cell function by UV irradiation. Keratinocyte-derived IL-10 modulates antigen-presenting cell function of splenic adherent cells. *J. Immunol.*, 152, 3410, 1994.
53. Beissert, S. et al., Impaired immunosuppressive response to ultraviolet radiation in interleukin-10-deficient mice. *J. Invest. Dermatol.*, 107, 553, 1996.
54. Ullrich, S.E., Does exposure to UV radiation induce a shift to a Th-2-like immune reaction? *Photochem. Photobiol.*, 64, 254, 1996.
55. Schwarz, A. et al., Interleukin-12 prevents ultraviolet B-induced local immunosuppression and overcomes UVB-induced tolerance. *J. Invest. Dermatol.*, 106, 1187, 1996.
56. Schmitt, D.A., Owen-Schaub, L., and Ullrich, S.E., Effect of IL-12 on immune suppression and suppressor cell induction by ultraviolet radiation. *J. Immunol.*, 154, 5114, 1995.
57. Schmitt, D.A., Walterscheid, J.P., and Ullrich, S.E., Reversal of ultraviolet radiation-induced immune suppression by recombinant interleukin-12: suppression of cytokine production. *Immunology*, 101, 90, 2000.
58. Beissert, S. et al., Supernatants from UVB radiation-exposed keratinocytes inhibit Langerhans cell presentation of tumor-associated antigens via IL-10 content. *J. Leukocyte Biol.*, 58, 234, 1995.
59. Hart, P.H. et al., Dermal mast cells determine susceptibility to ultraviolet B-induced systemic suppression of contact hypersensitivity responses in mice. *J. Exp. Med.*, 187, 2045, 1998.
60. Alard, P. et al., Local ultraviolet B irradiation impairs contact hypersensitivity induction by triggering release of tumor necrosis factor-alpha from mast cells. Involvement of mast cells and Langerhans cells in susceptibility to ultraviolet B. *J. Invest. Dermatol.*, 113, 983, 1999.
61. Alard, P. et al., Hapten-specific tolerance induced by acute, low-dose ultraviolet B radiation of skin requires mast cell degranulation. *Eur. J. Immunol.*, 31, 1736, 2001.
62. Kang, K. et al., $CD11b^+$ macrophages that infiltrate human epidermis after *in vivo* ultraviolet exposure potently produce IL-10 and represent the major secretory source of epidermal IL-10 protein. *J. Immunol.*, 153, 5256, 1994.
63. Buckman, S.Y. et al., COX-2 expression is induced by UVB exposure in human skin: implications for the development of skin cancer. *Carcinogenesis*, 19, 723, 1998.
64. Shreedhar, V. et al., A cytokine cascade including prostaglandin E2, IL-4, and IL-10 is responsible for UV-induced systemic immune suppression. *J. Immunol.*, 160, 3783, 1998.
65. Walterscheid, J.P., Ullrich, S.E., and Nghiem, D.X., Platelet-activating factor, a molecular sensor for cellular damage, activates systemic immune suppression. *J. Exp. Med.*, 195, 171, 2002.
66. Hart, P.H. et al., Mast cells, neuropeptides, histamine, and prostaglandins in UV-induced systemic immunosuppression. *Methods*, 28, 79, 2002.
67. Takahara, M. et al., iC3b arrests monocytic cell differentiation into CD1c-expressing dendritic cell precursors: a mechanism for transiently decreased dendritic cells *in vivo* after human skin injury by ultraviolet B. *J. Invest. Dermatol.*, 120, 802, 2003.
68. Hammerberg, C. et al., Activated complement component 3 (C3) is required for ultraviolet induction of immunosuppression and antigenic tolerance. *J. Exp. Med.*, 187, 1133, 1998.
69. Fisher, M.S. and Kripke, M.L., Systemic alteration induced in mice by ultraviolet light irradiation and its relationship to ultraviolet carcinogenesis. *Proc. Natl. Acad. Sci. U.S.A.*, 74, 1688, 1977.
70. Fisher, M.S. and Kripke, M.L., Suppressor T lymphocytes control the development of primary skin cancers in ultraviolet-irradiated mice. *Science*, 216, 1133, 1982.
71. Elmets, C.A. et al., Analysis of the mechanism of unresponsiveness produced by haptens painted on skin exposed to low dose ultraviolet radiation. *J. Exp. Med.*, 158, 781, 1983.
72. Ullrich, S.E. and Kripke, M.L., Mechanisms in the suppression of tumor rejection produced in mice by repeated UV irradiation. *J. Immunol.*, 133, 2786, 1984.
73. Noonan, F.P., De Fabo, E.C., and Kripke, M.L., Suppression of contact hypersensitivity by UV radiation and its relationship to UV-induced suppression of tumor immunity. *Photochem. Photobiol.*, 34, 683, 1981.
74. Ullrich, S.E., McIntyre, B.W., and Rivas, J.M., Suppression of the immune response to alloantigen by factors released from ultraviolet-irradiated keratinocytes. *J. Immunol.*, 145, 489, 1990.
75. Shreedhar, V.K. et al., Origin and characteristics of ultraviolet-B radiation-induced suppressor T lymphocytes. *J. Immunol.*, 161, 1327, 1998.

76. Moodycliffe, A.M. et al., Immune suppression and skin cancer development: regulation by NKT cells. *Nat. Immunol.*, 1, 521, 2000.
77. Hill, L.L. et al., A critical role for Fas ligand in the active suppression of systemic immune responses by ultraviolet radiation. *J. Exp. Med.*, 189, 1285, 1999.
78. Schwarz, A. et al., Ultraviolet light-induced immune tolerance is mediated via the Fas/Fas-ligand system. *J. Immunol.*, 160, 4262, 1998.
79. Schwarz, A. et al., Evidence for functional relevance of CTLA-4 in ultraviolet-radiation-induced tolerance. *J. Immunol.*, 165, 1824, 2000.
80. Groux, H. et al., A CD4+ T-cell subset inhibits antigen-specific T-cell responses and prevents colitis. *Nature*, 389, 737, 1997.
81. Dandie, G.W. et al., Effects of UV on the migration and function of epidermal antigen presenting cells. *Mutat. Res.*, 422, 147, 1998.
82. Cruz, P.D., Jr., Tigelaar, R.E., and Bergstresser, P.R., Langerhans cells that migrate to skin after intravenous infusion regulate the induction of contact hypersensitivity. *J. Immunol.*, 144, 2486, 1990.
83. Simon, J.C. et al., Ultraviolet B radiation converts Langerhans cells from immunogenic to tolerogenic antigen-presenting cells. Induction of specific clonal anergy in CD4+ T helper 1 cells. *J. Immunol.*, 146, 485, 1991.
84. Simon, J.C. et al., Low dose ultraviolet B-irradiated Langerhans cells preferentially activate CD4+ cells of the T helper 2 subset. *J. Immunol.*, 145, 2087, 1990.
85. Kitazawa, T. and Streilein, J.W., Studies on delayed systemic effects of ultraviolet B radiation on the induction of contact hypersensitivity, 3. Dendritic cells from secondary lymphoid organs are deficient in interleukin-12 production and capacity to promote activation and differentiation of T helper type 1 cells. *Immunology*, 99, 296, 2000.
86. Kitajima, T. et al., Ultraviolet B radiation sensitizes a murine epidermal dendritic cell line (XS52) to undergo apoptosis upon antigen presentation to T cells. *J. Immunol.*, 157, 3312, 1996.
87. Ansel, J.C., Luger, T.A., and Green, I., The effect of *in vitro* and *in vivo* UV irradiation on the production of ETAF activity by human and murine keratinocytes. *J. Invest. Dermatol.*, 81, 519, 1983.
88. Avalos-Diaz, E., Alvarado-Flores, E., and Herrera-Esparza, R., UV-A irradiation induces transcription of IL-6 and TNF alpha genes in human keratinocytes and dermal fibroblasts. *Rev. Rhum. Engl. Ed.*, 66, 13, 1999.
89. Leverkus, M., Yaar, M., and Gilchrest, B.A., Fas/Fas ligand interaction contributes to UV-induced apoptosis in human keratinocytes. *Exp. Cell Res.*, 232, 255, 1997.
90. Ouhtit, A. et al., Loss of Fas-ligand expression in mouse keratinocytes during UV carcinogenesis. *Am. J. Pathol.*, 157, 1975, 2000.
91. Gniadecki, R., Hansen, M., and Wulf, H.C., Resistance of senescent keratinocytes to UV-induced apoptosis. *Cell. Mol. Biol.* (Noisy-le-grand), 46, 121, 2000.
92. Hart, P.H., Grimbaldeston, M.A., and Finlay-Jones, J.J., Sunlight, immunosuppression and skin cancer: role of histamine and mast cells. *Clin. Exp. Pharmacol. Physiol.*, 28, 1, 2001.
93. Hart, P.H. et al., A critical role for dermal mast cells in *cis*-urocanic acid-induced systemic suppression of contact hypersensitivity responses in mice. *Photochem. Photobiol.*, 70, 807, 1999.
94. Hart, P.H. et al., Histamine involvement in UVB- and *cis*-urocanic acid-induced systemic suppression of contact hypersensitivity responses. *Immunology*, 91, 601, 1997.
95. Blum, A., *Carcinogenesis by Ultraviolet Light*, Princeton University Press, Princeton, NJ, 1959.
96. Protection against Depletion of Stratospheric Ozone by Chlorofluorocarbons, National Academy of Sciences, Washington, D.C., 1979, Appendix F, 325.
97. Nghiem, D.X. et al., Ultraviolet A radiation suppresses an established immune response: implications for sunscreen design. *J. Invest. Dermatol.*, 117, 1193, 2001.
98. Ullrich, S.E., Kripke, M.L., and Ananthaswamy, H.N., Mechanisms underlying UV-induced immune suppression: implications for sunscreen design. *Exp. Dermatol.*, 11(Suppl. 1), 13, 2002.
99. Nghiem, D.X. et al., Mechanisms underlying the suppression of established immune responses by ultraviolet radiation. *J. Invest. Dermatol.*, 119, 600, 2002.
100. Setlow, R.B. et al., Wavelengths effective in induction of malignant melanoma. *Proc. Natl. Acad. Sci. U.S.A.*, 90, 6666, 1993.
101. Ley, R.D., Ultraviolet radiation A-induced precursors of cutaneous melanoma in *Monodelphis domestica. Cancer Res.*, 57, 3682, 1997.

102. Klein-Szanto, A.J., Silvers, W.K., and Mintz, B., Ultraviolet radiation-induced malignant skin melanoma in melanoma-susceptible transgenic mice. *Cancer Res.*, 54, 4569, 1994.
103. Atillasoy, E.S. et al., UVB induces atypical melanocytic lesions and melanoma in human skin. *Am. J. Pathol.*, 152, 1179, 1998.
104. Ananthaswamy, H.N. et al., Sunlight and skin cancer: inhibition of p53 mutations in UV-irradiated mouse skin by sunscreens. *Nat. Med.*, 3, 510, 1997.
105. Ananthaswamy, H.N. et al., Inhibition of solar simulator-induced p53 mutations and protection against skin cancer development in mice by sunscreens. *J. Invest. Dermatol.*, 112, 763, 1999.
106. Damian, D.L., Halliday, G.M., and Barnetson, R.S., Broad-spectrum sunscreens provide greater protection against ultraviolet-radiation-induced suppression of contact hypersensitivity to a recall antigen in humans. *J. Invest. Dermatol.*, 109, 146, 1997.
107. Moyal, D.D. and Fourtanier, A.M., Broad-spectrum sunscreens provide better protection from the suppression of the elicitation phase of delayed-type hypersensitivity response in humans. *J. Invest. Dermatol.*, 117, 1186, 2001.
108. Fourtanier, A. et al., Improved protection against solar-simulated radiation-induced immunosuppression by a sunscreen with enhanced ultraviolet A protection. *J. Invest. Dermatol.*, 114, 620, 2000.
109. Bito, T. et al., Reduction of ultraviolet-induced skin cancer in mice by topical application of DNA excision repair enzymes. *Photodermatol. Photoimmunol. Photomed.*, 11, 9, 1995.
110. Yarosh, D. et al., Effect of topically applied T4 endonuclease V in liposomes on skin cancer in xeroderma pigmentosum: a randomised study. Xeroderma Pigmentosum Study Group. *Lancet*, 357, 926, 2001.
111. Pentland, A.P. et al., Reduction of UV-induced skin tumors in hairless mice by selective COX-2 inhibition. *Carcinogenesis*, 20, 1939, 1999.
112. Fischer, S.M. et al., Chemopreventive activity of celecoxib, a specific cyclooxygenase-2 inhibitor, and indomethacin against ultraviolet light-induced skin carcinogenesis. *Mol. Carcinogenesis*, 25, 231, 1999.
113. Fischer, S.M. et al., Celecoxib and difluoromethylornithine in combination have strong therapeutic activity against UV-induced skin tumors in mice. *Carcinogenesis*, 24, 945, 2003.
114. Afaq, F. et al., Botanical antioxidants for chemoprevention of photocarcinogenesis. *Front. Biosci.*, 7, d784, 2002.

# 22 The Skin Immune System and Tumor Immunosurveillance

*H. Konrad Muller, Gary M. Halliday, and Gregory M. Woods*

## CONTENTS



## I. INTRODUCTION

The concept of immunosurveillance was originally proposed by Lewis Thomas and F. Macfarlane Burnet.[1] They postulated that the cellular immune system was largely concerned with eliminating aberrant cells, thus preventing the development of cancer. Somatic cell mutations were considered to occur repeatedly throughout life and the resulting aberrant cells were destroyed by thymic-derived T lymphocytes (T cells). For immunosurveillance to have a substantial role in host–tumor interactions, the transformed cells would have to express new antigens.

Over the past 30 years immunosurveillance has remained controversial. Support for this hypothesis comes from the increased incidence of tumors in immunocompromised individuals, e.g., renal transplant recipients and patients with acquired immune deficiency syndrome (AIDS), those on immunosuppressive drugs, and the aged. In the aged individuals there is a general decrease in cell-mediated immunity accompanied by increased rates of skin neoplasia.[2] While increased incidences of skin cancer with age might reflect prolonged exposure to ultraviolet (UV) light, immunity also declines with age contributing to this trend. Other issues associated with age-related cancer include the combined effects across time of mutation load, epigenetic regulation, altered telomeres, and the role of the stroma.[3]

Immunosuppressive therapy used to prolong graft survival has been linked to the development of cutaneous neoplasia, which increases with time after transplantation. Marshall[4] in Melbourne, Australia, found that 8% of his transplant patients surviving after 1 year had skin tumors. This increased to 17% after 4 years or more. Sheil and colleagues,[5] also reported a high incidence of

0-8493-1959-5/05/$0.00+$1.50

skin tumors in transplant patients; for those surviving 5, 8, and 10 years, 34, 39, and 57% developed cancer, respectively.

Skin tumors found in transplant patients, reviewed by Penn,[6] include squamous cell carcinoma (SCC), basal cell carcinoma (BCC), Kaposi's sarcoma, malignant melanoma, and a small number with Bowen's disease. With immunosuppression in renal transplant patients the usual BCC:SCC ratio is reversed, and metastases are more prevalent. Penn reported multiple lesions were present in 43% of patients and also included actinic keratoses, keratoacanthomas, and multiple viral warts. Walder and colleagues[7] suggested that hyperkeratoses in transplant patients more frequently undergo malignant transformation.

Because the increased incidence of skin tumors in immunosuppressed transplant patients occurs in sun-exposed areas, it is possible that UV light also contributes to the development of these tumors. It may be that immunosuppressive agents enhance photocarcinogenesis.[2,8] This relationship is strengthened by evidence that azathioprine enhances UV light–induced skin cancer in hairless mice.[9] A further possibility is the role of viruses, as immunosuppressed transplant patients have an increased incidence of papilloma virus infection.[10,11]

Immunosuppressive therapy of patients with diseases, such as psoriasis, and autoimmunity has also been associated with an increase in skin neoplasia.[6] In psoriasis, patients treated with methotrexate, corticosteroids, tar, and solar radiation, an increased incidence of skin tumors has been reported including actinic keratoses, multiple keratoacanthomas, and *in situ* and invasive SCC.[12–14]

An increased incidence of skin cancer has also been reported in diseases where the immune system is compromised. Such diseases include lymphocytic lymphoma or leukemia, which suppress the immune system. The skin tumors are usually SCC and often develop on sun-exposed areas.[15,16] In patients with AIDS who have defective T-helper-cell function, a high incidence of Kaposi's sarcoma occurs.[17,18]

While at the clinical level an impaired immune system resulting from the use of immunosuppressive therapy or primary disease has been linked to an increased incidence of skin neoplasia, further support for immunosurveillance comes from experimental carcinogenesis studies with UVB radiation and chemical carcinogenesis.[19]

## II. TUMOR ANTIGENS

Because the prime assumption of immunosurveillance is that tumor cells possess antigens, which enable recognition of tumor, but not normal cells by the immune system, there has been extensive investigation into tumor-associated antigens. The cloning of genes that code for tumor antigens could lead to the development of a successful antitumor vaccine. An important aspect of these studies is to determine whether each tumor expresses a distinct tumor antigen or antigens common to all other tumor cells. This latter group of antigens could provide immunity against a large number of tumors and hence are important to characterize.

### A. Animal Studies

Tumor antigens were first shown to exist in experimental animal systems, and there is now convincing evidence that human tumors possess tumor-associated antigens. While the early experiments of Prehn and Main[20] made it highly likely that tumor-specific antigens exist, Klein and colleagues[21] provided definitive evidence that tumor-specific immunity against methylcholanthrene-induced sarcomas could be generated in primary autologous hosts.

Transplantation experiments in mice revealed that many chemically induced squamous tumors express individually tumor-specific antigens, which are not shared by other histologically similar tumors induced by the same carcinogen.[20,22,23] Cross-reacting tumor antigens have been only occasionally reported with chemically induced tumors.[24,25] Characteristics of these unique tumor-specific antigens include large antigenic diversity and the possible expression of multiple tumor-specific antigens within a single tumor. At present little is known on the molecular nature of these antigens or the genetic basis for their large antigenic diversity. Further, all of these antigens may not be immunogenic, and some may more readily activate immune defense mechanisms than others.[26] Even when multiple tumors are found on one animal, these tumors contain antigens that are all individually distinct.[27]

Unique tumor-specific transplantation antigens have also been described in UV-radiation-induced squamous tumors in mice. These skin tumors are immunologically rejected when transplanted into syngeneic recipients, but will grow if the host is immunosuppressed.[28] The immune response generated against each tumor is specific for the particular tumor transplanted.[29] Hong and Roberts[30] have suggested that UV-induced tumor antigens may be expressed prior to the appearance of visible skin tumors and that these antigens may activate cytotoxic T lymphocytes (CTL). In contrast to these studies with murine nonmelanoma skin cancers, melanomas induced in mice by initiation with UV radiation and promotion with croton oil, or initiation with 7,12-dimethylbenz[*a*]anthracene and promotion with 12-*O*-tetradecanoyl-phorbol-13-acetate (TPA) have been shown to induce an immune response that provided some protection against other melanomas.[31] Hence, expression of cross-reactive antigens may be dependent on the tumor type as well as the carcinogen primarily responsible for tumor formation.

The development of a new experimental melanoma model utilizing neonatal HGF/SF-transgenic mice and UV irradiation should allow further exploration of melanoma antigens.[32]

The development of CTL clones specific for tumor lines has extended our understanding of tumor antigens. By using cytotoxic T-cell lines specific for particular tumors but not normal cells, multiple independent tumor antigens have been shown to be present on UV-induced squamous tumors.[33] Thus, T cells can recognize specific antigens on tumor cells.

An elegant approach for the identification of tumor rejection antigens came from studies with mouse tumor cell variants expressing $tum^-$ antigens in response to treatment with mutagens *in vitro* (reviewed by Boon[34]). CTL clones used to analyze different $tum^-$ antigens demonstrated that different tumor cell variants expressed individual $tum^-$ antigens, which did not cross-react, demonstrating the presence of many different tumor antigens. By use of the CTL clones to select tumor cell variants, it was shown that loss of $tum^-$ antigens was associated with an inability of host mice to reject the tumors upon transplantation into syngeneic mice. This provided direct evidence that these tumor antigens recognized by CTL could act as tumor rejection antigens *in vivo*.[35]

## B. Human Studies

In humans, there are many descriptions of altered expression of various proteins by tumor cells, including melanomas.[36] However, in most cases it is not clear whether these molecules can be targets for immune-mediated destruction, or whether they are an altered expression of normal molecules, which occur as a result of the cellular changes associated with tumor development. In nonmelanoma skin cancer the latter include mutated p53 found in greater than 90% of SCC and in most BCC.[37] While CD8 CTL responses to p53 have been described and p53 specific CTL shown to recognize and kill SCC tumor lines, their effectiveness in controlling tumor growth is in doubt.[38] In nonmelanoma skin cancer the cancer-testis antigen NY-ESO-1 could be a target for CTL.[37]

Antigens expressed by human malignant melanoma have been more extensively studied than those of any other human skin tumor, probably because of the large volume of evidence that the immune system can control melanoma growth, and the clinical importance of this tumor. A wide number of antigens have now been identified in melanomas; some are expressed in other tumor cells, e.g., breast and prostate cancers.[39] Of these the MAGE gene family has received major attention.[40]

Acid extraction of peptides from major histocompatibility complex (MHC) class I molecules on human melanomas has eluted peptides that can be recognized by melanoma-specific tumor-infiltrating lymphocytes (TILs) and CTL from tumor-involved lymph nodes.[41,42] Multiple epitopes have been eluted that are present on different melanoma lines, demonstrating that single tumors express a range of antigens that are presented by tumor cells in an appropriate way for recognition by T lymphocytes. It has also been shown that $CD4^+$ T lymphocytes isolated from TILs are able to recognize a product of the tyrosinase gene associated with MHC class II.[43] Thus melanoma antigens associated with both MHC class I and II proteins can be involved in antitumor immunity.

CTL lines derived from the peripheral blood of patients with melanoma have been used to study melanoma tumor antigens.[44] By using this approach, an antigen, MZ2-E, encoded by the gene MAGE-1 was first identified and found to be expressed by a large proportion of melanomas but not normal tissues with the exception of testis.[45] This antigen was a nonapeptide, which, in association with HLA-A1, is recognized by CTL.[46] The MAGE family was initially considered to contain three members located on the human X chromosome.[47] Extensive characterization using data-based screening has identified a wider family (at present 13 subfamilies) encoded by genes predominantly on the X chromosome, but also on chromosomes 3 and 5. Some of these subfamilies are expressed in normal tissues,[40] including human skin during wound healing.[48]

The MAGE-2 gene is expressed in a higher proportion of melanomas than MAGE-1.[49] MAGE-3 codes for the tumor antigen MZ2-D, a nonapeptide segment that is presented in association with HLA-A1 on 69% of melanomas.[50]

Other tumor antigens recognized by CTL have been identified on melanocytes and melanomas. These include the differentiation antigens MART-1 (Melan-A), gp100, tyrosinase, tyrosinase-related protein 1 and 2, and melanocyte-stimulating hormone receptor[51–56]

The majority of these melanoma antigens are not new tumor-specific proteins but are either developmental antigens that are not expressed by normal adult cells or are differentiation antigens of the melanocyte lineage.[57] Undoubtedly, other antigens recognized by the immune system will be discovered on melanoma and other skin tumors.

While the early studies of antigen reactive T cells to melanoma antigens used CTL as an approach to evaluate antitumor immunity, the development of tetramer technology has allowed the more precise determination of responding T cells. However, the frequency of melanoma-specific antigen reactive T cells is low. For example, studies on patients with malignant melanoma have shown that only 0.01% of peripheral blood lymphocytes recognized Melan-A, while tyrosinase, gp100, MAGE-3, and NY-ESO-1 were not detected at all.[58] This has implications for mounting effective antitumor immunity in patients.

## III. ANTITUMOR IMMUNITY

### A. Induction

Whereas there is considerable information regarding the induction of skin immunity to contact sensitizers, little is known about the cellular or molecular events involved in induction of antitumor immunity in the skin. The developmental process of tumor formation complicates this. In tumor initiation, genetic changes in normal cells give the cell the potential to develop into a tumor. Such cells need to be promoted into growth, and the hyperplastic dividing cells must undergo further multiple genetic changes to progress toward malignancy. This will result in cells that have undergone different genetic changes and those tumor cells with a growth advantage will predominate.[59] There are many stages in this process where tumors could start to express tumor antigens. At present, it is unknown at which stage this may occur. Tumors also produce many different cytokines some of which can induce the activation of immunological suppressor mechanisms.[60] Ultimately, the individual characteristic of tumors including antigen expression and cytokine production will govern the immune response against the tumor.

Most human skin tumors arise within the epidermis, and hence cells with an immunological function in the epidermis will be important for the induction of antitumor immunity. The components of the skin immune system have been reviewed in other chapters of this book. Langerhans cells (LC) are dendritic antigen-presenting cells that are likely to play a role in the initiation of antitumor immunity. Dendritic epidermal T cells (DETC) are found in murine but not human epidermis, and could be involved in the early stages of immune responses to murine tumors. Additionally the dermis contains many cells with immune functions, including dermal dendritic cells, macrophages, mast cells, and T cells, which could be important in the early stages of antitumor immunity.

It has been convincingly demonstrated that LC are able to initiate protective immunity against a murine tumor line that was established from a chemically induced skin tumor.[61] This ability of LC to induce antitumor immunity was dependent on prior culture of the LC with granulocyte-macrophage colony-stimulating factor (GM-CSF), and this was abrogated if the LC were exposed to tumor necrosis factor-α (TNF-α) after GM-CSF.[62] It has also been shown that LC are able to stimulate proliferation of tumor antigen-specific lymphocytes.[63] GM-CSF and TNF-α modulate LC function,[64,65] and hence it is likely that production of these cytokines by developing tumors would influence the ability of LC to induce antitumor immunity.

Developed human and murine tumors are infiltrated with large numbers of LC. Using anti-S100 antibodies and the indirect immunoperoxidase technique, we have studied LC infiltrating a range of human skin tumors.[66] The LC density in lesional epithelium of Bowen's disease (11 cases), keratoacanthoma (13 cases), SCC (18 cases), and actinic keratoses (16 cases) were all significantly increased compared to untanned control skin (11 cases). In keratoacanthoma, SCC, and BCC, the LC concentrated at the interface between normal and neoplastic tissue, while in actinic keratoses and Bowen's disease the LC were evenly distributed throughout the lesions. In all of these lesions except actinic keratosis, the number of LC in epidermis adjacent to the lesions was also increased. LC are also observed in large numbers within cervical intraepithelial neoplasia. The number of LC was reduced in 14 cases of cervical condyloma but increased in 21 cases of cervical intraepithelial neoplasia, suggesting that wart virus infection may decrease the number of LC, compromising immunosurveillance; as the tumors develop LC may migrate into the lesions.[67]

The observation that LC can be identified in skin tumors indicates that, as these cells are primarily involved in the initiation of an immune response, induction of antitumor immunity can occur at this level. Nonetheless, their presence within tumors does not indicate a functional role and very little work has been undertaken on extracting these cells and performing a functional analysis. One such study, prior to the identification of dendritic cells, extracted macrophages from tumors and determined that these cells did have some antitumor activity but it was apparent from this early study that there was substantial heterogeneity in the responses including evidence for nonprotective effects.[68] On reflection, it is not surprising that the function of LC or DC that infiltrate tumors may not reflect their true function as, by definition, once a tumor has formed it has avoided the immune system, including the initiation phase, and its function may therefore be altered. Whereas it is probable that LC are involved in the initiation of antitumor immunity, by the time the tumors have developed into macroscopically visible lesions the immune response controlling tumor growth should have become well established. The role of LC at this advanced stage is debatable. For example, with squamous lung tumors a high LC dendritic cell population is associated with enhanced patient survival.[69] Likewise, Becker[70] has summarized a substantial literature supporting the notion that dendritic cells have a major prognostic role in cancer management. In contrast, spontaneously regressing human melanoma,[71] BCC,[72] and keratoacanthoma[73] are all infiltrated with similar numbers of LC to non-regressing tumors suggesting that LC may not play a major role in tumor regression. This is supported by murine studies. Skin tumors transplanted into athymic mice were found to increase the number of LC in the epidermis overlying the tumor, and no relationship was observed between the immune status of mice and LC density.[74] Weakly immunogenic tumor cell lines lead to an accumulation of LC in immunocompetent and incompetent mice, whereas a highly immunogenic regressor skin tumor was observed not to effect LC.[75] While skin tumor–produced factors may alter LC numbers,[76] a central issue is the functional status of dendritic cells in tumors.

Nonetheless, there is indirect evidence linking dendritic cells and LC with the induction of effective antitumor immunity. We have shown that patients with larger numbers of dendritic cells in their tumors have a better prognosis,[69] that LC migration to the local lymph nodes is reduced in progressor but not regressor skin tumors,[77] and that regressor tumors were infiltrated by a greater number of dendritic cells, which appeared to have the major phagocytic role.[78] Furthermore, immunotherapy with dendritic cells has shown promising signs[79] indicating that these cells are likely to initiate antitumor immunity.

For an immune response to be effective against a tumor it is necessary to activate CTL, usually $CD8^+$CTL. Consequently tumor antigens need to be presented to $CD8^+$ T cells via MHC-I, but if this occurs only by direct tumor cell contact, an ineffective immune response will occur. This is overcome by a process known as cross-priming, which is when exogenous antigens (e.g., tumor antigen or apoptotic tumor cells) are processed by an antigen-presenting cell and presented in association with MHC-I, rather than MHC-II, which usually occurs following the exogenous processing pathway.[80,81] Dendritic cells, which are known to infiltrate tumors and are highly efficient at cross-priming due to their unique ability to "shuttle" the processed tumor antigen from the endosome (class II pathway) to the cytosol (class I pathway),[82,83] can therefore present tumor antigens to $CD4^+$ cells and $CD8^+$ CTL in order to initiate an effective antitumor immune response.

Recently, plasmacytoid dendritic cells, or type I interferon-producing cells (I IFN) have been identified as being recruited to tumors, including ovarian carcinomas[84] and primary cutaneous melanomas,[85] where they have been shown to produce type I IFN.[86] This production of type I IFN suggests an antitumor role for these cells as this cytokine has antitumoral activity. However, its production is reduced,[87] as is the expression of MxA (the IFN-α inducible particle) associated with tumors.[86] Tumor production of interleukin-10 (IL-10) also decreases the T-cell stimulatory capacity of these cells.[84] Hence the role of plasmacytoid dendritic cells in tumors has yet to be resolved and may be more important in tumor invasion.

## B. Effector Cellular Mechanisms

The major cellular killing mechanisms involve MHC-restricted cytotoxic T and lymphocytic-secreting T lymphocytes as well as natural killer cells (NK cells). The first definitive evidence to support the role of activated cytotoxic T cells in the immunological regression of UV-induced skin tumors was provided by Lill and Fortner.[88] They demonstrated cytotoxic T cell activity *in vitro* against autologous tumor cells. *In vivo* depletion of CD8 T cells from mice transplanted with a range of UV-induced regressor skin tumors has been shown a requirement for $CD8^+$ T cells in skin tumor regression.[28]

NKT cells are generally regarded as T cells that share some of the features of NK cells. They do not express CD3 and are $CD4^-/CD8^-$ double negative, $CD8^+$, or $CD4^+$ T cells, which express the αβ T cell receptor with a limited repertoire and CD1d restricted.[89] In addition to a regulatory role, they have cytotoxic activity and antitumor properties.[90]

These cytotoxic cells can kill their target cells by either an intrinsic Fas/FasL pathway, or an extrinsic perforin/granzyme-mediated pathway to induce apoptosis in the target cells.[91] The Fas/FasL pathway requires the activation of the cytotoxic cell to express FasL. Contact between the effector cells and target cells through FasL-Fas induces apoptosis in the target cell by activating FADD that, in turn, initiates the caspase pathway and ultimately DNA degradation. Activation of FasL on CTLs requires 2 to 3 h of T-cell receptor stimulation, but once it is expressed it remains on the surface for 2 to 3 h. During this period the killing of any nearby cells that may express Fas expression can occur, which accounts for promiscuous killing.[92] Although this killing pathway operates in all cytotoxic cell lineages, its role is often secondary to the extrinsic pathway. In this pathway it is the combination of perforin and granzymes that leads to apoptosis of the target cells.

The initial view of the combined actions of perforin and granules (granzymes A and B) was that perforin, which had clearly been shown to induce complement-like pores in cell membranes, formed a transmembrane channel allowing the granules to enter the cell and cause target cell death. It was also believed that the membrane damage caused by perforin itself was sufficient to cause cell death.[93] The current view of cytotoxicity via the granule exocytosis pathway is a modification of this earlier perspective. Following recognition of the target cells, a tight junction is formed between the effector and target cells and the granules reorientate in the cytotoxic cells to the point of contact. This allows a controlled and directed secretion of perforin and the granules toward the target cells.[91] As the pore produced by perforin is too small to allow granzymes to pass,[94] it is likely that perforin binds to a receptor on the target cells[95] resulting in endocytosis of granzymes[96] and the induction of target cell death. Granzymes have also been shown to enter the cell directly via the mannose-6-phosphate receptor (MRP).[97] Once inside the cell the granzymes are activated and transported to the nucleus where they initiate the apoptotic process via a caspase-dependent[98] or -independent pathway involving mitochondrial activation.[99]

## C. Evidence for Antitumor Immunity and Tumor Destruction

There are two lines of direct evidence that the immune response is capable of causing destruction of human skin tumors: the increased incidence of skin tumors in pharmacologically immunosuppressed patients, and observations on spontaneously regressing skin tumors.

Transplant patients who are therapeutically immunosuppressed to prevent their immune systems from rejecting the grafts have an increased incidence of skin cancers.[100] They have increased incidences of all types of skin cancers, including BCC, SCC, melanoma, and Kaposi's sarcoma. The increase in risk of skin cancer is related to the degree of immunosuppression and the length of time the patient has been on immunosuppressive therapy, but not to any particular drug used to cause the immunosuppression.[101,102] The type of organ transplanted is not a predisposing factor.[103] In some instances the tumors regress upon withdrawal of the immunosuppressive drug.[104]

A recent large study of 5356 patients concluded that the risk of developing skin cancer in transplant recipients, like patients without a transplant, is higher on sun-exposed skin.[105] This suggests that in addition to drug-mediated immunosuppression, mutations induced by UV radiation are required to augment the level of skin cancer. Transplant patients have an increased incidence of some, but not all, internal malignancies in addition to the vast increase in skin cancers,[106] further suggesting that UV-induced genetic mutations in addition to drug-induced immunosuppression contribute to the high incidence of skin cancers in these patients.

There are also reports that skin tumors can arise from organs transplanted into patients who are immunosuppressed and that these can regress upon cessation of immunosuppressive therapy.[107,108] Presumably the transplanted organ contained a metastasis, which was controlled by the immune system. Upon transfer into an immunosuppressed host, the tumor was able to grow. Nevertheless, the large volume of clinical data now available on immunosuppressed patients all indicate that the immune response is able to control clinical development of skin tumors, and that a reduction in immune function, regardless of how that was caused, enables the outgrowth of skin tumors.

The other piece of evidence that the immune system causes destruction of human skin tumors comes from studies into spontaneous regression. Spontaneous regression occurs when a clinically identifiable cancer disappears, or regresses, in the absence of therapy capable of causing regression. It is now clear that spontaneous regression is due to the immune response to that tumor gaining sufficient momentum to cause clearance of the tumor. This has been reviewed in detail.[109] A dramatic example of this has recently been documented where a patient with biopsy-proven melanoma declined therapy and the melanoma then spontaneously regressed.[110]

Spontaneous regression, which is more common than frequently believed, can be either complete where the entire lesion is destroyed, or partial, where the immune system destroys part of the tumor before tumor escape mechanisms protect the remainder of the tumor. In 4% of melanomas there is a secondary lesion without a primary,[111] implying that at least 4% of primary melanomas spontaneously regress completely after they have metastasized. The incidence of complete regression of primary melanomas prior to metastatic spread is unknown. The incidence of complete regression in SCC and BCC has not been documented. Partial regression is more common, with 25% of melanomas[71] and 30% of BCC[112] having areas of partial regression at the time of therapeutic excision.

The evidence that the immune response is involved comes from studies that show that regressing melanomas,[71] BCC,[112] and keratoacanthomas[73] are all infiltrated with significantly larger numbers of CD4+ T lymphocytes compared to nonregressing lesions. These lymphocytes were activated as they expressed receptors for IL-2 and histologically appeared to be disrupting nests of tumor cells. The higher number of CD4+ T cells was only observed within the tumors themselves, and not in surrounding tissues adding further weight to the probability that these CD4+ T lymphocytes were mediating the tumor destruction as they needed to infiltrate the tumors. There were no differences between regressing and nonregressing tumors in numbers of CD8+ T cells or macrophages. These CD8+ T cells or macrophages could have been playing a role in the regression but were not present in limiting numbers in nonregressing tumors. This supports a role for CD4+ T cells in mediating tumor destruction.[113] The mechanism by which CD4+ T cells cause tumor destruction is unknown; however, it has been shown that CD4+ cytotoxic T cells kill melanoma cells by a mechanism independent of FasL[114] but dependent on TNF-related apoptosis-inducing ligand (TRAIL).[115]

Spontaneously regressing melanomas and BCC have increased levels of the Th1 cytokines IFN-γ, IL-2, and lymphotoxin[116,117] supporting conclusions that spontaneous regression is immunologically mediated. In these studies there were no changes in Th2 cytokines or pro-inflammatory cytokines suggesting that skin tumors are most effectively destroyed by cell-mediated immunity involving CD4 T cells and Th1-like immunity.

Further evidence that spontaneous regression is a clinical feature of immune destruction of human tumors comes from studies showing that T cells infiltrating regressing melanomas have a restricted T-cell receptor usage.[118,119] In another study, patients with multiple primary melanomas were found to have increased spontaneous regression consistent with immunization resulting from the multiple primaries augmenting regression. This was associated with changes in melanoma-specific cytotoxic T cells.[120] Human leukocyte antigen (HLA) associations with spontaneous regression of melanoma[121] further show that spontaneous regression is immunologically mediated.

Recent studies in mouse models have indicated that skin tumors that do not regress express high levels of MHC II but not co-stimulatory molecules, in association with FasL. This suggests that these skin tumors may present antigen to CD4+ T cells in the absence of co-stimulation so that the tumor cells can kill the partially activated CD4+ T cells in an FasL-dependent manner. Regressing tumors did not express MHC II or FasL, indicating that they could not partially activate and then kill CD4+ T cells by this mechanism.[122] It is possible that loss of MHC II or FasL expression by tumors could therefore cause them to regress by enabling the survival of tumor reactive CD4+ T cells; however, this issue remains to be resolved. Key questions are "What triggers spontaneous regression?" and "Why does a skin tumor that has evaded immunological destruction suddenly lose this capability so that the immune response gains control?"

In summary, the data of increased tumor incidence in pharmacologically immunosuppressed patients and demonstrations that spontaneous regression is immunologically mediated provide direct evidence that the immune response is able to recognize and destroy human skin tumors.

## IV. FAILURE OF TUMOR IMMUNITY

While immune responses to cutaneous tumors can be demonstrated, ultimately tumors such as melanoma frequently escape the immune system and spread widely in the body. However, even during the period of tumor development, immune mechanisms may be deviated to favor the growth of tumors, thus avoiding effective tumor immunosurveillance. This is now well described in UVB and chemical carcinogenesis.[19]

### A. Induction

Investigations over the past two decades have concentrated on changes in LC during the early stages of tumor development. Initial studies in this area were on UV-induced tumors and the associated immune events. These investigations are fully described elsewhere in this book. Our own studies concentrated on the immune system during chemical carcinogenesis.

Agents that cause tumor promotion such as DMBA and TPA deplete LC from the epidermis leading to an impaired immune response.[123,124] In contrast, tumor initiators, e.g., urethane, do not impair LC numbers and function — the immune response remains intact.[125] Experimental carcinogenesis with DMBA applied to murine skin is an ideal model to study these events. DMBA (1%) depletes epidermal LC reducing the density to about 50% after 3 days. This LC depletion persists for up to 8 weeks during which time squamous tumors develop. Repopulation of LC in the epidermis after this time parallels tumor regression.[124] Other studies by Zeid and Muller[126] have confirmed these observations using tobacco smoke condensate applied to murine skin.

A major feature of DMBA carcinogenesis is that the LC depletion is a tumor promotional event. DMBA doses that fail to cause LC depletion (0.1%), also fail to cause tumor promotion. Using a range of tumor-promoting agents we have shown a consistent correlation between LC depletion and tumor development.[127] A central issue of DMBA carcinogenesis has been the mechanism of DMBA-induced depletion. Possibilities include cell destruction, loss of cell membrane markers, or LC migration. Initial ultrastructural studies of DMBA-treated skin failed to demonstrate significant LC injury. Likewise, the key cell membrane markers remain intact, e.g., MHC class II. To answer the LC migration question, an alternative experimental model was required. Sheep provided an elegant model as DMBA could be applied to the skin, the migrating cells collected by lymphatic cannulation, and the LC enumerated by flow cytometry.[128] In these experiments DMBA produced a 100-fold increase in LC migration, which peaked 4 to 5 days following DMBA application.[129–131] In general, these findings parallel the LC depletion time course observed in DMBA-treated murine skin. It is worth adding that the tumor promoter TPA but not the tumor initiator urethane also enhanced LC migration.[132]

The effects of carcinogen-induced depletion of LC on cutaneous immunity were initially assessed by contact sensitivity responses. Mice did not develop a contact sensitivity response to 2,4-dinitroflurobenzene (DNFB) when sensitized through DMBA-treated dorsal trunk skin. Mice treated with DMBA on their dorsal trunk but sensitized on untreated abdominal skin gave a response, which did not differ from that of the controls, indicating that the effect of the carcinogen on the induction of cutaneous immunity is local, not systemic. This inability to induce contact sensitivity during chemical carcinogenesis was due to suppressor cell activation, as spleen cells from these mice inhibited immune hosts from responding to challenge with the antigen in adoptive transfer experiments. Other experiments have shown that these suppressor cells are long-lived and are antigen specific. Thus, the chemical carcinogen DMBA disrupts the function of the skin immune system so that suppressor cells rather than cells that mediate immunity are activated in response to antigenic challenge.[132,133]

Further analysis of the LC draining DMBA-treated skin has shown that 4 days after DMBA treatment the residual LC have lost their ability to induce antigen-specific T-lymphocyte proliferation.[134] The LC from DMBA-treated skin carry less antigen to the draining lymph nodes, fail to produce IL-Iβ, and have reduced expression of the co-stimulatory molecule B7-2.[135,136] They also form fewer clusters with $CD4^+$ T cells, but not $CD8^+$ T cells (unpublished observations). Further evaluation of the LC remaining in the skin after DMBA treatment has revealed that these cells are morphologically different from LC from normal skin; they are smaller, tend to be round with limited dendrites, and are similar to LC in neonatal skin. The latter have a limited capacity to carry antigens to the local lymph node and initiate antigen-specific immune responses; they trigger immunosuppression and a tolerance response.[137] Double-labeling experiments have shown that the LC in the skin post-DMBA are newly arrived cells similar in morphology and function to neonatal LC (Doherty et al., manuscript in preparation) Thus, the cells found in the epidermis after carcinogen treatment are functionally immature and unable to mount an effective antitumor response. Precisely how these cells drive the generation of immune suppressive mechanisms and suppressor cells awaits clarification.

It is worth noting that UVB also induces similar changes to DMBA in the cutaneous immune system. UVB decreases epidermal LC,[138] enhances cell migration,[139] reduces cluster formation with CD4+ T cells,[140] and generates suppressor cells.[141,142] Other effects of UVB that contribute to immunosuppression and not yet demonstrated with DMBA include DNA damage[143] and the mediating roles of urocanic acid[144,145]and IL-10.[146,147] Hence, both UVB and chemical carcinogens disrupt local immune function via LC, resulting in the generation of tolerance, thus favoring the growth of tumor cells.

## B. Tumor Destruction

Whereas skin tumors express tumor antigens that are recognized by the immune system leading to cell-mediated immunity and tumor destruction, in many cases escape mechanisms prevail allowing tumor cells to grow and evade immune destruction.

Downregulation of MHC class I molecules and modulation of tumor antigen expression provide important mechanisms of tumor escape. Melanoma cell variants that have lost the capacity to express MHC molecules on their surface will avoid destruction by CTL.[148] It is now recognized that components of the endogenous MHC-I processing pathway may be defective, resulting in the failure to express endogenous tumor peptides on the cell surface for T-cell recognition.

The nonclassical HLA class-I molecule HLA-G, known to play a major role in maintaining the immune barrier at the maternofetal interface, may be expressed on cells of malignant melanoma providing a mechanism of escape from immunosurveillance. HLA-G may act by blocking tumor-infiltrating NK cells.[149] In renal transplant recipients, HLA-G may be expressed in nonmelanoma skin cancers — 35% of SCC, 47% of *in situ* carcinoma, and 14% of BCC, but not in benign lesions.[150] The role of HLA-G in tumor escape from the immune response warrants further study.

With modulation of tumor antigens, antibody induces loss of the corresponding antigens from the cell surface, e.g., thymic leukemic cells. For breast cancer this phenomenon has been described in association with escape from antitumor immunity.[151] The role of antigenic modulation in the escape of cutaneous tumors remains unresolved.

Defects in Fas/Fas-ligand (FasL) interaction may play an important role in the development of UV-induced skin cancer and immune evasion. Loss of Fas expression has been shown to correlate with disease progression in melanoma[152] and melanoma cells may evade immune-mediated Fas-triggered apoptosis via a selective blockade of the Fas apoptotic pathway.[153] Interestingly, soluble Fas plasma levels are increased in metastatic melanoma and may be associated with poor prognosis.[154]

While loss of FasL expression in mouse keratinocytes has been shown during UV carcinogenesis,[155] the expression of FasL may contribute to the immune privilege of tumors. As noted already in experimental skin tumor studies, activated CD4+ T cells can be killed by tumor cells using Fas L.[122] Likewise, in lesions of metastatic melanoma, Fas-expressing T-cell infiltrates were proximal to FasL positive tumor cells; *in vivo* rapid tumor formation resulted from the injection of FasL positive mouse melanoma cells in mice.[156] In mycosis fungoides, tumor escape may also involve FasL-mediated apoptosis of infiltrating CD8+ CTL.[157] At this time the Fas/FasL system does not appear to play a major role as a trigger of apoptosis in Kaposi's sarcoma lesions.[158] Clearly, each cutaneous skin tumor requires its own analysis of Fas/FasL expression and its link to metastasis and immune escape.

Tumors may produce blocking factors that inhibit immune recognition of the tumor. These include antigen shedding,[159] which may curtail lymphocytes from recognizing antigen on the surface of the tumor. Shed antigen with antibody in antigen–antibody complexes may also act as blocking factors.[160,161] Such complexes may block the cytotoxic effect of lymphocytes when attached to the target cells and inhibit lymphocytes by attaching to the receptors on their surface via the antigen portion of the complex.[162] Currie and Alexander[163] showed that rat tumors that spontaneously shed antigen are more prone to metastasize than similar tumors that did not. Antibody alone binding to tumor antigens may also curtail tumor cell death. Blocking factors have been found in melanoma, providing a basis for lack of tumor destruction.[164]

A further mechanism of tumor escape may be linked to immunosuppressive factors secreted by the tumor cells or the host. These include prostaglandins[29] and other immunosuppressive factors found in the plasma of cancer patients — suppressive E-receptor factor,[165] normal immunosuppressive protein α-globulin,[166,167] α-1-acid glycoprotein,[168] haptoglobin,[169] α-1-anti-trypsin,[170] and important immune regulatory cytokines.

IL-10 has been shown to be secreted by melanomas[171] providing a potential to downregulate LC function, thereby curtailing cell-mediated immunity. IL-10 production by mycosis fungoides cells may also block dendritic cell maturation leading to tumor tolerance.[172] Interestingly, IL-10 gene polymorphisms and IL-10 production capability may contribute to the development of skin SCC after renal transplantation.[173] Further, IL-10 triggered during transplantation may induce expression of HLA-G already implicated in skin tumor development and its immune escape.[150]

Transforming growth factor-beta (TGF-β) is another immunosuppressive cytokine that can be produced by a range of tumors including carcinomas[174] and has also been shown to be produced in skin following treatment with the tumor promoter TPA.[175] Like IL-10, TGF-β can inhibit the ability of LC to mature into potent allostimulators. Halliday and Le[176] have found that TGF-β from progressively growing skin tumors can inhibit LC migration and keep these cells in an immature form, again providing an important mechanism of tumor escape from the immune system.

An issue of current importance is the status of dendritic cells in human tumors. A recent study on primary cutaneous melanomas concluded that the dendritic cells recruited into lesional and peritumor areas were predominantly immature plasmacytoid and myeloid dentritic cells.[86] Human melanoma cells have been reported to inhibit the differentiation of LC precursors.[177] Hence, defective maturation of primary cutaneous melanoma-associated dentritic cells would result in a lack of T-cell priming, explaining why melanomas may continue to grow despite the presence of infiltrating immune-related cells.[86] Clearly, a detailed assessment is required on the maturation and migratory status of dentritic cells in cutaneous tumors and the precise definition of the factors governing these events.

Finally, in the advanced stages of tumor growth with metastases, nonspecific immunosuppression remains a common clinical problem.

## V. THERAPEUTIC MANIPULATION OF ANTITUMOR IMMUNITY

As the immune system is able to limit the growth of skin cancers, and in some cases cause tumor regression, considerable attention has been focused on the potential of immunotherapy for skin tumor treatment. Multiple different approaches have been investigated for harnessing the immune system as a therapy for skin cancer. In recent years there has been resurgence in interest in this, largely due to the development of more effective biological tools and some promising results. At this stage it still remains largely experimental.

One of the most promising approaches for immunotherapy of skin cancer is the use of dendritic cells. Pioneering work by Knight and colleagues[178] and Grabbe et al.[61,179] showed that dentritic cells were capable of inducing antitumor immunity in animal models. Since then, many other studies have shown that dentritic cells are capable of presenting tumor antigens *in vivo* and of inducing antitumor immunity.[180,181] The development of techniques enabling the large-scale generation of dentritic cells in culture,[182] along with the identification of tumor rejection antigens, particularly for melanoma, made it feasible to investigate whether dentritic cells could be used for immunotherapy of humans.

The first study using human blood monocytes differentiated into dentritic cells in culture was promising, with some patients with melanoma showing objective measures of clinical responses and antitumor immunity.[183] This sparked a large number of different clinical trials into this form of immunotherapy, many with promising results.[184,185] In this approach human blood monocytes were *in vitro* differentiated into dentritic cells in the presence of cytokines, pulsed with tumor antigens, and injected into the patient. While promising, this form of immunotherapy is at early stages of development. Further research is needed to determine the optimal immunization regimen, form of antigen for dentritic cell pulsing, and the optimal stage of maturation of the DC.

Another major development in immunotherapy of skin cancer has been the introduction of pharmacological immune response modifiers. Imiquimod appears to be the first of a new generation of anticancer drugs, which activate antitumor immunity. It binds to Toll-like receptors, inducing migration of dentritic cells from the skin to local lymph nodes[186] and stimulating the production of Th1 cytokines[187] and IFN-$\alpha$.[188] Since clinical trials have demonstrated Imiquimod to be effective for treatment of BCC,[189,190] it has become a standard form of therapy for this type of skin cancer. There are also reports of successful treatment of melanoma,[191,192] actinic keratosis,[193] and SCC.[194] Imiquimod has demonstrated that it is possible to pharmacologically harness the immune system to treat skin cancer, and it is likely that there will be further major advances in this field in the future.

A number of other approaches to augment antitumor immunity, including cytokine gene modification of tumor cells,[195] cytokine injection into patients,[39] vaccination with antigen, and adoptive transfer of cytotoxic T cells,[196] are likely to be beneficial under some circumstances and have all been shown to have some degrees of success.

Improvements in the isolation and characterization of tumor antigens, understanding of the cellular and molecular signals that initiate tumor immunity, and the development of procedures for activating immunity and overcoming tumor evasion of the immune system[197] will lead to improvements in the immunotherapy of skin cancer.

## VI. CONCLUSIONS

The clinical and experimental observations reviewed in this chapter show that immunosurveillance plays a role in host defense against skin tumors. We now recognize that the immune system is much more complex than that envisaged by Burnet[1] when the concept of immunosurveillance was first proposed.

Activation of an effective immune response to tumor antigens requires initial presentation of antigens to T-helper lymphocytes in an MHC-restricted manner. The antigen-presenting cells take up and process antigen for presentation at the cell surface in association with MHC-II glycoproteins. It is only this form of the antigen that the T-helper lymphocyte recognizes. Activation of the T cells is further dependent on co-stimulatory signals, e.g., B7-CD28 interaction and cytokine production. Failure of any of these signals can result in an impaired immune response.

The skin immune system contains its own unique populations of antigen-presenting cells, with the most well characterized the LC. In addition, epidermal cells produce a range of cytokines, which enhance cutaneous immune events. Disruption of this system by chemical carcinogens and UV light results in defective LC function and impaired immunosurveillance. Ultimately, this defective response is associated with impaired T-cell activation. In general, these changes in the skin immune system result in T-suppressor rather than T-helper cell activation and this favors tumor escape rather than immune destruction. By the time many tumors are investigated, the response of the host is already compromised. The manipulation of T-cell activation pathways by cytokines, purified tumor antigens, and gene therapy offers potential approaches to enhance tumor cell destruction.

## REFERENCES


1. Burnet, F.M., The concept of immunological surveillance. *Prog. Exp. Tumour Res.*, 13, 1, 1970.
2. Smith, E.B. and Brysk, M.M., Immunity and skin cancer. *South. Med. J.*, 74, 44, 1981.
3. DePinho, R.A., The age of cancer. *Nature.*, 408, 248, 2000.
4. Marshall, V., Premalignant and malignant skin tumours in immunosuppressed patients. *Transplantation*, 17, 272, 1974.

5. Sheil, A.G. et al., Cancer and survival after cadaveric donor renal transplantation. *Transplant. Proc.*, 11, 1052, 1979.
6. Penn, I., Immunosuppression and skin cancer. *Clin. Plast. Surg.*, 7, 361, 1980.
7. Walder, B.K., Robertson, M.R. and Jeremy, D., Development and incidence of cancer following cyclosporine therapy. *Transplant. Proc.*, 18(Suppl. 1), 210, 1971.
8. Hoxtell, E.O. et al., Incidence of skin carcinoma after renal transplantation. *Arch. Dermatol.*, 113, 436, 1977.
9. Koranda, F.C. et al., Accelerated induction of skin cancers by ultraviolet radiation in hairless mice treated with immunosuppressive agents. *Surg. Forum*, 26, 145, 1975.
10. Hardie, I.R. et al., Skin cancer in Caucasian renal allograft recipients living in a subtropical climate. *Surgery*, 87, 177, 1980.
11. Lutzner, M.A., Immunopathology of papillomavirus-induced warts and skin cancers in immunodepressed and immunosuppressed patients. *Springer Semin. Immunopathol.*, 5, 53, 1982.
12. Claudy, A. and Thivolet, J., Multiple keratoacanthomas: association with deficient cell mediated immunity. *Br. J. Dermatol.*, 93, 593, 1975.
13. Clendenning, W.E. and Auerbach, R., Keratoacanthomata in generalised pustular psoriasis. *Acta Derm. Venereol.*, 43, 68, 1963.
14. Maddin, W.S. and Wood, W.S., Multiple keratoacanthomas and squamous cell carcinomas occurring at psoriatic treatment sites. *J. Cutaneous Pathol*, 6, 96, 1979.
15. Weimar, V.M., Ceilley, R.I., and Goeken, J.A., Aggressive biologic behavior of basal- and squamous-cell cancers in patients with chronic lymphocytic leukemia or chronic lymphocytic lymphoma. *J. Dermatol. Surg. Oncol.*, 5, 609, 1979.
16. Manusow, D. and Weinerman, B.H., Subsequent neoplasia in chronic lymphocytic leukemia. *J. Am. Med. Assoc.*, 232, 267, 1975.
17. Guarda, L.A. et al., Acquired immune deficiency syndrome: postmortem findings. *Am. J. Clin. Pathol*, 81, 549, 1984.
18. Moskowitz, L.B. et al., Frequency and anatomic distribution of lymphadenopathic Kaposi's sarcoma in the acquired immunodeficiency syndrome: an autopsy series. *Hum. Pathol.*, 16, 447, 1985.
19. Muller, H.K., Bucana, C.D., and Kripke, M.L., Antigen presentation in the skin: modulation by u.v. radiation and chemical carcinogens. *Semin. Immunol.*, 4, 205, 1992.
20. Prehn, R.T. and Main, J.M., Immunity to methylcholanthrene-induced sarcomas. *J. Natl. Cancer Inst.*, 18, 769, 1957.
21. Klein, G. et al., Demonstration of resistance against methylcholanthrene-induced sarcomas in the primary autochthonous host. *Cancer Res.*, 20, 1561, 1960.
22. Foley, E.J., Antigenic properties of methylcholanthrene-induced tumours in mice of the strain of origin. *Cancer Res.*, 13, 835, 1953.
23. Baldwin, R.W., Immunity to methylcholanthrene-induced tumours in inbred rats following implantation and regression of implanted tumours. *Br. J. Cancer*, 9, 652, 1955.
24. Koldofsky, P., Tumour-specific transplant antigens, recent results. *Cancer Res.*, 22, 1, 1969.
25. Basombrio, M.A., Search for common antigenicities among twenty-five sarcomas induced by methylcholanthrene. *Cancer Res.*, 30, 2458, 1970.
26. Wortzel, R.D. et al., The complexity of unique tumor-specific antigens, in *Cancer and Immunology*, Kripke, M.L. and Frost, P., Eds., University of Texas Press, Austin, 1986, 161.
27. Rogers, M.J., Tumour-associated antigens of chemically-induced tumours: new complexities. *Immunol. Today*, 5, 167, 1984.
28. Kripke, M.L., T cell suppressors in ultraviolet carcinogenesis. *Transplant. Proc.*, 16, 474, 1974.
29. Kripke, M.L., The immunology of skin cancer. *Symp. Fundam. Cancer Res.*, 38, 113, 1986.
30. Hong, S.R. and Roberts, L.K., Cross-reactive tumor antigens in the skin of mice exposed to subcarcinogenic doses of ultraviolet radiation. *J. Invest. Dermatol.*, 88, 154, 1987.
31. Donawho, C. and Kripke, M.L., Immunogenicity and cross-reactivity of syngeneic murine melanomas. *Cancer Commun.*, 2, 101, 1990.
32. Noonan, F.P. et al., Neonatal sunburn and melanoma in mice. *Nature*, 413, 271, 2001.
33. Urban, J.L. and Schreiber, H., Tumor antigens. *Annu. Rev. Immunol*, 10, 617, 1992.
34. Boon, T., Toward a genetic analysis of tumor rejection antigens. *Adv. Cancer Res.*, 58, 177, 1992.

35. Maryanski, J.L. et al., Immunogenic variants obtained by mutagenesis of mouse mastocytoma P815. III. Clonal analysis of the syngneic cytolytic T lymphocyte response. *Eur. J. Immunol.*, 12, 401, 1982.
36. Carrel, S. and Rimoldi, D., Melanoma-associated antigens. *Eur. J. Cancer*, 29A, 1903, 1993.
37. Urosevic, M. and Dummer, R., Immunotherapy for nonmelanoma skin cancer: does it have a future? *Cancer*, 94, 477, 2002.
38. Black, A.P. and Ogg, G.S., The role of p53 in the immunobiology of cutaneous squamous cell carcinoma. *Clin. Exp. Immunol.*, 132, 379, 2003.
39. Rosenberg, S.A., Progress in human tumour immunology and immunotherapy. *Nature*, 411, 380, 2001.
40. Chomez, P. et al., An overview of the MAGE gene family with the identification of all human members of the family. *Cancer Res.*, 61, 5544, 2001.
41. Storkus, W.J. et al., Identification of human melanoma peptides recognized by class I restricted tumor infiltrating T lymphocytes. *J. Immunol*, 151, 3719, 1993.
42. Slingluff, C.L., Jr., et al., Recognition of human melanoma cells by HLA-A2.1-restricted cytotoxic T lymphocytes is mediated by at least six shared peptide epitopes. *J. Immunol*, 150, 2955, 1993.
43. Topalian, S.L. et al., Human $CD4^+$ T cells specifically recognize a shared melanoma-associated antigen encoded by the tyrosinase gene. *Proc. Natl. Acad. Sci. U.S.A.*, 91, 9461, 1994.
44. Degiovanni, G. et al., Antigens recognized on a melanoma cell line by autologous cytolytic T lymphocytes are also expressed on freshly collected tumor cells. *Eur. J. Immunol*, 20, 1865, 1990.
45. van der Bruggen, P. et al., A gene encoding an antigen recognized by cytolytic T lymphocytes on a human melanoma. *Science*, 254, 1643, 1991.
46. Traversari, C. et al., A nonapeptide encoded by human gene MAGE-1 is recognized on HLA-A1 by cytolytic T lymphocytes directed against tumor antigen MZ2-E. *J. Exp. Med.*, 176, 1453, 1992.
47. Oaks, M.K., Hanson, J.P., Jr., and O'Malley, D.P., Molecular cytogenetic mapping of the human melanoma antigen (MAGE) gene family to chromosome region Xq27-qter: implications for MAGE immunotherapy. *Cancer Res.*, 54, 1627, 1994.
48. Becker, J.C., Gillitzer, R., and Brocker, E.B., A member of the melanoma antigen-encoding gene (MAGE) family is expressed in human skin during wound healing. *Int. J. Cancer*, 58, 346, 1994.
49. De Smet, C. et al., Sequence and expression pattern of the human MAGE2 gene. *Immunogenetics*, 39, 121, 1994.
50. Gaugler, B. et al., Human gene MAGE-3 codes for an antigen recognized on a melanoma by autologous cytolytic T lymphocytes. *J. Exp. Med.*, 179, 921, 1994.
51. Brichard, V. et al., The tyrosinase gene codes for an antigen recognized by autologous cytolytic T lymphocytes on HLA-A2 melanomas. *J. Exp. Med.*, 178, 489, 1993.
52. Coulie, P.G. et al., A new gene coding for a differentiation antigen recognized by autologous cytolytic T lymphocytes on HLA-A2 melanomas [see comments]. *J. Exp. Med.*, 180, 35, 1994.
53. Kawakami, Y. et al., Identification of a human melanoma antigen recognized by tumor-infiltrating lymphocytes associated with *in vivo* tumor rejection. *Proc. Natl. Acad. Sci. U.S.A.*, 91, 6458, 1994.
54. Bakker, A.B. et al., Melanocyte lineage-specific antigen gp100 is recognized by melanoma-derived tumor-infiltrating lymphocytes. *J. Exp. Med.*, 179, 1005, 1994.
55. Wang, R.F. et al., Identification of a gene encoding a melanoma tumor antigen recognized by HLA-A31-restricted tumor-infiltrating lymphocytes. *J. Exp. Med.*, 181, 799, 1995.
56. Salazar-Onfray, F. et al., Synthetic peptides derived from the melanocyte-stimulating hormone receptor MC1R can stimulate HLA-A2-restricted cytotoxic T lymphocytes that recognize naturally processed peptides on human melanoma cells. *Cancer Res.*, 57, 4348, 1997.
57. Pardoll, D.M., Tumour antigens. A new look for the 1990s [news; comment]. *Nature*, 369, 357, 1994.
58. Palmowski, M. et al., The use of HLA class I tetramers to design a vaccination strategy for melanoma patients. *Immunol. Rev.*, 188, 155, 2002.
59. Pitot, H.C. and Dragan, Y.P., Facts and theories concerning the mechanisms of carcinogenesis. *FASEB J.*, 5, 2280, 1991.
60. Young, M.R. et al., Tumor-derived cytokines induce bone marrow suppressor cells that mediate immunosuppression through transforming growth factor beta. *Cancer Immunol. Immunother.*, 35, 14, 1992.
61. Grabbe, S. et al., Tumor antigen presentation by murine epidermal cells. *J. Immunol.*, 146, 3656, 1991.
62. Grabbe, S., Bruvers, S., and Granstein, R.D., Effects of immunomodulatory cytokines on the presentation of tumor-associated antigens by epidermal Langerhans cells. *J. Invest. Dermatol.*, 99, 66S, 1992.

63. Cohen, P.J. et al., Murine epidermal Langerhans cells and splenic dendritic cells present tumor-associated antigens to primed T cells. *Eur. J. Immunol.*, 24, 315, 1994.
64. Heufler, C., Koch, F., and Schuler, G., Granulocyte/macrophage colony-stimulating factor and interleukin 1 mediate the maturation of murine epidermal Langerhans cells into potent immunostimulatory dendritic cells. *J. Exp. Med.*, 167, 700, 1988.
65. Koch, F. et al., Tumor necrosis factor alpha maintains the viability of murine epidermal Langerhans cells in culture, but in contrast to granulocyte/macrophage colony-stimulating factor, without inducing their functional maturation. *J. Exp. Med.*, 171, 159, 1990.
66. McArdle, J.P. et al., Quantitative assessment of Langerhans cells in actinic keratosis, Bowen's disease, keratoacanthoma, squamous cell carcinoma and basal cell carcinoma. *Pathology*, 18, 212, 1986.
67. McArdle, J.P. and Muller, H.K., Quantitative assessment of Langerhans' cells in human cervical intraepithelial neoplasia and wart virus infection. *Am. J. Obstet. Gynecol.*, 154, 509, 1986.
68. McBride, W.H., Phenotype and functions of intratumoral macrophages. *Biochim. Biophys. Acta*, 865, 27, 1986.
69. Zeid, N.A. and Muller, H.K. S100 positive dendritic cells in human lung tumors associated with cell differentiation and enhanced survival. *Pathology*, 25, 338, 1993.
70. Becker, Y., Dendritic cell activity against primary tumors: an overview. *In Vivo*, 7, 187, 1993.
71. Tefany, F.J. et al., Immunocytochemical analysis of the cellular infiltrate in primary regressing and non-regressing malignant melanoma. *J. Invest. Dermatol.*, 97, 197, 1991.
72. Hunt, M.J. et al., Regression in basal cell carcinoma: an immunohistochemical analysis. *Br. J. Dermatol.*, 130, 1, 1994.
73. Patel, A. et al., Evidence that regression in keratoacanthoma is immunologically mediated: a comparison with squamous cell carcinoma. *Br. J. Dermatol.*, 131, 789, 1994.
74. Bergfelt, L., Bucana, C., and Kripke, M.L., Alterations in Langerhans cells during growth of transplantable murine tumors. *J. Invest. Dermatol.*, 91, 129, 1988.
75. Halliday, G.M., Reeve, V.E., and Barnetson, R.S., Langerhans cell migration into ultraviolet light-induced squamous skin tumors is unrelated to anti-tumor immunity. *J. Invest. Dermatol.*, 97, 830, 1991.
76. Halliday, G.M., Lucas, A.D., and Barnetson, R.S., Control of Langerhans' cell density by a skin tumour-derived cytokine. *Immunology*, 77, 13, 1992.
77. Lucas, A.D. and Halliday, G.M., Progressor but not regressor skin tumours inhibit Langerhans' cell migration from epidermis to local lymph nodes. *Immunology*, 97, 130, 1999.
78. Byrne, S.N. and Halliday, G.M., Phagocytosis by dendritic cells rather than MHC II$^{high}$ macrophages is associated with skin tumour regression. *Int. J. Cancer.*, 106, 736, 2003.
79. Svane, I.M. et al., Clinical application of dendritic cells in cancer vaccination therapy. *APMIS*, 111, 818, 2003.
80. Heath, W.R. and Carbone, F.R., Cytotoxic T lymphocyte activation by cross-priming. *Curr. Opin. Immunol.*, 11, 314, 1999.
81. Heath, W.R. and Carbone, F.R., Cross-presentation, dendritic cells, tolerance and immunity. *Annu. Rev. Immunol.*, 19, 47, 2001.
82. Kovacsovics-Bankowski, M. and Rock, K.L., Presentation of exogenous antigens by macrophages: analysis of major histocompatibility complex class I and II presentation and regulation by cytokines. *Eur. J. Immunol.*, 24, 2421, 1994.
83. Shen, Z. et al., Cloned dendritic cells can present exogenous antigens on both MHC class I and class II molecules. *J. Immunol.*, 158, 2723, 1997.
84. Zou, W. et al., Stromal-derived factor-1 in human tumors recruits and alters the function of plasmacytoid precursor dendritic cells. *Nat. Med.*, 7, 1339, 2001.
85. Salio, M. et al., Plasmacytoid dendritic cells prime IFN-gamma-secreting melanoma-specific CD8 lymphocytes and are found in primary melanoma lesions. *Eur. J. Immunol.*, 33, 1052, 2003.
86. Vermi, W. et al., Recruitment of immature plasmacytoid dendritic cells (plasmacytoid monocytes) and myeloid dendritic cells in primary cutaneous melanomas. *J. Pathol.*, 200, 255, 2003.
87. Colonna, M., Krug, A.. and Cella, M., Interferon-producing cells: on the front line in immune responses against pathogens. *Curr. Opin. Immunol.*, 14, 373, 2002.
88. Lill, P.H. and Fortner, G.W., Identification and cytotoxic reactivity of inflammatory cells recovered from progressing or regressing syngeneic UV-induced murine tumours. *J. Immunol.*, 121, 1854, 1978.
89. Godfrey, D.I. et al., NKT cells: facts, functions and fallacies. *Immunol. Today*, 21, 573, 2000.

90. Smyth, M.J. et al., Differential tumor surveillance by natural killer (NK) and NKT cells. *J. Exp. Med.*, 191, 661, 2000.
91. Russell, J.H. and Ley, T.J., Lymphocyte-mediated cytotoxicity. *Annu. Rev. Immunol.*, 20, 323, 2002.
92. Wang, R. et al., CD95-dependent bystander lysis caused by $CD4^+$ T helper 1 effectors. *J. Immunol.*, 157, 2961, 1996.
93. Kagi, D. et al., Molecular mechanisms of lymphocyte-mediated cytotoxicity and their role in immunological protection and pathogenesis *in vivo*. *Annu. Rev. Immunol.*, 14, 207, 1996.
94. Browne, K.A. et al., Cytosolic delivery of granzyme B by bacterial toxins: evidence that endosomal disruption, in addition to transmembrane pore formation, is an important function of perforin. *Mol. Cell. Biol.*, 19, 8604, 1999.
95. Tschopp, J. et al., Phosphorylcholine acts as a $Ca^{2+}$-dependent receptor molecule for lymphocyte perforin. *Nature*, 337, 272, 1989.
96. Podack, E.R., How to induce involuntary suicide: the need for dipeptidyl peptidase I. *Proc. Natl. Acad. Sci. U.S.A.*, 96, 8312, 1999.
97. Motyka, B. et al., Mannose 6-phosphate/insulin-like growth factor II receptor is a death receptor for granzyme B during cytotoxic T cell-induced apoptosis. *Cell*, 103, 491, 2000.
98. Darmon, A.J., Nicholson, D.W., and Bleackley, R.C., Activation of the apoptotic protease CPP32 by cytotoxic T-cell-derived granzyme B. *Nature*, 377, 446, 1995.
99. Pinkoski, M.J. et al., Granzyme B-mediated apoptosis proceeds predominantly through a Bcl-2-inhibitable mitochondrial pathway. *J. Biol. Chem.*, 276, 12060, 2001.
100. Sheil, A.G.R., Development of malignancy following renal transplantation in Australia and New-Zealand. *Transplant. Proc.*, 24, 1275, 1992.
101. Jensen, P. et al., Skin cancer in kidney and heart transplant recipients and different long-term immunosuppressive therapy regimens. *J. Am. Acad. Dermatol.*, 40, 177, 1999.
102. Caforio, A.L.P. et al., Skin cancer in heart transplant recipients — risk factor analysis and relevance of immunosuppressive therapy. *Circulation*, 102, 222, 2000.
103. Fortina, A.B. et al., Skin cancer in heart transplant recipients: Frequency and risk factor analysis. *J. Heart Lung Transplant.*,19, 249, 2000.
104. Abgrall, S. et al., Tumors in organ transplant recipients may give clues to their control by immunity. *Anticancer Res.*, 22, 3597, 2002.
105. Lindelof, B. et al., Incidence of skin cancer in 5356 patients following organ transplantation. *Br. J. Dermatol.*, 143, 513, 2000.
106. Penn, I. Post-transplant malignancy — the role of immunosuppression [review]. *Drug Saf.*, 23, 101, 2000.
107. Kavouni, A., Shibu, M., and Carver, N., Squamous cell carcinoma arising in transplanted skin. *Clin. Exp. Dermatol.*, 25, 302, 2000.
108. Elder, G.J., Hersey, P., and Branley, P., Remission of transplanted melanoma — clinical course and tumour cell characterisation. *Clin. Transplant.*, 11, 565, 1997.
109. Halliday, G.M. and Barnetson, R.S.C., Spontaneous regression, in *Malignant Tumors of the Skin*, Edelson, R.L., Ed., Arnold, London, 1999, 411.
110. Menzies, S.W. and McCarthy, W.H., Complete regression of primary cutaneous malignant melanoma. *Arch. Surg.*, 132, 553, 1997.
111. Milton, G., Shaw, H., and McCarthy, W., Occult primary malignant melanoma: factors influencing survival. *Br. J. Surg.*, 64, 805, 1985.
112. Hunt, M.J. et al., Regression in basal cell carcinoma — an immunohistochemical analysis. *Br. J. Dermatol.*, 130, 1, 1994.
113. Halliday, G.M. et al., Spontaneous regression of human melanoma/non-melanoma skin cancer: association with infiltrating $CD4^+$ T cells. *World J. Surg.*, 19, 352, 1995.
114. Thomas, W.D. and Hersey, P., CD4 T cells kill melanoma cells by mechanisms that are independent of Fas (CD95). *Int. J. Cancer*, 75, 384, 1998.
115. Thomas, W.D. and Hersey, P., TNF-related apoptosis-inducing ligand (Trail) induces apoptosis in Fas ligand-resistant melanoma cells and mediates CD4 T cell killing of target cells. *J. Immunol.*, 161, 2195, 1998.
116. Lowes, M.A. et al., T helper 1 cytokine mRNA is increased in spontaneously regressing primary melanomas. *J. Invest. Dermatol.*, 108, 914, 1997.

117. Wong, D.A. et al., Cytokine profiles in spontaneously regressing basal cell carcinomas. *Br. J. Dermatol.*, 143, 91, 2000.
118. Ferradini, L. et al., Analysis of T-cell receptor variability in tumor-infiltrating lymphocytes from a human regressive melanoma — evidence for *in situ* T-cell clonal expansion. *J. Clin. Invest.*, 91, 1183, 1993.
119. Mackensen, A. et al., Evidence for *in situ* amplification of cytotoxic T-lymphocytes with antitumor activity in a human regressive melanoma. *Cancer Res.*, 53, 3569, 1993.
120. Saleh, F.H. et al., Primary melanoma tumour regression associated with an immune response to the tumour-associated antigen Melan-A/MART-1. *Int. J. Cancer*, 94, 551, 2001.
121. Lowes, M.A. et al., Regression of melanoma, but not keratoacanthoma, is associated with increased HLA-B22 and decreased HLA-B27 and HLA-DR1. *Melanoma Res.*, 9, 539, 1999.
122. Byrne, S.N. and Halliday, G.M., High levels of Fas ligand and MHC class II in the absence of CD80 or CD86 expression and a decreased $CD4^+$ T cell infiltration, enables murine skin tumours to progress. *Cancer Immunol. Immunother.*, 52, 396, 2003.
123. Halliday, G.M., MacCarrick, G.R., and Muller, H.K., Tumour promotors but not initiators deplete Langerhans cells from murine epidermis. *Br. J. Cancer*, 56, 328, 1987.
124. Muller, H.K., Halliday, G.M., and Knight, B.A., Carcinogen-induced depletion of cutaneous Langerhans cells. *Br. J. Cancer*, 52, 81, 1985.
125. Halliday, G.M. et al., Suppressor cell activation and enhanced skin allograft survival after tumor promotor but not initiator induced depletion of cutaneous Langerhans cells. *J. Invest. Dermatol.*, 90, 293, 1988.
126. Zeid, N.A. and Muller, H.K., Tobacco smoke condensate cutaneous carcinogenesis: changes in Langerhans' cells and tumour regression. *Int. J. Exp. Pathol*, 76, 75, 1995.
127. Woods, G.M. et al., Chemical carcinogens and antigens induce immune suppression via Langerhans cell depletion. *Immunology*, 88, 134, 1996.
128. Dandie, G.W., Ragg, S.J., and Muller, H.K., Migration of Langerhans cells from carcinogen-treated sheep skin. *J. Invest. Dermatol.*, 99, 51S, 1992.
129. Muller, H.K. et al., Langerhans cell alterations in cutaneous carcinogenesis. *In Vivo*, 7, 293, 1993.
130. Dandie, G.W. et al., The migration of Langerhans cells into and out of lymph nodes draining normal, carcinogen and antigen treated sheep skin. *Immunol. Cell Biol.*, 72, 79, 1994.
131. Ragg, S.J. et al., Langerhans cell migration patterns from sheep skin following topical application of carcinogens. *Int. J. Exp. Pathol.*, 75, 23, 1994.
132. Halliday, G.M. and Muller, H.K., Sensitization through carcinogen induced Langerhans cell deficient skin activates long lived suppressor cells for both cellular and humoral immunity. *Cell. Immunol.*, 109, 206, 1987.
133. Halliday, G.M. and Muller, H.K., Induction of tolerance via skin depleted of Langerhans cells by a chemical carcinogen. *Cell. Immunol.*, 99, 220, 1986.
134. Ragg, S.J. et al., Abrogation of afferent lymph dendritic cell function after cutaneously applied chemical carcinogens. *Cell. Immunol.*, 162, 80, 1995.
135. Ragg, S.J. et al., Failure of carcinogen-altered dendritic cells to initiate T cell proliferation is associated with reduced IL-1 beta secretion. *Cell. Immunol*, 178, 17, 1997.
136. Woods, G.M. et al., Carcinogen-modified dendritic cells induce immunosuppression by incomplete T-cell activation resulting from impaired antigen uptake and reduced CD86 expression. *Immunology*, 99, 16, 2000.
137. Dewar, A.L. et al., Acquisition of immune function during the development of the Langerhans cell network in neonatal mice. *Immunology*, 103, 61, 2001.
138. Toews, G.B. et al., Epidermal Langerhans cell density determines whether contact hypersensitivity or unresponsiveness follows skin-painting with DNFB. *J. Immunol.*, 124, 445, 1980.
139. Dandie, G.W. et al., Migration of Langerhans cells and gammadelta dendritic cells from UV-B-irradiated sheep skin. *Immunol. Cell Biol.*, 79, 41, 2001.
140. Muller, H.K. et al., Ultraviolet irradiation of murine skin alters cluster formation between lymph node dendritic cells and specific T lymphocytes. *Cell. Immunol*, 157, 263, 1994.
141. Okamoto, H. and Kripke, M.L., Effector and suppressor circuits of the immune response are activated *in vivo* by different mechanisms. *Proc. Natl. Acad. Sci. U.S.A.*, 84, 3841, 1987.
142. Noonan, F.P. and De Fabo, E.C., Immune suppression by ultraviolet radiation and its role in ultraviolet radiation induced carcinogenesis in mice. *Aust. J. Derm.*, 26, 4, 1985.

143. Kripke, M.L. et al., Pyrimidine dimers in DNA initiate systemic immunosuppression in UV-irradiated mice. *Proc. Natl. Acad. Sci. U.S.A.*, 89, 7516, 1992.
144. Noonan, F.P., De Fabo, E.C., and Morrison, H., *cis*-Urocanic acid, a product formed by ultraviolet B irradiation, initiates an antigen presentation defect in splenic dendritic cells *in vivo*. *J. Invest. Dermatol.*, 90, 92, 1988.
145. Noonan, F.P. et al., Mechanism of systemic immune suppression by UV irradiation *in vivo*. II. The UV effects on number and morphology of epidermal Langerhans cells and the UV-induced suppression of contact hypersensitivity have different wavelength dependencies. *J. Immunol.*, 132, 2408, 1984.
146. Rivas, J.M. and Ullrich, S.E., Systemic suppression of delayed-type hypersensitivity by supernatants from UV-irradiated keratinocytes. An essential role for keratinocyte-derived IL-10. *J. Immunol.*, 149, 3865, 1992.
147. Rivas, J.M. and Ullrich, S.E., The role of IL-4, IL-10, and TNF-alpha in the immune suppression induced by ultraviolet radiation. *J. Leukocyte Biol.*, 56, 769, 1994.
148. Boon, T., Gajewski, T.F., and Coulie, P.G., From defined human tumor antigens to effective immunization. *Immunol. Today*, 16, 334, 1995.
149. Ugurel, S., Reinhold, U., and Tilgen, W., HLA-G in melanoma: a new strategy to escape from immunosurveillance? *Onkologie*, 25, 129, 2002.
150. Aractingi, S. et al., Selective expression of HLA-G in malignant and premalignant skin specimens in kidney transplant recipients. *Int. J. Cancer*, 106, 232, 2003.
151. Chatenoud, L. and Bach, J.-F. Antigenic modulation — a major effector mechanism of antibody action. *Immunol. Today*, 5, 20, 1984.
152. Owen-Schaub, L.B. et al., Fas and Fas ligand interactions suppress melanoma lung metastasis. *J. Exp. Med.*, 188, 1717, 1998.
153. Ferrarini, M. et al., Blockade of the Fas-triggered intracellular signaling pathway in human melanomas is circumvented by cytotoxic lymphocytes. *Int. J. Cancer*, 81, 573, 1999.
154. Redondo, P. et al., Fas and Fas ligand: expression and soluble circulating levels in cutaneous malignant melanoma. *Br. J. Dermatol.*, 147, 80, 2002.
155. Ouhtit, A. et al., Loss of Fas-ligand expression in mouse keratinocytes during UV carcinogenesis. *Am. J. Pathol.*, 157, 1975, 2000.
156. Hahne, M. et al., Melanoma cell expression of Fas(Apo-1/CD95) ligand: implications for tumor immune escape.[comment]. *Science*, 274, 1363, 1996.
157. Ni, X. et al., Fas ligand expression by neoplastic T lymphocytes mediates elimination of $CD8^+$ cytotoxic T lymphocytes in mycosis fungoides: a potential mechanism of tumor immune escape? *Clin. Cancer Res.*, 7, 2682, 2001.
158. Fernandez-Figueras, M.T. et al., Absence of Fas (CD95) and FasL (CD95L) immunohistochemical expression suggests Fas/FasL-mediated apoptotic signal is not relevant in cutaneous Kaposi's sarcoma lesions. *J. Cutaneous Pathol.*, 26, 417, 1999.
159. Currie, G.A. and Basham, C., Serum mediated inhibition of the immunological reactions of the patient to his own tumour: a possible role for circulating antigen. *Br. J. Cancer*, 26, 427, 1972.
160. Hellstrom, I. and Hellstrom, K.E., Studies on cellular immunity and its serum mediated inhibition in Moloney-virus-induced mouse sarcomas. *Int. J. Cancer*, 4, 587, 1969.
161. Sjogren, H.O. et al., Suggestive evidence that the "blocking antibodies" of tumor-bearing individuals may be antigen–antibody complexes. *Proc. Natl. Acad. Sci. U.S.A.*, 68, 1372, 1971.
162. Bansal, S.C., Bansal, B.L., and Boland, J.P. Blocking and unblocking serum factors in neoplasia. *Curr. Top. Microbiol. Immunol*, 75, 45, 1976.
163. Currie, G.A. and Alexander, P., Spontaneous shedding of TSTA by viable sarcoma cells: its possible role in facilitating metastatic spread. *Br. J. Cancer*, 29, 72, 1974.
164. Murray, E. et al., Analysis of serum blocking factors against leukocyte dependent antibody in melanoma patients. *Int. J. Cancer*, 21, 578, 1978.
165. Oh, S.K. et al., Role of a SER immune suppressor in immune surveillance. *Immunology*, 64, 73, 1988.
166. Glaser, M., Ofek, I., and Nelken, D., Inhibition of plaque formation, rosette formation and phagocytosis by alpha globulin. *Immunology*, 23, 205, 1972.
167. Cooperband, S.R. et al., Transformation of human lymphocytes: inhibition by homologous alpha globulin. *Science*, 159, 1243, 1968.

168. Bennett, M. and Schmid, K., Immunosuppression by human plasma alpha 1-acid glycoprotein: importance of the carbohydrate moiety. *Proc. Natl. Acad. Sci. U.S.A.*, 77, 6109, 1980.
169. Baseler, M.W. and Burrell, R., Purification of haptoglobin and its effects on lymphocyte and alveolar macrophage responses. *Inflammation*, 7, 387, 1983.
170. Breit, S.N. et al., The role of alpha 1-antitrypsin deficiency in the pathogenesis of immune disorders. *Clin. Immunol. Immunopathol.*, 35, 363, 1985.
171. Chen, Q.Y. et al., Production of IL-10 by melanoma cells: examination of its role in immunosuppression mediated by melanoma. *Int. J. Cancer*, 56, 755, 1994.
172. Luftl, M. et al., Dendritic cells and apoptosis in mycosis fungoides. *Br. J. Dermatol.*, 147, 1171, 2002.
173. Alamartine, E. et al., Interleukin-10 promoter polymorphisms and susceptibility to skin squamous cell carcinoma after renal transplantation.[comment]. *J. Invest. Dermatol.*, 120, 99, 2003.
174. Alleva, D.G., Burger, C.J., and Elgert, K.D., Tumor-induced regulation of suppressor macrophage nitric oxide and TNF-alpha production. Role of tumor-derived IL-10, TGF-beta, and prostaglandin E2. *J. Immunol.*, 153, 1674, 1994.
175. Akhurst, R.J., Fee, F., and Balmain, A., Localised production of TGF-b mRNA in tumour promoter-stimulated mouse epidermis. *Nature*, 331, 363, 1988.
176. Halliday, G.M. and Le, S., Transforming growth factor-beta produced by progressor tumors inhibits, while IL-10 produced by regressor tumors enhances, Langerhans cell migration from skin. *Int. Immunol.*, 13, 1147, 2001.
177. Berthier-Vergnes, O. et al., Human melanoma cells inhibit the earliest differentiation steps of human Langerhans cell precursors but failed to affect the functional maturation of epidermal Langerhans cells. *Br. J. Cancer*, 85, 1944, 2001.
178. Knight, S.C. et al., Influence of dendritic cells on tumor growth. *Proc. Natl. Acad. Sci. U.S.A.*, 82, 4495, 1985.
179. Grabbe, S. et al., Tumor antigen presentation by epidermal antigen-presenting cells in the mouse: modulation by granulocyte-macrophage colony-stimulating factor, tumor necrosis factor alpha, and ultraviolet radiation. *J. Leukocyte Biol.*, 52, 209, 1992.
180. Cavanagh, L.L. et al., Epidermal Langerhans cell induction of immunity against an ultraviolet-induced skin tumour. *Immunology*, 87, 475, 1996.
181. Porgador, A., Snyder, D., and Gilboa, E., Induction of antitumor immunity using bone marrow-generated dendritic cells. *J. Immunol.*, 156, 2918, 1996.
182. Inaba, K. et al., Generation of large numbers of dendritic cells from mouse bone marrow cultures supplemented with granulocyte/macrophage colony-stimulating factor. *J. Exp. Med.*, 176, 1693, 1992.
183. Nestle, F.O. et al., Vaccination of melanoma patients with peptide- or tumor lysate-pulsed dendritic cells. *Nat. Med.*, 4, 328, 1998.
184. Nestle, F.O., Banchereau, J., and Hart, D., Dendritic cells: On the move from bench to bedside. *Nat. Med.*, 7, 761, 2001.
185. O'Rourke, M.G. et al., Durable complete clinical responses in a phase I/II trial using an autologous melanoma cell/dendritic cell vaccine. *Cancer Immunol. Immunother.*, 52, 387, 2003.
186. Suzuki, H. et al., Imiquimod, a topical immune response modifier, induces migration of Langerhans cells. *J. Invest. Dermatol.*, 114, 135, 2000.
187. Garland, S.M. Imiquimod. *Curr. Opin. Infect. Dis.*, 16, 85, 2003.
188. Witt, P.L. et al., Phase-I trial of an oral immunomodulator and interferon inducer in cancer patients. *Cancer Res.*, 53, 5176, 1993.
189. Geisse, J.K. et al., Imiquimod 5% cream for the treatment of superficial basal cell carcinoma: a double-blind, randomized, vehicle-controlled study. *J. Am. Acad. Dermatol.*, 47, 390, 2002.
190. Marks, R. et al., Imiquimod 5% cream in the treatment of superficial basal cell carcinoma: results of a multicenter 6-week dose-response trial. *J. Am. Acad. Dermatol.*, 44, 807, 2001.
191. Wolf, I.H. et al., Topical imiquimod in the treatment of metastatic melanoma to skin. *Arch. Dermatol.*, 139, 273, 2003.
192. Ugurel, S. et al., Topical imiquimod eradicates skin metastases of malignant melanoma but fails to prevent rapid lymphogenous metastatic spread. *Br. J. Dermatol.*, 147, 621, 2002.
193. Stockfleth, E. et al., Successful treatment of actinic keratosis with imiquimod cream 5%: a report of six cases. *Br. J. Dermatol.*, 144, 1050, 2001.

194. Orengo, I., Rosen, T., and Guill, C.K., Treatment of squamous cell carcinoma *in situ* of the penis with 5% imuquimod cream: a case report. *J. Am. Acad. Dermatol.*, 47, S225, 2002.
195. Ellem, K.A.O. et al., A case report — immune responses and clinical course of the first human use of granulocyte/macrophage-colony-stimulating-factor-transduced autologous melanoma cells for immunotherapy. *Cancer Immunol. Immunother.*, 44, 10, 1997.
196. Rosenberg, S.A. et al., Immunizing patients with metastatic melanoma using recombinant adenoviruses encoding MART-1 or gp100 melanoma antigens. *J. Natl. Cancer Inst.*, 90, 1894, 1998.
197. Hersey, P., Impediments to successful immunotherapy [review]. *Pharmacol. Ther.*, 81, 111, 1999.

# Part V

## Immunodermatological Diseases

# 23 Some Congenital Immunodeficiencies and Their Dermatological Manifestations

*J. Henk Sillevis Smitt*

## CONTENTS



0-8493-1959-5/05/$0.00+$1.50

## I. INTRODUCTION

The skin is not only a physical and mechanical barrier, but also constitutes an immunological line of defense. This is further substantiated by the concept of the skin immune system (SIS). Congenital immunodeficiencies comprise a great number of serious and rather rare diseases. They are usually recognized by clinical symptoms (Table 23.1),[1] in combination with abnormalities of cellular and/or humoral immunity as well as by biochemical parameters (Table 23.2 and Table 23.3).[2,3] In a growing number of primary immunodeficiency diseases the abnormal gene that corresponds to the particular deficiency has been identified. In recent years long-term survival of patients with congenital immunodeficiencies has been described by the use of hematopoietic stem cell transplantations.[4]

The skin, as an immunological line of defense, is one of the organs in which an immunodeficiency presents rather early in life.

## II. CLASSIFICATION OF THE PRIMARY IMMUNODEFICIENCIES

The primary immunodeficiencies are subdivided into several groups (Table 23.2 and Table 23.3).[2,3] For details concerning the different diseases belonging to each group, see References 5 and 6. To show the impact of immunodeficiencies on the skin, in this chapter some immunodeficiencies are dealt with in more detail.

**TABLE 23.1**
**Clinical Features in Immunodeficiencies**

**A. Features frequently present and highly suspicious:**
1. Chronic infection (caused by inadequate clearing or incomplete response to treatment)
2. Recurrent infection (more than expected)
3. Unusual infecting agents

**B. Features frequently present and moderately suspicious:**
1. Skin rash (eczema, candidiasis, etc.)
2. Diarrhea (chronic)
3. Failure to thrive
4. Hepatosplenomegaly
5. Evidence of autoimmunity

**C. Features associated with specific immunodeficiency disorders:**
1. Ataxia
2. Teleangiectasia
3. Short-limbed dwarfism
4. Cartilage-hair hypoplasia
5. Idiopathic endocrinopathy
6. Partial albinism
7. Thrombocytopenia
8. Eczema
9. Tetany

*Source:* Modified from Amman, A. and Wara, D., *Curr. Probl. Pediatr.*, 5, 3, 1975.

**TABLE 23.2**
**Primary Immunodeficiencies Associated with Known Genetic Lesions[2]**

1. Combined ID (B and T cells):
    - Severe Combined Immunodeficiency Disease (SCID)
        - Defective cytokine signaling [IL2RG (cytokine receptor common gamma chain), ILRA (IL2R(eceptor)A(lpha)), IL7RA (IL7R(eceptor)A(lpha)), JAK3 (JA(nus)K(inase)3)]
        - Defective T-cell receptor signaling [PTPRC (P(rotein)T(yrosinase)- P(hoshatase)R(eceptor)C(D45)), CD3G(amma), CD3E(psilon), ZAP70 Z(eta)A(ssociated)P(rotein)70)]
        - Defective receptor gene recombination [RAG1 (R(ecombinase)A(ctivating) G(ene)1), RAG2]
        - Defective nucleotide salvage pathway [ADA (A(denosine)D(e)A(minase)), PNP (P(urine)N(ucleotide)P(hosphorylase)]
        - Defective MHC class I expression [TAP1 (T(ransporters of)A(ntigenic) P(eptides)1), TAP2)
        - Defective MHC class II transcription [MHCIIT(rans)A(ctivator), RFXANK, RFX5, RFXAP)
        - Others [DCCRE1C (ARTEMIS), WHN [W(inged)H(elix)N(ude transcription factor)]
    - DiGeorge syndrome [del 22q11]
    - Ataxia teleangiectasia group [ATM(utated)RE11A]
    - Wiskott–Aldrich syndrome [WASP(rotein)]
    - Hyper-IgM syndrome [TNFSF5(T(umor)N(ecrosis)F(actor)S(uperfamily member)5), TNFR(eceptor)SF5, IKBKG (I(nhibitor)K(appa)BK(inase)G(amma)]
    - X-linked lymphoprolerifative syndrome [SH2D1A] (a signal transducing protein)
2. Antibody deficiencies (B cells):
    - The agammaglobulinemias [BTK (B(ruton)T(yrosine)K(inase)), IGHM (IGH(eavy chain)M), CD79A(Ig-alpha component B-cell-receptor), CD179B(components of surrogate light chain), BLNK (B-cell linker protein)]
    - Hyper-IgM syndrome, autosomal recessive [AICDA (A(ctivation)I(nduced)C(ytidine) D(e)A(minase))]
3. Cellular deficiencies:
    - Interferon gamma interleukin 12 axis [IFNGR1 (I(interF(ero)N G(amma)R(eceptor)1(alpha)), IFNGR2(beta), IL12B(eta), IL12R(eceptor)B(eta)1, STAT1 (S(ignal)T(ransducing)AT1)]
    - Autoimmune polyglandular syndrome type 1 [AIRE (A(uto)I(mmune)RE(gulator))]
    - Defective NK function [CD16 deficiency] [FcG(amma)RIIIa]
4. Defects of phagocytic function:
    - Chronic granulomatous disease [CYBA (CY(tochrome)BA(alpha)), CYBB(eta), NCF1 (N(eutrophil)C(ytosolic)F(actor)1), NCF2]
    - Chronic granulomatous disease variant [RAC2]
    - Leukocyte adhesion deficiency [ITBG2 (I(n)T(e)G(rin)B(eta)2), FLJ11320])
    - Chediak Higashi syndrome [LYST (LYS(osomal)T(ransport)protein)]
    - Neutrophil specific granule deficiency [CEBPE (a transcription factor)]
    - Cyclic neutropenia [ELA(stase)2]
    - Congenital agranulocytosis (Kostmann syndrome) [G-CSF3R (G(ranulocyte)-C(olony)S(timulating)F(actor)3R]
5. Complement defects:
    - All soluble complement components except factor B

*Source:* Modified from Bonilla, F.A. and Geha, R.S., *J. Allergy Clin. Immunol.*, 111, S571, 2003.

## III. COMBINED IMMUNODEFICIENCY (T AND B CELLS)

### A. Adenosine Deaminase Deficiency

#### 1. Introduction

Adenosine deaminase (ADA) accounts for 15% of patients with severe combined immunodeficiency (SCID),[7] and is an autosomal recessive enzyme defect in the nucleotide salvage pathway. The gene encoding ADA has been mapped to chromosome 20q13.2-11. Patients show a severe lymphopenia (counts of lymphocytes less than 500/mm$^3$) in combination with a variable degree of hypogamma-

**TABLE 23.3**
**Primary Immunodeficiencies Associated with Unknown Genetic/Molecular Mechanisms[3]**

| |
|---|
| Common variable immunodeficiency and IgA deficiency (autosomal recessive) both expressions of the same entity |
| Hyper-IgE syndrome |
| Chronic mucocutaneous candidiasis |
| Idiopathic CD-4 T-cell lymphopenia |
| Reticular dysgenesis |
| Some SCID patients |
| Omenn syndrome [RAG-1 and -2 in combination with additional factors] |

*Source:* Modified from Fischer, A., *Lancet,* 357, 1863, 2001.

globulinemia.[8] Analysis of lymphocyte subpopulations has demonstrated a marked heterogeneity among patients.[9] The severity of immunodeficiency varies from complete absence of T- and B-cell immunity to mild abnormalities of B- and T-cell function. As a result, considerable variation in the age of onset, the severity of symptoms, and the eventual outcome is observed. ADA deficiency causes depletion of thymocytes by an apoptotic mechanism, which is p53 dependent.[10] Deficient antibody–antigen interaction may result in impaired complement activation, depressed chemotaxis, and deficient opsonization and phagocytosis of particulate organisms; moreover, T-cell deficiency predisposes to infections with bacteria, viruses, protozoa, and fungi. The killing of these organisms is dependent on the interactions between macrophages and T cells, the secretion of lymphokines from T cells, and the activation of cytotoxic cells.

## 2. Skin Infections

Most patients tend to have recurrent infections of the skin and other organs and failure to thrive by 3 to 6 months of age. One of the first clinical signs is often a *Candida* infection of the skin. It starts in the skin folds and on the perineum and may become rather extensive, covering the skin with red and scaling often pustular lesions. The eruption is reminiscent of an extensive seborrheic dermatitis or acrodermatitis enteropathica, may evolve into an erythroderma (see below), and often is very resistant to treatment.[11]

Herpes viruses (cytomegalo, Epstein–Barr, herpes simplex, and herpes zoster/varicella) are among the most common viral skin infections encountered in T-cell-deficient patients.[12] The symptoms are often impressive and severe.

## 3. Erythroderma and Graft vs. Host Disease

Erythroderma in neonates and infants might be a presenting sign of immunodeficiency and has been described in SCID as well as in the Omenn syndrome, the Wiskott–Aldrich syndrome, and secretory IgA deficiency.[13] Skin induration is often present in erythroderma caused by immunodeficiency, as is pruritus.

The skin is one of the important targets in graft vs. host disease. In newborns with cellular immunodeficiencies a graft vs. host reaction may occur after *in utero* maternofetal transfusion,[14] by postnatal blood transfusion with non-irradiated donor blood,[15] or by bone marrow transplants that contain T cells. It may present as an erythroderma. The skin problems due to a graft vs. host reaction in infants after maternofetal transfusion may represent the first symptom of the immunodeficiency. The occurrence of graft vs. host disease is explained by the lack of cellular defense against maternal allogeneic lymphocytes, and these lymphocytes will subsequently attack fetal tissues including the skin. It may be very difficult to distinguish this eruption from dermatoses caused by infections. In acute graft vs. host disease of the skin the inflammatory infiltrate consists of lymphocytes predominantly of the CD8+ subgroup,[16] surrounding the blood vessels of the superficial plexus. The presence of these CD8+ cells is consistent with the hypothesis that cytotoxic cells are responsible for the graft vs. host reaction. This is further substantiated by the fact that only a few natural killer cells are present in the skin infiltrate.[16,17] In chronic graft vs. host disease the lymphocyte-rich infiltrate consists of a variable ratio of CD4+ and CD8+ lymphocytes.[18] Langerhans cells may be present in higher as well as in lower quantities.[18] Definite proof for a graft vs. host reaction is a chimerism of lymphocytes, from both donor (mother) and patient, in the blood and in the skin infiltrates. The presence of chimeric cells can be ascertained by karyotyping, human leukocyte or other antigenic typing, and a mixed lymphocyte reaction.[17]

## IV. PREDOMINANTLY ANTIBODY DEFECTS

### A. Selective IgA Deficiency

#### 1. Introduction

In antibody-deficient immunodeficiencies skin infections are regularly seen. Selective IgA deficiency is the most common antibody defect with an incidence of 0.03 to 0.97%;[11] fortunately the deficiency rarely causes symptoms.[19] IgA deficiency and common variable immunodeficiency (CVID) are now considered to be two expression patterns of the same entity, further substantiated by the fact that within the same family isolated IgA deficiency and CVID are found. Autosomal dominant inheritance with highly variable expression has been shown; however, no susceptibility gene has been identified yet. Symptomatic IgA deficiency accounts for 10 to 15% of the immunodeficient cases with clinical symptoms.[20] In most IgA-deficient persons, B cells are found that express membrane-bound IgA. These B cells are immature, however, and show IgM coexpression. They cannot be stimulated to become mature plasma cells and secrete IgA.[21]

In the skin IgA is secreted by the sweat glands and the sebaceous follicles, thus protecting the opening of the follicles into the pilosebaceous ducts and the pores of the sweat ducts.[22]

#### 2. Dermatitis Resembling Atopic Dermatitis

Dermatitis resembling atopic eczema is one of the most notable skin symptoms in IgA-deficient patients. This dermatitis has never been checked for the atopic dermatitis criteria defined by Hanifin and Rajka.[23] The atopic-like dermatitis can be accompanied by asthma. Multiple allergies particularly to bovine serum and milk proteins are often present. This is probably because in the absence of IgA in the gastrointestinal tract intact proteins are easily absorbed, giving a higher chance for sensitization and allergic symptoms. Whether or not this also results in dermatitis by deposition of these proteins in the skin with a subsequent inflammatory reaction remains to be established.

#### 3. Relation between Atopic Dermatitis and IgA Deficiency

Two intriguing theories have been hypothesized concerning atopic dermatitis:

1. A high IgE level in atopic patients is a response to the excessive absorption of allergens through mucosal surfaces, caused by a transient IgA deficiency.[24]
2. The exposure of the human immune system to low levels of xenogeneic antibodies (anti-idiotypic) to specific allergens may have primed the immune system, resulting in a deleterious and inappropriate response on exposure to these allergens (atopens).[25]

Considering that in IgA-deficient patients the specific IgE serum levels are most often normal, in contrast to the specific IgE levels in atopic dermatitis, the first atopic dermatitis hypothesis seems at least very questionable.[26] In the IgA-deficient state the human immune system is considerably exposed to xenogeneic antibodies, as they penetrate easily through the relatively unprotected gastrointestinal mucosa, suggesting the second hypothesis may play a role in allergic individuals with a selective IgA deficiency. It could thus be a factor in atopic dermatitis as well.

Another factor enhancing the occurrence of atopic dermatitis in IgA-deficient patients might be a higher rate of *Staphylococcus aureus* on the skin due to the absence of protecting IgA. Although a proof of the causal role of bacteria in atopic dermatitis has not been given, there are clinical observations that show a relation between *S. aureus* and the dermatitis.[27] In atopic patients it was shown that the secretion of IgA to the skin surface is greatly reduced while high IgE levels in the sweat are found.[28] Moreover, in atopic dermatitis the colonization with *S. aureus* in acute dermatitis is 100%.[28] The *S. aureus* colonization density in general, as well as the superantigen-producing *S. aureus* colonization in particular, is correlated with the severity of the eczema.[29]

As bacterial skin infections are not that common in IgA-deficient patients without dermatitis, it is feasible that local production of compensatory secretory IgM, which has been demonstrated to protect the nasal mucosa in IgA-deficient patients,[30] is also produced in the skin.

#### 4. Psoriasis and IgA Deficiency

The degree of neutrophil chemotaxis inhibition, caused by serum of patients with psoriasis, is positively correlated with the serum IgA level.[31] This suggests that a high serum IgA might be an antipsoriatic factor. Although it has not been found that many patients with psoriasis have an IgA deficiency, it was reported that patients with psoriasis and selective IgA deficiency have an unfavorable prognosis concerning their psoriasis.[32]

#### 5. Autoimmune Diseases and IgA Deficiency

In a 4-year period about 2.6% of patients seen at the National Institutes of Health with systemic lupus erythematosus (SLE) showed an IgA deficiency, representing a tenfold higher incidence of IgA deficiency in this population than in the general population.[33] One can speculate that the enhanced and prolonged exposure to antigens from viral, bacterial, and other origin results in a more intense formation of antibodies, in this case, autoantibodies. Moreover, a particular genetic predisposition, i.e., the increased prevalence of HLA-A1, B8, and DR3 is found in a number of patients.[34,35] These two factors might explain the development of autoimmune diseases.

## V. DEFECTS OF PHAGOCYTIC FUNCTION

### A. Chronic Granulomatous Disease

#### 1. Introduction

Chronic granulomatous disease (CGD) is a congenital immunodeficiency caused by a defect in the phagocyte oxidase complex that affects approximately 1:500,000 persons. The phagocytes in CGD are able to phagocytose microorganisms normally, but are unable to kill these organisms intracellularly due to a deficiency in oxygen radical production. This leads to chronic recurrent bacterial infections of skin, lymph nodes, liver, spleen, bone, and lungs. Several subtypes of CGD have been identified with distinct molecular defects, all showing more or less the same clinical picture. Based on the enzyme system that produces $O_2$-(NADPH oxidase), which consists of several components, the following CGD variants are known:[36,37]

- The X-linked variant (±67% of CGD cases) gene defect localized on Xp21.1, in which the large b-subunit of the membrane bound cytochrome-$b_{558}$ (gp91) is abnormal or absent

- The autosomal recessive variants, showing either absence of the cytosolic protein p47-phox (accounting for ±33% of CGD cases, gene defect found on chromosome 7q11.23), or defects in the small subunit of cytochrome b558 (p22-phox) (accounting for ±5% of CGD cases, gene defect found on chromosome 16q24), or the cytosolic component p67-phox (accounting for ±5% of CGD cases, gene defect found on chromosome 1q25)

## 2. Skin Lesions in X-Linked Cytochrome $b_{558}$ Negative Patients

The patients (boys) with the X-linked cytochrome $b_{558}$ negative form show the most severe infections, mostly with staphylococci and other catalase-positive bacteria. Skin symptoms are chronic pyoderma, abscesses, paronychia, and unspecific inflammatory reactions of the skin, sometimes granulomatous. Moreover, scarring lesions above lymph nodes can be found following spontaneous or surgical drainage of lymph node abscesses, resembling scrofuloderma.

In addition, these boys have seborrheic eczema-like skin lesions mostly around the orificia, showing an acute or chronic sometimes psoriasiform inflammatory reaction and subcorneal pustules.[38] One child with SLE has been reported.[39]

## 3. Skin Lesions in Carriers of X-Linked Cytochrome *b* Negative CGD

The female carriers who can be detected by subnormal hydrogen peroxide production and oxygen consumption during stimulation of their granulocytes, as well as by mosaicism of negative and positive cells in the nitroblue tetrazolium slide test after granulocyte stimulation show skin symptoms, as well.

Discoid lupus erythematosus (DLE)-like skin symptoms are common in this population.[40] The clinical picture of the skin lesions consists of demarcated red scaling lesions with slight atrophy, some teleangiectasias, together with hypo- and hyperpigmentation. Biopsies from these patients show some characteristics of DLE, and immunofluorescence studies, staining for IgG, IgM, IgA, C3, and fibrin, are usually negative.[41] Immunophenotyping of the cellular infiltrate in the skin lesions with the use of monoclonal antibodies showed perivascular and perifollicular infiltration with mainly $CD3^+$ T-cells, mostly of the $CD4^+$ subset with sporadic B cells and sparsity of dendritic cells in the epidermis. A massive human leukocyte antigen (HLA)-DR expression of keratinocytes in proximity of dermal infiltrates was noted.[41] This was in accord with the findings in idiopathic CDLE. It is tempting to speculate on the origin of the CDLE-like skin lesions in these females and on the cause of the absence of the dendritic cells in the lesional epidermis.

An intact respiratory burst is necessary for killing of bacteria and fungi and for intracellular digestion of elder or ruined cells.[42] In the suboptimally functioning granulocytes, biological active remnants may persist and thus become neoantigens. These antigens may induce autoimmune processes thus leading to CDLE-like skin reactions. Moreover, the T-lymphocyte population may be enhanced by the inadequate functioning of the phagocytes.

Generally, in lupus erythematosus, two hypotheses concerning its origin are contemplated: a membrane attack theory[43] and an antibody-dependent cellular cytotoxicity theory.[44] The fact that direct immunofluorescence is negative in CGD carriers does not seem to support the first hypothesis, in which local deposition of immunoglobulins, antigens, and complement factors is necessary to generate a membrane attack complex. When lymphocytes derived from lesional skin are cytotoxic, it is tempting to suggest that in CGD the abnormal phagocytes, unable to degrade cells damaged by ultraviolet light or other factors, are replaced by cytotoxic T cells.

Concerning the relative absence of dendritic cells in the lesional skin of the carriers it would be of interest to know whether these dendritic cells are lost by the just mentioned cytotoxic pathway and whether the density of these cells in the nonlesional skin of the same person is abnormal, as well.

# VI. OTHER WELL-DEFINED IMMUNODEFICIENCIES

Wiskott–Aldrich syndrome (WAS) and ataxia teleangiectasia (AT) are immunodeficiency diseases that are recognized by their particular combination of symptoms in which the skin plays an important role.

## A. Wiskott–Aldrich Syndrome (WAS)

### 1. Introduction

This X-linked recessive disorder (1:250,000 in Europe) is clinically characterized by a combination of thrombocytopenia with small thrombocytes, increased susceptibility to infection, and dermatitis. As a consequence of the thrombocytopenia, nasal or other hemorrhages occur early in life. Bacterial skin infections causing furunculosis, pyodermas, and abscesses are common. Viral (in particular cytomegalo and herpes virus) and fungal infections do occur often and Epstein–Barr virus infection is associated with the occurrence of B-cell lymphoma.

Scanning electron microscopy has revealed that the cytoskeleton of lymphocytes and platelets in affected boys is deranged. The gene for WAS is located on chromosome Xp11.23, and is called the WASP gene.[45] WASP is found only in blood cells and all WASP-related proteins (the WASP family) are involved in the transduction of signals to, and the organization of, the actin skeleton[46] and thus in the conformational change that is necessary for interaction with other cells and microbial agents. Quantitative abnormalities of total immunoglobulin levels develop in many patients, which are manifested by low levels of immunoglobulin M and increased levels of IgA, IgD, and IgE.

### 2. Atopic Eczema-Like Dermatitis

The eczematous lesions in patients with the WAS fulfill the diagnostic criteria for atopic dermatitis[23] as was shown by Saurat.[47] The eczematous lesions mostly begin in the second month of life or later but sometimes do not appear at all. When the children scratch themselves heavily, they induce linear purpuric streaks due to the thrombocytopenia.

Interestingly enough, complete clearance of the eczema is reported after successful bone marrow grafting.[48] This suggests that there is a causal relationship between the immunodeficiency and atopic eczema.

### 3. Vasculitis and Other Autoimmune Phenomena

In WAS, defects are observed in polarization, chemotaxis, and migration of cells involved in the immune system, among others leading to a disturbance of phagocytosis of apoptotic cells. The defective clearance of cellular debris might have important implications for the pathophysiology of clinical disease,[49] in particular of autoimmune phenomena and immune complex formation.

Vasculitis has been described in around 20% of the patients, and in particular cerebral vasculitis may be life-threatening.[50] In WAS, the immunological response to polysaccharide antigens is deficient. It seems possible that the biologic action of certain antigens, not processed normally by the reticuloendothelial system, results in progressive disorganization of the immune system. The presence of vasculitis may reflect a phase in this progressive disorganization, where the initial abnormality is increased susceptibility to infection and the terminal derangement results in malignancy.

## B. Ataxia Teleangiectasia (AT)

### 1. Introduction

AT is an autosomal recessively inherited chromosomal instability syndrome with progressive cerebellar degeneration, immunodeficiency, gonadal dysgenesis, ocular and cutaneous teleangiectasia, and high serum α-fetoprotein. An excess of lymphoid tumors and a modest increase in epithelial tumors has been noted. AT cells fail to execute cell cycle checkpoints immediately after DNA strand-break damage and exhibit excessive apoptotic cell death. The ATM gene has been mapped to chromosome 11q22-23.[51] It is involved in cell cycle control, intracellular protein transport, and DNA damage response. There is still much confusion in the literature regarding the exact biological functions of the ATM protein. A great variation in immunodeficiency has been observed, but a combination of decreased IgA, IgG2, and IgG4 levels and a more or less defective cellular immunity is often present.[52]

#### 2. Vascular and Pigment-Related Skin Lesions

The neurological symptoms are very impressive but are not dealt with in this chapter. The patients show teleangiectasias in particular on sun-exposed areas.[53] The origin of these teleangiectasias is not yet fully understood. Pigment disturbances are often found, e.g., café au lait spots, vitiligo, hypopigmented macules, and poliosis. Possibly the pigment disorders have something to do with the sensitivity to X-irradiation, or with defective clearance of autoimmunity-inducing cell remnants of partly cleared apoptotic cells, leading to autoimmune phenomena in the skin.

#### 3. Dermatitis (Atopic?)

In some reports on the skin changes in patients with AT, eczematous eruptions are described,[54] but in others these changes are not mentioned.[55] One can conclude that eczematous changes are not very common in this disease. Moreover an atopic syndrome is denied by several authors.[47,53]

#### 4. Other Findings

Progeroid findings are regularly reported consisting of: lipoatrophy and sclerodermatous changes of the face. Skin infections include impetigo, viral and mycotic infections. Mucous membrane lesions as recurrent herpetic stomatitis and oral candidiasis can be seen regularly.[53]

Several cases have been reported that exhibit granuloma formation in the skin and in some patients also in internal organs.[55] In none of the cases could an infectious microorganism be found. Probably the granuloma formation is the result of abnormal cytokine production profiles. For example, interleukin- 4(IL-4) and interferon-gamma (IFN-γ), cytokines mainly produced by T lymphocytes (defective in AT), have a downregulating effect,[56] whereas IL-1 and tumor necrosis factor-alpha (TNF-α), secreted by monocytes/macrophages, have an enhancing effect on granuloma formation.[57]

## VII. COMPLEMENT DEFICIENCIES

Most patients with complement deficiencies do not show clinical symptoms. If symptoms occur, recurrent infections and lupus erythematosus-like syndromes are most frequently encountered.[58] As a rule of thumb, early component deficiencies (C1, C4, C2) of the classical complement cascade are most often associated with lupus erthematosus, whereas deficiencies of the membrane attack pathway (C5 to C9) predispose to recurrent *Neisseria* infections and rheumatic disease.[58]

Complement deficiencies are rather rare. Probably the most frequent deficiency is a C2 deficiency.[59]

### A. C2 Deficiency

#### 1. Introduction

C2 complement deficiency is an autosomal recessive inherited disease. Homozygous C2 deficiency is seen in 1 in 10,000 to 1 in 40,000 individuals.[60] In some C2-deficient patients skin infections, mostly by bacteria, are found. Complement is necessary for normal opsonization, an important step in chemotaxis and bacterial killing by neutrophils. This explains the greater susceptibility to bacterial infections.

Autoimmune disorders occur in half the patients with the homozygous form of C2 deficiency. Systemic and DLE are the most frequent and are particularly common in females. Other diseases with skin symptoms, e.g., juvenile rheumatoid arthritis, dermatomyositis, vasculitis, Henoch Schönlein purpura, atrophoderma, cold urticaria, and linear scleroderma, may be associated with C2 deficiency, too, but mostly isolated observations were reported.

#### 2. Systemic and Discoid Lupus Erythematosus

Lupus erythematosus-like skin lesions occur from puberty onward in homozygous and heterozygous patients. The lupus can be rather fulminant. Patients with lupus erythematosus and C2 deficiency are unique in regard to the high prevalence of subacute lupus erythematosus and DLE, the photosensitivity and the frequent presence of anti-Ro (SSA) antibodies.[61] Photosensitivity is a prominent feature and might be related to the anti-Ro (SSA) autoantibodies, because it is known that ultraviolet radiation increases binding of Ro (SSA) autoantibodies to the surface of keratinocytes. Although in the past it was hypothesized that there were characteristics that may suggest a C2 deficiency in a patient with lupus erythematosus, such as an early age of onset, extensive cutaneous lesions, the occurrence of infections, mild or occult renal disease, absent or low ANA and anti-DNA titer, negative lupus band test, and rather mild systemic symptoms,[62] this is not confirmed by others.[61] Unfortunately, in recent studies it appeared that the prognosis for patients with lupus erythematosus with C2 deficiency is not better than that for patients with lupus erythematosus in general.[61] Why lupus-like illness is present in such a high frequency in C2 deficiency is not clear. It has recently been suggested that early complement components could be important cosignals in the negative selection of autoreactive B cells,[63] and in the absence of C2, autoreactive B cells are thus present in large quantities. Moreover, it can be hypothesized that organisms that can trigger LE have a better chance to do so because the defense system against them is disturbed. Another hypothesis suggests that since viral neutralization and clearance is deficient viral-antiviral complexes remain in the circulation thereby increasing the risk of immune complex disease.[64]

## VIII. IMMUNODEFICIENCY ASSOCIATED WITH OR SECONDARY TO OTHER DISEASES

### A. Hyper-IgE Syndrome

#### 1. Introduction

The hyper-IgE syndrome can be defined by recurrent infection from the skin (abscesses) and sinopulmonary tract from childhood and an IgE level of at least 2000 IU/ml.[63] It is a multisystem disorder with non-immunological abnormalities of dentition, bones, and connective tissue. Linkage to chromosome 4q has been reported in several families.[64] A strict definition is necessary because of the inconsistencies in the literature of what constitutes the syndrome.

By using the above-mentioned definition, atopic children with a very high IgE are excluded because these patients do not show recurrent sinopulmonary tract infections or abscesses from childhood onward.

#### 2. Characterization of the Defects Involved

The laboratory characteristics of patients with the hyper-IgE syndrome consists, apart from an IgE above 2000 IU/ml (per definition), of a high percentage of specific IgE binding to staphylococci, an increased urinary histamine excretion in some patients, a variable abnormality of the chemotactic responsiveness of patient's neutrophils, and a spontaneous production by monocytes of an inhibitor of neutrophil chemotaxis, accompanied by the production of a second inhibitor on exposure to staphylococci.[64]

### 3. Dermatological Features of the Syndrome

In the neonatal period a vesiculopustular skin eruption may be present. This rash predominantly affects the flexural surfaces of the body as well as the ears, the face, and the scalp, resembling in some aspects atopic dermatitis. Histologically there is an intraepidermal vesicle with eosinophils and a rather diffuse eosinophilic infiltrate in the dermis.[65,66]

Later in life eczematoid rashes occur that impetiginize rather easily. This eczematous eruption can be distinguished from atopic dermatitis by the accentuation of intertriginous, retroauricular, and hairline lesions. Hyper-IgE patients themselves lack, however, a history of asthma, hay fever, or hives.

Skin infections are rather frequent and present as nonpainful cold abscesses without any sign of inflammation due to a decreased influx of neutrophils and monocytes. They are always caused by *S. aureus*. Furunculosis, paronychia, cellulitis, and cheilitis can be observed, as well. Apart from *S. aureus* infections, many patients have frequent cutaneous infections from *Candida* species or streptococci.

Patients commonly have a coarse face with frontal bossing, hypertelorism, and wide alar bases.[67] Probably also due to the severe skin infections most patients develop the already mentioned rather coarse facial characteristics sometimes reminiscent of the facies leontina in patients with lepromatous leprosy. The primary immune defect is unknown. The sequence of events leading to the skin disorder remains hypothetical.

The hallmark of the disease is the elevated serum IgE level, especially antistaphylococcal IgE antibodies. A disorder in immune regulation involving different T-cell subsets and possibly B cells remains to be proved. There are reports showing a decreased number of suppressor T cells, which have a subnormal activity.[68] This immunodysregulation leads to high IgE production, which in turn, can release histamine by basophils and or mast cells. Histamine is known to suppress neutrophil chemotaxis and moreover is one of the mediators involved in itchy skin conditions.

## IX. CONCLUSION

In this chapter on primary immunodeficiencies and their impact on the SIS, it is noted that the immunodeficiencies offer an intriguing field in which much remains to be elucidated. Although a great deal of immunological parameters are rather well defined and understood, the skin is only sporadically integrated in the knowledge and relatively little research activity has been done to gain more insight into the consequences of these deficiencies on the SIS. It would be worthwhile to focus immunological research in immunodeficiencies more on the skin. By doing this the "experiments of nature" can be used to gain more insight into rather common dermatological problems such as atopic dermatitis and such autoimmune diseases as lupus erythematosus.

## REFERENCES

1. Amman, A. and Wara, D., Evaluation of infants and children with recurrent infections, *Curr. Probl. Pediatr.*, 5, 3, 1975.
2. Bonilla F.A. and Geha R.S., Primary immunodeficiency diseases, *J. Allergy Clin. Immunol.*, 111, S571, 2003.
3. Fischer, A., Primary immunodeficiency diseases: an experimental model for molecular medicine, *Lancet,* 357, 1863, 2001.

4. Antoine C., Müller S., Cant A. et al., Long-term survival and transplantation of haematopoietic stem cells for immunodeficiencies: report of the European experience 1968–99, *Lancet,* 361,553, 2003.
5. Stiehm, E.R., *Immunologic Disorders in Infants and Children,* 4th ed., W.B. Saunders, Philadelphia, 1996.
6. Amman, A.J., Immunodeficiency diseases, in *Basic and Clinical Immunology,* 8th ed., Stites, D.P., Iter, A., and Parslow, T.G., Eds., Appleton & Lange, Norwalk, CT, 1994.
7. Buckley, R.H., Primary immunodeficiency diseases: dissectors of the immune system, *Immunol. Rev.,* 185, 206, 2002.
8. Giblett, E.R., Anderson, J.E., Cohen, F., Pollara, B., and Meuwissen, H.J., Adenosine deaminase deficiency in two patients with severely impaired cellular immunity, *Lancet*, 2, 1067, 1972.
9. Markert, M.L., Hershfield, M.S., Schiff, R.I., and Buckley, R.H., Adenosine deaminase and purine nucleoside phosphorylase deficiencies: evaluation of therapeutic interventions in eight patients, *J. Clin. Immunol.*, 7, 389, 1987.
10. Benveniste, P. and Cohen A., p53 expression is required for thymocyte apoptosis induced by adenosine deaminase deficiency, *Proc. Natl. Acad. Sci. U.S.A.*, 92, 8373, 1995.
11. Buckley, R.H., Immunodeficiency diseases, *J. Am. Med. Assoc.*, 258, 2841, 1987.
12. Stiehm, E.R., Chin, T.W., Haas, A., and Peerless, A.G., Infectious complications of the primary immunodeficiencies, *Clin. Immunol. Immunopathol.*, 40, 69, 1986.
13. Pruszkowski, A., Bodemer, C., Fraitag, S., Teillac-Hamel, D., Amoric, J.-C., and de Prost, Y., Neonatal and infantile erythrodermas, *Arch. Dermatol.,* 136, 875, 2000.
14. Grogan, T.M., Odom, R.B., and Burgess, J.H., Graft vs. host reaction, *Arch. Dermatol.,* 113, 806, 1977.
15. Burns, L.J., Westberg, M.W., Burns, C.P., Klassen, L.W., Goeken, N.E., Ray, T.L., and Macfarlane, D.E., Acute graft versus host disease resulting from normal donor blood transfusions, *Acta Haematol.* (Basel), 71, 270, 1984.
16. Schmitt, D. and Thivolet, J., Use of monoclonal antibodies specific for T cell subsets in cutaneous disorders: II. Immunomorphologic studies in blood and skin lesions, *J. Clin. Immunol.*, 2(Suppl.), 111s, 1982.
17. Saurat, J.H., Cutaneous manifestations of graft versus host disease, *Int. J. Dermatol.*, 20, 249, 1981.
18. Sloane, J.P., Thomas, J.A., Imrie, S.F., Easton, D.F., and Powles, R.L., Morphological and immunohistological changes in the skin in allogeneic bone marrow transplants, *J. Clin. Pathol.*, 37, 919, 1984.
19. Hammarstrom, L., Vorechevsky, I., and Webster, D., Selective IgA deficiency (SigAD) and common variable immunodeficiency (CVID), *Clin. Exp. Immunol.,* 120, 225, 2000.
20. Rosen, F.S., Cooper, M.D., and Wedgwood, R.J.P., The primary immunodeficiencies (first part), *N. Engl. J. Med.*, 311, 235, 1984.
21. Conley, M.E. and Cooper, M.D., Immature IgA B cells in IgA deficient patients, *N. Engl. J. Med.*, 305, 495, 1981.
22. Gebhart, W., Metze, D., Jurecka, W., Schmidt, J.B., and Niebauer, G., IgA in human appendages, in *Immunodermatology,* Caputo, R., Ed., CIC Edizioni Internazionali, Rome, 1987, 185.
23. Hanifin, J.M. and Rajka, G., Diagnostic features of atopic dermatitis, *Acta Derm. Venereol.*, Suppl. 92, 44, 1980.
24. Taylor, B., Norman, A.P., Orgel, H.A., Stokes, C.R., Turner, M.W., and Soothill, J.F., Transient IgA deficiency and pathogenesis of infantile atopy, *Lancet,* 2, 111, 1973.
25. Collins, A.M., Xenogeneic antibodies and atopic disease, *Lancet*, 1, 734, 1988.
26. Out, T.A., Munster van, P.J.J., Graeff de, P.A., Thé, T.H., Vossen, J.M., and Zegers, B.J.M., Immunologic investigations in individuals with selective IgA deficiency, *Clin. Exp. Immunol.,* 64, 510, 1986.
27. Imayama, S., Shimozono, Y., Hoashi, M., Yasumoto, S., Ohta, S., Yoneyama, K., and Hori, Y., Reduced secretion of IgA to the skin surface of patients with atopic dermatitis, *J. Allergy Clin. Immunol.*, 94, 195, 1994.
28. Zollner, T.M., Wichelhaus, T.A., and Hartung, A. et al., Colonization with superantigen-producing *Staphylococcus aureus* is associated with increased severity of atopic dermatitis, *Clin. Exp. Allergy,* 30, 994, 2000.
29. Brockow K., Grabenhorst P., Abeck D. et al., Effect of gentian violet, corticosteroid and tar preparations in *Staphylococcus-aureus*-colonized atopic dermatitis, *Dermatology,* 199, 231, 1999.

30. Brandtzaeg, P., Karlsson, G., Hansson, G., Petruson, B., Björklander, J., and Hamson, L.A., The clinical condition of IgA deficient patients is related to the proportion of IgD- and IgM-producing cells in their nasal mucosa, *Clin. Exp. Immunol.*, 67, 626, 1986.
31. Schröder, J.M., Szperalski, B., Ko, Ch.J., and Christophers, E., IgA-associated inhibition of polymorphonuclear leucocyte chemotaxis in neutrophil dermatoses, *J. Invest. Dermatol.*, 77, 464, 1981.
32. Kerkhof, P.C.M. and van der, Steijlen, P.M., IgA deficiency and psoriasis: relevance of IgA in the pathogenesis of psoriasis, *Dermatology*, 191, 46, 1995.
33. Gershwin, M.E., Blaese, R.M., Steinberg, A.D., Wistar, R., and Strober, W., Antibodies to nucleic acids in congenital immune deficiency states, *J. Pediatr.*, 89, 377, 1976.
34. Oen, K., Petty, R.E., and Schroeder, M.L., Immunoglobulin A deficiency: genetic studies, *Tissue Antigens*, 19, 174, 1982.
35. Hammarström, L. and Smith, C.I.E., HLA A, B, C and DR antigens in immunoglobulin A deficiency, *Tissue Antigens*, 21, 75, 1983.
36. Roos, D., The genetic basis of chronic granulomatous disease, *Immunol. Rev.*, 138, 121, 1994.
37. Lekstrom-Himes, J.A. and Gallin, J.I., Immunodeficiency diseases caused by defects in phagocytes, *N. Engl. J. Med.*, 343, 1703, 2000.
38. Dohill, M., Prendiville, J.S., and Crawford, R.I., Cutaneous manifestations of chronic granulomatous disease; a report of four cases and review of the literature, *J. Am. Acad. Dermatol.*, 36, 899, 1997.
39. Manzi, S., Urbach, A.H., McCune, A.B. et al., Systemic lupus erythematosus in a boy with chronic granulomatous disease: case report and review of the literature, *Arthritis Rheum.*, 34, 101, 1991.
40. Brandrup, F., Koch, C., Petri, M., Schiödt, M., and Johansen, K.S., Discoid lupus erythematosus-like skin lesions and stomatitis in female carriers of X-linked chronic granulomatous disease, *Br. J. Dermatol.*, 104, 495, 1981.
41. Sillevis Smitt, J.H., Weening, R.S., Krieg, S., and Bos, J.D., Skin changes in carriers of X-linked chronic granulomatous disease, *Br. J. Dermatol.*, 122, 643, 1990.
42. Katz, P., Recent advances in chronic granulomatous disease: abnormalities of antibody-dependent cellular cytotoxicity, *Ann. Intern. Med.*, 99, 667, 1983.
43. Bieseker, G., Lavin, L., Ziskind, M., and Koffler, D., Cutaneous localization of the membrane attack complex in discoid and systemic lupus erythematosus, *N. Engl. J. Med.*, 306, 264, 1982.
44. Norris, D.A., New evidence pertaining to the mechanisms of cutaneous lupus erythematosus, in *Immunodermatology*, Macdonald, D.M., Ed., Butterworth, Kent, U.K., 267, 71, 1988.
45. Derry, J.M.J., Ochs, H.D., and Francke, U., Isolation of a novel gene mutated in Wiskott-Aldrich syndrome, *Cell*, 78, 635, 1994.
46. Snapper, S.B., and Rosen, F.S., A family of WASPs, *N. Engl. J. Med.*, 348, 350, 2003.
47. Saurat, J.H., Woodley, D., and Helfer, N., Cutaneous symptoms in primary immunodeficiencies, *Curr. Probl. Dermatol.*, 13, 50, 1985.
48. Parkman, R., Rappeport, J., Geha, R., Belli, J., Cassady, R., Levey, R., Nathan, D.G., and Rosen, F.S., Complete correction of the Wiskott-Aldrich syndrome by allogeneic bone marrow transplantation, *N. Engl. J. Med.*, 298, 921, 1987.
49. Thrasher, A.J., WASp in immune-system organization and function, *Nat. Rev.*, 2, 635, 2002.
50. Dupuis-Girod S., Medioni J., Haddad E., Quartier P., Cavazzana-Calvo M. et al., Autoimmunity in Wiskott-Aldrich syndrome: risk factors, clinical features and outcome in a single-center cohort of 55 patients, *Pediatrics*, 111, e622, 2003.
51. McConville, C.M., Woods, C.G., Farral, M. et al., Analysis of 7 polymorphic markers at chromosome 11q22-23 in 35 ataxia-teleangiectasia families: further evidence of linkage, *Hum. Genet.*, 85, 215, 1990.
52. Grumach, A.S., Moraes-Vasconcelos, D., Jacob, C.M.A., Kok, F., and Duarte, A.J.S., Immunological evaluation in Brazilian ataxia teleangiectasia patients, *ACI Int.*, 14, 102, 2002.
53. Cohen, L.E., Tanner, D.J., Schaefer, H.G., and Levis, W.R., Common and uncommon cutaneous findings in patients with ataxia teleangiectasia, *J. Am. Acad. Dermatol.*, 10, 431, 1984.
54. Reed, W.B., Epstein, W.L., Broder, E., and Sedgwick, R., Cutaneous manifestations of ataxia-teleangiectasia, *J. Am. Med. Assoc.*, 195, 746, 1996.
55. Paul, C., Teillac-Hamel, D., Fraitag, S. et al., Lésions granulomateuses cutanées au cours des déficits immunitaires congénitaux, *Ann. Derm. Venereol.*, 122, 501, 1995.

56. Sato, I.Y., Modulation of granuloma formation *in vitro* by endogenous mediators, *Immunopharmacology,* 221, 73, 1991.
57. Kasahara, K., The role of monokines in granuloma formation in mice: the ability of interleukin- and tumor necrosis factor alpha to induce lung granulomas, *Clin. Immunol. Immunopathol.,* 51, 419, 1989.
58. Voigtländer, V., Inherited complement deficiencies and skin diseases, in *Pediatric Dermatology,* Happle, R. and Grosshans, E., Eds., Springer-Verlag, Berlin, 1987, 89.
59. Agnello, V., Complement deficiency state, *Medicine*, 57, 1, 1978.
60. Agnello, V., Association of systemic lupus erythematosus and SLE-like syndromes with hereditary and acquired complement deficiency states, *Arthritis Rheum.*, 21(Suppl.), 146, 1978.
61. Lipsker, D., Schreckenberg-Gilliot, C., Uring-Lambert, B., Meyer, A., Hartmann, D., Grosshans, E.M., and Hauptmann, G., Lupus erythematosus associated with genetically determined deficiency of second component of the complement, *Arch. Dermatol.*, 136, 1508, 2000.
62. Rynes, R.I., Inherited complement deficiency states in SLE, *Clin. Rheum. Dis.*, 8, 28, 1982.
63. Carroll, M.C., The lupus paradox, *Nat. Genet.,* 19, 3, 1998.
64. Miller, M.E., Cutaneous infections and disorders of inflammation, *J. Am. Acad. Dermatol.,* 2, 1, 1980.
65. Donabedian, H. and Gallin, J.I., The hyperimmunoglobulin E recurrent-infection (Job's) syndrome, a review of the NIH experience and the literature, *Medicine*, 62, 195, 1983.
66. Grimbacher, B., Schaffer, A.A., Holland, S.M. et al., Genetic linkage of hyper-IgE syndrome to chromosome 4, *Am. J. Hum. Genet.,* 65, 735, 1999.
67. Kamei, R. and Honig, P.J., Neonatal Job's syndrome featuring a vesicular eruption, *Pediatr. Dermatol.,* 5, 75, 1988.
68. Chamlin, S.L., McCalmont, T.H., Cunningham, B.B., Esterly, N.B., Lai, C-H., Mallory, S.B., Mancini, A.J., Tamburro, J., and Frieden, I.J., Cutaneous manifestations of hyper-IgE syndrome in infants and children, *J. Pediatr.,* 141, 572, 2002.
69. Dahl, M.V., Hyper-IgE syndrome revisited, *Int. J. Dermatol.*, 41, 618, 2002.
70. Geha, R.S., Reinherz, E., Leung, D., McKee, K.T., Schlossmann, S., and Rosen, F.S., Deficiency of suppressor T-cells in the hyperimmunoglobulin E syndrome, *J. Clin. Invest.,* 68, 783, 1981.

# 24 Immunobullous Diseases

*Graham S. Ogg, Samantha Winsey, Sarah Wakelin, and Fenella Wojnarowska*

## CONTENTS



## I. INTRODUCTION

The immunobullous diseases are a group of acquired dermatoses that give rise to chronic blistering and erosions of the skin and mucous membranes. These uncommon diseases have an autoimmune etiology and are characterized by *in vivo* deposition of immunoreactants within the epidermis or at the cutaneous basement membrane zone (BMZ). In pemphigus there is interepidermal antibody deposition and intraepidermal blistering, whereas pemphigoid (bullous, mucous membrane, and gestationis variants), linear IgA disease, and epidermolysis bullosa acquisita show BMZ antibody deposition and subepidermal blistering. Knowledge of the structure and function of many molecular components of the cutaneous BMZ has advanced over the past decade, and the ultrastructural localization and molecular composition of target antigens have now been defined for most immunobullous diseases (Figure 24.1). There is increasing evidence that autoantibodies play a major pathogenic role in skin blistering. Other humoral and cellular immune mechanisms also appear to be involved in the pathogenesis of these diseases, although the precise sequence of events and interactions that ultimately cause blister formation have not been determined.

Genetic factors appear to influence susceptibility to these diseases and human leucocyte antigen (HLA) associations have now been reported for all. However, the events that lead to the induction

0-8493-1959-5/05/$0.00+$1.50

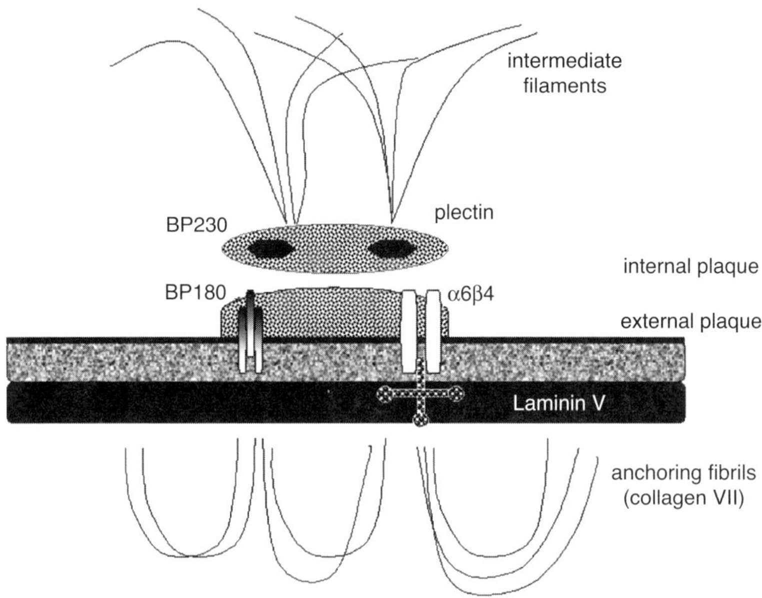


**FIGURE 24.1** Schematic diagram of the cutaneous BMZ showing target antigens of the subepidermal immunobullous diseases.

of immunobullous diseases and the mechanisms by which immunogenetic factors influence and modulate the disease process remain unknown. In a minority of patients, drug ingestion or infection may trigger disease onset, but in most cases there is no obvious precipitant. Some immunobullous diseases are associated with an increased risk of other autoimmune diseases, suggesting that immune dysregulation plays a role in their etiology.

Although they are classified as discrete entities, the immunobullous diseases exhibit overlapping clinical and immunological features, and it is likely that they share common immunopathological mechanisms. Most research on the humoral and cellular mechanisms of skin blistering in these diseases has been carried out on bullous pemphigoid (BP) and pemphigus, and this aspect of other bullous diseases remains relatively unexplored.

## II. CELLULAR MECHANISMS

The immunobullous diseases are accompanied by varying degrees of skin inflammation, and early lesions of most of these conditions are characterized histologically by perivascular and subepidermal infiltrates of inflammatory cells. The relative importance of humoral and cellular mediators in producing tissue injury appears to vary from one disease to another, and different cellular mechanisms appear to be involved in different diseases.

Mast cells have been proposed to link the early cellular and immune components in developing lesions of BP.[1] These cells have been observed in early lesional BP skin, and more advanced lesions demonstrate progressive hypogranulation of mast cells and influx of eosinophils.[2] After appropriate stimuli such as IgE, C3a, and C4a, mast cells can release a number of pro-inflammatory mediators including histamine, eosinophil chemotactic factor (ECF), high-molecular-weight neutrophil chemotactic factor, platelet-activating factor, and proteolytic enzymes. These may initiate BMZ damage and lead to the subsequent influx of eosinophils, which constitute the predominant inflammatory cell in BP.

Degranulated eosinophils are seen in close association with the basal epidermis in the early stages of blister formation, and deposition of eosinophil-derived enzymes has been demonstrated in the BMZ in perilesional skin, supporting the proposal that proteolytic enzymes of eosinophils play a role in the early stages of blister formation.[3] Elevated levels of eosinophil cationic protein (ECP) have been demonstrated in BP blister fluid and serum, and this may exert cytotoxic effects. An eosinophil-derived metalloprotease 92-kDa gelatinase has also been suggested to contribute significantly to the tissue damage in BP, as this enzyme is able to cleave the extracellular domain of BP180 in addition to acting on other BMZ components.[4] Eosinophilic infiltration may also be an early histological feature of pemphigus, and inflammatory cell infiltration may augment antibody-mediated tissue damage in this disease, but does not appear to play a primary role in cell dysadhesion.

A mixed inflammatory cell infiltrate consisting of neutrophils, macrophages, Langerhans cells/dendritic cells, and T lymphocytes has been noted in the conjunctiva in the acute stage of mucous membrane pemphigoid, with a T-lymphocytic infiltrate characterizing the chronic stage of this disease.[5] It is probable that these inflammatory cells produce fibrogenic cytokines such as transforming growth factor-β (TGF-β) and platelet-derived growth factor PDGF, which stimulate fibroblasts and give rise to the severe scarring that characterizes this condition. T cells from patients with BP have been shown to recognize recombinant BP180, and T-cell lines generated from such patients may produce the cytokines interferon-γ (IFN-γ; Th1), interleukin-5 (IL-5), and IL-13 (Th2) and display a $CD4^+$ phenotype. Multiple T-cell recognition sites have been defined within the BP180 molecule, including a large number within the NC16A domain. NC16A-domain-specific T cells have also been identified in the peripheral blood of individuals with herpes gestationis and linear IgA disease, suggesting that this region may be an important immunogenic site for the subepidermal blistering diseases.

Cellular events also appear to be involved in the pathogenesis of dermatitis herpetiformis (DH) with increasing evidence for the importance of T cells and neutrophils. Perivascular infiltrates of T lymphocytes are characteristic of developing DH lesions (as induced by potassium iodide application), and further investigation has shown lesional skin to contain increased numbers of activated T-helper cells.[6] It is possible that these cells induce inflammatory cell infiltration by release of cytokines such as IL-2, tumor necrosis factor (TNF), and IFN-γ. They have been shown to express HLA DR antigens, and have been documented in close association with Langerhans cells in involved skin, suggesting that a cell-mediated immune response is taking place. Neutrophils are the predominant cell present in the bullae and papillary tip microabscesses in this disease, and it has been proposed that keratinocyte-derived IL-8 acts as an important chemoattractant for these cells.[7] It remains to be determined whether T cells or neutrophils are the initial infiltrating cell in DH lesions.

Little is known about the cellular events in linear IgA disease (LAD), although neutrophils from patients with LAD have been shown to produce increased amounts of oxygen free radicals, and the patients' serum can stimulate increased production of free radicals from normal neutrophils and may contribute to recruitment of the latter to the dermoepidermal junction.[8,9]

The relative importance of cellular mechanisms may vary within a disease entity, as, for example, in epidermolysis bullosa acquisita (EBA). The mechanobullous form of EBA lacks inflammatory features both clinically and histologically, whereas the BP-like inflammatory variant is characterized by a neutrophil-rich infiltrate.[10] This may reflect alternative pathogenic mechanisms within this disease. EBA has been reported in a patient following treatment with granulocyte-macrophage colony-stimulating factor (GM-CSF).[11] Skin biopsies showed an inflammatory infiltrate composed predominantly of eosinophils, and this case supports the idea that activated granulocytes may mediate blister formation in some cases of EBA.

## III. HUMORAL MECHANISMS

### A. Autoantibodies

The presence of tissue-bound and circulating skin autoantibodies is characteristic of the immunobullous diseases, and documenting their presence is fundamental to establishing a diagnosis.

Tissue-bound antibodies can be demonstrated in all diseases by direct immunofluorescence (IMF) or direct immunoelectron microscopy (IEM) of perilesional skin. Circulating autoantibodies can also be demonstrated by indirect IMF, Western immunoblotting, or indirect IEM in all diseases with the exception of DH, and there is increasing evidence that these antibodies play a major role in disease pathogenesis.

The role of antibodies has been most clearly defined in the pemphigus group of diseases, and there is strong evidence that the antibodies found in pemphigus patients' sera are pathogenic. The earliest observations to demonstrate this were *in vitro* studies of human skin in organ culture, which showed that histological changes identical to those of pemphigus could be elicited by addition of pooled sera or purified IgG from patients with pemphigus vulgaris (PV).[12] These changes were complement independent.[13] Passive transfer studies subsequently showed that neonatal mice developed skin blistering and erosions following parenteral injection of pemphigus IgG, with binding of IgG to the epidermis of lesional and perilesional skin.[14] Neonatal mice have also been shown to develop clinical and immunopathological features of pemphigus following injection of a specific antiserum raised in rabbit against purified human PV antigen,[15] again supporting the concept of antibody pathogenicity.

Further evidence that antibody alone can induce acantholysis has come from work on pemphigus foliaceus (PF). In both PV and endemic PF, the major IgG antibody subclass is IgG4, and this is thought to be incapable of complement activation. Passive transfer of the IgG4 fraction of PF patients' sera, or PF IgG4 Fab′ fragments to neonatal mice has been shown to induce characteristic PF lesions without evidence of complement activation.[16] Transplacental passage of maternal PV antibodies is believed to cause neonatal pemphigus, which has been observed in the offspring of affected mothers, and provides evidence of antibody pathogenicity.

Desmogleins 1 and 3 are transmembrane glycoprotein components of the desmosome and are believed to represent the dominant targets for pathogenic antibodies in individuals with pemphigus. Desmoglein 1 is expressed throughout the epidermis but more intensely in the superficial layers, whereas desmoglein 3 is predominantly expressed in the lower parts of the epidermis. However, in the mucous membranes, desmogleins 1 and 3 are present throughout the epithelia, but desmoglein 1 is expressed at significantly lower amounts. These findings may partly explain the differential clinical phenotype of individuals with predominant circulating anti-desmoglein 1 and/or 3 antibodies.[17–19] Individuals with mucosal dominant PV have predominant circulating anti-desmoglein 3 antibodies, but those with mucocutaneous PV have both anti-desmoglein 1 and anti-desmoglein 3 antibodies. In contrast individuals with PF are thought to have predominant circulating anti-desmoglein 1 antibodies. Neonatal epidermis has an expression of desmoglein 3 in a pattern resembling that of adult mucous membranes, which may explain why mothers with PF rarely have neonates with disease. Furthermore, the *Staphylococcus aureus*–derived exfoliative toxins associated with staphylococcal scalded skin syndrome ETA and ETB are now known to cleave desmoglein 1 through their trypsin-like serine protease activity, generating further insight into mechanisms of cell–cell adhesion and blister formation.[20,21]

The pathogenicity of BP antibodies has been more difficult to demonstrate, due to species specific differences in the major antigenic epitopes. However, Liu et al.[22] have recently demonstrated that pemphigoid can be reproduced in mice by passive transfer of antibodies, raised against murine BP180 antigen fusion proteins, but not with those raised against human BP180 fusion proteins. It has been suggested that antibodies against the BP180 antigen could play a direct pathogenic role by disturbing the formation of hemidesmosomes, and thereby making the basal cells more fragile and prone to blister.[23] Anhalt et al. have also demonstrated that purified IgG from patients with BP can induce inflammatory lesions with visible blisters when injected into the cornea of rabbits. The intensity of the inflammation in this model correlated with the complement fixation titer of the BP IgG, supporting a role for complement in mediating production of BP lesions.[3]

In addition to IgG class anti-BMZ antibodies, raised levels of total IgE and BMZ-specific IgE antibodies have been noted in some patients with BP, and the elevated levels of serum IgE have been shown to correlate with disease activity.[24] This IgE diathesis appears to be unique to BP, and has not been noted in other immunobullous diseases. Low-affinity IgE receptor (FceRII)-expressing cells have been documented in lesional BP skin, and these are believed to correspond to macrophages, eosinophils, and T cells. It is possible that these FceRII-expressing cells react with IgE-antigen complexes and release inflammatory mediators, thereby contributing to the pathogenesis of BP.[25] The mononuclear infiltrate of the dermis in BP is composed mainly of CD3,CD4$^+$ T cells; B cells and plasma cells are seldom found in BP lesions.[26] As the titers of antibody in BP blister fluid and serum correlate, it is likely that blister fluid antibodies arise by diffusion from serum rather than local production. Evidence for antibody in the pathogenesis of mucous membrane pemphigoid comes from the subtype of individuals with antibodies directed to laminin 5. Passive transfer of rabbit antilaminin 5 IgG or Fab fragments to neonatal mice induced subepithelial mucocutaneous blistering consistent with the laminin 5 mucous membrane pemphigoid clinical phenotype.[27,28] Furthermore, circulating antibodies to β4 integrin have been identified in individuals with mucous membrane pemphigoid and may promote basement membrane zone separation in conjunctival and oral mucosal organ culture models.[29,30]

It has been proposed that DH is a gluten-sensitive immune-complex disease, as it is often associated with raised levels of circulating IgA immune complexes containing dimeric IgA, which is thought to be gut derived. However, IgA is found in uninvolved skin in DH, and drug treatment does not alter the IgA deposits. Although after many years of dietary (gluten-free) treatment the IgA deposits may diminish and eventually disappear, their role in the disease pathogenesis remains unresolved.[31] Tissue transglutaminase (TGc, transglutaminase 2) is believed to be a predominant autoantigen in individuals with celiac disease. TGc is a member of the transglutaminase (TG) family, which in humans consists of at least nine distinct proteins present in a wide variety of cell types. TG family members show conservation especially of certain enzymatically relevant domains and the active members catalyze a post-translational modification linking low-molecular-weight amines to proteins, or induce an isopeptide bond between or within polypeptide chains leading to a cross-linked supramolecular protein network. Further, under special circumstances they are also able to deamidate glutamine residues. Recent studies have shown that antibodies in patients with DH show a markedly higher avidity for epidermal TG (TGe, TG 3) than in those with celiac disease. These findings suggest that TGe, rather than TGc, is the dominant autoantigen in DH and may explain why skin symptoms appear in a proportion of patients having gluten-sensitive disease.[32]

Passive transfer of EBA antibodies has provided evidence for their pathogenic role in this disease. Following injection into mice, purified human IgG EBA antibodies have been reported to induce inflammatory histological changes and complement fixation, although blistering was not observed.[33] The antibodies in LAD have also been shown to have pathogenic action. An *in vitro* study has demonstrated that LAD antibodies can induce dermoepidermal separation.[34] Possible transient neonatal disease has also been documented in the offspring of a mother affected by LAD.[35]

The circulating autoantibody titer correlates with disease activity for pemphigus, but not for other immunobullous diseases. It is possible that locally bound antibody, other inflammatory mediators, and cellular mechanisms play a relatively greater role in these diseases. Although antibodies have been demonstrated to exert a direct pathogenic role *in vitro*, the immunological milieu is far more complicated *in vivo*. Additional factors are required to explain how, in pemphigus, BP, LAD, and DH, antibody can be demonstrated in clinically uninvolved skin, and circulating antibodies can persist during clinical remission. Nevertheless, beneficial therapeutic effects following removal of circulating antibody by plasmapheresis have been reported in recalcitrant BP, PG, and EBA as well as pemphigus.

The initial trigger that stimulates autoantibody production is unknown. An alteration in epidermal or BMZ molecules, leading to enhanced antigenicity, or enhanced autoreactivity of B-cell clones, leading to autoantibody production, are some current ideas, but these remain speculative at present. Similarly, the factors that bring about disease remission are also poorly understood. It has been proposed that for BP, a shift in antibody subclass from IgG1 to IgG4 may play a role in disease remission in BP.[36] The target antigens of several immunobullous diseases are molecules that appear to be important in maintaining cell-to-cell or dermoepidermal cohesion, and antibodies may cause skin blistering by directly interfering with the function of these molecules, e.g., antibodies against desmosomal glycoproteins in pemphigus and antibodies against the anchoring fibrils of the sublamina densa region in EBA.

## B. Complement

Following the binding of autoantibodies to their target antigens, complement activation may be triggered, and this in turn may lead to inflammatory injury and blister formation. This is supported by the findings of studies on pemphigoid. Pemphigoid gestationis (PG) antibodies avidly fix complement *in vitro*, and C3 can be demonstrated in the BMZ of perilesional skin by direct IMF in almost all cases of BP and PG. Presence of C3 within the lamina lucida of BP blisters has also been documented by immunoelectron microscopy, and activation of both the classical and alternative pathways of complement may be involved in lesional skin.[3]

Direct evidence of the pathogenic role of complement in BP has been demonstrated by the inability of mice depleted of complement (either genetically or with cobra venom factor) to develop blistering disease following injection of pathogenic anti-BP180 antibodies.[37] Furthermore F(ab)2 fragments of these pathogenic antibodies did not induce disease in the mice. In addition to inducing an inflammatory cell infiltrate, the presence of the membrane attack complex at the BMZ in BP lesions suggests that complement may also have direct cytopathic actions.[38]

The role of the complement system in pemphigus is controversial at present. Pemphigus antibodies can fix complement, and complement deposition has been observed in acantholytic lesions, but not in the adjacent clinically normal appearing skin of patients with pemphigus. Complement-fixing antibodies may mediate the development of inflammatory changes by the release of C5a, which induces the chemotaxis and activation of leukocytes, and by deposition of C3b at the intercellular space, which mediates the attachment and stimulation of leukocytes.[39] It could provide a mechanism to augment epidermal cell acantholysis in addition to the plasminogen-plasmin system (*vide infra*).[1]

In the inflammatory variant of EBA, neutrophil infiltration and tissue injury appear to be dependent on the generation of complement-derived chemotactic factors, and the BMZ immune complexes in this disease appear to be heterogeneous in their ability to mediate neutrophil adherence. A study on complement deposits in EBA and BP showed that complement activation in EBA proceeded to activation of the terminal complement components, and EBA antibodies appeared to be more potent activators of C5 than BP antibodies.[40] In LAD, complement does not appear to be necessary for antibody-induced dermoepidermal separation. Deposition of C3 is found in early lesional skin in DH, and complement components may be important as neutrophil chemoattractants in this disease. However, the presence of both complement and immune complexes in uninvolved skin suggests that other mechanisms are important in generating skin lesions. On treatment with a gluten-free diet, the prevalence of C3 in uninvolved skin falls progressively as the quantity of IgA falls, suggesting that less complement is being activated.[31]

## C. Proteases

Investigation of the mechanisms of complement-independent antibody-mediated acantholysis in pemphigus provided evidence for the role of proteases in causing cell dysadhesion in this disease. *In vitro* studies showed that pemphigus antibody-mediated acantholysis could be blocked by the addition of a general protease inhibitor, $\alpha$2-macroglobulin, or a serine protease inhibitor.[41] Subsequent studies showed that addition of pemphigus IgG to human epidermal cells in culture led to a specific increase in synthesis of the protease plasminogen activator (PA). It has been hypothesized that enhanced PA production by pemphigus antibodies leads to local generation of the broad-spectrum protease plasmin from its proenzyme plasminogen. Plasmin then cleaves epidermal cell adhesion molecules leading to increased fragility and blistering.[42] The mechanism by which binding of pemphigus antibody leads to increased synthesis of PA is unknown, but recent studies suggest that the inositol triphosphate pathway and phospholipase C may be involved in signal transduction.[43]

Mice depleted of neutrophils by pretreatment with an anti-neutrophil serum become resistant to the pathogenic effects of BP 180 antibodies,[44] indicating that neutrophils may contribute to the inflammatory response in BP. The role of proteases in blister formation has been shown using mouse models either genetically deficient for neutrophil elastase or with elastase inhibitors, and by demonstrating that elastase can cleave BP180 *in vitro* and *in vivo*.[45] Furthermore, mice genetically deficient for gelatinase B did not produce blisters after infusion with antibodies to BP180, unless reconstituted with neutrophils from normal mice.[46] The role of proteases in the pathogenesis of blistering in other bullous diseases is less well defined. High levels of collagenase and elastase activity have been documented in the blister fluid of DH. It is possible that these are derived from the abundant neutrophils present in lesional skin, and play an important role in blister formation. Alternatively, the basal keratinocyte in DH may be the source of proteases including collagenase, stromelysin-1, and plasminogen activator.[47] Release of proteases from neutrophils may be stimulated by local deposits of IgA immune complexes.[48] *In vitro* studies in LAD and BP suggest that proteases are important in antibody-mediated dermoepidermal separation. In BP it has been suggested that proteases are released from inflammatory cells secondary to complement activation, which in turn follows antibody–target antigen interaction.[49]

### D. Cytokines and Other Inflammatory Mediators

The immunobullous diseases are inflammatory conditions, and in addition to antibodies, complement, and proteases, it is likely that other humoral mediators play a role in both generating and controlling inflammation. BP blister fluid has been shown to contain platelet-activating factor, eosinophil chemotactic factor (ECF), leukotrienes B4 and C4, and increased levels of IL-6, TNF, and soluble CD23. Activated keratinocytes have been shown to release IL-1, IL-6, and TNF in response to various stimuli, and keratinocyte-derived cytokines may participate in the induction of skin blistering. It has also been speculated that the raised serum IgE and induction of IgG4 and IgE class antibodies and FceRII expressing cells in BP are attributable to excessive IL-4 activity.[25] However, the role of cytokines in the pathogenesis of bullous diseases has yet to be studied in detail.

Increased microvascular permeability permits inflammatory cell recruitment into lesional skin, leads to dermal edema and fibrin deposition, and contributes to blister formation. Recent evidence suggests that vascular permeability factor/vascular endothelial growth factor (VPF), which has a potency some 50,000 times that of histamine on a molar basis, may be an important mediator of increased microvascular permeability in bullous diseases. Overexpression of VPF expression by keratinocytes has been demonstrated in lesional skin of BP, DH, and erythema multiforme.[50]

Cytokine alterations that have been documented in lesional DH skin include increased expression of endothelial leucocyte adhesion molecule 1 (ELAM-1) in the deep dermis, IL-8 by basal keratinocytes, and GM-CSF by dendritic cells at the dermoepidermal junction.[7] These adhesion molecules and cytokines are known to promote the infiltration and activation of neutrophils, and may play an important role in the generation of DH lesions. A range of mechanisms must also exist to limit inflammation and tissue damage in the immunobullous diseases, and these have yet to be defined. For example, although the level of immunoreactive TNF is elevated in BP blisters, studies have shown that there is no actual increase in bioactivity of such fluid compared with suction blisters from unaffected controls. Increased levels of soluble TNF receptor have been demonstrated in BP blister fluid and these might neutralize the biological activity of TNF.[51]

## IV. IMMUNOBULLOUS DISEASES

### A. Pemphigus

Pemphigus is an intraepidermal blistering disease characterized by loss of epidermal cell cohesion (acantholysis). It presents with fragile blisters and erosions of the skin and mucous membranes.

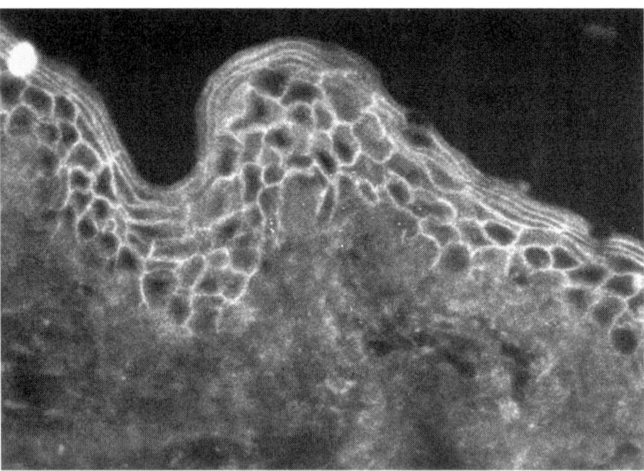

**FIGURE 24.2** Direct immunofluorescence of PV skin showing intercellular IgG deposition. (Original magnification × 200.)

The subtypes of pemphigus are pemphigus vulgaris (PV), pemphigus vegetans (PVe), pemphigus foliaceus (PF), pemphigus erythematosus (PE), and the newly described entities paraneoplastic pemphigus and IgA pemphigus. The target antigens of PV and PF antibodies have recently been defined, and are members of the desmoglein subfamily of the cadherin supergene family. The major PV and PF antigens are a 130-kDa desmosomal glycoprotein now thought to be desmoglein (Dsg)3 and 160-kDa Dsg1, respectively. These molecules are complexed with plakoglobin, a desmosomal plaque protein, and play an important role in cell adhesion.[52] There appears to be heterogeneity in the composition of desmosomes at different levels in the epidermis, and this may explain how acantholysis occurs at a suprabasal level in PV, and relatively higher in the epidermis in PF.[53] It has been suggested that circulating antibodies to desmoglein 3 are associated with mucosal dominant PV, whereas the presence of both anti-desmoglein 1 and 3 is associated with mucocutaneous PV. Antibody binding is noted throughout the epidermis in all variants of pemphigus (Figure 24.2), and it has been suggested that antibodies cause cell separation where the target antigen is the chief adhesion molecule. Paraneoplastic pemphigus antibodies recognize multiple antigens including those derived from nonstratified epithelia, and this may represent a cross-reactive phenomenon with tumor-associated antigens.

Immunogenetic studies have shown an association of pemphigus with HLA DR4, DQ8, DR6, and DQ5, and affected patients have an increased incidence of other autoimmune diseases. Endemic Brazilian PF may be triggered by an infective environmental factor, possibly borne by the Simulium black fly, and a minority of cases are drug induced or possibly diet associated. Penicillamine and sulfydryl drugs are most commonly implicated, and *in vitro* studies show that the latter may directly mediate acantholysis. There appears to be a correlation of antibody subclass with disease activity in PV: low levels of pemphigus IgG1 have been demonstrated in patients in remission and in their unaffected relatives, whereas patients with active disease have both IgG1 and IgG4 subclass antibodies.[54]

## B. Bullous Pemphigoid (BP)

BP is the most common immunobullous disease, and characteristically affects elderly people. It presents with tense blisters and pruritic urticated plaques (Figure 24.3) and may have a nonbullous prodromal phase. There usually is no identifiable trigger for this condition, and sufferers do not appear to be prone to develop other autoimmune diseases. Our recent immunogenetic studies have shown an increased incidence of HLA DQ7 in affected individuals.

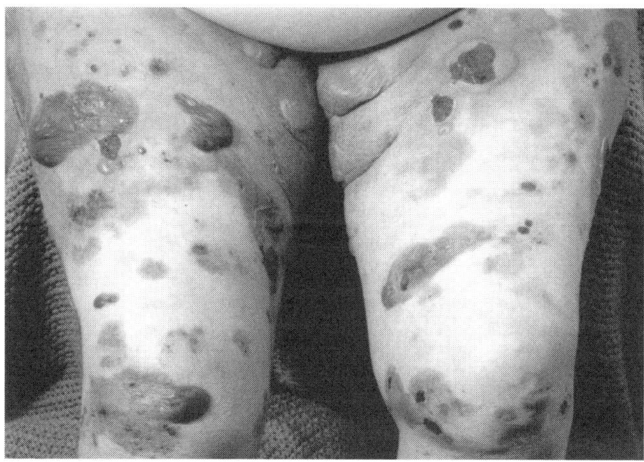

**FIGURE 24.3** BP: tense hemorrhagic blisters and urticated plaques. (Original magnification × 200.)

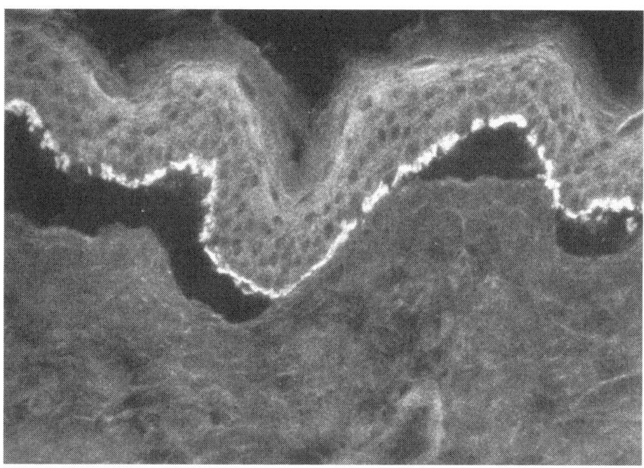

**FIGURE 24.4** Indirect immunofluorescence of BP serum on salt-split human skin substrate showing IgG labeling to the epidermal (roof) aspect of the split. (Original magnification × 200.)

In the majority of cases, circulating IgG anti-BMZ antibodies can be demonstrated in addition to tissue-bound antibodies. These antibodies bind to the epidermal (roof) aspect of a split skin substrate, which has been split through the lamina lucida (Figure 24.4). Two major target antigens, BP180 and BP230, have been identified by Western immunoblotting of BP sera against skin extracts. BP180 is a transmembrane molecule of the basal keratinocyte, which has a long collagenous extracellular tail.[55] BP230 is a major plaque protein of hemidesmosomes and has an intracellular localization. Although originally referred to as the minor BP antigen, BP180 is now believed to be of major antigenic significance in BP, as its immunodominant domains are extracellular and therefore accessible to antibody binding prior to cell disruption.

## C. Mucous Membrane Pemphigoid

Mucous membrane pemphigoid (MMP) is a chronic blistering disease with a predilection for mucosal surfaces and a propensity to produce severe scarring (Figure 24.5). Low titer circulating anti-BMZ antibodies of both IgG and IgA class occur in this disease, and may be detected more easily by use of a split skin substrate. MMP antibodies target BP180 and BP230. Recent studies have also demonstrated antibodies against laminin V, $\alpha 6\beta 4$ integrin, and collagen VII. The reason

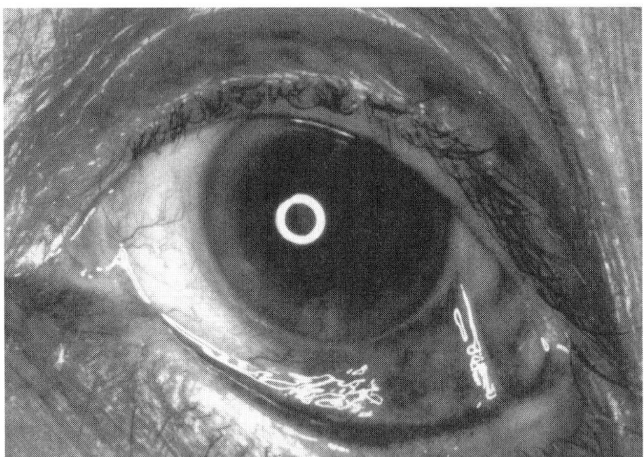

**FIGURE 24.5** Adhesions of the occular mucosa in MMP.

scarring is such a characteristic feature of MMP remains unknown at present, but increased amounts of fibrogenic growth factors are demonstrable by immunohistochemistry.[5] There is an association with HLA DQ7 (DQB1*0301), and affected patients are at an increased risk of developing other autoimmune diseases.

## D. Pemphigoid Gestationis

Pemphigoid gestationis (PG) is a rare autoimmune disease of pregnancy and the puerperium, and clinically resembles BP. It is characterized by intense linear deposition of C3 at the BMZ, and circulating IgG1 antibodies, which have strong complement fixing ability. Transplacental passage of antibody occurs and may produce transient mild neonatal disease. Aberrant expression of major histocompatibility complex (MHC) class II antigens in the placenta appears to trigger the immune response. Cytotoxic anti-HLA antibodies against both class I and class II antigens are a characteristic feature of this disease in addition to antibodies against BP180. Affected individuals have an increased incidence of autoimmune disease, especially Grave's disease, and this appears to be related to the immunogenetic association with HLA DR3 and DR4. Studies of complement polymorphisms have also shown that 90% of PG cases have a C4 null allele, and this may account for the abnormal handling of circulating immune complexes which is found in this condition.[56]

## E. Linear IgA Disease

This uncommon bullous dermatosis is characterized by linear deposition of IgA with or without other immunoreactants at the cutaneous BMZ. Circulating IgA BMZ antibodies may also be detected, and these are of the IgA1 subclass. The disease presents with grouped vesicles or bullae and there is often symptomatic involvement of the mucous membranes. It is now generally accepted that chronic bullous disease of childhood (CBDC) and adult LAD represent the same disease entity, these groups differing only in their age of disease onset. Unlike DH, LAD does not show any response to withdrawal of dietary gluten, and the trigger for disease onset is unknown in most cases, although infection or drug ingestion have been documented to precipitate some cases. There appears to be considerable heterogeneity in the target antigens recognized by LAD antibodies.[57] Target antigens so far identified include BP230, BP180 and its shed ectodomain, and a poorly characterized molecule of 285 kDa. Other potential target antigens include anchoring fibril and anchoring filament associated molecules.

Immunogenetic studies have identified HLA predispositions including an association with the HLA Cw7, B8, and DR3 haplotype. An association with the unusual allele of the TNF promoter region (TNF 2) and a prolonged disease duration have been demonstrated for LAD. TNF has several pro-inflammatory effects including neutrophil activation, and a heightened TNF response may play a role in the neutrophilic infiltrates that characterize LAD and DH.

### F. Epidermolysis Bullosa Acquisita

Epidermolysis bullosa acquisita (EBA) is one of the rarest immunobullous diseases and it is characterized by acquired skin fragility, with blistering and scarring of trauma-prone sites. This may be preceded by a BP-like inflammatory phase.[10] The major antigenic epitopes recognized by EBA antibodies are in the noncollagenous domain of collagen VII in the anchoring fibrils of the sublamina densa zone. These peptides show sequence homology with fibronectin, and may be important sites for interaction with other BMZ molecules.[58] Antibodies against these epitopes could directly affect anchoring fibril function and lead to enhanced BMZ fragility. EBA shares many clinical features with dystrophic EB, in which there is a genetic abnormality in collagen VII production, and the same target antigen is recognized by antibodies in bullous systemic lupus erythematosus (SLE).

Both EBA and bullous SLE have been reported to share a common genetic predisposition with an increased incidence of HLA DR2 in affected individuals, and this may predispose to collagen autoimmunity.

Although only one target antigen has been identified in EBA, this disease shows great clinical heterogeneity, and the factors that determine disease expression are unknown. It is usually a treatment-resistant disease and may fail to respond to potent immunosuppressants.

### G. Dermatitis Herpetiformis

Dermatitis herpetiformis (DH) presents with an intensely pruritic papulovesicular rash, and is characterized immunohistologically by the presence of granular IgA deposits in the dermal papillae of uninvolved skin. The disease usually starts in early adult life, and is associated with a subclinical gluten-sensitive enteropathy. Both the skin disease and enteropathy resolve on withdrawal of dietary gluten, and relapse on its reintroduction, but it remains undetermined how gluten produces lesions at either site. It has been hypothesized that adenoviral infection or high exposure to cereals may trigger gluten allergy.[59] Familial and genetic studies have shown that the susceptibility to develop DH or celiac diseases (CD) is genetically determined, and both DH and CD are associated with HLA alleles DQ A1*0501 and B1*0201. There is also an association with other autoimmune diseases.

The optimum treatment of DH is with a strict gluten-free diet, and this has been shown to reduce the risk of affected patients developing a small-bowel lymphoma. Alternatively, treatment with the antineutrophil drug dapsone can be used and provides prompt symptomatic control.

It has been suggested that the IgA immune complexes in the skin represent a gluten–antigluten immune complex, but this has not yet been confirmed. Circulating antigliadin antibodies are present in about half of the patients with DH, and their presence correlates well with gut pathology, but the titer does not correlate with the severity of the rash. IgA antibodies that bind to human skin have not been detected in the serum of patients with DH, but IgA antibodies against reticulin and endomysium may be detected in both the sera and gastrointestinal secretions of affected individuals. Recent data suggest that TGe is a dominant autoantigen in DH and differential recognition of TG family members may explain why skin symptoms appear in only a proportion of patients with gluten sensitivity.[32]

## V. IMMUNODIAGNOSIS

As the immunobullous diseases share common clinical features, further investigations are required to establish a diagnosis and exclude other bullous disorders. Histology of a fresh blister will

**TABLE 24.1**
**Immunofluorescent Features of the Immunobullous Diseases**

| Disease | Direct IMF* | Indirect IMF-Intact Skin and Split Skin | Target Antigens |
|---|---|---|---|
| Pemphigus | Intercellular IgG throughout epidermis | Intercellular IgG | Desmosomal plaque proteins — desmoglein 1 (160 kDa), desmoglein 3 (130 kDa), desmocollins, plakins (paraneoplastic) |
| Bullous pemphigoid | Linear IgG + C3 at BMZ | Linear IgG and C3 | BP1 (230 kDa), BP2 (180 kDa), 200 kDa |
| Mucous membrane pemphigoid | Linear IgG + C3 at BMZ | Linear IgG and C3 in low titer | BP1, BP2 as above. Laminin 5, α6β4 integrin, ?205kDa, ?45 kDa, collagen VII |
| Pemphigoid gestationis | Linear C3 | Linear C3 binding | BP2 180 kDa, BP1 230 kDa |
| Linear IgA disease | Linear IgA at BMZ | Linear IgA at BMZ | BP1 (230 kDa), BP2 (180 kDa), BP2 ectodomain (97 kDa), 285 kDa, collagen VII |
| Epidermolysis bullosa acquisita | Linear IgG ± C3 at BMZ | Linear IgG at BMZ | NC1 domains of collagen VII |
| Dermatitis herpetiformis | Granular IgA at BMZ | -ve | ?Epidermal transglutaminase |

differentiate intraepidermal and subepidermal bullous diseases by identifying the level of skin cleavage. The composition of any associated inflammatory infiltrate sometimes provides an additional diagnostic clue, and in the majority of cases the results of histology, direct IMF, and indirect IMF yield sufficient information to establish a diagnosis.

IMF investigations are the mainstay of diagnosis, and the IMF findings of different immunobullous diseases are summarized in Table 24.1. Direct IMF should be performed on perilesional skin or mucosa to demonstrates tissue-bound immunoreactants, antibodies, and complement components.

Indirect IMF of the patients' serum detects circulating antibodies against BMZ antigens or epidermal cells. Human skin or animal-derived epithelia such as monkey esophagus can be used as a substrate, but the former gives more reliable results. Indirect IMF can also be performed on split skin, and this is generally a more sensitive substrate for antibody detection. It also provides further information about the sites of antibody binding, and this may be of diagnostic value. Molar sodium chloride, calcium chloride, heat, suction, and proteolytic enzymes can be used to split the skin substrate, with the former used widely.

Western immunoblotting of the patient's serum against epidermal and dermal extracts obtained from salt split skin can be performed to estimate the molecular mass of the target antigen(s) against which circulating antibodies have formed. This also identifies whether antibodies react with epidermal or dermal associated antigens, and can be of help in differentiating dermal-binding antibodies that may occur in a minority of cases of BP and MMP in addition to EBA. Immunoprecipitation studies provide similar information, but involve use of proteins extracted from cultured epidermal cells or fibroblasts. One advantage of this procedure is that the antigen is less denatured. Immunoprecipitation can also be carried with monoclonal antibodies to document the presence and quantity of a specific antigen in a tissue extract.

Other specialized investigations include IEM to localize the ultrastructural site of *in vivo* antibody deposition and circulating antibody binding. The more recently developed immunogold technique provides greater definition of the site of immunoreactant labeling than immunoperoxidase techniques, but these remain research-based procedures, and are not routinely available outside specialized centers.

## VI. IMMUNOTHERAPY

The immunobullous diseases are chronic dermatoses, but some cases go into remission after several years. A range of anti-inflammatory drugs may be used to achieve control of active disease phases and maintain remission. Systemic corticosteroids such as oral prednisone and prednisolone are the mainstay of therapy for acute pemphigus and BP, and are usually effective in establishing disease control. They are usually started at a high dose, then tapered gradually to a lower maintenance dose. Pulsed therapy with intravenous steroids has been used to treat resistant pemphigus. Azathioprine is frequently used as a steroid-sparing drug, although there is a delay of several weeks in the onset of its effects. Other steroid-sparing agents that have been reported to be of use in immunobullous diseases include cyclophosphamide and cyclosporine. Cyclophosphamide may be given in a pulsed regimen with steroids or as a lower dose continuous therapy for pemphigus and in recalcitrant BP, and has been shown to be one of the most effective forms of treatment for severe ocular MMP. These drugs may cause serious adverse effects and require close monitoring. Widespread or severe disease usually requires prolonged systemic therapy, but in patients with mild or localized BP or MMP, a very potent topical corticosteroid alone may suffice.

The IgA-mediated diseases DH and LAD, the rare bullous variant of SLE and IgA pemphigus, respond to treatment with dapsone or the sulfonamides sulfapyridine and sulfamethoxypyridazine. These diseases are characterized by neutrophilic infiltrates and the drugs are presumed to act by modulating neutrophil function, although their precise mechanism of action is unknown.

Recent evidence suggests that a combination of tetracyclines and niacinamide may provide a useful alternative to systemic steroids in the treatment of BP and LAD, and tetracyclines alone have been used successfully in the treatment of MMP.[60] Colchicine has been reported to be of use in LAD and EBA, but the mechanobullous variant of EBA is typically a recalcitrant disease and therapeutic trials are hampered by its apparent rarity.

Plasmapheresis has been used as an adjuvant to corticosteroids in BP, PG, and pemphigus. This treatment must be given in conjunction with other agents to suppress the rebound increase in antibody synthesis that occurs post-plasmapheresis. In view of the serious potential risks associated with this therapy, it is reserved for severe, treatment-resistant disease. Adjuvant therapy with high doses of intravenous gamma globulins has been used with great success in several autoimmune disorders, and there have been a few recent reports of improvement in resistant cases of pemphigus and EBA with this treatment. However, the patients who fail to respond to these treatments are generally not reported.

## VII. CONCLUSION

The immunobullous diseases are rare inflammatory skin diseases that share overlapping clinical and immunological features. There is increasing evidence that both humoral and cellular immune mechanisms play a role in their pathogenesis, but their relative importance may differ from one disease to another. In the majority of cases, the cause of these diseases is unknown, but identification of the target antigens and immunogenetic factors provides advances in our understanding. Future ideas for therapy may be based on more specific modulation of the immune system, e.g., by recombinant cytokines.

## REFERENCES

1. Jordan, R.E., Kawana, S., and Fritz, K.A., Immunopathological mechanisms in pemphigus and bullous pemphigoid. *J. Invest. Dermatol.*, 85, 72s, 1985.
2. Wintroub, B.U., Mihm, M.C., and Goetzl, E.J., Morphologic and functional evidence for release of mast-cell products in bullous pemphigoid. *N. Engl. J. Med.*, 298, 417, 1978.

3. Anhalt, G. and Lazarus, G.S., Pemphigus and pemphigoid: autoantibody mediated dermatoses, in *Inflammation: Basic Principles and Clinical Correlates,* Galin, J.I., Goldstein, I.M., and Snyderman, R., Eds., Raven Press, New York, 1992, chap. 45.
4. Ståhle-Bäckdahl, M., Inoue, M., Guidice, G.J., and Parks, W.C., 92-kDa gelatinase is produced by eosinophils at the site of blister formation in bullous pemphigoid and cleaves the extracellular domain of recombinant 180-kDa bullous pemphigoid antigen. *J. Clin. Invest.,* 93, 2022, 1994.
5. Elder, M.J. and Lightman, S., The immunological features and pathophysiology of ocular cicatricial pemphigoid. *Eye,* 8, 196, 1994.
6. Garioch, J.J., Baker, B.S., Leonard, J.N., and Fry, L., T-lymphocytes in lesional skin of patients with dermatitis herpetiformis. *Br. J. Dermatol.,* 131, 822, 1994.
7. Graeber, M., Baker, B.S., Garioch, J.J., Valdimarsson, H., Leonard, J.N., and Fry, L., The role of cytokines in the generation of skin lesions in dermatitis herpetiformis. *Br. J. Dermatol.,* 129, 530, 1993.
8. Niwa, Y., Sakane, T., Shingu, M., Yanagida, I., Komura, J., and Miyachi, Y., Neutrophil-generated active oxygens in linear IgA bullous dermatosis. *Arch. Dermatol.,* 121, 73, 1985.
9. Hendrix, J.D., Mangum, K.L., Zone, J.J., and Gammon, W.R.. Cutaneous IgA deposits in bullous diseases function as ligands to mediate adherence of activated neutrophils. *J. Invest. Dermatol.,* 94, 667, 1990.
10. Gammon, W.R. and Briggaman, R.A., Epidermolysis bullosa acquisita and bullous systemic lupus erythematosus. *Dermatol. Clin.,* 11, 535, 1993.
11. Ward, J.C., Gitlin, J.B., Garry, D.J., Jatoi, A., Luikart, S.D., Zelickson, B.D., Dahl, M.V., and Skubitz, K.M., Epidermolysis bullosa acquisita induced by GM-CSF: a role for eosinophils in treatment related toxicity. *Br. J. Haematol.,* 81, 27, 1992.
12. Schiltz, J.R. and Michel, B., Production of epidermal acantholysis in normal human skin *in vitro* by the IgG fraction from pemphigus serum. *J. Invest. Dermatol.,* 67, 254, 1976.
13. Schiltz, J.R., Michel, B., and Papay, R., Pemphigus antibody interaction with human epidermal cells in culture. *J. Clin. Invest.,* 62, 778, 1978.
14. Anhalt, G.J., Labib, R.S., Voorhees, J.J., Beald, T.F., and Diaz, L.A., Induction of pemphigus in neonatal mice by passive transfer of IgG from patients with the disease. *N. Engl. J. Med.,* 306, 1189, 1982.
15. Peterson, L.L. and Wuepper, K.D., Isolation and purification of pemphigus vulgaris antigen from human epidermis. *J. Clin. Invest.,* 73, 1113, 1984.
16. Rock, B., Martins, C.R., Theofilopoulos, A.N., Balderas, R.S., Anhalt, G.J., Labib, R.S., Futamura, S., Rivitti, E.A., and Diaz, L.A., The pathogenic effect of IgG4 antibodies in endemic pemphigus foliaceus. *N. Engl. J. Med.,* 320, 1463, 1989.
17. Amagai, M., Tsunoda, K., Zillikens, D., Nagai, T., and Nishikawa, T., The clinical phenotype of pemphigus is defined by the anti-desmoglein autoantibody profile. *J. Am. Acad. Dermatol.,* 40, 167, 1999.
18. Komai, A., Amagai, M., Ishii, K., Nishikawa, T., Chorzelski, T., Matsuo, I., and Hashimoto, T., The clinical transition between pemphigus foliaceus and pemphigus vulgaris correlates well with the changes in autoantibody profile assessed by an enzyme-linked immunosorbent assay. *Br. J. Dermatol.,* 144, 1177, 2001.
19. Harman, K.E., Seed, P.T., Gratian, M.J., Bhogal, B.S., Challacombe, S.J., and Black, M.M., The severity of cutaneous and oral pemphigus is related to desmoglein 1 and 3 antibody levels. *Br. J. Dermatol.,* 144, 775, 2001.
20. Amagai, M., Matsuyoshi, N., Wang, Z. H., Andl, C., and Stanley, J.R., Toxin in bullous impetigo and staphylococcal scalded-skin syndrome targets desmoglein 1. *Nat. Med.,* 6, 1275, 2000.
21. Amagai, M., Yamaguchi, T., Hanakawa, Y., Nishifuji, K., Sugai, M., and Stanley, J.R., Staphylococcal exfoliative toxin B specifically cleaves desmoglein 1. *J. Invest. Dermatol.,* 118, 845, 2002.
22. Liu, Z., Diaz, L.A., and Giudice, G.A., Autoimmune response against the bullous pemphigoid 180 autoantigen. *Dermatology,* 189, 34, 1994.
23. Kitajima, Y., Hirako, Y., Owaribe, K., and Yaoita, H., A possible cell biologic mechanism involved in blister formation of bullous pemphigoid: anti-180 kDa BP antibody is an initiator. *Dermatology,* 189(Suppl. 1), 46, 1994.
24. Asbrink, E. and Hovmar, K.A., Serum IgE levels in patients with bullous pemphigoid and its correlation to the activity of the disease and anti-basement membrane zone antibodies. *Acta Derm. Venereol.* (Stockholm), 64, 243, 1984.

25. Soh, H., Hosokawa, H., and Asada, Y., IgE and its related phenomena in bullous pemphigoid. *Br. J. Dermatol.,* 128, 371, 1993.
26. Nestor, M.S., Cochrane, A.J., and Ahmed, A.R., Mononuclear cell infiltrates in bullous diseases. *J. Invest. Dermatol.,* 88, 172, 1987.
27. Lazarova, Z., Yee, C., Darling, T., Briggaman, R.A., and Yancey, K.B., Passive transfer of anti-laminin 5 antibodies induces subepidermal blisters in neonatal mice. *J. Clin. Invest.,* 98, 1509, 1996.
28. Lazarova, Z., Hsu, R., Briggaman, R.A., and Yancey, K.B., Fab fragments directed against laminin 5 induce subepidermal blisters in neonatal mice. *Clin. Immunol.,* 95, 26, 2000.
29. Chan, R.Y., Bhol, K., Tesavibul, N., Letko, E., Simmons, R.K., Foster, C.S., and Ahmed, A.R., The role of antibody to human beta4 integrin in conjunctival basement membrane separation: possible *in vitro* model for ocular cicatricial pemphigoid. Invest. *Ophthalmol. Vis. Sci.,* 40, 2283, 1999.
30. Bhol, K.C., Colon, J.E., and Ahmed, A.R., Autoantibody in mucous membrane pemphigoid binds to an intracellular epitope on human beta4 integrin and causes basement membrane zone separation in oral mucosa in an organ culture model. *J. Invest. Dermatol.,* 120, 701, 2003.
31. Fry, L., Dermatitis herpetiformis in *Management of Blistering Diseases,* Wojnarowska, F. and Briggaman, R.A., Eds., Chapman & Hall Medical, London, 1990, chap. 11.
32. Sardy, M., Karpati, S., Merkl, B., Paulsson, M., and Smyth, N., Epidermal transglutaminase (TGase 3) is the autoantigen of dermatitis herpetiformis. *J. Exp. Med.,* 195, 747, 2002.
33. Borrradori, L., Caldwell, J.B., Briggaman, R.A., Burr, C.E., Gammon, W.R. James, W.D., and Yancey, K.B., Passive transfer of autoantibodies from a patient with mutilating epidermolysis bullosa acquisita induces specific alterations in the skin of neonatal mice. *Arch. Dermatol.,* 131, 590, 1995.
34. Akahoshi, Y., Kanda, G., Anan, S., and Yoshida, H., Dermo-epidermal blister formation by linear IgA dermatosis sera in normal human skin in organ culture. *J. Dermatol.,* 14, 352,1987.
35. Collier, P.M., Kelley, S.E., and Wojnarowska, F., Linear IgA disease and pregnancy. *J. Am. Acad. Dermatol.,* 30, 407, 1994.
36. Modre, B., Allen, J., and Wojnarowska, F., Is class switching a mechanism of disease remission in bullous pemphigoid. *Br. J. Dermatol.,* 132, 654, 1995.
37. Liu, Z., Guidice, G.J., Swartz, S.J., Fairley, J.A., Till, G.O., Troy, J.L., and Diaz, L.A., The role of complement in experimental bullous pemphigoid. *J. Clin. Invest.,* 95, 1539, 1995.
38. Dahl, M.V., Falk, R.J., Carpenter, R., and Michael, A.F., Deposition of membrane attack complex of complement in bullous pemphigoid. *J. Invest. Dermatol.,* 82, 132, 1984.
39. Tagami, H., The role of complement-derived mediators in inflammatory skin diseases. *Arch. Derm. Res.,* 284(Suppl.), 2, 1992.
40. Mooney, E., Falk, R.J., and Gammon, W.R., Studies on complement deposits in epidermolysis bullosa acquisita and bullous pemphigoid. *Arch. Dermatol.,* 128, 58, 1992.
41. Farb, R.M., Dykes, R., and Lazarus, G.S., Anti-epidermal cell surface pemphigus antibody detaches viable epidermal cells from culture plates by activation of proteinase. *Proc. Natl. Acad. Sci. U.S.A.,* 75, 459, 1978.
42. Morioka, S., Lazarus, G.S., and Jensen, P.J., Involvement of urokinase type plasminogen activator in acantholysis induced by pemphigus IgG. *J. Invest. Dermatol.,* 89, 474, 1987.
43. Esaki, C., Seshima, M., Yamada, T., Osada, K., and Kitajima, Y., Pharmacologic evidence for involvement of phospholipase C in pemphigus IgG-induced inositol 1,4,5 triphosphate generation, intracellular calcium release, and plasminogen activator secretion in DJM-1 cells, a squamous cell carcinoma line. *J. Invest. Dermatol.,* 105, 329, 1995.
44. Liu, Z., Giudice, G.J., Zhou, X., Swartz, S.J., Troy, J.L., Fairley, J.A., Till, G.O., and Diaz, L.A., A major role for neutrophils in experimental bullous pemphigoid. *J. Clin. Invest.,* 100, 1256, 1997.
45. Liu, Z., Shapiro, S.D., Zhou, X., Twining, S.S., Senior, R.M., Giudice, G.J., Fairley, J.A., and Diaz, L.A., A critical role for neutrophil elastase in experimental bullous pemphigoid. *J. Clin. Invest.,* 105, 113, 2000.
46. Liu, Z., Shipley, J.M., Vu, T.H., Zhou, X., Diaz, L.A., Werb, Z., and Senior, R.M., Gelatinase B-deficient mice are resistant to experimental bullous pemphigoid. *J. Exp. Med.,* 188, 475, 1998.
47. Airola, K., Vaalamo, M., Reunala, T., and Saarialho-Kere, U., Enhanced expression of interstitial collagenase, stromelysin-1, and urokinase plasminogen activator in lesions of dermatitis herpetiformis. *J. Invest. Dermatol.,* 105, 184, 1995.

48. Oikarinen, A.I., Zone, J.J., Ahmed, A.R., Kiistala, U., and Uitto, J., Demonstration of the collagenase and elastase activities in the blister fluid from bullous skin diseases. Comparison between dermatitis herpetiformis and bullous pemphigoid. *J. Invest. Dermatol.*, 81, 261, 1983.
49. Takamori, K., Yoshiike, T., Morioka, S., and Ogawa, H., The role of proteases in the pathogenesis of bullous dermatoses. *Int. J. Dermatol.*, 27, 533, 1988.
50. Brown, L.F., Harrist, T.J., Yeo, K.-T., Ståhle-Bäckdahl, M., Jackman, R.W., Berse, B., Tognazzi, K., Dvorak, H.F., and Detmar, M., Increased expression of vascular permeability factor (vascular endothelial growth factor) in bullous pemphigoid, dermatitis herpetiformis and erythema multiforme. *J. Invest. Dermatol.*, 104, 744, 1995.
51. Zentner, A.., Rendl, J., Grelle, I., Dummer, R., Brocker, E.B., and Zillikens, D., Elevated levels of soluble tumour necrosis factor receptor I in blister fluids of bullous pemphigoid and suction blisters. *Arch. Derm. Res.*, 286, 355, 1994.
52. Amagai, M., Autoantibodies against cell adhesion molecules in pemphigus. *J. Dermatol.*, 21, 833, 1994.
53. Shimizu, H., Masunaga, T., Ishiko, A., Kikuchi, A., Hashimoto, T., and Nishikawa, T., Pemphigus vulgaris and pemphigus foliaceus sera show an inversely graded binding pattern to extracellular regions of desmosomes in different layers of human epidermis. *J. Invest. Dermatol.*, 105, 153, 1995.
54. Bohl, K., Mohimen, A., and Razzaque Ahmed, A., Correlation of subclass of IgG with disease activity in pemphigus vulgaris. *Dermatology,* 189 (Suppl. 1) 85, 1994.
55. Guidice, G.J., Emery, D.J., and Diaz, L.A., Cloning and primary structural analysis of the bullous pemphigoid autoantigen BP180. *J. Invest. Dermatol.*, 99, 243, 1992.
56. Black, M.M., New observations on pemphigoid "herpes" gestationis. *Dermatology,* 189(Suppl.), 50, 1994.
57. Wojnarowska, F., Allen, J., and Collier, P., Linear IgA disease: a heterogeneous disease. *Dermatology,* 189(Suppl. 1), 52, 1994.
58. Jones, S.A., Hunt, S.W., Prisayanh, P.S., Briggaman, R.A., and Gammon, W.R., Immunodominant domains of type VII collagen are short, paired peptide sequences within the fibronectin type III homology region of the non-collagenous domain. *J. Invest. Dermatol.*, 104, 231, 1995.
59. Lähdeaho, M., Parkkonen, B., and Renuala, T., Antipeptide antibodies to adenovirus E1B protein indicate enhanced risk of coeliac disease and dermatitis herpetiformis. *Int. Arch. Allergy Immunol.*, 101, 272, 1993.
60. Huigol, S.C. and Black, M.M., Management of the immunobullous disorders. I pemphigoid. *Clin. Exp. Dermatol.*, 20, 189, 1995.

# 25 Lichen Planus and Graft-vs.-Host Disease

*Henry J.C. de Vries, Bhupendra Tank, and Rick Hoekzema*

## CONTENTS



## I. INTRODUCTION

Lichen ruber planus is an inflammatory, pruritic disease of the skin and mucous membranes, which can be either generalized or localized. It is characterized by distinctive purplish, flat-topped papules, which have a predilection for the trunk and flexor surfaces. The lesions may be discrete or coalesce to form plaques. Histopathologically, there is a "saw-tooth" pattern of epidermal hyperplasia and vacuolar alteration in the basal layer of the epidermis along with a dense upper dermal inflammatory infiltrate composed predominantly of T cells. The etiology is unknown.

Lichen planus usually affects middle-aged adults. In general, its course is self-limiting and varies from some months to years, but sometimes it persists beyond this period. The lifetime prevalence is estimated less than 1%, but exact figures are not available. It is slightly more prevalent in females than in males.[1] No racial predilection has been observed to date.[2,3]

The cause of lichen planus remains to be elucidated. Immunological and genetic factors seem to play a role in the pathogenesis. Exogenous factors like drugs, ultraviolet (UV) radiation, contact allergens, and microbiological agents have been proposed.

Apart from the "classical" clinical lichen planus there is a range of skin disorders with a similar histopathological substrate. These lichenoid reactions are often associated with drugs (lichenoid drug eruptions), contact allergens (amalgam induced oral lichen planus), autoimmune diseases (LE overlap syndrome), and graft-vs.-host disease.

## II. CLINICAL FEATURES

Lichen planus is characterized by small, flat-topped, shiny, polygonal, violaceous, pruritic papules, which may coalesce to form plaques. A network of fine white lines known as Wickham's

0-8493-1959-5/05/$0.00+$1.50

striae may be observed in the lesions.[4] Although patients with lichen planus often complain of intense itch, excoriations are rarely seen. Linear lesions may also be observed as a result of isomorphism or Koebner's phenomenon. The flexor surfaces of the wrists and the forearms, legs, penile glans, and oral mucosa are the predilection sites. The lower back, trunk, and neck are less commonly affected. The eruption is usually symmetrical and limited to a few areas, although extensive lesions may be present in incidental cases.

Secondary scaling may be present in plaques and lesions of prolonged duration, whereas lesions on the lower legs may become hypertrophic to verrucous. Lichen planus is usually self-limiting and may persist for several months or years and eventually leave behind intense hyperpigmentation.

Apart from skin, the nails are affected in about 10% of patients, with longitudinal ridging, grooving, and splitting due to involvement of the nail matrix and pterygium formation. In severe and chronic cases this may lead to permanent nail loss (secondary anonychia).

Oral lichen planus is a distinct group that often appears without further cutaneous manifestations. Lesions on the oral mucosa were reported in up to 65% of patients with cutaneous lichen planus,[5] whereas simultaneous cutaneous involvement was observed in 20 to 34% of patients with oral lichen planus.[6] However, in a number of Scandinavian studies, it was reported that oral involvement alone was eight times more common than cutaneous involvement.[7]

Clinically, oral lichen planus consists of (1) white, (2) bilateral, and (3) symmetrical lesions. The diagnosis oral lichen planus is doubtful if these three criteria are not present and other causes of leukoplakia should then be considered.[8] The sites mostly affected are the buccal mucosa and the tongue. Sometimes oral lichen planus involves the esophagus.[9] Six variants of oral lichen planus, i.e., reticular, plaque-like, atrophic, papular, erosive, and bullous have been identified.[10] The reticular form, presenting as lace-like, white linear macules, is the most common variety and is not seen as a precancerous lesion.[11] In contrast, the erosive forms are said to be associated with malignant transformation into spinous cellular carcinoma but the premalignant potential of oral lichen planus remains controversial.[12] Premalignant leukoplakia lesions are often misdiagnosed (i.e., clinician's error and pathologist's error) as oral lichen planus and may be responsible for the acclaimed premalignant potential of oral lichen planus.[13] On the one hand, at present there is no sound evidence that oral lichen planus is a *premalignant condition* leaning toward malignant change.[14] On the other hand, certain forms of oral lichen planus have a *malignant potential* as described in many case reports justifying close follow-up.[15] In women a distinct variant of erosive lichen planus of the gingiva and genitalia is known as the vulval-vaginal-gingival syndrome.[16,17] More recently, the peno-gingival syndrome was reported in men.[18]

Lichen planus has been reported to be associated with various unrelated disorders such as malignancies,[19] gastrointestinal diseases, primary biliary cirrhosis, chronic active hepatitis, ulcerative colitis, diabetes mellitus, and an array of different autoimmune diseases, but a direct relationship remains doubtful.[4] Lichen planus is uncommon in children, but was reported in two studies involving 50 and 87 children, respectively.[20,21] In these studies it was observed that the course of the disease and response to treatment were similar to that in adults.

## III. HISTOPATHOLOGY

At light microscopic level, classical lichen planus papules show moderate hyperkeratosis with few if any parakeratotic cells.[22] The granular layer shows alternating wedge-shaped hypergranulosis which corresponds clinically to the formation of Wickham's striae.[23] Acanthosis is usually present and involves the rete ridges as well as the stratum malphigii. The rete ridges show irregular lengthening and pointing, which gives them a "saw-tooth" appearance. The dermoepidermal junction is obscured by inflammatory cells that extend from the dense, bandlike dermal infiltrate. There is vacuolar degeneration of the basal layer, which, in severe cases, leads to the formation of subepidermal clefts known as the Caspary-Joseph spaces (formerly known as Max Joseph spaces), which were reported in 17% of biopsies.[24,25] In addition, homogeneous eosinophilic bodies referred to as colloid bodies, cytoid bodies, or Civatte's bodies are often observed in the papillary dermis at the dermoepidermal junction and within the epidermis.[26] Characteristically there are clustered lymphocytes adjacent to these dyskeratotic and/or dead keratinocytes, a phenomenon referred to as satellite cell necrosis.[27] Ultrastructurally, point contact between lymphocytes and keratinocytes in the epidermis was reported, and it is suggested that adjacent lymphocytes induce apoptosis in these keratinocytes.[28] The colloid bodies originate from basal keratinocytes that have become apoptotic after which fragments have been extruded into the papillary dermis. They contain keratin and are composed of tight aggregates of tonofilaments.[29,30] Colloid bodies are observed in 37 to 100% of the biopsies and are considered to be among the earliest pathological changes.[24,31,32] Langerhans cells and melanocytes are often increased in numbers.[31,33] The principal dermal feature in lichen planus is the presence of a bandlike inflammatory infiltrate consisting almost entirely of lymphocytes, intermingled with a few macrophages and melanophages.[34] In contrast to what is observed in erythema multiforme, there is little infiltration into the epidermis. Lesions of drug-induced lichen planus tend to show more parakeratosis than lesions of idiopathic disease.[35] Parakeratosis may also be observed more often in oral involvement.[36]

## IV. IMMUNOHISTOPATHOLOGICAL FEATURES

Lichen planus-specific antigen (LPSA) was identified in 1983 by Olsen et al.[37] LPSA was observed in 80% of the patients with lichen planus in the stratum granulosum and stratum spinosum, but absent in stratum corneum and stratum basale.[38] LPSA was not detected in the skin of normal individuals and patients with other dermatoses.[39] However, LPSA was not present in all lichen planus lesions of a given patient. LPSA is not as prevalent in oral lichen planus, but patients may have anti-LPSA antibodies.[39] It is now believed that LPSA is a marker for lichen planus rather than its cause.

Antinuclear antibodies have been detected in patients with lichen planus using indirect immunofluorescent tests on rat esophagus.[40] Autoantibodies have been detected in half of patients. The frequency of antinuclear antibodies was higher in erosive oral lichen planus compared with non-erosive forms.[41] There is a significant association between the concomitance of hepatitis C virus infection and oral lichen planus and the presence of autoantibodies to epithelial antigens.[42]

Colloid bodies were observed using direct immunefluorescence microscopy in 87% of the patients affected by lichen planus.[32] Various amounts of immunoglobulins IgM, IgG, and IgA and complement components C1 and C5 were detected on colloid bodies.[34] Immunoglobulin IgM is believed to be deposited in the early stages during the formation of colloid bodies, and both fibrin[29] and albumin[34] were also noted. Moreover, colloid bodies in lichen planus lesions express cytokeratins 10/11, markers of accelerated epidermal differentiation, and fetal cytokeratins 8/18 and -13, markers of epidermal dedifferentiation.[43] It is speculated that these alterations in epithelialization may trigger T-cell activation and thus cause the onset of lichen planus. Nevertheless, colloid bodies are observed in many other diseases such as lupus erythematosus and are more likely the product of apoptotic keratinocytes due to the destruction of the basal cell layer.

Linear deposits of fibrin and fibrinogen in the basement membrane zone (BMZ) of cutaneous[29] and oral[44] lesions have been reported. Immunoglobulin IgM, but not IgA, was observed in the BMZ of all cutaneous lesions.[29] In only 4% of the oral lesions, IgM but not IgA or IgG was observed.[25] Complement components C3, C4, and C5 were also observed in the BMZ of both cutaneous[34] and oral[44] lesions. Whether these immune deposits are the effect or the cause of lichen planus remains unclear. Metalloproteinases may play a concurrent role in the destruction of the basement membrane.[45] Consequently, the absence of an intact basement membrane may induce keratinocyte apoptosis.

The characteristic dermal infiltrate in lichen planus consists predominantly of T lymphocytes and few or no B cells.[31,46] Recruitment of lymphocytes to the papillary dermis may be attributed by monokines induced by interferon-gamma, or IFN-$\gamma$ (MIG).[47] Several studies report a predominance of T-helper/inducer CD4+ lymphocytes.[31,46] It was found that in concordance with increased influx of T-helper cells in lesional tissue, the percentage of total lymphocytes and T-helper cells in peripheral blood of patients with lichen planus was decreased.[48] Moreover, patients with a longer duration of the disease showed a significant decrease of T helper/T cytotoxic ratio (CD4/CD8 ratio). However, in oral lichen planus a predominance of cytotoxic/suppressor CD8+ lymphocytes has been reported.[49-51] In early lesions, T-helper cells and macrophages were predominant, but in older lesions T-suppressor cells were mainly observed.[44] These T-suppressor cells also expressed HLA-DR antigens.[44,46] A unique subclass of cytotoxic gamma-delta T lymphocytes has been found in lichen planus.[52] This subpopulation is known to recognize bacterial peptides and autoantigens.[53] Keratinocytes in the skin lesions expressed HLA-DR antigens.[54] Keratinocytes in the oral lesions expressed HLA-DR but not HLA-DP or HLA-DQ antigens.[55] Such changes could have been induced indirectly by IFN-γ.[54] The levels of epidermal glucose-6-phosphate dehydrogenase in keratinocytes were inconsistent, whereas the levels of respiratory enzymes were reduced.[56]

In early lichen planus lesions an increased number of Langerhans cells is observed in the epidermis, prior to the dense dermal infiltration of lymphocytes.[22] This indicates a role of Langerhans cells in the pathogenesis, but there is no direct evidence that Langerhans cells take up, process, or present antigen in (oral) lichen planus. The results on the quantity of Langerhans cells in lichen planus are conflicting.[57,58] In oral lichen planus lesions fewer Langerhans cells expressed less CD45RO.[59] Possibly, CD45RO-positive (CD45RO+) Langerhans cells migrate to the lymph nodes and are replaced by incoming CD45RO-negative (CD45RO−) Langerhans cells.

The immunohistopathological changes that are typical in lichen planus may also be observed in the other lichenoid tissue reactions, namely, damage to the BMZ and the epidermal basal cells. A common element among these reactions is the dermal infiltrate, which consists mainly of T-helper cells and occasional suppressor/cytotoxic T cells.[60] Destruction of basal cells ultimately leads to the detachment of the basal cell plasma membrane from the lamina densa and causes vacuolar changes.[61] One cannot distinguish between lichen planus and lichenoid tissue reactions purely on the basis of (immuno)histopathology.

## V. PATHOGENESIS

To date, the exact cause of lichen planus remains unknown. A number of etiological factors and associated mechanisms have been put forward, but none of them provides a satisfactory unifying explanation regarding the underlying antigenic trigger that ultimately leads to the histopathological changes that are observed in this disease.

A virologically triggered autoimmune process has been proposed.[41,43] Studies on hepatitis C virus (HCV) in endemic areas like the Mediterranean countries, India, but also the United States, reported a weak epidemiological correlation between lichen planus and HCV infections.[62–65] However, such a correlation was not confirmed in other studies from different countries.[66–69] Apart from epidemiological evidence, HCV RNA was detected in lichen planus lesions of chronically HCV-infected patients.[70,71] In HCV-infected patients, co-existing oral lichen planus does not seem to be affected by the IFN therapy, even though HCV RNA was not detected in the serum after treatment.[72] This finding indicates that the pathogenesis of lichen planus in HCV-infected patients involves host factors induced by HCV infection rather than its direct viral participation. Intraspousal transmission of HCV in cases of erosive oral and vaginal lichen planus has been suggested.[73]

Several case reports have been published on hepatitis B virus vaccination and the onset of lichen planus.[74,75] Similar cases, 13 pediatric and 15 adult, have been reported from various countries in the last 5 years.[76] The pediatric cases are particularly noteworthy because lichen planus is uncommon in children. An autoimmune reaction may be triggered by the viral S epitope of the vaccine.

Abnormal keratinocyte metabolism, impaired production of tonofilaments, and defects in the assembly of desmosomes have also been implicated as etiological factors.[77] Basal keratinocytes are believed to behave more like transient amplifying cells and terminally differentiated keratinocytes because of decreased metabolic and regenerative capacity. This also explains the increased production of granular cells.[78] Although immunological involvement in the pathogenesis of lichen planus was demonstrated in previous studies, [31,46,79] the primary event in the disease has not yet been identified.

There are contradictory reports on the levels of immunoglobulins IgM, IgA, IgG, IgD, and IgE in the sera of patients with lichen planus.[80–82] The levels of complement were reported to be normal.[81] The incidence of autoimmune diseases, the frequency of autoantibodies, and the levels of serum immunoglobulins were observed not to be increased in patients with lichen planus.[83] Circulating immune complexes were reported in patients with oral lichen planus.[84] The exact role of humoral (auto)immunity in lichen planus still remains obscure and its contribution appears to be minor as compared with that of cellular immunity.

The pathogenic mechanism responsible for lichen planus has been mainly attributed to the dermal T cells. Evidence for the central role of T cells in the evolution of epidermal lichen planus has been reported in various studies. T-cell receptor gene and rearrangement studies indicated that clonal T cells are present in lichen planus tissue.[52,85,86] T-cell clones derived from T-cell lines from lesional lichen planus tissue showed significantly more cytotoxic capacity against autologous lesional keratinocytes than clones from nonlesional T-cell lines.[87] Most cytotoxic clones were CD8 positive. The histopathological abnormalities observed in lichen planus disappeared when lesional skin was transplanted onto athymic mice (lacking functional T cells).[88] Similar changes were reported to occur in explants of lesional skin maintained in organ cultures.[89] These findings indicated that the migration of T cells and other components of the cellular immune response is a crucial factor in the pathogenesis of lichen planus. This view is supported by animal studies in which it was demonstrated that lichen-planus-like lesions could be evoked in syngeneic mice by local transfer of autoreactive $CD4^+$ T-cell clones with cytotoxic potential.[88,90,91]

Although there is some evidence for humoral autoimmunity[39] and cellular hypersensitivity[92,93] in some cases of oral lichen planus, the exact contribution of cell-mediated autoimmunity in this condition still remains to be established. A diagrammatic representation of the hypothetical events leading to the evolution of lichen planus is shown in Figure 25.1.

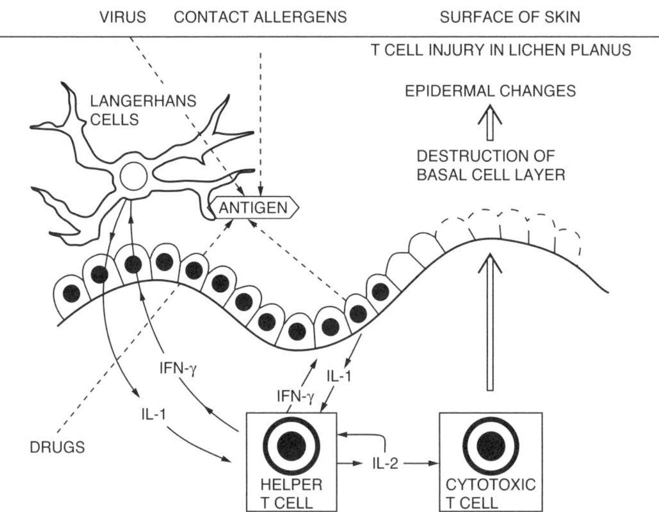


**FIGURE 25.1** Hypothetical pathogenesis of lichen planus (endogenous liberation of yet unidentified neoantigen from basal keratinocytes and lichenoid reactions triggered by the drugs and contact allergens. Keratinocytes as target cells for T-cell-mediated injury.

Oral lichen planus lesions contain increased numbers of Langerhans cells compared with normal oral mucosa.[94] It has been postulated that the primary event in classical (idiopathic) lichen planus is a delayed-type hypersensitivity reaction in which an unidentified neoantigen of basal keratinocytes is processed in the Langerhans cells followed by the recruitment of T cells.[22,95] This process is mediated via adhesive interactions between specific cell surface molecules[96,97] and directed by chemotactic cytokines produced by epithelial cells.[98] Calprotectin is upregulated in oral epithelium in many oral diseases including lichen planus and has potent antibacterial and antifungal effect through humoral and cell-mediated immunologic processes.[99] Cutaneous lymphocyte antigen (CLA), involved in skin homing of T lymphocytes, is upregulated both in oral and in cutaneous lichen planus.[100] Oral lichen planus lesions differ from cutaneous lichen planus lesions in the expression of alpha e beta 7 integrin, which is upregulated in the former but not in the latter tissue.[100] A subsequent study by the same authors reported an increase in the circulating "memory" subset ($CD45RO^+$) of T-helper cells in oral lichen planus patients while the naive T-helper subset ($CD45RA^+$) was increased in diseased epithelium.[59] Vascular cellular adhesion molecule 1 (VCAM-1) produced by endothelial and dendritic cells is upregulated in cutaneous lichen planus under the influence of IFN-$\gamma$.[101] Expression of tumor necrosis factor alpha (TNF-$\alpha$) receptor is significantly increased both in the lesional lichen planus keratinocytes and as the soluble form in serum from patients with lichen planus.[102] TNF-$\alpha$ receptor is known to play an important role in apoptosis, which is one of the main criteria in the histopathological diagnosis of lichen planus.[103,104] The numbers of T cells and Langerhans cells are significantly increased in intercellular adhesion molecule-1 (ICAM-1) expressing areas of the epithelium. In addition, keratinocyte ICAM-1 expression appeared to be associated with the accumulation of infiltrating T lymphocytes and Langerhans cells.[59] Interaction of ICAM-1 (CD54) on Langerhans cells[105] and lymphocyte function-associated antigen-1 (LFA-1, CD11a) on T cells[106] results in the generation, among others, of either $CD8^+$ (major histocompatibility complex, or MHC, class 1 restricted) or $CD4^+$ (MHC class II restricted) cytotoxic T cells.[107] Other specific adhesive interactions include CD3/T-cell receptor: antigen, CD8: MHC class I and CD4: MHC class II.[96,97] These data indicated that there is a selective recruitment of T cells in oral lichen planus. The cell-mediated response initiated by Langerhans cells thus includes cytotoxic T cells, which are directed against the "altered" keratinocytes and which may also be responsible for damaging cells of other organ systems such as hepatocytes.[108]

Cytokines are soluble protein mediators that play an important role in inflammation and may also influence the expression of lichen planus. As shown in Figure 25.1, interaction of an antigen (drugs, virus, and/or contact allergens) with either keratinocyte or Langerhans cell results in the production of interleukin-1 (IL-1). This IL-1, in turn, stimulates the production of IL-2 by T cells.[109] In addition, $HLA\text{-}DR^+$ keratinocytes produce pro-inflammatory cytokines.[60] Both the production of IFN-$\gamma$ and interleukin-6 (IL-6) are increased by activated lesional T cells as well as lesional keratinocytes but not in the nonlesional tissue.[110] This in turn induces the expression of HLA-DR on keratinocytes, which then progress into lesional cells.[109] The expression of LFA-1 on monocytes was observed to be induced by IFN-$\gamma$ produced by T cells, thereby facilitating the attachment of these cells to keratinocytes.[60] Helper T cells ($CD4^+$) and cytotoxic T cells ($CD8^+$) destroy keratinocytes via interaction with HLA-DR (MHC class II) and MHC class I antigens, respectively. Lymphokines may also directly damage basal cells or downregulate ($CD8^+$) cytotoxic/suppressor cells.[51] It was also suggested that activated T cells may recognize keratinocytes as "target cells" and interact directly with them.[46] A normal amount of $\beta 2$ microglobulin was reported to be produced by activated lymphocytes in patients with lichen planus.[111] The activity of natural killer (NK) cells was reported to be decreased in lichen planus and appeared to be related to the severity of the disease.[112] As the lesions evolve, cytokines derived from lymphocytes (IFN-$\gamma$) and keratinocytes (IL-1, IL-6) influence the behavior of the lesional cells and the overlying epidermis.

Certain individuals may be genetically susceptible to the immunological reactions described above and to acquiring lichen planus. Familiar lichen planus has been reported.[113,114] Significant association of certain HLA alleles of both MHC class I[115,116] and class II,[117,118] particularly of the HLA-DR1 and the HLA-B7 alleles, and family studies[113,119,120] indicate a genetic predisposition to lichen planus. However, the associations reported in the literature are inconsistent and could have been due to the different size, composition, and ethnic background of the patients. Genetic heterogeneity in lichen planus was investigated by La Nasa et al.[121] These authors reported that the frequency of HLA-DR1 and HLA-DQ1 was significantly increased, but that of HLA-DR3 was significantly decreased in cutaneous idiopathic lichen planus with or without mucosal lesions, thereby demonstrating that idiopathic lichen planus was influenced by HLA-associated genetic susceptibility.

## VI. LICHEN PLANUS-LIKE SKIN DISEASES

A variety of lichen planus subtypes are distinguished and include actinic lichen planus that is associated with sunlight and is especially reported in Middle Eastern countries.[122] The onset is primarily seen in the spring and summer with remission in the fall and winter. Bullous lichen planus is defined as the formation of blisters in preexisting lichen planus lesions and is caused by severe basal cell degeneration. It should be distinguished from lichen planus pemphigoides, a disease with bullous pemphigoid characteristics such as the occurrence of blisters in unaffected skin and linear deposits of IgG and C3 in the basement membrane zone.[123] IgM and IgA may also be present in the basement membrane zone.[124] Immunoelectron microscopic investigations into the relationship between bullous pemphigoid and lichen planus pemphigoides indicated that the locations of bullous pemphigoid antigen and lichen planus pemphigoides antigen were different[125] and that the target antigen in lichen planus pemphigoides was not the same as bullous pemphigoid antigen, but may be unique.[126] This was not supported by a case report where serum of a patient with lichen planus pemphigoides reacted with the 180-kDa bullous pemphigoid antigen (BPAg2, type XVII collagen), which is characteristic for bullous pemphigoid. It was speculated that this antigen was also an immunopathological clue for lichen planus pemphigoides.[127] Possibly, these different clinical phenotypes are associated with an autoimmune response to the same autoantigen, yet the immunoglobulin subclass of the autoantibody and the epitope that is recognized may be different.[128]

Lichen planopilaris affects the hair-bearing areas with involvement of hair follicles. The end stage of lichen planopilaris is loss of hair follicles, fibrosis, and baldness. Clinically, it is identical to pseudopelade of Broq, a hair disease also leading to baldness of unknown cause. Histopathologically, a lichenoid lymphocytic infiltrate surrounds and destroys the hair infundibulum and shaft. The interfollicular skin is relatively unaffected. The pathogenesis is believed to be initiated by a disruption of the immune privilege of the hair follicle leading to an immunologic reaction that is limited to the follicle.[129] In contrast to lichen planus with colloid bodies in large numbers, lichen planopilaris is said to be characterized by the absence of colloid bodies.[130] Furthermore, IgG and IgA deposits in lichen planopilaris lesions were restricted to hair follicles and were more linear and less fibrillar than in lichen planus lesions. Based on these findings the authors suggested that lichen planopilaris was a different disease entity from lichen planus. Nevertheless, it should be noted that the lichen planopilaris lesions under investigation in that study were long-standing (3 to 7 years). In contrast, Smith et al.[131] detected colloid bodies containing IgG and IgM adjacent to involved follicles in lichen planopilaris lesions.

Lichenoid eruptions may resemble classical lichen planus in many respects and may be induced by contact, inhalation, or ingestion of a large number of drugs and chemicals. Lichenoid drug eruptions have a less typical distribution and a more polymorphic appearance than classical lichen planus.[132] Usually, oral mucosa are not involved. Lupus erythematosus–lichen planus overlap syndrome represents a heterogeneous group of patients with skin lesions that have clinical, histological, and/or immunological features that are common in both diseases.[133,134] It has been suggested that the overlap syndrome is a lichen planus-like manifestation of discoid lupus erythematosus with distinct extracellular matrix protein expression.[135]

Chronic graft-vs.-host disease resembles idiopathic lichen planus both clinically and histologically. It is induced by hematopoietic stem cell transplantation and is discussed in detail below. Other clinical variants of lichen planus are reviewed in detail elsewhere.[2]

## VII. GRAFT-VS.-HOST DISEASE

At present, bone-marrow transplantation is a well-established therapy for severe hematological diseases. However, the potential threat of graft-vs.-host disease (GVHD) remains a major obstacle for successful transplantation.[136] Although GVHD usually occurs in patients undergoing bone-marrow transplantation,[137] it may also be seen in fetuses receiving leukocytes via maternal-fetal transfusion[138] and in otherwise healthy patients receiving blood transfusions after heart surgery.[139] GVHD has been reported incidentally after solid organ transplantation.

Graft-vs.-host disease occurs when lymphoid cells from an immunocompetent donor are introduced into a host not capable of rejecting these cells. The main targets of GVHD in humans are the skin, the gastrointestinal tract, and the liver. The severity of the cutaneous eruption often parallels that of the GVHD. There are two main forms of GVHD, the acute and the chronic forms.

In the acute disease, a morbilliform, blanchable, erythematous lichenoid-like rash arises on the trunk, neck, hands, and feet during 3 months after transplantation/transfusion.[140–142] Chronic disease occurs beyond the 3 months after transfusion/transplantation and is not necessarily preceded by the acute phase. Chronic GVHD may mimic scleroderma or lichen planus.[143]

The acute disease is histologically characterized by vacuolar changes in the basement membrane, decreased number of Langerhans cells, and a mononuclear inflammatory infiltrate in the papillary and reticular dermis.[142,144] Complement and immunoglobulins were reported to be either present[145] or absent.[146] In chronic GVHD, essentially a similar histologic pattern to that in idiopathic lichen planus is seen.[146] It was observed that the number of infiltrating T cells in chronic GVHD was lower as compared with oral lichen planus.[147] Increased number of ($CD1^+$) Langerhans cells was observed in both.

The acute form appears to be caused by the attack of immunocompetent donor T cells and null cells against incompatible host histocompatibility antigens,[141] whereas the chronic disease is thought to be caused by an attack on the host immune cells by the donor cells.[142] The development of GVHD after transfusion in otherwise healthy cardiac surgery patients may be due to incompatibilities in the HLA antigens.[144] Minor histocompatibility antigens are also thought to be involved in chronic eruption. Cutaneous GVHD provides an excellent model in which interactions between lymphocytes and the skin can be investigated. In GVHD, damage to the epithelial cells seems to be predominantly mediated by cytotoxic T cells in which Langerhans cells are selectively lost.[148] Various lymphokines such as IFNs and IL-2 may be released by T cells that have become sensitized via interaction with host cells and activate both donor and host mononuclear cells.[142]

As T cells appear to play a prominent role in the pathogenesis of GVHD, any attempts at preventing this disease must be targeted to these cells. Transplantation of bone marrow that has been depleted of T cells by the use of a cocktail of anti-T-cell monoclonal antibodies[149] has made a major contribution in the prevention of GVHD.

## VIII. IMMUNOTHERAPY IN LICHEN PLANUS

Lichen planus is self-limiting in most cases. Adequate treatment is often required because many patients have extensive lesions and suffer from severe itching. Only symptomatic treatment is available. General considerations include treatment of infections (like hepatitis C virus infection) and avoiding drugs that may cause lichenoid eruptions.

To date, sound evidence-based data on the treatment of lichen planus are not available and most reports are based on personal experience of the treating physician. In an evidence-based medical analysis on the efficacy of lichen planus treatment modalities 83 clinical trials were analyzed.[150] Apart from one trial evaluating the effect of oral acitretin on cutaneous lichen planus[151] and two studies on the effect of local corticosteroid on oral lichen planus,[152,153] the remainder of the trials were uncontrolled, observational, and/or retrospective. Recommendations on therapy were based only on the three randomized trials because of the low quality of the latter studies. This could have led to publication bias. The authors state that the first-line therapy in cutaneous lichen planus is oral acitretin. All other therapeutic modalities are of uncertain efficacy. Based on clinical experience, systemic corticosteroid therapy is recommended by many authors and could be classified as second-line therapy, but should be used with caution because of the systemic side effects when administered for a prolonged period. The first-line therapy in oral lichen planus is topical corticosteroid. It is evident that more randomized controlled studies are required to obtain sound evidence-based information on the effective treatment of lichen planus.

Retinoids have been used in cutaneous and oral lichen planus. Retinoids possess anti-inflammatory properties and may also alter keratinocyte cell surface antigens[154] and interact with T-lymphocytes in the lesion.[155] At present, acitretin is the only drug investigated in a controlled study in which it was noted to be effective in cutaneous lichen planus.[151] Oral etretinate and isotretinoin (25 to 50 mg daily) and topical tretinoin have been used in uncontrolled trials. Topical retinaldehyde[157] and tazarotene[157] have been used for oral lichen planus.

Topical or intralesional corticosteroids are effective in relieving pruritus and in inducing remission. Systemic corticosteroids should be used with caution. Antimicrobial drugs have been widely used. Administration of griseofulvin 500 mg/day for 4 weeks was said to produce improvement, especially in cases of oral lesions. Isoniazid, 400 mg daily, has been used and there are a number of reports documenting a beneficial effect of drugs such as trimethoprim/sulfamethoxazole and metronidazole. Dapsone has been used successfully in bullous lichen planus and in erosive lichen planus of the skin and oral mucosa. Oral photo-chemotherapy (PUVA)[158] and UVA[159] alone are believed to be effective and prolonged remission has been reported. Rarely, PUVA may induce lichen planus.[160]

Cyclosporine was used with varying degree of success in lichen planus. Ho et al.[161] reported in an anecdotal article complete clearing of severe chronic lichen planus in two patients after 8 weeks of treatment with oral cyclosporine at a dose of 6 mg/kg/day. Pigatto et al.[162] reported in an uncontrolled small trial clearing of the disease after 1 to 2 weeks in seven of eight patients who were treated with cyclosporine at a dose of 3 mg/kg/day. The primary target of cyclosporine appears to be T-helper/inducer cells and antigen-presenting cells.[163,164] Topical cyclosporine has shown no conclusive efficacy in oral lichen planus.[164–166]

Topical tetracycline,[167] topical cyclosporin,[166] and more recently topical tacrolimus[168,169] were investigated for their effect in the treatment of oral and erosive forms of lichen planus in noncontrolled studies. At present, oral drugs like thalidomide,[170] mycophenolate mofetil,[171] metronidazol,[172] azathioprine,[173] and low-molecular-weight heparin[174,175] have been investigated for treating several forms of lichen planus in uncontrolled studies.

Because adhesive interactions play a pivotal role in the migratory and cytotoxic events in lichen planus, modulating or abrogating the expression of adhesion molecules may provide an effective means of therapeutic intervention. Several approaches may be considered. Antibodies against inducing cytokines such as IFN-$\gamma$ and TNF-$\alpha$ may be valuable. Antibodies to IFN-$\gamma$ were reported to partially abrogate experimentally induced epidermal lichenoid reactions in mice.[176] Antibodies such as anti-ICAM-1, which impair the adhesion of leukocytes to endothelium, may reduce tissue infiltration and damage in chronic inflammation.[177] Investigations into agents that are able to prevent the release of TNF-$\alpha$ by stabilizing (preventing degranulation) mast cells may also be another fruitful approach. Cytokines that are able to downregulate the expression of adhesion molecules and interfere with the trafficking of leukocytes generally may be of therapeutic value and include IL-8,[178] transforming growth factor-beta,[179] and inhibitors of IL-1.[180] To date, Basiliximab, a monoclonal antibody directed at the IL-2 receptor and directly able to prevent T-cell activation, is the only therapeutic agent that has been used to treat erosive lichen planus.[181]

## IX. CONCLUSIONS

The present views in classical (idiopathic) lichen planus and lichenoid skin reactions due to exogenous stimuli are focused on immunologic and HLA-associated genetic susceptibility. Tissue damage and subsequent abnormal epidermal proliferation leading to acanthosis and hypergranulation are most likely to be the primary consequence of abundant T-cell activation *in situ* directed against "altered" keratinocytes. The exact contribution of T-cell-mediated immunity and the nature of the "altered" keratinocytes still remain important fields for future investigations. Hepatitis C virus infection may be the trigger in some but not all cases of lichen planus. Other key factors in the pathogenesis of lichen planus still remain to be elucidated. Graft-vs.-host disease resembling lichen planus or lichen planus-like reactions both clinically and histologically are mediated by host T cells. The use of anti-T-cell monoclonal antibodies may contribute to alleviate these disorders in the future.

## REFERENCES


1. Schmidt, H., Frequency, duration and localization of lichen planus, *Acta Derm. Venereol.* (Stockholm), 41, 164, 1961.
2. Arndt, K.A., Lichen planus, in *Dermatology in General Medicine*, 3rd ed., Fitzpatrick, T.B., Fisen, A.Z., Wolff, K. et al., Eds., McGraw-Hill, New York, 1987, 967.
3. Camisa, C., Lichen planus and related conditions, *Adv. Dermatol.,* 25, 47, 1987.
4. Boyd, A.S. and Neldner, K.M., Lichen planus, *J. Am. Acad. Dermatol.,* 25, 593, 1991.
5. Strauss, R.A., Fattore, L., and Soltani, K., The association of mucocutaneous lichen planus and chronic liver disease, *Oral Surg. Oral Med. Oral Pathol.,* 68, 406, 1989.
6. Silverman, S., Gorsky, M., and Lozada-Nur, F., A prospective follow-up study of 570 patients with oral lichen planus: persistence, remission, and malignant association, *Oral Surg. Oral Med. Oral Pathol.,* 60, 30, 1985.
7. Conklin, R.J. and Blasberg, B., Oral lichen planus, *Dermatol. Clin.,* 5, 663, 1987.
8. Meij, van der E.H. and Waal, van der I., Lack of clinicopathological correlation in the diagnosis of oral lichen planus based on the presently available diagnostic criteria and suggestions for modifications, *J. Oral Pathol. Med.,* 32, 507, 2003.
9. Ukleja, A., DeVault, K.R., Stark, M.E., and Achem, S.R., Lichen planus involving the esophagus, *Dig. Dis. Sci.,* 46, 2292, 2001.
10. Andreasen, J.O., Oral lichen planus. 1. A clinical evaluation of 115 cases, *Oral Surg. Oral Med. Oral Pathol.,* 25, 31, 1968.
11. Rode, M. and Kogoj-Rode, M., Malignant potential of the reticular form of oral lichen planus over a 25-year observation period in 55 patients from Slovenia, *J. Oral Sci.,* 44, 109, 2002.
12. Van Der Meij, E.H., Schepman, K.P., and Van Der Waal, I., The possible premalignant character of oral lichen planus and oral lichenoid lesions: a prospective study, *Oral Surg. Oral Med. Oral Pathol. Oral Radiol. Endod.,* 96, 164, 2003.
13. Bromwich, M., Retrospective study of the progression of oral premalignant lesions to squamous cell carcinoma: a South Wales experience, *J. Otolaryngol.,* 31,150, 2002.
14. Eisenberg E., Oral lichen planus: a benign lesion, *J. Oral Maxillofac. Surg.,* 58, 1278, 2000.
15. Silverman, S., Jr., Oral lichen planus: a potentially premalignant lesion, *J. Oral Maxillofac. Surg.,* 58, 1286, 2000.
16. Pelisse, M., The vulvo-vaginal-gingival syndrome. A new form of erosive lichen planus, *Int. J. Dermatol.,* 28, 381, 1989.
17. Eisen, D., The vulvovaginal-gingival syndrome of lichen planus. The clinical characteristics of 22 patients, *Arch. Dermatol.,* 130, 1379, 1994.
18. Rogers, R.S., III and Eisen, D., Erosive oral lichen planus with genital lesions: the vulvovaginal-gingival syndrome and the peno-gingival syndrome, *Dermatol. Clin.,* 21, 91, 2003.
19. Patel, G.K., Turner, R.J., and Marks, R., Cutaneous lichen planus and squamous cell carcinoma, *J. Eur. Acad. Dermatol. Venereol.,* 17, 98, 2003.

20. Sharma, R. and Maheshwari, V., Childhood lichen planus: a report of fifty cases, *Pediatr. Dermatol.*, 16, 345, 1999.
21. Handa, S. and Sahoo, B., Childhood lichen planus: a study of 87 cases, *Int. J. Dermatol.*, 41, 423, 2002.
22. Ragaz, A. and Ackerman, A.B., Evolution, maturation, and regression of lesions of lichen planus. New observations and correlations of clinical and histologic findings, *Am. J. Dermatopathol.*, 3, 5, 1981.
23. Ryan, T.J., Lichen planus, Wickham's striae and blood vessels, *Br. J. Dermatol.*, 85, 497, 1971.
24. Ellis, F.A., Histopathology of lichen planus based on analysis of one hundred biopsy specimens, *J. Invest. Dermatol.*, 48, 143, 1967.
25. Ross, T.H., Caspary-Joseph spaces: a comment on priority, *Int. J. Dermatol.*, 16, 842, 1977.
26. Taaffe, A., Current concepts in lichen planus, *Int. J. Dermatol.*, 18, 533, 1979.
27. Weedon, D., Lichenoid (interface) dermatoses, in *Skin Pathology*, 2nd ed., Weedon, D., Ed., Churchill Livingstone, London, 2002, 34.
28. Röcken, M., Zur pathogenese des lichen ruber planus — ein modernes konzept, *Z. Hautkr.*, 63, 911, 1988.
29. Konrad, K., Pehamberger, H., and Holubar, K., Ultrastructural localization of immunoglobulin and fibrin in lichen planus, *J. Am. Acad. Dermatol.*, 1, 233, 1979.
30. Burkhart, C.G., Ultrastructural study of lichen planus: an evaluation of the colloid bodies, *Int. J. Dermatol.*, 20, 188, 1981.
31. Bhan, A.K., Harrist, T.J., Murphy, G.F. et al., T cell subsets and Langerhans cells in lichen planus: *in situ* characterization using monoclonal antibodies, *Br. J. Dermatol.*, 105, 617, 1981.
32. Abell, R., Presbury, D.G., Marks, R. et al., The diagnostic significance of immunoglobulin and fibrin deposition in lichen planus, *Br. J. Dermatol.*, 93, 17, 1975.
33. Fernandez-Busey, R.A., Schmitt, D., Gaucherand, M. et al., Lichen planus: evaluation of cells in skin lesions and of T-lymphocyte subsets in blood, *J. Dermatol.* (Tokyo), 10, 17, 1983.
34. Baart de la Faille-Kuyper, E.H. and Baart de la Faille, H., An immunofluorescence study of lichen planus, *Br. J. Dermatol.*, 90, 365, 1974.
35. Fellner, M.J., Lichen planus, *Int. J. Dermatol.*, 19, 71, 1980.
36. Scully, G., El-Kom, M., Lichen planus: review and update on pathogenesis, *J. Oral Pathol.*, 14, 431, 1985.
37. Olsen, R.G., Du Plessis, D.P., Barron, C. et al., Lichen planus dermopathy: demonstration of a lichen planus-specific epidermal antigen in affected patients, *J. Clin. Lab. Immunol.*, 10, 103, 1983.
38. Olsen, R.G., Du Plessis, D.P., Schulz, E.J. et al., Indirect immunofluorescence microscopy of lichen planus, *Br. J. Dermatol.*, 110, 9, 1984.
39. Camisa, C., Allen, C.M., Bowen, B. et al., Indirect immunofluorescence of lichen planus, *J. Oral Pathol.*, 15, 218, 1986.
40. Lin, S.C., Sun, A., Wu, Y.C., and Chiang, C.P., Presence of anti-basal cell antibodies in oral lichen planus, *J. Am. Acad. Dermatol.*, 26, 943, 1992.
41. Carrizosa, A.M., Elorza, F.L., and Camacho, F.M., Antinuclear antibodies in patients with lichen planus, *Exp Dermatol.*, 6, 54, 1997.
42. Lodi, G., Olsen, I., Piattelli, A., D'Amico, E., Artese, L., and Porter, S.R., Antibodies to epithelial components in oral lichen planus (OLP) associated with hepatitis C virus (HCV) infection, *J. Oral Pathol. Med.*, 26, 36, 1997.
43. Biermann, H. and Rauterberg, E.W., Expression of fetal cytokeratins in epidermal cells and colloid bodies in lichen planus, *J. Cutaneous Pathol.*, 25, 35, 1998.
44. Schødt, M., Holmstrup, P., Dobelsteen, E. et al., Deposits of immunoglobulin, complement, and fibrinogen in oral lupus erythematosus, lichen planus and leukoplakia, *Oral Surg. Oral Med. Oral Pathol.*, 51, 603, 1981.
45. Zhou, X.J., Sugerman, P.B., Savage, N.W., and Walsh, L.J., Matrix metalloproteinases and their inhibitors in oral lichen planus, *J. Cutaneous Pathol.*, 28, 72, 2001.
46. De Panfilis, G., Manara, G.C., Sansoni, P. et al., T-cell infiltrate in lichen planus. Demonstration of activated lymphocytes using monoclonal antibodies, *J. Cutaneous Pathol.*, 10, 52, 1983.
47. Spandau, U., Toksoy, A., Goebeler, M., Brocker, E.B., and Gillitzer, R., MIG is a dominant lymphocyte-attractant chemokine in lichen planus lesions, *J. Invest. Dermatol.*, 111, 1003, 1998.
48. al-Fouzan, A.S., Habib, M.A., Sallam, T.H., el-Samahy, M.H., and Rostom, A.I., Detection of T lymphocytes and T lymphocyte subsets in lichen planus: *in situ* and in peripheral blood, *Int. J. Dermatol.*, 35, 426, 1996.

49. Takeuchi, Y., Tehnai, I., Kaneda, T. et al., Immunohistochemical analysis of cells in mucosal lesions of oral lichen planus, *J. Oral Pathol.,* 17, 367, 1988.
50. Matthews, J.B., Scully, C.M., and Potts, A.J.C., Oral lichen planus: an immunoperoxidase study using monoclonal antibodies to lymphocyte subsets, *Br. J. Dermatol.,* 111, 587, 1984.
51. Ishii, T., Immunohistochemical demonstration of T cell subsets and accessory cells in oral lichen planus, *J. Oral Pathol.,* 16, 356, 1987.
52. Gadenne, A.S., Strucke, R., Dunn, D., Wagner, M., Bleicher, P., and Bigby, M., T-cell lines derived from lesional skin of lichen planus patients contain a distinctive population of T-cell receptor gamma delta-bearing cells, *J. Invest. Dermatol.,*103, 347, 1994.
53. Owen, M., T-cell receptors and MHC molecules, in *Immunology,* 5th ed., Roitt, I., Brostoff, J., and Male, D., Eds., Mosby, St. Louis, MO, 2000, 85.
54. Simon, M., Lesional keratinocytes express OKM5, Leu-8 and Leu-11b antigens in lichen planus, *Dermatologica,* 177, 152, 1988.
55. Farthing, P.M. and Cruchley, A. T., Expression of MHC class II antigens (HLA DR, DP, and DQ) by keratinocytes in oral lichen planus, *J. Oral Pathol. Med.,* 18, 305, 1989.
56. Heyden, G., Arwill, T., and Gisslén, H., Histochemical studies on lichen planus, *Oral Surg. Oral Med. Oral Pathol.,* 37, 239, 1974.
57. Regezi, J.A., Stewart, J.C., Lloyd, R.V., and Headington, J.T., Immunohistochemical staining of Langerhans cells and macrophages in oral lichen planus, *Oral Surg Oral Med Oral Pathol.,* 60, 396, 1985.
58. Farthing, P.M., Matear, P., and Cruchley, A.T., Langerhans cell distribution and keratinocyte expression of HLA-DR in oral lichen planus, *J. Oral Pathol. Med.,* 21, 451, 1992.
59. Walton, L.J., Macey, M.G., Thornhill, M.H., and Farthing, P.M. Intra-epithelial subpopulations of T lymphocytes and Langerhans cells in oral lichen planus, *J Oral Pathol Med.,* 27, 116, 1998.
60. Shiohara, T., Moriya, N., and Nagashima, M., The lichenoid tissue reaction, *Int. J. Dermatol.,* 27, 365, 1988.
61. Weedon, D., The lichenoid tissue reaction, *Int. J. Dermatol.,* 21, 203, 1982.
62. Mokni, M., Rybojad, M., Puppin, D., Jr., Catala, S., Venezia, F., Djian, R., and Morel, P., Lichen planus and hepatitis C virus, *J. Am. Acad. Dermatol.,* 24, 792, 1991.
63. Sanchez-Perez, J., De Castro, M., Buezo, G.F., Fernandez-Herrera, J., Borque, M.J., and Garcia-Diez, A., Lichen planus and hepatitis C virus: prevalence and clinical presentation of patients with lichen planus and hepatitis C virus infection, *Br. J. Dermatol.,* 134, 715, 1996.
64. Chuang, T.Y., Stitle, L., Brashear, R., and Lewis, C., Hepatitis C virus and lichen planus: a case-control study of 340 patients, *J. Am. Acad. Dermatol.,* 41, 787, 1999.
65. Mahboob, A., Haroon, T.S., Iqbal, Z., Iqbal, F., and Butt, A.K., Frequency of anti-HCV antibodies in patients with lichen planus, *J. Coll. Physicians Surg. Pak.,* 13, 248, 2003.
66. Imhof, M., Popal, H., Lee, J.H., Zeuzem, S., and Milbradt, R., Prevalence of hepatitis C virus antibodies and evaluation of hepatitis C virus genotypes in patients with lichen planus, *Dermatology,* 195, 1, 1997.
67. Erkek, E., Bozdogan, O., and Olut, A.I., Hepatitis C virus infection prevalence in lichen planus: examination of lesional and normal skin of hepatitis C virus-infected patients with lichen planus for the presence of hepatitis C virus RNA, *Clin. Exp. Dermatol.,* 26, 540, 2001.
68. Daramola, O.O., George, A.O., and Ogunbiyi, A.O., Hepatitis C virus and lichen planus in Nigerians: any relationship? *Int. J. Dermatol.,* 41, 217, 2002.
69. van der Meij, E.H. and van der Waal, I., Hepatitis C virus infection and oral lichen planus: a report from the Netherlands, *J. Oral Pathol. Med.,* 29, 255, 2000.
70. Kurokawa, M., Hidaka, T., Sasaki, H., Nishikata, I., Morishita, K., and Setoyama, M., Analysis of hepatitis C virus (HCV) RNA in the lesions of lichen planus in patients with chronic hepatitis C: detection of anti-genomic- as well as genomic-strand HCV RNAs in lichen planus lesions, *J. Dermatol. Sci.,* 32, 65, 2003.
71. Lazaro, P., Olalquiaga, J., Bartolome, J., Ortiz-Movilla, N., Rodriguez-Inigo, E., Pardo, M., Lecona, M., Pico, M., Longo, I., Garcia-Morras, P., and Carreno, V., Detection of hepatitis C virus RNA and core protein in keratinocytes from patients with cutaneous lichen planus and chronic hepatitis C, *J. Invest. Dermatol.,* 119, 798, 2002.
72. Nagao, Y., Sata, M., Ide, T., Suzuki, H., Tanikawa, K., Itoh, K., and Kameyama, T., Development and exacerbation of oral lichen planus during and after interferon therapy for hepatitis C, *Eur. J. Clin. Invest.,* 26, 1171, 1996.

73. Nagao, Y., Tomonari, R., Kage, M., Komai, K., Tsubone, K., Kamura, T., and Sata, M., The possible intraspousal transmission of HCV in terms of lichen planus, *Int. J. Mol. Med.,* 10, 569, 2002.
74. Rebora, A., Rongioletti, F., Drago, F., and Parodi, A., Lichen planus as a side effect of HBV vaccination, *Dermatology,* 198, 1, 1999.
75. Schupp, P. and Vente, C., Lichen planus following hepatitis B vaccination, *Int. J. Dermatol.,* 38, 799, 1999.
76. Limas, C. and Limas, C.J., Lichen planus in children: a possible complication of hepatitis B vaccines, *Pediatr. Dermatol.,* 19, 204, 2002.
77. Clausen, J., Kjaergaad, J., and Bierring, F., Ultrastructure of the dermo-epidermal junction in lichen planus, *Acta. Derm. Venereol.* (Stockholm), 61, 101, 1981.
78. Black, M.M., The pathogenesis of lichen planus, *Br. J. Dermatol.,* 86, 302, 1972.
79. Walsh, L.J., Savage, N.W., Ishii, T. et al., Immunopathogenesis of oral lichen planus, *J. Oral Pathol. Med.,* 19, 389, 1990.
80. Stankler, L., Deficiency of circulating IgA and IgM in adult patients with lichen planus, *Br. J. Dermatol.,* 93, 25, 1975.
81. Sklavounova, A.D., Laskaris, G., and Angelopoulos, A.P., Serum immunoglobulins and complement (C¢3) in oral lichen planus, *Oral Surg. Oral Med. Oral Pathol.,* 55, 47, 1983.
82. Scully, C., Serum IgG, IgA, IgD, and IgE in lichen planus: no evidence for a humoral immunodeficiency, *Clin. Exp. Dermatol.,* 7, 163, 1982.
83. Shuttleworth, D., Graham-Brown, R.A.C., and Campbell, A.C., The autoimmune background in lichen planus, *Br. J. Dermatol.,* 115, 199, 1986.
84. Sallay, K., Kövesi, G., and Döri, F., Circulating immune complex studies on patients with oral lichen planus, *Oral Surg. Oral Med. Oral Pathol.,* 68, 567, 1989.
85. Zhou, X.J., Savage, N.W., Sugerman, P.B., Walsh, L.J., Aldred, M.J., and Seymour, G.J., TCR V beta gene expression in lesional T lymphocyte cell lines in oral lichen planus, *Oral Dis.,* 295, 1996.
86. Schiller, P.I., Flaig, M.J., Puchta, U., Kind, P., and Sander, C.A., Detection of clonal T cells in lichen planus. *Arch. Dermatol. Res.,* 292, 568, 2000.
87. Sugerman, P.B., Satterwhite, K., and Bigby, M., Autocytotoxic T-cell clones in lichen planus. *Br. J. Dermatol.,* 142, 449, 2000.
88. Gilhar, A., Pillar, T., Winterstein, G. et al., The pathogenesis of lichen planus, *Br. J. Dermatol.,* 120, 541, 1989.
89. Tammi, R., Hyyrylainen, A., and Fraku, J.E., Histologic characteristics of lichen planus transplanted onto nude mice and cultured *in vitro, Arch. Dermatol. Res.,* 280, 23, 1988.
90. Shiohara, T., Moriya, N., Tsuchiya, K. et al., Lichenoid tissue reaction induced by local transfer of Ia-reactive T-cell clones, *J. Invest. Dermatol.,* 87, 33, 1986.
91. Shiohara, T., The lichenoid tissue reaction. An immunological perspective, *Am. J. Dermatopathol.,* 10, 252, 1988.
92. Holmstrup, P. and Söberg, M., Cellular hypersensitivity and oral lichen planus lesions *in vitro, Acta Allergologica.,* 32, 304, 1977.
93. Laeijendecker, R. and Van Joost, Th., Oral manifestations of gold allergy, *J. Am. Acad. Dermatol.,* 30, 205, 1994.
94. van Loon, L.A., Krieg, S.R., Davidson, C.L., and Bos, J.D., Quantification and distribution of lymphocyte subsets and Langerhans cells in normal human oral mucosa and skin, *J. Oral Pathol. Med.,* 18, 197, 1989.
95. Lacy, M.F., Reade, P.C., and Hay, K.D., Lichen planus: a theory of pathogenesis, *Oral Surg. Oral Med. Oral Pathol.,* 56, 521, 1983.
96. Walsh, L.J., Lavker, R.M., and Murphy, G.F., Determinants of immune cell trafficking in the skin, *Lab. Invest.,* 63, 592, 1990.
97. Nickoloff, B.J., Role of interferon gamma in cutaneous trafficking of lymphocytes with emphasis on molecular and cellular adhesion events. *Arch. Dermatol.,* 124, 1835, 1989.
98. Kupper, T.S., Production of cytokines by epithelial tissues. A new model for cutaneous inflammation, *Am. J. Dermatopathol.,* 11, 69, 1989.
99. Eversole, L.R., Miyasaki, K.T., and Christensen, R.E., Keratinocyte expression of calprotectin in oral inflammatory mucosal diseases, *J. Oral Pathol. Med.,* 22, 303, 1993.

100. Walton, L.J., Thornhill, M.H., Macey, M.G., and Farthing, P.M., Cutaneous lymphocyte associated antigen (CLA) and alpha e beta 7 integrins are expressed by mononuclear cells in skin and oral lichen planus, *J. Oral Pathol. Med.,* 26, 402, 1997.
101. Groves, R.W., Ross, E.L., Barker, J.N., and MacDonald, D.M., Vascular cell adhesion molecule-1: expression in normal and diseased skin and regulation *in vivo* by interferon gamma, *J. Am. Acad. Dermatol.,* 29, 67, 1993.
102. Simon, M., Jr. and Gruschwitz, M.S., *In situ* expression and serum levels of tumour necrosis factor alpha receptors in patients with lichen planus, *Acta Derm. Venereol.,* 77, 191, 1997.
103. Rook, G. and Balkwill, F., Cell-mediated immune reactions, in *Immunology,* 5th ed., Roitt, I., Brostoff, J., and Male, D., Eds., Mosby, St. Louis, MO, 2000, 131.
104. Sklavounou, A., Chrysomali, E., Scorilas, A., and Karameris A., TNF-alpha expression and apoptosis-regulating proteins in oral lichen planus: a comparative immunohistochemical evaluation, *J. Oral Pathol. Med.,* 29, 370, 2000.
105. De Panfilis, G., Manara, G.C., Ferrari, C. et al., Adhesion molecules on the plasma membrane of epidermal cells. II. The intercellular adhesion molecule-1 is constitutively present on cell surface of human resting Langerhans cells, *J. Invest. Dermatol.,* 94, 317, 1990.
106. King, P.D. and Katz, D.R., Human tonsillar dendritic cell-induced T-cell responses: analysis of molecular mechanisms using monoclonal antibodies, *Eur. J. Immunol.,* 19, 581, 1989.
107. Stingel, G., Katz, S. I., Clement, L. et al., Immunologic functions of Ia bearing epidermal Langerhans cells, *J. Immunol.,* 121, 2005, 1978.
108. Korkij, W., Chuang, T.Y., and Soltani, K., Liver abnormalities in patients with lichen planus, *J. Am. Acad. Dermatol.,* 11, 609, 1984.
109. Morhenn, V.B., Etiology of lichen planus, *Am. J. Dermatopathol.,* 8, 154, 1986.
110. Fayyazi, A., Schweyer, S., Soruri, A., Duong, L.Q., Radzun, H.J., Peters, J., Parwaresch, R., and Berger, H., T lymphocytes and altered keratinocytes express interferon-gamma and interleukin 6 in lichen planus, *Arch. Dermatol. Res.,* 291, 485, 1999.
111. Scully, C. and Boyle, P., β2 microglobulin in lichen planus, *J. Dent. Res.,* 61, 758, 1982.
112. Simon, M., Hunyadi, J., Fickentscher, H. et al., Basic and interleukin-2-augmented natural killer cell activity in lichen planus, *Dermatologica,* 178, 141, 1989.
113. Kofoed, M.L. and Wantzin, G.L., Familial lichen planus. More frequent than previously suggested? *J. Am. Acad. Dermatol.,* 13, 50, 1985.
114. Sandhu, K., Handa, S., and Kanwar, A.J., Familial lichen planus, *Pediatr Dermatol.,* 20, 186, 2003.
115. Lowe, N.T., Cudworth, A.G., and Woodrow, J.C., HLA antigens in lichen planus. *Br. J. Dermatol.,* 95, 169, 1976.
116. Veien, N.K., Risum, G., Jørgensen, H.P. et al., HLA antigens in patients with lichen planus, *Acta. Derm. Venereol.* (Stockholm), 59, 205, 1979.
117. Powell, F.C., Rogers, R.S., Dickson, E.R. et al., An association between HLA-DR1 and lichen planus, *Br. J. Dermatol.,* 114, 473, 1986.
118. Valsecchi, R., Bontempelli, M., Ross, A. et al., HLA-DR and DQ antigens in lichen planus, *Acta. Derm. Venereol.* (Stockholm), 68, 77, 1988.
119. Mahood, J.M., Familial lichen planus. A report of nine cases from four families, with a brief review of the literature, *Arch. Dermatol.,* 119, 292, 1983.
120. Copeman, P.W., Tan, R.S., Timlin, D., and Samman, P.D., Familial lichen planus. Another disease or a distinct people? *Br. J. Dermatol.,* 98, 573, 1978.
121. La Nasa, G., Cottoni, F., Mulargia, M. et al., HLA antigen distribution in different clinical subgroups demonstrates genetic heterogeneity in lichen planus, *Br. J. Dermatol.,* 132, 897, 1995.
122. Niles, H., Lichen planus atrophicus annularis, *Arch. Dermatol. Syphilol.,* 44, 1125, 1941.
123. Zillikens, D., Caux, F., Mascaro, J.M., Wesselmann, U., Schmidt, E., Prost, C., Callen, J.P., Brocker, E.B., Diaz, L.A., and Giudice, G.J., Autoantibodies in lichen planus pemphigoides react with a novel epitope within the C-terminal NC16A domain of BP180, *J. Invest. Dermatol.,* 113, 117, 1999.
124. Mora, R.G., Nesbitt, L.T., and Brantley, L., Lichen planus pemphigoides: clinical and immunofluorescent findings in four cases, *J. Am. Acad. Dermatol.,* 8, 331, 1983.
125. Prost, C., Tesserand, F., Laroche, L. et al., Lichen planus pemphigoides: an immuno-electron microscopic study, *Br. J. Dermatol.,* 113, 31, 1985.

126. Davis, A., Boghal, B.S., Whitehead, P. et al., Lichen planus pemphigoides: its relationship to bullous pemphigoid, *Br. J. Dermatol.,* 125, 263, 1991.
127. Hsu, S., Ghohestani, R.F., and Uitto, J., Lichen planus pemphigoides with IgG autoantibodies to the 180 kd bullous pemphigoid antigen (type XVII collagen), *J. Am. Acad. Dermatol.,* 42, 136, 2000.
128. Zillikens, D., BP180 as the common autoantigen in blistering diseases with different clinical phenotypes, *Keio J. Med.,* 51, 21, 2002.
129. Smith, K.J., Crittenden, J., and Skelton, H., Lichen planopilaris-like changes arising within an epidermal nevus: does this case suggest clues to the etiology of lichen planopilaris? *J. Cutaneous Med. Surg.,* 4, 30, 2000.
130. Ioannides, D. and Bystryn, J.C., Immunofluorescence abnormalities in lichen planopilaris, *Arch. Dermatol.,* 128, 214, 1992.
131. Smith, W.B., Grabski, W.J., McCollough, M.L., and Davis, T.L., Immunofluorescence findings in lichen planopilaris: a contrasting experience, *Arch. Dermatol.,* 128, 1405, 1992.
132. Almeyda, J. and Levantine, A., Lichenoid drug eruptions, *Br. J. Dermatol.,* 85, 604, 1971.
133. Copeman, P.W.M., Schroeter, A.L., and Kierland, R.R., An unusual variant of lupus erythematosus or lichen planus, *Br. J. Dermatol.,* 83, 269, 1970.
134. Grabbe, S. and Kolde, G., Coexisting lichen planus and subacute cutaneous lupus erythematosus, *Clin. Exp. Dermatol.,* 20, 249, 1995.
135. de Jong, E.M., van der Vleuten, C.J., and van Vlijmen-Willems, I.M., Differences in extracellular matrix proteins, epidermal growth and differentiation in discoid lupus erythematosus, lichen planus and the overlap syndrome, *Acta Derm. Venereol.,* 77, 356, 199.
136. Barrett, A.J., Graft versus host disease: a review, *J. R. Soc. Med.,* 80, 368, 1987.
137. Horwitz, L.J. and Dreizen, S., Acral erythema induced by chemotherapy and graft-versus-host disease in adults with hematogenous malignancies, *Cutis,* 46, 397, 1990.
138. Morhenn, V.B. and Maibach, H.I., Graft vs. host reaction in a newborn, *Acta Derm. Venereol.* (Stockholm), 54, 133, 1974.
139. Sakakibara, T. and Juji, T., Post-transfusion graft-versus-host disease after open-heart surgery, *Lancet,* 2, 1099, 1986.
140. Aractingi, S. and Chosidow, O., Cutaneous graft-versus-host disease, *Arch. Dermatol.,* 134, 602, 1998.
141. Farmer, E.R. and Hood, A.F., Graft-versus-host disease, in *Dermatology in General Medicine,* 3rd ed., Fitzpatrick, T.B., Fisen, A.Z., Wolff, K. et al., Eds., McGraw-Hill, New York, 1987, 1344.
142. Harper, J.J., Cutaneous graft versus host disease, *Br. Med. J.,* 295, 401, 1987.
143. Van Joost, Th., Vuzevski, V.D., Ten Kate, F. et al., Localized oral and perioral lesions in chronic graft-versus-host disease, *J. Am. Acad. Dermatol.,* 16, 138, 1987.
144. Ray, T.L., Blood transfusions and graft-vs-host disease, *Arch. Dermatol.,* 126, 1347, 1990.
145. Tsoi, M.S., Strob, R., Jones, E. et al., Deposition of IgM and complement at the dermoepidermal junction in acute and chronic cutaneous graft-versus-host disease in man, *J. Immunol.,* 120, 1485, 1978.
146. Sauret, J.H., Bonnetblance, J.M., Gluckman, E. et al., Skin antibodies in bone marrow transplanted patients, *Clin. Exp. Dermatol.,* 1, 377, 1976.
147. Mattsson, T., Sundqvist, K.G., Heimdahl, A. et al., A comparative immunological analysis of the oral mucosa in chronic graft-versus-host disease and oral lichen planus, *Arch. Oral Biol.,* 37, 539, 1992.
148. Breathnach, S.M. and Katz, S.I., Immunopathology of cutaneous graft-versus-host disease, *Am. J. Dermatopathol.,* 9, 343, 1987.
149. Prentice, H.G., Blacklock, H.A., Janossy, G. et al., Use of anti-T-cell monoclonal antibody OKT3 to prevent acute graft-versus-host disease in allogeneic bone marrow transplantation for acute leukemia, *Lancet,* 1, 700, 1982.
150. Cribier, B., Frances, C., and Chosidow, O., Treatment of lichen planus. An evidence-based medicine analysis of efficacy, *Arch. Dermatol.,* 134, 1521, 1998.
151. Laurberg, G., Geiger, J.M., Hjorth, N., Holm, P., Hou-Jensen, K., Jacobsen, K.U., Nielsen, A.O., Pichard, J., Serup, J., Sparre-Jorgensen A. et al., Treatment of lichen planus with acitretin. A double-blind, placebo-controlled study in 65 patients, *J. Am. Acad. Dermatol.,* 24, 434, 1991.
152. Voute, A.B., Schulten, E.A., Langendijk, P.N., Kostense, P.J., and van der Waal, I., Fluocinonide in an adhesive base for treatment of oral lichen planus. A double-blind, placebo-controlled clinical study, *Oral Surg. Oral Med. Oral Pathol.,* 75, 181, 1993.

153. Thongprasom, K., Luangjarmekorn, L., Sererat, T., and Taweesap, W., Relative efficacy of fluocinolone acetonide compared with triamcinolone acetonide in treatment of oral lichen planus, *J. Oral Pathol. Med.,* 21, 456, 1992.
154. Guistina, T.A., Stewart, J.C.B., Ellis, C.N. et al., Topical application of isotretinoin gel improves oral lichen planus, *Arch. Dermatol.,* 122, 534, 1986.
155. Ferguson, M.M., Simpson, N.B., and Hammersley, N., The treatment of erosive lichen planus with a retinoid — etretinate, *Oral Surg. Oral Med. Oral Pathol.,* 58, 283, 1984.
156. Boisnic, S., Licu, D., Ben Slama, L., Branchet-Gumila, M.C., Szpirglas, H., and Dupuy, P., Topical retinaldehyde treatment in oral lichen planus and leukoplakia, *Int. J. Tissue React.,* 24, 123, 2000.
157. Petruzzi, M., De Benedittis, M., Grassi, R., Cassano, N., Vena, G., and Serpico, R., Oral lichen planus: a preliminary clinical study on treatment with tazarotene, *Oral Dis.,* 8, 291, 2002.
158. Gonzales, E., Montaz, T.K., and Freedman, S., Bilateral comparison of generalized lichen planus treated with psoralens and ultraviolet, *J. Am. Acad. Dermatol.,* 10, 958, 1984.
159. Chen, H.R., A newly developed method for treatment of oral lichen planus with ultraviolet radiation, *Taiwan I Hsueh Hui Tsa Chih,* 88, 248, 1989.
160. Nanda, S., Grover, C., and Reddy, B.S., PUVA-induced lichen planus, *J. Dermatol.,* 30, 151, 2003.
161. Ho, V.C., Gupta, A.K., Ellis, C.N. et al., Treatment of severe lichen planus with cyclosporine, *J. Am. Acad. Dermatol.,* 22, 64, 1990.
162. Pigatto, P.D., Chiappion, G., Bigardi, A. et al., Cyclosporin A for treatment of severe lichen planus, *Br. J. Dermatol.,* 122, 121, 1990.
163. Mozzanica, N., Catloaneo, A., Legori, A. et al., Immunohistologic evaluation of the effect of cyclosporin treatment on lichen planus immune infiltrate, *J. Am. Acad. Dermatol.,* 24, 550, 1991.
164. Francès, C., Boisnic, S., Etienne, S. et al., Effect of local application of cyclosporine on chronic erosive lichen planus of the oral cavity, *Dermatologica,* 177, 194, 1988.
165. Sieg, P., Von Domarus, H., Von Zitzewitz, V. et al., Topical cyclosporin in oral lichen planus: a controlled randomized prospective trail, *Br. J. Dermatol.,* 132, 790, 1995.
166. Demitsu, T., Sato, T., Inoue, T., Okada, O., and Kubota, T., Corticosteroid-resistant erosive oral lichen planus successfully treated with topical cyclosporine therapy, *Int. J. Dermatol.,* 39(1), 79, 2000.
167. Walchner, M., Messer, G., Salomon, N., Plewig, G., and Rocken, M., Topical tetracycline treatment of erosive oral lichen planus, *Arch. Dermatol.,* 135, 92, 1999.
168. Vente, C., Reich, K., Rupprecht, R., and Neumann, C., Erosive mucosal lichen planus: response to topical treatment with tacrolimus. *Br. J. Dermatol.,* 140, 338, 1999.
169. Olivier, V., Lacour, J.P., Mousnier, A., Garraffo, R., Monteil, R.A., and Ortonne, J.P., Treatment of chronic erosive oral lichen planus with low concentrations of topical tacrolimus: an open prospective study, *Arch. Dermatol.,* 138, 1335, 2002.
170. Camisa, C. and Popovsky, J.L., Effective treatment of oral erosive lichen planus with thalidomide, *Arch. Dermatol.,* 136, 1442, 2000.
171. Nousari, H.C., Goyal, S., and Anhalt, G.J., Successful treatment of resistant hypertrophic and bullous lichen planus with mycophenolate mofetil, *Arch. Dermatol.,* 135, 1420, 1999.
172. Buyuk, A.Y. and Kavala, M., Oral metronidazole treatment of lichen planus, *J. Am. Acad. Dermatol.,* 43, 260, 2000.
173. Verma, K.K., Sirka, C.S., and Khaitan, B.K., Generalized severe lichen planus treated with azathioprine, *Acta Derm. Venereol.,* 79, 493, 1999.
174. Stefanidou, M.P., Ioannidou, D.J., Panayiotides, J.G., and Tosca, A.D., Low molecular weight heparin; a novel alternative therapeutic approach for lichen planus, *Br. J. Dermatol.,* 141, 1040, 1999.
175. Graham-Brown, R.A., Low molecular weight heparin for lichen planus, *Br. J. Dermatol.*, 141, 1002, 1999.
176. Shiohara, T., Nickoloff, B.J., Moriya, N. et al., *In vivo* effects of interferon-gamma and anti-interferon-gamma antibody on the experimentally induced lichenoid tissue reaction, *Br. J. Dermatol.,* 119, 199, 1988.
177. Wegner, C.D., Gundel, R.H., Reilly, P. et al., Intercellular adhesion molecule-1 (ICAM-1) in the pathogenesis of asthma, *Science,* 247, 456, 1990.
178. Gimbrone, M.A., Obin, M.S., Luis, E.A. et al., Endothelial interleukin-8: a novel inhibitor of leukocyte-endothelial interactions, *Science,* 246, 1601, 1989.

179. Gamble, J.R. and Vadas, M.A., Endothelial adhesiveness for blood neutrophils is inhibited by transforming growth factor-b, *Science,* 242, 97, 1988.
180. Walsh, L.J., Au, T.W., and Seymour, G.J., Inhibition of the induction of contact hypersensitivity by an epithelial cell-derived interleukin-1 inhibitor, *Aust. J. Dermatol.,* 30, 48, 1989.
181. Rebora, A., Parodi, A., and Murialdo, G., Basiliximab is effective for erosive lichen planus, *Arch. Dermatol.,* 138, 1100, 2002.

# 26 Lupus Erythematosus

*Jan D. Bos and Menno A. de Rie*

## CONTENTS



## I. INTRODUCTION

The existence of skin diseases related to sun exposure is an ancient observation, as exemplified by the description of a condition inflicted by sun and called *herpes esthiomenos* by Hippocrates. The distinction between different photodermatoses came in the 19th century, when Casenave was the first to use the term *lupus erythemateux* for a skin disease characterized by scarring, violaceous lesions especially in sun-exposed parts of the face. Kaposi (1872) recognized that this was not only a skin disease but that systemic manifestations may also occur (*lupus erythematosus disseminatosus et aggregatus*).[1] The recognition of circulating antinuclear factors in 1958 by Friou[2] and the subsequent detection of immunoglobulin deposition at the dermoepidermal junction (DEJ)[3,4] both resulted in the concept of lupus erythematosus (LE) as a disease resulting from autoimmune processes.

At present, we are aware of the existence of a heterogenous group of diseases belonging to the LE spectrum. These may be categorized as cutaneous LE, subacute LE, systemic LE, drug-induced LE, ANA-negative SLE, lupus-like syndrome in homozygous C2 and C4 deficiency, late onset systemic LE (SLE), Japanese LE, and neonatal LE.[5] In the scope of this chapter, emphasis is on pathomechanisms, clinical immunology, and immunotherapy of the specific cutaneous manifestations of LE.

## II. MAJOR CLINICAL CHARACTERISTICS OF CUTANEOUS LE

LE is now seen as a spectrum disease with systemic manifestations that may occur in almost any organ and in any combination. Criteria for the diagnosis of systemic SLE have become widely accepted and are of use in clinical practice[6] (Table 26.1). These criteria for SLE from the American College of Rheumatology were updated in 1997. The criterion "positive LE cell preparation" was deleted, and the item "false-positive test for syphilis" was expanded to "positive finding of antiphospholipid antibodies," including IgG or IgM anticardiolipin antibodies and lupus anticoagulant.

In cutaneous LE, a primary distinction is made between specific and nonspecific dermatological abnormalities.[7,8] The term *specific* refers to the histopathology of the lesion. Characteristic microscopic signs of specific cutaneous LE include epidermal atrophy; hydropic degeneration of cells

0-8493-1959-5/05/$0.00+$1.50

**TABLE 26.1**
**Criteria for the Diagnosis of SLE: A Patient Is Said to Have SLE If Any Combination of 4 of the Following Characteristics Occurs, Either Simultaneously or Subsequently**

1. Malar rash (fixed malar erythema)
2. Discoid rash (CDLE)
3. Photosensitivity
4. Oral ulcers (or nasopharyngeal)
5. Arthritis (non-erosive; >2 joints)
6. Serositis (pleuritis, pericarditis)
7. Renal disorder (proteinuria > 0.5 g/day, cellular casts)
8. Neurologic disorder (seizures, psychosis)
9. Hematologic disorder (anemia, leukopenia, lymphopenia, thrombocytopenia)
10. Immunologic disorder (LE cells, anti-dsDNA, anti-Sm, antiphospholipid antibodies)
11. Antinuclear antibody (ANA)

**TABLE 26.2**
**Clinical Forms of Histopathologically Specific Cutaneous LE**

| Clinical Types | Acute LE | Subacute LE | Chronic LE |
|---|---|---|---|
| Subtypes | Butterfly rash | Annular | Localized (face) |
| | Disseminated erythema | Psoriasiform | Cutaneous disseminated |
| | Bullous LE | Exanthematous | LE profunda and others |
| Photosensitivity | high | Medium to high | Medium |
| SLE association | >95% | 50% | <5% |
| Natural course | Days to weeks | Months | Years |

of the epidermal basal layer (apoptosis); follicular plugging; thickening of the basal membrane zone; a mononuclear cellular infiltrate localized subepidermally, around the postcapillary venules, and around the (capillary venules of) skin appendages; and, finally, dilatation of vascular capillaries. All these histopathological signs may occur in variable intensity. A secondary distinction in the group of specific LE is made by recognizing acute, subacute and chronic forms and variants (Table 26.2). Rare clinical manifestations of chronic cutaneous LE include LE profundus (Kaposi-Irgang), hypertrophic discoid LE, lupus tumidus, and mucosal LE. These variants are not further discussed.

Nonspecific cutaneous LE then is a collection of dermatological abnormalities that do not show the specific histopathological signs described above. Included in this group are vascular abnormalities such as Raynaud's phenomenon, (necrotizing) vasculitis, livedo reticularis, erythromelalgia, perniones, thrombophlebitis, diffuse (frontal) alopecia, sclerodactylia, hyper- or hypopigmentation, calcinosis cutis, urticaria, rheumatoid nodules, and, finally, oral ulcers. Nonspecific dermatoses are especially common in SLE. Overlap syndromes such as mixed connective tissue disease (MCTD), pemphigus erythematosus, and sclerodermatomyositis, in which some of these abnormalities may also be encountered exemplify the complexity and wide spectrum of pathogenic events that form part of the SLE syndrome.

## III. CELLULAR AND HUMORAL IMMUNITY IN LE

A basic finding in lupus erythematosus is the occurrence of a wide variety of circulating autoantibodies (Table 26.3). It is unclear whether these autoantibodies are primarily or secondarily formed.

**TABLE 26.3**
**Autoantibodies and Their Specificity in SLE**

| | |
|---|---|
| Antinuclear antibodies | |
| Single-stranded DNA (ssDNA): | Membrane pattern |
| Native double-stranded DNA (dsDNA, nDNA): | *Crithidia lucilae* |
| Histones | Exclude drug-induced SLE |
| Extractable nuclear antigens (ENA) | |
| Sm antibodies | Marker for SLE |
| RNP | SLE, MCTD, scleroderma |
| SSA (Ro)/SSB (La) | SLE, Sjögren, SCLE |
| Scl 70 | Scleroderma |
| Jo-1 | Polymyositis |
| PCNA | SLE with proliferative glomerulonephritis |
| Ku (K1) | SLE, polymyositis/scleroderma |
| Anticytoplasmatic antibodies | |
| Mitochondria | |
| Lysosomes | |
| Microsomes | |
| Ribosomes | |
| Glycoproteins | |
| Antiphospholipid antibodies | |
| Cardiolipin | |
| BFP | |
| Lupus anticoagulant | |
| Antibodies against blood cells | |
| Erythrocytes | |
| Leukocytes | |
| Thrombocytes | |
| Antibodies against various antigens | |
| Gastric mucosa | |
| Thyroglobulin | |
| Muscle sarcolemna | |
| Neurons | |

*Source:* Mutasim, D.F. and Adams, B.B., *J. Am. Acad. Dermatol.*, 42, 159, 2000. With permission.

Primary autoantibody formation may be the result of intrinsic dysregulation of antibody formation or, alternatively, may be triggered by exogenous antigens, such as from retroviruses.[9,10] Secondary autoantibody formation may occur as a result of tissue damage with the subsequent release of previously hidden autoantigens. In NZB/NZW mice that develop anti-DNA antibodies and glomerulonephritis, anti-DNA titers precede the development of renal disease.[11] In patients, anti-DNA titers rise before exacerbation of systemic disease occurs. The phenomenon of neonatal LE, in which autoantibodies are passively acquired from the mother, and in whom cutaneous disease disappears when these autoantibodies fade away from the child's circulation, also emphasizes the primary role of autoantibodies in LE pathogenesis. These findings indicate that autoantibody formation is not secondary to tissue damage in LE.

The presence of autoantibodies is said to be the result of B-cell hyperactivity. Essential for our understanding of the pathogenesis of SLE then is why these autoantibodies are produced. B-cell hyperactivity may be intrinsic, antigen-driven, or T-cell dependent.[12] Subsequently, it is believed that T-cell-directed autoantibody formation is the result of failure to eliminate autoreactive T cells. At present, disposal of autoaggressive T cells is thought to take place in the thymus, where new bone marrow–derived immature T cells are selected and autoreactivity is recognized with subsequent induction of apoptosis of these cells.[13] Clonal deletion is mediated through the T-cell antigen receptor, CD28, and Fas. SLE may be seen as an autoimmune disease characterized by loss of T-cell tolerance to nuclear antigens.[14]

In addition, it is believed that autoimmune diseases characterized by autoantibody formation have an underlying abnormality at the level of type 1 T-cell/type 2 T-cell balance. A shift to type 2 T-cell dominance is associated with B-cell help and formation of autoantibodies, through the production of a subset of cytokines — interleukin-1 (IL-1), IL-4, IL-5, IL-13 — that can induce B-cell production of immunoglobulins.

SLE-like disease may, however, also occur without the presence of autoantibodies, most notoriously in homozygous complement deficiencies.[15] SLE-like disease is very common in deficiencies of the earlier components of the complement system (C1q,r,s, C4, C2) but may occur in deficiencies of later components in the cascade (C5, 6, 7, and 8). In general, later component deficiencies are associated with severe infections. It is thought that earlier components play a role in natural immune complex clearing. Their deficiency thus leads to immune complex disease with many characteristics overlapping with SLE.

At this moment, it is difficult to draw a complete picture of SLE pathogenesis, in which complement deficiencies, type 1/2 T-cell imbalance, and insufficient killing of autoreactive T cells are included. Other undiscussed phenomena in SLE, such as abnormalities at the level of natural killer cells, monocytes, and macrophages, hormonal influences, and MHC associations, confound to the development of a simple model. Even exposition to ultraviolet (UV) irradiation may lead to exacerbations of SLE. In this regard, it is of note that autoantibodies in SLE tend to cluster in two populations of surface structures in apoptotic keratinocytes.[16] As UV irradiation leads to apoptosis of keratinocytes, exposition of the immune system to thereby induced surface structures may trigger it and enhance T-cell help for autoantibody production. Of course, it must be that different underlying mechanisms occur in various combinations, differing from patient to patient.

## IV. MODELS OF CUTANEOUS LE IMMUNOPATHOGENESIS

The spectrum of cutaneous LE, including neonatal LE lesions, specific LE and variants, and nonspecific LE is large and difficult to describe in general immunopathological terms. Vasculitis resulting from immune complex deposition (leukocytoclastic) may be found in some of these conditions. The best-studied form of cutaneous LE is the histopathologically specific type of lesion, where two main hypotheses have been formulated and tested. In one, emphasis is on immunoglobulin deposition at the DEJ, with complement activation and formation of the membrane attack complex (MAC) C5b–C9. In the other, emphasis is on cytotoxic T cells, which, through their Fc receptors for immunoglobulins, may recognize autoantibodies bound to epidermal cells (antibody-dependent cellular cytotoxicity, or ADCC).[17]

The presence of immunoglobulins and complement factors at the DEJ is highly suggestive for the presence of immune complex (IC) formation at that site. Thus, a pathogenetic model of cutaneous LE based on initial IC deposition, complement activation, acute inflammation, followed by a chronic inflammatory state was proposed soon after the recognition of the lupus band. Such a model was further supported by the identification of C5–C9 in LE skin lesions as soon as antibodies specific for MAC became available.[18] In a direct immunofluorescence study of cutaneous LE, granular MAC deposition at the DEJ was found in 29 of 38 biopsies (76%).[19]

Complement activation and deposition of MAC thus are common events in cutaneous lesions of LE. In view of the existence of complement regulatory proteins, both in soluble form as well as inserted in cell membranes, it is interesting to note what studies have been preformed in this area. At least clusterin and S-protein have been found to be colocalized with MAC, indicating inhibition of complement activation as part of MAC formation.[20] A major problem with the complement activation model of cutaneous LE pathogenesis is that acute inflammation, starting with influx of polymorphonuclear granulocytes, is not a feature in any stage of skin lesions. Also,

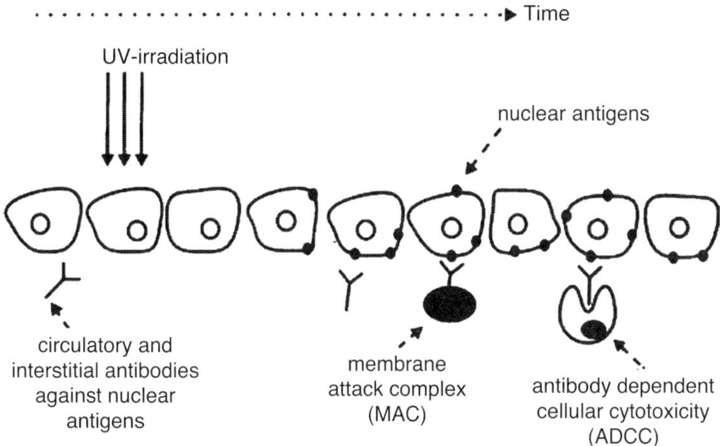


**FIGURE 26.1** In specific cutaneous LE, UV irradiation leads to expression of previously hidden nuclear antigens on keratinocyte cell membranes. These antigens become available for binding with antibodies to nuclear antigens that these patients have circulating as well as in interstitial fluid. Antigen–antibody complex formation may then lead to membrane attack complex formation and cellular cytotoxicity leading to keratinocyte degeneration.

human intact keratinocytes have been found to be resistant to complement-mediated lysis,[21] probably because they express membrane-inserted complement regulatory proteins (CRP) decay accelerating factor (DAF), membrane cofactor protein (MCP), and CD59.

The ADCC hypothesis has been worked out by Norris and co-workers.[22] It is based on the lesional presence of immunoglobulins and effector cells, mainly of the T-cell type.[23] These lymphocytes may act in ADCC *in vitro*.[24] The damage to epidermal cells with keratinocyte necrosis might follow influx of $CD8^+$ cyctotoxic T cells which can adhere to increased numbers of adhesion molecules (ICAM-1) expressed on keratinocytes as a result of stimulation by interferon-$\gamma$ (IFN-$\gamma$) secreted by cutaneous activated $CD4^+$ Th1 cells. The intraepidermal cytotoxic T cells would exert their effect through production of perforins or tumor necrosis factor-$\alpha$ (TNF-$\alpha$).[25]

The ADCC hypothesis is especially interesting in view of the photosensitivity in LE. In general, the action spectrum of photosensitivity is in the UVB (280 to 320 nm) range, but UVA (320 to 400 nm) may also lead to flares,[26] and testing has shown sensitivity to UVA, UVB, as well as to visible light in most patients.[27] After UV exposure, certain autoantigens are expressed on keratinocyte cell membranes, including Ro/SSA and nRNP.[28] These autoantigens then become available for binding by their specific antibodies in the extracellular fluid. Subsequently Fc receptors on effector lymphocytes recognize these keratinocyte-bound immune complexes, with subsequent lysis of these cells.[29] It may be that both membrane attack formation and cytotoxicity may occur due to UV induction of nuclear antigen expression on basal keratinocyte membranes and subsequent binding of interstitial antibodies directed against (some of) these nuclear antigens (Figure 26.1).

## V. IMMUNODIAGNOSIS OF CUTANEOUS LE

The recognition of immunoglobulin deposition in the skin of cutaneous lesions of LE, independently by Burnham and Cormane, was a breakthrough. The lupus band, detected by direct immunofluorescence in frozen skin tissue, has subsequently been developed as a diagnostic and investigative tool. A positive lupus band is almost always present in untreated involved discoid LE. It may contain IgG, IgM, IgA, properdin, C3, C4,and C1q. In SLE, uninvolved and sun-unexposed skin show a lupus band in 37 vs. 87% in uninvolved sun-exposed skin.[30] In questionable cases, the lupus band can thus be of help, with C4 the most SLE-specific finding. Immunoglobulin deposition at the DEJ may also be encountered in other diseases such as rheumatoid arthritis, but never is the fluorescence so linear, intense, and obtainable with antibodies against various parts of MAC as it is in SLE.[31]

In view of the possibility that patients with cutaneous specific LE may have simultaneous SLE or may later develop it, it is common practice to examine patients for systematization at regular, yearly intervals. The chance that a patient with CDLE will develop SLE during his or her lifetime is estimated to be 5%.[32] Routine laboratory tests including urinanalysis should be accompanied by LE-specific serological tests (ANA, LE cascade).

## VI. IMMUNOTHERAPY IN CUTANEOUS LE

Therapy in cutaneous LE varies with the severity of the condition. General measures including comforting the patient and underlining the need for rest form the basis, in addition to which rules for the avoidance of UV exposure are given. Topical sunscreens with good UVA and UVB filters are essential.

Typically, specific therapy starts with topical steroids, stronger ones to be preferred over weaker preparations. Often these are given in pulsed schemes, once daily for 4 subsequent days, with a rest period of 3 days thereafter, during which emollients may be given. Sometimes, such as in panniculitis (LE profunda), intralesional corticosteroids are of help.[33]

When topical measures are not sufficient, a wide variety of systemic agents are available.[34] Good clinical studies in which these different modalities are compared in prospective randomized trials with outcome parameters such as efficacy, induction of remission, adverse events, cost–benefit analysis, and analysis of quality of life indices are not available for cutaneous LE. Such studies are especially difficult to perform because patients differ so much from each other as to their place in LE spectrum, making randomized studies of comparable groups difficult. An overview of possible systemic therapy in (severe) cutaneous LE is given in Table 26.4.

## VII. CONCLUSIONS

Lupus erythematosus is a systemic disease with dominant cutaneous pathology. Each patient has unique clinical manifestations as well as a course that is unpredictable. The spectrum of systemic and cutaneous symptoms, signs, and abnormalities is so wide it can only be partly dealt with in the context of this chapter.

The immunopathogenesis of SLE can be described to a certain extent, but it is difficult to draw a complete picture of it. Complement deficiencies, type 1/2 T-cell imbalance, insufficient killing of autoreactive T cells, UV susceptibility, and many other characteristics should all be included in a definite pathogenetic model. For the specific cutaneous lesions of LE, the best model developed so far is that of the ADCC hypothesis. Especially in photosensitive LE, a series of events beginning with induction of nuclear antigen expression on keratinocytes after UV exposure, followed by binding of the antigens with circulating and interstitial autoantibodies, ending with Fc receptor-mediated lysis of keratinocytes by T cells, is most proximal to what may happen *in vivo*.

Immunodiagnosis and immunotherapy are constantly being refined, but a major breakthrough in the management of this disorder will depend on true insight into elementary steps in the formation of this disease in both its systemic and its cutaneous forms.[35]

**TABLE 26.4**
**Immunomodulating and Immunosuppressive Modalities in Use or in Development for the Systemic Treatment of Severe Cutaneous and/or SLE**

- Antimalarials
  - Chloroquine
  - Hydroxychloroquine
- Corticosteroids
  - Prednisone (oral)
  - Methylprednisolone (i.v.)
- Cyclosporine
- IVIG (intravenous immunoglobulins)
- Diaminodiphenylsulfon (DDS, Dapson)
- Retinoids
  - Isotretinoin
  - Acitretin
- Gold preparations
- Thalidomide[37]
- Clofazamine
- Cytotoxic agents
  - Azathioprine
  - Cyclophosphamide
  - Methotrexate
  - Mycophenolate mofetil
- Immunoablative therapy
- Autologous stem cell transplantation[38]

## REFERENCES


1. Kaposi, M.K., Neue Beiträge zur Kenntniss des Lupus erythematosus, *Arch. Dermatol. Syphilol.*, 4, 36, 1872.
2. Friou, G.J., The significance of the lupus globulin–nucleoprotein reaction, *Ann. Intern. Med.*, 49, 866, 1958.
3. Burnham, T.K., Neblett, T.R., and Fine, G., Application of fluorescent antibody technic to the investigation of lupus erythematosus and various dermatoses, *J. Invest. Dermatol.*, 41, 451, 1963.
4. Cormane, R.H., "Bound" globulin in the skin of patients with chronic discoid lupus erythematosus and systemic lupus erythematosus, *Lancet*, I, 534, 1964.
5. Sontheimer, R.D. and Provost, T.T., Lupus erythematosus, in *Immunologic Diseases of the Skin,* Jordon, R.E., Ed., Appleton & Lange, Norwalk, CT, 1991, 355.
6. Hochberg, M.C., Updating the American College of Rheumatology revised criteria for the classification of systemic lupus erythematosus, *Arthritis Rheum.*, 40, 1725, 1997.
7. Gilliam, J.N. and Sontheimer, R.D., Distinctive cutaneous subsets in the spectrum of lupus erythematosus, *J. Am. Acad. Dermatol.*, 4, 471, 1981.
8. Sontheimer, R.D., Madison, P.J., Reichlin, M., Jordon, R.E., Stastny, P., and Gilliam, J.N., Serologic and HLA associations in subacute cutaneous lupus erythematosus: a clinical subset of lupus erythematosus, *Ann. Intern. Med.*, 97, 664, 1982.
9. Talal, N., Garry, R.F., Schur, P.H. et al., A conserved idiotype and antibodies to retroviral protein in systemic lupus erythematosus, *J. Clin. Invest.*, 85, 1866, 1990.
10. Ranki, A., Kurki, P., Riepponen, S., and Stephansson, E., Antibodies to retroviral proteins in autoimmune connective tissue disease: relation to clinical manifestations and ribonucleoprotein autoantibodies, *Arthritis Rheum.*, 35, 1483, 1992.

11. Steinberg, A.D. and Reinertsen, J.L., Lupus in New Zealand mice and in dogs, *Bull. Rheum. Dis.*, 28, 940, 1977.
12. Smith, H.R. and Steinber, A.D., Autoimmunity: a perspective, *Annu. Rev. Immunol.*, 1, 175, 1983.
13. Tan, E.M., Autoimmunity and apoptosis, *J. Exp. Med.*, 179, 1083, 1994.
14. Kong, Ph.I., Odegard, J.M., Bouzahzah, F., Choi, J.-Y., Eardley, L.D., Zieinski, C.E., and Craft, J.E., Intrinsic T cell defects in autoimmunity, *Ann. N.Y. Acad. Sci.*, 987, 60, 2003.
15. Pickering, M.C., Botto, M., Lachmann, P.J., and Walport, M.J., Systemic lupus erythematosus, complement deficiency, and apoptosis, *Adv. Immunol.*, 76, 227, 2001.
16. Casciola-Rosen, L.A., Anhalt, G., and Rosen, A., Autoantigens targeted in systemic lupus erythematosus are clustered in two populations of surface structures on apoptotic keratinocytes, *J. Exp. Med.*, 179, 1317, 1994.
17. Norris, D.A. and Lee, L.A., Antibody dependent cellular cytotoxicity in skin disease, *J. Invest. Dermatol.*, 85, 165s, 1985.
18. Biesecker, G., Lavin, L., Ziskind, M., and Koffler, D., Cutaneous localization of the membrane attack complex in discoid and systemic lupus erythematosus, *N. Engl. J. Med.*, 306, 264, 170, 1982.
19. Helm, K.F. and Peters, M.S., Deposition of membrane attack complex in cutaneous lesions of lupus erythematosus, *J. Am. Acad. Dermatol.*, 31, 515, 1994.
20. French, L.E., Polla, L.L., Tschopp, J., and Schifferli, J.A., Membrane attack complex (MAC) deposits in skin are not always accompanied by S-protein and clusterin, *J. Invest. Dermatol.*, 98, 758, 1992.
21. Norris, D.A., Ryan, S.B., Kissinger, R.M., Fritz, K.A., and Boyce, S.T., Systematic comparison of antibody-mediated mechanisms of keratinocyte lysis *in vitro, J. Immunol.*, 135, 1073, 1985.
22. Norris, D.A., Pathomechanisms of photosensitive lupus erythematosus, *J. Invest. Dermatol.*, 100, 58s, 1993.
23. Bos, J.D., Emsbroek, J.A., and Krieg, S.R., T-cell subsets and Langerhans cells in cutaneous lupus erythematodes, in *Immunodermatology,* McDonald, D.M., Ed., Butterworths, London, 1984, 261.
24. Wahlin, B. and Perlmann, P., Characterization of human K cells by surface antigens and morphology at the single cell level, *J. Immunol.*, 131, 2340, 1983.
25. Nickoloff, B.J., Role of interferon-γ in cutabeous trafficking of lymphocytes with emphasis on molecular and cellular adhesion events, *Arch. Dermatol.*, 124, 1835, 1988.
26. Orteu, C.H., Sontheimer, R.D., and Dutz, J.P., The pathophysiology of photosensitivity in lupus erythematosus, *Photodermatol. Photoimmunol. Photomed.,* 17, 95, 2001.
27. Sanders, C.J.G., Van Weelden, H., Kazzaz, G.A.A., Sigurdsson, V., Toonstra, J., and Bruijnzeel-Koomen, C.A.F.M., Photosensitivity in patients with lupus erythematosus; a clinical and photobiological study of 100 patients using a prolonged phototest protocol, *Br. J. Dermatol.,* 149, 131, 2003.
28. LeFeber, W.P., Norris, D.A., Ryan, S.R., Huff, J.C., Lee, L.A., Kubo, M., Boyce, S.T., Kotzin, B.L., and Weston, W.L., Ultraviolet light induces binding of antibodies to selected nuclear antigens on cultured human keratinocytes, *J. Clin. Invest.*, 74, 1545, 1984.
29. Furukawa, F., Kanouchi, M., and Imamura, S., Susceptibility to UVB light in cultured keratinocytes of cutaneous lupus erythematosus, *Dermatology*, 189Suppl. 1), 18, 1994.
30. Ahmad, A.R. and Provost, T.T., Incidence of a positive lupus band test using sun-exposed and -unexposed skin, *Arch. Dermatol.*, 115, 228, 1979.
31. Smith, C.D., Marino, C., and Rothfield, N.F., The clinical utility of the lupus band test, *Arthritis Rheum.*, 27, 382, 1984.
32. Healy, E., Kieran, E., and Rogers, S., Cutaneous lupus erythematosus: a study of clinical and laboratory prognostic factors in 65 patients, *Ir. J. Med. Sci.*, 164, 113, 1995.
33. Rothe, M.J. and Kerdal, F.A., Treatment of cutaneous lupus erythematosus, *Lupus*, 1, 351, 1992.
34. Ruiz-Irastorza, G., Khamashta, M.A., Castellino, G., and Hughes, G.R.V., Systemic lupus erythematosus, *Lancet*, 357, 1027, 2001.
35. Bos, J.D., The skin immune system: lupus erythematosus as a paradigm, *Arch. Dermatol. Res.,* 287, 23, 1994.
36. Mutasim, D.F. and Adams, B.B., A practical guide for serologic evaluation of autoimmune connective tissue diseases, *J. Am. Acad. Dermatol.,* 42, 159, 2000.
37. Ordi-Ros, J., Cortes, F., Curucull, E., Mauri, M., Bujan, S., and Vilardell, M., Thalidomide in the treatment of cutaneous lupus refractory to conventional therapy, *J. Rheumatol.,* 27, 1429, 2000.
38. Sherer, Y. and Shoenfield, Y., Stem cells transplantation: a cure for autoimmune disease, *Lupus,* 7, 137, 1998.

# 27 Cutaneous Vasculitis

*Cord Sunderkötter and Gerhard Kolde*

## CONTENTS



## I. INTRODUCTION AND CLASSIFICATION

The term *vasculitis* denotes an inflammatory condition in which destruction of the wall of blood vessels by leukocytes is the primary event. This definition excludes conditions where blood vessels are destroyed by physical trauma associated with secondary inflammatory reactions (e.g., after laser therapy), and it also excludes vessel damage secondary to destructive inflammatory processes of the surrounding tissue, such as abscess formation. Vasculitic syndromes or vasculitides are histologically characterized by leukocytic infiltration and damage of the wall of blood vessels, often coupled with compromise of the lumen. In vasculitis of the small vessels, e.g., the postcapillary venules, infiltrating cells cannot be distinguished from transmigrating cells, but the inflammatory reaction usually results in necrosis of the vascular wall with subsequent extravasation of erythrocytes (hemorrhage), which therefore presents an important histological criterion. Damage of the surrounding tissue is usually not very marked, unless several neighboring vessels are involved and sufficient collateral blood flow is not available. By contrast, destruction of medium-sized vessels more often results in necrosis of the supplied tissue area, as there is usually no sufficient collateral blood flow available once the lumen of a medium-sized vessel is suddenly compromised.

The nomenclature and classification of the vasculitides have remained an evolving process since the first classification attempt by Zeek in 1952.[1] The reasons that make classification difficult are the various and only partially evolved pathogenetic mechanisms, the overlapping clinical features, and the few pathognomic signs and symptoms of individual vasculitic disorders. In spite of these difficulties, two classification systems have gained wide acceptance. In 1990, the American College of Rheumatology proposed clinical, histologic, and historical criteria to distinguish seven vasculitic entities.[2] Four years later, the Chapel Hill Consensus Conference (CHCC) on the nomenclature of systemic vasculitides published a working classification[3] that is based on the size of the

0-8493-1959-5/05/$0.00+$1.50

**TABLE 27.1**
**Classification of Vasculitic Syndromes**

A. Involving predominantly large blood vessels
   1. Takayasu's arteritis
   2. Giant cell arteritis (e.g., temporal arteritis)
   3. Aortitis of rheumatic connective tissue disease
   4. Aortitis related to other diseases (e.g., syphilitic aortitis)
B. Involving predominantly medium-sized blood vessels
   1. Polyarteritis nodosa (PAN) group
      a. Classic PAN
      b. Cutaneous PAN (benign, no systemic involvement)
      c. Infantile PAN (Kawasaki disease vasculitis)
C. Involving predominantly small blood vessels
   1. ANCA-associated pauci-immune vasculitis
      a. Wegener's granulomatosis
      b. Microscopic polyangiitis
      c. Churg–Strauss syndrome
   2. Vasculitis associated with vascular deposits of immune complexes (leukocytoclastic vasculitis)
      a. Leukocytoclastic vasculitis with predominant deposition of IgA
      b. Leukocytoclastic vasculitis with predominant deposition of IgG or IgM
      c. Essential mixed cryoproteinemias
      d. Urticarial vasculitis
      e. Serum sickness
   3. Vasculitis associated with connective tissue disease (as in rheumatoid arthritis, systemic lupus erythematosus, infectious disease, malignancies)
   4. Vasculitis associated with sepsis (Shwartzman phenomenon-like pathophysiology)
   5. Vasculitis associated with infection of endothelial cells

involved vessels, but also includes histopathologic features (e.g., granulomatous infiltrates in giant cell arteritis), immunohistologic findings (e.g., IgA-dominant vascular immune deposits in Schönlein–Henoch purpura), markers of immunodiagnostic significance (e.g., antineutrophil cytoplasmic antibodies in Wegener's granulomatosis), and clinical features such as the extent of the process with regard to the organs chiefly (e.g., the lung in Churg–Strauss syndrome) or exclusively affected (e.g., the skin in some forms of cutaneous vasculitis). As a result of its clear terms and definitions, the CHCC proposal has become a frequently used classification system, although it has not been developed for diagnostic purposes and may fail to differentiate one type of vasculitis from another in clinical settings. To overcome these problems, the definition of certain vasculitides needs to be supplemented with additional clinical criteria and surrogate laboratory markers.[4] However, there is yet no consensus how to integrate these parameters into the CHCC system. In Table 27.1, we present a modified CHCC classification that is currently used by most groups.

Vasculitic lesions in the skin either derive from inflammation restricted to the dermal vessels or they are part of a systemic vasculitis. Generally, nearly all types of vasculitis can affect the skin and thus present as a form of cutaneous vasculitis. The term cutaneous vasculitis is sometimes used only for cases in which the inflammation is confined exclusively to vessels in the dermis without involving other organs. One should, however, keep in mind that there could be involvement of noncutaneous vessels that remain undetected only because our diagnostic means (e.g., hemoccult) are not sensitive enough or because their involvement is transient. On the other hand, such minor systemic lesions may not become clinically relevant, therefore justifying the term *cutaneous vasculitis* for clinical use.

Vasculitis in the skin mostly involves the small vessels (postcapillary venules) and is then often associated with apoptosis of infiltrating granulocytes featuring fragmentation of the nuclei (karyorrhexis or leukocytoclasia). This feature has inspired the term *leukocytoclastic vasculitis*. Leukocytoclasia is also found in urticarial vasculitis, which represents a distinct form of chronic relapsing inflammation to the small vessels (see Chapter 28). There are other skin diseases with inflammatory changes involving the blood vessels such as Behcet's syndrome, and with inflammatory changes around the vasculature such as pyoderma gangrenosum and Sweet's syndrome, which by some authors have been subsumed under the term (cutaneous) vasculitis.[5] These conditions are better classified as neutrophilic vascular reactions[6] or neutrophilic dermatoses[7] because the vasculitic alterations represent a secondary rather than primary event. Whether purpura pigmentosa and other lymphocytic inflammations of the blood vessels represent a distinct group of vasculitides has not been clarified yet.[8] The erythrocyte extravasates observed in these diseases speak for lymphocyte-mediated damage of the vessel wall, but there is no fibrinoid necrosis and disappearance of the small blood vessels.

## II. MECHANISMS OF VASCULAR DAMAGE

Most forms of vasculitis in the skin are mediated by immunopathogenic mechanisms. These encompass the following: the formation of immune complexes, the production of antineutrophil cytoplasmic antibodies, or pathogenic T-cell responses and granuloma formation. Most vasculitides induced by infectious agents are also based on these mechanisms.[9] There are only few vasculitic syndromes that are caused by direct microbial invasion of endothelial cells (e.g., some forms of tick-bite fever caused by Rickettsia).

### A. Immune Complex Formation

#### 1. Deposition of Immunoglobulins

Deposition of circulating immune complexes at the wall of small vessels is a frequent cause for cutaneous leukocytoclastic vasculitis. The local Arthus reaction represents an experimental model for such a type III hypersensitivity class of immunological inflammation. Deposition of immunoglobulins has also been reported for vasculitic syndromes involving medium-sized and large vessels, but less consistently and as yet without a clearly defined role in their pathophysiology.

The presumed sequence of events in immune complex–induced vasculitis of small vessels encompasses formation of large lattices of immune complexes, their deposition at the vessel wall, their insufficient elimination, activation of the complement system, and the cytotoxic reaction of granulocytes while trying to phagocytose the complexes at the endothelial cells. Formation of immune complexes is a routine procedure of the immune system, which occurs, e.g., during chewing. It does not usually entail immune complex–mediated diseases, unless there are deviations in formation or elimination of immune complexes. The tendency of immune complexes to become deposited at the vessel wall depends on their physical properties (larger size, cationic charge that facilitates initial binding to basement membrane) and on a prolonged persistence in the circulation.[10–12] Only immune complexes large enough to precipitate are able to elicit the Arthus reaction. Formation of large lattices and persistence in the circulation is facilitated when a slight excess of multivalent antigens is present or a state of near equivalence between antibodies and antigens.[10,12] The immune system attempts to maintain them in a soluble form and to facilitate their uptake and clearance by rapid activation of the complement system. Initial binding of C1 to immunoglobulins delays Fc-Fc interactions and thus formation of large lattices. Subsequent binding of a large number of C3b or C4b molecules to immune complexes inhibits the formation of insoluble immune aggregates and even may disrupt those already formed.[11,12] Clearance of circulating immune complexes is performed by tissue macrophages, especially in the spleen and in the liver. They are transported to the liver by erythrocytes as these cells carry the complement receptor CR1 to which immune complexes bind via C3b.[11] In the liver immune complexes are released from CR1 with the help of complement factor I and taken up by phagocytes that express FcγR and complement receptors CR1 or CR3. Thus, the activated complement system is able to prevent damage, provided that the immune complexes have not yet been deposited at the vessel wall. When deposition has already occurred, the complement system has damaging effects by attracting and activating granulocytes. However, it is unlikely that it will destroy endothelial cells by going all the way to formation of the lytic C5b–C9 complex, because endothelial cells like all nucleated cells express protecting factors such as CR1, decay accelerating factor, and membrane cofactor.

Emergence of precipitable immune complexes is promoted when their formation and clearance are disturbed.[11] Immune complexes composed primarily of $IgG_4$ or IgA are less efficient in activating the classical complement pathway and subsequently in binding C3. They thus exhibit a greater tendency to become insoluble, and to persist in the circulation. This may facilitate and perpetuate vasculitic reactions in Henoch–Schönlein purpura. Deficiencies in CR1, C1qrs, C2, or null mutations of the gene for C4A as well as deficiencies in other complement components have been shown to correlate with increased incidence of vasculitis in patients suffering from rheumatoid arthritis or systemic lupus erythematosus.[11,13] Some infectious agents (streptococci, chlamydia, hepatitis B and C virus) appear to induce the formation and vascular deposition of pathogenic immune complexes more often than others. Antigens of hepatitis B and C virus have been found in mixed cryoglobulins, and are thus a common cause for so-called cryoglobulinemic vasculitis.[14,15] Antigens of hepatitis B are also implicated in the pathogenesis of polyarteritis nodosa.[16]

Lodging of large immune complexes along the vessel basement membrane is facilitated, e.g., by locally increased dilation and permeability of blood vessels.[17,18] This is achieved by mediators derived from mast cells or platelets such as eicosanoids, kinins, histamine, platelet-activating factors, or vascular endothelial growth factor,[18,19] and under certain circumstances even by complement.[20] In addition, turbulences at branching vessels or gravitational hydrostasis also favor deposition of immune complexes; the latter explains the predilection for lesions on the legs. Another factor directing the deposition of immune complexes at the vessel wall may be the exclusive expression of human FcγRIIa (CD32) on the luminal surface of endothelial cells of the superficial vascular plexus, but not of the deep vascular plexus.[21]

## 2. Recruitment of Granulocytes and Mechanisms of Granulocyte-Dependent Endothelial Damage

Once immune complexes have been deposited, mechanisms come into play that result in recruitment of granulocytes: the activation of chemotactic complement components (C3a, C5a), and the usual cascade of chemokines and adhesion molecules. Their induction involves IgG-induced activation of local mast cells via FcγRIII with release of tumor necrosis factor (TNF).[22] TNF is one of the main factors for inducing expression of adhesion molecules and chemotactic factors. Neutralization of one adhesion molecule such as E-selectin (CD62E) usually does not impair recruitment of granulocytes, but it does reduce the extent of hemorrhage.[23] Thus, there must be mechanisms that are specific for vasculitis, but that do not occur in nonvasculitic inflammation. This difference is essential for the understanding of leukocytoclastic vasculitis at the postcapillary venules: one has to distinguish between the processes that are common to all forms of granulocytic inflammations and those that only occur and are mandatory for simultaneous destruction of the corresponding vessels. As immune complexes apparently are one prerequisite for leukocytoclastic vasculitis, they must trigger such special processes.

Granulocytes are mandatory for the damaging effects in leukocytoclastic vasculitis,[23] as is their expression of receptors for Fcγ.[24] Activation of leukocytes by binding of immune complexes to their FcγRIII and FcγRI without the inhibitory effects of FcγRII is crucial for the Arthus reaction.[25–27] In contrast, the need for complement varies and partly depends on the tissue site (in immune complex–induced peritonitis less than in skin and lung), on species and inbred strains of species.[25,26,28] When particles opsonized by immunoglobulins or lattices of immune complexes are too large to be fully enclosed within phagocytic vesicle, this will result in release of cytotoxic products into the extracellular milieu, a process termed *frustrated phagocytosis*.[29,30]

Neutrophil-mediated injury of endothelial cells, in addition, requires interaction of products from both neutrophils and endothelial cells. Major cytotoxic agents are reactive oxygen radicals, followed by degrading enzymes from neutrophilic granula. Toxic oxygen radicals are generated in a complex cascade under participation of enzymatic events in both neutrophils and endothelial cells.[31] Briefly, elastase released from neutrophils can gain entry into endothelial cells, where it converts xanthine dehydrogenase into xanthine oxidase, a process finally resulting in the generation of superoxide anion ($O^{2-}$) and $Fe^{2+}$. The latter helps to reduce $H_2O_2$,which has diffused from neutrophils into the cytosol of endothelial cells, to the highly reactive oxygen radical $HO^-$, which is likely to execute the decisive cytotoxic blow to endothelial cells.

A specific feature in vasculitis may be the increased or prolonged adherence between neutrophils and endothelial cells due to deposited immune complexes and altered expression of adhesion molecules.[23,31] Damage of endothelial cells in response to granulocyte products has been shown to be also facilitated when endothelial cells are in a state of activation.[32]

In summary, leukocytoclastic vasculitis arises when there is a certain constellation consisting of altered adhesion processes coupled with activation of neutrophils at the vessel wall.[23] This principle also holds true when leukocytoclastic vasculitis is elicited without immune complexes as encountered in sepsis. A model of this is the Shwartzman reaction, which entails increased adherence of granulocytes to endothelial cells after first injection of lipopolysaccharide (LPS) coupled with degranulation and oxidative burst of granulocytes during a second injection of LPS.[23,33] There is evidence for mutual activating interactions between granulocytes and endothelial cells as stimulation of the latter with LPS results in release of factors that trigger degranulation of granulocytes. The altered adhesion processes in vasculitis appear to entail and to enable firm and perhaps prolonged clinging of granulocytes to the vessel wall so that release of their cytotoxic products directly enters or harms endothelial cells. Mediating such firm adhesion appears to be one feature also of antineutrophil cytoplasmic antibodies (ANCA).[34]

## B. Antineutrophil Cytoplasmic Antibodies

ANCA are a heterogenous group of autoantibodies. Most of them show specificity for either proteinase 3 (cANCA) or myeloperoxidase (pANCA). They are regularly found in a group of small vessel vasculitides, the so-called ANCA-associated vasculitides, such as Wegener's granulomatosis, microscopic polyangiitis, and Churg–Strauss syndrome. A well-described effector function of these autoantibodies is stimulation of neutrophils to produce reactive oxygen species and to release proteolytic enzymes, similarly as shown for immune complexes. However, neutrophil activation can be due to interaction of monomeric ANCA with PR3/MPO and Fc$\gamma$ receptors, while stimulation by ANCA-containing immune complexes cannot be excluded as an additional mechanism.[35,36]

In the meantime a direct causal link between ANCA and the development of glomerulonephritis and vasculitis has been demonstrated in an animal model where the passive transfer of ANCA was sufficient to induce disease.[35–37] According to a hypothetical sequence of events, transient activation, e.g., by infections, leads to activation of granulocytes with subsequent release of cytokines and movement of lysosomes to the cell membrane, thereby rendering their antigenic contents accessible to ANCAs. Cytokines such as TNF-$\alpha$ are able to upregulate local expression of adhesion molecules and, in concert with bound ANCAs, trigger enhanced adherence, while ANCAs additionally induce respiratory burst and degranulation of granulocytes with subsequent damage to the vessel wall.

## C. Pathogenic T-Cell Responses and Granuloma Formation

One of the histologic hallmarks of certain vasculitic syndromes with involvement of medium-sized and large vessels is the presence of granulomatous inflammation. In giant cell arteritis and Takayasu's arteritis, the granulomas are restricted to the vessel wall leading to destruction of the internal elastic lamina. The detection of clonally expanded CD4+ T cells of the Th1 type in the lesional tissue indicates that the granulomatous inflammation is due to an aberrant Th1 cell response to autoantigens and/or environmental insults, such as infections.[38] However, all current attempts to isolate an infectious agent from the lesional tissue have failed.[39] The local T-cell response was recently demonstrated to be initiated by activation and maturation of resident dendritic cell in the vascular wall.[40]

ANCA-associated Wegener's granulomatosis and Churg–Strauss syndrome are characterized by necrotizing granulomatous inflammation of the extravascular interstitial tissue. As in giant cell arteritis, the clonal and polyclonal CD4+ T cells derived from lesional tissue and peripheral blood of Wegener's granulomatosis exhibit a predominant Th1 profile, while a Th2 cytokine pattern had been reported for microscopic polyangiitis, which forgoes granulomas.[41–43] The transformation from localized to generalized disease is supposed to be accompanied by a shift of the Th1 pattern toward a Th0/Th2 granulomatous immune response.[44,45] There is evidence that the aberrant granuloma formation in Wegener's granulomatosis is secondary to necrotizing tissue inflammation that is caused by ANCA-induced activation of extravascular neutrophils and monocytes.[46] The mechanisms of the cell activation and tissue necrosis are probably similar to those that cause small vessel vasculitis. Granulomatous inflammation in Churg–Strauss syndrome appears to be due to comparable mechanisms.[47]

## III. CLINICAL HALLMARKS

The clinical features of vasculitis in the skin depend on the size of the blood vessels affected by the inflammatory process. The hallmark of cutaneous vasculitis of the small blood vessels, as seen in all types of leukocytoclastic vasculitis, are purpuric papules arising from red macules. The lesions may develop into ecchymoses, blisters, necroses, and even ulcerations. Sites of predilection are the lower legs and other skin areas with stasis or disturbed hemodynamic blood flow. In the vasculitic syndromes involving medium-sized vessels, the presenting symptoms are faint to intense red subcutaneous nodules, which usually undergo necrotic ulceration. The necrosis due to ischemia may involve the surrounding dermis, the subcutaneous fatty tissue, and even structures underlying the skin, such as the nasal septum and gingival palate in Wegener's granulomatosis.[48] Vasculitis of the medium-sized blood vessels that does not culminate in extensive necrosis may macroscopically present as livedo racemosa, a distinct type of livedo reticularis with a broken network of bluish discolorization due to disturbed blood flow with shunting of deoxygenated blood to the venular bed. It has been observed, e.g., in cutaneous polyarteritis nodosa or in cryoproteinemic vasculitis.[49,50] Necrotizing inflammation of medium-sized muscular arteries, especially of internal organs, may lead to aneurysmal dilatations as observed in classic polyarteritis nodosa. Cutaneous symptoms associated with vasculitis of large vessels may additionally encompass gangrene due to ischemia, although this is not a very frequent complication. In giant cell arteritis, tenderness and focal thickening of involved superficial temporal arteries present a common symptom, whereas acute gangrene in the scalp regions or on the tongue or legs is rare.[51,52] Takayasu's arteritis can be accompanied by erythema induratum, pyoderma gangrenosum or erythema nodosum,[53] but like other cutaneous symptoms occurring during vasculitic syndromes they are not always sequelas of vessel damage, but of other pathomechanisms underlying the systemic disease.

## IV. DIAGNOSIS

Assuming a cutaneous vasculitis is present, one has (1) to establish the diagnosis, (2) to evaluate the extent of systemic involvement, and (3) to determine a possible treatable cause of the inflammation. Definite diagnosis and pathological classification of the vascular inflammation require the histologic examination of the lesions. Biopsies should be taken from mature, but nonulcerated lesions to avoid histopathological pitfalls caused by alterations secondary to inflammatory damage of the blood vessels. Only deep punch or excisional biopsies are sufficient to include both the small- and medium-sized blood vessels and to determine the target and extent of the inflammatory process. Vascular immunoglobulin depositions as detected by immunofluorescence or immunohistochemistry on frozen biopsy material are found in more than 80% of the patients with cutaneous vasculitis.[14] The relevance of IgA fluorescence for differentiating Schönlein–Henoch disease from other immune complex vasculitides is high as IgA-associated vasculitis is more prone to systemic involvement and, in adults, presents a higher risk for severe complications such as renal failure. IgA depositions are not specific as they are also found in some nonvasculitic disorders such as alcoholic liver disease.[54] In patients with clinical signs of vasculitis, however, isolated IgA staining in a fresh or histamine-induced lesion provides a diagnostic hint on Schönlein–Henoch disease, and thus implies a higher risk for extracutaneous involvement of the renal, gastrointestinal, and musculoskeletal systems than vasculitides with only IgG-containing deposits. The frozen biopsies can additionally be used for special tests such as looking for vascular deposits of certain microbial antigens. The extent of systemic involvement is determined by checking for fever, hematuria, and other systemic symptoms, by careful clinical examination, and by clinical and laboratory examinations of the organ systems most often affected.[14,55] Particular emphasis should be given to the kidneys, the gastrointestinal tract, the lungs, and the central nervous system. Determining the cause of vasculitis is more difficult and in many cases cannot be achieved. In cutaneous leukoclastic vasculitis, there are three major categories of etiologic factors: infectious agents, drugs, and underlying diseases characterized by the presence of circulating immune complexes.[56] Nevertheless, in 50% of the cases, no clear cause can be identified.

In summary, basic blood tests should include sedimentation rate or C-reactive protein, repeated urine analysis for blood and protein, as well as hemoccult and blood pressure in order not to overlook severe systemic involvement. A differential blood count may be performed to gain hints on infections or leukemia. In severe or remittent forms of vasculitis a complete workup may become necessary in an attempt to determine the cause of the inflammatory process, taking into account the parameters mentioned above such as circulating immune complexes (including rheumatoid factor, cryoproteins, ANCA), levels of immunoglobulins or complement, paraproteins, autoantibodies, serological titers for microbes, etc.

## V. TREATMENT REGIMENS

An ideal treatment of vasculitis would be directed at eliminating or combating the cause of the inflammatory reaction. However, the cause often remains unknown or cannot be directly tackled. Because most vascular inflammations are mediated in part by immunopathogenic mechanisms, both cutaneous and systemic vasculitis are treated with drugs that modulate or even suppress the immune system.

Steroids are the treatment of first choice in systemic vasculitis. Numerous studies, including several controlled randomized trials, have shown that the continuous or pulsed administration of a steroid is effective in inducing remission of systemic polyarteritis nodosa, Takayasu's arteritis, giant cell arteritis, and Churg–Strauss syndrome.[57] In unresponsive or life-threatening disease and in ANCA-associated Wegener's granulomatosis and microscopic polyangiitis, steroids need to be complemented by cyclophosphamide, the most efficacious cytotoxic agent in the induction therapy of vascular inflammation.[57] Because of the severe side effects after long-term application of cyclophosphamide, maintenance therapy is now often performed with less toxic azathioprin,[58] methotrexate,[59] or mycophenolate mofetil.[60] The intravenous administration of high-dose immunoglobulins was found to be effective in ANCA-associated vasculitides refractory to or intolerant of conventional immunosuppressive treatments, but they should be considered an adjuvant.[61] New therapeutic regimens used for systemic vasculitides include hemopoietic stem cell transplantation[62] and the administration of the recently developed biologic agents that are capable of directly targeting selective components of the immune response[63] such as TNF-α. An example for treatment of the cause using a biologic agent is interferon-alpha (IFN-α) in the treatment of hepatitis virus-associated polyarteritis nodosa and cryoglobulinemic vasculitis[63]

In cutaneous vasculitis, the treatment is based mostly on experience as there are almost no controlled randomized therapeutic trials. Steroids and/or cytotoxic agents are of no scientifically proven benefit and are only advised for patients with significant systemic involvement or with significant cutaneous ulcerations,[56] and for patients with systemic hypocomplementemic vasculitis.[64] Uncomplicated cutaneous vasculitis is recommended to be treated symptomatically with compression stocking to prevent further deposition of immune complexes along dilated vessels and to be observed. In chronic or remittent forms anti-inflammatory and immunomodulatory agents can be tried, which are generally less toxic than immunosuppressive strategies. From the various agents used,[65] we found pentoxifylline effective, especially when combined with dapsone. The efficacy of pentoxifylline partially results from inhibiting the synthesis of TNF-α.[66] In our animal model of the Shwartzman reaction administration of pentoxifylline, especially in conjunction with dexamethasone, markedly suppressed the rise in serum TNF and simultaneously attenuated the formation of vasculitic lesions.[67] Dapsone may exert its therapeutic effects in vasculitis by suppressing lysosomal enzyme activity and oxygen-mediated cytotoxicity in granulocytes and by decreasing the influx of neutrophils.[68] It is also used as monotherapy, but the combination with pentoxifylline or colchicine seems more effective. Colchicine inhibits the migratory capacity of leukocytes by suppressing microtubule assembly, and it seems to interfere with neutrophil–endothelial interactions by diminishing quantitative and qualitative display of adhesion molecules (selectins) on endothelial cells.[69] Although several reports suggested an appreciable improvement in necrotizing leukocytoclastic vasculitis,[70] a randomized controlled trial[71] has failed to show an effect of colchicine monotherapy. In patients with leukocytoclastic vasculitis unresponsive to the anti-inflammatory and immunomodulatory therapy regimens, several case reports have demonstrated beneficial effects of low-dose methotrexate, azathioprine, or cyclosporine A.[55] Cyclosporine was, however, also reported to induce vasculitis.[72] Apart from systemic therapy, topical steroids are often used in cutaneous vasculitis, but no data support this practice.[56]

## VI. CONCLUDING REMARKS

The term *vasculitis* should be reserved only for primary inflammations of the blood vessels with subsequent vascular damage. Although the effector mechanisms of the endothelial cell damage have become rather clear, we still do not understand the events crucial for this type of inflammation. To evaluate which of the pathophysiological events are characteristic for vasculitis one has to carefully distinguish between the mechanisms common to all forms of acute inflammation and those that are found only during inflammations with marked vascular damage. The field of vasculitis thus still entails a number of riddles.

Dermatologists are regularly confronted with vasculitis, as the skin is among the organs most frequently involved in the manifestation of vasculitic syndromes. Symptoms of cutaneous vasculitis are most common in inflammation of the small-sized vessels, but generally all forms of vasculitis can affect the skin. Thus, the skin may alert patient and physician to an underlying severe systemic form. Since vasculitic lesions of the skin are easily accessible, the skin immune system offers an excellent field to learn more about the cause, the features, and the therapeutic possibilities of vasculitic syndromes.

## REFERENCES

1. Zeek, P.M., Periarteritis nodosa: a critical review, *Am. J. Surg. Pathol.*, 2, 777, 1952.

2. Hunder, G.G. et al., The American College of Rheumatology 1990. Criteria for the classification of vasculitis, *Arthritis Rheum.*, 33, 1065, 1990.
3. Jennette, J.C. et al., Nomenclature of systemic vasculitides, *Arthritis Rheum.*, 37, 187, 1994.
4. Luqmani, R.A. and Robinson, H., Introduction to, and classification of, the systemic vasculitides, *Best Pract. Res. Clin. Rheumatol.*, 15, 187, 2001.
5. Ryan, T.J., Cutaneous vasculitis, in *Textbook of Dermatology,* Vol. 3, Champion, R.H., Burton, J.L., and Ebling, F.J.G., Eds., Blackwell Scientific Publications. p 2155, 1998.
6. Jorizzo, J.L. et al., Neutrophilic vascular reactions, *J. Am. Acad. Dermatol.*, 19, 983, 1988.
7. Hunt, S.J. and Santa Cruz, D.J., Neutrophilic dermatoses, *Semin. Dermatol.*, 8, 266, 1989.
8. Kossard, S., Defining lymphocytic vasculitis, *Australas. J. Dermatol.*, 41, 149, 2000.
9. Tervaert, J.W., Infections in primary vasculitides, *Cleveland Clin. J. Med.,* 69, SII24, 2002.
10. Mannik, M., Development of immune complexes in the skin, *J. Invest. Dermatol.*, 93, 77S, 1989.
11. Schifferli, J.A., Ng, Y.C., and Peters, D.K., The role of complement and its receptor in the elimination of immune complexes, *N. Engl. J. Med.,* 315, 488, 1986.
12. Schifferli, J.A., Complement and immune complexes, *Res. Immunol.,* 147, 109, 1996.
13. Smiley, J.D. and Moore, S.E., Immune-complex vasculitis: role of complement and IgG-Fc receptor functions, *Am. J. Med. Sci.,* 298, 267, 1989.
14. Sais, G. et al., Prognostic factors in leukocytoclastic vasculitis: a clinicopathologic study of 160 patients, *Arch. Dermatol.,* 134, 309, 1998.
15. Trejo, O. et al., Cryoglobulinemia: study of etiologic factors and clinical and immunologic features in 443 patients from a single center, *Medicine* (Baltimore), 80, 252, 2001.
16. Guillevin, L. et al., Polyarteritis nodosa related to hepatitis B virus. A prospective study with long-term observation of 41 patients, *Medicine* (Baltimore), 74, 238, 1995.
17. Cochrane, C.G., Mechanisms involved in the deposition of immune complexes in tissues, *J. Exp. Med.*, 134, 75S, 1971.
18. Braverman, I.M. and Yen, A., Demonstration of immune complexes in spontaneous and histamine-induced lesions and in normal skin of patients with leukocytoclastic angiitis, *J. Invest. Dermatol.*, 64, 105, 1975.
19. Clauss, M. et al., A permissive role for TNF in VEGF-induced vascular permeability, *Blood,* 97, 1321, 2001.
20. Saadi, S. and Platt, J.L., Transient perturbation of endothelial integrity induced by natural antibodies and complement, *J. Exp. Med.,* 181, 21, 1995.
21. Groger, M. et al., Dermal microvascular endothelial cells express CD32 receptors *in vivo* and *in vitro, J. Immunol.*, 15, 1549, 1996.
22. Watanabe, N. et al., Mast cells induce autoantibody-mediated vasculitis syndrome through tumor necrosis factor production upon triggering FcR, *Blood,* 94, 3855, 1999.
23. Sunderkötter, C. et al., Different pathophysiological pathways converging on vessel damage in leukocytoclastic vasculitis, *Exp. Dermatol.,* 10, 391, 2001.
24. Ravetch, J.V. and Clynes, R.A., Divergent roles for Fc receptors and complement *in vivo, Annu. Rev. Immunol.*, 16, 421, 1998.
25. Ierino, F.L. et al., Recombinant soluble human Fc gamma RII: production, characterization, and inhibition of the Arthus reaction, *J. Exp. Med.,* 178, 1617, 1993.
26. Köhl, J. and Gessner, E., On the role of complement and Fc gamma-receptors in the Arthus reaction, *Mol. Immunol.,* 36, 893, 1999.
27. Szalai, A.J. et al., The Arthus reaction in rodents: Species-specific requirement of complement, *J. Immunol.,* 164, 463, 2000.
28. Hazenbos, W.L. et al., Impaired IgG-dependent anaphylaxis and Arthus reaction in Fc gamma RIII (CD16) deficient mice, *Immunity*, 5, 181, 1996.
29. Henson, P.M., The immunologic release of constituents from neutrophil leukocytes. II. Mechanisms of release during phagocytosis, and adherence to nonphagocytosable surfaces, *J. Immunol.,* 107, 1547, 1971.
30. Edwards, S.W., *Biochemistry and Physiology of the Neutrophil,* Cambridge University Press, Cambridge, U.K., 1994.
31. Lentsch, A.B. and Ward, P.A., Regulation of inflammatory vascular damage, *J. Pathol.,* 190, 343, 2000.

32. Westlin, W.F. and Gimbrone, M.A., Neutrophil-mediated damage to human vascular endothelium, *Am. J. Pathol.,* 142, 117, 1993.
33. Scholzen, T.E. et al., Alpha-melanocyte stimulating hormone prevents lipopolysaccharide-induced vasculitis by down-regulating endothelial cell adhesion molecule expression, *Endocrinology,* 144, 360, 2003.
34. Radford, D.J. et al., Antineutrophil cytoplasmic antibodies stabilize adhesion and promote migration of flowing neutrophils on endothelial cells, *Arthritis Rheum.*, 44, 2851, 2001.
35. Csernok, E., Anti-neutrophil cytoplasmic antibodies and pathogenesis of small vessel vasculitides, *Autoimmun. Rev.,* 2, 158, 2003.
36. Rarok, A.A., Limburg, P.C., and Kallenberg, C.G., Neutrophil-activating potential of antineutrophil cytoplasm autoantibodies, *J. Leukocyte Biol.*, 74, 3, 2003.
37. Xiao, H. et al., Antineutrophil cytoplasmic autoantibodies specific for myeloperoxidase cause glomerulonephritis and vasculitis in mice, *J. Clin. Invest.*, 110, 955, 2002.
38. Weyand, C.M. and Goronzy, J.J., Medium- and large-vessel vasculitis, *N. Engl. J. Med.,* 349, 160, 2003.
39. Sneller, M.C., Granuloma formation, implications for the pathogenesis of vasculitis, *Cleveland Clin. J. Med.,* 69, SII40, 2002.
40. Krupa, W. M. et al., Trapping of misdirected dendritic cells in the granulomatous lesions of giant cell arteritis, *Am. J. Pathol.,* 161, 1815, 2002.
41. Ludviksson, B.R. et al., Active Wegener's granulomatosis is associated with HLA-DR$^+$ CD4$^+$ T cells exhibiting an unbalanced Th1-type T cell cytokine pattern: reversal with IL-10, *J. Immunol.,* 160, 3602, 1998.
42. Csernok, E. et al., Cytokine profiles in Wegener's granulomatosis: predominance of type 1 (Th1) in the granulomatous inflammation, *Arthritis Rheum.,* 42, 742, 1999.
43. Komocsi, A. et al., Peripheral blood and granuloma CD4(+)CD28(–) T cells are a major source of interferon-gamma and tumor necrosis factor-alpha in Wegener's granulomatosis, *Am. J. Pathol.*, 160, 1717, 2002.
44. Muller, A. et al., Localized Wegener's granulomatosis: predominance of CD26 and IFN-gamma expression, *J. Pathol.,* 192, 113, 2000.
45. Balding, C.E. et al., Th2 dominance in nasal mucosa in patients with Wegener's granulomatosis, *Clin. Exp. Immunol.*, 125, 332, 2001.
46. Jennette, J.C., Implications for pathogenesis of patterns of injury in small- and medium-sized-vessel vasculitis, *Cleveland Clin. J. Med.*, 69, SII33, 2002.
47. Keine, M. et al., Elevated interleukin-4 and interleukin-13 production by T cell lines from patients with Churg-Strauss syndrome, *Arthritis Rheum.*, 44, 469, 2001.
48. Hoffman, G.S. et al., Wegener's granulomatosis: an analysis of 158 patients, *Ann. Intern. Med.,* 116, 488, 1992.
49. Baumgärtel, M.W. et al., Essentielle Kryofibrinogenämie mit generalisierter Livedo reticularis, *Hautarzt,* 45, 243, 1994.
50. Bauza, A., Espana, A. and Idoate, M., Cutaneous polyarteritis nodosa, *Br. J. Dermatol.*, 146, 694, 2002.
51. Levine, S.M. and Hellmann, D.B., Giant cell arteritis, *Curr. Opin. Rheumatol.*, 14, 3, 2002.
52. Monteiro, C. et al., Temporal arteritis presenting with scalp ulceration, *J. Eur. Acad. Dermatol. Venereol.*, 16, 615, 2002.
53. Skaria, A.M. et al., Takayasu arteritis and cutaneous necrotizing vasculitis, *Dermatology,* 200, 139, 2000.
54. Saklayen, M.G. et al., IgA deposition in the skin of patients with alcoholic liver disease, *J. Cutan. Pathol.,* 23, 12, 1996.
55. Fiorentino, D.F., Cutaneous vasculitis, *J. Am. Acad. Dermatol.*, 48, 311, 2003.
56. Lotti, T. et al., Cutaneous small-vessel vasculitis, *J. Am. Acad. Dermatol.,* 39, 667, 1998.
57. Langford, C.A., Management of systemic vasculitis, *Best Pract. Res. Clin. Rheumatol.,* 15, 281, 2001.
58. Jayne, D. et al., European Vasculitis Study Group. a randomized trial of maintenance therapy for vasculitis associated with antineutrophil cytoplasmic autoantibodies, *N. Engl. J. Med.,* 349, 36, 2003.
59. Reinhold-Keller, E. et al., High rate of renal relapse in 71 patients with Wegener's granulomatosis under maintenance of remission with low-dose methotrexate, *Arthritis. Rheum.,* 15, 326, 2002.

60. Nowack, R. et al., Mycophenolate mofetil for maintenance therapy of Wegener's granulomatosis and microscopic polyangiitis: a pilot study in 11 patients with renal involvement, *J. Am. Soc. Nephrol.,* 10, 1965, 1999.
61. Jayne, D.R. et al., Intravenous immunoglobulin for ANCA-associated systemic vasculitis with persistent disease activity, *Q. J. Med.,* 93, 433, 2000.
62. Bacon, P.A. and Carruthers, D., New therapeutic aspects: haemopoietic stem cell transplantation, *Best Pract. Res. Clin. Rheumatol.*, 15, 299, 2001.
63. Langford, C.A. and Sneller, M.C., Biologic therapies in the vasculitides, *Curr. Opin. Rheumatol.,* 15, 3, 2003.
64. Worm, M. et al., Hypocomplementaemic urticarial vasculitis: successful treatment with cyclophosphamide-dexamethasone pulse therapy, *Br. J. Dermatol.,* 139, 704, 1998.
65. Atzori, L., Ferreli, C., and Biggio, P., Less common treatment in cutaneous vasculitis, *Clin. Dermatol.*, 17, 641, 1999.
66. Samlaska, C.P. and Winfield, E.A., Pentoxifylline, *J. Am. Acad. Dermatol.*, 30, 603, 1994.
67. Sunderkötter, C., et al., Influence of steroids, pentoxifylline and cobra venom factor on *in vivo* models with inflammatory vascular damage, *J. Invest. Dermatol.,* 104, 651, 1995 (Abstr.).
68. Katz, S.I., Sulfones, in *Dermatology in General Medicine,* Vol. 2, Fifth, E., Fitzpatrick, T.B., Eisen, A.Z., Wolf, K., Freedberg, I.M., and Austen, K.F., Eds., McGraw-Hill, New York, 1999, chap. 253.
69. Cronstein, B.N. et al., Colchicine alters the quantitative and qualitative display of selectins on endothelial cells and neutrophils, *J. Clin. Invest.,* 96, 994, 1995.
70. Callen, J.P., Colchicine is effective in controlling chronic cutaneous leukocytoclastic vasculitis, *J. Am. Acad. Dermatol.*, 13, 193, 1985.
71. Sais, G. et al., Colchicine in the treatment of cutaneous leukocytoclastic vasculitis. Results of a prospective, randomized controlled trial, *Arch. Dermatol.*, 131, 1399, 1995.
72. Gupta, M.N., Sturrock, R.D., and Gupta, G., Cutaneous leucocytoclastic vasculitis caused by cyclosporin A (Sandimmun), *Ann. Rheum. Dis.,* 59, 319, 2000.

# 28 Urticarial Vasculitis

*Torsten Zuberbier, Norbert Haas, and Beate M. Henz*

## CONTENTS



## I. INTRODUCTION

Urticarial vasculitis is defined as a leukocytoclastic vasculitis presenting with clinical aspects of urticaria. The disease represents a transitional stage between ordinary urticaria and leukocytoclastic vasculitis in association with autoimmune processes.

The incidence of urticarial vasculitis among chronic urticaria patients varies from 2 to 29%.[1–3] Among our own series of 83 patients with chronic urticaria, 10 exhibited the clinical and histological features of urticarial vasculitis. In a subgroup of urticarial vasculitis patients (32%), hypocomplementhemia was present as well.[4] As with other autoimmune diseases, urticarial vasculitis affects preferably young to middle-aged women (range 6 to 68 years).[5]

## II. CLINICAL ASPECTS

As in chronic urticaria, the wheals in patients with urticarial vasculitis are typically generalized in distribution, and individual urticaria lesions are raised, indurated, faintly red or purplish red in color, with an occasional fine, punctate purpura within the lesions (Figure 28.1). Urticarial vasculitis wheals generally persist longer than those in chronic urticaria (up to 72 h) and resolve, leaving at times a mild residual hyperpigmentation or more often purpuric patches. Most patients experience pruritus at the sites of the lesions, but some also complain of a burning sensation.[5]

In addition to wheals, other types of skin lesions can coexist in urticarial vasculitis, such as angioedema (in 42%), macular erythemas, target lesions typical for erythema multiforme, or livedo reticularis lesions.[5] Furthermore, other organs may be involved, as summarized in Table 28.1. The clinical course of urticarial vasculitis is generally benign, with resolution of the disease within 1 year in 30 to 40% of patients. The situation changes when full-blown systemic lupus erythematosus (SLE) develops (Table 28.2).

Features of leukocytoclastic vasculitis can occasionally also be found in acute urticaria and in lesions of cold and delayed pressure urticaria.[5] Furthermore, they can be present in Muckle–Wells syndrome and are a major feature of Schnitzler's syndrome, which is characterized in addition by a monoclonal gammopathy (IgM, usually kappa light chain isotype), fever, arthralgias, weight loss, and bone pain in the absence of lymphoproliferative disease.[6–9] One case of Cogan's syndrome, characterized by bouts of acute keratitis and vestibuloauditory dysfunction, has also been described

0-8493-1959-5/05/$0.00+$1.50

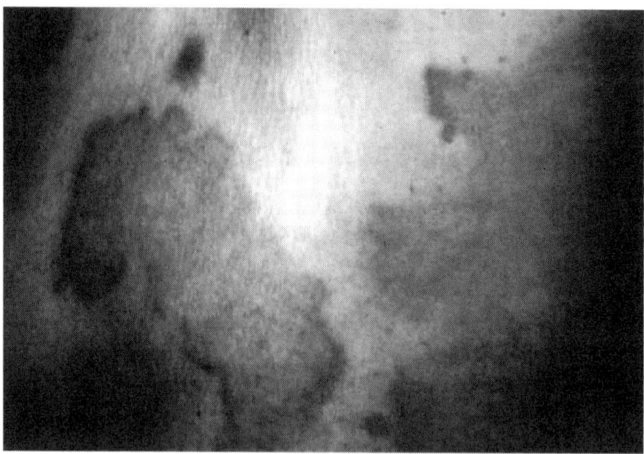

**FIGURE 28.1** Clinical aspect of urticarial whealing, with an elevated erythematous margin.

**TABLE 28.1**
**Clinical Symptoms of the Urticarial Vasculitis Syndrome**

| Organ | Frequency of Involvement | Clinical Manifestations |
|---|---|---|
| Skin | 100% | Pruritic or burning wheals (lasting >24 h), angioedema, bullae, erythema multiforme, livedo reticularis, Raynaud's phenomenon, purpura |
| Joints | 75% | Arthralgias, swelling, stiffness, arthritis of single or multiple joints |
| Kidneys | 60% | Hematuria, proteinuria, decreased creatinine clearance |
| Respiratory system | 55% | Chronic obstructive pulmonary disease, pleuritic chest pain, laryngeal edema |
| Eyes | 35% | Uveitis, episcleritis, conjunctivitis, loss of vision |
| Gastrointestinal tract | 30% | Nausea, vomiting, diarrhea, abdominal pain |
| Nervous system | 12% | Mononeuritis, myositis, seizures, pseudotumor cerebri, increased central nervous system pressure |
| Cardiovascular and hematological systems | 5% | Raynaud's syndrome, carditis, lymphadenopathy, leukopenia, thrombocytopenia, shock, anemia |
| General systemic | 10% | Fever |

*Source:* Based on data from References 5 and 11.

to present with urticarial vasculitis. This patient's disease was thought to have been caused by *Chlamydia trachomatis*.[10]

There are a number of other systemic diseases potentially associated with urticarial vasculitis, including serum sickness, SLE, Still's disease, Sjögren's syndrome, bacterial (Lyme disease), or viral (hepatitis B, mononucleosis) infections, neoplasms, food allergy, and drug reactions.[5,11,12–14] The associated clinical and laboratory changes range from features of ordinary urticaria to SLE.[3,11,15–22]

## III. HISTOPATHOLOGY AND LABORATORY CHANGES

The various histological and laboratory findings in urticarial vasculitis are summarized in Table 28.3. The most important diagnostic feature in histological sections is damage to walls of the small superficial venules, evidenced by endothelial swelling or obliteration of the vessel lumen, fibrinoid changes within the vessel walls, and extravasation of erythrocytes into the dermis (Figure 28.2).[1,5,11]

**TABLE 28.2**
**Clinical Signs of Urticarial Vasculitis, Ranging from Chronic Urticaria to Florid SLE**

| | Clinical Signs | Diagnosis |
|---|---|---|
| 1. | Idiopathic chronic urticaria, vessel damage, wheals lasting >24 h | Chronic urticaria |
| 2. | Leukocytoclastic vasculitis on histology | |
| 3. | Purpuric or erythema multiforme-like lesions | |
| 4. | Clinical signs of multisystem disease (see Table 28.1) | Urticarial |
| 5. | ESR, circulating immune complexes, positive direct immunofluorescence, Ø serum complement (see Table 28.3) | Vasculitis syndrome |
| 6. | Resistance to therapy with antihistamines | |
| 7. | Serologic evidence of connective tissue disease (+ double-stranded ANF; + lupus band on immunofluorescence) | SLE |

*Source:* Based on data from Reference 5.

**TABLE 28.3**
**Laboratory Changes in Patients with Urticarial Vasculitis (frequency is shown in parenthesis, if known)**

| | |
|---|---|
| Histopathology | Fibrinoid changes in vessel walls (88%) |
| | Tissue eosinophilia (63%) |
| | Leukocytoclastic vasculitis (61%) |
| | Erythrocyte extravasation (58%) |
| | Neutrophilic infiltration (58%) |
| | Edema of upper dermis (44%) |
| Immunopathology (direct IF) | Deposits of (a) IgM, IgG, IgA or (b) Clq, C4, C3 or (c) fibrinogen in vessel walls and at the dermoepidermal junction, 89% of specimens |
| Changes in peripheral blood | ESR (75%) |
| | CH50 (35%), Clq, C4, C3 (32%), C5 |
| | Circulating immune complexes, normal or decreased immunoglobulins, rarely positive: ANF, R, cryoglobulins, bacterial or viral antigens; rarely: leukopenia, thrombocytopenia |
| Autoantibodies against | Clq |
| | IL-1 |
| | IgE |
| | FcεRI |
| | Thyroid microsomal antigens |

*Abbreviations:* ESR, erythrocyte sedimentation rate; ANF, antinuclear factor; RF, rheumatoid factor; IF, immunofluorescence.

*Source:* Based on data in References 5 and 11.

Deposits of fibrinoid material in and around the vessel walls can be detected in most cases (Table 28.3). Evidence of leukocytoclasia and neutrophilic as well as eosinophilic infiltration is mostly present as well (Table 28.3). Edema of the upper dermis can be detected in about half of the sections. In less than 10% of sections, predominantly mononuclear cell infiltrates are seen, and in 30 to 40% these cells are admixed with neutrophils. These latter sections probably represent lesions that have persisted for a longer time period.[5]

On direct immunofluorescence, deposits of immunoglobulins, complement fragments, and fibrinogen can be detected in the majority of cases (Table 28.3).[14–19,21] Changes in laboratory findings

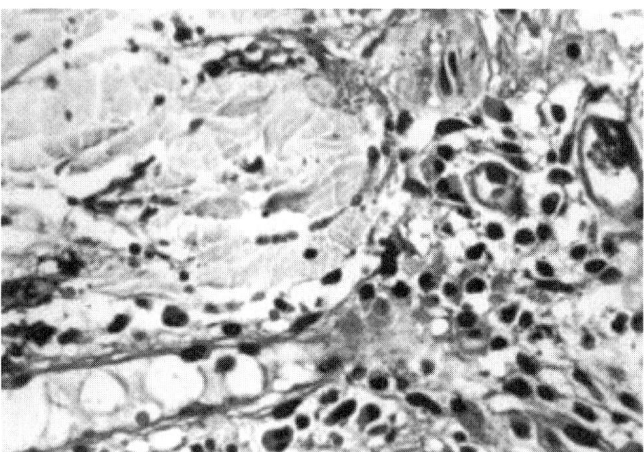

**FIGURE 28.2** Histopathology of urticarial vasculitis lesion, with necrosis of the upper dermis and leukocytoclastic features such as fibrinoid changes in vessel walls and perivascular tissue, eosinophilia, erythrocyte extravasation, neutrophilic infiltration, and nuclear dust (HE; original magnification × 400).

are noted in up to 75% of the patients, as summarized in Table 28.3. A variety of autoantibodies and bacterial or viral antigens have been described in individual cases (see above).

## IV. PATHOGENESIS

Vasculitis is a reaction pattern of the cutaneous vasculature caused by a wide variety of substances. Therefore, more than one pathogenetic mechanism is involved. There are a number of indications that immune complexes are invariably present during the induction phase of urticarial vasculitis. They are not always measurable, possibly because even in experimental immune complex disease, complexes are no longer detectable in the serum 2 and 18 h after their injection.[24,25] Variability in the severity of disease may be another reason; Pussell et al.[26] have noted a correlation between disease severity and detection and level of immune complexes.

The nature of the involved immune complexes is unknown so far. Autoantibodies to IgE, the high-affinity IgE receptor, thyroid microsomal antigens, C1q, interleukin-1 (IL-1), antinuclear factor, and antibodies to bacterial or food antigens are possible components (see above and Table 28.3).

Table 28.4 depicts the possible pathogenetic events that lead to immune complex vasculitis. Immune complexes stimulate various formed elements of the blood and the tissue, inducing secretion of histamine, serotonin, platelet-activating factor (PAF), prostaglandins, leukotrienes, other eicosanoids (HETEs), cytokines like tumor necrosis factor (TNF-α), and reactive oxygen species. Many of these mediators cause vasodilatation, increased vascular permeability, endothelial cell damage, the deposition of circulating immune complexes within the walls of the capillary venules, chemotaxis, and mediator secretion by various cell types.[5,27,28] Immune complexes also activate complement and cause the generation of vasoactive and leukotactic complement fragments, like C3a and C5a. Fluid- and cell-derived leukotactic factors in the blood induce integrin expression on leukocytes and adhesion molecules on endothelial cell, allowing for the emigration of leukocytes into the perivascular tissue. Thus, immune complexes initiate a complex sequence of events that results in the clinical and histopathological features seen in urticarial vasculitis, with endothelial damage by mediators and cellular components the key events. Induction of edema by mediator release from mast cells via immune complexes or complement fragments must be the major distinctive feature in this process, compared to ordinary leukocytoclastic vasculitis. While the pathogenetic features fit most closely with an Arthus-type vasculitis,[28] other underlying pathogenetic factors must be considered as well. Because the immune complexes have no pathological effects

**TABLE 28.4**
**Cells and Mediators Potentially Involved in the Immune Complex–Mediated Events within Vessels and in the Perivascular Location in Urticarial Vasculitis**

| A: Intravascular Immune Complexes | | B: Perivascular Immune Complexes | |
|---|---|---|---|
| Cells | Mediators | Cells | Mediators |
| Basophils | Histamine | Mast cells | Histamine |
| Platelets | PAF | Neutrophils | PAF |
| Neutrophils | Leukotrienes | Eosinophils | Prostaglandins |
| Monocytes | HETEs | Monocytes | Leukotrienes |
| | Serotonin | | HETEs |
| | Prostaglandins | | Proteases |
| | Cytokines | | Cytokines |
| | Proteases | | MBP, EDN |
| | Oxygen species | | Oxygen species |
| | C3a | | C3a |
| | C5a | | C5a |

*Abbreviations:* PAF, platelet-activating factor; HETE, hydroxyeicosatretraenoic acid; MBP, major basic protein; EDN, eosinophil-derived neurotoxin.

in normal circumstances, specific components of these complexes like their histamine-releasing properties might play a role. In addition, alterations of mast cell releasability may be involved. It has been shown that, e.g., increases in the ganglioside contents of the mast cell membrane enhances IgE -mediated mast cell mediator release.[29]

For the extreme aspect of urticarial vasculitis, namely, SLE, genetic factors and the sex of the individual may also play pathogenetic roles.[5] The same holds for intrinsic genetic defects of the complement system.[19]

Autoantibodies against the high-affinity IgE receptor, which have been observed in chronic urticaria, have also been described in urticarial vasculitis.[30] They probably have no pathophysiological relevance since IgE-dependent histamine release, which can cause ordinary wheals, is not a major cause for the evolution of wheals in urticarial vasculitis.

## V. TREATMENT

As histamine constitutes only one of the various pathogenetic components in urticarial vasculitis, most patients do not experience satisfactory relief from treatment with H1-receptor blockade.[5,11] Instead, systemically applied corticosteroids are effective in almost all cases,[11,31] but due to their side effects should not be chosen in the first place. Other possibilities are nonsteroidal anti-inflammatory drugs, antimalarials, cytostatic drugs like azathioprin or cyclophosphamide, and in occasional patients also colchicine.[11,32] We have recently reported on the excellent control of treatment-resistant urticarial vasculitis to interferon-alpha (IFN-$\alpha$), but not IFN-$\gamma$ in a patient with a lymphoproliferative disease,[33] and almost all of our patients respond to dapsone alone or in combination with pentoxiphyllin, a TNF-$\alpha$ antagonist.[34] Since the first edition of this chapter in 1997 only a few novel suggestions for treatment have been published. These include the successful use of mycophenolate mofetil[35] and the use of cyclophosphamide-dexamethasone pulse therapy.[36] Both treatments are based only on case reports and randomized double-blind controlled studies in the field of urticarial vasculitis are needed. However, these therapeutic observations fit overall with the proposed pathogenetic events in the disease, with specific mediators and immunological vs. inflammatory events predominating in individual patients.

## REFERENCES

1. Monroe, E.W., Schulz, C.I., Maize, J.C., and Jordon, R.E., Vasculitis in chronic urticaria: an immunopathologic study, *J. Invest. Dermatol.*, 76, 103, 1981.
2. Natbony, S.E., Phillips, M.E., Elias, J.M., Godfrey, H.P., and Kaplan, A.P., Histologic studies of chronic idiopathic uticaria, *J. Allergy Clin. Immunol.*, 71, 177, 1983.
3. Small, P., Barrett, D., and Champlin, E., Chronic urticaria and vasculitis, *Ann. Allergy,* 48, 172, 1982.
4. Jones, R.R., Bhogal, B., Dash, A., and Schifferli, J., Urticaria and vasculitis: a continuum of histological and immunopathological changes, *Br. J. Dermatol.*, 108, 695, 1983.
5. Czarnetzki, B.M., *Urticaria,* Springer, Berlin, 1986, chap. 8.
6. Schnitzler, L., Schubert, B., Boasson, M. et al., Urticaire chronique: lesions osseuses, macroglobulinemie IgM: maladie de Waldenström? *Bull. Soc. Fr. Dermatol. Syphiligr.*, 81, 363, 1974.
7. Saurat, J.H., Fournier, C., and Didierjean, L., Schnitzler's syndrome (urticaria and macroglobulinemia). Immunoreactivity of the IgM against interleukin 1 as shown by Western blot, *Dermatologica,* 177, 259, 1988.
8. Borradori, L., Rybojad, M., Puissant, A., Dallot, A., Verola, O., and Morel, P., Urticarial vasculitis associated with a monoclonal IgM gammopathy: Schnitzler's syndrome, *Br. J. Dermatol.*, 123, 113, 1990.
9. Janier, M., Bonvalet, D., Blanc, M.-F., Lemarchand, F., Cavelier, B., Ribrioux, A., Aguenier, B., and Cavatte, J., Chronic urticaria and macroglobulinemia (Schnitzler's syndrome): report of two cases, *J. Am. Acad. Dermatol.*, 20, 206, 1989.
10. Ochonisky, S., Chosidow, O., Kuentz, M., Man, N., Fraitag, S., Pelisse, J.M., and Revuz, J., Cogan's syndrome. An unusual etiology of urticarial vasculitis, *Dermatologica,* 183, 218, 1991.
11. Mehregan, D.R., Hall, M.J., and Gibson, L.E., Urticarial vasculities: a histopathologic and clinical review of 72 cases, *J. Am. Acad. Dermatol.*, 26, 441, 1992.
12. Lewis, J.E., Urticarial vasculitis occurring in association with visceral malignancy, *Acta Derm. Venereol.* (Stockholm), 70, 345, 1984.
13. Epstein, M.M., Watsky, K.L., and Lanzi, R.A., The role of diet in the treatment of a patient with urticaria and urticarial vasculitis, *J. Allergy Clin. Immunol.*, 90, 414, 1992.
14. Olson, J.C. and Esterly, N.B., Urticarial vasculitis and Lyme disease, *J. Am. Acad. Dermatol.*, 22, 1114, 1990.
15. Wisnieski, J.J. and Jones, S.M., Comparison of autoantibodies to the collagen-like region of Clq in hypocomplementemic urticarial vasculitis syndrome and systemic lupus erythematosus, *J. Immunol.*, 148, 1396, 1992.
16. Grattan, C.E.H., Francis, D.M., Hide, M., and Greaves, W.M., Detection of circulating histamine releasing autoantibodies with functional properties of anti-EgE in chronic urticaria, *Clin. Exp. Allergy,* 21, 695, 1991.
17. Gruber, B.L., Baeza, M.L., Marchese, M.J., Agnello, V., and Kaplan, A.P., Prevalence and functional role of anti-IgE autoantibodies in urticarial syndromes, *J. Invest. Dermatol.*, 90, 213, 1988.
18. Leznoff, A. and Sussman, G.L., Syndrome of idiopathic chronic urticaria and angioedema with thyroid autoimmunity: a study of 90 patients, *J. Allergy Clin. Immunol.*, 84, 66, 1989.
19. Agnello, W., Ruddy, S., Winchester, R.J., Christian, C.L., and Kunkel, H.G., Hereditary C2 deficiency in systemic lupus erythematosus and acquired complement abnormalities in an unusual SLE-related syndrome, *Birth Defects,* 2, 312, 1975.
20. Ballow, M., Ward, C.W., Jr., Geshwin, M.E., and Day, N.K., C1-bypass complement activation pathway in patients with chronic urticaria and angioedema, *Lancet,* 2, 248, 1975.
21. McLean, R.H., Weinstein, A., Chapitis, J., Lowenstein, M., and Rothfield, N.F., Familial partial deficiency of the third component of complement (3) and the hypocomplementaemic cutaneous vasculitis syndrome, *Am. J. Med.*, 68, 549, 1980.

22. Hide, M., Francis, D.M., Grattan, C.E.H., Hakimi, J., Kochan, J.P., and Greaves, M.W., Autoantibodies against the high-affinity IgE receptor as a cause of histamine release in chronic urticaria, *N. Engl. J. Med.,* 328, 1599, 1993.
23. Braverman, I.M. and Yen, A., Demonstration of immune complexes in spontaneous and histamine-induced lesions and in normal skin of patients with leukocytoclastic angiitis, *J. Invest. Dermatol.,* 64, 105, 1975.
24. Cream, J.J., Bryceson, A.D.M., and Ryder, G., Disappearance of immunoglobulin and complement from the Arthus reaction and its relevance to studies of vasculitis in man, *Br. J. Dermatol.,* 84, 106, 1971.
25. De Shazo, C.V., Henson, P.M., and Cochrane, C.G., Acute immunologic arthritis in rabbits, *J. Clin. Invest.,* 51, 50, 1972.
26. Pussell, B.A., Lockwood, C.M., Scott, C.M., Pinching, A.J., and Peters, D.K., Value of immune complex assay in diagnosis and management, *Lancet,* 2, 359, 1978.
27. Warren, J.S., Mandel, D.M., Johnson, K.J., and Ward, P.A., Evidence for the role of platelet-activating factor in immune complex vasculitis in the rat, *J. Clin. Invest.,* 83, 669, 1989.
28. Crawford, J.P., Movat, H.Z., Ranadive, N.S., and Hay, J.B., Pathways to inflammation induced by immune complexes: development of the Arthus reaction, *Fed. Proc.,* 41, 2583, 1982.
29. Zuberbier, T., Pfrommer, C., Beinhölzl, J., Hartmann, K., Ricklinkat, J., and Czarnetzki, B.M., Gangliosides enhance IgE receptor-dependent histamine and LTC4 release from human mast cells, *Biochem. Biophys. Acta,* 1269, 79, 1995.
30. Zuberbier, T., Fiebiger, E., Maurer, D., Stingl, G., and Henz, B.M., Anti-FcεRIα serum autoantibodies in different subtypes of urticaria, *Allergy,* 55, 951, 2000.
31. Goupille, P., Pizzuti, P., Diot, E., Jattiot, F., Guilmot, J.-L., and Valat, J.-P., Schnitzler's syndrome (urticaria and macroglobuliemia) dramatically improved with corticosteroids, *Clin. Exp. Rheumatol.,* 13, 95, 1995.
32. Werni, R., Schwarz, T., and Gschnait, F., Colchicine treatment of urticarial vasculitis, *Dermatologica,* 172, 36, 1986.
33. Czarnetzki, B.M., Algermissen, B., Jeep, S., Haas, N., Nürnberg, W., Müller, K., and Kropp, J.-D., Interferon treatment of patients with chronic urticaria and mastocytosis, *J. Am. Acad. Dermatol.,* 30, 500, 1994.
34. Nürnberg, W., Grabbe, J., and Czarnetzki, B.M., Urticarial vasculitis syndrome effectively treated with dapsone and pentoxifyllin, *Acta Derm. Venereol.* (Stockholm), 75, 43, 1995.
35. Worm, M., Sterry, W., and Kolde, G., Mycophenolate mofetil is effective for maintenance therapy of hypocomplementaeic urticarial vasculitis, *Br. J. Dermatol.,* 143, 1324, 2000.
36. Worm, M., Muche, M., Schulze, P., Sterry, W., and Kolde, G., Hypocomplementaric urticarial vasculitis: successful treatment with cyclophosphamide-dexamethasone pulse therapy, *Br. J. Dermatol.,* 139, 704, 1998.

# 29 Immunological Mechanisms of Cutaneous Adverse Drug Reactions

*Ewa Guigné, Jean Revuz, and Jean-Claude Roujeau*

## CONTENTS



## I. INTRODUCTION

Cutaneous adverse drug reactions (ADRs) manifest themselves in a variety of clinical diseases, and the exact pathomechanisms of most of them remain rather unclear. Many kinds of cutaneous ADRs are definitely not immunologically mediated, including phototoxic reactions, hyperpigmentation, anticoagulant skin necrosis, toxicity toward hairs or skin from anticancer drugs (and many others), antiretroviral agent–related lipodystrophy, effects on skin and appendages of corticosteroids and hormones. In recent years, however, increasing evidence has indicated that most acute drug eruptions are probably of immunological origin. Especially, histological and immunohistological studies of skin lesions and the analysis of drug-specific T-cell lines and clones assess that drug-specific T cells

0-8493-1959-5/05/$0.00+$1.50

are a key factor in most reactions and that their functional capacity, including cytokine production and cytotoxic function, plays an important role in many distinct forms of drug allergy.[1–7] It remains to be explicated why the skin is the principal target of adverse reactions to medications of systemic administration and what are the determinants of the clinical diversity of these reactions.

## II. GENERAL IMMUNOLOGICAL MECHANISM OF CUTANEOUS ADR

### A. How Drugs Are Recognized by the Immune System: The Reactive Metabolites Dogma

#### 1. The Hapten Theory

Most drugs are small chemical molecules that need to bind to larger molecules to be recognized by the immune system, according to the classical hapten theory. The binding can occur to many different molecules such as soluble proteins, cell-bound proteins (membrane receptors and adhesions molecules), and major histocompatibility complex (MHC) molecules. Some drugs, such as β-lactam antibiotics, are chemically active and able to covalently bind as haptens to proteins. These hapten–protein structures can then be recognized by the immune system, especially by immunoglobulins and by T cells after intracellular processing and MHC presentation.

#### 2. The Reactive Metabolite Hypothesis

Most medications are nonreactive in their native form. It has been believed for years that these so-called pro-haptens had first to be metabolized to an active reactive compound, which may then bind to a protein and behave as the hapten leading to drug recognition.[4,8,9] This "reactive metabolite hypothesis" provided the rationale for extensive investigation of alterations in the enzymes directing the detoxification of drugs, as a possible source of increased production of reactive compounds leading to a higher risk of reaction.[10] The best-known example is that of sulfamethoxazole and other sulfonamides. Slow acetylation of sulfonamides could lead to a relative increase in the oxidative pathway via cytochrome P4502C9, resulting in higher production of hydroxylamine and nitroso metabolites. It was proposed that patients suffering from hypersensitivity reactions to sulfonamides in addition to being slow acetylators had also some alteration in detoxification of reactive metabolites due to glutathion deficiency and/or genetic or acquired dysfunction of glutathion transferase. A need for combining alterations of several enzymes could explain the rarity of severe reactions. This metabolic track has been especially explored to explain the high frequency of reaction to sulfonamides in HIV-infected patients. After several publications pointing to an increased prevalence of slow acetylation phenotypes among patients with AIDS who had skin rashes to sulfonamides, several large prospective studies did not find any difference in acetylation, glutathion, and glutathion transferase among patients with HIV, who reacted or tolerated sulfonamides.[11,12]

#### 3. Recent Advances in Noncovalent Binding of Drugs to MHC Molecules

Sulfonamide reactive metabolites were shown to be strong immunogens in rats but in humans, with the notable exception of drug-induced hepatitis, there is little evidence that reactive metabolites are the primary antigen in drug reactions.[11–13]

On the contrary, more than 90% of the drug-specific T-cell clones derived from the blood lymphocytes of patients who experienced a drug reaction to sulfonamides reacted only to sulfamethoxazole and not to oxidative metabolites. It was also demonstrated that several "nonreactive drugs" such as the parent form of sulfamethoxazole, lidocaine, carbamazepine were able to bind in a noncovalent way to MHC molecules on the surface of antigen-presenting cells inducing T-cell reaction.[14] Effector cytotoxic cells were also shown to be specific of native sulfamethoxazole.[15]

Taken together, these recent data suggest that the native form of medications rather than reactive metabolites are the primary antigens in humans after direct noncovalent binding to MHC molecules.

### 4. The Danger Hypothesis

The reactive metabolite hypothesis has gained new interest anyhow with the "danger signals" theory.[16,17,18] This postulates that several mediators of inflammation resulting from any cell injury enhance the immune response. These mediators, including CD40-ligand, interferon-alpha (IFN-$\alpha$), tumor necrosis factor-alpha (TNF-$\alpha$), interleukin-1-beta (IL-1$\beta$), and heat-shock proteins can activate dendritic cells and upregulate their expression of co-stimulatory molecules, thus permitting a full response to antigens presented in this context. Conversely in the absence of inflammation, antigen presentation without co-stimulation could lead to unresponsiveness and tolerance. The endogenous danger signals are produced by stressed cells and by cells killed by necrosis. Reactive metabolites of many medications can actually cause necrotic cell death. According to this danger hypothesis, patients with increased production or impaired detoxification of reactive metabolites of medications would develop a stronger reaction, whether the antigen is the reactive metabolite itself or the inert parent drug. This could explain in part why drug administered for an acute infectious disease may be more prone to induce an adverse reaction than drugs used for chronic non-inflammatory conditions. The "danger signal" theory could also help to understand why some viral diseases, especially Epstein Barr virus (EBV), human herpes virus 6 (HHV6), and human immunodeficiency virus (HIV) infection, can lead to an increased rate of adverse reactions to antibiotics or sulfonamides.[19,20] In any case, this appealing theory is still lacking good experimental evidence and is far from being universally accepted.[21]

## B. Immunological Reaction to Drugs via Specific T Cells

### 1. Indirect Suggestions of Immune Mediation in Cutaneous ADRs

Accumulated clinical information indirectly suggested an immune mediation of cutaneous ADRs. The shortened latency period in the cases of drug rechallenge cannot be explained by toxicity but, rather, indicated immunological memory. Many case reports pointed to positive patch tests and lymphocyte transformation tests with the culprit drugs.[22] Associations with some human leukocyte antigens (HLA) phenotypes and an increased incidence of drug reactions in patients suffering from collagen diseases, especially systemic lupus, were also reported.[14]

### 2. Immunohistological Features of Cutaneous Lesions in ADRs

Immunohistological examination of the skin lesions of drug eruptions shows mild to important infiltrate of $CD4^+$ and $CD8^+$ T cells, the presence of apoptotic keratinocytes, and a variable amount of eosinophils and polymorphonuclears. In the most frequent "maculopapular" drug eruptions the infiltrate is so mild and there are so few apoptotic keratinocytes that it is often difficult to distinguish lesional from normal skin. In Stevens–Johnson syndrome and toxic epidermal necrolysis the massive apoptosis of epidermal cells contrast with a mild lymphocytic infiltrate.[23] The importance of the mononuclear cells infiltrate is a characteristic of the so-called hypersensitivity syndrome/drug reaction with eosinophilia and systemic symptoms (DRESS).[24] Infiltration of the epidermis by neutrophiles leading to subcorneal pustules is the hallmark of pustular drug eruptions/acute generalized exanthematous pustulosis (AGEP).[25]

In all instances the mononuclear cell infiltrate is mainly composed of T cells. $CD4^+$ lymphocytes predominate in the perivascular dermis, $CD8^+$ T cells predominate within the epidermis, when both $CD4^+$ and $CD8^+$ T cells in similar number are found at the dermoepidermal junction.[26] These T cells, particularly at the dermoepidermal junction, express markers of activation: CD25 (IL-2 receptor) and HLA-DR.[27] They also express adhesion molecules like CD11a-CD18 (leukocyte function-related antigen-1/LFA-1) and CD62-L (L-selectin).[28,29] Both $CD4^+$ and $CD8^+$ cells in dermal infiltrate have cytotoxic potential. The probable pathway leading to keratinocyte damage is a T-cell cytotoxicity via cytotoxic granule proteins: perforin and granzyme B.[30–33] Perforin and granzyme B positive cells are frequently located at the dermoepidermal junction zone and in the epidermis along with signs of keratinocyte damage.

Immunochemistry also evidenced activation of endothelial cells within the capillary of superficial dermis. Endothelial cells strongly express adhesion molecules, such as CD62E (E-selectin), CD62P (P-selectin), CD31 (platelet endothelial cell adhesion molecule-1), and CD54 (intercellular adhesion molecule-1), particularly at the sites of lymphocytic infiltration into the epidermis.[26]

Keratinocytes also are activated at the site of early lesions, as evidenced by the overexpression of MHC class I molecules, the expression of CD54/ICAM1 and of HLA-DR.[28]

### 3. Experimental Evidence of Immune Mediation in Cutaneous ADRs

Experimental data also supported the role of T cells in drug reactions. As an example, delayed-type hypersensitivity could be evoked in guinea pigs[34] and in mice[35] by repeated injections of β-lactam antibiotics emulsified with Freund's complete adjuvant. The passive transfer of splenocytes from primed animals into naive recipients transmitted the reactivity. Moreover, the reaction was diminished or abolished by the addition of anti-T-cell monoclonal antibody, indicating T-lymphocyte dependence of the drug reactivity in animals. In the same experiments, antibodies were detected in only 1 of 15 guinea pigs and the transfer of serum did not elicit any reaction to β-lactam in naive recipients.[34]

More recently, drug-specific human T-cell lines and T-cell clones were obtained after *in vitro* stimulation of peripheral blood lymphocytes (PBL) from patients who had experienced a drug reaction and had a positive "lymphocyte transformation test" to these drugs. Specific clones were obtained toward a variety of drugs including β-lactam antibiotics, lidocaine, sulfamethoxazole, phenytoin, carbamazepine, phenobarbital, lamotrigine.[36–40] These results not only definitely proved that drugs could be immunogenic in humans, but also provided many insights on how T cells recognize drugs. One of the most original findings was that the native form of "nonreactive" drugs could be recognized by T cells after noncovalently binding on MHC molecules of antigen-presenting cells. In contrast to classical T-dependent antigens, drugs were able to directly bind to MHC molecules expressed on the cell membrane of antigen-presenting cells, without need for prior internalization and processing. Most clones were highly drug specific, i.e., nonreactive with other drugs, but also nonreactive with metabolites of the parent drug. Drug recognition was usually MHC restricted but up to 25% of clones were also activated when the drug was presented by allogeneic antigen-presenting cells expressing different MHC.

For each drug, heterogeneous clones have been obtained, even from an individual patient. A majority was of CD4 lineage and MHC class II restricted. CD4 clones usually produced Th2 cytokines, including IL-5,[36,41–44] when CD8 clones most often produced Th1 cytokines and mainly IFN-γ.[37,38] Drug-specific reactive lymphocytes were detected at a very low frequency in the blood of patients with drug eruptions, explaining why the lymphocyte transformation test was generally unreliable as a diagnosis test, with a high rate of false negative results.[45]

T cells considered as the effectors of the skin lesions were also isolated from positive patch tests to drugs (pustular and maculopapular eruption), and less frequently directly from the original lesions in a few cases of blistering eruptions,[6] fixed drug eruption,[28] and toxic epidermal necrolysis.[15] In blistering eruptions these cells were always $CD8^+$, expressed activation markers, produced IFN-γ, and were cytotoxic toward autologous B cells or keratinocytes in a MHC-restricted fashion.

In the cases of maculopapular eruptions it has been proposed that effector cells could be drug-specific cytotoxic CD4 cells.[30]

## C. Why Drug Allergy Manifests Itself in the Skin

The mechanism of the preferential expression of drug allergy in the skin is rather unknown. Keratinocytes have the whole enzyme equipment needed to metabolize drugs. Coming back to the example of sulfonamides, epidermal cells were shown to produce both acetylated nonreactive metabolites and oxidated reactive metabolites.[46] This was proposed as an explanation for cutaneous ADRs. It was suggested that keratinocytes activated by reactive metabolites could either activate epidermal dendritic cells (by producing danger signals) or become capable of presenting antigens themselves through the expression of MHC class II antigens. This explanation does not sound highly plausible in any case, considering that the amount of reactive metabolites of sulfamethoxazole produced by keratinocytes is about $10^3$ lower than the amount produced by hepatocytes.[46]

The increase of the T-cell percentage expressing skin-homing receptors, such as the cutaneous lymphocyte-associated antigen (CLA), during acute cutaneous allergy may explain, at least in part, why the reaction predominates in the skin.[29] It remains to be understood why T lymphocytes express CLA. It was also proposed that skin resident lymphocytes might play a key role. Some evidence supporting this hypothesis has been provided for fixed drug eruption,[47] a very original kind of reaction, but not yet for other types.

## III. PECULIAR CHARACTERISTICS OF SPECIFIC CUTANEOUS DRUG ADVERSE REACTIONS

### A. Urticaria and Angioedema

Urticaria and angioedema are due either to immediate IgE-mediated specific activation (anaphylactic) or to direct nonspecific activation of a cascade of inflammatory mediators (anaphylactoid). The most frequent inducers of anaphylactic reactions are: foreign proteins, penicillins, erythromycin, carbamazepine, and some general anesthetics. Hyperosmolar contrast media, salicylates, nonsteroidal anti-inflammatory drugs, angiotensin-converting enzyme inhibitors, and angiotensin II receptor inhibitors are the most frequent causes of anaphylactoid reactions. The mechanisms of anaphylactic reaction are well deciphered. The culprit drug binds to a serum protein if small or acts as complete antigen if large. Drug–protein complex is recognized by IgE antibodies, produced by B cells. When cross-linked by antigen, specific IgE bound to mast cells or basophils induce degranulation and release of large quantities of inflammation mediators: histamine, leukotrienes B and D, prostaglandin $D_2$, platelet-activating factor; proteolytic enzymes.[48,49] Inflammation mediators release causes vasodilatation and blood pressure drops, resulting in the rapid onset of anaphylaxis.

### B. Drug-Induced Maculopapular Eruption

Maculopapular eruption is the most frequent pattern of skin reaction to drugs. Many medications including β-lactam antibiotics, anti-infectious sulfonamides, anticonvulsants, allopurinol, induce such benign eruptions in more than 3% of users.[1–3]

Both $CD4^+$ and $CD8^+$ cells in dermal infiltrate have cytotoxic potential as demonstrated by the presence of cytotoxic granule protein: perforin and granzyme B. In addition, eosinophils may contribute to tissue damage by the release of various toxic granule proteins such as eosinophilic cationic protein. Drug-specific T cells may also orchestrate skin inflammation through the release of type 1 and 2 cytokines as IFN-γ, IL-5, eotaxine, and RANTES, which induce the recruitment and activation of eosinophils, IL-6, IL-1β, TNF-α and to lesser degree of monocyte chemotactic protein (MCP)-3.[27,50–52]

### C. Toxic Epidermal Necrolysis and Stevens–Johnson Syndrome

Toxic epidermal necrolysis (TEN) and Stevens–Johnson syndrome (SJS) are severe, acute, life-threatening diseases characterized by extensive skin detachment and erosions of the mucous membranes. Sulfonamides, anticonvulsants, allopurinol, nevirapine, oxicam, nonsteroidal anti-inflammatory drugs are the major causes of TEN and SJS. The histology shows a widespread apoptosis of epidermal cells with few mononuclear cells in the dermis. These are CD8$^+$ T cells, present in the epidermis, at the dermoepidermal junction, and also in the fluid of the blisters.[53–23] Phenotypic analysis of the blister fluid CD8$^+$ T cells reveals a phenotype of memory T cells expressing TCR-αβ. These T cells were shown to exhibit an MHC class I restricted drug-specific cytotoxicity against autologous cells, including keratinocytes (References 15, 31, and unpublished data).

In addition to the direct killing of epidermal cells by CTL, it had been proposed that the overexpression of Fas/CD95 and its ligand by activated keratinocytes could disseminate the apoptotic process[32] T-cell cytotoxicity against keratinocytes was shown to be mediated by perforin/granzyme-B pathway in any case. In addition, keratinocytes are rather resistant to Fas/CD95-mediated apoptosis[33] and most clinical attempts to block the progression of TEN by using the fas-blocking properties of high-dose human immunoglobulins were disappointing.

## D. Hypersensitivity Syndrome or Drug Reaction with Eosinophilia and Systemic Symptoms

DRESS is a severe systemic disease characterized by fever, lymph node swelling, hepatitis, and exanthema. A peculiar feature of this syndrome is its rather long-lasting clinical courses. Anticonvulsants, minocycline, dapsone, allopurinol, and anti-infectious sulfonamides are the most common culprit drugs.[24] The pathogenesis of this disease is not yet clarified. Frequently, patients have an expansion of activated and sometimes oligoclonal T cells in the blood, concerning both CD4$^+$ and CD8$^+$ subsets and restricted to T-helper type 1 response.[36] The drug binding to T cells may have some characteristics of superantigen stimulation. The important percentage of eosinophils in the blood circulation is probably due to the release of IL-5 and eotaxin by activated cells.[54] In addition, several studies shed some light on the relationship between viral infection and DRESS. Specifically, it has been shown recently that HHV-6 reactivation was rather frequent after the onset of the reaction and might contribute to the relapse or chronic course of rash, hepatitis, or other manifestations.[55]

## E. Acute Generalized Exanthematous Pustulosis

AGEP is characterized by fever, appearance of multiple sterile pustules, elevated neutrophil counts, and sometimes eosinophilia. This disease is caused by drugs (such as aminopenicillins, pristiniamycine, diltiazem) in at least 90% of cases. Biopsy of acute lesions reveals the typical presence of intraepidermal pustules, infiltrated with neutrophils, an unusual feature for a drug allergic reaction.[25] However, immunolabeling also demonstrates the presence of activated HLA-DR$^+$ or CD25$^+$, CD4$^+$, and CD8$^+$ T cells in the epidermis and in the dermis.[56] These data suggest that T cells may be involved in AGEP. Moreover, prior studies in patients with AGEP have revealed a high rate of strongly positive patch tests to drugs compared with patients with other types drug eruptions.[22] The positive patch tests often mimic the morphology of original reaction, including pustule formation. Drug-specific T-cell lines and clones were generated from positive patch tests and from the blood of patients with drug-induced AGEP.[57] These cells produced significantly more IL-8 and RANTES than drug-specific clones obtained after reactions of different clinical types. AGEP is therefore a model for T cell–PMN interaction. Further work is required to better understand what is priming T cells in favor of preferential IL-8 production.

## F. Fixed Drug Eruption

Fixed drug eruption is a localized variant of drug-induced cutaneous ADR characterized by recurrence of a few round inflammatory and sometimes blistering plaques at identical sites when the patient is reexposed to the culprit drug. The eruption resolves in a few days, leaving pigmented areas. The causative drugs are principally pyrazolone analgesics, barbiturates, sulfonamides, and cyclines.[58]

Immunohistochemistry shows a dermal CD4$^+$ and CD8$^+$ T-cell infiltrate, whereas epidermal infiltrate is composed predominantly of CD8$^+$ cells. An unusual persistence of these epidermal CD8$^+$

T cells along the dermo epidermal junction has been observed in skin biopsy samples obtained from non-inflammatory, pigmented plaques, 3 weeks after the acute lesions, but these lymphocytes did not proliferate in the culture with the culprit drug.[59,60] The recurrence of skin lesions at identical sites could be due to the activation of skin-resident CD8 T cells with cytolytic potential, persisting in the epidermis. These T cells produce IFN-$\gamma$, which may activate keratinocytes.[29] Alternatively, drug-induced, TNF-$\alpha$-dependent, ICAM-1 expression by keratinocytes in the cutaneous lesions could provide a localized initiating stimulus for activation of the disease-associated epidermal T cells.[28,61]

## IV. CONCLUSION

Recent studies assess the decisive role of drug-specific T cells in the pathomechanisms of many cutaneous ADRs where these cells appear to orchestrate the inflammatory skin reaction. The many different pathways of T-cell activation and cytokine production probably explain the different clinical features of drug eruptions.

Future directions in drug allergy will be attempts to gain better understanding of the mechanisms governing (1) T-cell sensitization to medications as small nonreactive molecules, (2) regulation of the magnitude of the response, and (3) direction of effector cells toward the skin. That will allow better diagnosis, treatment, and prediction of cutaneous ADR.

## REFERENCES


1. Yawalkar, N. and Pichler, W.J., Immunohistology of drug-induced exanthema: clues to pathogenesis, *Curr. Opin. Allergy Clin. Immunol.*, 1, 303, 2001.
2. Pichler, W.J. and Yawalkar, N., Allergic reactions to drugs: involvement of T-cells, *Thorax,* 55 (Suppl. 2), S61, 2000.
3. Pichler, W.J. et al., Cellular and molecular pathophysiology of cutaneous drug reactions, *Am. J. Clin. Dermatol.,* 3, 229, 2002.
4. Pichler, W.J., Deciphering the immune pathomechanism of cutaneous drug reactions, *Allergy*, 57 (Suppl. 72), 34, 2002.
5. Gonzalez, F.J. et al., Participation of T lymphocytes in cutaneous allergic reaction to drugs, *Clin. Exp. Allergy*, 28 (Suppl. 4), 3, 1998.
6. Hertl, M. and Merk, H.F., Lymphocyte activation in cutaneous drug reaction, *J. Invest. Dermatol.,* 105, 95, 1995.
7. Merk, H.F. and Hertl, M., Immunologic mechanisms of cutaneous drug reaction, *Semin. Cutaneous Med. Surg.,* 15, 228, 1996.
8. Park, B.K., Pirmohamed, M., and Kitteringham, N.R., Role of drug disposition in drug hypersensitivity: a chemical, molecular, and clinical perspective, *Chem. Res. Toxicol.*, 11, 969, 1998.
9. Cribb, A.E. and Spielberg, S.P., Sulfamethoxazole is metabolized to the hydroxylamine in humans, *Clin. Pharmacol. Ther.,* 51, 522, 1992.
10. Knowles, S.R., Uetrecht, J., and Shear, N.H., Idiosyncratic drug reactions: the reactive metabolite syndromes, *Lancet,* 356, 1587, 2000.
11. Eliaszewicz, M. et al., Prospective evaluation of risk factors of cutaneous drug reactions to sulfonamides in patients with AIDS, *J. Am. Acad. Dermatol.,* 47, 40, 2002.
12. Pirmohamed, M. et al.. Direct and metabolism-dependent toxicity of sulphasalazine and its principal metabolites towards human erythrocytes and leucocytes, *Br. J. Clin. Pharmacol.,* 32, 303, 1991.
13. Wolkenstein, P., Charue, D., and Laurent, P., Metabolic predisposition to cutaneous adverse drug reactions. Role of toxic epidermal necrolysis caused by sulfonamides and anticonvulsants, *Arch. Dermatol.,* 131, 544, 1995.
14. Zanni, M.P. et al., HLA-restricted, processing and metabolism-independent pathway of drug recognition by human a T lymphocytes, *J. Clin. Invest.,* 102, 1591, 1998.
15. Nassif, A. et al., Drug-specific cytotoxic T lymphocytes in the skin lesions of a patient with toxic epidermal necrolysis, *Allergologie,* 24, 222, 2001.

16. Gallucci, S. and Matzinger, P., Danger signals: SOS to the immune system, *Curr. Opin. Immunol.*, 13, 114, 2001.
17. Matzinger, P., Tolerance, danger, and the extended family, *Annu. Rev. Immunol.*, 12, 991, 1994.
18. Pirmohamed, M.M. et al., The danger hypothesis -potential role in idiosyncratic drug reactions, *Toxicology*, 181, 55, 2002.
19. Heller, H.M., Adverse cutaneous drug reactions in patients with human immunodeficiency virus-1 infection, *Clin. Dermatol.*, 18, 485, 2000.
20. Suzuki, Y. et al., Human herpesvirus 6 infection as a risk factor for the development of severe drug-induced hypersensivity syndrome, *Arch. Dermatol.*, 134, 1108, 1996.
21. Vance, R.E., Cutting edge commentary: a Copernician revolution? Doubts about the danger, *J. Immunol.*, 165, 1725, 2000.
22. Wolkenstein, P. et al., Patch-testing in severe cutaneous adverse drug reactions including Stevens-Johnson syndrome and toxic epidermal necrolysis, *Contact Dermatitis*, 35, 234, 1996.
23. Correia, O. et al., Cutaneous T-cell recruitment in toxic epidermal necrolysis, *Arch. Dermatol.*, 129, 466, 1993.
24. Bocquet, H., Bagot, M., and Roujeau, J.C., Drug-induced pseudolymphoma and drug hypersensivity syndrome (drug rash with eosinophilia and systemic symptoms: DRESS), *Semin. Cutaneous Med. Surg.* 15, 250, 1996.
25. Roujeau, J.C., Bioulac-Sage, P., and Bourseau C., Acute generalized exanthematous pustulosis: analysis of 63 cases, *Arch. Dermatol.*, 127, 1333, 1991.
26. Barbaud, A. et al., Role of delayed cellular hypersensitivity and adhesion molecules in amoxicillin-induced morbilliform rashes, *Arch. Dermatol.*, 133, 481, 1997.
27. Yawalkar, N. et al., Infiltration of cytotoxic T cells in drug-induced cutaneous eruptions, *Clin. Exp. Allergy*, 30, 847, 2000.
28. Shiohara, T. et al., Fixed drug eruption. Expression of epidermal keratinocyte intercellular adhesion molecule-1 (ICAM-1), *Arch. Dermatol.*, 125, 1371, 1989.
29. Blanca, M. et al., Expression of the skin-homing receptor in peripheral blood lymphocytes from subjects with non immediate cutaneous allergic drug reactions, *Allergy*, 55, 998, 2000.
30. Schnyder, B. et al., T-cell mediated cytotoxicity against keratinocytes in sulfamethoxazole-induced skin reaction, *Clin. Exp. Allergy*, 28, 1412, 1998.
31. LeCleach, L. et al., Blister fluid T lymphocytes during toxic epidermal necrolysis are functional cytotoxic cells which express human natural killer (NK) inhibitory receptors, *Clin. Exp. Immunol.*, 119, 225, 2000.
32. Viard, I. et al., Inhibition of toxic epidermal necrolysis by blockade of CD95 with human intravenous immunoglobulin, *Science*, 282, 490, 1998.
33. Berthou, C., Michel, L., and Soulie, A., Acquisition of granzyme B and fas ligand proteins by human keratinocytes contributes to epidermal cell defense, *J. Immunol.*, 159, 5293, 1997.
34. Nagakura, N. et al., Immunological properties of cephalexin-induced delayed type hypersensitivity reaction in guinea pigs, *Chem. Pharm. Bull.* (Tokyo), 38, 3410, 1990.
35. Hattori, H. et al., Evaluation of delayed type hypersensitivity to beta-lactam antibiotics in mice, *J. Antimicrob. Chemother.*, 31, 739, 1993.
36. Mauri-Hellweg, D. et al., Activation of drug specific $CD4^+$ and $CD8^+$ T cells in individuals allergic to sulfonamides, phenytoin and carbamazepine, *J. Immunol.*, 155, 462, 1995.
37. Hertl, M. et al., Selective generation of $CD8^+$ T-cell clones from the peripheral blood of patients with cutaneous reactions to beta-lactam antibiotics, *Br. J. Dermatol.*, 128, 619, 1993.
38. Zanni, M.P. et al., Characterization of lidocaine-specific T cells, *J. Immunol.*, 158, 1139, 1997.
39. Naisbitt, D.J. et al., Characterization of drug-specific T cells in lamotrigine hypersensitivity, *J. Allergy Clin. Immunol.*, 111, 1393, 2003.
40. von Greyerz, S. et al., Degeneracy and additional alloreactivity of drug-specific human alpha beta(+) T cell clones, *Int. Immunol.*, 13, 877, 2001.
41. Yawalkar, N. et al., Evidence for a role for IL-5 and eotaxin in activating and recruiting eosinophils in drug-induced cutaneous eruptions, *J. Allergy Clin. Immunol.*, 106, 1171, 2000.
42. Hashizume, H., Takigawa, M., and Tokura, Y., Characterization of drug-specific T cells in Phenobarbital-induced eruption, *J. Immunol.*, 168, 5359, 2002.

43. Pichler, W.J. et al., High IL-5 production by human drug-specific T cell clones, *Int. Arch. Allergy Immunol.,* 113, 177, 1997.
44. Brugnolo, F. et al., Highly Th2-skewed cytokine profile of beta-lactam-specific T cells from nonatopic subjects with adverse drug reactions, *J. Immunol.*, 163, 1053, 1999.
45. Kalish, R.S. et al., Sulfonamide-reactive lymphocytes detected at very low frequency in the peripheral blood of patients with drug-induced eruptions, *J. Allergy Clin. Immunol.,* 94, 465, 1994.
46. Reilly, T.P. et al., A role for bioactivation and covalent binding within epidermal keratinocytes in sulfonamide-induced cutaneous drug reactions, *J. Invest. Dermatol.*, 114, 1164, 2000.
47. Mizukawa, Y. et al., Direct evidence for interferon-gamma production by effector-memory-type intraepidermal T cells residing at an effector site of immunopathology in fixed drug eruption, *Am. J. Pathol.*, 161, 1337, 2002.
48. Blanca, M. et al., New aspects of allergic reactions to betalactams: cross reactions and unique specificities, *Clin. Exp. Allergy,* 24, 407, 1994.
49. Vega, J. et al., Immediate allergic reactions to amoxicillin, *Allergy*, 49, 317, 1994.
50. Pichler, W.J. et al., High IL-5 production by human drug-specific T cell clones, *Int. Arch. Allergy Immunol.*, 113, 177, 1997.
51. Gutierrez-Ramos, J.C., Lloyd, C., and Gonzalo, J.A., Eotaxin from an eosinophilic chemokine to a major regulator of allergic reactions, *Immunol. Today,* 20, 500, 1999.
52. Barbaud, A.M. et al., Immunocompetent cells and adhesion molecules in 14 cases of cutaneous drug reactions induced with the use of antibiotics, *Arch. Dermatol.,* 134, 1040, 1998.
53. Miyauchi, H. et al., T-cell subsets in drug-induced toxic epidermal necrolysis. Possible pathogenic mechanism induced by CD8-positive T cells, *Arch. Dermatol.,* 127, 851, 1991.
54. Choquet-Kastylevsky, G. et al., Increased levels of Interleukin-5 are associated with the generation of eosinophilia in drug-induced hypersensivity syndrome, *Br. J. Dermatol.,* 139, 1026, 1998.
55. Descamps, V. et al., Association of human herpesvirus 6 infection with drug reaction with eosinophilia and systemic symptoms, *Arch. Dermatol.,* 137, 301, 2001.
56. Schmid, S. et al., Acute generalized exanthematous pustulosis: role of cytotoxic T cells in pustule formation, *Am. J. Pathol.,* 161, 2079, 2002.
57. Britschgi, M. et al., T cell involvement in drug-induced acute generalized exanthematous pustulosis, *J. Clin. Invest.,* 107, 1433, 2001.
58. Huff, J.C., Weston, W.L., and Tonnesen, M.G., Erythema multiforme: a critical review of characteristics, diagnostic criteria and causes, *J. Am. Acad. Dermatol.,* 8, 763, 1983.
59. Hidsen, M. et al., Fixed drug eruption: an immunohistochemical investigation of the acute and healing phase, *Br. J. Dermatol.,* 116, 351, 1987.
60. Komatsu, T. Moriya, N., and Shiohara, T., T cell receptor (TCR) repertoire and function of human epidermal T cells: restricted TCR V alpha-V beta genes are utilized by T cells residing in the lesional epidermis in fixed drug eruption, *Clin. Exp. Immunol.,* 104, 343, 1996.
61. Teraki, Y., Moriya, N., and Shiohara, T., Drug-induced expression of intercellular adhesion molecule-1 on lesional keratinocytes in fixed drug eruption, *Am. J. Pathol.,* 145, 550, 1994.

# 30 Atopic Dermatitis

*Kristian Thestrup-Pedersen*

## CONTENTS



## I. INTRODUCTION

This chapter summarizes known aspects of the "immunology" of atopic dermatitis (AD). It is deliberately brief. The main message is that we still do not know how the "immune inflammation" starts in AD. What is the primary contributor vs. secondary contributors initiating and sustaining the immune inflammation? And what are the genetic factors behind the changes? At the end of the chapter I suggest various hypotheses concerning AD to illustrate the complexity of this disorder. Likely, "one fault" is responsible for the development of the many changes, which — over time — develop in this common disease.

## II. EPIDEMIOLOGY

There are several epidemiological findings that are important for understanding AD. It develops early in life, when the immune system of the child meets the "environment." We observed that children, who later in life develop AD, are born "later," i.e., with an increased gestational age, than non-atopic children.[1] Further, children who develop insulin-dependent diabetes mellitus (IDDM), i.e., have a Th1 tilted immune system, have significantly less AD, even at a time before the expression of their IDDM.[2]

AD becomes clinically evident in approximately 90% of children before the age of 4 years.[3] And it disappears in two thirds of the children before the age of 12.[4] Thus, it is an "early life event." We still lack prospective studies, where children are followed over a long time period to obtain exact data on how many continue or redevelop AD in adulthood. Some studies claim that up to

0-8493-1959-5/05/$0.00+$1.50

75% will have eczema in adulthood, but there is likely a bias as the studies have been performed at university departments, where only the worst cases of AD are seen.[5]

Studies in rural areas of Africa have clearly shown that African school children aged 5 to 8 years do not have AD.[6] This is in sharp contrast to many well-conducted studies showing how AD reaches a cumulative prevalence between 15 and 20% in Europe and the United States.[7–10] Thus, in Africa AD is a very rare — to non-existent — disease. The microbiological exposure of African children is very different from a child in Europe.

## III. ANIMAL MODELS OF ATOPIC DERMATITIS

One mouse model is the Japanese "funny mouse" or NC/Nga mouse. These mice are healthy at birth and stay healthy, if kept in germ-free conditions. But, if exposed to the microbiology of normal animal facilities, they will develop "dermatitis" from week 8 with increased serum IgE. This happens at a time when TARC (T-cell activated and regulated chemokine) becomes upregulated in the keratinocytes.[11] TARC is one (of many) cytokines that can attract T lymphocytes.[12] Recent studies seem to indicate — although not quite convincingly — that if NC/Nga mice are treated with antibiotics, then the development of dermatitis is delayed.[13] These findings certainly indicate that the "microbiological exposure" to the immune system early in life is decisive for eczema development in a genetically predisposed animal. However, attempts to establish the NC/Nga mouse model at the LEO Pharmaceutical Company in Copenhagen turned out to be impossible (Christian Vestergaard, personal communication). So, the model is trickier than published. Also, STAT6$^{-/-}$ NC/Nga mice, which cannot make IgE and Th2 cytokines, develop AD-like skin lesions showing that a Th2-mediated immune response is not necessary for the AD phenotype of the mice.[14]

## IV. THE INNATE IMMUNE SYSTEM

Recent studies have clearly shown how the innate immune system of atopic dermatitis skin is deficient.[15] Thus, human defensin β2 and cathelicidins (LL-37) are clearly downregulated on both the mRNA and the protein levels in adults with AD. This is likely a major reason that AD skin is colonized by *Staphylococcus aureus*. This is important as "superantigens," which can stimulate T lymphocytes "multiclonally," can induce inflammation of the skin.[16] Clinically, we know that severe eczema improves when using either systemic or topical remedies to reduce the bacterial load on the skin.[17] However, the presence of superantigen-secreting *S. aureus* on skin is more complicated than expected. Thus, certain phage types may exist for a certain period with a sudden change of the phage type — without any relation to the clinical activity of the disease (Lomholt et al., in preparation). Thus, the presence of *S. aureus* can, at the least, augment the skin inflammation.[16,17]

There are IgE antibodies toward *S aureus* in patients with AD.[18] Whether these are important for elicitation of eczema via IgE on inflammatory dendritic cells (IDECs) is at present not certain.

Mannose-binding lectins found in plasma are another important part of the innate immune system, being important for optimal phagocytosis of bacteria. They have been found to be normal in adult patients with AD (M. Deleuran, personal communication).

## V. IgE ANTIBODIES AND ATOPIC DERMATITIS

It has been known for a century that "hypersensitivity" to environmental allergens is a very common finding among patients with AD.[19] In 1969, it was discovered that this "hypersensitivity" was mediated by IgE.[20] This led to a technical development, whereby IgE-mediated hypersensitivity could be measured. Thus, IgE became the focus of investigation in patients with AD, and "allergy" came into study as the primary cause for AD development. In a provocative paper the editor of

**TABLE 30.1**
**Prospective Allergoligical Analysis among a 1-Year Birth Cohort**

| | | |
|---|---|---|
| No. of children investigated | 562 | 46 developed atopic eczema at age of 18 months (8.2%) |
| At least one positive test at a given investigation | 80% of all infants had a positive histamine release, RAST or skin prick tests at one investigation | 450 infants had "type I allergy" during their growth; only 46 developed eczema |
| Cord blood IgE > 0.3 ng/l | 27% of boys | 15% of girls |
| Histamine release positive | 39% of boys | 35% of girls |
| RAST test positive | 24% of boys | 5% of girls |

this book and colleagues suggested that true "atopic eczema" is IgE mediated and suggested a new classification of this skin disorder.[21] The fact that up to 80% will have type I allergies certainly supports this view. However, the "extrinsic" vs. the "intrinsic" model of AD is not solved by the IgE definition of the disease, simply because neither clinically nor histologically is it possible to differentiate between extrinsic vs. intrinsic AD. Further, children who outgrow their "extrinsic" AD continue to have IgE-specific antibodies, but no eczema.

Normally, type I allergens are environmental allergens. In a recent study Novak and co-workers[22] found 90 patients with extrinsic AD and 24 with intrinsic AD, where all extrinsic patients had type I allergies to food or environmental allergens, whereas the 24 intrinsic AD patients did not. But, when type I allergies toward superantigens, *Candida,* and *Malasessia* were studied, 85 and 53%, respectively, had type I allergies to these allergens, shifting half of the 24 patients with intrinsic AD to become extrinsic.

A prospective study screened a birth cohort of 562 infants for total serum IgE, RAST, histamine release tests, and skin prick tests against a panel of allergens at birth, 3, 6, 9, 12, and 18 months of age. The study was conducted in Odense, Denmark.[23] A very brief summary is shown in Table 30.1.

The observations show how type I allergy is very common among infants. The allergies are of low-grade intensity and disappear in most infants. The infants did not develop eczema despite their IgE-mediated allergy or allergies. It is interesting to note that boys are more "reactive" than girls regarding increased cord blood and RAST test positivity. Boys develop AD earlier in life than girls (Olesen et al., in preparation), which could support the IgE importance for an "initiation" of the skewed immune system seen in AD.[21]

IgE increases over time both in its total serum concentration and regarding the occurrence of type I allergies. Studies show that up to 80% of children and adults with AD have specific IgE antibodies toward specific environmental antigens. There is a clear correlation between the ability to produce IgE and the occurrence of specific IgE antibodies to house dust mites.[24] Thus, the allergies develop "over time." This is important as they could be "secondary" to a changed immune system.

## VI. THE T LYMPHOCYTE SYSTEM AND ATOPIC DERMATITIS

The majority of cells present in skin of atopic eczema are T lymphocytes with a preponderance of $CD4^+$ T cells.[25] The T cells express activation markers. Immunosuppressive therapy specifically aimed at activated T cells, such as steroids, cyclosporine, pimecrolimus, and tacrolimus, stops or inhibits disease expression. Thus, based on clinical observations it is clear that T-cell "activity" is at the center of disease expression.

The number of T lymphocytes in adults with AD is increased. Using stereological counting we observed that adults with 30% of their skin affected with eczema have on average double the amount of T lymphocytes in their skin compared with peripheral blood.[26] Thus, patients with AD simply have "too many T lymphocytes" in their peripheral immune system. This then points to T-cell emission from the thymus. We have recently shown that the size of the thymus is significantly increased in infants with AD compared to healthy infants (Olesen et al., submitted for publication).

Phenotypic analysis have shown that there is an increased presence of $CD4^+CD8^+$ T lymphocytes in the peripheral blood and skin of patients with AD, more than in psoriasis and cutaneous T-cell lymphoma.[27,28] $CD4^+CD8^+$ T cells are frequent in the thymus, but not in the peripheral immune system. The most direct explanation would be that thymic emission is the default; i.e., the "thymus" in patients with AD sends out too many "immature" T cells. However, it needs to be shown, if the $CD4^+CD8^+$ phenotype exists of $\alpha/\alpha$ chains of the $CD8^+$ T-cell receptor in order to document whether these observed cells are "immature" or are activated $CD8^+$ T cells.[29]

The telomere length of various T-cell subsets is significantly decreased, indicating an increased turnover of T cells in AD. However, this is not unique to AD but is also observed in patients with psoriasis.[30] Further, studies on thymic receptor excision circles (TRECs) show that adults with AD can have increased and, with age, reduced TREC levels, supporting the theory that there is a significant turnover of T lymphocytes in the peripheral immune system of patients with AD (Just et al., in preparation).

Many studies have been performed to determine the cytokine profile of skin-homing T cells in AD. One of the most cited studies is the Th1 vs. Th2 study on house dust mite testing in AD.[31] It indicates that there is a Th2 to Th1 shift from acute to chronic AD. Other studies have clearly documented that there are "allergen-specific" T cells among the skin-infiltrating lymphocytes.[32] The clones mostly expressed a Th1 profile.[32] Of all skin-homing T lymphocytes two studies have shown extensive "oligoclonality,"[32,33] again indicating that the T cells of AD skin inflammation are much more complex than a "one-hit" allergen response. The multiplicity of different skin-homing T-cell clones could support that "superantigens," in combination with allergen-specific T cells are important for the skin inflammation.

Finally, it has been argued that decreased apoptosis of skin-homing T lymphocytes is involved in the chronic inflammation of AD.[34]

## VII. INFLUENCES ON THE DEVELOPMENT OF THE IMMUNE SYSTEM

AD develops early in life, when the peripheral immune system is shaped. Studies of African children show how AD is rare,[6] and how parasitic infections "prevent" atopy.[35] The "hygiene hypothesis" is prevailing, but not yet substantiated.[36] However, rural life in Africa,[6] anthroposophic lifestyle,[37] and probiotics[38,39]can inhibit AD expression early in life. Measles, mumps, and rubella vaccination and against morbilli and rubella seem to augment its frequency, at least in Scandinavia.[40]

However, antigen-avoidance e.g., house dust mite, does not diminish type I allergy or AD disease activity in either infants[41] or adults.[42–44]

## VIII. STATIONARY SKIN CELLS AND ATOPIC DERMATITIS

Keratinocytes, Langerhans cells, mast cells, fibroblasts, melanocytes could in principle play important roles in AD. The best evidence is that keratinocytes from patients with AD have an increased expression of granulocyte-macrophage colony-stimulating factor (GM-CSF).[45] It is quite likely that a change of ectodermal tissue could lead to AD as ectodermal tissue is so important for the proper maturation of the peripheral immune system.[46] However, there are no "hard data" to confirm this hypothesis except the findings of the Italian investigators.[45] Still, the genetic background of AD could be linked to ectodermal tissue as patients do suffer from "skin barrier problems."

Langerhans cells of epidermis are clearly changed in AD. The inflammatory dendritic epidermal cells (IDECs) are cells with an increased expression of receptors for IgE,[47] and they can beyond doubt augment "immune stimulation" of AD skin in an allergen-specific way. IDECs are not "specific" for AD, but can be observed in other inflammatory skin diseases.

Mast cells are slightly increased in AD.[48] But whether they are of primary importance for disease expression is not known. They do have receptors for IgE antibodies and they can secrete interleukin-4 (IL-4). Recent studies on "gain-of-function" mutations of their IL-4 receptor[49] has not been confirmed.

Melanocytes are not considered important in AD, although the number of nevi in children with AD is significantly less than in controls.[50] What it means for AD disease is speculative. Fibroblasts can release IL-4, but their contribution to AD is likely secondary. One could argue that the "lichenification" of the skin of patients with AD may related to changes of fibroblasts, but this, too, is speculative.

## IX. CYTOKINES/CHEMOKINES OF ATOPIC DERMATITIS

Many cytokines and chemokines have been demonstrated to be present in AD. Again, the question is whether this is because of "increased expression of cytokines from the stationary cells" like TARC[12] or whether it is it secondary to the T-cell activation i.e., release of interferon-gamma (IFN-$\gamma$) from activated T cells. As an example, IL-10, a cytokine known to be "anti-inflammatory" is highly overexpressed in AD skin.[51]

Recent studies of gene-differential displays confirm different cytokine and other protein expressions, but studying a skin biopsy or a blood sample means looking at a mixture of cells that are most likely secondarily activated.[52,53]

## X. HYPOTHESES OF ATOPIC DERMATITIS

First, it must be remembered that AD develops early in life and then disappears in the majority of patients. It is the interaction between the "immune system" and likely the "microbiological environment," which seems able elicit the phenotype of AD. Up to 80% of all infants will during their development exhibit type I "allergy," but only one in ten will develop AD.[23] At the moment the question is: Is AD a disease of "stationary cells," i.e., keratinocytes, or is it a "hematological/immune cell disease"?

### A. The Keratinocyte Hypothesis

This hypothesis is substantiated by the fact that AD keratinocytes express more GM-CSF than those of control subjects.[45] Likely, more and yet unknown cytokines could be involved, in particular TARC[11,12] and/or TSLP[46] and/or CLL27 (cTACK).[54]

In a recent mouse model epidermal tissue was rendered deficient of their IKK2-signaling pathway. The mice developed severe skin inflammation shortly after birth, and although T lymphocytes were attracted as inflammatory cells, these cells could be shown not to be present for their antigen specificity.[55] It could be documented that tumor necrosis factor-alpha (TNF-$\alpha$) was the responsible cytokine. Such evidence could clearly support that AD may arise as an "epidermal" disease likely linked to a genetic change of the tissue. Also, a changed apoptosis of keratinocytes have been observed in AD likely from an interplay with activated T lymphocytes.[56,57]

"Epidermal tissue" is very important for "thymic epithelium" as this derives from skin. Therefore, the important communication between a developing immune system could clearly be the reason for a "default" establishment of the immune system — including an increased presence of $CD4^+CD8^+$ T cells in the blood.[27] The increased size of thymus (Olesen et al., submitted for publication) and both the increase and decrease in TREC values (Just et al., in preparation) would support this theory.[58]

### B. The Inflammatory Dentritic Cell Hypothesis

IDECs are present in AD and are effective in stimulating an immune response — at least *in vitro*.[47] The significance of antigen-specific stimulations is, however, questioned by the fact that 80% of infants do have type I allergy or allergies during their growth and very few develop AD.[23] Second, house mite allergen avoidance is not helpful in patients with type I allergy to house dust mite.[41–44] Third, when children outgrow atopic eczema, they still have type I allergies as seen in children with asthma or hay fever. This, of course, places a large question mark on the role of type I allergies. Still, if IDECs could be found already in cord blood of children who later develop AD, then the IDEC hypothesis would be supported.

## XI. INFLAMMATORY CELLS OF ATOPIC DERMATITIS

Patients with extrinsic AD have increased eosinophil participation compared with patients with intrinsic AD.[25] Eosinophils are present and their increased stay and prolonged life may be caused by the increased IL-4 in the skin. However, eosinophils are nonspecific effector cells of the immune system and need T-lymphocyte activation to be present.

The most prominent cell type in AD is the T lymphocytes. Numerous studies have documented their presence and that they are activated (see above). There is evidence for allergen-specific activation and superantigen stimulation. Still, many clones are present among AD skin-homing T lymphocytes.[32,33]

Very preliminary findings suggest that there can be immune stimulation between skin-homing T lymphocytes and peripheral blood lymphocytes (J. Baumgartner-Nielsen et al., in preparation). If so, "immature, atopic T lymphocytes" may escape from the thymus into the peripheral immune system including the skin, where they eventually are removed by autocytotoxic $CD4^+CD8^+$ T lymphocytes. This is still speculative, but it would not contradict any previous findings of immunity and AD.

Within the last few years it has become increasingly clear that a subset of T regulatory cells exists. The data so far stem mostly from experiments in mice, where the activity of T regulatory cells can be clearly demonstrated. Mice lacking T regulatory cells develop chronic inflammatory and autoimmune diseases. T regulatory cells are within the group of CD4+CD25+ T cells. They also express CTLA and can upregulate glucocorticoid-induced receptors, which when stimulated can break self-tolerance.[59] The CD4+CD25+ subset has recently been found to be increased in blood of atopic patients, but its function seemed normal although its "suppressive" function was reduced after superantigen stimulation.[60] We have observed that markers for T regulatory cells are present in atopic eczema (unpublished), but their functionality and significance for not being able to dampen the skin inflammation remain to be shown.

## XII. THE FUTURE

A most important area is to find the genes responsible for or at least associated with AD development. This could focus future research on how the genetic changes lead to a disturbance or overreactivity seen in the immune system of patients with AD (Deleuran, M. et al., in preparation). Many of our observations so far may clearly be secondary to primary events leading to the AD immune deviation.

## REFERENCES

1. Olesen, A.B., Ellingsen, A.R., Olesen, H., Juul, S., and Thestrup-Pedersen, K., Atopic dermatitis and birth factors: historical follow up by record linkage. *Br. Med. J.*, 314, 1003, 1997.

2. Olesen, A.B., Juul, S., Birkebaek, N., and Thestrup-Pedersen, K., Association between atopic dermatitis and insulin-dependent diabetes mellitus: a case-control study. *Lancet,* 357, 1749, 2001.
3. Olesen, A.B., Ellingsen, A.R., Larsen, F.S., Larsen, P.Ø., Veien, N.K., and Thestrup-Pedersen, K., Atopic dermatitis may be linked to whether a child is first or second born. *Acta Derm. -Venereol.* (Stockholm), 76, 457, 1996.
4. Emerson, R.M., Williams, H.C., and Allen, B.R., Severity distribution of atopic dermatitis in the community and its relationship to secondary referral. *Br. J. Dermatol.*, 139, 73, 1998.
5. Wuthrich, B., Clinical aspects, epidemiology, and prognosis of atopic dermatitis. *Ann. Allergy, Asthma Immunol.*, 83, 464, 1999.
6. Shaheen, S.O., Aaby, P., Hall, A.J., Barker, D.J., Heyes, C.B., Shiell, A.W., and Goudiaby, A., Measles and atopy in Guinea-Bissau. *Lancet*, 347, 1792, 1996.
7. Olesen, A.B., Bang, K., Juul, S., and Thestrup-Pedersen, K., Stable incidence of atopic dermatitis among children in Denmark during the 1990s. *Acta Derm. Venereol.* (Stockholm), 2004; accepted for publication.
8. Mortz, C.G., Lauritsen, J.M., Bindslev-Jensen, C., and Andersen, K.E., Prevalence of atopic dermatitis, asthma, allergic rhinitis, and hand and contact dermatitis in adolescents. The Odense Adolescence Cohort Study on Atopic Diseases and Dermatitis. *Br. J. Dermatol.*, 144, 523, 2001.
9. Girolomoni, G., Abeni, D., Masini, C. et al., The epidemiology of atopic dermatitis in Italian school children. *Allergy*, 58, 420, 2003.
10. Laughter, D.. Istvan, J.A., Tofte, S.J., and Hanifin, J.M., The prevalence of atopic dermatitis in Oregon schoolchildren. *J. Am. Acad. Dermatol.*, 43, 649, 2000.
11. Vestergaard, C.. Yoneyama, H., Murai, M. et al., Overproduction of Th2-specific chemokines in NC/Nga mice exhibiting atopic dermatitis-like lesions. *J. Clin. Invest.*, 104, 1097, 1999.
12. Vestergaard, C., Bang, K., Gesser, B., Yoneyama, H., Matsushima, K., and Larsen, C.G., A Th2 chemokine, TARC, produced by keratinocytes may recruit $CLA^+CCR4^+$ lymphocytes into lesional atopic dermatitis skin. *J. Invest. Dermatol.*, 115, 640, 2000.
13. Hashimoto, Y., Kaneda, Y., Takahashi, N., Akashi, S., Arai, I., and Nakaike, S., Clarithromycin inhibits the development of dermatitis in NC/Nga mice. *Chemotherapy*, 49, 222, 2003.
14. Yagi, R., Nagai, H., Iigo, Y., Akimoto, T., Arai, T., and Kubo, M., Development of atopic dermatitis-like skin lesions in STAT6-deficient NC/Nga mice. *J. Immunol.*, 168, 2020, 2002.
15. Ong, P.Y., Ohtake, T., Brandt, C. et al., Endogenous antimicrobial peptides and skin infections in atopic dermatitis. *N. Engl. J. Med.*, 347, 1151, 2002.
16. Skov, L., Olsen, J.V., Giorno, R., Schlievert, P.M., Baadsgaard, O., and Leung, D.Y.M., Application of staphylococcal enterotoxin B on normal and atopic skin induces upregulation of T cells by a superantigen-mediated mechanism. *J. Allergy Clin. Immunol.*, 105, 820, 2000.
17. Breuer, K., Häussler, S., Kapp, A., and Werfel, T., *Staphylococcus aureus:* colonizing features and influence of an antibacterial treatment in adults with atopic dermatitis. *Br. J. Dermatol.*, 147, 55, 2002.
18. Breuer, K., Wittmann, M., Bosche, B., Kapp, A., and Werfel, T., Severe atopic dermatitis is associated with sensitisation to staphylococcal enterotoxin B (SEB). *Allergy*, 55, 551, 2000.
19. Nexmand, P.H., Clinical Studies of Besnier's Prurigo, dissertation, Rosenkilde & Bagger, Copenhagen, Denmark, 1948.
20. Berg, T. and Johansson, S.G., IgE concentrations in children with atopic diseases. A clinical study. *Int. Arch. Allergy Appl. Immunol.*, 36, 219, 1969.
21. Bos, J.D., Van Leent, E.J.. and Sillevis Smitt, J.H., The millennium criteria for the diagnosis of atopic dermatitis. *Exp. Dermatol.*, 7, 132, 1998.
22. Novak, N., Bieber, T., and Leung, D.Y., Immune mechanisms leading to atopic dermatitis. *J. Allergy Clin. Immunol.*, 112(6 Suppl.), S128, 2003.
23. Johnke, H., Environmental Factors and Atopic Predisposition as Predictors for the Development of Atopic Eczema in Childhood, Ph.D. thesis, Faculty of Health Sciences, University of Southern Denmark, Odense, 2003.
24. Hansen, S.K., Deleuran, M., Johnke, H., and Thestrup-Pedersen, K., House dust mite antigen exposure of patients with atopic dermatitis or psoriasis. *Acta Derm. Venereol.* (Stockholm), 78, 139, 1998.
25. Rho, N.K., Kim, W.S., Lee, D.Y., Lee, J.H., Lee, E.S., and Yang, J.M., Immunophenotyping of inflammatory cells in the lesional skin of extrinsic and intrinsic type of atopic dermatitis. *Br. J. Dermatol.*, in press.

26. Ellingsen, A.R., Sorensen, F.B., Larsen, J.O., Deleuran, M.S., and Thestrup-Pedersen, K., Stereological quantification of lymphocytes in skin biopsies from atopic dermatitis patients. *Acta Derm. Venereol.* (Stockholm), 81, 258, 2001.
27. Bang, K., Lund, M., Wu, K., Mogensen, S.C., and Thestrup-Pedersen, K. $CD4^+CD8^+$ (thymocyte-like) T lymphocytes present in blood and skin from patients with atopic dermatitis suggest immune dysregulation. *Br. J. Dermatol.*, 144, 1140, 2001.
28. Bang, K., Lund, M., Mogensen, S.C., and Thestrup-Pedersen, K., *In vitro* culture of skin-homing T lymphocytes from inflammatory skin diseases. *Exp. Dermatol.*, submitted.
29. Flamand, L., Crowley, R.W., Lusso, P., Colombini-Hatch, S., Margolis, D.M., and Gallo, R.C., Activation of $CD8^+$ T lymphocytes through the T cell receptor turns on CD4 gene expression: implications for HIV pathogenesis. *Proc. Natl. Acad. Sci. U.S.A.*, 95, 3111, 1998.
30. Wu, K.. Higashi, N., Hansen, E.R., Lund, M., Bang, K., and Thestrup-Pedersen, K., Telomerase activity is increased and telomere length shortened in T cells from blood of patients with atopic dermatitis and psoriasis. *J. Immunol.*, 165, 4742, 2000.
31. Grewe, M., Gyufko, K., Schopf, E., and Krutmann, J., Lesional expression of interferon-gamma in atopic eczema. *Lancet*, 343, 25, 1994.
32. Werfel, T., Morita, A., Grewe, M., Renz, H., Wahn, U., Krutmann, J., and Kapp, A., Allergen specificity of skin-infiltrating T cells is not restricted to a type-2 cytokine pattern in chronic skin lesions of atopic dermatitis. *J. Invest. Dermatol.*, 107, 871, 1996.
33. Tanaka, A., Takahama, H., Kato, T. et al., Clonotypic analysis of T cells infiltrating the skin of patients with atopic dermatitis: evidence for antigen-driven accumulation of T cells. *Hum. Immunol.*, 48, 107, 1996.
34. Orteu, C.H., Rustin, M.H., O'Toole, E., Sabin, C., Salmon, M., Poulter, L.W., and Akbar, A.N., The inhibition of cutaneous T cell apoptosis may prevent resolution of inflammation in atopic eczema. *Clin. Exp. Immunol.*, 122, 150, 2000.
35. van den Biggelaar, A.H., van Ree, R., Rodrigues, L.C., Lell, B., Deelder, A.M., Kremsner, P.G., and Yazdanbakhsh, M., Decreased atopy in children infected with *Schistosoma haematobium*: a role for parasite-induced interleukin-10. *Lancet*, 356, 723, 2000.
36. Flohr, C., Dirt, worms and atopic dermatitis. *Br. J. Dermatol.*, 148, 871, 2003.
37. Alm, J.S., Schwartz, J., Lilja, G., and Scheynius, A., Atopy in children of families with an anthroposophic lifestyle. *Lancet*, 359, 1485, 1999.
38. Kalliomaki, M., Salminen, S., Poussa, T., Arvilommi, H., and Isolauri, E., Probiotics and prevention of atopic disease: 4-year follow-up of a randomised placebo-controlled trial. *Lancet*, 361, 1869, 2003.
39. Rosenfeldt, V., Benfeldt, E., Nielsen, S.D., Michaelsen, K.F., Jeppesen, D.L., Valerius, N.H., and Paerregaard, A., Effect of probiotic *Lactobaccillus* strains in children with atopic dermatitis. *J. Allergy Clin. Immunol.*, 111, 389, 2003.
40. Olesen, A.B., Juul, S., and Thestrup-Pedersen, K., Atopic dermatitis is increased following vaccination for measles, mumps and rubella or measles infection. *Acta Derm. Venereol.* (Stockholm), 83, 445, 2003.
41. Koopmann, L.P., van Strien, R.T., Kerkhof, M. et al., Placebo-controlled trial of house dust mite-impermeable mattress covers. *Am. J. Respir. Crit. Care Med.*, 166, 307, 2002.
42. Ricci, G., Patrizi, A., Specchia, F., Menna, L., Bottau, P., D'Angelo, V., and Masi, M., Mite allergen (Der p1) levels in houses of children with atopic dermatitis: the relationship with allergometric tests. *Br. J. Dermatol.*, 140, 651, 1999.
43. Gutgesell, C., Heise, S., Seubert, S., Seubert, A., Domhof, S., Brunner, E., and Neumann, C., Double-blind placebo-controlled house dust mite control measures in adult patients with atopic dermatitis. *Br. J. Dermatol.*, 145, 70, 2001.
44. Holm, L., Bengtsson, A., van Hage-Hamsten, M., Ohman, S., and Scheynius, A., Effectiveness of occlusive bedding in the treatment of atopic dermatitis 6 a placebo-controlled trial of 12 months duration. *Allergy,* 56, 152, 2001.
45. Pastore, S.. Fanales-Belasio, E.. Albanesi, C., Chinni, L.M., Giannetti, A., and Girolomoni, G., Granulocyte macrophage colony-stimulating factor is overproduced by keratinocytes in atopic dermatitis. Implications for sustained dendritic cell activation in the skin. *J. Clin. Invest.*, 99, 3009, 1997.
46. Soumelis, V., Reche, P.A., Kanzler, H. et al., Human epithelial cells trigger dendritic cell mediated allergic inflammation by producing TSLP. *Nat. Immunol.*, 3, 673, 2002.

47. Wollenberg, A., Kraft, S., Hanau, D., and Bieber, T., Immunomorphological and ultrastructural characterization of Langerhans cells and a novel, inflammatory dendritic epidermal cell (IDEC) population in lesional skin of atopic eczema. *J. Invest. Dermatol.*, 106, 446, 1996.
48. Damsgaard, T.E., Olesen, A.B., Sorensen, F.B., Thestrup-Pedersen, K., and Schiotz, P.O., Mast cells and atopic dermatitis. Stereological quantification of mast cells in atopic dermatitis and normal human skin. *Arch. Dermatol. Res.*, 28, 256, 1997.
49. Pascale, E., Tarani, L., Meglio, P., Businco, L., Battiloro, E., Cimino-Reale, G., Verna, R., and D'Ambrosio, E., Absence of association between a variant of the mast cell chymase gene and atopic dermatitis in an Italian population. *Hum. Hered.,* 51, 177, 2001.
50. Broberg, A. and Augustsson, A., Atopic dermatitis and melanocytic naevi. *Br. J. Dermatol.*, 142, 306, 2000.
51. Ohmen, J.D., Hanifin, J.M., Nickoloff, B.J. et al., Overexpression of IL-10 in atopic dermatitis. Contrasting cytokine patterns with delayed-type hypersensitivity reactions. *J. Immunol.*, 154, 1956, 1995.
52. Nomura, I., Goleva, E., Howell, M.D. et al., Cytokine milieu of atopic dermatitis, as compared to psoriasis, skin prevents induction of innate immune response genes. *J. Immunol.*, 171, 3262, 2003.
53. Matsumoto, Y., Oshida, T., Obayashi, I. et al., Identification of highly expressed genes in peripheral blood T cells from patients with atopic dermatitis. *Int. Arch. Allergy Immunol.*, 129, 327, 2002.
54. Homey, B., Alenius, H., Muller, A. et al., CCL27-CCR10 interactions regulate T cell-mediated skin inflammation. *Nat. Med.*, 8, 157, 2002.
55. Pasparakis, M., Courtois, G., Hafner, M. et al., TNF-mediated inflammatory skin disease in mice with epidermis-specific deletion of IKK2. *Nature*, 417, 861, 2002.
56. Trautmann, A., Akdis, M., Kleemann, D. et al., T cell-mediated Fas-induced keratinocyte apoptosis plays a key pathogenetic role in eczematous dermatitis. *J. Clin. Invest.*, 106, 25, 2000.
57. Trautmann, A., Akdis, M., Schmid-Grendelmeier, P., Disch, R., Brocker, E.B., Blaser, K., and Akdis, C.A., Targeting keratinocyte apoptosis in the treatment of atopic dermatitis and allergic contact dermatitis. *J. Allergy Clin. Immunol.*, 108, 839, 2001.
58. Thestrup-Pedersen, K., Ellingsen, A.R., Olesen, A.B., Lund, M., and Kaltoft, K., Atopic dermatitis may be a genetically determined dysmaturation of ectodermal tissue, resulting in disturbed T-lymphocyte maturation. A hypothesis. *Acta Derm. Venereol.* (Stockholm), 77, 20, 1997.
59. Shimizu, J., Yamazaki, S., Takahashi, T., Ishida, Y., and Sakaguchi, S., Stimulation of CD25+CD4+ regulatory T cells through GITR breaks immunological self-tolerance. *Nature Immunol.*, 3, 135, 2002.
60. Liang-Shiou, O., Golvea, E., Hall, C., and Leung, D.Y.M., T regulatory cells in atopic dermatitis and subversion of their activity by superantigens. *J. Allergy Clin. Immunol.*, 113, 756–763, 2004.

# 31 Allergic Contact Dermatitis

*Pierre Saint-Mezard, Maya Krasteva, Frédéric Berard, Bertrand Dubois, Dominique Kaiserlian, and Jean-François Nicolas*

## CONTENTS



0-8493-1959-5/05/$0.00+$1.50

## I. INTRODUCTION

Contact dermatitis is one of the most common skin diseases, with a great socioeconomic impact.[1] As the outermost barrier of the human body, the skin is the first to encounter chemical and physical factors from the environment. According to the pathophysiological mechanisms involved, two main types of contact dermatitis may be distinguished. *Irritant contact dermatitis* is due to the pro-inflammatory and toxic effects of xenobiotics able to activate the skin innate immunity. *Allergic contact dermatitis* (ACD) requires the activation of antigen-specific acquired immunity leading to the development of effector T cells, which mediate the skin inflammation.

ACD is a T-cell-mediated inflammatory reaction occurring at the site of challenge with a contact allergen in sensitized individuals. It is characterized by redness, papules, and vesicles, followed by scaling and dry skin.[2] Knowledge of the pathophysiology of ACD is derived chiefly from animal models in which the skin inflammation induced by hapten painting of the skin is referred to as contact sensitivity (CS) or contact hypersensitivity (CHS). ACD and CS (CHS) are thus considered synonymous and define a hapten-specific T-cell-mediated skin inflammation.[3] The skin and the draining lymph nodes (LN) play a central role in the induction and triggering of a CS reaction. Three elements are necessary for the development of a CS reaction: antigen-presenting dendritic cells (DC), hapten-specific T cells, and the hapten itself.

## II. HAPTENS — CONTACT ALLERGENS

The origin and nature of the compounds able to induce a CS reaction are very diverse, but they share some common features. Contact allergens are low-molecular-weight chemicals, named haptens, that are not immunogenic by themselves and need to bind to epidermal proteins. These then act as carrier proteins to form the hapten–carrier complex that finally acts as the antigen. Most haptens bear lipophilic residues, which enable them to cross through the corneal barrier, and electrophilic residues, which account for covalent bonds to the nucleophilic residues of cutaneous proteins.[4–6]

Haptens often derive from unstable chemicals, named prohaptens, which require an additional metabolization step *in vivo* in the epidermis to be converted into an electrophilic hapten endowed with antigenic properties. This is the case of urushiol (poison ivy)[7] and of photosensitizers, which must be activated by ultraviolet (UV) light in order to bind to epidermal proteins. Metal salts do not bind covalently to cutaneous proteins but form complexes with these proteins through weak interactions. Some metal salts also undergo chemical conversions in the skin, as hexavalent chromium salts, which are turned into trivalent chromium, a highly reactive form binding to cutaneous proteins.[8] Evidence that conversion of the parent compound into a reactive metabolite is necessary for the development of CS was recently demonstrated for the polyaromatic hydrocarbon (PAH) dimethylbenz(*a*)anthracene (DMBA). CS to DMBA only occurred in strains of mice that could metabolize the compound and inhibitors of PAH metabolism reduced the magnitude of the reaction. Furthermore, among the PAHs, only those that could induce aryl hydrocarbon hydroxylase, the rate-limiting enzyme in the PAH metabolic pathway, were immunogenic.[9] The implications of these experiments are that at least for some contact allergens, the metabolic status of the host is a key determinant of individual susceptibility to the development of ACD.

Recent studies from several laboratories have shown that T cells recognize haptens as structural entities bound covalently to, or by complexation to, peptides anchored in the grooves of major histocompatibility complex (MHC) class I and class II molecules. Thus, the contact allergen is a chemical but the antigen able to activate hapten-specific T cells is a haptenated peptide.[10]

## III. PATHOPHYSIOLOGY OF CONTACT SENSITIVITY

Knowledge of the mechanisms by which a xenobiotic can induce CS responses comes from the study of strong haptens, also known as "experimental haptens," as they do not exist in the usual

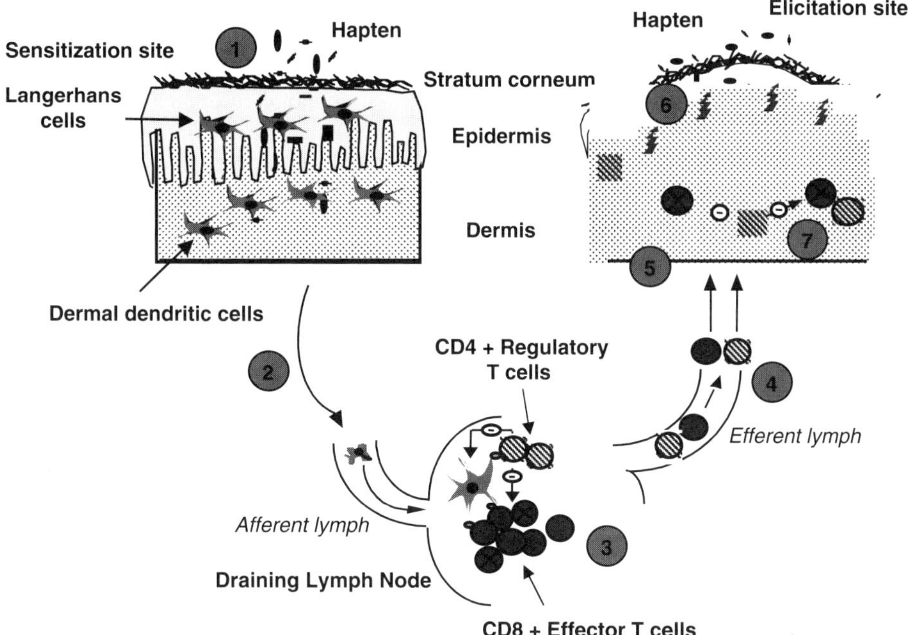


**FIGURE 31.1 (See color insert following page 304.)** Pathophysiology of CHS. *Sensitization step:* Haptens penetrate the stratum corneum. Hapten loading by skin DC (step 1) parallels activation and migration of DC through the afferent lymphatic vessels to the draining lymph nodes (step 2). Migrating DC are located in the paracortical area of the draining LN where they can present haptenated peptides on MHC class I and II molecules to CD8+ and CD4+ T cells, respectively (step 3). Specific T-cell precursors expand clonally in the draining LN and diffuse to the bloodstream through the efferent lymphatic vessels and the thoracic duct (step 4). During this process they acquire skin-specific homing antigens (CLA and CCR4) and become memory T cells. Primed T cells preferentially diffuse in the skin after transendothelial migration. At the end of the sensitization step everything is ready for the development of a CS reaction upon challenge with the relevant hapten. *Elicitation phase:* When the hapten is painted for a second (and subsequent) time, it diffuses through the epidermis and could be loaded by LC or other skin cells expressing MHC molecules, such as keratinocytes and dermal DC, which are then able to activate trafficking specific T cells (step 5). CD8+ cytotoxic T-cell activation initiates the inflammatory process through keratinocyte apoptosis and cytokine/chemokine production (step 6). This is responsible for the recruitment of leukocytes (including regulatory T cells) from the blood to the skin leading to the development of skin lesions (step 7).

environment of human beings. The pathophysiology of CS consists of two distinct phases (Figure 31.1), which are summarized below:

## Phase 1: Sensitization Phase (also referred to as afferent phase or induction phase of CS)

This occurs at the first contact of skin with the hapten and leads to the generation of hapten-specific T cells in the LN and their migration back to the skin. The ability of a hapten to induce sensitization relies on two distinct properties. Through their pro-inflammatory properties, haptens activate the skin innate immunity and deliver signals able to induce the migration and maturation of cutaneous DC. Through their binding to amino acid residues they modify self-proteins and allow the expression in the skin of new antigenic determinants.

Haptens or haptenated proteins are loaded by cutaneous DC and are expressed as haptenated peptides in the groove of MHC class I and class II molecules at the cell surface. Hapten-bearing DC migrate from the skin to the regional LN where specific CD8+ and CD4+ T lymphocytes are primed in the paracortical area. T cells proliferate and emigrate out of the LN to the blood where they recirculate between the lymphoid organs and the skin. The sensitization step lasts 10 to 15 days in humans, and 5 to 7 days in the mouse. This first step has no clinical consequence.

The theory of the first contact of a chemical being immunogenic for the host is true for the strong haptens but cannot be accepted for the vast majority of haptens responsible for ACD. Indeed, ACD to moderate or weak haptens almost never occurs after the first contact but may take years of permanent skin exposure to develop.

### Phase 2: Elicitation Phase (also known as efferent or challenge phase of CS)

Challenge of sensitized individuals with the same hapten leads in 24 to 72 h to the appearance of ACD/CS. Haptens diffuse in the skin and are taken up by skin cells that express MHC I and II/haptenated peptide complexes. Specific T lymphocytes are activated in the dermis and the epidermis, and trigger the inflammatory process responsible for the cutaneous lesions. Recent studies have demonstrated that $CD8^+$ cytotoxic T lymphocytes are the main effector cells of CHS to strong haptens and that they are recruited early after challenge before the massive infiltration of leukocytes, which contain the downregulatory cells of CHS, found in the $CD4^+$ T-cell subset.

The efferent phase of CS takes 72 h in humans, and 24 to 48 h in the mouse. The inflammatory reaction persists only for a few days and rapidly decreases following downregulatory mechanisms.

### Primary Allergic Contact Sensitivity

Although the development of CHS has been postulated to require two spatially and temporally dissociated phases, clinical evidence has demonstrated that ACD could develop after a single skin contact with a strong hapten in previously unsensitized patients. This phenomenon has been referred to as "primary ACD."[11] We have recently demonstrated, in a murine model, that the pathophysiology of this primary (one-step) ACD is identical to the classical (two-step) ACD reaction.[12] The afferent and efferent phases of primary ACD can be induced after a single skin contact with haptens due to the persistence of the hapten in the skin for long period of time, allowing the skin recruitment and the activation of T cells that have been primed in the lymphoid organs.

## A. The Central Role of Cutaneous Dendritic Cells

As elsewhere described in detail in this book, there are different subtypes of DC in the skin. Although they are all able to uptake haptens and to present haptenated peptides to T cells, two subsets of cutaneous DC seem crucial in the development of CS.

The basic role of epidermal Langerhans cells (LC) has been shown by two sets of experiments. On the one hand, animals painted with a hapten on cutaneous sites naturally or artificially depleted in LC are unable to mount a CS response.[13,14] On the other hand, sensitization of naive mice can be achieved by injection of *in vitro* haptenized total epidermal cells, purified LC or DC lines, whereas injection of total epidermal cells depleted in LC before haptenization is inefficient in inducing sensitization.[15–17]

Dermal DC could also participate in the induction phase of CS, even though their precise contribution and phenotype is not well known.[18] Recent studies by Geissmann et al.[20] have brought some insights in the turnover of macrophages and DC in the dermis in normal and inflammatory skin. Two different subsets of monocytes can be defined according to the expression of the chemokine receptor CCR2.[19,20] CCR2 monocytes appear to be involved in the physiological turnover of resident macrophages and DC, whereas $CCR2^+$ monocytes are recruited in inflammatory sites where they could differentiate into mature DC able to present exogenous antigens to T cells. Because hapten application is responsible for activation of skin innate immunity, it is possible that the $CCR2^+$ inflammatory monocytes that are recruited in the skin could uptake the hapten and participate in the afferent phase of CHS.[21]

### 1. Cutaneous DC Load Haptens in the Skin and Migrate to the Draining LN

Activation of naive specific T-cell precursors occurs in the regional draining LN upon presentation of haptenated peptides by cutaneous migrating DC. Initial observations showed that induction of a CS reaction requires an intact draining lymphatic system[22] and that, after skin painting with the hapten fluorescein isothiocyanate (FITC), DC bearing the hapten, some of which containing Birbeck granules, accumulate in the draining lymph nodes.[23,24]

Cutaneous DC continuously migrate out of the skin at a low rate, which dramatically increases after hapten exposure.[25] This phenomenon is the consequence of numerous factors including the secretion of inflammatory cytokines and chemokines induced by the pro-inflammatory properties of the hapten itself. At 15 min after hapten painting, LC start to synthesize interleukin-1β (IL-1β) mRNA and to release the protein. Then, keratinocytes are activated and release tumor necrosis factor (TNF-α) and granulocyte-macrophage colony-stimulating factor (GM-CSF).[26] In the epidermis, LC and keratinocytes are firmly associated by E-cadherin/E-cadherin junctions.[27] Binding of TNF-α and IL-1β on their cognate receptors (TNF-α RII and IL-1 RI and RII) expressed on LC is followed by a decreased expression of E-cadherin on the LC membrane, allowing their disentanglement from surrounding keratinocytes.[28–31] Furthermore, IL-1β and TNF-α inhibit the expression of chemokine receptors such as CCR1, CCR2, CCR5, and CCR6 on the LC membrane, inducing a loss of sensitivity to their cognate ligands, in particular to MIP-3α (CCL20), a chemokine produced by keratinocytes.[32] In parallel, TNF-α and IL-1β induce the expression of adhesive molecules such as CD54, α6 integrin, and different isoforms of CD44, which permit some interactions between LC and the extracellular matrix, allowing the migration of cutaneous DC.

To reach the lymphatic vessels, LC have to cross the dermoepidermal junction and the dermis. To this end, LC secrete different types of enzymes, such as metalloproteinase (MMP) 3 and 9,[33] which could cleave macromolecules of the dermoepidermal junction and of the extracellular matrix. They are also involved in the cleavage of E-cadherin and of pro-TNF-α in its biologically active form.[34] Once in the dermis, DC acquire sensitivity to the chemokines MIP-3β (CCL19) and SLC (CCL21) through the upregulation of the chemokine receptor CCR7.[32,35] CCL21 is expressed on endothelial cells from lymphatic vessels and by stromal cells from the T-cell area in LN.[36] The CCL21/CCR7 interaction is crucial during the sensitization phase of CS. Indeed, Endeman and colleagues[37] have described a strong inhibition of CS following injections of SLC-blocking antibodies before and during the sensitization phase. Moreover, TNF-α is able to induce a strong upregulation of CCL21 on the endothelial cells of skin lymphatic vessels. The overexpression of CCL21 is of critical importance in the migratory properties of peripheral DC and is able to increase, by a factor of 10, the number of cutaneous DC able to migrate from the skin to the LN and subsequently the magnitude of antigen-specific T-cell activation.[38]

### 2. Maturation of Cutaneous DC

The term *maturation* takes into account a group of morphological, phenotypic, and functional modifications that transform skin DC into professional antigen-presenting cells (APC) able to prime naïve specific T-cell precursors. Although the different steps of DC maturation and differentiation are well described *in vitro*,[18] correlation with the *in vivo* modifications is not yet totally achieved. Migration and maturation of cutaneous DC are intimately linked. Indeed, factors known to induce migration of DC are also able to engage DC in a maturation program. Presence of TNF-α and IL-1β in the skin leads to the upregulation of MHC class II molecules on DC membranes. In the first 3 h following application of the hapten, expression of MHC II molecules at the DC surface first decreases,[39] whereas their intracellular level increases, which probably reflects an endocytosis process triggered by hapten binding.[40] From hour 6 after hapten painting, synthesis of MHC II mRNA starts to increase to reach a maximum at around 18 h. This upregulation of mRNA synthesis, plus an increase in the half-life of membrane MHC II molecules,[41] is responsible for the strong

MHC class II expression observed after 24 h. In a similar way, the expression and stability of MHC class I molecules on DC increase.

DC maturation is also associated to the loss of capability to internalize and process exogenous antigens. Indeed, the expression of DC receptors such as mannose receptors or FcR receptors decreases during DC maturation. Birbeck granules disappear from LC and the intracellular machinery that controls macropinocytosis and phagocytosis is blocked.[42] Although this process was clearly demonstrated *in vitro*, recent *in vivo* data suggest that mature migratory skin DC recovered from LN may still be able, at least for a proportion of them, to internalize, process, and present some exogenous antigen.[43]

In parallel, during the maturation process, DC express co-stimulatory molecules such as CD80 (B7-1), CD86 (B7-2), CD40, CD83, adhesive molecules such as CD54 (ICAM-1) and CD58 (LFA-3), and chemokine receptors such as CCR4, CCR7, and CXCR4, which permit them to migrate through lymphatic vessels.

In summary, cutaneous DC uptake haptens in the skin and migrate to draining LN. This migration is associated with an upregulation of MHC and co-stimulatory molecules that confer a high efficiency in the priming of naive T cells to skin DC.

## B. Hapten-Specific T Lymphocytes

### 1. Hapten-Specific T-Cell Activation

CS reactions are dependent on the priming of effector T cells during the sensitization phase. Adoptive transfer of T cells from sensitized mice into naive recipients results in the transfer of sensitization. Moreover, T-cell depletion of sensitized mice totally removes the CS reaction. Finally, patients with thymic aplasia (Di George syndrome) cannot be sensitized.[44]

T-cell activation requires the combination of two distinct signals. The first signal involves the interaction of the T-cell receptor (TCR) and the MHC/peptide complex. The second signal requires co-stimulatory molecules and/or the secretion of cytokines and chemokines by DC. The absence of this second signal may lead to anergy or the death of the T cell, which has already engaged its TCR.

### 2. Hapten Determinants for T Cells Provide the First Signal

T lymphocytes usually recognize hapten-modified peptides in the groove of MHC molecules.[45] Most of the results were obtained with the strong hapten TNP (trinitrophenyl) in mouse models. *In vitro* experiments have shown that for MHC class I-restricted[10,46] as well as MHC class II-restricted determinants.[47,48] T cells react to MHC-associated TNP-peptides and not to covalently TNP-modified MHC molecules, whereas TCR would interact mainly with the hapten TNP and parts of the MHC molecule.[45] However, metal T-cell recognition may be different from the general scheme described above for nonmetal chemicals. Indeed, Weltzien and co-workers have recently shown that nickel may behave like a superantigen and could directly link TCR and MHC outside the groove of the MHC molecule, in a peptide-independent manner.[49]

The special nature of haptens may explain the different routes of processing that they could follow in APC. Haptens could bind to extracellular and cell surface proteins, which are internalized and processed into peptides via the endosomal/lysosomal compartments where they bind to the MHC class II groove. These haptenated peptides can eventually be recognized by class II-restricted $CD4^+$ T cells. In addition, because most haptens are lipid soluble molecules they may also enter the cell, conjugate with intracytoplasmic proteins, and after processing in the endogenous route may be presented to MHC class I-restricted $CD8^+$ T cells. Alternatively, direct binding of haptens, without processing, to a peptide in the groove of either MHC class I or class II molecules may also contribute to recognition by $CD8^+$ or $CD4^+$ T cells, respectively.[50] These different routes of hapten presentation have been demonstrated for the haptens TNP,[51] urushiol,[52] and arsonate.[53] These data point to the existence of both hapten-specific class I-restricted CD8+ T cells and class II-restricted CD4+ T cells.

## 3. The Second Signal Is Provided by Mature DC

During their maturation, DC upregulate the expression of CD80 and CD86, two ligands of CD28, constitutively expressed on T cells.[54,55] CD28 ligation is mandatory for the development of CS since mice deficient for the CD28 molecule present a strong reduction of CS.[56] CD86 seems to be the CD28 ligand involved in the second signal.[57] Indeed, injection of anti-CD86 blocking antibodies inhibits the activation of both CD4+ and CD8+ T cells and the development of CS.

TCR engagement induces the activation of the nuclear factor NF-AT, which regulates IL-2 gene transcription. The instability of the IL-2 mRNA limits the production of this cytokine, which is essential for the proliferation and activation of T cells. One of the effects of CD28 engagement is to stabilize the IL-2 mRNA, leading to a 20- to 30-fold increase in IL-2 production.[58] Moreover, through the activation of AP-1 and NF-κB, CD28 engagement induces an increase in IL-2 and antiapoptotic Bcl-XL gene transcription, which both protect T cells from the apoptotic signals received after TCR engagement.[59]

Circulating CD4+ and CD8+ T cells penetrate in the paracortical area of LN through the postcapillary high endothelial venules (HEV) in response to the chemokine DC-CK1, secreted by resident DC of this zone.[60] The rare specific T-cell precursors are activated by presentation of haptenated peptides by skin-derived DC and start a program of clonal expansion and differentiation. This process is initiated by physical contact between T cells and DC, which implicate cell membrane remodeling, allowing the engagement of TCR/MHC-peptide complexes and co-stimulatory molecules with their cognate ligands. This membrane juxtaposition, associated with transmission of the information, presents some analogy with the neural synapse and is called immune synapse.

The plasmic membrane of mature DC expresses a high level of adhesive molecules, which are essential for T-cell activation. It comprises integrins such as CD54 and CD58 and the lectin DC-SIGN. These molecules interact, respectively, with LFA-1 (CD11a/CD18), a β2 integrin, CD2, and ICAM-3/2 molecules, which are expressed on T cells.[61] In seconds following the T cell/DC interaction, a small number of TCR engagements lead to cytoskeleton rearrangement by actine polymerization, and activation of ZAP-70 and the adaptative protein Vav-1.[62] These modifications generate a central zone, rich in MHC-peptide/TCR complex surrounded by an integrin ring called SMAC (for supramolecular activation cluster). In this zone, CD4+ and CD8+ molecules are progressively replaced by CD28 and CTLA-4.[63]

Other couplings of co-stimulatory molecules from the TNF-TNF family receptors such as CD40/CD40-L or RANK/RANK-L participate in T-cell activation. Their interactions lead to the upregulation of OX40-L on DC membranes. Interaction between OX40-L and OX40, expressed on activated T cells, induces an overexpression of CD80 and CD86 and thus a better T-cell activation, which is relevant for CS because mice deficient for OX40-L display a dramatic decrease in CS reaction to oxazolone, DNFB, and FITC. This poor CS response was due to deficient T-cell priming as shown by decreased T-cell proliferation induced by DC from OX40-L-deficient mice.[64]

## 4. T-Cell Polarization and Constitution of CD4+ and CD8+ T-Cell Populations

Classically, two distinct roles have been attributed to CD4+ and CD8+ T-cell subsets in immunological responses. CD4+ T cells, or T helper (Th) cells, are considered as sources of cytokines and help establish B- and T-specific responses. CD8+ T cells are associated with cytotoxic functions, cleaning of potentially dangerous cells, and produce mainly interferon-gamma (IFN-γ) and TNF-α. However, more recent studies on T-cell subsets have revealed that CD8+ T cells can synthesize a pattern of cytokines as large as that produced by CD4+ T cells.[65] Moreover, CD4+ T cell functions are not restricted to T-cell help or cytokine secretion and may comprise cytotoxicity.[66]

Depending on the pattern of cytokine secretion, different functional subpopulations of T lymphocytes serve to determine the qualitative aspects of the adaptative immune response. CD4+ Th1 cells produce IFN-γ, IL-2, and TNF-α, and CD4+ Th2 cells produce IL-4, IL-10, IL-13, and IL-5. Similarly, Tc1 cells produce type 1 cytokines (IFN-γ, IL-2, and TNF-α) and Tc2 cells type 2 cytokines (IL-4, IL-10, IL-13, and IL-5). However, Tc2 cells could also produce TNF-α in some conditions.[65] A simplification of the nomenclature is the use of "type 1" and "type 2" cytokine pattern for either CD4+ or CD8+ T cells.

For CD4+ and CD8+ T cells, orientation through one or the other subtypes is dependent on comparable environmental factors.[67] *In vitro* treatment of APC/T-cell mixtures with IL-4 plus anti-IFN-γ mAb polarizes T cells to a type 2 phenotype, whereas IL-12 plus anti-IL-4 mAb treatment polarizes T cells to a type 1 phenotype. However, the mechanisms implicated during the T cell–DC dialogue *in vivo* responsible for the polarization of T cells are still poorly understood.

Two hypotheses have been recently proposed to explain the basis of the dichotomy of T-cell responses. The first hypothesis postulates the existence of distinct DC subpopulations (DC1 vs. DC2) involved in the polarization of the immune response (type 1 vs. type 2). After CD40 triggering, one subpopulation of DC, derived from monocytes in humans or expressing CD8α in mouse (myeloid), referred to as DC1, would provoke a type 1 response by producing high amounts of IL-12. The other subpopulation, derived from plasmacytoid DC in human and CD8α− in mouse (lymphoid) and defined as DC2, produces few IL–12 and might be able to induce a type 2 response.[68] However, CD8α− cells can prime both type 1 and type 2 responses depending on the activation signal they receive,[69,70] demonstrating that the phenotype of a given DC subset cannot be considered a marker of functionality for the activation of type 1 vs. type 2 T cells. The second hypothesis considers that environmental factors will influence the maturation process of a given DC enabling it to prime for type 1 or type 2 T cells.[71] Along this line, Soumelis et al.[72] have reported that human epithelial cells produce a cytokine, thymic stromal lymphopoietin (TSLP), that binds to specific receptors on CD11c+ DCs. This induces the production of Th2-attracting chemokines and primes naïve T cells for a Th2 phenotype.

Polarization of type 1 T cells is crucial to the development of specific effector T-cell populations and optimal CS reaction. CS to DNFB is due to CD8+ effector type 1 T cells and is regulated by CD4+ type 2 T cells.[73,74] Type 1 polarization by injection of IL-12 at the time of sensitization favors CD8+ T-cell differentiation and increases the CS reaction.[75] On the contrary, type 2 polarization using IL-4 (or anti-IFN-γ mAbs) leads to a diminished CS response associated with an altered CD8+ T-cell priming.[75]

## 5. Need for CD4+ Help in Hapten-Specific CD8+ Responses?

CS to strong haptens is mediated by CD8+ T cells and regulated by CD4+ T cells. More importantly, CD8+ effectors can develop in the absence of CD4+ T cells. This has been demonstrated by different sets of experiments: (1) mice depleted in CD8+ T cells or deficient in CD8+ T cells — MHC class I-KO (knockout) mice — cannot develop CS responses; (2) mice depleted in CD4+ T cells or genetically deficient in CD4+ T cells (MHC class II-KO mice) develop an enhanced CS response; (3) DC recovered from MHC class I-deficient mice cannot sensitize for CS in transfer experiments, whereas DC recovered from MHC class II-deficient mice are able to induce a normal CS reaction.[73,76–82]

That CD4+ T-cell help is not necessary for development of CHS is in keeping with recent studies showing that antigen-specific cytotoxic T lymphocyte (CTL) responses can be induced in the absence of help provided that (1) the immunogen has intrinsic pro-inflammatory properties (e.g., endotoxins and pathogenic microorganisms) able to generate a danger signal to the DC,[83] (2) the affinity of TCR for MHC/peptide complexes is high; (3) the frequency of specific CD8+ T-cell precursors is high.[84] Contact-sensitizing haptens have two important properties that may explain their immunogenicity in the absence of CD4+ help. First, they are pro-inflammatory xenobiotics through induction of chemokine and cytokine production by skin cells.[3] Second, covalent binding of haptens, such as DNFB or TNCB, on amino acid residues of proteins generates a high number of haptenated peptides allowing activation of high numbers of CTL precursors.[85]

### 6. Migration of Specific T Cells in the Blood and in the Skin

Once activated, T cells emigrate from the LN through the efferent lymphatic vessels and then circulate in the blood. Emigration of T cells outside the LN is associated with modifications in the expression of chemokine and adressine receptors. Different subsets of T cells are generated during an immune response. A subset of activated specific T cells downregulates the expression of CCR7 and then loses the ability to recirculate into the LN. The CCR7 T cells constitute the peripheral memory T-cell subsets able to enter peripheral tissues and especially the skin. CCR7-T cells constitute the other memory subset called central memory T cells, which has kept the ability to recirculate from the blood to LN, but which cannot be recruited in peripheral tissues.[86] Upon a subsequent antigen challenge, peripheral memory T cells may act as innate cells in respect to their quick and strong release of IFN-$\gamma$ and RANTES, which confer an increased efficiency in the T-cell response. The central memory T cells play a role in the preservation of relative high frequency of hapten-specific T cells.

$CD4^+$ and $CD8^+$ T cells found in the skin of sensitized mice express CCR4, $\alpha4\beta1$ integrin, and cutaneous lymphocyte antigen (CLA).[87] Skin-selective homing of primed T cells depends on tissue microenvironment and more specifically on skin DC.[88] Migration of T cells from the blood to the skin occurs at the site of postcapillary HEV through interactions of CLA and CCR4 with their respective ligands, E-, P-selectin, and TARC (CCL17), constitutively expressed on endothelial cells.[89–92] The passage of T cells in the dermis requires the sequential interaction of VLA-4 and LFA-1 receptors on T cells with VCAM-1 and ICAM-1 on endothelial cells.[93]

Thus, at the end of the afferent phase of CHS, specific T cells that have been activated by hapten-bearing DC are found in the LN (central memory cells), in the blood, and in the skin (peripheral memory cells). The skin has a normal looking appearance. Specific T cells will be activated directly in the skin and massively recruited upon a subsequent skin contact with the same hapten.

## C. Expression of Contact Sensitivity Reaction

Hapten skin painting in sensitized individuals induces the skin inflammatory reaction, which occurs in three steps. First, activation of the skin innate immunity recruits hapten-specific T cells. Second, T cells are activated, produce IFN-$\gamma$ and cytotoxicity, which results in the activation of skin resident cells and in the production of new mediators of the inflammatory reaction. Third, leukocytes (polymorphonuclears, monocytes, T cells) are recruited and progressively induce the morphological changes typical of contact dermatitis.

### 1. T-Cell Recruitment

Skin contact with the hapten induces, as during the sensitization phase, the release of TNF-$\alpha$ and IL-1$\beta$,[94,95] followed by the production of cytokines and chemokines. This first signal induces the recruitment of hapten-specific T cells from the blood to the dermis and the epidermis. One of characteristic features of CS consists of the early recruitment of type 1 $CD8^+$ effector T cells followed by a late arrival of the $CD4^+$ T-cell population, which contains the regulatory T cells responsible for the resolution of the inflammation.[96]

That $CD8^+$ and $CD4^+$ T cells are recruited at different times after hapten painting may be explained by the differential expression of chemokine receptors by T-cell subsets as well as by the sequential production of chemokines during the development of the skin inflammation. Even if it is still unclear which chemokines drive the initial influx of T cells, the recruitment of activated $CD8^+$ T cells seems under the control of the IP-10/CXCR3 chemokine/chemokine receptor pathway.[97–99] The contribution of IP-10 (CXCL10) has been recently suggested by a study showing that

IP-10-deficient mice present a deficient skin recruitment in IFN-γ-producing T cells and a diminished CS reaction.[100] The recruitment of CD4+ T cells is possibly under the control of the MDC (CCL22) and TARC (CCL17) chemokines and their receptor CCR4 expressed on activated CD4+ T cells.[92] These two chemokines are upregulated in the skin around 12 h after hapten exposure concomitantly with the infiltration of mononuclear cells. Another recently described chemokine, CTACK (CCL27), and its receptor CCR10 are also important in the traffic of activated T cells in the skin.[101,102] This chemokine is constitutively expressed by keratinocytes and its synthesis is upregulated following IL-1β and TNF-α exposure.

In parallel with chemokines and chemokine receptors, adhesion molecules (CLA, VLA-4, and LFA-1) are involved in the infiltration of T cells in the skin. Under the influence of TNF-α, endothelial cells upregulate their respective ligands (E-, P-selectin, VCAM-1, and ICAM-1) allowing a direct interaction with T cells and their extravasation in the dermis.

### 2. Characterization of Effector T Cells

During the 1980s, studies from Cher and colleagues[103] clearly established that classical delayed-type hypersensitivity (DTH) to nominal protein antigens was mediated by CD4+ T cells. The overrepresentation of CD4+ T cells in established ACD lesions and the presence of hapten-specific CD4+ T cells in the blood of sensitized patients[104,105] have led to the wrong conclusion that CS was mediated by CD4+ T cells.

Animals models have contributed to elucidate the nature of the effector T-cell population in CS. Mice deficient in CD8+ T cells, following the invalidation of the MHC class I β2 microglobulin gene, or mice depleted in CD8+ T cells are unable to develop a CS reaction to experimental haptens.[73] However, lack of CD8+ T cells in these mice does not affect the classical DTH to proteins. Alternatively, mice deficient in CD4+ T cells, following the invalidation of the MHC class II Aβ gene, or mice depleted in CD4+ T cells develop a stronger and sustained CS reaction, suggesting a regulatory function for the CD4+ T-cell compartment.[73] Thus, CS appears as very different from classical DTH reactions in term of T-cell subset involved in the effector pro-inflammatory functions. Recent studies on nickel ACD have confirmed that the pathophysiology of ACD in humans was similar to that of CS in mice and involved CD8+ effector T cells and CD4+ regulatory T cells.[106]

### 3. IFN-γ Production by CD8+ T Cells

Once in the skin, type 1 CD8+ T cells recognize hapten-modified peptides presented by cutaneous cells. In part due to their chemical properties, haptens are able to cross through plasmic cell membranes, to bind to intracellular proteins, and are then presented in an MHC class I context by resident skin cells. It is certainly by this mechanism, or by a direct binding to external MHC I/peptide complexes, that haptenated peptides are presented to CD8+ T cells.[10,51]

TCR engagement induces the release of type 1 cytokines such as IFN-γ, which in turn is responsible for the increased production in the skin of IP-10, IP-9, and Mig, of IL-1, IL-6, TNF-α, GM-CSF, and MIP-2 (CXCL8). This complex cytokine and chemokine production amplifies the inflammatory response initiated by the hapten (IL-1, TNF-α) and is responsible for the massive infiltration of leukocytes. Recruited cells comprise polynuclear neutrophils, T cells, and inflammatory monocytes able to differentiate into macrophages and DC.

Resident mast cells recently have been proposed to be key regulators of the amplification phase of skin inflammation.[107] Indeed, following CD8+ T-cell activation, mast cells produce TNF-α and MIP-2, which are both needed for the recruitment of neutrophils constitutively expressing CXCR1 and 2.

### 4. Cytotoxic Activity of CD8+ T Cells

IFN-γ release by CD8+ T cells is not sufficient for the full development of the CS reaction, since CS is only moderately impaired in mice deficient for IFN-γ receptors.[108] Recent studies have shown that CD8+ T-cell cytotoxicity was mandatory for the development of CS responses since mice deficient in the two cytotoxic pathways, i.e., Fas/Fas-L and perforin, were unable to develop a CS reaction, although IFN-γ-producing CD8+ T cells were detected at the site of hapten challenge.[109] Moreover, the two CD8+ CTL pathways are redundant since abrogation of CS occurs only when the two pathways are inactivated in the same animal. Thus, the CD8+ T cells are effectors of CHS through cytotoxicity.

Keratinocytes are the main targets of the cytotoxic effect of hapten-specific CD8+ T cells.[110] Keratinocyte apoptosis coincides with CD8+ T-cell arrival in the epidermis and increases proportionally with the number of infiltrating CD8+ T cells.[96] This epidermal damage facilitates the penetration of haptens present on the skin that may increase the inflammation.[111] Finally, perforin release by CD8+ T cell is associated to the production of RANTES, MIP-1α, and MIP-1β, which mediate the recruitment of CCR1+ and CCR5+ monocytes and granulocytes.[112]

In summary, hapten-specific type 1 T-cell activation leads to the production of a cascade of cytokines and chemokines by skin cells that induce a massive recruitment of leukocytes responsible for the cutaneous changes typical of CS. After a peak obtained at 24 to 48 h, the inflammation starts to resolve slowly by active downregulatory mechanisms, which limit the tissular damages and maintain skin integrity.

## D. Regulation of Contact Sensitivity

Downregulation of CS was initially attributed to clearance of the hapten from the skin in the few days following hapten painting. However, recent studies have shown that a hapten could stay in the epidermis for as long as 2 weeks after a single skin contact.[12] In parallel, several groups have reported that the downregulation of CS was an active immune phenomenon mediated by a subset of suppressor/regulatory CD4+ T cells.[73,81,113] Several CD4+ T cell subsets with downregulatory activities have been described in murine models and in human diseases, among which are Th2 cells, Th3 cells, Tr1 cells, and CD4+25+ cells, which could be involved in the resolution of the CS reaction.[114]

The regulation of CS could be divided into two phases, a central and peripheral phase.[115,116] The central regulatory phase controls the expansion and differentiation of CD8+ effector T cells in the LN while the peripheral phase limits the inflammatory process generated in the skin. CD4+CD25+ natural regulatory T cells seem to be involved in the first phase. Indeed, a recent study has shown that CD4+CD25+ T cells are necessary in the oral tolerance phenomenon to haptens through the total inhibition of the clonal expansion of hapten-specific CD8+ T cells.[114,117] Moreover, mice treated with an IL-2–IgG2b fusion protein showed a decreased CS reaction associated with an increase in the CD4+CD25+ T-cell subset.[118] Finally, depletion of CD4+25+ T cells by *in vivo* treatment of mice with an anti-CD25 mAb at the time of sensitization led to an enhanced CS reaction and an increased CD8+ T-cell priming (B. Dubois and D. Kaiserlian, unpublished data).

The mechanisms by which CD4+ T cells (CD4+25+ and/or CD4+25− T cells) limit the skin inflammatory reaction are still not understood and may involve IL-10 and other immunosuppressive cytokines.[106] The immunosuppressive effect occurs through the inhibition of production of IFN-γ, IL-6, IL-1, GM-CSF, and TNF-α. IL-10 plays a crucial role in the downregulation of CS reactions inasmuch as IL-10-deficient mice mount an exaggerated CS reaction to oxazolone, increased in both magnitude and duration as compared to wild-type mice. Moreover, IL-10 injection before challenge totally abrogated the CS response.[119] Finally, resolution of CS is associated with the recruitment in the skin of a regulatory CCR8+ T-cell population, which produces a large amount of IL-10 around 24 h postchallenge.[120] The production of IL-10 is not restricted to T cells and can be supplied locally by other cells such as keratinocytes, which synthesize the cytokine by 48 to 72 h after hapten painting.[121]

Other regulatory mechanisms may be involved in the resolution of CS. As an example, in the presence of a large quantity of IFN-γ, endothelial cells downregulate the expression of E- and P-selectins, thereby limiting the arrival of new infiltrating leukocytes in the dermis.[122]

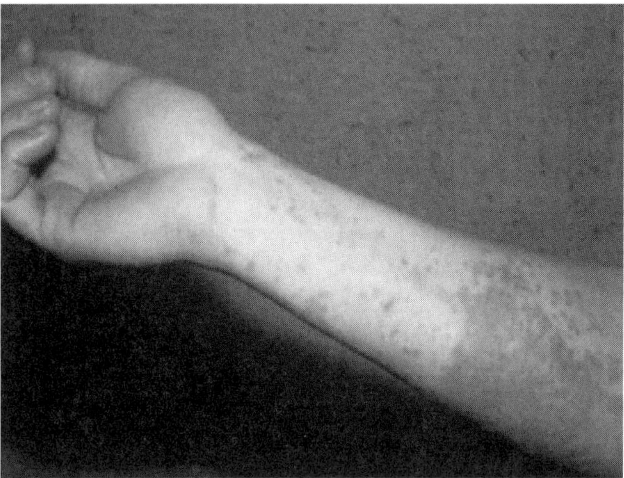

**FIGURE 31.2** Clinical aspect of ACD.

## IV. CLINICAL HALLMARKS

In a sensitized individual, ACD appears 24 to 96 h after contact with the causative allergen. Its initial localization is at the site of contact.[2] The edges of the lesions may be well demarcated, but unlike irritant contact dermatitis it may propagate in the immediate vicinity or to distant unrelated sites (Figure 31.2). In its acute phase, ACD is characterized by erythema and edema, followed by the appearance of papules, closely set vesicles, oozing, and crusting. In the chronic stages, the involved skin becomes lichenified, fissured, and pigmented, but new episodes of oozing and crusting may occur, usually as a consequence of a new exposure to the causative allergen. ACD is usually accompanied by intense pruritus. Systemically induced eczema or hematogenous contact dermatitis is induced by oral or parenteral application of certain contact allergens in previously sensitized individuals. The best-known example is the "flare-up" phenomenon at sites of previous eczematous skin changes following an experimental challenge by oral or parenteral application. Substances most often implicated in inducing hematogenous contact eczema are metal salts and drugs.

## V. HISTOPATHOLOGY OF ALLERGIC CONTACT DERMATITIS

The histopathologic findings are different in acute and chronic contact dermatitis and are dependent on the severity of the inflammatory reaction. The most common histologic feature is spongiosis, which results from intercellular edema (Figure 31.3). It is often limited to the lower epidermis but, if the reaction is severe, it may affect the upper layers. The clinical expression of intense fluid accumulation in the acute stage is the formation of vesicles that may rupture at the epidermal surface. The papillary vessels are dilated, with perivascular lymphohistiocytic infiltrate, and the upper dermis is edematous. The lymphohistiocytic infiltrate extends in the epidermis (exocytosis) and accumulates in the spongiotic vesicles. In subacute and chronic ACD the spongiotic pattern gradually fades out, the epidermis becomes hyperplastic, and parakeratosis develops.

## VI. DIAGNOSIS

The site and clinical appearance of the lesions frequently suggest the etiologic factor when the patient is first seen. Thus, sharply delineated geometric lesions are evocative of sensitivity to rosin in adhesive tape.[123] Dermatitis at the site of contact with jewelry, blue jeans buttons, wristwatches,

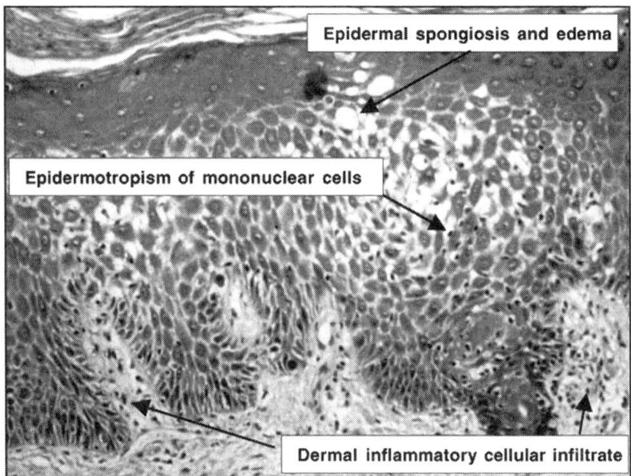


**FIGURE 31.3** Histopathologic features of ACD.

and other metallic objects are seen in nickel dermatitis. It is important to know the location of the initial skin changes and to try to establish a list of possible contactants that may have caused them. If the dermatitis has taken a chronic course, the patient's observations about factors causing relapses may be helpful. A search for possible sources should concentrate on occupation, hobbies, clothing and personal objects, home environment, and past and previous treatment. Inhalants, dust exposure, and ingestion have to be considered. A family history or a past history of atopy and psoriasis may be decisive, particularly when a diagnosis of hand eczema is discussed.

*Patch testing* is the universally accepted method for the detection of the causative contact allergens. The positive patch test reproduces an experimental contact dermatitis on a limited area of the skin. A good patch test indicates contact sensitization of past or present relevance and produces no false-positive reaction. Based on the principles of evidence-based medicine, patch testing is cost-effective only if patients are selected on the basis of a clear-cut clinical suspicion of contact allergy and only if patients are tested with chemicals relevant to the problem.[124] Finn chambers and several other tape methods are currently in use.[125] Most allergens used in patch testing are well-defined chemical substances. To save time, mixes of chemically related chemicals may be used. The most frequently encountered contact allergens have been selected by various international contact dermatitis groups and included in standard patch test series.[126] There are additional series aimed toward specific occupations and other spheres of activities. Most commercially available allergens supplied in syringes are incorporated in petrolatum. Considerable efforts have been made to standardize the concentration of the allergens to ensure comparable results worldwide. Great care must be taken in testing with nonstandardized chemicals not found in commercially available kits because testing with irritant concentrations may result in false-positive reactions.[127]

Patch tests are usually applied for 48 h on the upper half of the back. Patches are read at least 20 min after their removal. The method of recording recommended by the European and North American contact dermatitis groups is as follows:[128]

| | |
|---|---|
| + | Weak positive reaction: erythema, infiltration, possibly papules |
| ++ | Strong positive reaction: erythema, infiltration, papules, vesicles |
| +++ | Extreme positive reaction: intense erythema and infiltration, coalescing vesicles, bullous reaction |
| ? | doubtful reaction (weak erythema only) |
| IR | irritant reaction of different types |
| NR | negative reaction |
| NT | not tested |

Performing a second reading 24 or 48 h after patch test removal is recommended. In doing only a single reading, a large number of delayed reactions will be missed, while others due to early irritant effects will be considered allergic.[127] The type of positive reaction that can safely be interpreted as indicating allergic contact sensitivity exhibits erythema, edema, and small vesicles extending slightly beyond the patch border. Pruritus and reactivation of previous eczematous skin lesions at the time of testing indicate allergy.

When a positive patch test is considered to reveal a genuine contact sensitivity, a decision has to be made regarding its relevance. Current relevance is related to "current clinical symptoms, occurring in the last few days or weeks"; past relevance refers to older clinical events.[129] The major prerequisites for a contact allergy to be clinically relevant are (1) exposure to the sensitizer; (2) presence of a dermatitis that is understandable and explainable with regard to the exposure, on the one hand, and type, localization, and course of the dermatitis, on the other hand.[130]

## VII. COMMON CAUSES OF ALLERGIC CONTACT DERMATITIS

### A. Metals

Nickel is the most common cause of ACD in women in almost all countries. The greater exposure of women to high-nickel-content jewelry is a predisposing factor. Ear piercing is considered to be the principal inducer of nickel contact dermatitis. Hand eczema in nickel-sensitive patients is often of the dyshidrotic type and may be aggravated by nickel ingestion. A threshold of 0.5 μg of nickel/$cm^2$/week has been established to which only a small number of nickel-sensitive patients will react.[131] The Danish nickel exposure regulation and the nickel directive (European Union) regulating nickel content in objects that are in direct and prolonged contact with the skin have resulted in a significant decrease in nickel sensitization in young patients.[132,133]

Chromate is the most common contact allergen in men and sensitization to it is usually occupational. Occupational exposure is most frequent in construction workers who handle cement. Other common sources are chrome-tanned leather, bleaching agents, paints, and printing solutions.

### B. Cosmetics and Skin Care Products

Compulsory ingredient labeling of cosmetic products (excluding perfumes) has greatly facilitated the diagnosis and treatment of cosmetic contact dermatitis. Positive patch tests are found most frequently to preservatives, perfumes, active or category-specific ingredients, excipients/emulsifiers, and sunscreens.[134] The relevance of the positive patch tests is confirmed if the contact dermatitis disappears upon discontinuation of the use of the product. Most allergic reactions are caused by cosmetics that remain on the skin: "stay-on" or "leave-on" products.[135]

### C. Dermatitis from Clothes and Shoes

Contact dermatitis to clothes is usually located in the axillae, which is due to the release of allergens from the textile under the action of sweat and friction. Clothing dermatitis from formaldehyde is rare nowadays. Textile dye dermatitis is usually related to disperse dyes.[136] Leather articles contain several substances that may cause ACD: chrome, adhesives (paratertiary butyl phenol formaldehyde resin), and dyes. A number of accelerators and antioxidants used in the production of synthetic rubber may also cause contact dermatitis.

### D. Drug Dermatitis

Drug dermatitis may be elicited by the active ingredient of a topical drug, by the vehicle, or by a preservative. Contact sensitization to antibiotics, antiseptics, and anesthetics is relatively frequent, especially in patients with leg ulcer. ACD from topical corticosteroids has been reported with increasing frequency.[137,138] Systemic application of a drug to which an individual has been sensitized by a previous cutaneous exposure may cause systemic contact dermatitis.

### E. Plant Dermatitis

Plant dermatitis can manifest itself in a variety of ways, depending on the plant and the means of exposure. Airborne contact dermatitis mimicking photodermatitis may be caused by sesquiterpene lactones found in the Compositae family, while contact dermatitis to plants from the Liliaceae and Alstroemeriaceae families may present as a dry painful dermatitis of the fingers in bulb growers, called "tulip fingers." Urushiol, present in poison ivy and poison oak, is the most common cause of ACD in the United States, with 50% of the adult population clinically sensitive to it.

## VIII. TREATMENT

The only available etiologic treatment of ACD is elimination of the contact allergen. The patients should be informed about the identity of the offending agent and the possible sources of the sensitizer. Cross-reacting substances should be listed.

Topical steroids are used in the acute stage and are gradually replaced by ointments and cold creams as the skin lesions withdraw. If ACD is widespread and severe, systemic corticosteroids may be indicated for a short period of time.

Reducing the total body load of nickel has been attempted in nickel eczema by means of a nickel-restricted diet and by treatment with disulfiram. Trials have yielded conflicting results regarding the clinical effect of the treatment, and the application of the metal-chelator disulfiram was limited by serious side effects.[139] Oral hyposensitization to urushiol and nickel has been attempted but is not performed in practice.

Conventional immunosuppressive therapy is not appropriate in the management of ACD. New immunomodulating macrolactams have been successfully tested in clinical trials.[140–142] Perspectives in pharmacological intervention include new classes of immunosuppressors, inhibitors of cellular metabolic activity, inhibitors of cell adhesion molecules, targeted skin application of regulatory cytokines, and neutralization of pro-inflammatory cytokines (antisense oligonucleoides, anticytokine antibodies, soluble cytokine receptors).

## IX. CONCLUSION

Recent advances in the mechanisms by which haptens can generate a specific T-cell activation leading to ACD have strengthened the importance of hapten presentation by LC to specific T cells. The induction of ACD depends on the production by epidermal cells, within minutes or hours following hapten application, of a rather specific pattern of cytokines. This cytokine milieu seems necessary for efficient hapten handling by LC and for T-cell priming in the regional draining lymph nodes. More recently, it was demonstrated that LC have a dual function in the pathophysiology of ACD. On the one hand, LC activate effector cells that mediate the inflammatory reaction aimed at eliminating the potentially harmful haptens. On the other hand, LC are able to activate regulatory cells that limit the skin inflammation. These regulatory cells are extremely important for the outcome of ACD, since their absence will lead to a chronic skin inflammation with major tissue damage. Although $CD4^+$ T cells have been shown to comprise regulatory cells in ACD, the molecular mechanisms by which they exert their regulatory properties are at present unknown. Ongoing studies will undoubtedly provide more information on how $CD4^+$ regulatory T cells could be specifically activated and thus provide new ways of treating ACD.

## ACKNOWLEDGMENTS

This work was supported by the Region Rhône Alpes Grant 8HC07H and by Institutional Grants from INSERM. Pierre Saint-Mezard is supported by Laboratoire BIODERMA, Lyon, France.

## REFERENCES

1. Uter, W., Schnuch, A., Geier, J., and Frosch, P.J., Epidemiology of contact dermatitis. The information network of departments of dermatology (IVDK) in Germany. *Eur. J. Dermatol.* 8, 36–40, 1998.
2. Krasteva, M. et al., Contact dermatitis II. Clinical aspects and diagnosis. *Eur. J. Dermatol.* 9, 144–59, 1999).
3. Krasteva, M. et al., Contact dermatitis I. Pathophysiology of contact sensitivity. *Eur. J. Dermatol.* 9, 65–77, 1999.
4. Lepoittevin, J. and Leblond, I., Hapten-peptide T cell receptor interactions: molecular basis for the recognition of haptens by T lymphocytes. *Eur. J. Dermatol.* 7, 151–154, 1997.
5. Dupuis, G.B., Nature of hapten-protein interactions. Chemically reactive function in haptens and proteins, in *Allergic Contact Dermatitis to Simple Chemicals. A Molecular Approach,* C.D. Calnan and H.I. Maibach, Eds., Marcel Dekker, New York, 1982.
6. Berard, F., Marty, J.P., and Nicolas, J.F., Allergen penetration through the skin. *Eur. J. Dermatol.* 13, 324–330, 2003.
7. Dupuis, G., Studies on poison ivy. *In vitro* lymphocyte transformation by urushiol-protein conjugates. *Br. J. Dermatol.* 101, 617–624, 1979.
8. Saloga, J., Knop, J., and Kolde, G., Ultrastructural cytochemical visualization of chromium in the skin of sensitized guinea pigs. *Arch. Dermatol. Res.* 280, 214–219, 1988.
9. Anderson, C. et al., Metabolic requirements for induction of contact hypersensitivity to immunotoxic polyaromatic hydrocarbons. *J. Immunol.* 155, 3530–3537, 1995.
10. Martin, S., Ortmann, B., Pflugfelder, U., Birsner, U., and Weltzien, H.U., Role of hapten-anchoring peptides in defining hapten-epitopes for MHC-restricted cytotoxic T cells. Cross-reactive TNP-determinants on different peptides. *J. Immunol.* 149, 2569–2575, 1992.
11. Vigan, M., Girardin, P., Adessi, B., and Laurent, R. Late reading of patch tests. *Eur. J. Dermatol.* 7, 574–576, 1997.
12. Saint-Mezard, P. et al., Afferent and efferent phases of allergic contact dermatitis (ACD) can be induced after a single skin contact with haptens: evidence using a mouse model of primary ACD. *J. Invest. Dermatol.* 120, 641–647, 2003.
13. Toews, G.B., Bergstresser, P.R., and Streilein, J.W., Epidermal Langerhans cell density determines whether contact hypersensitivity or unresponsiveness follows skin painting with DNFB. *J. Immunol.* 124, 445–453, 1980.
14. Lynch, D.H., Gurish, M.F., and Daynes, R.A., Relationship between epidermal Langerhans cell density ATPase activity and the induction of contact hypersensitivity. *J. Immunol.* 126, 1892–1897, 1981.
15. Ptak, W., Rozycka, D., Askenase, P.W., and Gershon, R.K., Role of antigen-presenting cells in the development and persistence of contact hypersensitivity. *J. Exp. Med.* 151, 362–375, 1980.
16. Tamaki, K., Fujiwara, H., Levy, R.B., Shearer, G.M., and Katz, S.I., Hapten specific TNP-reactive cytotoxic effector cells using epidermal cells as targets. *J. Invest. Dermatol.* 77, 225–229, 1981.
17. Girolomoni, G. et al., Establishment of a cell line with features of early dendritic cell precursors from fetal mouse skin. *Eur. J. Immunol.* 25, 2163–2169, 1995.
18. Caux, C., Pathways of development of human dendritic cells. *Eur. J. Dermatol.* 8, 375–384, 1998.
19. Kurimoto, I., Grammer, S.F., Shimizu, T., Nakamura, T., and Streilein, J.W., Role of F4/80$^+$ cells during induction of hapten-specific contact hypersensitivity. *Immunology* 85, 621–629, 1995.
20. Geissmann, F., Jung, S., and Littman, D.R., Blood monocytes consist of two principal subsets with distinct migratory properties. *Immunity* 19, 71–82, 2003.
21. Taylor, P.R., and Gordon, S., Monocyte heterogeneity and innate immunity. *Immunity* 19, 2–4, 2003.
22. Frey, J.R. and Wenk, P., Experimental studies on the pathogenesis of contact eczema in the guinea-pig. *Int. Arch. Allergy Appl. Immunol.* 11, 81–100, 1957.

23. Macatonia, S.E., Edwards, A.J., and Knight, S.C., Dendritic cells and the initiation of contact sensitivity to fluorescein isothiocyanate. *Immunology* 59, 509–514, 1986.
24. Macatonia, S.E., Knight, S.C., Edwards, A.J., Griffiths, S., and Fryer, P., Localization of antigen on lymph node dendritic cells after exposure to the contact sensitizer fluorescein isothiocyanate. Functional and morphological studies. *J. Exp. Med.* 166, 1654–167, 1987.
25. Kamath, A.T., Henri, S., Battye, F., Tough, D.F., and Shortman, K., Developmental kinetics and lifespan of dendritic cells in mouse lymphoid organs. *Blood* 100, 1734–41, 2002.
26. Enk, A.H., Angeloni, V.L., Udey, M.C., and Katz, S.I., An essential role for Langerhans cell-derived IL-1 beta in the initiation of primary immune responses in skin. *J. Immunol.* 150, 3698–3704, 1993.
27. Borkowski, T.A. et al., Expression of E-cadherin by murine dendritic cells: E-cadherin as a dendritic cell differentiation antigen characteristic of epidermal Langerhans cells and related cells. *Eur. J. Immunol.* 24, 2767–2774, 1994.
28. Schwarzenberger, K., and Udey, M.C., Contact allergens and epidermal proinflammatory cytokines modulate Langerhans cell E-cadherin expression in situ. *J. Invest. Dermatol.* 106, 553–558, 1996.
29. Wang, B. et al., Tumour necrosis factor receptor II (p75) signalling is required for the migration of Langerhans' cells. *Immunology* 88, 284–288, 1996.
30. Wang, B. et al., Depressed Langerhans cell migration and reduced contact hypersensitivity response in mice lacking TNF receptor p75. *J. Immunol.* 159, 6148–6155, 1997.
31. Tang, A., Amagai, M., Granger, L.G., Stanley, J.R., and Udey, M.C., Adhesion of epidermal Langerhans cells to keratinocytes mediated by E-cadherin. *Nature* 361, 82–85, 1993.
32. Dieu, M.C. et al., Selective recruitment of immature and mature dendritic cells by distinct chemokines expressed in different anatomic sites. *J. Exp. Med.* 188, 373–386, 1998.
33. Kobayashi, Y., Matsumoto, M., Kotani, M., and Makino, T., Possible involvement of matrix metalloproteinase-9 in Langerhans cell migration and maturation. *J. Immunol.* 163, 5989–5993, 1999.
34. Gearing, A.J. et al., Processing of tumour necrosis factor-alpha precursor by metalloproteinases. *Nature* 370, 555–557, 1994.
35. Cyster, J.G., Chemokines and the homing of dendritic cells to the T cell areas of lymphoid organs. *J. Exp. Med.* 189, 447–450, 1999.
36. Ngo, V.N. et al., Lymphotoxin alpha/beta and tumor necrosis factor are required for stromal cell expression of homing chemokines in B and T cell areas of the spleen. *J. Exp. Med.* 189, 403–412, 1999.
37. Engeman, T.M., Gorbachev, A.V., Gladue, R.P., Heeger, P.S., and Fairchild, R.L., Inhibition of functional T cell priming and contact hypersensitivity responses by treatment with anti-secondary lymphoid chemokine antibody during hapten sensitization. *J. Immunol.* 164, 5207–5214, 2000.
38. Martin-Fontecha, A. et al., Regulation of dendritic cell migration to the draining lymph node: impact on T lymphocyte traffic and priming. *J. Exp. Med.* 198, 615–621, 2003.
39. Becker, D., Neiss, U., Neis, S., Reske, K., and Knop, J., Contact allergens modulate the expression of MHC class II molecules on murine epidermal Langerhans cells by endocytotic mechanisms. *J. Invest. Dermatol.* 98, 700–705, 1992.
40. Becker, D., Mohamadzadeh, M., Reske, K., and Knop, J., Increased level of intracellular MHC class II molecules in murine Langerhans cells following *in vivo* and *in vitro* administration of contact allergens. *J. Invest. Dermatol.* 99, 545–549, 1992.
41. Pierre, P., and Mellman, I., Developmental regulation of invariant chain proteolysis controls MHC class II trafficking in mouse dendritic cells. *Cell* 93, 1135–1145, 1998.
42. Garrett, W.S. et al., Developmental control of endocytosis in dendritic cells by Cdc42. *Cell* 102, 325–334, 2000.
43. Ruedl, C., Koebel, P., and Karjalainen, K., *In vivo*-matured Langerhans cells continue to take up and process native proteins unlike *in vitro*-matured counterparts. *J. Immunol.* 166, 7178–7182, 2001.
44. Waksman, B.H., in *Cellular Hypersensitivity Immunity: Inflammation and Cytotoxicity,* C.W. Parkers, Ed., W.B. Saunders, Philadelphia, 1978, 173–218.
45. Weltzien, H.U. et al., T cell immune responses to haptens. Structural models for allergic and autoimmune reactions. *Toxicology* 107, 141–151, 1996.
46. von Bonin, A., Ortmann, B., Martin, S., and Weltzien, H.U., Peptide-conjugated hapten groups are the major antigenic determinants for trinitrophenyl-specific cytotoxic T cells. *Int. Immunol.* 4, 869–874, 1992.

47. Kohler, J., Hartmann, U., Grimm, R., Pflugfelder, U., and Weltzien, H.U., Carrier-independent hapten recognition and promiscuous MHC restriction by CD4+ T cells induced by trinitrophenylated peptides. *J. Immunol.* 158, 591–597, 1997.
48. Cavani, A., Hackett, C.J., Wilson, K.J., Rothbard, J.B., and Katz, S.I., Characterization of epitopes recognized by hapten-specific CD4+ T cells. *J. Immunol.* 154, 1232–1238, 1995.
49. Gamerdinger, K. et al., A new type of metal recognition by human T cells: contact residues for peptide-independent bridging of T cell receptor and major histocompatibility complex by nickel. *J. Exp. Med.* 197, 1345–1353, 2003.
50. Sinigaglia, F., The molecular basis of metal recognition by T cells. *J. Invest. Dermatol.* 102, 398–401, 1994.
51. Martin, S., von Bonin, A., Fessler, C., Pflugfelder, U., and Weltzien, H.U., Structural complexity of antigenic determinants for class I MHC-restricted, hapten-specific T cells. Two qualitatively differing types of H-2Kb-restricted TNP epitopes. *J. Immunol.* 151, 678–687, 1993.
52. Kalish, R.S., Wood, J.A., and LaPorte, A., Processing of urushiol (poison ivy) hapten by both endogenous and exogenous pathways for presentation to T cells *in vitro*. *J. Clin. Invest.* 93, 2039–2047, 1994.
53. Nalefski, E.A. and Rao, A., Nature of the ligand recognized by a hapten- and carrier-specific, MHC-restricted T cell receptor. *J. Immunol.* 150, 3806–3816, 1993.
54. Reiser, H. and Schneeberger, E.E., Expression and function of B7-1 and B7-2 in hapten-induced contact sensitivity. *Eur. J. Immunol.* 26, 880–885, 1996.
55. Symington, F.W., Brady, W., and Linsley, P.S., Expression and function of B7 on human epidermal Langerhans cells. *J. Immunol.* 150, 1286–1295, 1993.
56. Kondo, S., Kooshesh, F., Wang, B., Fujisawa, H., and Sauder, D.N., Contribution of the CD28 molecule to allergic and irritant-induced skin reactions in CD28$^{-/-}$ mice. *J. Immunol.* 157, 4822–4829, 1996.
57. Xu, H., Heeger, P.S., and Fairchild, R.L., Distinct roles for B7-1 and B7-2 determinants during priming of effector CD8+ Tc1 and regulatory CD4+ Th2 cells for contact hypersensitivity. *J. Immunol.* 159, 4217–4226, 1997.
58. Fraser, J.D., Irving, B.A., Crabtree, G.R., and Weiss, A., Regulation of interleukin-2 gene enhancer activity by the T cell accessory molecule CD28. *Science* 251, 313–316, 1991.
59. Boise, L.H. et al., CD28 co-stimulation can promote T cell survival by enhancing the expression of Bcl-XL. *Immunity* 3, 87–98, 1995.
60. Adema, G.J. et al., A dendritic-cell-derived C-C chemokine that preferentially attracts naive T cells. *Nature* 387, 713–717, 1997.
61. Geijtenbeek, T.B. et al., Identification of DC-SIGN, a novel dendritic cell-specific ICAM-3 receptor that supports primary immune responses. *Cell* 100, 575–585, 2000.
62. Krawczyk, C. et al., Vav1 controls integrin clustering and MHC/peptide-specific cell adhesion to antigen-presenting cells. *Immunity* 16, 331–343, 2002.
63. Monks, C.R., Freiberg, B.A., Kupfer, H., Sciaky, N., and Kupfer, A., Three-dimensional segregation of supramolecular activation clusters in T cells. *Nature* 395, 82–86, 1998.
64. Chen, A.I. et al., Ox40-ligand has a critical costimulatory role in dendritic cell:T cell interactions. *Immunity* 11, 689–698, 1999.
65. Sad, S., Marcotte, R., and Mosmann, T.R., Cytokine-induced differentiation of precursor mouse CD8+ T cells into cytotoxic CD8+ T cells secreting Th1 or Th2 cytokines. *Immunity* 2, 271–279, 1995.
66. Hahn, S. et al., Down-modulation of CD4+ T helper type 2 and type 0 cells by T helper type 1 cells via Fas/Fas-ligand interaction. *Eur. J. Immunol.* 25, 2679–2685, 1995.
67. Li, L., Sad, S., Kagi, D., and Mosmann, T.R., CD8+Tc1 and Tc2 cells secrete distinct cytokine patterns *in vitro* and *in vivo* but induce similar inflammatory reactions. *J. Immunol.* 158, 4152–4161, 1997.
68. Maldonado-Lopez, R., Maliszewski, C., Urbain, J., and Moser, M., Cytokines regulate the capacity of CD8+alpha(+) and CD8+alpha(–) dendritic cells to prime Th1/Th2 cells *in vivo*. *J. Immunol.* 167, 4345–4350, 2001.
69. Cella, M., Facchetti, F., Lanzavecchia, A., and Colonna, M., Plasmacytoid dendritic cells activated by influenza virus and CD4+0L drive a potent TH1 polarization. *Nat. Immunol.* 1, 305–310, 2000.
70. MacDonald, A.S., Straw, A.D., Bauman, B., and Pearce, E.J., CD8+- dendritic cell activation status plays an integral role in influencing Th2 response development. *J. Immunol.* 167, 1982–1988, 2001.
71. Ardavin, C. et al., Origin and differentiation of dendritic cells. *Trends Immunol.* 22, 691–700, 2001.

72. Soumelis, V. et al., Human epithelial cells trigger dendritic cell mediated allergic inflammation by producing TSLP. *Nat. Immunol.* 3, 673–680, 2002.
73. Bour, H. et al., Major histocompatibility complex class I-restricted CD8+ T cells and class II-restricted CD4+ T cells, respectively, mediate and regulate contact sensitivity to dinitrofluorobenzene. *Eur. J. Immunol.* 25, 3006–3010, 1995.
74. Xu, H., DiIulio, N.A., and Fairchild, R.L., T cell populations primed by hapten sensitization in contact sensitivity are distinguished by polarized patterns of cytokine production: interferon gamma-producing (Tc1) effector CD8+ T cells and interleukin (Il) 4/Il-10-producing (Th2) negative regulatory CD4+ T cells. *J. Exp. Med.* 183, 1001–1012, 1996.
75. Gorbachev, A.V., DiIulio, N.A., and Fairchild, R.L., IL-12 augments CD8+ T cell development for contact hypersensitivity responses and circumvents anti-CD154 antibody-mediated inhibition. *J. Immunol.* 167, 156–162, 2001.
76. Gocinski, B.L. and Tigelaar, R.E., Roles of CD4+ and CD8+ T cells in murine contact sensitivity revealed by *in vivo* monoclonal antibody depletion. *J. Immunol.* 144, 4121–4128, 1990.
77. Bouloc, A., Cavani, A., and Katz, S.I., Contact hypersensitivity in MHC class II-deficient mice depends on CD8+ T lymphocytes primed by immunostimulating Langerhans cells. *J. Invest. Dermatol.* 111, 44–49, 1998.
78. Kolesaric, A., Stingl, G., and Elbe-Burger, A., MHC class I+/II- dendritic cells induce hapten-specific immune responses *in vitro* and *in vivo*. *J. Invest. Dermatol.* 109, 580–585, 1997.
79. Krasteva, M. et al., Dual role of dendritic cells in the induction and down-regulation of antigen-specific cutaneous inflammation. *J. Immunol.* 160, 1181–1190, 1998.
80. Martin, S. et al., Peptide immunization indicates that CD8+ T cells are the dominant effector cells in trinitrophenyl-specific contact hypersensitivity. *J. Invest. Dermatol.* 115, 260–266, 2000.
81. Xu, H., DiIulio, N.A., and Fairchild, R.L., T cell populations primed by hapten sensitization in contact sensitivity are distinguished by polarized patterns of cytokine production: interferon gamma-producing (Tc1) effector CD8+ T cells and interleukin (Il) 4/Il-10-producing (Th2) negative regulatory CD4+ T cells. *J. Exp. Med.* 183, 1001–1012, 1996.
82. Xu, H., Banerjee, A., Dilulio, N.A., and Fairchild, R.L., Development of effector CD8+ T cells in contact hypersensitivity occurs independently of CD4+ T cells. *J. Immunol.* 158, 4721–4728, 1997.
83. Matzinger, P., The danger model: a renewed sense of self. *Science* 296, 301–305, 2002.
84. Wang, B. et al., Multiple paths for activation of naive CD8+ T cells: CD4+-independent help. *J. Immunol.* 167, 1283–1289, 2001.
85. Martin, S. et al., A high frequency of allergen-specific CD8+ Tc1 cells is associated with the murine immune response to the contact sensitizer trinitrophenyl. *Exp. Dermatol.* 12, 78–85, 2003.
86. Sallusto, F., Lenig, D., Forster, R., Lipp, M., and Lanzavecchia, A., Two subsets of memory T lymphocytes with distinct homing potentials and effector functions. *Nature* 401, 708–712, 1999.
87. Santamaria-Babi, L.F., CLA+ T cells in cutaneous diseases. *Eur. J. Dermatol.* 14, 13–18, 2004.
88. Dudda, J.C., Simon, J.C., and Martin, S., Dendritic cell immunization route determines CD8+ T cell trafficking to inflamed skin: role for tissue microenvironment and dendritic cells in establishment of T cell-homing subsets. *J. Immunol.* 172, 857–863, 2004.
89. Berg, E.L. et al., The cutaneous lymphocyte antigen is a skin lymphocyte homing receptor for the vascular lectin endothelial cell-leukocyte adhesion molecule 1. *J. Exp. Med.* 174, 1461–1466, 1991.
90. Campbell, J.J. et al., The chemokine receptor CCR4 in vascular recognition by cutaneous but not intestinal memory T cells. *Nature* 400, 776–780, 1999.
91. Erdmann, I. et al., Fucosyltransferase VII-deficient mice with defective E-, P-, and L-selectin ligands show impaired CD4+ and CD8+ T cell migration into the skin, but normal extravasation into visceral organs. *J. Immunol.* 168, 2139–2146, 2002.
92. Reiss, Y., Proudfoot, A.E., Power, C.A., Campbell, J.J., and Butcher, E.C., CC chemokine receptor (CCR)4 and the CCR10 ligand cutaneous T cell-attracting chemokine (CTACK) in lymphocyte trafficking to inflamed skin. *J. Exp. Med.* 194, 1541–1547, 2001.
93. Santamaria, L.F., Perez Soler, M.T., Hauser, C., and Blaser, K., Allergen specificity and endothelial transmigration of T cells in allergic contact dermatitis and atopic dermatitis are associated with the cutaneous lymphocyte antigen. *Int. Arch. Allergy Immunol.* 107, 359–362, 1995.
94. Enk, A.H. and Katz, S.I., Early molecular events in the induction phase of contact sensitivity. *Proc. Natl. Acad. Sci. U.S.A.* 89, 1398–1402, 1992.

95. Heufler, C. et al., Cytokine gene expression in murine epidermal cell suspensions: interleukin 1 beta and macrophage inflammatory protein 1 alpha are selectively expressed in Langerhans cells but are differentially regulated in culture. *J. Exp. Med.* 176, 1221–1226, 1992.
96. Akiba, H. et al., Skin inflammation during contact hypersensitivity is mediated by early recruitment of $CD8^+$ T cytotoxic 1 cells inducing keratinocyte apoptosis. *J. Immunol.* 168, 3079–3087, 2002.
97. Albanesi, C. et al., A cytokine-to-chemokine axis between T lymphocytes and keratinocytes can favor Th1 cell accumulation in chronic inflammatory skin diseases. *J. Leukocyte Biol.* 70, 617–623, 2001.
98. Bonecchi, R. et al., Differential expression of chemokine receptors and chemotactic responsiveness of type 1 T helper cells (Th1s) and Th2s. *J. Exp. Med.* 187, 129–134, 1998.
99. Flier, J. et al., The CXCR3 activating chemokines IP-10, Mig, and IP-9 are expressed in allergic but not in irritant patch test reactions. *J. Invest. Dermatol.* 113, 574–578, 1999.
100. Dufour, J.H. et al., IFN-gamma-inducible protein 10 (IP-10; CXCL10)-deficient mice reveal a role for IP-10 in effector T cell generation and trafficking. *J. Immunol.* 168, 3195–3204, 2002.
101. Homey, B. et al., Cutting edge: the orphan chemokine receptor G protein-coupled receptor-2 (GPR-2, CCR10) binds the skin-associated chemokine CCL27 (CTACK/ALP/ILC). *J. Immunol.* 164, 3465–3470, 2000.
102. Homey, B. et al., CCL27-CCR10 interactions regulate T cell-mediated skin inflammation. *Nat. Med.* 8, 157–165, 2002.
103. Cher, D.J., and Mosmann, T.R., Two types of murine helper T cell clone. II. Delayed-type hypersensitivity is mediated by TH1 clones. *J. Immunol.* 138, 3688–3694, 1987.
104. Gawkrodger, D.J., Vestey, J.P., Wong, W.K., and Buxton, P.K., Contact clinic survey of nickel-sensitive subjects. *Contact Dermatitis* 14, 165–169, 1986.
105. Silvennoinen-Kassinen, S., Ikaheimo, I., Karvonen, J., Kauppinen, M., and Kallioinen, M., Mononuclear cell subsets in the nickel-allergic reaction *in vitro* and *in vivo*. *J. Allergy Clin. Immunol.* 89, 794–800, 1992.
106. Cavani, A., Albanesi, C., Traidl, C., Sebastiani, S., and Girolomoni, G., Effector and regulatory T cells in allergic contact dermatitis. *Trends Immunol.* 22, 118–120, 2001.
107. Biedermann, T. et al., Mast cells control neutrophil recruitment during T cell-mediated delayed-type hypersensitivity reactions through tumor necrosis factor and macrophage inflammatory protein 2. *J. Exp. Med.* 192, 1441–1452, 2000.
108. Saulnier, M., Huang, S., Aguet, M., and Ryffel, B., Role of interferon-gamma in contact hypersensitivity assessed in interferon-gamma receptor-deficient mice. *Toxicology* 102, 301–312, 1995.
109. Kehren, J. et al., Cytotoxicity is mandatory for $CD8^+$(+) T cell-mediated contact hypersensitivity. *J. Exp. Med.* 189, 779–786, 1999.
110. Traidl, C. et al., Disparate cytotoxic activity of nickel-specific $CD8^+$ and $CD4^+$ T cell subsets against keratinocytes. *J. Immunol.* 165, 3058–3064, 2000.
111. Trautmann, A., Akdis, M., Brocker, E.B., Blaser, K., and Akdis, C.A., New insights into the role of T cells in atopic dermatitis and allergic contact dermatitis. *Trends Immunol.* 22, 530–532, 2001.
112. Wagner, L. et al., Beta-chemokines are released from HIV-1-specific cytolytic T-cell granules complexed to proteoglycans. *Nature* 391, 908–911, 1998.
113. Gorbachev, A.V. and Fairchild, R.L. $CD4^+$(+) T cells regulate $CD8^+$(+) T cell-mediated cutaneous immune responses by restricting effector t cell development through a Fas ligand-dependent mechanism. *J. Immunol.* 172, 2286–2295, 2004.
114. Dubois, B., Chapat, L., Goubier, A., and Kaiserlian, D., $CD4^+CD25^+$ T cells as key regulators of immune responses. *Eur. J. Dermatol.* 13, 111–116, 2003.
115. Gorbachev, A.V. and Fairchild, R.L., Regulatory role of $CD4^+$ T cells during the development of contact hypersensitivity responses. *Immunol. Res.* 24, 69–77, 2001.
116. Gorbachev, A.V. and Fairchild, R.L., Induction and regulation of T-cell priming for contact hypersensitivity. *Crit. Rev. Immunol.* 21, 451–472, 2001.
117. Dubois, B., Chapat, L., Goubier, A., Papiernik, M., Nicolas, J.F., and Kaiserlian, D., Innate $CD4^+CD25^+$ regulatory T cells are required for oral tolerance and control $CD8^+$ T cells mediating skin inflammation. *Blood*, 102, 3295–3330, 2003.
118. Ruckert, R., Brandt, K., Hofmann, U., Bulfone-Paus, S., and Paus, R., IL-2-IgG2b fusion protein suppresses murine contact hypersensitivity *in vivo*. *J. Invest. Dermatol.* 119, 370–376, 2002.

119. Ferguson, T.A., Dube, P., and Griffith, T.S., Regulation of contact hypersensitivity by interleukin 10. *J. Exp. Med.* 179, 1597–1604, 1994.
120. Sebastiani, S. et al., Chemokine receptor expression and function in CD4+ T lymphocytes with regulatory activity. *J. Immunol.* 166, 996–1002, 2001.
121. Enk, A.H. and Katz, S.I., Identification and induction of keratinocyte-derived IL-10. *J. Immunol.* 149, 92–95, 1992.
122. Melrose, J., Tsurushita, N., Liu, G., and Berg, E.L., IFN-gamma inhibits activation-induced expression of E- and P-selectin on endothelial cells. *J. Immunol.* 161, 2457–2464, 1998.
123. Kanerva, L. and Alanko, K., Allergic contact dermatitis from 2-hydroxyethyl methacrylate in an adhesive on an electrosurgical earthing plate. *Eur. J. Dermatol.* 8, 521–524, 1998.
124. van der Valk, P.G., Devos, S.A., and Coenraads, P.J., Evidence-based diagnosis in patch testing. *Contact Dermatitis* 48, 121–125, 2003.
125. Suneja, T. and Belsito, D.V., Comparative study of Finn Chambers and T.R.U.E. test methodologies in detecting the relevant allergens inducing contact dermatitis. *J. Am. Acad. Dermatol.* 45, 836–839, 2001.
126. Lachapelle, J.M. et al., Proposal for a revised international standard series of patch tests. *Contact Dermatitis* 36, 121–123, 1997.
127. Loffler, H. et al., Evaluation of skin susceptibility to irritancy by routine patch testing with sodium lauryl sulfate. *Eur. J. Dermatol.* 11, 416–419, 2001.
128. Fregert, S., *Manual of Contact Dermatitis,* 2nd ed., Munksgaard, Copenhagen, 1981.
129. Lachapelle, J.M., A proposed relevance scoring system for positive allergic patch test reactions: practical implications and limitations. *Contact Dermatitis* 36, 39–43, 1997.
130. Bruze, M., What is a relevant contact allergy? *Contact Dermatitis* 23, 224–225, 1990.
131. Menne, T., Prevention of nickel allergy by regulation of specific exposures. *Ann. Clin. Lab. Sci.* 26, 133–138, 1996.
132. Jensen, C.S., Lisby, S., Baadsgaard, O., Volund, A., and Menne, T., Decrease in nickel sensitization in a Danish schoolgirl population with ears pierced after implementation of a nickel-exposure regulation. *Br. J. Dermatol.* 146, 636–642, 2002.
133. Schnuch, A., Geier, J., Lessmann, H., and Uter, W., [Decrease in nickel sensitization in young patients — successful intervention through nickel exposure regulation? Results of IVDK, 1992–2001]. *Hautarzt* 54, 626–632, 2003.
134. Goossens, A. et al., Adverse cutaneous reactions to cosmetic allergens. *Contact Dermatitis* 40, 112–113, 1999.
135. De Groot, A.C., Fatal attractiveness: the shady side of cosmetics. *Clin. Dermatol.* 16, 167–179, 1998.
136. Hatch, K.L. and Maibach, H.I., Textile dye allergic contact dermatitis prevalence. *Contact Dermatitis* 42, 187–195, 2000.
137. Rocha, N., Silva, E., Horta, M., and Massa, A., Contact allergy to topical corticosteroids 1995–2001. *Contact Dermatitis* 47, 362–363, 2002.
138. Corazza, M., Mantovani, L., Maranini, C., Bacilieri, S., and Virgili, A., Contact sensitization to corticosteroids: increased risk in long term dermatoses. *Eur. J. Dermatol.* 10, 533–535, 2000.
139. Veien, N.K., Hattel, T., and Laurberg, G., Low nickel diet: an open, prospective trial. *J. Am. Acad. Dermatol.* 29, 1002–1007, 1993.
140. Saripalli, Y.V., Gadzia, J.E., and Belsito, D.V., Tacrolimus ointment 0.1% in the treatment of nickel-induced allergic contact dermatitis. *J. Am. Acad. Dermatol.* 49, 477–482, 2003.
141. Ruzicka, T., Assmann, T., and Lebwohl, M., Potential future dermatological indications for tacrolimus ointment. *Eur. J. Dermatol.* 13, 331–342, 2003.
142. Marsland, A.M. and Griffiths, C.E., The macrolide immunosuppressants in dermatology: mechanisms of action. *Eur. J. Dermatol.* 12, 618–622, 2002.

# 32 Psoriasis

*Jörg Christoph Prinz*

## CONTENTS



## I. INTRODUCTION

Psoriasis vulgaris is a benign, principally nonlethal chronic inflammatory skin disease that may be associated with severe arthritis. Skin lesions are characterized by sharply demarcated erythematous plaques of variant size covered with silvery scaling. These changes result from intense skin inflammation with infiltration of inflammatory cells into the dermis and epidermis and strongly enhanced keratinocyte proliferation. Psoriasis has a prevalence of up 2% in Western populations. After onset it shows a chronically, often life-long relapsing course in the majority of patients. The disease is genetically determined, associated with particular human lymphocyte antigen (HLA) class I and II alleles, and there is substantial evidence that T-cell-mediated immune mechanisms play a major role in disease manifestation.

Psoriasis has been known since ancient times. Early descriptions are attributed to the *Encyclopedia of Medicine* written by Celsus (25 B.C.–A.D. 50), where it likely represents one of the subtypes of the "*impetigines*," and to the Third Book of Moses (Leviticus), chapter 13, where psoriasis is assumed behind the term *zaraath*.[1,2] It was only by the year 1801 that the thousands-of-years-old confusion of leprosy and psoriasis was resolved by the British dermatologist Robert Willan (1757–1812). He distinguished psoriasis as two disease types, "*Lepra graecorum*" and psoriasis, from leprosy; Ferdinand von Hebra finally recognized them as a common disease entity.[3]

The diagnosis of psoriasis stands for a particular skin pathology. Clinically, however, psoriasis shows marked heterogeneity, with nonpustular psoriasis of early or late onset, acute exanthematic (guttate) or chronic plaque psoriasis, localized or generalized pustular psoriasis, erythrodermic

0-8493-1959-5/05/$0.00+$1.50

psoriasis, palmo-plantar psoriasis, and psoriatic arthropathy all subsets under the main heading of psoriasis vulgaris. Polygenic predisposition and multifactorial environmental factors that influence disease onset and course add further to the complexity of the disease.

## II. EPIDEMIOLOGY AND GENETICS OF PSORIASIS

The true incidence of psoriasis is difficult to determine. The prevalence varies in different parts of the world between 0.1 and 3%. In Western industrialized nations psoriasis is estimated to affect 1.5 to 2% of the population.

Studies on families and twins clearly support a strong hereditary component of psoriasis.[4] Lomholt[5] in a comprehensive analysis on the population of the Faroe Islands observed that 91% of patients had affected relatives. The overall risk of first-degree relatives to acquire psoriasis is estimated at between 8 and 23%. The concordance in monozygotic twins is 65 to 70%, compared to 15 to 20% in dizygotic twins.[6,7]

The inherited predisposition has been mapped to several gene loci. They include PSORS1 (for *pso*riasis *s*usceptibility locus) on chromosome 6p21.3, PSORS2 on 17q, PSORS3 on 4q, PSORS4 on 1cen-q21, PSORS5 on 3q21, PSORS6 on 19p, PSORS7 on chromosome 1p, and PSORS9 on 4q31 (http://www.ncbi.nlm.nih.gov/Omim). Further potential psoriasis gene loci have been identified on chromosome 16q and 20p.[8] The loci PSORS1 on 6p21.3 and PSORS2 on 17q have been confirmed by more than one research group. Interestingly, some of these loci (PSORS2, PSORS4, and on chromosome 20p) overlap with the genetic linkage of childhood atopic eczema.[9] PSORS1 on chromosome 6 appears as the most relevant location. It carries the HLA region, which is known for its essential role in antigen presentation to T cells of the immune system, and it explains the association of psoriasis with HLA-Cw6, which appears as the major psoriatic risk allele.

The HLA-Cw*0602 allele seems to define particular psoriasis subtypes. It was present in all of 29 Caucasian patients with guttate psoriasis associated with streptococcal infection, while this allele was detected in only 20% of a control population of 604 random Caucasian donors.[10] Furthermore, it identifies type 1 psoriasis as one of two subtypes of nonpustular psoriasis that have been defined by the age of disease onset, family history, and HLA association. Type 1 psoriasis represents approximately two thirds of psoriasis patients. It is characterized by early disease onset usually before the age of 40 years, with a maximum at the age of 16 (females) or 22 (males) years. Type 1 patients express predominantly the HLA alleles HLA-Cw6, HLA-B57, and HLA-DRB1*0701 that often are inherited as an extended haplotype (HLA-Cw6-57-DRB1*0701-DQA1*0201-DQB1*0303), which is an evolutionarily conserved set of alleles that are inherited as a complex.[11] Type 2 psoriasis is characterized by a late onset with a maximum at the age of 60 (females) or 57 (males) years, and by an overrepresentation of HLA-Cw2. Other HLA alleles found more frequently in nonpustular psoriasis are A2, A24, B13, B27, B37, Cw7, Cw8, and Cw11.[12]

The association of psoriasis with the HLA-C region is not yet fully understood. Inheritance as an extended haplotype makes it difficult to assign a particular allele within this complex of alleles with a pathogenic function. Therefore, genes other than HLA-Cw6 itself, or a combination of genes within the HLA region, could actually carry the risk for psoriasis. Nair et al.[13] localized the PSORS1 locus to a 60-kb interval telomeric to HLA-C. As detected by the use of a transmission disequilibrium test, individual markers yielded significant linkage disequilibrium across most of the major histocompatibility complex (MHC). However, the strongest evidence for marker-trait disequilibrium was found in an approximately 300-kb region extending from the MICA gene to the CDSN gene.[13] Gonzalez et al.[14] suggested that the psoriasis susceptibility gene is located within a critical region of 147 kb, telomeric to HLA-C and centromeric to the corneodesmosin gene, and concluded that the association of HLA-Cw6 to psoriasis may be secondary to linkage disequilibrium. Polymorphisms of the S-gene, located 160 kb telomeric of HLA-C at 6p21.3 and coding for corneodesmosin, or of the HCR or the MICA gene have been discussed as potential candidates.[15–18] Increased expression of corneodesmosin and an altered expression of HCR within psoriatic plaques suggested that they might affect proliferation of keratinocytes.[19,20] The susceptibility to psoriasis is influenced further by polymorphisms of particular cytokine genes: interleukin-1 (IL-1), IL-6, IL-10, IL-12, tumor necrosis factor-alpha (TNF-$\alpha$).[21–24]

Together, these findings demonstrate that psoriasis is a polygenically determined disease with a major risk haplotype on chromosome 6p21.3 and various other contributing gene loci. Obviously, various genetic traits cooperate with environmental factors to produce a particular disease predisposition. This may explain why psoriasis develops in only 10% of HLA-Cw6-positive individuals, and why genome-wide linkage scans for psoriasis have not yet identified a distinct psoriasis gene.

## III. PSORIATIC SKIN LESIONS

### A. Histopathology

The common features of psoriatic skin changes are keratinocyte hyperproliferation with hyper- and parakeratosis, epidermal accumulation of neutrophilic granulocytes, and a mononuclear infiltrate with macrophages and T cells in the papillary dermis and in the epidermis. The precise histopathologic picture of psoriasis depends on stage and localization of the lesion. Early lesions display rather unspecific changes with dilatation of the papillary capillaries, edema, and an influx of T cells resembling delayed-type hypersensitivity reactions.[25] Infiltration of T cells is the earliest event within developing lesions. It is followed by epidermal changes that develop with parakeratosis (incomplete cornification) and disappearance of the granular layer. At this stage the phenomenon of the "squirting papillae" occurs, with release of neutrophilic granulocytes from the dermal capillaries.[26] The neutrophilic granulocytes may establish small, so-called Monroe microabscesses within the parakeratotic layer or, intermingled with epidermal cells, spongiform pustules of Kogoj beneath the parakeratotic stratum corneum.[27,28] Increased numbers of mast cells are observed in the dermis.[29]

The fully developed lesions are characterized by acanthosis (thickening of the epidermis), elongated rete ridges with often club-shaped dermal papillae and thinning of the suprapapillary layers of the epidermis, and elongated papillary capillaries. The granular layer is absent. Parakeratosis may be accompanied by orthohyperkeratosis. Only the intraepidermal pustules or microabscesses, however, represent fully pathognomonic features of psoriasis. A more pronounced accumulation of granulocyte is the basis of pustular psoriasis, with clinically visible spongiform macropustules in a degenerated epidermis.[30] As a particular functional alteration, lesional psoriatic keratinocytes produce antimicrobial peptides, so-called $\beta$-defensins.[31] The high concentration of $\beta$-defensins within psoriatic scales may explain the resistance of patients with psoriasis to bacterial infections, and they distinguish psoriasis from atopic eczema, where $\beta$-defensin production is virtually absent.[32,33]

### B. Gene Expression

Large-scale gene expression studies have identified more than 1300 genes with a potential role in psoriasis pathogenesis and maintenance of psoriatic inflammation.[34–36] When clustered according to biological process categories, the genes could be assigned to different functional groups. The major categories included cell organization and biogenesis, cell proliferation, mitotic cell cycle, epidermal differentiation, exocytosis, the JAK-STAT cascade, gene transcription, nitric oxide (NO) biosynthesis, neurogenesis, melanocyte biosynthesis, leukotriene metabolism, exocytosis of immune cells, and genes of the inflammatory response and of the immune response. Further analysis of immune system genes revealed the presence of many regulating cytokines and chemokines within involved skin, and markers of dendritic cell activation in uninvolved skin.[35]

Various of the lesionally expressed genes could be allocated to known psoriasis susceptibility loci: HCR, Corneodesmosin, P70, TNF: 6p21.3/PSORS1; CMRF35: 17Q25/PSORS2; chemokines, epidermal growth factors: 4q21/PSORS3; the "epidermal differentiation complex" including S100:

1q21/PSORS4; cystatin A: 3q21/PSORS5; and the leukocyte surface antigen CD37: 19p13/PSORS6.[36]

The gene clusters reflect many former approaches to the pathogenesis of psoriasis, which attributed its cause to a misregulated keratinocyte proliferation, neurogenic inflammation of the skin, misregulated eicosanoid production/metabolism, cyclic nucleotide (cAMP, cGMP) perturbations, or to autoimmune mechanisms. Recognition of the hierarchy of these events, however, came from treatment approaches that finally identified T-cell-mediated immune mechanisms as the main driving force of psoriatic skin perturbations.

## IV. PSORIASIS PATHOGENESIS: THE ROLE OF IMMUNE MECHANISMS

### A. Evidence for a Role of T Cells

The observation that cyclosporine, a generalized immunosuppressant, could dramatically alleviate severe psoriasis symptoms suggested that T cells were involved in the disease pathogenesis.[37,38] Exacerbation of psoriasis following therapeutic application of the pro-inflammatory cytokines IL-2, an essential lymphokine for T-cell activation, or of interferon-alpha (IFN-$\alpha$) or IFN-$\gamma$ furthermore suggested a role of immune mechanisms in psoriasis.[39–41] Reports that bone marrow allografts could either clear or transfer psoriasis reinforced the idea that the disease might have a primary immune basis.[42,43] This conclusion was confirmed by clinical trials with T-cell-directed immunosuppressive regimens such as FK506, monoclonal antibodies against cell surface molecules on T cells (CD3, CD4), or with a T-cell selective immunotoxin ($DAB_{389}$IL-2), and it initiated novel T-cell-directed treatment approaches using recombinant fusion molecules such as LFA3TIP or CTLA4Ig.[44,45] The therapeutic efficacy of these approaches emphasized that increased lesional keratinocyte proliferation, accumulation of neutrophilic granulocytes, as well as psoriatic inflammation in general are a sequel to the activation of T cells in the skin.[46]

In experiments with immunodeficient SCID mice receiving engrafted healthy skin from patients with psoriasis, the injection of blood-derived T cells from the same patients induced typical psoriatic alterations including epidermal hyperproliferation and accumulation of neutrophilic granulocytes.[47] The psoriasis-inducing effect could be attributed to $CD4^+$ T cells.[48] Together these data provide compelling evidence of aberrant T-cell involvement in producing the symptoms of chronic plaque psoriasis. They furthermore suggest a particular sensitivity of psoriatic keratinocytes to T-cell-derived signals.

### B. The Psoriatic T-Cell Infiltrate

Infiltration of T cells and macrophages is the earliest detectable histologic alteration in newly forming psoriatic lesions, and it precedes epidermal hyperproliferation.[25] The T cells accumulate mainly in clusters within the papillary dermis, from where fewer T cells exocytose into the epidermis. While the dermal T-cell infiltrate consists mainly of $CD4^+$ T cells, $CD8^+$ T cells constitute the majority of the epidermal infiltrate.[49] According to the expression of low-molecular-weight isoform of the tyrosine phosphatase CD45 ($CD45RO^+$) the lesional T cells belong to the memory-effector subset.[50] Many of the infiltrating T cells express markers of activation that suggest an active participation in the pathogenic inflammatory process.

Accumulation of activated memory T cells into psoriatic skin is initiated by a series of interaction of several glycoprotein ligands and chemokine receptors on the T-cell surface (cutaneous lymphocyte-associated antigen, or CLA, ICAM-1, CCR10) with a variety of adhesion factors on vascular endothelium (P-selectin, E-selectin, CCL27).[51–53] The expression of CLA and of the chemokine receptor CCR10 are quite unique to memory T cells involved in inflammatory skin diseases. Not only do CLA and CCR10 identify skin-specific T cells, they also mediate tethering of T cells to the endothelium in cutaneous venules and direct T-cell migration to the dermal extracellular matrix and basal keratinocytes.

P-selectin and E-selectin are upregulated on endothelial cells during cutaneous inflammation and bind to T cells through P-selectin glycoprotein ligand-1 (PSGL-1).[52] CLA is an inducible carbohydrate modification of PSGL-1. In fact, both lesional and nonlesional skin of patients with psoriasis shows an increased overall expression of several of these adhesion receptors. For example, E-selectin is increased on endothelial cells and ICAM-1 has been shown to be upregulated on T cells.[54] Furthermore, in psoriasis and other inflammatory disorders, CCL27 is highly upregulated by basal keratinocytes and secreted into the papillary dermis where it is immobilized on extracellular matrix and on the surface of endothelial cells.[53] Binding of CCR10 to the skin-associated chemokine CCL27 is considered essential for the migration of T cells into lesional skin, and neutralization of CCL27 in a mouse model of skin inflammation impairs lymphocyte recruitment.

## C. Cytokines in Psoriasis

Various studies support the contention that the lesional psoriatic T cells represent a particular regulatory T-cell subset that, indeed, is capable of inducing the alterations characteristic of psoriasis. T-cell clones established from psoriatic skin lesions had the select capacity of enhancing the proliferation of keratinocytes *in vitro*.[55–57] Furthermore, they exhibited a particular cytokine pattern that, according to its biological activities, should be able to mediate all the other features of psoriasis.[58] It includes IL-3, IL-6, and granulocyte-macrophage colony-stimulating factor (GM-CSF), which can enhance keratinocyte proliferation *in vitro*; IL-8, which is a key chemotactic cytokine for neutrophilic granulocytes; IL-5, which in combination with IL-3 promotes expansion and activation of mast cells; and IFN-γ, TNF-α, and TNF-β, which activate macrophages and enhance their microbicidal actions.[59] In addition, IFN-γ is involved in the mitogenic effect of T cells on keratinocytes.[56,57] TNF-α induces keratinocytes to produce β-defensins and IL-8.[60,61] By the production of IFN-γ and the lack of IL-4 the lesional psoriatic T cells yielded a predominantly Th1-pattern, which is usually associated both with effective cellular immune responses against bacteria and with T-cell-mediated autoimmune tissue injury.[59,62] The presence of IL-5 argues for a particular differentiation within the Th1 T-cell subset.[58] Keratinocytes may respond to several T-cell-derived cytokines with an increase in proliferation.[63] Yet, studies using engrafted skin in the SCID mouse model or purified keratinocytes from patients with psoriasis suggest that the psoriatic keratinocytes are particularly sensitive to the stimulatory signals from T cells.[47,57]

Within this cytokine pattern pro-inflammatory TNF-α appears as a key cytokine. Neutralizing TNF-α antibodies or soluble TNF-α receptors are most efficient in alleviating psoriasis and psoriasis arthritis.[64,65] This dramatic effect suggests that TNF-α production is an upstream event essential for psoriasis onset. Since virtually any cell compartment involved in psoriasis (keratinocytes, macrophages, mast cells, T cells) is capable of producing TNF-α, it is not yet clear which cell type actually starts the TNF-α-mediated inflammatory cascade.

Th1 T cells can be antagonized Th2 cytokines. Recent studies achieved a reduction of clinical psoriasis scores by subcutaneous injection of recombinant human IL-11, IL-10, or IL-4.[66–68] IL-4 treatment reduced the concentrations of IL-8 and IL-19, two cytokines directly involved in psoriasis, the number of chemokine receptor CCR5$^+$ Th1 cells, and the IFN-γ/IL-4 ratio. This effect was accompanied by a two- to threefold increase in the number of IL-4$^+$ CD4$^+$ T cells. Thus, Th2 cytokine therapy can induce a Th2 differentiation in human CD4$^+$ T cells and has promise as a potential treatment for psoriasis.[68]

Whether the T cells causing psoriasis belong principally to the CD4$^+$ or CD8$^+$ T-cell subset is uncertain. Both CD4$^+$- and CD8$^+$-activated T cells have been found in psoriatic plaques.[49] A major contribution of CD4$^+$ T cells to initiation and maintenance of psoriatic inflammation has been suggested by the efficacy of systemic treatment with monoclonal CD4 antibodies, even in severe cases of psoriasis.[69–71] Immunodeficient mice bearing xenografts of normal unaffected skin from patients with psoriasis developed psoriasis after intradermal injection with autologous CD4+ T cells.[48] However, psoriasis can worsen in patients with active human immunodeficiency virus (HIV) acquired immunodeficiency syndrome (AIDS) despite a falling CD4+ cell count.[72] It now appears that a functional interaction between both T-cell subsets in psoriasis seems most likely, with CD8+ T cells depending on CD4+ T-cell help to create an appropriate environment to permit activation and clonal expansion of additional dormant epidermal CD8+ cells.

## V. WHAT ACTIVATES T CELLS IN PSORIASIS?

### A. The Role of Streptococcal Throat Infection

The concept of a T-cell-mediated skin disease has prompted the need to clarify how the T cells become activated within the skin of patients to initiate a psoriatic lesion. Taking the classical case: in the majority of patients, the first psoriasis manifestations are preceded by upper respiratory tract infections with group A β-hemolytic streptococci (*Streptococcus pyogenes*). Streptococci are Gram-positive bacteria that induce a typical suppurative antimicrobial tissue reaction with diffuse or abscess-like accumulation of neutrophilic granulocytes and lymphohistiocytic infiltrates. The association of streptococcal infection with psoriasis was first observed by Winfield in 1916.[73] The incidence of preceding streptococcal infections ranges between ~60 and 97%.[74,75] This variability may in part be attributed to the difficulties of retrospective diagnosis of infection due to the delayed onset of psoriasis. Still, the close relationship between streptococcal infection and psoriasis is well accepted and has been interpreted to reflect a definite causal role of group A β-hemolytic streptococci in the initiation of disease.[76] The association of streptococcal infection with type 1 psoriasis or guttate psoriasis implies an inherited susceptibility of a distinct immune response pattern to streptococcal antigens as a key to understanding psoriasis pathogenesis.[10,77]

Against the background of a streptococcal trigger an explanation for psoriatic T-cell activation was rapidly at hand: bacterial superantigens.[76,78] These microbial toxins were accused because of two particular capabilities that could explain skin-selective disease. Bacterial superantigens polyclonally activate T cells by ligating particular T-cell receptor β chain variable regions (TCRBV) with major histocompatibility complex (MHC) class II molecules on antigen-presenting cells, and, at the same time, they induce on T cells the expression of the CLA, which functions as a skin-selective homing receptor.[79,80]

It is very tempting to employ streptococcal superantigens for explaining psoriatic T-cell activation. On closer sight, however, it is far from conclusive for two major reasons. First, the skin changes induced by superantigens from group A streptococci are different from those in psoriasis. Superantigens induce a transitory rash as seen in scarlet fever.[81] As with staphylococcal scalded skin disease, which is another superantigen-mediated disorder of the skin, scarlet rash clearly depends on the presence of superantigen-producing bacteria and vanishes upon successful antibiotic treatment of the triggering infection.[82,83] Thus, in psoriasis, superantigens might enhance migration of activated T cells into the skin, as suspected in other skin diseases such as atopic eczema, but beyond this there is no reason to believe that they are causally involved in an often lifelong lesional psoriatic immune response.[84]

### B. Analysis of the Lesional Psoriatic T-Cell Receptor Usage: Evidence of Clonal T-Cell Expansion

Molecular analysis of T-cell receptor (TCR) usage in psoriatic skin lesions has provided strong evidence in favor of an antigen-driven lesional T-cell response. TCR usage within psoriatic skin lesions appears highly restricted, with repetitive TCR rearrangements reflected by the presence of clonally expanded T-cell populations.[85,86] The same clonally expanded T-cell populations or repetitive TCR rearrangements were associated with the lesional psoriatic immune response over prolonged periods of time and in relapsing disease.[86–88] Extensive cloning and sequencing of TCR rearrangements of several BV gene families in repetitive biopsies from the same patients indicated that the lesional TCR usage is quite stable in general, with hardly any variations in the selected TCR rearrangements over time.[88] These results emphasize that the psoriatic immune response involves a restricted subset of clonally expanded T cells. It apparently becomes activated by antigens, which are continuously present within psoriatic skin lesions, and it shows no signs of epitope spreading. Instead, identification of a conserved TCR β-chain (TCRB) CDR3 motif within multiple lesions from different patients suggested that the psoriatic immune response is not only preserved within individual patients but that a common psoriatic antigen may be driving responses in different patients.[89] Identical TCR clonotypes were furthermore identified within skin and joints of patients suffering from both psoriasis and psoriasis arthritis indicating that T cells originating from the same T-cell clones are present at the two different sites of chronic inflammation.[90]

### C. Which Are the Psoriatic Antigens?

Streptococcal throat infections may provide a clue to identify the psoriatic autoantigens at least for the subtype of streptococci-induced psoriasis: molecular mimicry between streptococcal and keratinocyte proteins has been a controversial but highly intriguing hypothesis.[76] Molecular mimicry proposes that infecting pathogens express peptides that are similar in structure or sequence to a particular self-component and thus induce cross-reactive immune responses between pathogen and host.[91] The classical paradigm for antigen mimicry has been acute rheumatic fever induced by group A β-hemolytic streptococci. Immunologically relevant structural homologies of streptococcal M proteins, which are major streptococcal virulence factors, with various organ-specific proteins such as myosin have been identified by both cross-reacting serum antibodies and T cells from patients affected by rheumatic fever in numerous studies.[92]

Common epitopes are also shared between streptococcal antigens and keratinocyte proteins.[92] They can easily be demonstrated by cross-reactive antibodies.[93,94] Based on several amino acid sequence homologies with streptococcal M proteins that were identified by database searches, keratin 6, but also other keratins, were formerly suggested as psoriatic autoantigens.[95] And indeed, peripheral blood T cells of patients with psoriasis showed increased reactivity to several synthetic peptides corresponding to these homologous regions, when tested *in vitro*.[96,97] A particular relevance of these findings for the psoriatic T-cell response is suggested by increased lesional frequencies of streptococci-specific T cells.[98,99] Therefore, in a concept of molecular mimicry, by their homologies streptococcal M proteins might have the capacity to direct a primary antistreptococcal T-cell response to homologous organ-specific keratin peptides presented on keratinocytes or on dendritic cells that have taken up keratinocyte proteins from apoptotic keratinocytes. Dendritic cells isolated from psoriatic skin lesions are potent stimulators of autologous lymphocytes isolated from the peripheral blood of the patients.[100]

## VI. CONCLUSIONS

In summary, psoriasis may be considered as a paradigm of a T-cell-mediated autoimmune disease. On a polygenic predisposition, environmental factors may promote the formation of an immune response against yet unknown autoantigens in the skin. A particular sensitivity of psoriatic keratinocytes to respond to T-cell-derived cytokines may contribute to the formation of a typical, complex, and highly characteristic skin inflammation that contains central aspects of an antimicrobial skin reaction.[101] These include excessive epithelial hyperplasia with intense desquamation, which may be considered an expulsive mechanism of epithelial surfaces to combat microbial invasion;[102] production of human β-defensins that are antibacterial, keratinocyte-derived peptides;[31] increased numbers of mast cells that hold a pivotal position in antibacterial defense reactions;[29,103] and infiltration of neutrophilic granulocytes that are potent antimicrobial phagocytes.

Thus, T cells appear as the functional link between genetic predisposition and environmental factor in psoriasis. Although many open questions require further clarification, T-cell-directed immunosuppressive or immunomodulatory treatment modalities have already today changed the treatment approach remarkably.

## REFERENCES

1. Dirckx, J.H., Dermatologic terms in the *De Medicina* of Celsus. *Am. J. Dermatopathol.* 5, 363, 1983.
2. Glickman, F.S., Lepra, psora, psoriasis. *J. Am. Acad. Dermatol.* 14, 863, 1986.
3. Leach, D. and Beckwith, J., The founders of dermatology: Robert Willan and Thomas Bateman. *J. R. Coll. Physicians. Lond.* 33, 580, 1999.
4. Hoede, K., Zur Frage der Erblichkeit der Psoriasis. *Hautarzt* 8, 433, 1957.
5. Lomholt, G., Psoriasis: Prevalence, Spontaneous Course, and Genetics; A Census Study on the Prevalence of Skin Diseases on the Faroe Islands. Dissertation. G. E. C. Gad, Copenhagen, 1963.
6. Brandrup, F., Holm, N., Grunnet, N., Henningsen, K., and Hansen, H.E., Psoriasis in monozygotic twins: variations in expression in individuals with identical genetic constitution. *Acta Derm. Venereol.* 62, 229, 1982.
7. Farber, E.M., Nall, M.L., and Watson, W., Natural history of psoriasis in 61 twin pairs. *Arch. Dermatol.* 109, 207, 1974.
8. Nair, R.P., Henseler, T., Jenisch, S., Stuart, P., Bichakjian, C.K., Lenk, W., Westphal, E., Guo, S.W., Christophers, E., Voorhees, J.J., and Elder, J.T., Evidence for two psoriasis susceptibility loci (HLA and 17q) and two novel candidate regions (16q and 20p) by genome-wide scan. *Hum. Mol. Genet.* 6, 1349, 1997.
9. Cookson, W., Ubhi, B., Lawrence, R., Abecasis, G., Walley, A., Cox, H., Coleman, R., Leaves, N., Trembath, R., Moffatt, M., and Harper, J., Genetic linkage of childhood atopic dermatitis to psoriasis susceptibility loci. *Nat. Genet.* 27, 372, 2001.
10. Mallon, E., Bunce, M., Savoie, H., Rowe, A., Newson, R., Gotch, F., and Bunker, C., HLA-C and guttate psoriasis. *Br. J. Dermatol.* 143, 1177, 2000.
11. Schmitt Egenolf, M., Eiermann, T.H., Boehncke, W.H., Stander, M., and Sterry, W., Familial juvenile onset psoriasis is associated with the human leukocyte antigen (HLA) class I side of the extended haplotype Cw6-B57-DRB1*0701-DQA1*0201-DQB1*0303: a population- and family-based study. *J. Invest. Dermatol.* 106, 711, 1996.
12. Christophers, E. and Henseler, T., Characterization of disease patterns in nonpustular psoriasis. *Semin. Dermatol.* 4, 271, 1985.
13. Nair, R.P., Stuart, P., Henseler, T., Jenisch, S., Chia, N.V., Westphal, E., Schork, N.J., Kim, J., Lim, H.W., Christophers, E., Voorhees, J.J., and Elder, J.T., Localization of psoriasis-susceptibility locus PSORS1 to a 60-kb interval telomeric to HLA-C. *Am. J. Hum. Genet.* 66, 1833, 2000.
14. Gonzalez, S., Martinez Borra, J., Del Rio, J., Santos Juanes, J., Lopez Vazquez, A., Blanco Gelaz, M., and Lopez Larrea, C., The OTF3 gene polymorphism confers susceptibility to psoriasis independent of the association of HLA-Cw*0602. *J. Invest. Dermatol.* 115, 824, 2000.
15. Tazi Ahnini, R., Camp, N.J., Cork, M.J., Mee, J.B., Keohane, S.G., Duff, G.W., and di Giovine, F.S., Novel genetic association between the corneodesmosin (MHC S) gene and susceptibility to psoriasis. *Hum. Mol. Genet.* 8, 1135, 1999.
16. Jenisch, S., Koch, S., Henseler, T., Nair, R.P., Elder, J.T., Watts, C.E., Westphal, E., Voorhees, J.J., Christophers, E., and Kronke, M., Corneodesmosin gene polymorphism demonstrates strong linkage disequilibrium with HLA and association with psoriasis vulgaris. *Tissue Antigens* 54, 439, 1999.
17. Asumalahti, K., Veal, C., Laitinen, T., Suomela, S., Allen, M., Elomaa, O., Moser, M., de Cid, R., Ripatti, S., Vorechovsky, I., Marcusson, J., Nakagawa, H., Lazaro, C., Estivill, X., Capon, F., Novelli, G., Saarialho Kere, U., Barker, J., Trembath, R., and Kere, J., Coding haplotype analysis supports HCR as the putative susceptibility gene for psoriasis at the MHC PSORS1 locus. *Hum. Mol. Genet.* 11, 589, 2002.
18. Gonzalez, S., Martinez Borra, J., Torre Alonso, J., Gonzalez Roces, S., Sanchez del Rio, J., Rodriguez Perez, A., Brautbar, C., and Lopez Larrea, C., The MICA-A9 triplet repeat polymorphism in the transmembrane region confers additional susceptibility to the development of psoriatic arthritis and is independent of the association of Cw*0602 in psoriasis. *Arthritis Rheum.* 42, 1010, 1999.

19. Allen, M., Ishida Yamamoto, A., McGrath, J., Davison, S., Iizuka, H., Simon, M., Guerrin, M., Hayday, A., Vaughan, R., Serre, G., Trembath, R., and Barker, J., Corneodesmosin expression in psoriasis vulgaris differs from normal skin and other inflammatory skin disorders. *Lab. Invest.* 81, 969, 2001.
20. Kobayashi, H., Takahashi, M., Takahashi, H., Ishida Yamamoto, A., Hashimoto, Y., Sato, K., Tateno, M., and Iizuka, H., CD4+ T-cells from peripheral blood of a patient with psoriasis recognize keratin 14 peptide but not "homologous" streptococcal M-protein epitope. *J. Dermatol. Sci.* 30, 240, 2002.
21. Tsunemi, Y., Saeki, H., Nakamura, K., Sekiya, T., Hirai, K., Fujita, H., Asano, N., Kishimoto, M., Tanida, Y., Kakinuma, T., Mitsui, H., Tada, Y., Wakugawa, M., Torii, H., Komine, M., Asahina, A., and Tamaki, K., Interleukin-12 p40 gene (IL12B) 3′-untranslated region polymorphism is associated with susceptibility to atopic dermatitis and psoriasis vulgaris. *J. Dermatol. Sci.* 30, 161, 2002.
22. Reich, K., Mossner, R., Konig, I., Westphal, G., Ziegler, A., and Neumann, C., Promoter polymorphisms of the genes encoding tumor necrosis factor-alpha and interleukin-1beta are associated with different subtypes of psoriasis characterized by early and late disease onset. *J. Invest. Dermatol.* 118, 155, 2002.
23. Asadullah, K., Eskdale, J., Wiese, A., Gallagher, G., Friedrich, M., and Sterry, W., Interleukin-10 promoter polymorphism in psoriasis. *J. Invest. Dermatol.* 116, 975, 2001.
24. Arias, A., Giles, B., Eiermann, T., Sterry, W., and Pandey, J., Tumor necrosis factor-alpha gene polymorphism in psoriasis. *Exp. Clin. Immunogenet.* 14, 118, 1997.
25. Braun-Falco, O. and Christophers, E., Structural aspects of initial psoriatic lesions. *Arch. Dermatol. Forsch.* 251, 95, 1974.
26. Pinkus, H. and Mehregan, A.H., The primary histologic lesion of seborrheic dermatitis and psoriasis. *J. Invest. Dermatol.* 46, 109, 1966.
27. Ragaz, A. and Ackerman, A.B., Evolution, maturation, and regression of lesions of psoriasis. New observations and correlation of clinical and histologic findings. *Am. J. Dermatopathol.* 1, 199, 1979.
28. Gordon, M. and Johnson, W.C., Histopathology and histochemistry of psoriasis. I. The active lesion and clinically normal skin. *Arch. Dermatol.* 95, 402, 1967.
29. Harvima, I.T., Naukkarinen, A., Harvima, R.J., and Horsmanheimo, M., Enzyme- and immunohistochemical localization of mast cell tryptase in psoriatic skin. *Arch. Dermatol. Res.* 281, 387, 1989.
30. Shelley, W.B. and Kirschbaum, J.O., Generalized pustular psoriasis. *Arch. Dermatol.* 84, 73, 1961.
31. Harder, J., Bartels, J., Christophers, E., and Schroder, J.M., A peptide antibiotic from human skin. *Nature* 387, 861, 1997.
32. Henseler, T. and Christophers, E., Disease concomitance in psoriasis. *J. Am. Acad. Dermatol.* 32, 982, 1995.
33. Ong, P., Ohtake, T., Brandt, C., Strickland, I., Boguniewicz, M., Ganz, T., Gallo, R., and Leung, D., Endogenous antimicrobial peptides and skin infections in atopic dermatitis. *N. Engl. J. Med.* 347, 1151, 2002.
34. Oestreicher, J., Walters, I., Kikuchi, T., Gilleaudeau, P., Surette, J., Schwertschlag, U., Dorner, A., Krueger, J., and Trepicchio, W., Molecular classification of psoriasis disease-associated genes through pharmacogenomic expression profiling. *Pharmacogenomics J.* 1, 272, 2001.
35. Zhou, X., Krueger, J., Kao, M., Lee, E., Du, F., Menter, A., Wong, W., and Bowcock, A., Novel mechanisms of T-cell and dendritic cell activation revealed by profiling of psoriasis on the 63,100-element oligonucleotide array. *Physiol. Genomics* 13, 69, 2003.
36. Bowcock, A., Shannon, W., Du, F., Duncan, J., Cao, K., Aftergut, K., Catier, J., Fernandez Vina, M., and Menter, A., Insights into psoriasis and other inflammatory diseases from large-scale gene expression studies. *Hum. Mol. Genet.* 10, 1793, 2001.
37. Mueller, W. and Hermann, B., Cyclosporin A for psoriasis. *N. Engl. J. Med.* 301, 355, 1976.
38. Van Joost, T., Bos, J.D., Heule, F., and Meinardi, M.M., Low-dose cyclosporin A in severe psoriasis. A double-blind study. *Br. J. Dermatol.* 118, 183, 1988.
39. Quesada, J.R. and Gutterman, J.U., Psoriasis and alpha-interferon. *Lancet* 326, 1466, 1986.
40. Fierlbeck, G. and Rassner, G., Treatment of psoriasis and psoriatic arthritis with interferon gamma. *J. Invest. Dermatol.* 95, 138, 1990.
41. Lee, R.E., Gaspari, A.A., Lotze, M.T., Chang, A.E., and Rosenberg, S.A., Interleukin 2 and psoriasis. *Arch. Dermatol.* 124, 1811, 1988.
42. Eedy, D., Burrows, D., Bridges, J., and Jones, F., Clearance of severe psoriasis after allogenic bone marrow transplantation. *Br. Med. J.* 300, 908, 1990.

43. Gardembas Pain, M., Ifrah, N., Foussard, C., Boasson, M., Saint Andre, J., and Verret, J., Psoriasis after allogeneic bone marrow transplantation. *Arch. Dermatol.* 126, 1523, 1990.
44. Abrams, J.R., Lebwohl, M.G., Guzzo, C.A., Jegasothy, B.V., Goldfarb, M.T., Goffe, B.S., Menter, A., Lowe, N.J., Krueger, G., Brown, M.J., Weiner, R.S., Birkhofer, M.J., Warner, G.L., Berry, K.K., Linsley, P.S., Krueger, J.G., Ochs, H.D., Kelley, S.L., and Kang, S., CTLA4Ig-mediated blockade of T-cell costimulation in patients with psoriasis vulgaris. *J. Clin. Invest.* 103, 1243, 1999.
45. Ellis, C. and Krueger, G., Treatment of chronic plaque psoriasis by selective targeting of memory effector T lymphocytes. *N. Engl. J. Med.* 345, 248, 2001.
46. Prinz, J.C., Which T cells cause psoriasis? *Clin. Exp. Dermatol.* 24, 291, 1999.
47. Wrone Smith, T. and Nickoloff, B.J., Dermal injection of immunocytes induces psoriasis. *J. Clin. Invest.* 98, 1878, 1996.
48. Nickoloff, B.J. and Wrone Smith, T., Injection of pre-psoriatic skin with $CD4^+$ T cells induces psoriasis. *Am. J. Pathol.* 155, 145, 1999.
49. Bos, J.D., Hulsebosch, H.J., Krieg, S.R., Bakker, P.M., and Cormane, R.H., Immunocompetent cells in psoriasis. *In situ* immunophenotyping by monoclonal antibodies. *Arch. Dermatol. Res.* 275, 181, 1983.
50. Bos, J.D., Hagenaars, C., Das, P.K., Krie.g., S.R., Voorn, W.J., and Kapsenberg, M.L., Predominance of "memory" T cells ($CD4^+$, $CDw29^+$) over "naive" T cells ($CD4^+$, $CD45R^+$) in both normal and diseased human skin. *Arch. Dermatol. Res.* 281, 24, 1989.
51. Fuhlbrigge, R.C., Kieffer, J.D., Armerding, D., and Kupper, T.S., Cutaneous lymphocyte antigen is a specialized form of PSGL-1 expressed on skin-homing T cells. *Nature* 389, 978, 1997.
52. von Andrian, U. and Mackay, C., T-cell function and migration. Two sides of the same coin. *N. Engl. J. Med.* 343, 1020, 2000.
53. Homey, B., Alenius, H., Muller, A., Soto, H., Bowman, E., Yuan, W., McEvoy, L., Lauerma, A., Assmann, T., Bunemann, E., Lehto, M., Wolff, H., Yen, D., Marxhausen, H., To, W., Sedgwick, J., Ruzicka, T., Lehmann, P., and Zlotnik, A., CCL27-CCR10 interactions regulate T cell-mediated skin inflammation. *Nat. Med.* 8, 157, 2002.
54. de Boer, O., Wakelkamp, I., Pals, S., Claessen, N., Bos, J., and Das, P., Increased expression of adhesion receptors in both lesional and non-lesional psoriatic skin. *Arch. Dermatol. Res.* 286, 304, 1994.
55. Strange, P., Cooper, K.D., Hansen, E.R., Fisher, G., Larsen, J.K., Fox, D., Krag, C., Voorhees, J.J., and Baadsgaard, O., T lymphocyte clones from lesional psoriatic skin release growth factors that induce keratinocyte proliferation. *J. Invest. Dermatol.* 101, 695, 1993.
56. Prinz, J.C., Gross, B., Vollmer, S., Trommler, P., Strobel, I., Meurer, M., and Plewig, G., T cell clones from psoriasis skin lesions can promote keratinocyte proliferation *in vitro*. *Eur. J. Immunol.* 24, 593, 1994.
57. Bata-Csorgo, Z., Hammerberg, C., Voorhees, J.J., and Cooper, K.D., Kinetics and regulation of human keratinocyte stem cell growth in short-term primary *ex vivo* culture. Cooperative growth factors from psoriatic lesional T lymphocytes stimulate proliferation among psoriatic uninvolved, but not normal, stem keratinocytes. *J. Clin. Invest.* 95, 317, 1995.
58. Vollmer, S., Menssen, A., Trommler, P., Schendel, D., and Prinz, J.C., T lymphocytes derived from skin lesions of patients with psoriasis vulgaris express a novel cytokine pattern that is distinct from that of T helper type 1 and T helper type 2 cells. *Eur. J. Immunol.* 24, 2377, 1994.
59. Abbas, A.K., Murphy, K.M., and Sher, A., Functional diversity of helper T lymphocytes. *Nature* 383, 787, 1996.
60. Schroder, J.M. and Harder, J., Human beta-defensin-2. *Int. J. Biochem. Cell Biol.* 31, 645, 1999.
61. Nickoloff, B.J., Karabin, G.D., and Barker, J.N.W.N., Localization of IL-8 and its inducer TNF-$\alpha$ in psoriasis. *Am. J. Pathol.* 138, 129, 1991.
62. Schaible, U.E., Collins, H.L., and Kaufmann, S.H., Confrontation between intracellular bacteria and the immune system. *Adv. Immunol.* 71, 267, 1999.
63. Hancock, G.E., Kaplan, G., and Cohn, Z.A., Keratinocyte growth regulation by the products of immune cells. *J. Exp. Med.* 168, 1395, 1988.
64. Gottlieb, A.B., Chaudhari, U., Mulcahy, L.D., Li, S., Dooley, L.T., and Baker, D.G., Infliximab monotherapy provides rapid and sustained benefit for plaque-type psoriasis. *J. Am. Acad. Dermatol.* 48, 829, 2003.
65. Mease, P.J., Goffe, B.S., Metz, J., VanderStoep, A., Finck, B., and Burge, D.J., Etanercept in the treatment of psoriatic arthritis and psoriasis, a randomised trial. *Lancet* 356, 385, 2000.

66. Trepicchio, W., Ozawa, M., Walters, I., Kikuchi, T., Gilleaudeau, P., Bliss, J., Schwertschlag, U., Dorner, A., and Krueger, J., Interleukin-11 therapy selectively downregulates type I cytokine proinflammatory pathways in psoriasis lesions. *J. Clin. Invest.* 104, 1527, 1999.
67. Asadullah, K., Sterry, W., Stephanek, K., Jasulaitis, D., Leupold, M., Audring, H., Volk, H.D., and Docke, W.D., IL-10 is a key cytokine in psoriasis. Proof of principle by IL-10 therapy, a new therapeutic approach. *J. Clin. Invest.* 101, 783, 1998.
68. Ghoreschi, K., Thomas, P., Breit, S., Dugas, M., Mailhammer, R., Van Eden, W., Van der Zee, R., Biedermann, T., Prinz, J.C., Mack, M., Mrowietz, U., Christophers, E., Schloendorf, D., Plewig, G., Sander, C.A., and Roecken, M. Interleukin-4 therapy of psoriasis induces TH2 responses and improves human autoimmune disease. *Nat. Med.* 9, 40, 2003.
69. Prinz, J.C., Braun-Falco, O., Meurer, M., Daddona, P., Reiter, C., Rieber, E.P., and Riethmüller, G., Chimeric CD4 monoclonal antibody in the treatment of generalized pustular psoriasis. *Lancet* 338, 320, 1991.
70. Gottlieb, A., Lebwohl, M., Shirin, S., Sherr, A., Gilleaudeau, P., Singer, G., Solodkina, G., Grossman, R., Gisoldi, E., Phillips, S., Neisler, H., and Krueger, J., Anti-CD4 monoclonal antibody treatment of moderate to severe psoriasis vulgaris, results of a pilot, multicenter, multiple-dose, placebo-controlled study. *J. Am. Acad. Dermatol.* 43, 595, 2000.
71. Bachelez, H., Flageul, B., Dubertret, L., Fraitag, S., Grossman, R., Brousse, N., Poisson, D., Knowles, R., Wacholtz, M., Haverty, T., Chatenoud, L., and Bach, J., Treatment of recalcitrant plaque psoriasis with a humanized non-depleting antibody to CD4. *J. Autoimmun.* 11, 53, 1998.
72. Myskowski, P.L. and Ahkami, R., Dermatologic complications of HIV-infection. *Med. Clin. North Am.* 80, 1415, 1996.
73. Winfield, J.M., Psoriasis as sequel to acute inflammations of the tonsils, clinical note. *J. Cutaneous Dis.* 34, 441, 1916.
74. Whyte, H.J. and Baughman, R.D., Acute guttate psoriasis and streptococcal infection. *Arch. Dermatol.* 89, 350, 1964.
75. Telfer, N.R., Chalmers, R.J.G., Whale, K., and Colman, J., The role of streptococcal infection in the initiation of guttate psoriasis. *Arch. Dermatol.* 128, 39, 1992.
76. Valdimarsson, H., Baker, B.S., Jonsdottir, I., Powles, A.V., and Fry, L., Psoriasis, a T-cell-mediated autoimmune disease induced by streptococcal superantigens? *Immunol. Today* 16, 145, 1995.
77. Weisenseel, P., Laumbacher, B., Besgen, P., Ludolph-Hauser, D., Herzinger, T., Roecken, M., Wank, R., and Prinz, J.C., Streptococcal infection distinguishes different types of psoriasis. *J. Med. Genet.* 39, 767, 2002.
78. Leung, D.Y.M., Travers, B.J., Giorno, R., Norris, D.A., Skinner, R., Aelion, J., Kazemi, L.V., Kim, M.H., Trumble, A.E., Kotb, M., and Schlievert, P.M., Evidence for a streptococcal superantigen-driven process in acute guttate psoriasis. *J. Clin. Invest.* 96, 2106, 1995.
79. Kappler, J., Kotzin, B., Herron, L., Gelfand, E.W., Bigler, R.D., Boylston, A., Carrel, S., Posnett, D.N., Choi, Y., and Marrack, P., V beta-specific stimulation of human T cells by staphylococcal toxins. *Science* 244, 811, 1989.
80. Leung, D.Y., Gately, M., Trumble, A., Ferguson Darnell, B., Schlievert, P.M., and Picker, L.J., Bacterial superantigens induce T cell expression of the skin-selective homing receptor, the cutaneous lymphocyte-associated antigen, via stimulation of interleukin 12 production. *J. Exp. Med.* 181, 747, 1995.
81. Braun, M.A., Gerlach, D., Hartwig, U.F., Ozegowski, J.H., Romagne, F., Carrel, S., Kohler, W., and Fleicher, B., Stimulation of human T cells by streptococcal "superantigen" erythrogenic toxins (scarlet fever toxins). *J. Immunol.* 150, 2457, 1993.
82. Ladhani, S., Joannou, C.L., Lochrie, D.P., Evans, R.W., and Poston, S.M., Clinical, microbial, and biochemical aspects of the exfoliative toxins causing staphylococcal scalded-skin syndrome. *Clin. Microbiol. Rev.* 12, 224, 1999.
83. Barnett, B.O. and Frieden, I.J., Streptococcal skin diseases in children. *Semin. Dermatol.* 11, 3, 1992.
84. Leung, D.Y., Travers, J.B., and Norris, D.A., The role of superantigens in skin disease. *J. Invest. Dermatol.* 105, 37S, 1995.
85. Chang, J.C.C., Smith, L.R., Froning, K.J., Schwabe, B.J., Laxer, J.A., Caralli, L.L., Kurland, H.H., Karasek, M.A., Wilkinson, D.I., Carlo, D.J., and Brostoff, S.W., $CD8^+$ T cells in psoriatic lesions preferentially use T-cell receptor V$\beta$3 and/or V$\beta$13.1 genes. *Proc. Natl. Acad. Sci. U.S.A.* 91, 9282, 1994.

86. Menssen, A., Trommler, P., Vollmer, S., Schendel, D., Albert, E., Gürtler, L., Riethmüller, G., and Prinz, J.C., Evidence for an antigen-specific cellular immune response in skin lesions of patients with psoriasis vulgaris. *J. Immunol.* 155, 4078, 1995.
87. Chang, J.C., Smith, L.R., Froning, K.J., Kurland, H.H., Schwabe, B.J., Blumeyer, K.K., Karasek, M.A., Wilkinson, D.I., Farber, E.M., Carlo, D.J., and Brostoff, S.W., Persistence of T-cell clones in psoriatic lesions. *Arch. Dermatol.* 133, 703, 1997.
88. Vollmer, S., Menssen, A., and Prinz, J.C., Dominant lesional T cell receptor rearrangements persist in relapsing psoriasis but are absent from nonlesional skin. Evidence for a stable antigen-specific pathogenic T cell response in psoriasis vulgaris. *J. Invest. Dermatol.* 117, 1296, 2001.
89. Prinz, J.C., Vollmer, S., Boehncke, W.-H., Menssen, A., Laisney, I., and Trommler, P., Selection of conserved TCR-VDJ-rearrangements in chronic psoriatic plaques indicates a common antigen in psoriasis vulgaris. *Eur. J. Immunol.* 29, 3360, 1999.
90. Borgato, L., Puccetti, A., Beri, R., Codella, O., Frigo, A., Simeoni, S., Pacor, M., Corrocher, R., and Lunardi, C., The T cell receptor repertoire in psoriatic synovitis is restricted and T lymphocytes expressing the same TCR are present in joint and skin lesions. *J. Rheumatol.* 29, 1914, 2002.
91. Oldstone, M.B., Molecular mimicry and autoimmune disease. *Cell* 50, 819, 1987.
92. Robinson, J.H. and Kehoe, M.A., Group A streptococcal M proteins, virulence factors and protective antigens. *Immunol. Today* 13, 362, 1992.
93. Swerlick, R.A., Cunningham, M.W., and Hall, N.K., Monoclonal antibodies crossreactive with group A streptococci and normal and psoriatic human skin. *J. Invest. Dermatol.* 87, 367, 1986.
94. McFadden, J.H., Valdimarsson, H., and Fry, L., Cross-reactivity between streptococcal M surface antigen and human skin. *Br. J. Dermatol.* 125, 443, 1991.
95. Valdimarsson, H., Baker, B.S., Jonsdottir, I., and Fry, L., Psoriasis, a disease of abnormal keratinocyte proliferation induced by T lymphocytes. *Immunol. Today* 7, 256, 1986.
96. Sigmundsdottir, H., Sigurgeirsson, B., Troye Blomberg, M., Good, M.F., Valdimarsson, H., and Jonsdottir, I., Circulating T cells of patients with active psoriasis respond to streptococcal M-peptides sharing sequences with human epidermal keratins. *Scand. J. Immunol.* 45, 688, 1997.
97. Gudmundsdottir, A.S., Sigmundsdottir, H., Sigurgeirsson, B., Good, M.F., Valdimarsson, H., and Jonsdottir, I., Is an epitope on keratin 17 a major target for autoreactive T lymphocytes in psoriasis? *Clin. Exp. Immunol.* 117, 580, 1999.
98. Baker, B.S., Powles, A.V., Malkani, A.K., Lewis, H., Valdimarsson, H., and Fry, L., Altered cell-mediated immunity to group A haemolytic streptococcal antigens in chronic plaque psoriasis. *Br. J. Dermatol.* 125, 38, 1991.
99. Baker, B.S., Bolith, S., Powles, A.V., Valdimarsson, H., and Fry, L., Streptococcal antigen-specific T lymphocytes in skin lesions of guttate psoriasis. *J. Invest. Dermatol.* 98, 535, 1992.
100. Nestle, F.O., Turka, L.A., and Nickoloff, B.J., Characterization of dermal dendritic cells in psoriasis. Autostimulation of T lymphocytes and induction of Th1 type cytokines. *J. Clin. Invest.* 94, 202, 1994.
101. Prinz, J.C., Disease mimicry, a pathogenetic concept for T cell-mediated autoimmune disorders triggered by molecular mimicry? *Autoimmun. Rev.* 3, 10, 2004.
102. McCarty, M., Host-parasite relations in bacterial diseases, in *Microbiology*, B.D. Davis, R. Dulbecco, H.N. Eisen, H.S. Ginsberg, W.B. Wood, and M. McCarty, Eds., Harper & Row, Hagerstown, NY, 1973, 627–665.
103. Prodeus, A.P., Zhou, X., Maurer, M., Galli, S.J., and, Carroll, M.C., Impaired mast cell-dependent natural immunity in complement C3-deficient mice. *Nature* 390, 172, 1997.

# 33 Viral Infections

*Mary Norval*

## CONTENTS



## I. INTRODUCTION

Viruses belonging to a range of families are associated with infections of the skin, and a number of these are widespread in the human population; the most important are outlined in Table 33.1, which also illustrates some of their characteristics. There can be replication of the virus solely in the epidermis at the site of inoculation or, in contrast, spread from the dermis or subdermal tissues to local blood vessels, lymphatics, and the nervous system. Other viruses reach the skin via a systemic route from a primary infection at a distant body site. Not all are shed from the skin. There is also variation in the type of infection caused, ranging from subclinical or acute, with effective elimination from the body thereafter, to ones that remain persistent or latent for the lifetime of the host. Differences in the host immune response, and the paucity of information for many of these viruses, preclude presentation of a unified scheme to explain the mechanisms of cutaneous immunity

0-8493-1959-5/05/$0.00+$1.50

**TABLE 33.1**
**Common Viral Infections of Human Skin**

| Virus | Classification: Family/Genus | Skin Lesions (Disease) | Sites of Initial Infection | Shedding of Virus from Skin Lesions | Systemic Spread | Main Routes of Transmission |
|---|---|---|---|---|---|---|
| Human papillomaviruses | Papova/*Papillomavirus* | Warts | Cutaneous, mucocutaneous | + | – | Close contact/sexual |
| Molluscum contagiousum | Poxviridae/*Molluscipoxvirus* | Papules | Cutaneous | + | – | Close contact |
| Orf | Poxviridae/*Parapoxvirus* | Papulovesicles | Cutaneous | + | – | Close contact (zoonosis) |
| Herpes simplex virus | Herpesviridae/*Simplexvirus* | Vesicles | Cutaneous, mucocutaneous | + | + | Close contact/sexual |
| Varicella zoster virus | Herpesviridae/*Varicellavirus* | Vesicles (varicella, zoster) | Respiratory tract | + | + | Respiratory secretions/ contact |
| Various Coxsackie serotypes | Picornaviridae/*Enterovirus* | Vesicles (hand, foot, and mouth disease), macular rash | Respiratory and gastrointestinal tracts | + | + | Respiratory secretions/ fecal-oral |
| Human parvovirus B19 | Parvoviridae/*Parvovirus* | Macropapules (erythema infectiosum) | Respiratory tract | – | + | respiratory secretions |
| Human herpesvirus-6 | Herpesviridae/*Roseolovirus* | Macular rash (exanthem subitum), erythematous papules (pityriasis rosea?) | Respiratory tract | – | + | Respiratory secretions/ contact |
| Human herpesvirus-7 | Herpesviridae/*Roseolovirus* | Erythematous papules (pityriasis rosea?) | Respiratory tract | – | + | Respiratory secretions/ contact |
| Human herpesvirus-8 (Kaposi's sarcoma-associated herpesvirus) | Herpesviridae/*Rhadinovirus* | Multiple plaques and nodules (Kaposi's sarcoma?) | ? | – | + | Close contact/sexual |
| Rubella | Togaviridae/*Rubivirus* | Macropapules (German measles) | Respiratory tract | – | + | Respiratory secretions/ congenital |
| Various Echovirus serotypes | Picornaviridae/*Enterovirus* | Maculopapules | Respiratory tract | – | + | Respiratory secretions/ fecal-oral |
| Hepatitis C virus | Flaviviridae/*Hepacavirus* | Vasculitis, porphyria cutanea tarda, cutaneous/ mucocutaneous lichen planus | Liver, peripheral blood | – | + | Blood, i.v. drug abuse, perinatal |

to viral infections. Therefore, in this chapter, three virus types, human papillomaviruses (HPV), herpes simplex virus (HSV), and measles virus (MV), are chosen as examples to illustrate the varied aspects of cutaneous viral infections; in each case, emphasis is placed on the local immune responses generated in the skin. New, and frequently controversial, evidence linking the human herpesviruses-6, 7, and 8 (HHV-6, 7, and 8) with particular cutaneous diseases is summarized. The skin manifestations of human immunodeficiency virus (HIV) infection are covered briefly. The chapter starts with an outline of viral replication cycles including a brief assessment of the possible outcomes on host cells.

## II. VIRAL REPLICATION AND EFFECTS ON HOST CELLS

The first and critical interaction of the virus with the host cell is the attachment phase in which a receptor-binding protein on the virion adsorbs to a specific receptor on the surface of a specific cell type. Both the receptor-binding protein and its ligand have been identified for some of the viruses infecting the skin, mainly from *in vitro* studies, although it has become clear in recent years that there is frequently more than one specific cell receptor involved in the attachment process. Following adsorption, the virus penetrates into the cell, by receptor-mediated endocytosis or fusion, then is uncoated and begins to synthesize viral mRNA. On translation, these first viral proteins tend to have nonstructural regulatory or enzymatic functions. The early phase of protein synthesis is followed by a late phase, where the structural components of the viral capsid are synthesized predominantly and there is also synthesis of new viral genomes. The strategies involved in the synthesis of these macromolecules vary among the different virus families, but there is always strict temporal control of each phase. The final stages of the replication cycle consist of assembly of the capsid and release of the newly formed virions. Release is either by nonspecific lysis of the infected cell or by budding from the cytoplasmic or, more infrequently, the nuclear membrane, giving the new virus particles an envelope, modified from the host cell's membrane by the insertion of viral glycoproteins. The budding process is not generally cytolytic.

The effect of a virus infection on the host cell is varied, especially when considered *in vivo* with the contribution of immune mechanisms. Some viruses are cytopathic, either by producing specific factors early in the replication cycle that inhibit host cell macromolecular synthesis, as is the case for HSV, or by more nonspecific means, presumably by using cellular metabolites preferentially for the synthesis of new viral components rather than for the maintenance of the cell. For the cytopathic viruses, immune responses that recognize viral antigens in infected cells before the assembly stage are advantageous in preventing the production of new viral particles, local and systemic spread, or transmission to a new host. For the viruses causing persistent infections, continuing for several weeks, months, or for the lifetime of the host, the virus can be present in an infectious form throughout or it can be latent, with little or no expression of viral proteins. A number of viral infections of the skin are persistent, which may be one reason for the high prevalence of such diseases in the human population. A varied range of strategies has evolved to maintain persistence, some of which are only now being recognized. These include frequent antigenic changes and integration of the viral genome, plus many mechanisms for rendering the immune response less effective. Thus, while the skin immune system (SIS) is capable of eradicating some cutaneous viral infections and of preventing future infections with the same virus, in other cases it is not, and may even heighten the clinical symptoms.

## III. HUMAN PAPILLOMAVIRUSES

### A. Virus Types and Diseases

Papillomaviruses are naked icosahedral particles about 55 nm in diameter, which contain circular double-stranded DNA of about 8000 base pairs (Figure 33.1). They infect many species and are

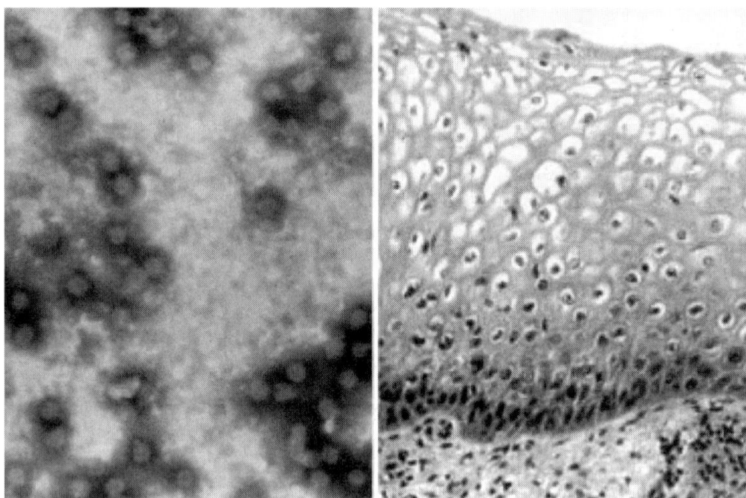

**FIGURE 33.1** (Left) HPV particles purified from plantar warts (negative stain, original magnification × 110,000); (right) section of a cervical biopsy showing koilocytes (hematoxylin and eosin, original magnification × 250).

thought to be species specific. There are more than 130 different human types that are closely related but distinguished, unusually for viruses, by the nucleotide sequence of part of the genome coding for some structural and nonstructural proteins (reviewed in Reference 1). There is also divergence in the regulatory region including sites controlling viral replication and assembly. The variations contribute to the species specificity of papillomaviruses and to their range of clinical associations and pathogenicity.

HPV infect stratifying epithelium and some types induce hyperproliferation, leading to the formation of benign papillomas or warts. In some instances they are associated with malignant transformation. There is an apparent preference of certain HPV types for either cutaneous or mucocutaneous sites. The first class contains the common skin types, including HPV-1, 2, 3, and 4, causing warts most frequently on the hands, feet, and face. The second class contains the types causing infections of the urogenital and anorectal systems (condylomata acuminata and flat warts) (HPV-6 and 11, the "low-risk" genital types) and the upper respiratory tract (HPV-6 and 11). The DNA of several HPV types, most notably HPV-16, 18, and 33 ("high-risk" genital types), has been found in dysplastic and malignant lesions of the cervix, vulva, and penis,[2,3] and the DNA of HPV-6 and 11 has been found in various oral malignancies, particularly tonsillar cancer.[4,5] There is a third class, including HPV-5 and 8, present predominantly in patients with epidermodysplasia verruciformis (EV). EV is a genetic disease with an underlying defect in cell-mediated immunity in which individuals develop multiple skin warts from an early age; there is a high risk of conversion of these lesions to squamous cell carcinomas (SCC) on sun-exposed sites of the body several decades later.[6] Finally immunosuppressed patients, such as renal allograft recipients, have a high prevalence of HPV infection, this increasing with time post-transplantation. Within these HPV lesions on sun-exposed body sites, there is frequent development of SCC, and an additional increased risk of genital dysplasia.[7]

Much attention has focused on the function of the gene products of HPV, synthesized during replication (reviewed in Reference 1). In brief, there are two structural proteins comprising the capsid, L1 and L2, and about seven other open reading frames, which can be variably spliced. Two of these encode the proteins E6 and E7, which are probably the most relevant for the oncogenic process. They complex with the tumor suppressor gene products, p53 and retinoblastoma protein (pRb), respectively, abrogating their function, and cooperate together in the immortalization of primary human keratinocytes. They are expressed in genital dysplasia and malignancies (see, for example, Reference 8), and the mRNA of E7 is abundant in genital warts.[9]

## B. Viral Replication

Although the exact prevalence of HPV infections in the general population is unknown, most people are thought to have come in contact with HPV at some times in their lives. Infections are spread by contact, either person to person or via an inanimate object. Successful transmission depends on there being a break in the surface of the skin or mucosa so that the virus can gain entry to the basal layers of the epidermis. One specific receptor to which the virus adsorbs has been identified as α6-integrin.[10] Differences in genetic susceptibility may exist and there is some evidence of viral latency where infection occurs without the development of a clinically apparent lesion.

Following infection of a few cells in the stratum basale, the virus is found in the form of non-integrated genomic DNA. As the keratinocytes migrate upward through the stratum spinosum to the stratum granulosum, there is amplification of the viral DNA, and synthesis of viral proteins begins with the expression of E6 and E7 proteins in the suprabasal layer first; then E1, E2, and E5 are expressed, promoting the synthesis of viral DNA rather than cellular DNA. Finally L1, L2, and E4 proteins are found, linked to the terminal differentiation of the keratinocytes. Assembly of new viral particles takes place in the stratum corneum, with minimal disruption to the skin architecture and function. In cutaneous warts these particles can be seen as crystalline arrays in the nucleus of the degenerating cells and they are presumably released to the environment with dead squames. This rather unusual pattern of host–virus interaction has consequences for the generation of an effective immune response, not least the sparse expression of most viral proteins in the lower layers of the epidermis (see section below). In genital warts only a few viral particles are found. In cervical HPV infections and low grade dysplasia of the cervix, characteristic keratinocytes with vacuoles surrounding dense nuclear chromatin are seen in the suprabasal layers (Figure 33.1); these are called koilocytes and, although most are not associated with viral particles or proteins, they are considered pathognomonic of HPV infection. In high-grade cervical intraepithelial neoplasia (CIN) or carcinomas, no viral particles are observed and the viral DNA is almost always integrated into the host cell DNA. Integration associated with transformation results in the disruption of the E2 gene while the E6 and E7 genes remain intact. E2 protein is necessary for efficient viral DNA synthesis and normally represses the transcriptional expression of the E6 and E7 genes.

Studies of the interaction of HPV with epidermal cells have been hampered by the lack of both an *in vitro* cell culture permissive for viral replication and suitable animal models. This has also meant that the preparation of reagents for immunological assays and testing of immune function have been unusually difficult. However, advances have been made in recent years with the development of an organotypic culture for differentiating epithelial cells, the validation of several transplantation strategies in animal models, and the availability of capsid proteins by overexpression in various heterologous systems including vaccinia virus and baculovirus (reviewed in Reference 11). Virus-like particles (VLPs) have proved particularly useful. They are formed by the *in vitro* assembly of recombinant HPV capsid proteins, either L1 alone or L1 plus L2.[12] Chimeric VLPs can accommodate only small quantities of HPV nonstructural proteins.

## C. Immune Responses

It has proved difficult to monitor both local and systemic immune responses in HPV infections for several reasons. The initiation of the infection is almost invariably unknown so that early host responses cannot be measured; there is a wide variety of HPV types involved, which may, or may not, cross-react immunologically, and may cause a range of lesions or subclinical infection. The interaction of HPV types with the host is thought to be dynamic so it is almost impossible to distinguish a recent HPV exposure from past HPV exposures that have become persistent. In addition, as already indicated above, it is not straightforward to obtain relevant viral antigens or epitopes for use in immunological assays.

There is abundant clinical evidence to support a critical role for cell-mediated immunity in the control of HPV infections. Patients with depressed cell-mediated immunity, either hereditary or secondary to drugs, tumors, or HIV infection, frequently develop extensive and disabling warts. In contrast, individuals with defective antibody production do not suffer multiple or persistent warts. Despite the contribution of the immune response to the control of HPV infections, the majority of cutaneous warts tend to persist for several weeks or months before regression. Occasionally, they do not regress and can be recalcitrant to treatment, even in subjects who appear fully immunocompetent. Genital HPV infections seem to persist for many years in certain individuals and this provides a very high risk factor for the progression of cervical dysplasia.[13] These observations suggest that HPV are not strongly antigenic or that they may have developed strategies to evade the normal SIS. Although some early reports indicate that patients with chronic HPV infections demonstrate depressed systemic immune function,[14] these have not been corroborated more recently[15] and any viral immunomodulation is likely to be confined to the lesion itself.

Systemic antibody and T-cell responses to HPV antigens are reviewed by Tindle and Frazer[16] and Konya and Dillner.[17] In brief, seroconversion may not occur for several months (estimated at 6 to 12 months in one study[17]) after HPV DNA has been detected and is not found in all individuals known to be infected with HPV. The antibody response, primarily IgG1 and IgA, is type specific and is known to be neutralizing. Lymphoproliferation in response to HPV has been shown and may favor resolution of the infection but the type specificity of the stimulation is not clear at the present time. Cytotoxic T-cell responses, specific for HPV, can also be detected in a proportion of infected subjects (usually less than 50%) although their role in viral clearance and at what stage remains to be established.

## 1. Local Immunity

As HPV infections do not spread from the initial site of inoculation in the epidermis, the first immune responses are likely to be innate, such as those mediated by macrophages and natural killer (NK) cells. However, histological examination of skin warts and genital HPV lesions shows a lack of inflammatory cells.[19] As outlined above, the unusual pattern of host–HPV interaction in the epidermis has consequences for the generation of an effective immune response in that the expression of most HPV proteins in the basal layers is low and there is little cell death locally. In addition, as is the case for many other viruses, HPV have evolved strategies to avoid the normal SIS, despite their small size and limited genome capacity. Some of these have been recognized in recent years (see Table 33.2) and help to explain the frequent persistence of HPV infections for long periods of time in immunocompetent individuals. Indeed, O'Brien and Campo have suggested that the ability to avoid the host's immune defenses may be linked to the oncogenic potential of the individual HPV types.[22] Despite these evasion mechanisms, in most instances skin warts resolve in a matter of months and, in the cervix, the virus is eliminated in the majority of subjects before malignancy develops.

The cells most likely to act as antigen-presenting cells for HPV are the Langerhans cells (LC),[23] which are thought to take up viral antigens derived from HPV-infected keratinocytes and present them. LC can also bind and internalize free HPV particles, but recently it was shown that such a process does not activate LC, cultured *in vitro*, and no stimulation of T cells occurs.[20] The amount of viral antigen and inflammatory signals necessary for the activation of the LC within the HPV-infected epidermis are limited, helping to explain the frequently delayed and restricted immune response generated.

There is a decrease in the density of epidermal LC in many cutaneous[24] and mucosal[25] HPV lesions and this reduction is more marked in the lesions of immunosuppressed allograft recipients.[26] The mRNA of CD1a, a phenotypic marker for human LC, is also decreased in genital warts

**TABLE 33.2**
**Summary of Immune Evasion Mechanisms of HPV Types[20–22]**

| Immune Function Affected | HPV Type and Protein | Immune Consequences |
|---|---|---|
| **IFN** | | |
| Iinhibition of IFN-α activity | HPV-16 and 18 E7 | Loss of anti-viral activity, loss of MHC class I enhancement, loss of NK cell activation |
| Inhibition of IFN-β promoter | HPV-11 and 16 E7 | |
| Inhibition of IFN-responsive genes | HPV-16 E6 | |
| **MHC Class I** | | |
| Repression of MHC heavy chain promoter | HPV-6/11, 16, and 18 E7 | Loss of cytotoxic T-cell activity |
| Repression of MHC class I transcription and transport | HPV-16 E5 | |
| **MHC Class II** | | |
| Repressed antigen presentation through endosomal pathway | HPV-16 E5 and E7? | Loss of antigen presentation to CD4+ T cells |
| **IL-18** | | |
| Downregulation of expression | HPV-16 E6 and E7 | Loss of Th1 and NK cell stimulation through IFN-γ promotion of Th2 activity |
| **Langerhans Cells** | | |
| Loss of activation | HPV-16 L1/L2 VLP | Loss of IL-12 secretion, loss of migration from the epidermis, loss of ability to stimulate T cells |

compared with normal skin.[27] Another study reported a reduction in the numbers of immature epidermal dendritic cells in cervical dysplasia and HPV infection.[28] However, the depletion in LC is found to be similar in regressing and progressing warts, suggesting that the density of this cell type is not a critical factor in determining immunity to HPV.[29,30]

Changes in major histocompatibility complex (MHC) class II expression have been reported in the epidermis of genital warts,[31] CIN, and cervical carcinomas[32] with a general upregulation on both dysplastic keratinocytes and the remaining LC.[33] It should be noted that interferon-gamma (IFN-γ) tends not to induce MHC class II or intercellular adhesion molecule-1 (ICAM-1) expression on cervical cell lines *in vitro*,[34] and the upregulation is not a generalized response to cytokines as there is no correlation with the number of inflammatory cells in the lesions.[35] On the other hand, Mota et al.[36] showed that CIN progression was associated with *de novo* expression of HLA-DR and ICAM-1 on keratinocytes and no adhesion/co-stimulation molecules were detected on the epithelial LC in cervical lesions. In addition Hilders et al.[37] and Markey et al.[38] have reported evidence to suggest that HLA-DR is the MHC class II antigen most likely to be involved in HPV immunity as its expression correlates with the extent of lymphocyte infiltration. A meta-analysis has been performed recently to establish if any HLA-DR allele specificities confer altered susceptibility to HPV-related cervical diseases: it was shown that HLA-DR13 was protective regardless of the infecting HPV type, HLA-DR15 led to increased susceptibility only when HPV-16 was involved and HLA-DR7 was protective when the type was other than HPV-16 and was a susceptibility factor for HPV-16-associated cervical neoplasia.[17]

Studies of T-cell numbers in the epidermis of cutaneous warts indicate that they are not increased compared with normal skin;[39] in cervical HPV infection and CIN, they are greatly depleted, with CD8+ in the majority.[40] In condylomata acuminata, a very low level of interleukin-2 (IL-2) mRNA is found which may also reflect the small numbers of lymphocytes within such lesions. Jackson et al.[39] examined T cells and adhesion molecule expression in cutaneous warts and have shown that the dermis below the lesion contained more T cells than normal skin, almost all of the memory phenotype. It was striking that ICAM-1 and E-selectin expression was increased in the dermis of warts compared with normal skin, with no expression of either molecule in the epidermis. The lack of adhesion molecules may help to explain the paucity of T cells in the epidermis as the ICAM-1–LFA-1 pathway is thought to be critical in adhesion of keratinocytes to T cells, at least *in vitro*, although other candidate molecules for the recruitment of leukocytes into the epidermis have been proposed. Among these are IL-8 and monocyte chemotactic and activating factor or the adhesion molecule, LFA-3, present on epidermal LC and keratinocytes in normal skin and whose ligand on T cells is CD2. In one of the few studies to monitor virus-specific T cells in cervical tumors, cytotoxic T lymphocytes were demonstrated to infiltrate the carcinoma, and may be important in the immune control of tumor progression.[41]

It is of interest to extend these phenotypic observations to the measurement of cytokine expression in HPV lesions and here various studies frequently report conflicting results, which may reflect the stage of the HPV infection, the site involved, or the HPV type. The mRNAs of 11 cytokines were assessed by reverse-transcription polymerase chain reaction (RT-PCR) in cutaneous warts, and compared with normal skin: of these, only IL-10 mRNA was downregulated in warts while IL-1$\alpha$ mRNA was upregulated, and warts expressing IL-1$\alpha$ mRNA also expressed amphiregulin.[42] In studies of condylomata acuminata, caused by HPV-6 and 11 infection, the mRNAs of tumor necrosis faction-alpha (TNF-$\alpha$), transforming growth factor-beta-1 (TGF-$\beta$1), and IFN-$\gamma$ were reduced compared with normal skin.[9] However, the first two of these cytokines was reported to increase in EV lesions,[43] a difference suggested to be due to some immune dysfunction in EV such as a cytokine receptor defect or the influence of products induced by the special EV HPV types. The mRNAs of IL-1$\alpha$ and IL-1$\beta$ in condylomata were also reduced.[27] The downregulation in genital lesions may have a cascade effect on immune responses locally by influencing HLA class I and II expression and perhaps affecting antigen expression. In addition, in the condylomata, the mRNAs of various growth-inhibitory products like p53 were decreased and growth-stimulating products increased, which may be a direct effect of HPV infection.[27] The end result of all these changes could be keratinocyte proliferation without differentiation. It has also been reported that the production of TNF-$\alpha$ by basal keratinocytes is downregulated in CIN, while the production of IL-10 is upregulated, in comparison with the normal cervical epithelium.[36] This may indicate a tendency toward a Th2 type of adaptive immunity rather than a Th1 response in cases where the HPV infection is not cleared.

One further and very interesting mechanism concerns the expression of HLA class I molecules in HPV-associated lesions. It has been reported that 60% of cervical tumors show complete or heterogeneous (allele-specific) loss of HLA class I antigens.[44] The downregulation was also observed in metastatic cells, and patients with early-stage cervical carcinoma, exhibiting the change, had a worse prognosis. Disturbed class I expression is also found in CIN I to III.[32] These data suggest a selection of HLA class I-negative cells during tumor progression. The E7 of HPV-16 and 18 and the E5 of HPV-16 are known to inhibit the expression of HLA class I molecules (Table 33.2). In addition, HPV could influence class I molecule expression in other ways, such as by altering cellular oncogene products or by affecting different cytokines that then regulate class I synthesis.

## 2. Regression

The specific viral proteins or epitopes that are critical in stimulating effective immunity, leading to regression of HVP infections, have not been identified, and it is possible that there are contributions from a range of the early proteins, in addition to L1 and L2. It is thought that regression and the resistance to reinfection are probably type specific. It is also known that, in subjects with multiple warts, treatment of one can lead to the regression of not only that lesions but of the others too. This might imply that viral antigens or virus released from the treated wart can stimulate an effective immune response against other HPV infections.

When common warts regress spontaneously, infiltrating lymphocytes and macrophages are found and keratinocytes show evidence of cytopathic effects. Plane warts, which are caused frequently by HPV-3 infection and tend to regress more readily than other warts, have a mononuclear cell infiltrate, expressing mainly $CD4^+$, in the dermis during regression.[45] Coleman et al.[30] have monitored phenotypic changes in regressing genital warts. Clearance was characterized by an active cell-mediated immune response with an influx of T cells and macrophages. The T cells were in both the stroma and the epidermis at a $CD4^+$:$CD8^+$ ratio of about 1:0.9, while in nonregressing warts the ratio was 1:1.5. The macrophages were in the stroma only and represented 20% of the mononuclear cells in that site. There was evidence of activation in regressing warts by expression of CD25 on the T cells, induction of HLA-DR and ICAM-1 on keratinocytes, and expression of E-selectin and VCAM-1 on endothelial cells. These changes are indicative of a delayed-type hypersensitivity (DTH) response. However, much remains unclear and the factors inducing the initiation of spontaneous regression are not characterized. It is not known, for example, whether $CD4^+$ cells might mediate cytotoxic activity or might release cytokines that could inhibit the proliferation of infected keratinocytes or stimulate infiltrating macrophages. It is also unclear if antigen presentation occurs via the LC, either locally or in the draining lymph node, or if keratinocytes or macrophages might fulfill this role in regression. It is possible that the keratinocytes modulate the cytokine environment in the HPV-infected site, thus activating immune effector cells and LC. The subsequent recruitment and activation state of the local dendritic cells may be decisive in viral clearance to promote the homing of HPV-specific $CD4^+$ and $CD8^+$ T cells plus antibody-producing B cells to the infected area.[46] In support of this hypothesis, imiquimod, a synthetic molecule used as a topical therapy for genital warts, has been shown to stimulate a range of proinflammatory cytokines, particularly IFN-α, IL-6, and IL-8, from keratinocytes.[47] It also activates macrophages and LC to induce Th1 cytokines including IL-12[48] and increases the number of T cells infiltrating into the lesions.

The intraepithelial memory T lymphocytes generated as a result of HPV infection are likely to be critical in effective resistance to reinfection.[46] Also, memory Th responses to HPV-16 E2 and E6 have been detected, using a IFN-γ ELISPOT assay, in the blood of 60% of healthy people while T-cell reactivity against HPV-16 E7 is rarely found.[49] Thus, peripheral blood memory T cells, producing IFN-γ in response to some nonstructural HPV-16 proteins, may play a major role in protection against persistent infection and the HPV-associated malignancies.

## IV. HERPES SIMPLEX VIRUS TYPE 1 AND 2

### A. The Viruses and Their Diseases

HSV-1 and 2 belong to the *Alphaherpesvirinae* subfamily of herpesviruses and infect mucoepithelial cells, the former commonly in the orolabial region and the latter in the genital region. They are among the most widespread of the human viral pathogens, HSV-1 infecting approximately 80% of the world's population and HSV-2 30%. The virions contain a core of double-stranded linear DNA capable of coding for at least nine viral-encoded glycoproteins, with the tegument between the nucleocapsid and the envelope (Figure 33.2). It is thought that the viral glycoproteins gB or gC attach to heparin sulfate proteoglycans present on many cell types. This is followed by binding of glycoprotein D to specific receptors, yet to be fully identified, that are present on lymphocytes, epithelial cells, and some neuronal cells. After the adsorption stage, gB and gD are involved in fusion of the viral envelope with the cytoplasmic membrane, thus allowing the nucleocapsid to enter the cell and it is then transported to the nucleus. At least two viral proteins are involved in the transactivation of gene expression and one in the shutoff of host macromolecular synthesis. A regulatory cascade of viral protein synthesis in three phases follows, called immediate early (α), expressed without any prior synthesis of viral proteins; early (β), mostly proteins involved in nucleic acid metabolism; and late (γ), primarily structural polypeptides. Assembly of the capsid occurs

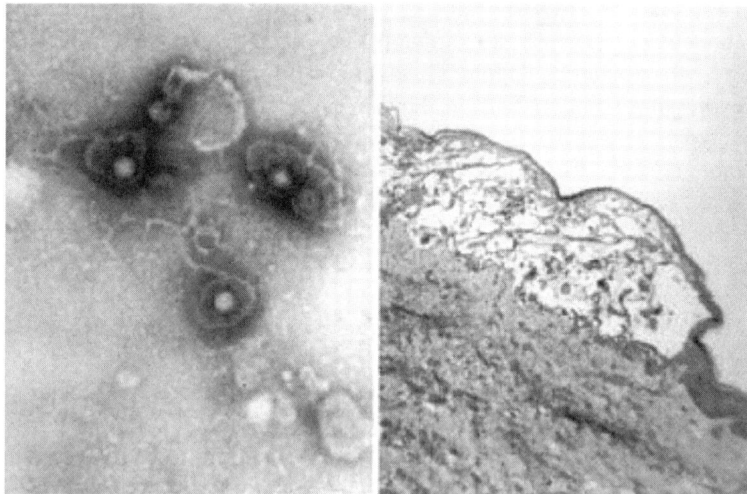

**FIGURE 33.2** HSV particles in vesicular fluid (negative stain, original magnification × 50,000) on the left side, and section of a herpetic vesicle (hematoxylin and eosin, original magnification × 250) on the right side.

with budding from the nuclear membrane and transport to the external environment, probably through the Golgi apparatus.

In human subjects, HSV replicates in keratinocytes in skin and mucous membranes, entering through abrasions. It causes subclinical infections or vesicular lesions, which are generally limited to the portal of entry of the virus. The lesions are caused by a combination of virally infected cell death and the inflammatory response. The vesicles usually heal without leaving scars. At the time of the primary infection, HSV infects axonal nerve terminals in the local site before retrograde transport to neuronal cell bodies where latency is established. Latency is a life-long state and the virus is thought to persist in the form of concatamers of non-integrated DNA in the nucleus of the neuron, without viral protein expression but with limited mRNA expression in the form of latency-associated transcripts. Reactivation of the viral genome can occur at intervals, frequently triggered by a recognizable stimulus such as ultraviolet (UV) exposure (see section below), which leads to the return of the virus to the site of the original infection. The precise mechanism responsible for reactivation in the ganglia is unknown but may involve changes in factors important in the regulation of neural gene transcription. Keratinocytes in that neurodermatome then become infected, resulting in a clinically inapparent lesion called a recurrence or a lesion called a recrudescence. The primary and recrudescent lesions progress from erythema through the stages of papules, vesicles, erosions, or ulcers before healing in about 14 days. Palpable local lymphadenopathy often develops as clinical symptoms appear.

Several studies have been conducted on individuals with recrudescent HSV infections to examine their immune responses to the virus. However, the majority of the work to identify the role of individual viral proteins and glycoproteins and the contribution of various immune effector mechanisms in controlling primary and recurrent HSB infection has been accomplished in animal models, most notably the mouse, although it has proved more difficult to develop a reliable model of recrudescence in rodents.

## B. Immune Responses

During primary HSV infections, the immune response becomes activated and controls the extent of the lesions and the production of new viral particles. However, it does not prevent the establishment of latency or eliminate a latent infection, or, in some individuals, prevent intermittent recrudescences. The intensity of the inflammatory response generally declines in the recrudescent lesions so that they are less severe and of shorter duration than in the primary infection. Several reviews cover the role of different arms of the innate and acquired systemic immunity in the control of HSV,[50,51] and in this chapter only the immunological events in the local cutaneous site of HSV-1 infection are considered.

## 1. Local Immunity to HSV-1

In most human HSV-1 infections, the virus is confined to the epidermis where it induces the formation of multinucleated giant cells and is cytopathic for keratinocytes. There is intraepidermal vesicle formation as demonstrated in Figure 33.2, with the vesicular fluid composed of virus particles, inflammatory cells, and cell debris. Infected keratinocytes have been reported to express the mRNA for IL-1β, TNF-α, and IL-6, maximal 24 h after infection,[52] and, recently, we have shown that they are also induced to synthesis IL-10, a cytokine that may help to downregulate immune responses locally.[53] One of the few phenotypic studies of recrudescent lesions has revealed that viral glycoproteins are present in the nuclei and cytoplasm of necrotic cells at 1 to 3 days postinfection only.[54] At this early stage, an inflammatory cell infiltrate is found in the dermis, consisting of T cells primarily with smaller numbers of NK cells and B cells. $CD4^+$ T cells are seen three to six times more frequently than $CD8^+$ cells and most are activated. Later, monocytes and macrophages are prominent with the $CD4^+$:$CD8^+$ ratio reducing to 2.5:1. The local immunological events following HSV infection are complex, and Table 33.3 outlines one possible temporal sequence.

Several studies have tried to elucidate the mechanism of immune induction to HSV-1 and the picture at present is not clear. One of the most recent and convincing reports indicates that, following subcutaneous infection of mice with HSV-1, the only cell type capable of presenting an immuno-

**TABLE 33.3**
**Suggested Stages in the Generation of Local Immune Responses to HSV-1 Infection**

| Temporal Sequence of Events | Consequences |
|---|---|
| Infection of keratinocytes | Inhibition of host cell protein synthesis, downregulation MHC class I synthesis, production of IFN-α and β, then β-chemokines, IL-12, IL-1, IL-6, IL-10, and TGF-β |
| Infection of Langerhans cells | Production of IL-1β and TNF-α, ?maturation or cell death |
| Infection of mature dendritic cells | Downregulation of CD83, no production of virus particles, (poor T cell stimulation) |
| Infection of immature dendritic cells | Inhibition of dendritic cell maturation, cell death |
| Transport of viral antigens via antigen-presenting cells (APC) to draining lymph node, or as virally infected APC | Antigen presentation in draining lymph node |
| T cells in draining lymph node | Antigen-specific activation and proliferation, expression of CLA homing or other homing receptors, extravasation via upregulated E-selectin on vascular endothelium |
| Infiltrating cells in vesicle: | |
| NK cells | Cytotoxic, production of IFN-γ, macrophage activation, upregulation MHC class I and ICAM-1 |
| $CD4^+$ T cells | Production of Th1 cytokines especially IFN-γ, cytotoxic (MHC class II) restricted, upregulation MHC class I and E-selectin |
| $CD8^+$ T cells | Cytotoxic (MHC class I restricted), cytokine production |
| B cells | Antibodies involved in cytotoxicity and neutralization |
| Monocytes/macrophages | Cytotoxic, production of IL-12, TNF-α, and TGF-β, resistant to HSV infection, ?local antigen presentation |
| **Prevention of HSV spread and resolution of lesion** | |

dominant epitope of HSV-1 gB to prime cytotoxic T cells is the CD11c$^+$CD8α$^+$CD45RA$^-$ dendritic cell.[55] The priming occurs in the local lymph node within 6 h postinfection. This cell population differs from the CD11b$^+$ submucosal dendritic cells shown to be involved in priming the Th response to HSV-2.[56] The dendritic cells are not thought to contain infectious virus but most likely acquire HSV antigens from virally infected apoptotic keratinocytes and then undergo class I restricted cross-presentation. Mikloska et al.[57] have found that immature monocyte-derived dendritic cells that resemble LC could be infected productively with HSV-1, with sequential expression of immediate-early, early, and late viral proteins. Up to 80% of the dendritic cells could be infected and about half of these were killed within 2 days of infection. The expression of HLA class I and II molecules was not affected by the infection but there was downregulation of CD1a, ICAM-1, CD80, and CD86. The virus may employ this interaction with immature dendritic cells to inhibit their maturation and subsequent T-cell stimulation. Mature dendritic cells, which are able to induce strong T-cell responses, can also be infected with HSV. In this case, only the immediate-early and early transcripts are found and no virus particles are produced.[58] CD83, a surface marker of mature dendritic cells, is downregulated within 10 h postinfection.[58] Other surface markers are not affected. HSV-1 interferes with mature dendritic cell-mediated T-cell proliferation and the loss in CD83 coincides with the reduced T-cell stimulation so that the virus may have evolved this route as a further means to evade the immune response.[59]

The above results describe the role of various dendritic cell populations in the initiation of immune responses in HSV-1 infections, and the involvement of LC, which form the major dendritic cell network in the epidermis, remains uncertain. There is evidence from experimental mice that the density of LC at the site of intradermal inoculation of HSV affects the severity of the infection. Thus, sites with lower densities of LC, for example, the eye or footpad, are more severely affected.[60] HSV is able to enter LC, and LC are capable of acting as antigen-presenting cells for HSV in lymphoproliferation tests of human cells *in vitro*.[61] Williams et al.[62] have shown that a murine epidermal cell population containing LC is not able to stimulate primary T-cell responses to HSV *in vitro*, although it could induce secondary responses to HSV. Thus, the LC may require maturation *in vivo* by migration to the draining lymph node before they are competent to present HSV to unprimed T cells.

As mentioned above, HSV has evolved a remarkable range of immune evasion mechanisms and one of these thought to be important in the initial stages in the skin is the ability to downregulate the expression of HLA class I molecules on the surface of infected keratinocytes and fibroblasts. This is due to the function of the immediate-early protein ICP47 that binds to the peptide transporter TAP, thus preventing the translocation of the peptides into the endoplasmic reticulum.[63] Posavad et al.[64] have suggested that the suppression in HLA class I molecules may allow the infected cells to escape temporarily from the cytotoxic activity of the CD8$^+$ T cells. However, as IFN-γ is produced by activated NK and CD4$^+$ T cells, which are the first lymphocyte populations to migrate into the lesions, the expression of HLA class I is soon upregulated. Thus, by day 2 following reactivation, the infected keratinocytes are subsequently lysed by specific CD8$^+$ T cells, helping to prevent any further spread of the virus locally. Spread is also controlled early in the lesion development by IFN-α, produced by the infected keratinocytes, by a direct antiviral effect.[65]

An increase in the size of the lymph nodes draining the site of human HSV infections is seen frequently and is also found after intradermal or epicutaneous infections of mice. This is due to the proliferation of both CD4$^+$ and CD8$^+$ T cells. The CD4$^+$ T cells can transfer DTH to infected recipient mice and also, as shown in a transfer experiment, have the ability to clear infectious virus from the epidermis.[66] Various viral proteins elicit T cells mediating DTH, including gG, gC, and gD. The viral-specific CD4$^+$ T cells have the general properties of the Th1 subset. They are probably important in the control of both primary and recrudescent infections, and may also act as cytotoxic cells, recognizing viral antigens in association with MHC class II antigens expressed on dendritic cells in the skin and on macrophages and keratinocytes following upregulation. Human keratinocytes infected with HSV have been shown to act as targets for such cells *in vitro*.[67] Homing receptors for CD4$^+$ T cells have not been defined as yet.

CD8+ cytotoxic T cells, which, in the past, were not thought to play as critical a role in the local control of HSV infections as CD4+ T cells, have more recently been shown in herpetic lesion infiltrates.[68] In the context of MHC class I antigens, the CD8+ cells recognize gB and the immediate-early protein ICP27, in particular. At the peak of the response to a cutaneous footpad infection of mice, up to 5% of the CD8+ T cells in the draining lymph node and 10% in the spleen are specific for one immunodominant epitope of gB, indicating a huge expansion in this population.[69] The gB-specific CD8+ T cells are activated by 6 to 8 h postinfection and begin to proliferate by 24 h postinfection — a remarkably prompt response to the HSV.[70] Koelle et al. have shown that the activated HSV-specific CD8+ T cells found in the lesions express the skin-homing receptor cutaneous lymphocyte-associated antigen (CLA), which interacts with upregulated E-selectin in venular endothelial cells in the infected site.[71] The CLA may be induced locally by IL-12 or TGF-β, or cells expressing the CLA may be selectively recruited to the lesion.

Macrophages also play an important role as local effector cells. They exhibit intrinsic resistance to HSV replication due mainly to their arginase activity as arginine is required for HSV replication. In addition, they exhibit extrinsic resistance by producing complement, interferons, and other mediators such as TNF-α, which enhance the local inflammatory response. Their effectiveness has been demonstrated in a mouse model where an antibody against CD3 receptor that blocks emigration of monocytes into the skin was shown to reduce clearance of virus from the epidermis.[72] IFN-γ is also involved at this stage so that activation of the recruited macrophages may be necessary. It is not known if macrophages can present HSV antigens during reinfections or recrudescences.

Antibody-mediated immune responses in HSV infections probably play a minor role in primary infection but may contribute to the control of recrudescences or reinfections by the mechanism of antibody-dependent cell-mediated cytotoxicity (ADCC) and neutralization.[73] The cell types mediating ADCC include macrophages, NK cells, and neutrophils, and neutralization may be particularly important at the stage of viral entry into, or exit from, nerve endings. However, as already explained, HSV has developed multiple strategies by which it can evade immune responses. In the context of antibodies, the gC of HSV-1 is able to bind complement factors; this inhibits the complement cascade and protects against both complement-mediated destruction of infected cells and viral neutralization. Also gE and gI bind the Fc receptor of IgG so that recognition of bound antibody by complement and ADCC is reduced. It is not known what effect such modulation to the immune response may have in local sites *in vivo*.

## 2. The Effects of UVB Radiation on HSV-1 Infection

Exposure to sunlight is a common triggering factor for HSV-1 recrudescence. In one report 33% of subjects who suffered from herpes labialis recognized that UV radiation was the stimulus for the reappearance of the vesicular lesion.[74] The importance of UV radiation was first shown experimentally by Wheeler[75] and several studies since have confirmed the initial observation. For example, Rooney et al.[76] used a sunscreen in a double-blind, placebo-controlled crossover trial of 38 patients with recurrent herpes labialis. The individuals were UV-irradiated with a burning dose on two occasions on the usual site of the their lesions. On one occasion, a sunblock was applied before the exposure and, on the other, a placebo cream. It was discovered that 70% of the subjects treated with the placebo plus UV radiation developed HSV recrudescences, while 0% developed lesions when protected by the sunblock.

Details concerning the immunological events that follow UV radiation have been obtained from several models of primary HSV infection in mice. Howie et al.[77] have shown that UVB irradiation with a single suberythemal dose prior to epidermal or subcutaneous infection of mice with HSV-1 resulted in a suppressed DTH when the mice were challenged subsequently with inactivated virus. Antigen-specific T cells were generated in the spleens of the irradiated animals capable of transferring the immune suppression to mice already infected with the virus.[78] It was also shown that the initial presentation of HSV by LC in the epidermis could determine whether DTH itself or specific cells that suppressed DTH were generated.[79] Yasumoto et al.[80] have provided evidence that UV exposure before subcutaneous infection of mice with HSV resulted in a switch in cytokine production by lymph node cells and spleen cells on culture *in vitro* in the presence of HSV antigens. The synthesis of IFN-$\gamma$ and IL-2 was suppressed while that of IL-4 was enhanced. Thus, the Th2 subset of T cells may be preferentially activated in the UV-irradiated mice. This could occur through the generation of T-regulatory cells, as has been shown in other systems.[81,82]

A model of cutaneous HSV-1 reactivation in SKH-1 hairless mice was described recently.[83] Following epidermal infection of the mice on abraded skin, and resolution of the lesions, the mice were irradiated with two minimal inflammatory doses from a source which approximated to the solar spectrum. Recrudescent lesions were induced in about 60% of the animals. The effect of the UV was local, as irradiation of the uninvolved side did not result in recrudescence. The mechanism leading to this modulation of memory responses to HSV has not been evaluated yet. However, van der Molen et al.[84] have shown that UV radiation reduces the ability of human epidermal cells to present HSV-1 to autologous memory T cells. Thus, one direct effect of the UV may be to modulate the activity of the antigen-presenting cells locally in the epidermis.

The events that follow the irradiation have not been worked out in detail but could be twofold. First, the virus has to reactivate in the neurons of the ganglia, perhaps through the transactivation of viral UV-response elements, and then it replicates in the periphery. Second, the immune response locally is likely to be suppressed temporarily by the UV exposure, but sufficiently to allow some viral replication and the generation of clinically apparent lesions. Recovery of the immune system following the delayed influx of effector cells into the infected site would then curtail the extent of the lesion and promote healing.

## V. HUMAN HERPESVIRUSES-6, -7, AND -8

### A. The Viruses

Like the other members of the Herpesviridae family, HHV-6, -7, and -8 are thought to persist for the lifetime of the host following the initial infection and the main route of transmission is probably by contact (reviewed in References 85 and 86). Some properties of these newly discovered viruses are outlined in Table 33.4 but many others, including their precise clinical associations, mechanisms of latency, and extent of asymptomatic shedding are uncertain at the present time.

HHV-6 is divided into two variants, A and B, defined by differences in serological reactions and DNA sequences. Variant A has not been shown to cause any specific disease while B can be asymptomatic or cause a common disease of young children (6 months to 2 years) called exanthem subitum or roseaola infantum. This is a mild, febrile illness with a rash, lasting 24 to 48 h, in about 10% of cases. The site of primary viral replication is not known. The transient rash might be caused by the presence of infected T cells in the skin or by the activation of T cells mediating DTH. The virus itself may be present in skin keratinocytes as well as in mononuclear cells infiltrating the skin. HHV-6 is probably spread via infected saliva, and most children in developed countries are seropositive by the age of two. The illness is controlled by cell-mediated immune mechanisms and the virus thereafter establishes a latent infection in $CD4^+$ T cells, monocytes,[87] and bone marrow progenitors. In adults, HHV-6 can cause symptoms resembling infectious mononucleosis, which can be serious in immunocompromised subjects. RT-PCR for the mRNA of a major structural gene expressed late in the replication cycle of HHV-6 can be used to differentiate latent and replicating virus in clinical specimens.[88]

Underlying viral infections may predispose patients to develop severe cutaneous reactions to drugs: for example, patients with AIDS are at a 1000 time higher risk than immunocompetent subjects in this regard.[89] It has been reported recently that HHV-6 can reactivate during severe drug-induced hypersensitivity syndrome, characterized by being multiorgan and potentially fatal. This

**TABLE 33.4**
**Characteristics of HHV-6, -7, and -8**

| | HHV-6 | HHV-7 | HHV-8 |
|---|---|---|---|
| First discovered | 1986 | 1989 | 1993 |
| Subfamily | Betaherpesvirinae | Betaherpesvirinae | Gammaherpesvirinae |
| Prevalence | Ubiquitous | Ubiquitous | Limited to certain geographical areas, and AIDS patients |
| Cell receptor | CD46 | CD4 and others (undefined) | $\alpha3\beta1$ integrin (CD49c/29) and others (undefined) |
| Infects: | | | |
| Preferentially | $CD4^+$ T cells | $CD4^+$ T cells | $CD19^+$ B cells |
| Also | B cells, NK cells, monocytes, endothelial cells | Epithelial cells | Null cells, endothelial cells, perivascular spindle cells, dorsal root ganglia, monocytes, fibroblasts, keratinocytes |
| Latent infection | $CD4^+$ T cells, monocytes, bone marrow progenitors | $CD4^+$ T cells | $CD19^+$ B cells |

was shown by a large increase in IgG specific for HHV-6, HHV-6 viraemia in some cases,[90] and the presence of HHV-6 in mononuclear cells infiltrating the skin in other cases.[91] If an immunological mechanism is proposed here, it is possible that cytotoxic T lymphocytes directed against HHV-6 antigens are polyreactive, recognizing a broad range of antigens, including those displayed on keratinocytes modified by the drugs.[92]

HHV-7 is found in some cases of exanthem subitum, although less commonly than HHV-6 and in slightly older children. It may be associated with symptoms of infectious mononucleosis, and reactivation of HHV-7, like HHV-6, may also be involved in some cases of cutaneous adverse drug reaction.[92] Most people have developed antibodies to HHV-7 by late childhood and, as the virus is shed from salivary glands, it is probably transmitted in saliva. Viral antigens are also detected in skin.[93] It has been suggested that the immune response generated to HHV-6 might protect to some extent against infection with HHV-7,[94] thus helping to explain why clinical disease due to HHV-7 is less frequent than that due to HHV-6. There is evidence that either HHV-6 or HHV-7, or both, acting synergistically, might cause pityriasis rosea. This disease association is discussed in Section V.B.

HHV-8 is also referred to as Kaposi's sarcoma-associated herpesvirus (KSHV) (reviewed in Reference 86). Most primary infections with HHV-8 are asymptomatic and the virus remains latent thereafter, most probably in the $CD19^+$ B cells of the peripheral blood.[95] Unlike the other human herpesviruses, infection with HHV-8 is not ubiquitous, especially in developed countries. HHV-8 is limited to certain geographical areas and there are genetic and behavioral risk factors. For example, the seroprevalence in blood donors in northern Europe is less than 5% while it is greater than 50% in many African populations.[96] Homosexual men can have asymptomatic infection rates approaching 40%.[96] Transmission is probably sexual in low-prevalence countries and may be by casual contact in Africa. The virus has come to prominence recently due to its association with Kaposi's sarcoma: more details regarding this aspect can be found in Section V.C.

## B. Pityriasis Rosea

Pityriasis rosea is a common acute disease with a very characteristic rash (shown in Figure 33.3) appearing in a "T-shirt" distribution (rarely extending beyond the mid-upper arms or neck) with the lesions following the lines of the dermatomes. A herald patch with a pink rim of scaling is

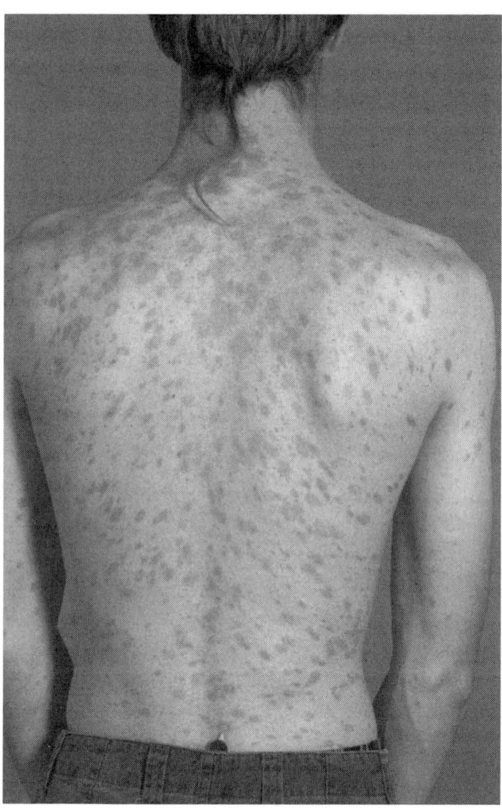

**FIGURE 33.3** The rash of pityriasis rosea showing the "T-shirt" distribution: the lesions are oval and their long axes tend to lie along dermatomal lines. (From Kavanagh, G.M. and Savin, J.A., *Dermatology: Self-Assessment Picture Tests,* Mosby International, St. Louis, MO, 1998, 46. With permission from Elsevier).

frequently seen first. New lesions can occur over a period of several weeks and then the condition gradually resolves. Pityriasis rosea is usually found in children or young adults.

A virus has been suspected as the etiological agent in pityriasis rosea due to the rapid clinical onset of the disease, some clustering of cases, the rarity of recurrences, and the seasonal variation in incidence. Such a role for HHV-6 or HHV-7 has been suggested, although it is difficult to define a causal relationship between a virus and a clinical disease, particularly when the virus is ubiquitous and reactivation rather then a primary infection might be involved. A further complication lies in the possible interaction of one virus with another. In one of the most recent and most convincing studies to date, Watanabe et al.[97] used nested PCR to test for viral DNA in lesional and nonlesional skin, saliva, peripheral blood mononuclear cells, and serum, as well as *in situ* hybridization for viral mRNA in skin lesions.[97] Both HHV-6 and -7 DNA was found in a high percentage of all the tissues tested but was rarely found in similar samples from control subjects or patients with psoriasis. The mRNAs of HHV-6 and -7 were detected in the majority of skin samples from the pityriasis rosea cases. It was concluded that pityriasis rosea is associated with a systemic active infection with both HHV-6 and -7, presumably due to the reactivation from latency of these viruses acquired in early childhood. Although herpes viral particles were not seen by electron microscopy in lesional skin in this study, they have been reported previously in 71% of pityriasis rosea lesional skin samples.[98] It should be noted that not all studies conclude that HHV-6 and/or -7 is involved in pityriasis rosea,[99,100] but there is at least the intriguing possibility that these two viruses could cooperate, for example, by HHV-7 providing a transactivating factor that then promotes the reactivation of HHV-6.[101,102]

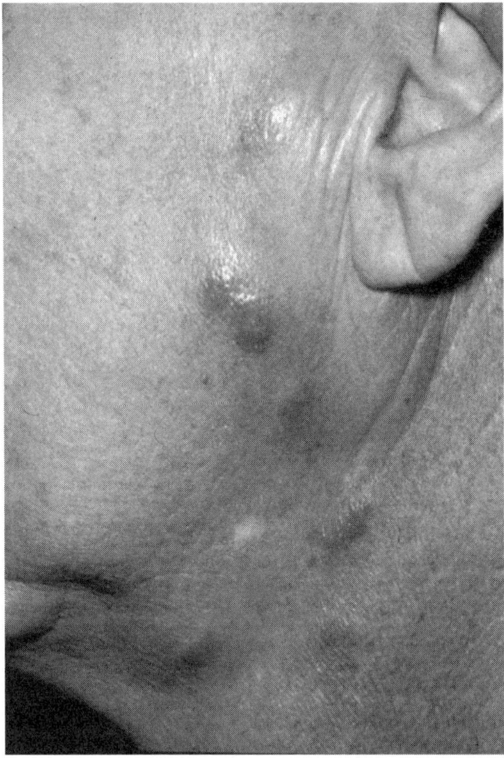

**FIGURE 33.4** Multiple nodular lesions of Kaposi's sarcoma on the face and neck. (From Kavanagh, G.M. and Savin, J.A., *Dermatology: Self-Assessment Picture Tests,* Mosby International, St. Louis, MO, 1998, 46. With permission from Elsevier).

## C. Kaposi's Sarcoma

Kaposi's sarcoma is one of the most frequent skin cancers in immunosuppressed Mediterranean subjects who have had transplants, and an aggressive epidemic form is a common feature of HIV-infected homosexual males. The tumors consist of endothelial cells with characteristic spindle shape, arranged in bundles. They are frequently multiple, occurring in the skin where they are visible as blue-pink or red-brown plaques or nodules (Figure 33.4), as well as occurring in lymph nodes and the gastrointestinal tract. The discovery of HHV-8 in a Kaposi's sarcoma skin lesion was by PCR-based subtractive hybridization,[103] and its identification led to the suggestion that HHV-8 might play a role in oncogenesis. The initial interaction of the virus with the host is not known, but clinical life-long latency results with the virus present in $CD19^+$ B cells. This latency is controlled by cytotoxic T lymphocytes in immunocompetent subjects.[104] The Kaposi's sarcoma may develop many years after the primary infection (thought to be at least 2 to 6 years) and may coincide with the onset of AIDS, when the associated decrease in immune function presumably leads to the reactivation of HHV-8. It has been shown recently that NK cells are also critical in controlling HHV-8 latent infections and the development of Kaposi's sarcoma.[105] In the tumor itself, the spindle cells contain viral DNA and express some viral proteins, implying that these viral gene products impart a growth advantage, although most of the cells do not produce virus.[106,107] A recent study has examined patterns of the viral mRNA expression, present in latent and lytic infections, in Kaposi's sarcoma lesions at different clinical stages but no clear differences emerged.[108]

HHV-8 is known to synthesize several proteins that have homology to human proteins, some promoting the replication of the infected cells and those cells adjacent to them, and others preventing apoptosis. A number act through the same cell-signaling pathways used by other herpesviruses, especially Epstein–Barr virus. The factors identified thus far are multiple and include a secreted IL-6 homologue that is a growth promoter, antiapoptotic, and induces VEGF,[109] a Bcl-2 analogue that is antiapoptotic, a caspase 8 inhibitory protein that inhibits Fas-mediated apoptosis and induces cellular IL-6 expression,[110] at least three chemokines belonging to the macrophage inflammatory protein family that initiate chemotactic signaling and inhibit the Th1 response,[111] a chemokine receptor, and several proteins reducing MHC class I expression,[112] thereby downregulating cytotoxic T-cell activity. It is also possible that HHV-8 is not involved directly in initiating Kaposi's sarcoma but inflammatory cytokines may attract virus-infected cells into the lesions.[113] In support of this view, the suggestion has been made that HIV *tat* could be a key factor in provoking the local inflammation.[114]

## VI. HUMAN IMMUNODEFICIENCY VIRUS

### A. HIV-Related Skin Diseases

Following an incubation period of 1 to 2 months, the primary infection with HIV is characterized frequently by headache, fever, symptoms of infectious mononucleosis, malaise, lymphadenopathy, and a fine morbilliform rash that may resemble that of pityriasis rosea, syphilis, or erythema multiforme. The patient seroconverts at this stage, is highly infectious, and the blood $CD4^+$ count may drop dramatically, then recover within a week or so. Subsequently, the virus persists and the subject can remain asymptomatic, or with persistent generalized lymphadenopathy, for an average of 8 to 10 years before symptoms of AIDS develop, with profound suppression of both cell-mediated and humoral immune responses. Death results, frequently from a secondary infectious disease, secondary cancer, or neurological disease.

Almost half of HIV-infected subjects exhibit a weak DTH response to common antigens during the asymptomatic phase. The majority then becomes anergic to skin tests when the blood $CD4^+$ drops to less than $200/mm^3$. It has been proposed that DTH skin testing is an independent predictor of progression to AIDS in HIV-infected patients,[115] and that it can predict survival time.[116] In addition, it could be useful in monitoring the success of antiviral therapy[117] and in determining whether patients should be offered preventative therapy for infectious diseases, such as tuberculosis.[118]

Almost all patients infected with HIV develop a skin-associated disease, most commonly Kaposi's sarcoma (see Section V.C.), psoriasis, and pruritis associated with eosinophilic folliculitis.[119] The causes of these last two conditions have not been identified. In addition, various infections of the skin, such as mucosal candidiasis, are very frequent. A shift from the Th1 to a Th2 cytokine response in the periphery may lead to an atopic state.[120] The atopic reaction could be triggered by a variety of factors including mites or staphylococci. It is supposed that the HIV is causing immune dysfunction leading to altered cytokine expression and so to the inflammatory cutaneous diseases. A recent study analyzed the expression of various cytokines in lesional and nonlesional skin of HIV-infected subjects with Kaposi's sarcoma, psoriasis, and pruritis due to eosinophilic folliculitis.[121] It was shown that the lesional skin from these three diseases has distinct and distinguishable levels and patterns of cytokine expression, with the same, but lower, intensity in the matched normal skin. These host reaction patterns may be determined by the genetic polymorphisms of the individual, which could result in differences in the quantity and type of inflammatory skin cytokines produced in response to antigenic stimuli in the skin.[121]

### B. The Involvement of HIV with the Skin

Several studies since the discovery of HIV in 1983 have tried to investigate its association with the skin. The mucous membrane, which lacks the stratum corneum but is rich in LC and macrophages, is thought to be the main route by which HIV enters the body. With regard to the skin rash occurring at the time of primary infection, LC were found to be a major site of HIV replication in the epidermis as they contain mRNA for the multiply spliced regulatory genes.[122] Simonitsch et al.[123] studied a skin biopsy from an erythematous plaque in a primary HIV infection and showed that there was vacuolization of the basal keratinocytes with an inflammatory infiltrate consisting of CD8+ T cells and CD68+ histiocytes/dendritic cells. Numbers of LC were decreased and the remaining LC co-expressed CD1a and HIV p24, and were in close proximity to the cytotoxic T lymphocytes. These results provide further evidence for skin involvement at the acute stage of the infection.

*In vitro*, LC were the first cutaneous cell type shown to be capable of infection with HIV[124] (M-tropic forms), and immature monocyte-derived dendritic cells are susceptible to productive infection with M-tropic, but not T-tropic, forms of HIV.[125] Mature dendritic cells are not susceptible due to a reduction in the receptor for the M-tropic forms and to a block at the transcriptional level. Epidermal sheets, obtained from uninfected subjects, can be inoculated with HIV and a proportion of the dendritic cells migrating from the explants become strongly positive for the viral structural protein p24.[126]

Published results from *in vivo* studies of the skin following the acute phase of HIV infection are frequently inconsistent. For example, in the 1980s, both immunohistochemistry and electron microscopy were used with some groups reporting HIV-infected LC (for example, Reference 127) and others not (for example, Reference 128). A subsequent PCR-based study of patients infected with HIV at different stages of the disease revealed both viral DNA and viral RNA in the skin in many samples, with detection more frequent in the dermis than in the epidermis.[129] There was no correlation of the presence of viral nucleic acid with the stage of the HIV infection, the number of peripheral CD4+ cells, or whether the skin appeared normal or diseased. In contrast, another report involving immunohistochemistry, electron microscopy, *in situ* hybridization, PCR, and co-culturing did not indicate a latent or productive infection in the epidermis of patients with HIV.[130]

The reasons for these controversial results may lie in the sensitivity of the detection protocols (reviewed in Reference 131). First, LC could die as a result of the infection with HIV or produce only low quantities of viral RNA. Second, the dendritic cells may be latently infected *in vivo* and only become activated when contact with T cells takes place. Third, the dendritic cells could act as antigen-presenting cells but virus-specific cytotoxic T lymphocytes could lyse them very effectively. However, it is still thought that the dendritic cells might be critical in carrying infectious HIV to the lymph nodes and, once there, to activate T cells for permissive viral production. Dendritic cells express DC-SIGN (CD209), which is required for HIV sequestration, protection, and transmission to T cells.[132] LC do not express DC-SIGN and may use alternative C-type molecules, such as Langerin.[131]

The treatment of subjects infected with HIV, suffering from psoriasis, eosinophilic folliculitis, or pruritis, with UVB phototherapy or PUVA chemotherapy has been a matter of some debate in recent years as it is known that HIV can be activated in cell culture and in transgenic mice by UV radiation (reviewed in Reference 133). Several investigations have revealed no deleterious effect of such therapies on clinical state or immunological responses and little effect on plasma viral load (reviewed in Reference 134). However, when the skin was assessed following UVB phototherapy by RT-PCR and RT-PCR *in situ* hybridization, there was a six- to tenfold increase in HIV expression.[135] This appeared to be due to activation of HIV by NF-κB. It is possible that the UV-induced apoptosis of infected T cells may negate this upregulatory effect of UV radiation on cells such as the LC so that there is no overall change in HIV status. An increased photosensitivity to UVB radiation does not occur in individuals infected with HIV.[136]

## VII. MEASLES VIRUS

### A. The Virus and the Disease

Human subjects represent the only natural reservoir for measles virus, and the infection occurs globally, representing a leading cause of childhood mortality. A coordinated control program including vaccination policies seeks to eradicate measles. This has been largely successful in industrialized countries but there are still more than 40 million cases of measles annually in developing countries with more than 1 million deaths, mostly of young children.

MV contains a single-stranded minus-sense RNA genome, packaged in a nucleocapsid, together with the virus-encoded RNA-dependent RNA polymerase, necessary for infectivity. The hemagglutinin and two subunits of the fusion protein are found as integral envelope proteins. The matrix protein lies on the inner surface of the envelope. Only one serotype has been described although more than 20 genotypes are now recognized. CD46, the complement membrane cofactor that is expressed on all human nucleated cells, was the first receptor identified for MV but is used mainly by attenuated vaccine and tissue culture-adapted MV strains. The clinical MV strains adsorb to the human signaling lymphocyte activation molecule (SLAM, CD150), which is expressed on activated T and B cells, memory cells, immature thymocytes, and mature monocytes. How the virus enters unstimulated monocytes, its major target, or endothelial and epithelial cells remains uncertain.[137] Penetration is by fusion, a process requiring both the fusion and hemagglutinin proteins. The nucleocapsid is released into the cytoplasm where replication takes place. Release is by budding from the cytoplasmic membrane without cell lysis.

MV is transmitted by the respiratory route, is highly infectious, and the incubation period is 7 to 13 days. After replication in the respiratory mucosa and lungs, the virus spreads to the local lymphoid tissue, most likely in tissue-resident macrophages or dendritic cells from the basolateral side of epithelial cells.[138] This stage is followed by a cell-associated viraemia with circulation of the virus systemically to other organs and to endothelial and epithelial cells in many sites, including the skin. In the skin the virus is thought to replicate in endothelial cells lining the capillaries, and a characteristic macropapular rash occurs, which marks the onset of the acquired immune response. A few days after the appearance of the rash, the virus is cleared from the skin and long-term immunity is induced. However, during the generation of immunity and for several weeks thereafter, defects in immune function develop. These contribute to the morbidity and mortality of MV infection, particularly to the development of secondary infections and autoimmune encephalomyelitis. There is a marked lymphopoenia, affecting mainly the T-cell population, and a loss of DTH to recall antigens. In addition, antigen-specific and polyclonal stimulation of lymphocytes *in vitro* are severely depressed. Furthermore, the initial Th1 cytokine profile in the blood changes to a Th2 profile, marked by the presence of IL-4 (reviewed in Reference 139).

Much research recently has concentrated on the pivotal role of dendritic cells in the generation of immunity to MV. MV can infect dendritic cells and such cells are probably critical in the induction of the early virus-specific immunity. However, the dendritic cells are also thought to be central in the general immunosuppression that follows MV infection. Various mechanisms for this have been proposed including the inhibition of IL-12 production from virally infected dendritic cells thus downregulating Th1 cytokine responses, the inhibition of T cell proliferation by the viral glycoprotein complex expressed at high level on infected dendritic cells, and T-cell depletion by dendritic cell–T-cell fusion or TRAIL-mediated induction of apoptosis (reviewed in Reference 140).

## B. Local Immunity

Little information is available on events in cutaneous sites before, during, and after the measles rash, except infiltration of lymphocytes and monocytes into local areas of viral replication has been noted. A light and electron microscope study showed multinucleated giant cells in the epidermis at the maximum stage of the rash, thought to be formed by hyper- or parakeratosis.[141] Viral inclusions and nucleocapsids were not visible in the epidermis. Dermal edema occurred with nucleocapsids present in the endothelium of the dermal capillaries. LC, derived *in vitro* from $CD34^+$ cord blood progenitors, are susceptible to infection with MV and are able to block naive allogeneic $CD4^+$ T-cell proliferation in response to uninfected LC.[142] The inhibition is not HLA restricted and not antigen specific. Such a response by the LC to MV may contribute to the immunosuppression that follows infection, although the interaction of LC with MV *in vivo* has not been established as yet.

The types of cells involved in the mononuclear infiltrate have not been identified, but it is assumed that $CD8^+$ cytotoxic T cells are present and act by an HLA class I restricted cytotoxic mechanism. That subjects with severe defects in cell-mediated immunity can develop progressive measles in the absence of a rash suggested that T-cell immunopathology is a critical factor in the rash. It is thought that the synthesis of IFN-$\alpha/\beta$, and subsequent activation of NK cells, is not an important component of the local response. Circulating antibodies are first detectable at the time of the rash and titers rise thereafter. Virus-specific IgM and IgA antibodies are produced initially, followed by IgG. Probably these immunoglobulins play a role in controlling viral replication by preventing virus-induced membrane fusion, lysing infected cells, modulating viral antigens, and suppressing synthesis of viral components. Their contribution, if any, to the resolution of the skin rash is uncertain.

It is known that $CD4^+$ T cells proliferate systemically during the rash, despite minimal DTH and *in vitro* lymphoproliferative responses at this time. Some of these cells have class II-restricted cytotoxic activity and may lyse infected cells in local sites; however, they are thought more likely to release an array of cytokines, which attract or activate macrophages, B cells, and T cells. At approximately the time of the rash, IFN-$\gamma$ and IL-2 levels increase in the plasma, indicative of Th1 CD4 and perhaps CD8 cytotoxic activities, but this is followed by a rise in IL-4 production that remains elevated for several weeks, suggesting the switch to the Th2 cytokine profile already mentioned above (reviewed in Reference 140).

## VIII. CONCLUSIONS

In this chapter, an overview has been given indicating the range of common viral infections of human skin, many of which can be regarded as "successful" in that they affect the majority of people at some time in their lives and are global in their distribution. Several cause persistent infections, either with or without periods of latency. The replication strategies of some of these viruses plus their local immune evasion mechanisms are now becoming apparent. Three very different viruses, HPV, HSV, and measles, were selected to illustrate aspects of local immunological control in the skin. Controversial evidence linking HHV-6, 7, and 8 with particular human cutaneous diseases and associating HIV with cells in the skin has also been included.

Rapid advances are being made at the present time in determining the initial steps in antigen presentation in the skin that prime the appropriate T-cell responses. Thus, the interaction between a particular virus and LC/dendritic cells/macrophages is becoming clearer, at least for some of the cutaneous infections, although has rarely been investigated *in vivo* as yet. Epitopes that stimulate protective antiviral immune responses are also being identified. With this knowledge may come the development of novel methods to control viral diseases affecting the skin, perhaps at the initiation of the infection. However, at the moment, the highest likelihood of success in the management of these diseases may lie in further advances in prophylactic and therapeutic vaccine design so that the most appropriate responses are elicited to provide protective immunity in the cutaneous or mucocutaneous site. More limited clinical success may also come from the future use of selected immunostimulants, which could be administered cutaneously or epicutaneously.

## REFERENCES

1. Howley, P.M., Papillomavirinae: the viruses and their replication, in *Field's Virology*, 4th ed., D.M. Knipe and P.M. Howley, Eds., Lippincott/Williams & Wilkins, Baltimore, MD, 2001, 946.
2. Ho, G.Y., Burk, R.D., Klein, S., Kadish, A.S., Chang, C.J., Palan, P., Basu, J., Tachezy, R., Lewis, R., and Romney, S., Persistent genital human papillomavirus infection as a risk factor for persistent cervial dysplasia, *J. Natl. Cancer Inst.*, 87, 1365, 1995.

3. Koutsky, L.A., Holmes, K.K., Critchlow, C.W., Stevens, C.E., Paavonen, J., Beckmann, A.M., De Rouen, T.A., Galloway, D.A., Vernon, D., and Kiviat, N.B., A cohort study of the risk of cervical intraepithelial neoplasia grade 2 or 3 in relation to papillomavirus infection, *N. Engl. J. Med.*, 327, 1272, 1992.
4. Gillison, M.L., Koch, W.M., Capone, R.B. et al., Evidence for a causal association between human papillomavirus and a subset of head and neck cancers, *J. Natl. Cancer Inst.*, 92, 709, 2000.
5. Snijders, P.J., Steenbergen, R.D., Meijer, C.J., and Walboomers, J.M., Role of human papillomaviruses in cancer of the respiratory and upper digestive tract, *Clin. Dermatol.*, 15, 415, 1997.
6. Majewski, S. and Jablonska, S., Epidermodysplasia verruciformis as a model of human papillomavirus-induced genetic change, *Arch. Dermatol.*, 131, 1312, 1995.
7. Proby, C., Storey, A., McGregor, J. et al., Does papillomavirus infection play a role in non-melanoma skin cancer? *Papillomavirus Rep.*, 7, 53, 1996.
8. Jeon, S. and Lambert, P.F., Integration of human papillomavirus type 16 DNA into the human genome leads to increased stability of E6 and E7 mRNAs: implications for cervical carcinogenesis, *Proc. Natl. Acad. Sci. U.S.A.*, 92, 1654, 1995.
9. Arany, I., Rady, P., and Tyring, S.K., Alterations in cytokine antioncogene expression in skin lesions caused by "low risk" types of human papillomaviruses, *Viral Immunol.*, 6, 255, 1993.
10. Evander, M., Frazer, I.H., Payne, E., Qi, Y.M., Hengst, K., and McMillan, N.A., Identification of the alpha 6 integrin as a candidate receptor for papillomaviruses, *J. Virol.*, 71, 2449, 1997.
11. Meyers, C. and Laimins, L.A., *In vitro* systems for the study and propagation of human papillomaviruses, *Curr. Top. Microbiol. Immunol.*, 186, 199, 1994.
12. Schiller, J. and Lowry, D., Papillomavirus-like particle vaccines, *J. Natl. Cancer Inst. Monogr.*, 28, 50, 2001.
13. Remmink, A.J., Walboomers, J.M., Helmerhorst, T.J., Voorhorst, F.J., Rozendaal, L, Risse, E.K., Meijer, C.J., and Kenemans, P., The presence of persistent high risk HPV genotypes in dysplastic cervical lesions is associated with progressive disease: natural history up to 36 months, *Int. J. Cancer*, 61, 4, 1995.
14. Carson, L.F., Twiggs, L.B., Fokishima, M., Ostrow, R.S., and Faras, A.J., Human genital papilloma infections: an evaluation of immunologic competence in the genital neoplasia-papilloma syndrome, *Am. J. Obstet. Gynecol.*, 155, 784, 1986.
15. Mohanty, K.C., Scott, C.S., Limbert, H.J., and Master, P.S., Circulating B and T lymphocyte subpopulations in patients with genital warts, *Br. J. Clin. Pract.*, 41, 601, 1987.
16. Tindle, R.W. and Frazer, I.H., Immune responses to human papillomaviruses and the prospects for human papillomavirus-specific immunization, *Curr. Top. Microbiol. Immunol.*, 186, 218, 1994.
17. Konya, J. and Dillner, J., Immunity to oncogenic human papillomaviruses, *Adv. Cancer. Res.*, 82, 205, 2001.
18. Carter, J.J. and Galloway, D.A., Humoral immune response to human papillomavirus infection, *Clin. Dermatol.*, 249, 259, 1997.
19. Rogozinski, T.T., Jablonska, S., and Jarzabek-Chorzelska, M., Role of cell-mediated immunity in spontaneous regression of plane warts, *Int. J. Dermatol.*, 27, 322, 1988.
20. Fausch, S.C., Da Silva, D.M., Rudolf, M.P., and Kast, W.M., Human papillomavirus-like particles do not activate Langerhans cells: a possible immune escape mechanism used by human papillomaviruses, *J. Immunol.*, 169, 3242, 2002.
21. O'Brien, P.M. and Campo, M.S., Evasion of host immunity directed by papillomavirus-encoded proteins, *Virus Res.*, 88, 103, 2002.
22. O'Brien, P.M. and Campo, M.S., Papillomaviruses: a correlation between immune evasion and oncogenicity? *Trends Microbiol.*, 11, 300, 2003.
23. Nestle, F.O. and Burg, G., Dendritic cells: role in skin diseases and therapeutic applications, *Clin. Exp. Dermatol.*, 24, 204, 1999.
24. Chardonnet, Y., Viac, J., and Thivolet, J., Langerhans cells in human warts, *Br. J. Dermatol.*, 115, 669, 1986.
25. Tay, S.K., Jenkins, D., Maddox, P., Campion, M., and Singer, A., Subpopulations of Langerhans cells in cervical neoplasia, *Br. J. Obstet. Gynaecol*, 94, 10, 1987.
26. Viac, J., Chardonnet, Y., Euvrard, S., Chignol, M.C., and Thivolet, J., Langerhans cells, inflammation markers and human papillomavirus infections in benign and malignant epithelial tumours from transplant patients, *J. Dermatol.*, 19, 67, 1992.

27. Memar, O.M., Arany, I., and Tyring, S.K., Skin-associated lymphoid tissue in human immunodeficiency virus-1, human papillomavirus and herpes simplex virus infections, *J. Invest. Dermatol.*, 105, 99s, 1995.
28. Connor, J.P., Ferrer, K., Kane, J.P., and Goldberg, J.M., Evaluation of Langerhans cells in the cervical epithelium of women with cervical intraepithelial neoplasia, *Gynecol. Oncol.*, 75, 130, 1999.
29. Bishop, P.E., McMillan, A., and Fletcher, S., An immunohistochemical study of spontaneous regression of condylomata acuminata, *Genitourin. Med.*, 66, 79, 1990.
30. Coleman, N., Birley, H.D., Renton, A.M., Hanna, N.F., Ryait, B.K., Bryne, M., Taylor-Robinson, D., and Stanley, M.A., Immunological events in regressing genital warts, *Am. J. Clin. Pathol.*, 102, 768, 1994.
31. Viac, J., Soleer, C., Chardonnet, Y., Euvrard, S., and Schmitt, D., Expression of immune associated surface antigens of keratinocytes in human papillomavirus-derived lesions, *Immunobiology*, 188, 392, 1993.
32. Cromme, F.V., Meijer, C.J., Snijers, P.J., Uyterlinde, A., Kenemans, P., Helmerhorst, T., Stern, P.L., van den Brule, A.J., and Walboomers, J.M., Analysis of MHC Class I and II expression in relation to presence of HPV genotypes in premalignant and malignant cervical lesions, *Br. J. Cancer*, 67, 1372, 1993.
33. Hughes, R.G., Norval, M., and Howie, S.E.M., Expression of MHC Class II antigens by Langerhans cells in cervical intraepithelial neoplasia, *J. Clin. Pathol.*, 41, 253, 1988.
34. Woodworth, C.D. and Simpson, S., Comparative lymphokine secretion by cultured human cervical keratinocytes, papillomavirus-immortalised, and carcinoma cell lines, *Am. J. Pathol.*, 142, 1544, 1993.
35. Glew, S.S., Conner, M.E., Snijders, P.J., Stanbridge, C.M., Buckley, C.H., Walboomers, J.M., Meijer, C.J., and Stern, P.L., HLA expression in preinvasive cervical neoplasia in relationship to human papillomavirus infection, *Eur. J. Cancer*, 29A, 1963, 1993.
36. Mota, F., Rayment, N., Chong, S., Singer, A., and Chain, B., The antigen-presenting environment in normal and human papillomavirus (HPV)-related premalignant cervical epithelium, *Clin. Exp. Immunol.*, 116, 33, 1999.
37. Hilders, C.G., Houbiers, J.G., van Ravenswaay Claasen, H.H., Veldhuizen, R.W., and Fleuren, G.J., Association between HLA-expression and infiltration of immune cells in cervical carcinoma, *Lab. Invest.*, 69, 651, 1993.
38. Markey, A.C., Churchill, L.J., and MacDonald, D.M., Altered expression of major histocompatibility complex (MHC) antigens by epidermal tumours, *J. Cutaneous Pathol.*, 17, 65, 1990.
39. Jackson, M., Benton, E.C., Hunter, J.A.A., and Norval, M., Local immune responses in cutaneous warts: an immunocytochemical study of Langerhans cells, T cells and adhesion molecules, *Eur. J. Dermatol.*, 4, 389, 1994.
40. Tay, S.K., Jenkins, D., Maddox, P., and Singer, A., Lymphocyte phenotypes in cervical intraepithelial neoplasia and human papillomavirus infection, *Br. J. Obstet. Gynaecol.*, 94, 16, 1987.
41. Evans, E.M., Man, S., Evans, A.S., and Borysiewicz, L.K., Infiltration of cervical cancer tissue with human papillomavirus-specific cytotoxic T-lymphocytes, *Cancer Res.*, 57, 2943, 1997.
42. Jackson, M., McKenzie, R.C., Benton, E.C., Hunter, J.A., and Norval, M., Cytokine mRNA expression in cutaneous warts: induction of interleukin-1 alpha, *Arch. Dermatol. Res.*, 289, 28, 1996.
43. Majewski, S., Hunzelmann, N., Nischt, R., Eches, B., Rudnicka, L., Orth, G., Kreig, T., and Jablonska, S., TGF-beta-1 and TNF alpha expression in the epidermis of patients with epidermodysplasia verruciformis, *J. Invest. Dermatol.*, 97, 862, 1991.
44. Duggan-Keen, M., Keating, P.J., Cromme, F.V., Walboomers, J.M., and Stern, P.L., Alterations in major histocompatibility complex expression in cervical cancer: possible consequences for immunotherapy, *Papillomavirus Rep.*, 5, 3, 1994.
45. Rogozinski, T.T., Jablonska, S., and Jarzabek-Chorelska, M., Role of cell-mediated immunity in spontaneous regression of plane warts, *Int. J. Dermatol.*, 27, 322, 1988.
46. Offringa, R., de Jong, A., Toes, R.E.M., van der Burg, S.H., and Melief, C.J.M., Interplay between human papillomaviruses and dendritic cells, *Curr. Top. Microbiol. Immunol.*, 276, 215, 2003.
47. Kono, T., Kondo, S., Pastore, S., Shivji, G.M., Tomai, M.A., McKenzie, R.C., and Sauder, D.N., Effects of a novel topical immunomodulator, imiquimod, on keratinocytes cytokine gene expression, *Lymphokine Cytokine Res.*, 13, 71, 1994.
48. Wagner, T.L., Ahonen, C.L., Couture, A.M., Gibson, S.J., Miller, R.L., Smith, R.M., Reiter, M.J., Vasilakos, J.P., and Tomai, M.A., Modulation of $T_H1$ and $T_H2$ cytokine production with the immune response modifiers R-848 and imiquimod, *Cell. Immunol.*, 191, 10, 1999.

49. Welters, M.J., de Jong, A., van den Eeden, S.J., van der Hulst, J.M., Kwappenberg, K.M., Hassane, S., Franken K.L., Drijfhout, J.W., Fleuren, G.J., Kenter, G., Melief, C.J., Offringa, R., and van der Burg, S.H., Frequent display of human papillomavirus type 16 E6-specific memory T-helper cells in the healthy population as witness of previous viral encounter, *Cancer Res.*, 63, 636, 2003.
50. Whitley, R.J., HSV infections, in *Field's Virology*, 4th ed., D.M. Knipe and P.M. Howley, Eds., Lippincott/Williams & Wilkins, Baltimore, MD, 2001, 2461.
51. Mester, J.C. and Rouse, B.T., The mouse model and understanding immunity to herpes simplex virus, *Rev. Inf. Dis.*, 13(Suppl.), 935s, 1991.
52. Sprecher, E. and Becker, Y., Detection of IL-1β, TNF-α and IL-6 gene transcription by polymerase chain reaction in keratinocytes, Langerhans cells and peritoneal exudate cells during infection with herpes simplex virus-1, *Arch. Virol.*, 126, 253, 1992.
53. Zak-Prelich, M., Halliday, K.E., Walker, C., Norval, M., and McKenzie, R.C., Infection of murine keratinocytes with herpes simplex virus type 1 induces the expression of interleukin-10 but not interleukin-1α or TNF-α, *Immunology*, 104, 468, 2001.
54. Cunningham, A.L., Turner, R.R., Miller, A.C., Para, M.F., and Merigan, T.C., Evolution of recurrent herpes simplex lesions. An immunohistologic study, *J. Clin. Invest.*, 75, 226, 1985.
55. Smith, C.M., Belz, G.T., Wilson, N.S., Villadangos, J.A., Shortman, K., Carbone, F.R., and Heath, W.R., Conventional CD8α+ dendritic cells are preferentially involved in CTL priming after footpad infection with herpes simplex virus-1, *J. Immunol.*, 170, 4437, 2003.
56. Zhao, X., Deak, E., Soderberg, K., Linehan, M., Spezzano, D., Zhu, J., Knipe, D.M., and Iwasaki, A., Vaginal submucosal dendritic cells, but not Langerhans cells, induce protective Th1 responses to herpes simplex virus-2, *J. Exp. Med.*, 197, 153, 2003.
57. Mikloska, Z., Bosbjak, L., and Cunningham, A.L., Immature monocyte-derived dendritic cells are productively infected with herpes simplex virus type 1, *J. Virol.*, 75, 5958, 2001.
58. Kruse, M., Rosorius, M., Kratzer, F., Bevec, D., Kuhnt, C., Steinkasserer, A., Schuler, G., and Hauber, J., Inhibition of CD83 cell surface expression during dendritic cell maturation by interference with nuclear export of CD83 mRNA, *J. Exp. Med.*, 191, 1581, 2000.
59. Kobelt, D., Lechmann, M., and Steinkasserer, A., The interaction between dendritic cells and herpes simplex virus-1, *Curr. Top. Microbiol Immunol.*, 276, 145, 2003.
60. Sprecher, E. and Becker, Y., Langerhans cell density and activity in mouse skin and lymph nodes affect herpes simplex virus type 1 (HSV-1) pathogenicity, *Arch. Virol.*, 107, 191, 1989.
61. Yasumoto, S., Okabe, M., and Mori, R., Role of epidermal Langerhans cells in resistance to herpes simplex virus infection, *Arch. Virol.*, 90, 261, 1986.
62. Williams, N.A., Hill, T.J., and Hooper, D.C., Murine epidermal antigen-presenting cells in primary and secondary T-cell proliferative responses to herpes simplex virus *in vitro*, *Immunology*, 72, 34, 1991.
63. Hill, A. Jugovic, P., York, I., Russ, G., Bennink, J., Yewdell, J., Pleogh, H., and Johnson, D., Herpes simplex virus turns off the TAP to evade host immunity, *Nature*, 375, 411, 1995.
64. Posavad, C.M., Koelle, D.M., and Corey, L., Tipping the scales of herpes simplex virus reactivation: the important responses are local, *Nat. Med.*, 4, 381, 1998.
65. Mikloska, Z. and Cunningham, A.L., Alpha and gamma interferons inhibit herpes simplex virus type 1 infection and spread in epidermal cells after axonal transmission, *J. Virol.*, 75, 11821, 2001.
66. Seid, J.M., Leung, K.N., Pye, C., Phelan, J., Nash, A.A., and Godfrey, H.P., Clonal analysis of the T cell response of mice to herpes simplex virus: correlation between lymphokine production *in vitro* and induction of DTH and anti-viral activity *in vivo*, *Viral Immunol.*, 1, 35, 1987.
67. Cunningham, A.L. and Noble, J.R., Role of keratinocytes in human recurrent herpetic lesions. Ability to present herpes simplex virus antigen and act as a target for T lymphocyte cytotoxicity *in vitro*, *J. Clin. Invest.*, 83, 490, 1989.
68. Koelle, D.M., Posavad, C.M., Barnum, G.R., Johnson, M.L., Frank, J.M., and Corey, L., Clearance of HSV-2 from recurrent genital lesions correlates with infiltration of HSV-specific cytotoxic T lymphocytes, *J. Clin. Invest.*, 101, 1500, 1998.
69. Coles, R.M., Mueller, S.N., Heath, W.R., Carbone, F.R., and Brooks, A.G., Progression of armed CTL from draining lymph node to spleen shortly after localised infection with herpes simplex virus 1, *J. Immunol.*, 168, 834, 2002.

70. Mueller, S.N., Jones, C.M., Smith, C.M., Heath, W.R., and Carbone, F.R., Rapid cytotoxic T lymphocyte activation occurs in the draining lymph nodes after cutaneous herpes simplex virus infection as a result of early antigen presentation and not the presence of the virus, *J. Exp. Med.*, 195, 651, 2002.
71. Koelle, D.M., Lui, Z., McClurkan, C.M., Topp, M.S., Riddell, S.R., Pamer, E.G., Johnson, A.S., Wald, A., and Corey, L, Expression of cutaneous lymphocyte-associated antigen by $CD8^+$ T cells specific for a skin-tropic virus, *J. Clin. Invest.*, 110, 537, 2002.
72. Nash, A.A. and Cambouropoulos, P., The immune response to herpes simplex virus, *Semin. Virol.*, 4, 181, 1993.
73. Kohl, S., The role of antibody in herpes simplex virus infection in humans, *Curr. Top. Microbiol. Immunol.*, 179, 75, 1992.
74. Vestey, J.P., Norval, M., Howie, S., Maingay, J., and Neill, W.A., Variation in lymphoproliferative responses during recrudescent orofacial herpes simplex virus infections, *Clin. Exp. Immunol.*, 77, 384, 1989.
75. Wheeler, C.E., Pathogenesis of recurrent herpes simplex infections, *J. Invest. Dermatol.*, 65, 341, 1975.
76. Rooney, J.F., Bryson, Y., Mannix, M.L., Dillon, M., Wohlenberg, C.R., Bamks, S., Wallington, C.J., Notkins, A.L., and Straus, S.E., Prevention of ultraviolet-light-induced herpes labialis by sunscreen, *Lancet*, 338, 1419, 1991.
77. Howie, S., Norval, M., and Maingay, J.P., Exposure to low dose ultra-violet B light suppresses delayed type hypersensitivity to herpes simplex virus in mice, *J. Invest. Dermatol.*, 86, 125, 1986.
78. Howie, S.E., Norval, M., Maingay, J., and Ross, J.A., Two phenotypically distinct T cells ($Ly1^+2^-$ and $Ly1^-2^+$) are involved in ultra-violet-B-light induced suppression of the efferent DTH to HSV-1 *in vivo*, *Immunology*, 58, 653, 1986.
79. Howie, S.E.M., Ross, J.A., Norval, M., and Maingay, J.P., *In vivo* modulation of antigen presentation generates $T_s$ rather than $T_{DH}$ in HSV-1 infection, *Immunology*, 60, 419, 1987.
80. Yasumoto, S., Moroi, Y., Koga, T., Mitsuyama, M., and Hori, Y., Ultraviolet-B irradiation alters cytokine production by immune lymphocytes in herpes simplex virus-infected mice, *J. Dermatol. Sci.*, 8, 218, 1994.
81. Moodycliffe, A.M., Nghiem, D., Clydesdale, G., and Ullrich, S.E., Immune suppression and skin cancer development: regulation by NKT cells, *Nat. Immunol.*, 1, 521, 2000.
82. Schwarz, A., Beissert, S., Grosse-Heitmeyer, K., Gunzer, M., Bluestone, J.A., Grabbe, S., and Schwarz, T., Evidence for functional relevance of CTLA-4 in ultraviolet-radiation-induced tolerance, *J. Immunol.*, 165, 1824, 2000.
83. Goade, D.E., Nofchissey, R.A., Kusewitt, D.F., Hjelle, B., Kreisel, J., Moore, J., and Lyons, C.R., Ultraviolet light induces reactivation in a murine model of cutaneous herpes simplex virus-1 infection, *Photochem. Photobiol.*, 74, 108, 2001.
84. van der Molen, R.G., Out-Luiting, C., Claas, F.H., Norval, M., Koerten, H.K., and Mommaas, A.M., Ultraviolet-B radiation induces modulation of antigen presentation of herpes simplex virus by human epidermal cells, *Hum. Immunol.*, 62, 589, 2001.
85. Yamanish, K., Human herpesvirus 6 and human herpesvirus 7, in *Field's Virology*, 4th ed., D.M. Knipe and P.M. Howley, Eds., Lippincott/Williams & Wilkins, Baltimore, MD, 2001, 2785.
86. Moore, P.S. and Chang, Y., Kaposi's sarcoma-associated herpesvirus, in *Field's Virology*, 4th ed., D.M. Knipe and P.M. Howley, Eds., Lippincott/Williams & Wilkins, Baltimore, MD, 2001, 2803.
87. Kondo, K., Kondo, T., Okuno, T., Takahashi, M., and Yamanishi, K., Latent human herpesvirus 6 infection of human monocytes/macrophages. *J. Gen. Virol.*, 72, 1401, 1991.
88. Norton, R.A., Caserta, M.T., Hall, C.B., Schnabel K., Hocknell, P., and Dewhurst, S., Detection of human herpes virus-6 by reverse-transcription-PCR. *J. Clin. Microbiol.*, 37, 3672, 1999.
89. Rzany, B., Mockenhaupt, M., Stoker, U., Hamouda, O., and Schopf, E., Incidence of Stevens-Johnson syndrome and toxic epidermal necrolysis in patients with the acquired immunodeficiency syndrome in Germany. *Arch. Dermatol.*, 129, 1059, 1993.
90. Tohyama, M., Yahata, Y., Yasukawa, M., Inagi, R., Urano, Y., Yamanishi, K., and Hashimoto, K., Severe hypersensitivity syndrome due to sulfasalazine associated with reactivation of human herpesvirus 6. *Arch. Dermatol.*, 134, 1113, 1998.
91. Suzuki, Y., Inagi, R., Aono, T., Yamanishi, K., and Shiohara, T., Human herpesvirus 6 infection as a risk factor for the development of severe drug-induced hypersensitivity syndrome. *Arch. Dermatol.*, 134, 1108, 1998.

92. Le Cleach, L., Fillet, A.M., and Chosidow, O., Human herpesviruses 6 and 7 — new roles yet to be discovered? *Arch. Dermatol.*, 134, 1155, 1998.
93. Kempf, W., Adams, V., Mirandola P., Menotti, L., DiLuca, D., Wey, N., Muller, B., and Campadelli-Fiume, G., Persistence of human herpes virus 7 in normal tissues detected by expression of a structural antigen, *J. Infect. Dis.*, 178, 841, 1998.
94. Yasukawa, M., Yakushijin, Y., Furukawa, M., and Fujita, S., Specificity analysis of human CD4+ T-cell clones directed against human herpesvirus 6 (HHV-6), HHV-7, and human cytomegalovirus, *J. Virol.*, 67, 6259, 1993.
95. Ambroziak, J.A., Blackbourn, D.J., Herndier, B.G., Glogau, R.G., Gullett, J.H., McDonald, A.R., Lennette, E.T., and Levy, J.A., Herpes-like sequences in HIV-infected and uninfected Kaposi's sarcoma patients, *Science*, 268, 582, 1995.
96. Buonaguro, F.M., Tomesello, M.L., Buonaguro, L., Satriano, R.A., Ruocco, E., Castello, G., and Ruocco, V., Kaposi's sarcoma: aetiopathogenesis, histology and clinical features, *J. Eur. Acad. Dermatol. Venereol.*, 17, 138, 2003.
97. Watanabe, T., Kawamura, T., Jacob, S.E., Aquilino, E.A., Orenstein, J.M., Black, J.B., and Blauvelt, A., Pityriasis rosea is associated with systemic active infection with both human herpesvirus-7 and human herpesvirus-6, *J. Invest. Dermatol.*, 119, 779, 2002.
98. Drago, F., Malaguti, F., Ranieri, E., Losi, E., and Rebora, A., Human herpes virus-like particles in pityriasis rosea lesions: an electron microscope study, *J. Cutaneous Pathol.*, 29, 359, 2002.
99. Karabulut, K.A., Kocak, M., Yilmaz, N., and Eksioglu, M., Detection of human herpesvirus 7 in pityriasis rosea by nested PCR, *Int. J. Dermatol.*, 41, 563, 2002.
100. Kempf, W., Adams, V., Kleinhans, M., Burg, G., Panizzon, R., Campadelli-Fiume, G., and Nestle, F., Pityriasis rosea is not associated with human herpesvirus 7, *Arch. Dermatol.*, 135, 1070, 1999.
101. Katsafanas, G., Schirmer, E., Wyatt, L., and Frenkel, N., *In vitro* activation of human herpesvirus 6 and 7 from latency, *Proc. Natl. Acad. Sci. U.S.A.*, 93, 9788, 1996.
102. Tanaka-Taya, K., Kondo, T., Nakagawa, N., Inagi, R., Miyoshi, H., Sunagawa, T., Okada, S., and Yamanishi, K., Reactivation of human herpesvirus 6 by infection of human herpesvirus 7, *J. Med. Virol.*, 60, 284, 2000.
103. Chang, Y., Cesarman, E., Pessin, M.S., Lee, F., Culpepper, J., Knowles, D.M., and Moore, P.S., Identification of herpesvirus-like DNA sequences in AIDS-associated Kaposi's sarcoma, *Science*, 265, 1865, 1994.
104. Osman, M., Kubo, T., Gill, J., Neipel, F., Becker, M., Smith, G., Weiss, R., Gazzard, B., Boshoff, C., and Gotch, F., Identification of human herpesvirus 8-specific cytotoxic T-cell responses, *J. Virol.*, 73, 6136, 1999.
105. Sirianni, M.C., Vincenzi, L., Topino, S., Giovannetti, A., Mazzetta, F., Libi, F., Scaramuzzi, D., Andreoni, M., Pinter, E., Barrarrini, S., Rezza, G., Monini, P., and Ensoli, B., NK cell activity controls human herpesvirus 8 latent infection and is restored upon highly active antiretroviral therapy in AIDS patients with regressing Kaposi's sarcoma, *Eur. J. Immunol.*, 32, 2711, 2002.
106. Boshoff, C., Schulz, T.F., Kennedy, M.M., Graham, A.K., Fisher, C., Thomas, A., McGee, J.O., Weiss, R.A., and O'Leary, J.J., Kaposi's sarcoma-associated herpesvirus infects endothelial and spindle cells, *Nat. Med.*, 1, 1274, 1995.
107. Staskus, K.A., Zhong, W., Gebhard, K., Mohanraj, D., Twiggs, L.B., Carson, L.F., and Ramakrishnan, S., Kaposi's sarcoma-associated herpesvirus gene expression in endothelial (spindle) tumour cells, *J. Virol.*, 71, 715, 1997.
108. Polstra, A.M., Goudsmit, J., and Cornelissen, M., Latent and lytic HHV-8 mRNA expression in PBMCs and Kaposi's sarcoma skin biopsies of AIDS Kaposi's sarcoma patients, *J. Med. Virol.*, 70, 624, 2003.
109. Moore, P.S., Boshoff, C., Weiss, R.A., and Chang, Y. Molecular mimicry of human cytokine and cytokine response pathway genes by Kaposi's sarcoma herpesvirus, *Science*, 274, 1739, 1996.
110. An, J., Sunm Y., Sun, R., and Rettig, M.B., Kaposi's sarcoma-associated herpesvirus encoded vFLIP induces cellular IL-6 expression: the role of the NK-kappaB and JNK/Ap1 pathways, *Oncogene*, 22, 3371, 2003.
111. Sozzani, S., Luini, W., Bianchi, G., Allavena, P., Wells, T.N., Napolitano, M., Bernardini, G., Vecchi, A., D'Ambrosio, D., Mazzeo, D., Sinigaglia, F., Santoni, A., Maggi, E., Romagnani, S., and Mantovani, A., The viral chemokine macrophage inflammatory protein-II is a selective Th2 chemoattractant, *Blood*, 62, 4036, 1998.

112. Coscoy, L. and Ganem, D., Kaposi's sarcoma associated herpesvirus encodes two proteins that block cell surface display of MCH Class I chains by enhancing their endocytosis, *Proc. Natl. Acad. Sci. U.S.A.*., 94, 8051, 2000.
113. Enroli, B. and Sturzl, M., Kaposi's sarcoma: a result of the interplay among inflammatory cytokines, angiogenic factors and viral agents, *Cytokine Growth Factor Rev.*, 9, 63, 1998.
114. Barillari, G., Gendelman, R., Gallo, R.C., and Ensoli, B., The Tat protein of human immunodeficiency virus type 1, a growth factor for AIDS Kaposi's sarcoma and cytokine-activated vascular cells, induces adhesion of the same cell types by using integrin receptors recognizing the RGD amino acid sequence, *Proc. Natl. Acad. Sci. U.S.A.*, 90, 7941, 1993.
115. Blatt, S.P., Hendrix, C.W., Butzin, C.A., Freeman, T.M., Ward, W.W., Hensley, R.E., Melcher, G.P., Donovan D.J., and Boswell, R.N., Delayed-type hypersensitivity skin testing predicts progression to AIDS in HIV-infected patients, *Ann. Intern. Med.*, 119, 177, 1993.
116. Dolan, M.J., Clerici, M., Blatt, S.P., Hendrix, C.W., Melcher, G.P., Boswell, R.N., Freeman, T.M., Ward, W., Hensley, R., and Shearer, G.M., *In vitro* T cell function, delayed-type hypersensitivity skin testing, and $CD4^+$ T cell subset phenotyping independently predict survival time in patients infected with human immunodeficiency virus, *J. Infect. Dis.*, 172, 79, 1995.
117. Meroni, L., Marchetti, G., Monforte, A., and Galli, M., Delayed-type hypersensitivity skin testing can predict CD4 count increase in HIV patients with poor immunologic responses to HAART, *JAIDS*, 33, 278, 2003.
118. Moreno, S., Baraia-Etxaburu, J., Bouza, E., Parras, F., Parez-Tascon, M., Miralles, P., Vicente T., Alberdi, J.C., Cosin, J., and Lopez-Gay, D., Risk for developing tuberculosis among anergic patients infected with HIV, *Ann. Intern. Med.*, 119, 194, 1993.
119. Duvic, M., Human immunodeficiency virus and the skin: selected controversies, *J. Invest. Dermatol.*, 105, 117s, 1995.
120. Clerici M., Wynn, T.A., Berzofsky, J.A., Blatt, S.P., Hendrix, C.W., Sher, A., Coffman, R.L., and Shearer, G.M., Role of IL-10 in T helper dysfunction in asymptomatic individuals infected with human immunodeficiency virus, *J. Clin. Invest.*, 93, 768, 1994.
121. Beuer-McHam, J.N., Ledbetter, L.S., Sarris, A.H., and Duvic, M., Cytokine expression patterns distinguish HIV associated skin diseases, *Exp. Dermatol.*, 9, 341, 2000.
122. Henry, M., Uthman, A., Ballaun, C., Stingl, G., and Tschachler, E., Epidermal Langerhans cells of AIDS patients express HIV-1 regulatory and structural genes, *J. Invest. Dermatol.*, 103, 593, 1994.
123. Simonitsch, I., Geusau, A., Chott, A., and Jurecka, W., Cutaneous dendritic cells are main targets in acute HIV-1-infection, *Mod. Pathol.* 13, 1232, 2000.
124. Berger, R., Gartner, S., Rappersberger, K., Foster, C.A., Wolff, K., and Stingl, G., Isolation of human immunodeficiency virus type 1 from human epidermis: virus replication and transmission studies, *J. Invest. Dermatol.*, 99, 271, 1992.
125. Granelli-Piperno, A., Zhong, L., Haslett, P., Jacobson, J., and Steinman, R.M., Dendritic cells infected with VSV-pseudotyped HIV-1 present antigens to $CD4^+$ and $CD8^+$ T cells from HIV-1 infected individuals, *J. Immunol.*, 165, 6620, 2000.
126. Kawamura, T., Cohen, S., Borris, D.L., Aquilino, E.A., Glushakova, S., Margolis, L.B., Orenstein, J.M., Offord, R.E., Neurath, A.R., and Blauvelt, A., Candidate microbiocides block HIV-1 infection of human immature Langerhans cells within epithelial tissue explants, *J. Exp Med.*, 192, 1491, 2000.
127. Tschachler, E., Groh, V., Popovic, M., Mann, D.L., Konrad, K., Safai, B., Eron, L., diMarzo Veronese, F., Wolff, K., and Stingl, G., Epidermal Langerhans cells — a target for HTLV-III/LAV infection, *J. Invest. Dermatol.*, 88, 233, 1987.
128. Kanitakis, J., Marchand, C., Su, H., Trivolet, J., Zambruno, G., Schmitt, D., and Gazzolo, L., Immunohistochemical study of normal skin of HIV-infected patients shows no evidence of infection of epidermal Langerhans cells by HIV, *AIDS Res. Hum. Retroviruses*, 5, 293, 1989.
129. Kanitakis, J, Escaich, S., Trepo, C., and Thivolet, J., Detection of human immunodeficiency virus-DNA and RNA in the skin of HIV-infected patients using polymerase chain reaction, *J. Invest. Dermatol.*, 97, 91, 1991.
130. Kalter, D.C., Greenhouse, J.J., Orenstein, J.M., Schnittman, S.M., Gendelman, H.E., and Meltzer, M.S., Epidermal Langerhans cells are not principal reservoirs of virus in HIV disease, *J. Immunol.*, 146, 3396, 1991.

131. Steinman, R.M., Granelli-Piperno, A., Pope, M., Trumfheller, C., Ignatius, R., Arrode, G., Racz, P., and Tenner-Racz, K. The interaction of immunodeficiency viruses with dendritic cells, *Curr. Top. Microbiol. Immunol.*, 276, 1, 2003.
132. Kwon, D.S., Gregario, G., Bitton, N., Hendrickson, W.A., and Littman, D.R., DC-SIGN mediated internalisation of HIV is required for *trans*-enhancement of T cell infection, *Immunity*, 16, 135, 2002.
133. Zmudzka, B.Z., Miller, S.A., Jacobs, M.E., and Beer, J.Z., Medical UV exposures and HIV activation, *Photochem. Photobiol.*, 64, 246, 1996.
134. Akaraphanth, R. and Lim, H.W., HIV, UV and immunosuppression, *Photodermatol. Photoimmunol. Photomed.*, 15, 28, 1999.
135. Beuer-McHam, J., Simpson, E., Dougherty, I., Bonkobara, M., Arizumi, K., Lewis, D.E., Dawson, D.B., Duvic, M., and Cruz, P.D., Activation of HIV in human skin by ultraviolet B radiation and its inhibition by NFκB blocking agents, *Photochem. Photobiol.*, 74, 805, 2001.
136. Kaporis, A., Lim, H.W., Moy, J., Soter, N.A., and Sanchez, M., Skin response to ultraviolet B light in patients infected with human immunodeficiency virus, *Photodermatol. Photoimmunol. Photomed.*, 11, 188, 1996.
137. Andres, O., Obojes, K., Kim, K.S., ter Meulen, V., and Schneider-Schaulies, S., CD46- and CD150-independent endothelial infection with wild-type measles viruses, *J. Gen. Virol.*, 84, 1189, 2003.
138. Naim, H.Y., Ehler, E., and Billeter, M.A., Measles virus matrix protein specifies apical viral release and glycoprotein sorting in epithelial cells, *EMBO J.*, 19, 3576, 2000.
139. Griffin, D.E., Immune responses during measles virus infection, *Curr. Top. Microbiol. Immunol.*, 191, 117, 1995.
140. Schneider-Schaulies, S. and ter Meulen, V., Modulation of immune functions by measles virus, *Springer Semin. Immunopathol.*, 24, 127, 2002.
141. Kimura, A., Tosaka, K., and Nakao, T., Measles rash. I. Light and electron microscopic study of skin eruptions, *Arch. Virol.*, 47, 295, 1975.
142. Steineir, M.P., Grosjean, I., Bella, C., and Kaiserlian, D., Langerhans cells are susceptible to measles virus infection and actively suppress T cell proliferation, *Eur. J. Dermatol.*, 8, 413, 1998.

# 34 Fungal Infections

*Roderick J. Hay*

## CONTENTS



## I. INTRODUCTION

The normal skin is home to scores of bacteria and lipophilic yeasts whose presence is tolerated without triggering an inflammatory response. How pathogens are distinguished from commensals, when both are antigenic and actively metabolizing, remains an unsolved mystery. Although the mechanisms of host resistance to organisms that infect the epidermis are necessarily different than those deployed against infections in other sites,[1] they are clearly effective in many instances. Yet, in some common skin infections such as dermatophytosis and human papilloma virus infections, there appears to be modulation of the host defense mechanisms. This is not due, as originally thought, to an intrinsic lack of immunologically active cells. Within the epidermis there are specific afferent and efferent pathways for immunologically mediated responses. Reception and processing of microbial antigens are largely performed by modified dendritic cells, Langerhans cells, as well as other cellular elements such as dermal macrophages. Likewise, keratinocytes play an active role in antifungal defense and can be activated to express class II antigens or release cytokines as well as other inflammatory mediators such as tumor necrosis factors (TNF) and interleukins 1 and 8 (IL-1, IL-8). They also express other factors involved in the development of inflammatory responses such as adhesion molecules. In addition, this network communicates actively with other cellular and humoral arms of the immunological system including subsets of B and T lymphocytes and neutrophils. The importance of these changes that occur in response to fungal antigens is that the epidermis is activated at the site of antigenic challenge, a feature that helps localize effector cells at one particular site and where it is possible to reactivate the system at some later event should the need arise.

Perhaps the least well understood aspect of this epidermal activity is the means by which antigen reception and lymphocyte activation, accomplished during an infection of the epidermis,

0-8493-1959-5/05/$0.00+$1.50

is translated into an effector response. It is clear that certain effector mechanisms such as the migration of polymorphonuclear leukocytes to the site of invasion or cytokine-regulated increased epidermal cell turnover may act to remove foreign substances, such as fungi, from the skin surface. The overall effectiveness of such mechanisms in epidermal infection is not known; nor is it clear whether immunological efficacy varies from site to site on the skin surface, thereby creating "microbial safe areas." However, it is possible that there are skin locations where immunological detection and, in particular, the effector paths are less efficient than others.

The fungal infections affecting the skin are common diseases seen in both temperate and tropical environments. This chapter is concerned with the superficial mycoses, dermatophytosis, cutaneous candidosis, and *Malassezia* infections. Little is known about host defense against the more rarely seen superficial fungal diseases, such as black and white piedra, and these are not discussed further.

## II. DERMATOPHYTOSIS

Among the superficial fungal pathogens, most is known about host defense against dermatophytosis, in which a range of different clinical and host inflammatory responses are seen. At one end of this spectrum of responsiveness, there are dermatophyte infections that are self-limited, elicit an inflammatory reaction, and that generally respond to minimal therapy and seldom recur.[2] Zoophilic dermatophytosis, infections of animal origin occurring in humans, are frequently highly inflammatory and are followed by long-lasting immunity. For example, second infections in humans with the cattle ringworm fungus, *Trichophyton verrucosum*, are rare.[3] By contrast, human anthropophilic dermatophytoses are becoming increasingly common and are often persistent, sometimes despite therapy.[4] Relapse after treatment is also frequent. Examples include *T. rubrum* infections affecting the feet, *T. tonsurans* in the scalp,[5] and *T. concentricum*,[6] which causes widespread tinea corporis in remote areas of the humid tropics. Persistence of these infections, in some cases despite treatment, is common and dermatophytosis accounts for high proportions of patients seeking treatment in temperate and tropical areas. In certain occupational groups, persistent dermatophyte infections are equally problematic. In the United Kingdom workers in heavy industry such as coal mining are susceptible to chronic foot infections, tinea pedis, leading to moderate disability as well as significant economic loss through illness and industrial compensation.[7]

### A. Early Stages of Dermatophytosis

Dermatophyte fungi grow in the form of long chains of cells, hyphae, and generally do not penetrate farther than the granular layer of the stratum corneum. The first phase of epidermal invasion consists of adherence between the fungal cell and the keratinocyte.[8] This has been shown to be a time-dependent adhesion process in which the invading arthrospore is attached to an underlying keratinocyte over a 2 to 3 h period before germination. The process is accompanied by structural changes in the organism such as swelling of arthrospores and the expression of an extracellular fibrillar layer. The adhesion process is readily inhibited by low antifungal drug concentrations. It is likely that carbohydrate-specific adhesins on the conidial surface that recognize mannose and galactose are involved in this process.[9] Experiments to elucidate the mechanisms of this adherence phenomenon in dermatophyte infections have been limited by the difficulty of producing isolated arthrospores rather than using microconidia, which are produced in large quantities in culture and the fact that, in a real infection, interaction between clumps of shed human keratinocytes carrying the fungi and host stratum corneum is the most likely earliest phase of the infection.

Once adherence has occurred, the dermatophyte arthroconidia can germinate and the infection is established in the outer stratum corneum.[10] In experimentally infected mice, this process may well be limited by the rapid recruitment of neutrophils to the site of attack.[11] However, in humans there is little evidence of early mobilization of neutrophils in dermatophytosis. Neutrophil accumulation is a feature of infections in which there is penetration of the hair follicle.[12]

Skin invasion by dermatophytes involves the production of proteases, some of which are inducible in the presence of amino acid residues. While at least three low-molecular-weight proteases have also been isolated from *T. mentagrophytes,*[13] a number of different proteases have been extracted from *T. rubrum.* These range in size from 34 to 77 to 105 kDa. In addition, this dermatophyte produces a secreted metalloprotease with a molecular weight of about 200 kDa, which shows specificity for collagen and elastin. In *Microsporum canis* metalloproteases are produced by invading organisms at the site of hair shaft infection.[14]

Human dermatophyte infections can be classified as inflammatory or noninflammatory; the former infections are often caused by zoophilic fungi, the latter by anthropophilic organisms. Defense against dermatophytes depends on the activation of both immune and nonimmune mechanisms. The principle pathways of defense that have been identified are the interaction between fungi and unsaturated transferrin, migration of polymorphonuclear leukocytes into the area of infection, and T-lymphocyte activation.[1] There has been little work on the so-called nonspecific mechanisms of defense against dermatophytosis. Generally, the fungi are inhibited in a number of different ways. Unsaturated transferrin inhibits the growth of dermatophytes by a direct mechanism involving its binding to the fungal cell membrane.[15] Lactoferrin also enhances resistance in experimental infections, possibly through an effect on mononuclear cell function.[16] Other inhibitory mechanisms include the production in sebum of medium chain length fatty acids, which are inhibitory to dermatophyte growth.[1] The speed of growth of the epidermis, as measured by the uptake of tritiated thymidine into the basal layer, is also increased in human dermatophytosis; a similar phenomenon has been shown in experimental dermatophytosis using guinea pig skin grafted onto athymic mice.[17] In this experimental model, increased epidermal proliferation occurs early, within 48 h, in the course of infection and in the absence of T lymphocytes. This suggests that there is a direct and T-cell-independent mechanism for increasing epidermal growth in response to fungal invasion. It is still possible, however, that immunological activation provides a means of amplifying this epidermal proliferative response.

Killing of dermatophytes by both murine and human neutrophils and macrophages can be demonstrated. The chief effector cells that are active against dermatophyte fungi are neutrophils (PMN) and, to a lesser extent, macrophages.[18] The former are important components of the histological response to hair follicle invasion in humans and animals. Human PMN have been shown to destroy up to 60% of *T. rubrum* and *T. quinckeanum* germlings within 2 h; macrophages kill up to 20% in a similar time. PMN killing is enhanced by concanavalin-A or phorbol myristate acetate.[19] The effects of PMNs have been reproduced by an *in vitro* system using lactoperoxidase, hydrogen peroxidase, and potassium iodide and can be abrogated with catalase, superoxide dismutase, and histidine, which are known scavengers of hydrogen peroxide, superoxide anion, and singlet oxygen, respectively.[19] Killing can proceed even in the absence of ingestion of fungal hyphae by neutrophils. The existence of a second non-oxidative method of phagocyte-mediated defense via a peptide mechanism, as occurs with *Candida,* for dermatophytes has not been investigated. *Trichophyton rubrum* produces a catalase and a secreted superoxide dismutase, both of which may interfere with the outcome of phagocyte-mediated defense.[19]

Neutrophils are attracted to the site of infection both by production of epidermally derived chemotactic factors such as leukotriene derivatives and also by certain dermatophyte cell wall antigens, which activate the alternate pathway of complement.[20]

## B. Immunity and Dermatophytosis

The majority of patients with dermatophytosis are healthy and have no obvious predisposing factors. Previous studies have occasionally revealed a number of underlying diseases in patients with dermatophytosis, notably hereditary palmoplantar keratoderma[21] and Raynaud's phenomenon.[4] A high proportion of chronically infected individuals, over 40% in some surveys, are atopic on personal or family history.[22] Patients with chronic mucocutaneous candidosis (CMC) (see Section

IV) are also particularly susceptible to widespread intractable dermatophytosis as well as candidosis; individuals infected with human immunodeficiency virus (HIV) may also have chronic ringworm. These studies suggest that patients with impaired immunological defense mechanisms, in particular those affecting T-lymphocyte function, are prone to chronic infection.

However, in all these examples, whereas the clinical expression of infection may be modified by the patients' underlying condition, the prevalence of dermatophytosis in compromised patients is not significantly different from that seen in healthy subjects. In patients with AIDS, the prevalence of infection has been no higher in some studies than in members of "at risk" groups without HIV infection,[23] but there is an association in that it correlates with low CD4 counts.[24] Also, as stated previously, with the exception of atopy, underlying disease is not seen in the majority of patients with dermatophytosis.[25] This is in sharp distinction to patients with infections due to *C. albicans* where there is usually some predisposing abnormality ranging from occlusion of the skin surface to defects in neutrophil or T-lymphocyte function.

In experimental dermatophytosis in a mouse model using the natural murine pathogen, *T. quinckeanum,* transfer of T lymphocytes bearing the Thy-1 helper phenotype from immune animals to naive recipients is the key event in determining immunity. During primary infection in mice, there is evidence of polyclonal suppression of lymphocyte activation during the phase of activation of lymphocytes reactive with dermatophyte antigens.[26] Immunity to infection can be transferred to irradiated naive animals with lymphocytes bearing the Thy-1 phenotype, but not Ly-2.2.[27] Passive transfer of antibody will also not convey resistance on recipients.

In humans, there is a correlation among inflammatory responses, T-lymphocyte activation, and recovery. In experimental infections, recovery occurs at the same time as lesions become inflamed and delayed-type hypersensitivity to the fungal antigen develops. Patients with persistent foot infections (*T. rubrum*) or tinea corporis (*T. concentricum*) have reduced levels of lymphocyte blastogenesis to dermatophyte antigen.[28,29] In chronic infections caused by *T. rubrum* compared to those infections due to *T. mentagrophytes*, for example, the lymphocyte transformation responses of peripheral blood lymphocytes from infected patients are weak. There is little clinical inflammatory reaction and relapse or persistence of infection is common. In less than 15% of cases is there evidence of an underlying disease affecting the immune system to explain these findings. There is also evidence that some immune responses such as absent delayed-type hypersensitivity to trichophytin can be reversed by successful therapy.[30] In the rare disseminated forms of dermatophytosis where there is involvement of internal organs there may also be evidence of disturbance of immune function.[31,32]

Although immunological mechanisms provide potential methods of defense, the persistence of infection in many apparently healthy individuals suggests that these are either ineffective or inoperative in some patients. It has been shown that some patients with persistent dermatophytosis have defective lymphocyte blastogenesis to T-cell mitogens and dermatophyte antigen and that this can be reversed either by substituting heterologous (fetal calf) for autologous serum or after successful antifungal treatment.[31,33] This suggests that an inhibitory factor is present in serum. Dermatophyte antigen has been identified in such infected serum employing an immunoradiometric assay using the mouse antidermatophyte IgM monoclonal TQ-1.[34] Antigen derived from *Trichophyton* species containing TQ-1 reactive epitopes increases susceptibility of Balb/c mice to dermatophyte infection and interferes with T-cell-mediated immunity.[26] TQ-1 antibody reacts with phosphoryl-choline (PC) and immunoreactivity can be abrogated by pretreatment with PC. Phosphoryl-choline hapten is found in other parasites including filaria and also affects expression of immune responses in these infections. Another, probably different, factor has also been identified. Oligosaccharides derived from glycoproteins present in the dermatophyte cell wall may interfere with both T- and B-lymphocyte activation. This is a reversible process *in vitro*, but preexposure of lymphocytes to dermatophyte inhibitory factor (DIF) will prevent proliferation of T cells in response to mitogens such as phytohemagglutinin (PHA), as well as dermatophyte antigens.[35,36]

The fungal components that are most closely identified with host resistance via T-cell activation are glycopeptides. The possibility that dermatophytes interfere with the process of immunological activation in the skin is supported by immunohistochemical studies of biopsies from chronically infected skin. In acute dermatophyte infections, immunophenotypic techniques can be used to demonstrate the presence of numbers of effector lymphocytes in the vicinity of the infection.[37] Work has now shown that the dermal infiltrate mainly contains cells that are Leu2a positive (that is, T-helper cells).[37,38] Conversely, few express CD-8 (T-suppressor markers). HLA-DR is strongly expressed and most biopsies show Langerhans cells using a variety of different cell markers. However, in chronically infected patients, despite the presence of an infiltrate, adhesion molecules, such as ICAM-1, are poorly expressed in epidermis.[38] This may reflect suppression of the expression of these integrins in the epidermis despite intact cell-mediated immunity. Suppression of this aspect of immune activation by DIF produced by dermatophytes *in situ* is a possible explanation, which may account for the success of dermatophytes such as *T. rubrum* in causing persistent infections.

There are still a number of unexplained findings, particularly the relationship between atopy and infection. There is evidence from a number of studies that atopic subjects are more susceptible to persistent infections, particularly if they are not involved in occupations where exposure to infection occurs frequently. Patients with persistent foot infections due to *T. rubrum* are more likely to have positive immediate-type immune responses to skin testing with trichophytin. It has also been shown that this occurs with chronic anthropophilic infections in other sites such as the body and the groin. It is not clear, however, whether this occurs because of a defect in T-cell responsiveness developed specifically in atopic individuals, e.g., through a Th2 path, or whether the production of specific IgE and consequent release of mediators such as histamine affect the expression of an effective immunological response. Support for the latter hypothesis has come from a study that has shown that high IgE levels are accompanied by raised specific IgG4. In the same study, a higher level of delayed-type hypersensitivity to intradermal trichophytin but similar lymphocyte transformation responses were seen in patients with *T. rubrum* compared to controls.[39] It is clear that interferon-gamma (IFN-γ)-producing cells[40] are found in the infiltrate of dermatophyte lesions. However, at present a correlation between dry or chronic type infection and defective IFN-γ production is not established.[41] Variations in IgE production in response to successful therapy would again indicate a fluctuating relationship between Th1 and Th2 pathways.[42]

In summary, in dermatophytosis an active immunological response develops under model conditions. However, in some human infections, particularly those caused by *T. rubrum*, there is little inflammation and the infections tend to be chronic. There is evidence that the immunological response in such cases may be poorly developed either because of immunoregulation by the host or through the intervention of fungally mediated suppression. Chronic dermatophytosis is only seldom a marker of a severe immunodeficiency state.

## III. CUTANEOUS CANDIDOSIS

Superficial *Candida* infections of the skin are uncommon except in occluded areas such as in the groin or between the digits. Although there is now a considerable body of information about the relationship between the immune system and systemic *Candida* infections or oropharyngeal candidosis and AIDS,[43] less is known about the immunology of *Candida* skin infections. The exception to this is a rare syndrome, chronic mucocutaneous candidosis (CMC), which has been the subject of a considerable amount of immunological investigation over the years. However, it is still not clear whether, and which of, the different immunological abnormalities described in patients with CMC are causal and which are epiphenomena secondary to the infection itself. In part, the difficulty in defining immunological abnormalities has been compounded by a growing realization that patients with CMC comprise a heterogeneous group, consisting of at least five different disorders. It is likely that these do not share a common immunological defect. A clinical classification of CMC is shown in Table 34.1. A further problem is that immunological defects discovered in individual patients with CMC may vary with time. The clinical and immunological features of CMC are described below.

**TABLE 34.1**
**Chronic Mucocutaneous Candidosis**

1. Childhood Onset
   Inherited CMC without endocrinopathy:
   a. Autosomal recessive
   b. Autosomal dominant
   Inherited CMC with endocrinopathy:
   a. CMC with autosomal recessive endocrinopathy syndrome (hypoadrenalism, hypoparathyroidism, etc.)
   b. Autosomal dominant CMC with hypothyroidism
   CMC associated with keratitis
   Sporadic CMC
2. Adult onset
   CMC with thymoma
   CMC with other disease states

## IV. CHRONIC MUCOCUTANEOUS CANDIDOSIS

Chronic mucocutaneous candidosis is a disease that is characterized by the development of persistent superficial infection, notably oropharyngeal or cutaneous candidosis, as well as dermatophytosis and papilloma virus infection. The condition is a syndrome that comprises a number of different diseases with specific genetic or metabolic defects. The classification shown in Table 34.1 should not be regarded as exclusive and it is likely that other distinct forms of CMC may exist.

### A. Clinical Features

With some variations, the syndrome consists of a number of characteristic clinical features. The disorder usually, but not exclusively, starts in infancy or early childhood. Most patients have persistent oral candidosis, which responds only partially to conventional antifungal therapy, or relapses soon after apparently successful treatment. Chronic hypertrophic and dysplastic changes may develop on the tongue and buccal mucosa. Cutaneous *Candida* infection occurs in many patients. This may involve flexural skin as well as the face and the hands, and sometimes it is widespread over the trunk and limbs. In long-standing lesions, the cutaneous changes may resemble ringworm. Gross hyperkeratosis, previously referred to as *Candida* granuloma, may develop. Paronychia are common and are often accompanied by gross nail-plate infection and hyperkeratosis with nail destruction. This leads to total dystrophic onychomycosis with secondary involvement of the skin of the terminal phalanx.

There have been recent advances in our understanding of the genetics of this disorder. For example, in a detailed study of a family in whom dominant hypothyroidism was associated with CMC it was found that there was a putative linkage association with a locus on chromosome 2p.[44] Further, with an increasing understanding of the importance of mutations in the autoimmune regulator (AIRE) gene and the autoimmune polyendocrinopathy syndrome that is associated with CMC in some cases, two siblings who had CMC and hypoparathyroidism were found to have specific mutations in the AIRE gene accompanied by altered expression of the T-cell V $\beta$ receptor.[45]

### B. Immunological Defects in Chronic Mucocutaneous Candidosis

At this stage, it is not possible to state with any degree of certainty that the underlying immune defect in CMC has been identified.[46] There are a large number of different abnormalities that have been described in patients with this condition, but it is not clear whether these are primary or secondary to the infection.[47,48] They have included absent delayed-type hypersensitivity both to

*Candida* and other antigens, defective lymphocyte transformation and defects in neutrophil killing of yeasts, leukocyte migration, and cytokine production as well as selective antibody deficiency.[49] In one study,[50] IL-2 production was found to be defective in many of the patients investigated when *Candida* polysaccharide, but not cytoplasmic, antigen was used for stimulation. The interpretation of this finding is difficult; but clearly the nature of the antigen used for immunological investigation of patients is a further source of variation. By contrast, IL-6 was found to increase on stimulation with either antigen. Production of IFN-γ was variable with some patients producing none at all.

It has also not been possible to group the different forms of CMC according to immune defect as many of the patients have had a variable response whereas others have shown reversal of the immune defect with successful antifungal chemotherapy.[51,52] However, there is clearly a change in T-cell immunoregulation, which appears to be associated with defective memory responses to antigens. In some cases there are increased levels of IL-4 and a decrease in Th1-mediated cell-mediated immunity.[53]

Attempts to reverse potential immunological impairment with specific immune therapy using transfer factor, thymopoietin, or leukocyte transfusions have met with variable degrees of success.[54] Unfortunately, the clinical responses are seldom sustained for long periods, although there are often temporary improvements. In addition, it is known that certain antigenic components of *C. albicans*, such as mannan, as well as some glycoproteins are immunomodulatory.[55] As reversal of immune defects such as absent delayed-type hypersensitivity to *Candida* antigens has been seen with successful clearance of candidosis in patients with CMC, it is possible that some immunological changes may be secondary to the infection itself. There are intriguing parallels here with the situation described for dermatophytosis. Patients with chronic mucocutaneous candidosis may also have severe and persistent dermatophyte infections in addition to *Candida* infection.

A detailed study of the skin-specific nature of the immune defect in CMC may provide further clues as to the underlying immunological problem in these patients.

In summary, although a wide variety of different immunological defects have been described in patients with CMC, methodological problems ranging from difficulties with the adoption of an appropriate clinical classification to variation in test results after successful antifungal therapy have obscured their interpretation.

## V. VAGINAL CANDIDOSIS

The other superficial *Candida* infection, for which there has been recent progress in understanding the nature of immunological mechanisms, is vaginal candidosis. In this disease, which is a common condition affecting many women, few of whom have any overt immunological defect, relapse and persistent infection occur in a significant number of cases, again suggesting failure of the development of an adequate immune response. Attention has focused on the localized nature of defense against candidosis of the vaginal mucosa.[56] For example, in experimental vaginal infections in mice there is an increase in the numbers of lymphocytes that can be eluted from local secretions during infection, particularly $CD8^+$ lymphocytes.[57] However, another group of investigators found that protection from infection was significantly greater if eluted $CD3^+$ or $CD4^+$ cells were transferred to naive animals, subsequently challenged with *Candida*.[58] Likewise, attempts to protect animals from *Candida* infection show that mucosal immunity can be enhanced by rectal but not intranasal immunization,[59] again emphasizing the importance of local immunity. However, the expression of local responses immunity is variable and, for example, it appears in experimental murine infections that, although vaginal epithelium expresses adhesion molecules such as VCAM 1, the infiltrating mucosal lymphocytes and those in draining lymph nodes show little evidence of corresponding integrin expression.[60] The relationship between immune responses and human infection remains unclear at present.

## VI. INFECTIONS DUE TO *MALASSEZIA* SPP.

Lipophilic yeasts, *Malassezia* spp., are common skin commensals occurring in large numbers around the orifices of the sebaceous follicles. Their classification is complicated although it is now known that there are at least five genetically distinct species that are either commensal or pathogenic in humans. The main diseases associated with these organisms are pityriasis versicolor, *Malassezia* folliculitis, and seborrheic dermatitis.

Pityriasis versicolor is a superficial fungal infection characterized by the development of hypo- or hyperpigmented scaly patches, which become confluent over the upper trunk.[61] It is a common disease, particularly in the tropics. Pityriasis versicolor is an infection of otherwise healthy individuals although it has been associated with idiopathic and iatrogenic Cushing's syndrome,[62] and possibly malnutrition. It is not, however, more common in patients with AIDS[63] in contrast to seborrheic dermatitis.

There have been few investigations of the nature of the immune response in this infection. There is, for example, evidence that healthy subjects have antibodies to *Malassezia* species but that these do not differ significantly in titer to patients with pityriasis versicolor.[64] There is evidence that patients with pityriasis versicolor have only weak cellular immune responses, assessed by lymphocyte blastogenesis, to the specific *Malassezia* antigen,[65] and this has been associated with low numbers of specifically reactive T cells in their peripheral blood.[66] Another explanation is that *Malassezia* species elaborate a lipid-rich layer external to the cell wall, removal of which is associated with significantly improved *in vitro* T-cell-mediated responses.[67] Fungus-mediated immunomodulation may therefore play a role in the persistence of infection.[68]

Seborrheic dermatitis (SD) is a common chronic, scaly, and erythematous skin disease usually confined to parts of the face, scalp, and the front of the chest. Less commonly, flexural sites are involved. The majority of patients with this condition are otherwise healthy individuals, although there is often a high frequency of SD in patients with chronic neurological disease as well as AIDS. SD may be particularly florid in HIV-positive patients.

The pathogenesis of this condition and its relationship to lipophilic yeasts is still controversial. The evidence that the two are associated is largely based on the observation that patients with SD respond to antifungal chemotherapy and that when these are discontinued the condition relapses.[69] These clinical changes are mirrored by the behavior of the organisms themselves, which disappear from the skin surface with clinical response but reappear with relapse.

However, there are many features of the relationship between lipophilic yeasts and SD, which are difficult to explain. For example, there are marked variations in the colonization rates by lipophilic yeasts in healthy individuals and SD patients with or without AIDS. Although in some cases this may be due to differences in the methods used for assessing colonization, in SD patients without AIDS the numbers of organisms present in lesions are not only highly variable but the counts are also often similar or lower than those found in uninvolved skin.[70] In AIDS patients with SD, there are large variations in colonization rates in both unaffected and lesional skin.[71,72] There does, however, appear to be a relation between SD, disease severity, and the severity of immunosuppression as judged by CD4 lymphocyte counts,[71] with low counts associated with the most severe forms of SD. These data do not provide evidence that SD is an infection due to *Malassezia* where invasion of the stratum corneum would occur; rather, the presence of normal numbers of yeast appears to be concerned with triggering an inflammatory response.

The evidence that SD is very common in patients with AIDS might suggest that immunological mechanisms may be involved directly in its pathogenesis. However, investigations of the relationship between immune responses and SD have proved to be inconclusive. There is no evidence to show that patients with SD have defective delayed-type hypersensitivity to antigens of *Malassezia* species or that there is reduced lymphocyte transformation to these organisms. SD patients without AIDS do not have contact sensitization to *Malassezia* antigens on skin sites from which the epidermis has been stripped by tape.[73] These data must be weighed against the observation that the application of killed organisms to skin sites can lead to clinical changes similar to those seen with SD[74] and that scaling can be produced on rabbit skin exposed to killed yeasts.[75]

In skin biopsies from some patients with SD, there is a predominance of lymphocytes that bear the CD4 phenotype in the inflammatory infiltrate.[76] The numbers of CD1a$^+$ epidermal cells are similar in both normal and lesional skin. Also, high numbers of circulating Leu 7 and Leu 11 positive lymphocytes have been found in certain patients suggesting increased numbers of natural killer cells. There are no similar studies in patients with AIDS.

There is also conflicting evidence whether patients with SD have excessive antibody responses to *Malassezia* species. Some, but not all groups, have found raised antibody levels of the IgG class but without evidence of abnormal IgA or IgE responses.[64,76] Midgley and Hay[64] found that by using Western blotting many patients with SD had a dominant antibody reaction to a *Malassezia* antigen with a molecular weight of 35 kDa. Control atopic patients also sometimes had raised antibody titers to whole *Malassezia* yeast antigen but reacted to a different antigenic band at about 65 kDa. Similar results have not been found by other investigators who have either found no difference between antibody titers in patients and controls or even diminished titers in the SD group. While these findings may simply reflect different methods of assessing antibody titers, such as immunofluorescence vs. ELISA, or even the use of different antigen preparations, the evidence for the involvement of an immunological mechanism as the direct cause of inflammation leading to SD has not been established. However, patients with SD appear more likely to produce an inflammatory response to the presence of apparently normal numbers of *Malassezia* yeasts on the skin, and therefore it is possible that there is a defect in immunoregulation such as failure to suppress an immunological signal from a "normal" skin surface antigen.

At present, there is insufficient evidence to support either a direct toxic or immunological mechanism as the primary cause of SD, although failure to suppress a normal inflammatory response is a possible explanation.

The other conditions related to *Malassezia* yeasts include an irritant folliculitis and a form of head and neck eczema seen in atopic individuals. Nothing is known about the immune responses in the former. In the latter, there is usually a clinical response to topically applied azole antifungals and patients also show immediate-type hypersensitivity to extracts of *Malassezia*.[77] Atopic individuals with head and neck dermatitis are also more likely to have specific IgE to *Malassezia*.[78] Atopic individuals with positive prick test reactions to *Malassezia* are more likely to show enhanced production of the Th2-related cytokines such as IL-4 and 13 compared with the Th1-related cytokines such as IFN-$\gamma$.[79] There has been considerable work on the characterization of the allergen-associated antigens, and *M. globosa*, for example, produces one glycoprotein strongly associated with IgE reactivity: Malg46b.[80] It has also been found using a cDNA library cloned from *Malassezia* that the yeast produces a number of different IgE-binding proteins.[81] Uptake of yeast antigens is thought to be mediated through dendritic cells, and immature monocyte-derived dendritic cells are highly effective at internalizing *Malassezia* antigen even in the absence of IgE.[82] This work strongly points to an association in some atopic individuals between exposure to *Malassezia* and the pathogenesis of eczema.

## VII. CONCLUSION

The evidence from a study of the immunological responses to superficial fungal infections would suggest that although mechanisms exist to combat these invasive infections the means of circumventing normal immunological responses also exist. These include immunomodulation by the host or by the organism itself. At present, studies of immunoregulation in skin have concentrated on diseases such as leprosy and psoriasis. However, a closer study of infections such as dermatophytosis may provide a new model for furthering our understanding of the methods involved in evasion of the immune system in the epidermis. Other fungi, apart from dermatophytes, including *Candida* may also evade host responses in a similar manner. In the case of *Malassezia*, the problem at first appears to be different in that the organism is tolerated as a commensal yet also appears to be associated with inflammatory skin disease such as SD or a genuine infection, pityriasis versicolor. However, once again fungus-mediated immunomodulation appears to play a key role. Also in the case of dermatophytosis and *Malassezia* in atopic individuals the intervention of Th2-type immunological responses plays an important role in determining the outcome of immune interaction, chronic disease with the former and an allergic response with the latter.

## REFERENCES

1. Sohnle, P.G., Dermatophytosis, in *Immunology of the Fungal Diseases*, Cox, R.A., Ed., CRC Press, Boca Raton, FL, 1989, 1–27.
2. Tagami, H., Kudoh, K., and Takematsu, H., Inflammation and immunity in dermatophytosis. *Dermatologica,* 179(Suppl. 1), 1–8, 1989.
3. Hall, F.R., Ringworm contracted from cattle in western New York State. *Arch. Dermatol.*, 94, 35–37, 1962.
4. Hay, R.J., Chronic dermatophyte infections. I: Clinical and mycological features. *Br. J. Dermatol.*, 106, 1–9, 1982.
5. Rasmussen, J.E. and Ahmed, A.R., Trichophytin reactions in children with tinea capitis. *Arch. Dermatol.*, 114, 371–372, 1978.
6. Serjeantson, S. and Lawrence, G., Autosomal recessive inheritance of susceptibility to tinea imbricata. *Lancet,* 1, 13–15, 1977.
7. Hay, R.J., Campbell, C.K., Wingfield, R., and Clayton, Y.M., A comparative study of dermatophytosis in coal miners and dermatological outpatients. *Br. J. Ind. Med.,* 40, 353–355, 1983.
8. Zurita, J. and Hay, R.J., The adherence of dermatophyte microconidia and arthroconidia to human keratinocytes *in vitro. J. Invest. Dermatol.*, 89, 529–534, 1987.
9. Esquenazi, D., de Souza, W., Alviano, C.S., and Rozental, S., The role of surface carbohydrates on the interaction of microconidia of *Trichophyton mentagrophytes* with epithelial cells. *FEMS Immunol. Med. Microbiol.*, 35, 113–123, 2003.
10. Kligman, A.M., The pathogenesis of tinea capitis due to *Microsporum audouinii* and *Microsporum canis. J. Invest. Dermatol.*, 18, 231–246, 1952.
11. Hay, R.J., Calderon, R.A., and Mackenzie, C.D., Experimental dermatophytosis in mice; correlation between light and electron microscopic changes in primary, secondary and chronic infection. *Br. J. Exp. Pathol.*, 45, 56–63, 1988.
12. Graham, J.H. and Barrosos-Tobila, C., Dermatophytosis, in *The Pathologic Anatomy of the Mycoses*, Baker, R.D., Ed., Springer, Berlin, 1971, 211–235.
13. Yu, R.J., Harmon, S.R. et al., Two cell bound keratinases of *Trichophyton mentagrophytes. J. Invest. Dermatol.* 56, 27–32, 1971.
14. Brouta, F., Descamps, F., Monod, M. et al., Secreted metalloprotease gene family of *Microsporum canis. Infect. Immun.*, 70, 5676–5683, 2002.
15. King, R.D., Khan, H.A., Foye, J.C. et al., Transferrin, iron and dermatophytes 1. Serum dermatophyte inhibitory component definitely identified as unsaturated transferrin. *J. Lab. Clin. Med.*, 86, 204–212, 1975.
16. Wakabayashi, H., Takakura, N., Yamauchi, K. et al., Effect of lactoferrin feeding on the host antifungal response in guinea-pigs infected or immunised with *Trichophyton mentagrophytes. J. Med. Microbiol.,* 51, 844–850, 2002.
17. Green, F., Lee, K.W., and Balish, E., Chronic *T. mentagrophytes* dermatophytosis of guinea pig skin grafts on nude mice. *J. Invest. Dermatol.,* 79, 125–131, 1982.
18. Calderon, R.A. and Hay, R.J., Fungicidal activity of human neutrophils and monocytes on dermatophyte fungi, *Trichophyton quinckeanum* and *T. rubrum. Immunology,* 61, 289–296, 1987.
19. Calderon, R.A. and Shennan, G.I., Susceptibility of *Trichophyton quinckeanum* and *T. rubrum* to products of oxidative metabolism. *Immunology,* 61, 283–288, 1987.
20. Davies, R.R. and Zaini, F., Drugs affecting *Trichophyton rubrum* induced neutrophil chemotaxis *in vitro. Clin. Exp. Dermatol.,* 13, 228–231, 1988.

21. Elmros, T. and Liden, S., Hereditary palmoplantar keratoderma; incidence of dermatophyte infections and the results of topical treatment with retinoic acid. *Acta Derm. Venereol.*, 63, 254–257, 1983.
22. Jones, H.E., Reinhardt, J.H., and Rinaldi, M.G., A clinical, mycological and immunological survey of dermatophytosis. *Arch. Dermatol.*, 108, 61–68, 1973.
23. Torssander, J., Karlsson, A., Morfeldt-Mason, L. et al., Dermatophytosis and HIV infection — study in homosexual men. *Acta Derm. Venereol.*, 68, 53–59, 1988.
24. Munoz-Perez, M.A., Rodriguez-Pichardo, A., Camacho, F. et al., Dermatological findings correlated with CD4 lymphocyte counts in a prospective 3 year study of 1161 patients with human immunodeficiency virus disease predominantly acquired through intravenous drug abuse. *Br. J. Dermatol.*, 139, 33–39, 1998
25. Svejgaard, E., Immunologic investigations of dermatophytes and dermatophytosis. *Semin. Dermatol.*, 4, 201–221, 1985.
26. Calderon, R.A. and Hay, R.J., Cell-mediated immunity in experimental murine dermatophytosis. I: T-suppressor activity elicited in dermatophyte infections caused by *T. quinckeanum*. *Immunology*, 53, 457–464, 1984.
27. Calderon, R.A. and Hay, R.J., Cell-mediated immunity in experimental murine dermatophytosis. II. Adoptive transfer of immunity in dermatophyte infection by lymphoid cells from donors with acute or chronic infections. *Immunology*, 53, 465–472, 1984.
28. Jones, H.E., Reinhardt, J.H., and Rinaldi, M.G., Model dermatophytosis in naturally infected subjects. *Arch. Dermatol.*, 110, 369–374, 1974.
29. Hay, R.J., Reid, S., Talwat, E., and MacNamara, K., Immune responses of patients with tinea imbricata. *Br. J. Dermatol.*, 108, 581–586, 1983.
30. Elewski, B.E., El Charif, M., Cooper, K.D. et al., Reactivity to trichophytin antigen in patients with onychomycosis: effect of terbinafine. *J. Am. Acad. Dermatol.*, 46, 371–375, 2002.
31. Allen, D.E., Snyderman, R., Meadows, L. et al., Generalized *Microsporum audouinii* infection and depressed cellular immunity associated with a missing plasma factor required for lymphocyte blastogenesis. *Am. J. Med.*, 63, 991–1000, 1977.
32. Liautaud, B. and Marill, F.G., La maladie dermatophytique. Observations Algeriennes recentes. *Bull. Soc. Fr. Pathol. Exotique*, 77, 637–648, 1984.
33. Mayou, S.C., Calderon, R.A., Goodfellow, A., and Hay, R.J., Deep (subcutaneous) dermatophyte infection presenting with unilateral lymphoedema. *Clin. Exp. Dermatol.*, 12, 358–388, 1987.
34. Calderon, R.A., Hay, R.J., and Shennan, G.I., Circulating antigens and antibodies in human and mouse dermatophytosis. Use of monoclonal antibody reactive to phosphorylcholine-like epitopes. *J. Gen. Microbiol.*, 133, 2699–2705, 1987.
35. Dahl, M.V., Dermatophytosis and the immune response. *J. Am. Acad. Dermatol.*, 31, S34–41, 1994.
36. McGregor, J.M., Hamilton, A.J., and Hay, R.J., Possible mechanisms of immune modulation in chronic dermatophytoses: an *in vitro* study. *Br. J. Dermatol.*, 127, 233–238, 1992.
37. Brasch, J. and Sterry, W., Immunophenotypical characterization of inflammatory cellular infiltrates in tines. *Acta. Derm. Venereol.*, 72, 345–347, 1992.
38. Schectman, R.C., Allen, M.H., McGregor, J.M., and Hay, R.J., Skin inflammation in chronic dermatophyte infections caused by *Trichophyton rubrum* — lack of epidermal expression of ICAM-1. *J. Med. Vet. Mycol.*, 31, 459–462, 1993.
39. Leibovici, V., Evron, R., Axelrod, O. et al., Imbalance of immune responses in patients with chronic and widespread fungal skin infection. *Clin. Exp. Dermatol.*, 20, 390–394, 1995.
40. Koga, T., Duan, H., Urabe, K., et al., Immunohistochemical detection of interferon-gamma-producing cells in dermatophytosis. *Eur. J. Dermatol.*, 11, 105ñ107, 2001.
41. Koga, T., Shimizu, A., and Nakayama, J., Interferon-gamma production in peripheral lymphocytes of patients with tinea pedis: comparison of patients with and without tinea unguium. *Med. Mycol.* 39, 87–90, 2001.
42. Escalante, M.T., Sanchez-Borges, M. Capriles-Hulett, A. et al., *Trichophyton*-specific IgE in patients with dermatophytosis is not associated with aeroallergen sensitivity. *J. Allergy Clin. Immunol.*, 105, 547–551, 2000.
43. Odds, F.C., *Candida and Candidosis,* Bailliere Tindall, London, 1992, 252–278.

44. Atkinson, T.P., Schaffer, A.A., Grimbacher, B. et al., An immune defect causing dominant chronic mucocutaneous candidiasis and thyroid disease maps to chromosome 2p in a single family. *Am. J. Hum. Genet.*, 69, 791–803, 2001.
45. Kogawa, K., Kudoh, J., Nagafuchi, S. et al., Distinct clinical phenotype and immunoreactivity in Japanese siblings with autoimmune polyglandular syndrome type 1 (APS-1) associated with compound heterozygous novel AIRE gene mutations. *Clin. Immunol.,* 103, 277–283, 2002.
46. Kirkpatrick, C.H., Rich, R.B., and Bennett, J.E., Chronic mucocutaneous candidiasis; model building in cellular immunology. *Ann. Intern. Med.,* 74, 955–978, 1971.
47. Lilic, D. and Gravenor, I., Immunology of chronic mucocutaneous candidiasis. *J. Clin. Pathol.*, 54, 81ñ83, 2001.
48. Domer, J.E. and Carrow, E.W., Candidiasis, in *Immunology of the Fungal Diseases,* Cox, R.A., Ed., CRC Press, Boca Raton, FL, 1989, 57–92.
49. Kalfa, V.C., Roberts, R.L., and Stiehm, E.R., The syndrome of chronic mucocutaneous candidiasis with selective antibody deficiency. *Ann. Allergy Asthma Immunol.,* 90, 259–264, 2003.
50. Lilic, D., Cant, A.J., Abinun, M. et al., Chronic mucocutaneous candidiasis. I. Altered antigen-stimulated IL-2, IL-4, IL-6 and interferon-gamma (IFN-gamma) production. *Clin. Exp Immunol.,* 105, 205–212, 1996.
51. Drouhet, E. and Dupont, B., Laboratory and clinical assessment of ketoconazole in deep-seated mycoses. *Am. J. Med.,* 74(Suppl. 1B), 30–45, 1983.
52. Kennedy, C.T., Valdimarsson, H., and Hay, R.J., Chronic mucocutaneous candidiasis with a serum-dependent neutrophil defect: response to ketoconazole. *J. R. Soc. Med.,* 74, 158–162, 1981.
53. Kobrynski, L.J., Tanimune, L., Kilpatrick, L. et al., Production of T-helper cell subsets and cytokines by lymphocytes from patients with chronic mucocutaneous candidiasis. *Clin. Diagn. Lab. Immunol.,* 3, 740–745, 1996.
54. Dwyer, J.M., Chronic mucocutaneous candidiasis. *Annu. Rev. Med.,* 32, 491–497, 1981.
55. Durandy, A., Fischer, A., Le Deist, F. et al., Mannan specific and mannan induced T-cell suppressive activity in patients with chronic mucocutaneous candidosis. *J. Clin. Immunol.*, 7, 400–410, 1987.
56. Fidel, P.L., Jr., The protective immune response against vaginal candidiasis: lessons learned from clinical studies and animal models. *Int. Rev. Immunol.,* 21, 515–548, 2002.
57. Ghaleb, M., Hamad, M., and Abu-Elteen, K.H., Vaginal T lymphocyte population kinetics during experimental vaginal candidosis: evidence for a possible role of $CD8^+$ T cells in protection against vaginal candidosis. *Clin. Exp. Immunol.,* 131, 26–33, 2003.
58. Santoni, G., Boccanera, M., Adriani, D. et al., Immune cell-mediated protection against vaginal candidiasis: evidence for a major role of vaginal CD4(+) T cells and possible participation of other local lymphocyte effectors. *Infect. Immun.,* 70, 4791–4797, 2002.
59. Cardenas-Freytag, L. Steele, C., Wormley, F.L., Jr. et al., Partial protection against experimental vaginal candidiasis after mucosal vaccination with heat-killed *Candida albicans* and the mucosal adjuvant LT(R192G). *Med. Mycol.*, 40, 291–299, 2002.
60. Fidel, P.L., Jr., Luo, W., Steele, C. et al., Analysis of vaginal cell populations during experimental vaginal candidiasis. *Infect. Immun.,* 67, 3135–3140, 1999.
61. Faergemann, J., Lipophilic yeasts in skin disease. *Semin. Dermatol.*, 4, 173–184, 1985.
62. Burke, R.C., Tinea versicolor. Susceptibility factors and experimental infections in human beings. *J. Invest. Dermatol.*, 36, 398–402, 1961.
63. Mathes, B.M. and Douglas, M.C., Seborrheic dermatitis in patients with acquired immunodeficiency syndrome. *J. Am. Acad. Dermatol.,* 13, 947–951, 1985.
64. Midgley, G. and Hay, R.J., Serological responses to *Pityrosporum* (*Malassezia*) in seborrhoeic dermatitis demonstrated by ELISA and Western blotting. *Bull. Soc. Fr. Med. Mycol.,* 17, 267–278, 1983.
65. Sohnle, P.G. and Collins-Lech, C., Cell mediated immunity to *Pityrosporum orbiculare* in pityriasis versicolor. *J. Clin. Invest.,* 62, 45–50, 1978.
66. Sohnle, P.G. and Collins-Lech, C., Analysis of the lymphocyte transformation response to *Pityrosporum orbiculare* in patients with tinea versicolor. *Clin. Exp. Immunol.*, 49, 559–564, 1982.
67. Kesavan, S., Holland, K.T., and Ingham, E., The effects of lipid extraction on the immunomodulatory activity of *Malassezia* species *in vitro. Med. Mycol.*, 38, 239–247, 2000.
68. Ashbee, H.R. and Evans, E.G., Immunology of diseases associated with *Malassezia* species. *Clin. Microbiol. Rev.*, 15, 21–57, 2002.

69. Shuster, S., The aetiology of dandruff and mode of action of therapeutic agents. *Br. J. Dermatol.*, 111, 235–242, 1984.
70. Bergbrant, I.M. and Faergemann, J., Seborrhoeic dermatitis and *Pityrosporum ovale:* a cultural and immunological study. *Acta. Derm. Venereol.*, 69, 332–335, 1989.
71. Shectman, R., Midgley, G., and Hay, R.J., Colonization rates by *Malassezia* species of normal and affected skin of HIV positive seborrhoeic dermatitis patients. *Br. J. Dermatol.*, 133, 694–698, 1995.
72. Wikler, J.R., Nieboer, C., and Willemze, R., Quantitative skin cultures of *Pityrosporum* yeasts in patients seropositive for the human immunodeficiency virus with and without seborrhoeic dermatitis. *J. Am. Acad. Dermatol.*, 27, 37–39, 1992.
73. Nicholls, D., Midgley, G.M., and Hay, R.J., Patch testing against *Pityrosporum* antigens. *Clin. Exp. Dermatol.*, 15, 75, 1990.
74. Moore, M., Kile, R.L., Engman, M.F., and Engman, M.F., *Pityrosporum ovale* (Bottle Bacillus of Unna, spore of Malassez). Cultivation and possible role in seborrhoeic dermatitis. *Arch. Derm. Syphilol.*, 33, 457–472, 1936.
75. Rosenberg, E.W., Belew, P., and Bale, G., Effect of topical applications of heavy suspensions of killed *Malassezia ovalis* on rabbit skin. *Mycopathologia,* 72, 147–154, 1980.
76. Bergbrant, I.M., Johanssen, S., Robbins, D. et al., The evaluation of various methods and antigens for the detection of antibodies against *Pityrosporum ovale* in patients with seborrhoeic dermatitis. *Clin. Exp. Dermatol.*, 16, 339–343, 1991.
77. Hjorth, N. and Clemmensen, O.J., Treatment of dermatitis of the head and neck with ketoconazole in patients with type 1 hypersensitivity for *Pityrosporum orbiculare. Semin. Dermatol.,* 2, 26–29, 1983.
78. Mayser, P. and Gross, A., IgE antibodies to *Malassezia furfur, M. sympodialis* and *Pityrosporum orbiculare* in patients with atopic dermatitis, seborrheic eczema or pityriasis versicolor, and identification of respective allergens. *Acta Derm. Venereol.*, 80, 357–361, 2002.
79. Johansson, C., Eshaghi, H., Linder, M.T. et al., Positive atopy patch test reaction to *Malassezia furfur* in atopic dermatitis correlates with a T helper 2-like peripheral blood mononuclear cells response. *J. Invest. Dermatol.,* 118, 1044–1051, 2002.
80. Koyama, T., Kanbe, T., Ishiguro, A. et al., Isolation and characterization of a major antigenic component of *Malassezia globosa* to IgE antibodies in sera of patients with atopic dermatitis. *Microbiol. Immunol.*, 44, 373–379, 2000.
81. Rasool, O., Zargari, A., Almqvist, J. et al., Cloning, characterization and expression of complete coding sequences of three IgE binding *Malassezia furfur* allergens, Mal f 7, Mal f 8 and Mal f 9. *Eur. J. Biochem.,* 267, 4355–4361, 2000.
82. Buentke, E., Zargari, A., Heffler, L.C. et al., Uptake of the yeast *Malassezia furfur* and its allergenic components by human immature $CD1a^+$ dendritic cells. *Clin. Exp. Allergy,* 30, 1759–1770, 2000.

# 35 Parasitic Infections

*Raúl M. Cabrera, Rubén T. Guarda, Francis E. Palisson, and Sergio B. González*

## CONTENTS



## I. INTRODUCTION

All types of immune responses to parasites have been described. The chronicity of most parasitic infections is due to weak natural immunity and the ability of parasites to evade or resist elimination by specific immune response. The parasite can evade the immune response by antigenic variation (*Trypanosoma brucei, T. rhodesiense*), host molecule acquisition, loss of surface antigens, intrinsic membrane changes (schistosomes), specific T-cell suppression (filariasis, leishmaniasis), inactivation of antibodies (schistosomes), immune blockade by soluble antigen liberation, immune complex, IgG2c blockade antibodies (schistosomes, *Trichinella*), anatomic location (scabies mite), antigen masking (*Schistosomiasis mansoni*), and evasion of macrophage killing (*Toxoplasma gondii, T. cruzi*).[1]

Parasites have a large amount of antigens. Some of them are structural (somatic antigens) and others are metabolic products (metabolic antigens), e.g., secretions and enzymes. The antigenic diversity of pathogenic parasites is reflected in the variety of specific immune response they elicit. Medical parasitology has three main divisions: (1) diseases due to protozoa (single-celled animals), (2) helminths (worms), and (3) arthropods.[2]

We discuss limited but representative types of immune reactions due to parasitic infections of the skin.

0-8493-1959-5/05/$0.00+$1.50

## II. PROTOZOAL INFECTIONS

Leishmania infection produces a spectrum of illnesses that depends on both the species of the infecting organism and the host immune response. The bite of an infected female sandfly of the Phlebotomiae subfamily produces the inoculation of the flagellated protozoa (promastigotes) of the genus *Leishmania* into the epidermis and dermis. The mature promastigotes, bearing surface antigens of 116,000 Dam, bind C3 and then attach to C3b receptors of macrophages thus becoming internalized. Inside the macrophages the promastigotes lose their flagella and become amastigotes. The infected macrophage ruptures, releasing its population of amastigotes, which in turn infects other macrophages.[3] It has recently been shown that, in addition to macrophage, murine epidermal Langerhans cells (LC) are able to phagocytose *L. major* and serve as host cells for the parasite, both *in vitro* and *in vivo*, in the infected skin. LC migrate from the epidermis into the dermis prior to the uptake of *L. major*. In the course of the infection with *L. major*, a dramatic change in the distribution of LC is observed. A considerable loss of NLDC-45$^+$ (non-lymphoid dendritic cells) LC in the segment of the epidermis overlying the parasite-containing infiltrate is concomitant with the appearance of NLCD-45$^+$ cells in the dermal layer of the lesion, some of which contain *L. major*. The LC of the epidermis are not parasitized. The migration of epidermal LC into the regional lymph node (LN) has been demonstrated by irreversible labeling of LC with fluorescent cell linker and *in vivo* tracking. A small number of *L. major*-laden LC appear to leave the site of cutaneous infection homing to the LN, since only 0.1 to 0.5% of the *L. major*-infected LC labeled with fluorescent cell linker have been recovered from the draining LN. The great efficiency of the migratory LC is based on their capacity of binding and activating large numbers of antigen-specific T cells in the draining LN. As a result, activated T cells migrate via the blood into the lesions, where infected macrophages and LC that remain in the dermis regulate their effector activity through several mechanisms including cytokine secretion. The signals promoting the migration of LC have not been defined although the involvement of tumor necrosis factor-alpha (TNF-$\alpha$) and interleukin-1$\beta$ (IL-1$\beta$) has been suggested.[4,5] In the lymph node, dendritic cells (DC) have a remarkable capacity to present very low amounts of persistent *L. major* antigen to specific T cells, and allow the sustained stimulation of protective memory cells.[6] This potency is based on the unusual stability of major histocompatibility complex (MHC) class II antigen complexes in DC.[7] LC can also secrete IL-12, which is known to promote the development of Th1 cells.[8] In mice, LC loaded with *L. major* antigen *in vitro* are highly efficient in inducing protective immunity against cutaneous leishmaniasis when applied intravenously. They migrate into the spleen, where they first cause a primary cytokine response and over weeks induce a characteristic shift toward development of T helper cell type 1 (Th1) cells mediated by LC-derived IL-12.[9]

Chemokines and their receptors regulate the movement and interaction of antigen DC and T cells and additionally have direct immunological effects. In (CCR)2 null mice the migration of LC to draining lymph nodes is markedly impaired, with lower numbers of DC in the spleen due to a reduction in the CD8$\alpha$(1) Th1-inducing subset of DC. Absence of CCR2 in mice shifts the *L. major*-resistant phenotype to a susceptible state dominated by Th2 cytokines, B-cell outgrowth, and sustained neutrophilic inflammation.[10]

Opposing dermal chemokine profiles can be observed in self-healing localized cutaneous leishmaniasis (LCL) (*L. mexicana*) (CCL2/MCP-1, CXCL9/MIG, CXCL10/IP-10) associated with a protective CCL2/MCP-1 with leishmanicidal activities in human monocytes, in contrast to lesions of chronic diffuse cutaneous leishmaniasis DCL (*L. mexicana*) (CCL3/MIP-1alpha) without protective functions.[11] *Leishmania* infections are associated with the development of circulating antibodies. However, the level of antibodies or its class is not related to the type or stage of infections. Passive transfer of antibodies has failed to protect experimental animals against infections.[12] Systemic leishmaniasis (Kala-Azar) is associated with high levels of IgG and IgM, but they do not have any protective role.[13] Circulating antigen (51-kDa *Leishmania* antigen), among circulating immune complexes, has been found in the sera of 30% of people with visceral leishmaniasis. It has also been detected in the sera of patients with cutaneous leishmaniasis, and persists in the sera of clinically cured patients.[14] In *localized Leishmania lymphadenitis,* the parasite elimination mechanism appears to be similar to that in cutaneous leishmaniasis, in which immunologically mediated lysis of the host macrophages containing amastigotes is the main elimination mechanism. The lysis is associated with and may be caused by the formation of *in situ* immune complexes of leishmanial antigen and antibody. High extracellular levels of complement components C3, C1q, and C3d have been reported after necrosis in cutaneous leishmaniasis.[15]

Natural killer (NK) cells are active participants in the defense against the intracellular protozoan parasite *L. major.* NK cells participate in the early, nonspecific phase of anti-leishmanial activity. Depletion of NK cells, *in vivo,* reduces the resistance of C57BL/6 mice, and *in vivo* activation of NK cells can induce resistance in BALB/c mice. It has not been possible to demonstrate measurable cytotoxicity against *Leishmania*-infected cells by using infected macrophages as target cells in the NK cytotoxicity assay. It is most likely that the role of NK cells involves immunoregulatory mechanisms rather than cytotoxic activity against *Leishmania*-infected cells.[16] The contact of *Leishmania* parasites with the cutaneous immunocompetent cells is crucial for understanding the more specific immune response and the elimination of the parasite. The cutaneous form of leishmaniasis in the New World is termed American cutaneous leishmaniasis (ACL) and represents a good model of the complex cellular immune response. Murine models of ACL have shown that in localized cutaneous leishmaniasis (LCL) an adequate cell-mediated immune (CMI) response is mounted, and leishmaniasis is restricted to well-defined skin lesions. Histologically, granulomas are composed of prominent infiltration of lymphocytes, variable numbers of epithelioid cells, and few parasites. DCL is characterized by a selective anergy in CMI response with extensive involvement of the skin, nasobucopharyngeal mucosal tissue, and LN. Numerous undifferentiated macrophages laden with parasites, few lymphocytes, and plasma cells are present in DCL. Mucocutaneous leishmaniasis (MCL) represents a very destructive form, due to exacerbated CMI response with granuloma containing a mixture of lymphocytes and macrophages with few parasites.[17] The epidermal compromise in ACL is summarized in Table 35.1.

In LCL and MCL, a selective accumulation of T cells toward the basal layer of the epidermis has been observed. These $CD3^+$ T cells are either $CD4^+$ or CD $8^+$. Most infiltrating T cells express the $\alpha\beta$ T-cell receptor (TCR), with only few cells expressing the $\gamma\delta$ TCR (3.6%). In DCL, one observes more $\gamma\delta$ T cells in the granulomas than in LCL lesions; however, few of these cells are observed in the epidermis (Table 35.1).[18,19]

During infection by *L. major*, $CD4^+$ $25^+$ regulatory T cells accumulate in the dermis, where they suppress — by both IL-10-dependent and IL-10-independent mechanisms — the ability of $CD4^+$ $CD25^-$ effector T cells to eliminate the parasite from the site. The capacity of lesions derived from $CD4^+$ $CD25^+$ and $CD4^+$ $CD25^-$ T-cell subsets to produce IL-10 and interferon-gamma (IFN-

**TABLE 35.1**
**Epidermal Compromise in American Cutaneous Leishmaniasis[18]**

| | LCL | MCL | DCL |
|---|---|---|---|
| Epidermal LC ($CD1a^+$) | +++ | – | + |
| Epidermal T cells (basal layer) | ++ | ++ | +/– |
| Keratinocytes HLA-DR (+) | +++ | +++ | – |
| Keratinocytes ICAM-1 (+) | Patches | Universal | – |

**TABLE 35.2**
**Cytokine Profile in American Cutaneous Leishmaniasis[16]**

| | CL | MCL | DCL |
|---|---|---|---|
| IFN-γ | ↑↑↑ | ↑↑↑ | ↑↑↑ |
| IL-1β | ↑↑↑ | ↑↑↑ | ↓ |
| IL-2 | ↑↑ | ↑↑↑ | ↑↑ |
| IL-4 | ↓ | ↑↑ | ↑↑↑ |
| IL-5 | ↓ | ↑↑ | ↑↑↑ |
| IL-6 | ↑↑↑ | ↑↑ | – |
| IL-8 | ↑↑ | – | – |
| IL-10 | ↓ | ↑↑↑ | ↑ |
| TNF-α | ↑↑ | ↑↑↑ | ↓ |
| TNF-β | ↑ | ↑↑↑ | ↑ |

*Symbols:* ↓ very low expression, ↑↑ high expression, ↑↑↑ very high expression, – not found.

γ), respectively, increased the possibility that a delicate balance exists between suppressor and effector T-cell functions within chronically infected skin.[20]

Disease resistance and susceptibility appear to depend on the cytokine profile secreted by particular subsets of CD4+ lymphocytes. In mouse strains that develop small localized lesions (C57Bl/6 mouse), resistance is preferentially associated with the presence of IFN-γ-producing CD4+ cells of the Th1 subset. In mice that develop a progressive and ultimately fatal infection (BALB/c mouse), susceptibility is preferentially associated with the presence of IL-4-producing T cells of the Th2 subset. It has been directly demonstrated by adoptive transfer of specific Th1 and Th2 cell lines that these T-cell subsets mediate disease resistance or susceptibility. Anti-IL-4 treatment attenuates disease in susceptible mice, while anti-IFN-γ antibody treatment induces susceptibility in otherwise resistant mice.[21] Cross-regulation of Th1 and Th2 cells has been performed *in vitro*. In BALB/c mice infected with *L. major*, the Th1 cell function is actively inhibited when Th2 cells produce IL-4. Differences in the role of IL-4 and IL-10 in the suppression of Th1 response to *L. major* have been evident in the *in vivo* studies. Administration of anti-IL-4, but not anti-IL-10, to *L. major*-infected *scid* mice, restored with a mixture of $CD45RB^{high}$ (naive, Th1) and $CD45RB^{low}$ (memory, Th2) cells, led to the development of protective Th1 response. These data suggest that $CD45RB^{low}$ population inhibits the Th1 response to *L. major* by an IL-4-dependent mechanism.[22]

Using the polymerase chain reaction technique, two different groups of investigators have been able to determine the range of cytokines produced in human lesions of ACL (Table 35.2). These cytokine patterns suggest that most T cells present in MCL and DCL secrete a mixture of Th1 and Th2 cytokines patterns, but in DCL granuloma type a Th2 cytokine pattern predominates. In LCL, the cytokine patterns show a mixture of Th1 and Th0 patterns with preponderance of IFN-γ over IL-4, and low levels of IL-5 and IL-10.[21] IL-12, also known as NK- stimulating factor (NKSF), and cytotoxic lymphocyte maturation factor (CLMF) cytokine produced by monocytes and B cells can promote the development of Th1 cells in leishmaniasis. Treatment with recombinant murine IL-12 during the first week of infection has been able to cure 89% of normally susceptible BALB/c mice. Cure is associated with depressed production of IL-4 by lymph node cells cultured with antigens or mitogens, and unchanged or increased production of IFN-γ.[23]

A critical period exists for establishing curative Th1 response during the first week after infection. Disease development may depend on a transient dysregulation of T-cell response during the initial phase of infection in which a downregulation of Th1 type response in early human ACL may allow the parasite to survive and multiply. Lymphocyte blastogenesis assay and cytokine production in patients with *L. braziliensis* infection of less than 60 days (early cutaneous leishmaniasis) showed absent or low lymphocyte proliferation after stimulation with *Leishmania* antigen, and low levels of IFN-γ and high levels of IL-10 are found in the lymphocyte supernatant. In contrast, in patients with late cutaneous leishmaniasis (illness duration > 2 months), intradermal skin tests with leishmanial lysate prepared from an *L. amazonensis* strain became positive and IFN-γ production was high. IL-10 levels were low or absent.[24]

Genetic factors can control the Th cell development. A difference in maintaining a responsiveness of T cells to IL-12 exists between BALB/c (Th2 response to *L. major*) and B10.D2 (Th1 response *to L. major*) mice. Although *in vitro* naive T cells from both strains initially responded to IL-12, purified naive T cells from resistant B10.D2 mice strains maintained IL-12 responsiveness after development in BALB/c-nonresistant predominant cocultures, whereas BALB/c cells derived from the same coculture lost IL-12 responsiveness. These findings indicate that endogenous differences allow B10.D2 T cells to differentially maintain IL-12 responsiveness. This model supports the hypothesis that *L. major* resistance is probably dependent on maintenance of the IL-12 signaling pathway and not on differential regulation of IL-4 production.[25]

Current treatment of leishmaniasis is expensive and toxic, and an efficient vaccine has not been described.[26] Nitric oxide (NO) released by skin macrophage is critical for parasite elimination. A new and inexpensive form of treatment is under study. In MCL, immunostimulatory DNA (specific DNA sequences containing oligodeoxynucleotides CpG-ODN) has been able to convert ineffective anti-*Leishmania* vaccines into effective vaccines capable of aborting MCL. It is also involved in the development of protective immunity by reducing the initial parasite burden (by induction of NO production in local skin macrophages) and also by allowing for the development of Th1-predominant immune responses via induction of IL-12 from local macrophages and dendritic cells.[27–30]

## III. HELMINTHIC INFECTIONS

### A. Schistosomiasis

Schistosomes are parasitic worms that are a prime example of a complex multicellular pathogen that flourishes in the human host despite the development of a pronounced immune response.

In the skin, a granulomatous and fibrotic infection is produced by *S. mansoni and S. hematobium.* IgA markedly impairs schistosome fecundity by limiting both the egg laying of mature worms and the hatching capacity of a schistosome egg into viable miracidia. FcεRI is expressed in eosinophils from hypereosinophilic patients, and the eosinophil degranulation participates in eosinophil-mediated cytotoxicity against *S. mansoni*, playing a major role in the defense against the parasite.[31] Circulating immune complexes downregulate granulomatous hypersensitivity to *S. mansoni* eggs in patients with chronic intestinal schistosomiasis.[32]

Leukocytes of patients with *S. mansoni* respond with a Th2 pattern of cytokine production to egg antigens and a Th0 pattern to worm antigens.[33] *Schistosomiasis mansoni* eggs produce a rapid and pronounced Th0 response, which rapidly transforms into a Th2 response.[34] Th2 cells producing IL-4 play a major role in egg-induced granuloma formation and induction. Downmodulation of Th2-like responses is influenced by non-T-cell-derived cytokines.[35] *Schistosomiasis mansoni* granulomas constitutively make IL-5, which originates from granuloma CD4+ T lymphocytes. Eosinophils produce a soluble substance that, along with IL-2 and ongoing class II MHC/TCR interaction, enhances lymphocyte IL-5 output.[36] Macrophages from individuals infected with schistosoma induce unresponsiveness in specific Th1 lymphocytes resulting in the immunologic downregulation of egg-induced granulomatous inflammation characteristically seen in this disease, although they are able to stimulate Th2 type responses.[37] IL-12 suppresses schistosome egg-induced Th2 responses by decreasing IL-4, IL-5, and IL-10 secretion and by increasing the production of Th1 cytokines and IFN-γ.[38] This results in a decrease of the granulomatous inflammation and reduction of fibrosis, thus reducing local damage. Egg antigen-stimulated lymphoid cell culture supernatants from schistosome-infected mice can significantly inhibit antigen-specific, MHC-restricted proliferate responses of cloned schistosomal egg antigen (SEA)-specific $CD4^+$ (Th1 type) lymphocytes.[39] Macrophage inflammatory protein 1 alpha contributes to cellular recruitment during schistosome egg granuloma formation.[40] TNF and ICAM-1 participate in *S. mansoni* egg granuloma formation by activating lymphocytes, suggesting that one mechanism of TNF in granuloma development is inducing ICAM-1 expression.[41] ICAM-1 can perform a co-stimulatory function in antigen-presenting cell/T-cell interactions. It is possible that ICAM-1 shedding in the granuloma microenvironment interrupts proper co-stimulation, leading to unresponsive SEA-specific T cells. In this way, soluble ICAM-1 contributes to the modulation of cellular responses to SEA in chronic human schistosomiasis.[42]

Reflecting the complexity of the host–parasite relationship and the need to more fully understand both immune response development and parasite biology, an effectively designed antischistosome vaccine has yet to be produced.

## B. Filariasis

### 1. Onchocerciasis

This type of filariasis subset is viewed as an immune-mediated disease, in which the host response to the parasite, particularly microfilariae in the skin and ocular tissues, leads to tissue damage. Infection in humans begins with inoculation of infective *Onchocerca volvulus* larvae into the skin by female blackfly (*Simulium* sp.) bites. Over a period of months to years, infective larvae develop into adult worms and become encased in a rim of host tissue, thus forming characteristic subcutaneous nodules (onchocercomata). During this period, there is a polyclonal B-cell activation with generation of antibodies (mostly IgG, IgM, and IgE) against multiple parasite antigens.[43] The mean levels of serum total IgE are extremely high in *O. volvulus* infection and may contribute to acute inflammatory complications. Serum antigen–antibody complexes are found in a high percentage of people infected with *O. volvulus*; immune complex deposits may lead to acute inflammation and tissue damage.[44] Degranulation of eosinophils *in vivo* in skin areas surrounding microfilariae suggests that eosinophils may be major effector cells in antibody-dependent killing of microfilariae.[45]

Individuals infected with *Onchocerca volvulus* also have decreased reactivity to tuberculin skin tests and increased prevalence of lepromatous leprosy, suggesting an impaired cell-mediated immunity.[46] Proliferation of peripheral blood mononuclear cells and production of IL-4 in response to both helminth and mycobacterial antigens decreased dramatically with increasing microfilarial density.[47]

In contrast to most infected people with low-active or inactive onchodermatitis, individuals with severe hyperreactive onchodermatitis have enhanced peripheral cell-mediated immune responses to onchocercal antigens and an extensive inflammatory cell infiltrate of the upper dermis composed of plasma cells, eosinophils, and lymphocytes. These individuals also have an increased number of activated lymphocytes in peripheral blood, as assessed by the expression of HLA-DR, transferring receptors, and IL-2 receptors, when compared with individuals with positive microfilariae without disease. Increased numbers of $CD4^+$ cells and cells with the NK phenotype, together with an increased $CD4^+/CD8^+$ ratio, were found in hyperreactive oncodermatitis patients.[48]

T-regulatory-1 (Tr1) cells — a subset of $CD4^+$ T cells — are characterized by suppressor functions *in vitro* and *in vivo* and by a predominant production of IL-10 and/or TGF-β. In patients with chronic onchocerciasis and few signs of dermatitis despite the presence of millions of small worms in the skin, skin-derived T cells that bear characteristics of Tr1 cells were found, producing no IL-2 or IL-4 but substantial amounts of IL-10, variable amounts of IL-5, and some IFN-γ.[49]

DNA immunization has good potential for induction of humoral responses against nematode infections in mice,[50] and could be a promising model in future human trials.

### 2. Loiasis

*Loa loa* is a filarial parasite that causes a chronic infection characterized by the migration of adult worms in subcutaneous tissues and across the eye and occasional angioedematous swelling. Humans are the only significant reservoir of these parasites, although nonhuman primates can also be infected.[51]

*Loa loa* can survive in the host for a long period of time. Chronic infection causes a great release of parasite antigens capable of inducing immediate- and delayed-type hypersensitivity reactions including host tissue damage mediated by immune complex deposits. Hypergammaglobulinemia is common in *L. loa*-endemic areas and polyclonal serum IgE elevation is found in the majority of patients.[52] Eosinophilia is an almost constant finding in loiasis; eosinophils adhere to and kill *L. loa* microfilariae *in vitro*, suggesting a probable role in antibody-dependent killing of microfilariae. Infective stage larvae of *L. loa* upon *in vitro* incubation with normal human serum activated the alternative complement pathway. C3 conversion products are detected on larval cuticles by eosinophil adherence and by immunofluorescence with C3c antiserum. No evidence for cuticle binding of IgG, IgA, IgM, Clq, or C4 is found by immunofluorescence. Larval viability is unaffected by complement activation or by adherence of eosinophils.[53] Using adult antigen from *L. loa* in immunoblotting, there is a difference in the antigen recognition patterns between amicrofilaremic (occult or "resistant") patients and those with asymptomatic microfilaremia. Those individuals who are able to clear their microfilariae recognized a high-molecular-weight antigen (~160 kDa), which is not recognized by those with microfilaremia. Conversely, microfilaremic individuals exclusively recognized an 18-kDa antigen.[54] The proliferation and cytokine profiles of peripheral blood mononuclear cells from microfilaremic subjects infected by *L. loa*, in response to antigens of several parasitic stages, were compared with those from amicrofilaremic individuals. While a strong lymphoproliferative response and consistent levels of both Th1-(IL-2), IFN-γ, and Th2-(IL-4, IL-5) type cytokines were observed in response to adult worms and microfilariae antigens in amicrofilaremic individuals; microfilaremic subjects were characterized by T-cell unresponsiveness, including decreased T-cell proliferation and low IL-2 mRNA expression.[55] By using flow cytometry for the intracellular detection of cytokines, increased frequency of Th2-type cytokine-producing T cells in microfilaremic loiasis compared with the amicrofilaremic group was noted.[56]

## IV. ARTHROPODS

### A. Arthropod Bites: General Aspects

The most frequent hypersensitivity reactions in humans are induced by arthropods through bites, stings, or direct contact. We will refer only to those induced by arthropod bites, with particular emphasis in mosquito bites as these are the most frequent cause of this worldwide problem. Arthropod bites introduce antigenic materials, usually oral secretions (salivary proteins) and, less frequently, mouthpieces in animal or human skin. Those antigens elicit antibody- and cell-mediated hypersensitivity reactions expressed in well-characterized clinicopathological reaction patterns. A typical chronological sequence of skin clinical reactivity to consecutive bites of the same arthropod (Table 35.3) has been evidenced in animals and humans for many arthropods including mosquitoes,[57,58] fleas,[59] and bedbugs.[60] In individuals without previous exposure, the first bites do not cause visible reactions (stage I). The following bites induce a delayed reaction (an erythematous papule) after 24 h (stage II). Subsequent bites cause a biphasic reaction: an immediate but transient reaction (an erythematous macule or papular wheal) after 10 to 15 min and later a delayed reaction after 12 to 24 h (stage III). The latency between both reactions shortens with subsequent bites due to a gradual anticipation of the delayed reaction, later showing only immediate reactions (stage IV). Finally, with prolonged exposure to multiple bites, a nonreactive status is reached (stage V).[61] Constant antigenic stimulation produces changing balances between cell- and antibody-mediated effector immune responses, ending in immunological tolerance. These responses are generally

**TABLE 35.3**
**Chronological Sequence of Clinical Cutaneous Reactivity to Arthropod Bites[57,58]**

| Stages | Skin Reactions | |
|---|---|---|
| | Immediate | Delayed |
| I | – | – |
| II | – | + |
| III | + | + |
| IV | + | – |
| V | – | – |

specific as shown by clinical reactivity or tolerance to bites limited to a particular species; nevertheless cross-reactivity or cross-tolerance between species and genus has been shown by clinical responses and serum antibody characterization presumably due to common antigens.[62]

Arthropod bite-induced clinical reactions may be cutaneous or systemic and represent mostly immediate IgE-mediated, IgE-dependent late-phase allergic and delayed cell-mediated reactions. Local reactions in bite sites include papules, wheals, vesicles, bullae, necrotic Arthus-type reactions, eosinophilic cellulitis (Wells' syndrome), and chronic prurigo (strophulus or nodularis). Generalized cutaneous reactions include extensive papular urticaria, generalized typical urticaria, serum sickness-like syndrome, erythema multiforme, and anaphylactoid purpura. Anaphylaxis, although much more frequent with Hymenoptera stings, has seldom been described with insect bites.[58]

Individuals may be nonreactive, hyporeactive, or hyperreactive to arthropod bites depending on constitutional and acquired factors. Exaggerated cutaneous reactions may appear in patients with atopic conditions,[63] AIDS/HIV infection,[64,65] alfa-1-antitrypsin deficiency,[66] congenital agammaglobulinemia,[67] chronic lymphocytic leukemia,[68] and T/NK lymphocytosis.[69]

## B. Mosquito Bites

The mechanisms of mosquito bite hypersensitivity are only partially understood. Salivary protein antigens are introduced in mammals through adult female mosquito blood-sucking bites causing antibody- and cell-mediated hypersensitivity. In normal individuals, mosquito hypersensitivity is expressed as both immediate and delayed, cutaneous or systemic reactions. Bite-site reactions include: papules, wheals, vesicles, large bullae, local angioedema, and febrile large inflammatory reactions ("skeeter syndrome").[70,71] Generalized cutaneous and systemic reactions include extensive papular urticaria,[72] generalized urticaria, and, more rarely, recurrent serum-sickness-like syndrome,[73] asthma,[74] and anaphylaxis.[75–77]

Exaggerated local and systemic reactions to mosquito bites include fever, lymphadenopathy, chronic excoriating papular eruption, large bullae, plaques or nodules, necrotic Arthus-like type reaction, and atypical hydroa vacciniformis. These reactions may be seen in patients with lymphoid cell disorders: AIDS/HIV infection[64,65] (including patients receiving zidovudine),[78] chronic lymphocytic leukemia,[68,79] and a particular T-cell/NK-cell (T/NK) disorder first identified by Tokura in 1990.[80] The latter, now called Epstein–Barr virus-associated T/NK lymphoproliferative disease, is more often seen in Asian countries, characteristically associated with severe hypersensitivity to mosquito bites (HMB) expressed in abnormal local as well as systemic reactions. Local reactions, previously described as "Arthus-type reaction," are mainly large plaques or bullae that develop into necrosis at bite sites, and an atypical hydroa vacciniforme presented as an extensive papulovesicular and edematous facial eruption. Systemic reactions are high fever, general malaise, and subsequently lymphadenopathy and hepatosplenomegaly. HMB is associated with chronic Epstein–Barr virus (EBV) infection and NK leukemia/lymphoma. NK cells are infected with monoclonal or biclonal

EBV and may be the crucial factor for HMB since they are found primarily in lesional skin. Isolated blood CD56+ cells exhibit a twofold increase in *in vitro* proliferation in response to mosquito extracts. Most patients have IgE levels > 1000 IU/ml. Half of patients have died of hemophagocytic syndrome (malignant histiocytosis), granular lymphocyte proliferative disorder, or lymphomas.[69]

Saliva is the source of mosquito allergens. Mosquitoes in which the salivary duct is cut do not induce reactions after feeding.[81] Intradermal injection of oral secretion of *Aedes aegypti* induces a positive immediate cutaneous reaction in sensitized humans, and sensitizes previously nonsensitized guinea pigs.[82] Although whole-body extract and salivary glands may bind serum IgE from allergic individuals, binding antigens most probably pertain solely to saliva secretion.[62,70,81,83–86] Salivary protein antigens have been reported in most mosquito species, including *Aedes* species (*aegypti, communis, vexans, albopictus, albifasciatus, togoi*), *Culex* species (*pipiens, pipiens pallens, quinquefasciatus, tritaeniorhynchus*), and *Anopheles stephensi*.[62,83,87–92] Some salivary antigens are common to several mosquito species and others are species specific.[62,91] Among the former, a 68-kDa apyrase (Aed a 1) is common to several *Aedes* species (*aegypti, vexans,* and *albopictus*) and *C. quinquefasciatus*;[62] a 36-kDa antigen is shared by *A. communis* and *A. aegypti*.[87] The saliva of *A. aegypti* adult females contains up to 20 proteins,[93] 8 of which are allergens that bind serum IgE from hypersensitive subjects.[62,94,95] The cDNA encoding for three major salivary allergens has been cloned and sequenced to obtain recombinant proteins named rAed a 1, rAed a 2, and rAed a 3. The rAed a 1 is a 68-kDa protein identical to apyrase (a saliva diphosphohydrolase) and able to induce both skin immediate and delayed reactions in previously sensitized humans.[86] Intradermal injection of rAed a 2 in mice induced significant serum IgE and IgG1 increases and immediate but not delayed skin reactions.[96]

Antibody-mediated mosquito bite hypersensitivity is dependent on salivary antigen-specific IgE and IgG antibodies and is primarily mediated by Th2 lymphocytes. Mice sensitized by *A. aegypti* bites showed dominant Th2-dependent IgE and IgG1 responses but no Th1-dependent IgG2a response.[97] Similarly, mice repeatedly exposed to *A. albopictus* bites doubled serum levels of total IgE and IgG1 but not IgG2a.[98] In humans exposed to *A. vexans* bites, serum salivary gland-specific IgE and IgG levels correlate with skin immediate and delayed reactions and are higher in individuals with immediate reactions.[99] High titers of IgE and IgG antibodies specific to mosquito salivary gland extracts were present in hypersensitive subjects.[100] In mosquito bite-sensitive children, human IgE and IgG4 antibodies bind to the same saliva proteins as antibodies from immunized mice.[88] IgE and IgG antibodies induced by some mosquito antigens seem not to alter the biting behavior of mosquitoes.[101]

IgE antibody production is the main animal and human humoral response to most salivary antigens from many mosquito species.[62,88,91,96,99,102] This IgE response correlates with immediate reactions.[87,96,99,103] Serum IgE cross-reactivity between species may occur due to common salivary antigens or common epitopes in different salivary antigens.[89] Passive transfer of immediate reactions by serum (Prausnitz–Küstner test) has been demonstrated in animals[104] and humans.[102] A late-phase allergic cutaneous reaction that is IgE- and mast cell-dependent has been suggested as a response mechanism to mosquito bites[105] supported by frequent early eosinophil infiltrates[106] and delayed reactions persisting up to 6 h after a positive Prausnitz–Küstner test with serum containing *A. aegypti* saliva-specific IgE antibodies.[102] No salivary eosinophil chemotactic activity has yet been identified, but a 200-kDa neutrophil chemotactic factor was recently shown in *Anopheles stephensi* saliva.[107] Intradermal tests with *A. stephensi* whole-body extracts in Indian volunteers showed a specific and significantly higher positivity (47.8%) in the asthma/rhinitis group (6% in the control group). Some had positive bronchial provocation tests with such extracts, suggesting a role of mosquito particles in IgE-mediated respiratory disorders.[108]

Specific IgG antibody responses against whole-body extract, salivary glands, and saliva antigens have also been shown.[83–85] They are mostly Th2-dependent IgG1 and IgG4 but not Th-1-dependent IgG2a.[96,97] IgG4 antibodies to 36- and 22-kDa *Aedes communis* salivary antigens are present in most individuals hypersensitive to *A. communis* bites.[87] While antisaliva IgE antibodies are important in the pathogenesis of the immediate reactions, IgG4 antibodies seem to be markers of both intense prolonged exposure[87] and natural desensitization to bites.[102]

Evidence supporting cell-mediated immune response is limited. Passive transfer of delayed hypersensitivity by leukocytes has been shown in guinea pigs.[104] Of six patients, two with strong delayed reactions to mosquito bites showed positive lymphocyte transformation assay with *A. communis* whole-body extracts.[109] A girl with congenital agammaglobulinemia and blood eosinophilia developed severe delayed (but not immediate) cutaneous reactions to naturally occurring mosquito bites (10 to 20 h later) and to intradermal injection of whole-body extracts from two mosquito species (48 h later). A lesional skin biopsy taken 24 h after a natural bite showed a perivascular infiltrate of lymphocytes and histiocytes with few eosinophils and neutrophils.[67]

A seasonally intense pruritic equine dermatitis (sweet itch) is induced by hypersensitivity to *Culicidae* mosquitoes and is an important animal model for mosquito allergy. Skin biopsies show a mixed inflammatory infiltrate (predominantly eosinophils and lymphocytes), and increased numbers of mast cells in the dermis, plus LC and T cells in the dermoepidermal junction.[110,111] Mast cells and basophils are involved, presumably through the generation of histamine, platelet-activating factor, and sulfidoleucotrienes.[112,113] Increased numbers of epidermal and dermal IgE-bearing cells, tryptase-positive cells, and double-labeled tryptase/IgE cells have been shown.[114] IgE and IgG serum antibodies to *Culicoides* salivary gland antigens have been detected.[115] Ponies with sweet itch had a significantly increased number of circulating $CD5^+$ and $CD4^+$ T lymphocytes. They showed increased numbers of eosinophils and $CD4^+$ lymphocytes in the skin after intradermal injection of *Culicoides* antigen extract.[116] Upregulation of eotaxin and monocyte chemoattractant protein-1 (MCP-1) in skin biopsies suggests their role in the dermal influx of eosinophils and mononuclear cells.[117] Similar *Culicoides*-induced hypersensitivity is present in cattle and sheep.[118]

Hypersensitivity to mosquitoes may be detected through prick or intradermal tests using commercial whole-body extract or saliva antigenic preparations, ELISA or RAST techniques for serum specific IgE or IgG subclasses, immunoblotting, and lymphocyte transformation tests (exposure to mosquito bites is not recommended). Skin tests using whole-body extracts are not reliable or standardized, often showing false-negative results due to low content of relevant mosquito saliva antigens or false-positive results due to irritating non-allergenic proteins.[85] Recombinant salivary allergens will certainly improve *in vitro* and *in vivo* diagnostic test standardization and specificity.[119]

Human natural desensitization commonly occurs through years of exposure.[57,120] Desensitization with mosquito allergenic extracts has conflicting results due to lack of standardized antigens. Delayed-type reactions are easier to desensitize[58,61] as occurs naturally in stage IV of clinical reactivity (Table 35.3). In sera of tolerant individuals, only mosquito-saliva-specific IgG4 (but not IgE) antibodies are present.[102] Intravenous injections of mosquito extracts in rabbits induce tolerance to natural mosquito bites.[58] The hope is that desensitization immunotherapy will improve with the introduction of recombinant antigens.[119]

## C. Flea Bites

Flea-induced dermatitis is the most common veterinary allergic condition in the world.[121] The most common species affecting humans are *Cnetocephalides* (*felis* and *canis*) and *Pulex irritans*.[122] Experimental flea bites in humans induced positive cutaneous reactions in 166 of 269 bites, an extremely high proportion (63%) consisting only of delayed reactions.[81] Oral secretion sensitizes guinea pigs only when combined with complete Freund's adjuvant, suggesting that the antigen is a hapten.[123] It has been recently suggested that the putative allergens responsible for flea bite hypersensitivity are salivary proteins of 40 and 12-8-kDa.[124]

In dogs, flea bites induce IgG and IgE antibody response to flea antigens.[125] IgE antibodies from canine serum bind to at least 15 different allergens (from 14 to 150 kDa) from cat fleas,[126] and passive transfer of immediate hypersensitivity to flea bites by serum has been shown among guinea pigs,[61] suggesting that immediate hypersensitivity is a main mechanism in animal flea bite allergy. All flea-sensitive dogs had positive skin tests to flea antigen and high serum titers of flea-specific serum IgE and IgG antibodies. Significantly higher numbers of chimase and/or tryptase/anti-IgE double-labeled mast cells were found in skin biopsies of flea-sensitized dogs. A selective release of mast cell tryptase was shown after flea exposure.[127]

In humans, Croce[128] and Croce and De Almeida[129] have suggested that Hebra's prurigo is a hypersensitivity expression of atopic individuals (mainly children) to flea bites, mediated by IgE and local immune complexes (Arthus-type reaction). They were able to reproduce, both clinically and histologically, typical lesions of Hebra's prurigo using experimental flea bites (with immediate reaction in 94%, and delayed reaction in 88% of 36 patients) and intradermal injections of flea extracts (with immediate reaction in 97% and delayed reaction in 76% of cases). A positive reactivity passive transfer by serum was demonstrated in 25% of the 36 patients. Precipitin lines in agar double diffusion assay using flea extracts against concentrated patients' sera were found in 76% of the patients studied, and a markedly elevated total IgE (ranging from 1950 and 26000 IU/ml) was found in all patients. A deep dermal perivascular infiltrate of lymphocytes, neutrophils, and eosinophils, plus a vasculitis with granular deposits of IgG, IgM, and C3 in the papillary dermis vessels were found in natural lesions and experimental lesions produced by experimental bites and extracts.[128,129]

## D. Other Arthropod Bites

In addition to local skin reactions, bite-induced anaphylaxis can be induced by several other insects including *Tabanidae* species, tsetse fly, kissing-bugs, and ticks.[130–133] Saliva components may be advantageous for the host or the arthropod. Effective host immune response can be mounted against ticks, which need several days to complete their blood meals.[134] Antibodies, induced in hamsters by *Phlebotomus argentipes* sandfly salivary antigens, may play a role in inhibiting the migration of *Leishmania donovani* to the sandfly esophagus and may cause the death of the insect.[135] On the contrary, *P. papatasi* sandfly (the vector of *L. major*) fed better in the strong $CD4^+$-dependent delayed-type hypersensitivity sites induced by intradermal injections of salivary gland homogenates in mice, taking advantage of host immunity.[136] Hematophagous arthropod saliva may have immunosuppressive activity to hosts as has been reported with *Lutzomia longipalpis* sandflies[137] and ticks,[138] which may result in a dramatic increase in *Leishmania* infectivity.[139] Hemiptera species, particularly *Reduviidae* (kissing-bugs), the *Tripanosoma* vectors, also showed saliva immunosuppressive activity on mice lymphocytes that could aid *Rhodnius prolixus* bugs in successful repeated feedings.[140] Kissing-bugs are a cause of frequent human hypersensitivity in some U.S. areas and may induce severe systemic reactions including fever, dyspnea, syncopes, hypotension, laryngeal and glossal edema, gastrointestinal disorders, and convulsions.[141] Procalin, the salivary 20-kDa major triatomine allergen, has recently been identified, cloned, and recombined, promising to improve diagnosis and immunotherapy.[142]

## E. Furuncular Cutaneous Myasis

Antibodies have been found in rabbits immunized with *Dermatobia hominis* extract or experimentally infested with *D. hominis* larvae. During primary infestation the antibody response is high during the first larval stage and decreases during the second and third larval stages. In previously immunized hosts, the infestation induces a stronger antibody and cellular immune response.[143,144] Lymphocyte blastogenesis in response to *Cordylobia anthropophaga* larval soluble extracts has been demonstrated by tritiated thymidine assay.[145] Immunohistochemical studies from a patient with a *D. hominis* lesion have shown a lymphocytic infiltrate (with some immunoblasts) in the dermis and hipodermis, predominantly helper T cells with a high HLA-DR expression. Electron microscopy shows an intimate association among lymphocytes, eosinophils, and activated fibroblasts.[146]

## F. Scabies

After the fertilized female excavates a sloping burrow in the stratum corneum, the chamber becomes cluttered with abandoned eggshells, fecal pellets, cement that glues the eggs, and dead female mites at the end of the burrow. All of these can act as potential antigens. The antigens responsible for the immune reactions in scabies are mostly undefined, but cross-antigenicity between the *Sarcoptes scabiei* (Ss) mite and house dust mite *Dermatophagoides pteronyssinus*[147] and *D. farinae*[148] have been demonstrated. The recent construction of cDNA libraries from *S. sabiei* var. *hominis* and the isolation of Ss antigen 1 (Ssag1) and antigen 2 (Ssag2) have failed to show any protective efficacy in rabbits after subcutaneous immunization.[149]

When the potential antigens of Ss reach the dermis, humoral and cellular responses are activated. Some patients develop increased serum IgE levels at the time of clinical presentation, and decrease their concentration after treatment.[150] Indirect evidence of IgE role has been found. Intracutaneous skin tests with extracts of adult female mites show a wheal reaction in individuals with scabies, and passive transfer of this reaction by a serum factor (Prausnitz–Künstner test) has been demonstrated. Serum of patients with crusted scabies (CS), a special clinical form of overwhelming infestation with thousands of mites infesting the epidermis, causes histamine release (basophil degranulation test), and patients with CS may have high levels of IgE.[151] One third of all patients have IgE deposits in the vessel walls of the upper dermis, from papules in biopsies containing mites and biopsies of inflammatory papules with no mites. The fluorescence is more pronounced in biopsies containing mites.[152] Significant increases in IgG and IgM serum are found in serum of patients with scabies, and regression of these increases is observed after treatment. IgA levels significantly decrease during infestation,[153] and CS has been described in a patient with acquired selective IgA deficiency.[154] A classical humoral immune response to primary and secondary infestations has been demonstrated.[155] In dogs, the challenge infestations are characterized by resistance to reinfestation and by rapid development of increased IgE and IgG to Ss var. *canis* protein.[156] The role of immune complexes is still unknown. *In vitro,* addition of mite or human unparasitized scale extracts to the serum of patients with scabies does not modify the fixation of $I^{125}$-$C_1$ q as compared with control tubes (serum with physiological saline). This suggests that antigens or substances derived from scabies mite are not involved in the immune complexes present in the serum of the parasitized patients.[157] Indirect evidence of a possible role for immune complexes is demonstrated in some patients with scabies who develop bullous lesions concomitantly with or subsequent to the occurrence of scabietic lesions. At least some of the bullous eruptions occurring in scabies are true bullous pemphigoid.[158] The humoral immune response, although activated during infestation, does not seem to play an essential role in the control of the disease.

The role for cell-mediated immune response is supported by several findings, including a delayed-type hypersensitivity reaction[159] and the presence of papules and nodules, days or weeks after infestation. Patients with primary immunodeficiencies (Bloom's syndrome)[160] or secondary immunodeficiencies (topical steroid therapy),[161] immunosuppressive therapy,[162] acquired immunodeficiency syndrome,[163] and bone marrow transplant[164] have been associated with CS. Although recent studies with monoclonal antibodies for T-cells ($CD2^+$) and T-cell-subset (CD4, CD8) blood counts do not differ from normal, a progressive recruitment of mononuclear cells (especially T cells) in the skin has been demonstrated. The density of the infiltrate is related to the type of lesion, presence of mites or debris, and persistence of the antigenic components in the skin. In young lesions like scabies burrows and papules, $CD4^+$ lymphocytes predominate. Scabies burrows with mites, eggshells, and fecal pellets have $CD4^+$ lymphocytes in the lower third of the malpighian stratum in the proximity of the burrow. Scabies papules have $CD4^+$ lymphocytes in the papillary dermis and those containing mites have a higher infiltration pattern. Tissue cytotoxic/suppressor T lymphocytes ($CD8^+$) are fewer in number so that the ratio of helper to suppressor lymphocytes in tissue is 4:1. Monocyte and B-lymphocyte infiltration is minimal. Nodules are found in 5% of infested patients but often persist for weeks or months despite therapy. Monocytes constitute 30 to

40% of the mononuclear infiltrate of nodules, and the mononuclear infiltration mainly based on $CD4^+$ lymphocytes and $CD14^+$ monocytes is dense and fills the upper dermis, reticular dermis, and adnexal structures.[165] Mites and their eggs were thought to be rarely found in nodular lesions of scabies. However, serial sections from 27 scabietic scrotal papules or nodules revealed mite parts in 22%. This supports the contention that scabietic nodules may result from persisting antigens of mite parts.[166] Persistent antigens can also explain the findings of indeterminate cells ($CD1^+$, $S\text{-}100^+$, $HLA\text{-}DR^+$) in nodular scabies.[167]

Using glycerinated extracts of *Dermatophagoides farinae* and *D. farinae* mixed with *D. pteronyssinus* (Hollister-Stier, Elkhart, IN), we have shown that lymphocytes of patients with vulgar scabies have a significantly high lymphoproliferation test response in comparison with normal controls. Lymphocytes from patients with CS do not respond to these antigens. These data support the hypothesis of a possible failure of the cellular immune response in patients with CS. The role of the cellular immune response seems to be more important than the humoral immune response in the rejection of the scabies mite.[168]

## V. CONCLUSION

The immune response plays different roles in the control of parasitic diseases according to the nature of the parasite. It can be part of a successful response toward the elimination of the parasite (LCL) or, on other occasions, the strong immune response of the host can produce a more serious disease than the parasite itself. Good examples of this latter condition are the hepatic granulomas of *schistosomiasis* and the mucosal granulomas of MCL. In some cases, the ability of the parasite to adapt to the host using several mechanisms to evade the immunological immune response is part of a successful parasitism. When the parasitic infection occurs, the entire immune system is induced to respond. Some parasitic infections can trigger predominantly a humoral immune response (mosquito bites, flea bites); others induce predominantly a cellular immune response (leishmaniasis, schistosomiasis). The final outcome of the infection is the result of a delicate balance of many biological variables between the parasite and the host, but one of the principal biological variables is the host immune response. A feature of recent work has been the elucidation of the regulatory role of the T cells and their clones (Th0, Th1, Th2), cytokine profiles that have provided a valuable framework for investigating the immune regulatory mechanisms associated with host resistance and susceptibility of some parasitic infections (leishmaniasis, schistosomiasis). The future challenge is to convert this scientific knowledge into therapeutic strategies, for the benefit of hundreds of millions still suffering from diseases caused by parasites.

## REFERENCES

1. Castells Rodellas, A., Luelmo, J., and Roca, M., Inmunología de las parasitosis, *Piel*, 8, 80, 1993.
2. Orkin, M., Maibach, H.Y., and Dahl, M.V., Parasitic infections and infestations, in *Dermatology*, Orkin, M., Maibach, H.Y., and Dahl, M.V., Eds., Appleton & Lange, Norwalk, CT, 1991, chap. 18.
3. Kubba, R. and Al-Gindan, Y., Leishmaniasis, in *Dermatologic Clinics*, Vol. 7, Tomecki, K.J., Ed., W.B. Saunders, Philadelphia, 1989, 331.
4. Moll, H., Fuchs, H., Blank, C., and Rollinghoff, M., Langerhans cell transport *Leishmania major* from the infected skin to draining lymph mode for presentation to antigen-specific T cells, *Eur. J. Immunol.*, 23, 1595, 1993.
5. Moll, H., Epidermal Langerhans cells are critical for immunoregulation of cutaneous leishmaniasis, *Immunol. Today*, 14, 383, 1993.
6. Moll, H., Flohe, S., and Rollinghoff, M., Dendritic cells in *Leishmania major*-immune mice harbors persistent parasites and mediate an antigen-specific T cell immune response, *Eur. J. Immunol.*, 25, 693, 1995.

7. Flohe, S., Lang, T., and Moll, H., Major histocompatibility complex class II molecules in Langerhans cells infected with *Leishmania major:* synthesis, stability and subcellular distribution, *Infect. Immun.*, 65, 3444, 1997.
8. Hufler, C., Koch, F., Stanzi, U., Topar, G., Wysocka, M., Trienchieri, G., Enk, A., Steinman, R.M., Romani, N., and Schuler, G., Interleukin-12 is produced by dendritic cells and mediates T helper 1 development as well as interferon-γ production by helper 1 cells, *Eur. J. Immunol.*, 26, 659, 1996.
9. Flohe, S.B., Bauer, C., Flohe, S., and Moll, H., Antigen-pulsed epidermal Langerhans cells protect susceptible mice from infection with the intracellular parasite *Leishmania major, Eur. J. Immunol.*, 28, 3800, 1998.
10. Sato, N., Ahuja, S.K., Quinones, M., Kostecki, V., Reddick, R.L., Melby, P., Kuziel, W.A., and Ahuja, S., CC Chemokine receptor (CCR) 2 is required for Langerhans cell migration and localization of T helper cell type (Th1)-inducing dendritic cells: absence of CCR2 shifts the *Leishmania major*-resistant phenotype to a susceptible state dominated by Th2 cytokines, B cell outgrowth, and sustained neutrophilic inflammation, *J. Exp. Med.*, 192, 205, 2000.
11. Ritter, U. and Korner, H., Divergent expression of inflammatory dermal chemokines in cutaneous leishmaniasis, *Parasite Immunol.*, 24, 295, 2002.
12. Preston, P.M. and Dumonde, D.C., Experimental cutaneous leishmaniasis, protective immunity in subclinical and self-healing infection in the mouse, *Clin. Exp. Immunol.*, 23, 126, 1976.
13. Musumeci, S., Fisher, A., and Pizzarelli, C., Dysproteinemia in kala-azar, *Trans. R. Soc. Trop. Med. Hyg.*, 1, 176, 1977.
14. Mary, C., Ange, S., Dunan, S., Lamouroux, D., and Quilici, M., Characterization of circulating antigen involved in immune complexes in visceral leishmaniasis patients, *Am. J. Trop. Med. Hyg.*, 49, 492, 1993.
15. Azadeh, B., Sells, P.G., Ejeckam, G.C., and Rampling, D., Localized *Leishmania* lymphadenitis: immunohistochemical studies, *Am. J. Clin. Pathol.*, 102, 11, 1994.
16. Laskay, T., Rollinghoff, M., and Solbach, W., Natural killer cells participate in the early defense against *Leishmania major* infection in mice, *Eur. J. Immunol.*, 23, 2237, 1993.
17. Tapia, F.J., Cáceres-Dittmar, G., and Sanchez, M.A., Inadequate epidermal homing leads to tissue damage in human cutaneous leishmaniasis, *Immunol. Today*, 15, 160, 1994.
18. Cáceres-Dittmar, G., Sanchez, M.A., Oriol, O., Kraal, G., and Tapia, F.J., Epidermal compromise in American cutaneous leishmaniasis, *J. Invest. Dermatol.*, 99, 95s, 1992.
19. Lima, H.C., Vasconcelos, A.W., David, J.R., and Lerner, E.A., American cutaneous leishmaniasis: *in situ* characterization of the cellular immune response with time, *Am. J. Trop. Med. Hyg.*, 50, 743, 1994.
20. Belkaid, Y., Piccirillo, C.A., Mendez, S., Shevach, E.M., and Sacks, D., $CD4^+$ $25^+$ regulatory T cells control *Leishmania major* persistence and immunity, *Nature*, 420, 502, 2000.
21. Sypek, J.P., Chung, C.L., Mayor, S.E., Subramanyan, J.M., Goldman, S.J., Sierbuth, D.S., Wolf, S.F., and Schaub, R.G., Resolution of cutaneous leishmaniasis: interleukin 12 initiates a protective T helper type 1 immune responses, *J. Exp. Med.,* 177, 1797, 1993.
22. Powrie, F., Correa-Oliveira, R., Mauze, S., and Coffman, R., Regulatory interaction between $CD45RB^{high}$ and $CD45RB^{low}$ $CD4^+$ T cells are important for the balance between protective and pathogenic cell-mediated immunity, *J. Exp. Med.*, 179, 589, 1994.
23. Heinzel, F.P., Schoenhaut, D.S., Rerko, R.M., Rosser, L.E., and Gately, M.K., Recombinant interleukin 12 cures mice infected with *Leishmania major, J. Exp. Med.*, 177, 1505, 1993.
24. Rocha, P.N., Almeida, R.P., Bacellar, O., De Jesus, A.R., Filho, A.C., Barral, A., Coffman, R.L., and Carvalho, E.M., Down-regulation of Th1 type of response in early human American cutaneous leishmaniasis, *J. Infect. Dis.*, 180, 1731, 1999.
25. Guler, M.L., Gorham, J.D., Hsieh, C.S, Mackey, A.J., Steen, R.G., Dietrich, W.F., and Murphy, K.M., Genetic susceptibility to *Leishmania:* IL12 responsiveness in Th1 cell development, *Science,* 271, 984, 1996.
26. Handman, E., Leishmaniasis: current status of vaccine development, *Clin. Microbiol. Rev.*, 14, 229, 2001.
27. Stacey, K.J. and Blackwell, J.M., Immunostimulatory DNA as an adjuvant in vaccination against *Leishmania major, Infect. Immun.*, 67, 3719, 1999.
28. Stacey, K.J., Sweet, M.J., and Hume, D.A., Macrophages ingest and are activated by bacterial DNA, *J. Immunol.,* 157, 2116, 1996.

29. Walker, P.S., Scharton-Kersten, T., Kriegg, A.M., Love-Homan, L., Rowton, E.D., Udey, M.C., and Vogel, J.C., Immunostimulatory oligodeoxynucleotides promote protective immunity and provide systemic therapy for leishmaniasis via IL-12 and IFN-gamma–dependent mechanisms, *Proc. Natl. Acad. Sci. U.S.A.,* 96, 6970, 1999.
30. Von Stebut, E., Belkaid, Y., Nguyen, B., Wilson, M., Sacks, D.L., and Udey, M., Skin-derived macrophages from *Leishmania major*–susceptible mice exhibit interleukin-12-and interferon-$\gamma$ independent nitric oxide production and parasite killing after treatment with immunostimulatory DNA, *J. Invest. Dermatol.,* 119, 621, 2002.
31. Gounni, A.S., Lamkhioued, B., Ochiai, K., Tanaka, Y., Delaporte, E., Capron, A., Kinet, J.P., and Capron, M., High-affinity IgE receptor on eosinophils is involved in defence against parasites, *Nature,* 367, 183, 1994.
32. Rezende, S.A., Miranda, T.C., Ferreira, M.G., and Goes, A.M., *In vitro* granuloma modulation induced by immune complexes in human *Schistosomiasis mansoni, Braz. J. Med. Biol. Res.,* 26, 207, 1993.
33. Williams, M.E., Montenegro, S., Domingues, A.L., Wynn, T.A., Teixeira, K., Mahanty, S., Coutinho, A., and Sher, A., Leukocytes of patients with *Schistosoma mansoni* respond with a Th2 pattern of cytokine production to mitogen or egg antigens but with a Th0 pattern to worm antigens, *J. Infect. Dis.,* 170, 946, 1993.
34. Vella, A.T. and Pearce, E.J., Schistosoma mansoni egg-primed Th0 and Th2 cells: failure to downregulate IFN-gamma production following *in vitro* culture, *Scan. J. Immunol.,* 39, 12, 1994.
35. Wynn, T A., Eltoum, I., Cheever, A.W., Lewis, F.A., Gause, W.C., and Sher, A., Analysis of cytokine mRNA expression during primary granuloma formation induced by eggs of *Schistosoma mansoni, J. Immunol.,* 151, 1430, 1993.
36. Metwali, A., Elliott, D., Blum, A.M., and Weinstock, J.V., Granuloma eosinophils enhance IL-5 production by lymphocytes from mice infected with *Schistosoma mansoni, J. Immunol.,* 151, 7048, 1993.
37. Flores-Villanueva, P.O., Harris, T.S., Ricklan, D.E., and Stadecker, M.J., Macrophages from schistosomal egg granulomas induce unresponsiveness in specific cloned Th1 lymphocytes *in vitro* and downregulate schistosomal granulomatous disease *in vivo, J. Immunol.,* 152, 1847, 1994.
38. Oswald, Y.P., Caspar, P., Jankovic, D., Wynn, T.A., Pearce, E.J., and Sher, A., IL-12 inhibits Th2 cytokine responses induced by eggs of *Schistosoma mansoni, J. Immunol.,* 153, 1707, 1994.
39. Flores-Villanueva, P.O., Chikunguwo, S.M., Harris, T.S., and Stadecjker, M.J., Role of IL-10 on antigen presenting cell function for schistosomal egg-specific monoclonal T helper cell responses *in vitro* and *in vivo, J. Immunol.,* 151, 3192, 1993.
40. Lukacs, N.W., Kunkel, S.L., Strieter, R.M., Warmington, K., and Chensue, S.W., The role of macrophage inflammatory protein 1 alpha in *Schistosoma mansoni* egg-induced granulomatous inflammation, *J. Exp. Med.,* 177, 1551, 1993.
41. Lukacs, N.W., Chensue, S.W., Strieter, R.M., Warmington, K., and Kunkel, S.L., Inflammatory granuloma formation mediated by TNF-alpha inducible intercellular adhesion molecule-1, *J. Immunol.,* 152, 5883, 1994.
42. Secor, W.E., dos-Reis, M.G., Ramos, E.A., Matos, E.P., Reis, E.A., do-Carmo, T.M., and Harn, D.A., Jr., Soluble intercellular adhesion molecules in human schistosomiasis: correlations with disease severity and decreased responsiveness to egg antigens, *Infect. Immun.,* 62, 2695, 1994.
43. Garraud, O., Nkenfou, C., Bradley, J.E., Perler, FB., and Nutman, T.B., Identification of recombinant filarial proteins capable of inducing polyclonal and antigen-specific IgE and IgG4 antibodies, *J. Immunol.*, 155, 1316, 1995.
44. Sisley, B.M., Mackenzie, C.D., Steward, M.W., Williams, J.F., O'Day, J., Luty, A.J., Braga, M., and el Sheikh, H., Associations between clinical disease, circulating antibodies and C1q-binding immune complexes in human onchocerciasis, *Parasite Immunol.*, 9, 447, 1987.
45. Gutierrez-Pena, E.J., Knab, J., and Buttner, D.W., Immunoelectron microscopic evidence for release of eosinophil granule matrix protein onto microfilariae of *Onchocerca volvulus* in the skin after exposure to amocarzine, *Parasitol. Res.*, 84, 607, 1998.
46. Rougemont, A., Boisson-Pontal, M.E., Pontal, P.G., Gridel, F., and Sangare, S., Tuberculin skin tests and B.C.G. vaccination in hyperendemic area of onchocerciasis, *Lancet*, 1, 309, 1977.
47. Stewart, G.R., Boussinesq, M., Coulson, T., Elson, L., Nutman, T., and Bradley, J.E., Onchocerciasis modulates the immune response to mycobacterial antigens, *Clin. Exp. Immunol.*, 117, 517, 1999.

48. Brattig, N.W., Tischendorf, F.W., Albiez, E.J., Buttner, D.W., and Berger, J., Distribution pattern of peripheral lymphocyte subsets in localized and generalized form of onchocerciasis, *Clin. Immunol. Immunopathol.*, 44, 149, 1987.
49. Satoguina, J., Mempel, M., Larbi, J., Badusche, M., Loliger, C., Adjei, O., Gachelin, G., Fleischer, B., and Hoerauf, A., Antigen-specific T regulatory-1 cells are associated with immunosuppression in a chronic helminth infection (onchocerciasis), *Microbes Infect.*, 4, 1291, 2002.
50. Harrison, R.A. and Bianco, A.E., DNA immunization with *Onchocerca volvulus* genes, Ov-tmy-1 and OvB20: serological and parasitological outcomes following intramuscular or GeneGun delivery in a mouse model of onchocerciasis, *Parasite Immunol.*, 22, 249, 2000.
51. Ungeheuer, M., Elissa, N., Morelli, A., Georges, A.J., Deloron, P., Debre, P., Bain, O., and Millet, P., Cellular responses to *Loa loa* experimental infection in mandrills (*Mandrillus sphinx*) vaccinated with irradiated infective larvae, *Parasite Immunol.*, 22, 173, 2000.
52. Nutman, T.B., Miller, K.D., Mulligan, M., and Ottesen, E.A., *Loa loa* infection in temporary residents of endemic regions: recognition of a hyperresponsive syndrome with characteristic clinical manifestations, *J. Infect. Dis.*, 154, 10, 1986.
53. Yates, J.A., Higashi, G.I., Lowichik, A., Orihel, T.C., Lowrie, R.C., Jr., and Eberhard, M.L., Activation of the alternative complement pathway in normal human serum by *Loa loa* and *Brugia malayi* infective stage larvae, *Acta Trop.*, 42, 157, 1985.
54. Egwang, T.G., Dupont, A., Leclerc, A., Akue, J.P., and Pinder, M., Differential recognition of *Loa loa* antigens by sera of human subjects from a loiasis endemic zone, *Am. J. Trop. Med. Hyg.*, 41, 664, 1989.
55. Baize, S., Wahl, G., Soboslay, P.T., Egwang, T.G., and Georges, A.J., T helper responsiveness in human *Loa loa* infection; defective specific proliferation and cytokine production by $CD4^+$ T cells from microfilaraemic subjects compared with amicrofilaraemics, *Clin. Exp. Immunol.*, 108, 272, 1997.
56. Winkler, S., Willheim, M., Baier, K., Aichelburg, A., Kremsner, P.G., and Graninger, W., Increased frequency of Th2-type cytokine-producing T cells in microfilaremic loiasis, *Am. J. Trop. Med. Hyg.*, 60, 680, 1999.
57. Mellanby, K., Man's reaction to mosquito bites, *Nature*, 158, 554, 1946.
58. McKiel, J.A. and West, A.S., Nature and causation of insect bite reactions, *Pediatr. Clin. North Am.*, 8, 795, 1961.
59. Benjamini, E., Feingold, B.F., and Kartman, L., Skin reactivity in guinea pigs sensitized to flea bites: the sequence of reactions, *Proc. Soc. Exp. Biol. Med.*, 108, 700, 1961.
60. Sansom, J.E., Reynolds, N.J., and Peachey, R.D., Delayed reaction to bed bug bites, *Arch. Dermatol.*, 128, 272, 1992.
61. Feingold, B.F., Benjamini, E., and Michaeli, D., The allergic responses to insect bites, *Annu. Rev. Entomol.*, 13, 137, 1968.
62. Peng, Z., Li, H., and Simons, F.E.R., Immunoblot analysis of salivary allergens in 10 mosquito species with worldwide distribution and the human IgE responses to these allergens, *J. Allergy Clin. Immunol.*, 101, 498, 1998. Erratum, *J. Allergy Clin. Immunol.*, 101, 746, 1998.
63. Killby, V.A. and Silverman, P.H., Hypersensitive reactions in man to specific mosquito bites, *Am. J. Trop. Med. Hyg.*, 16, 374, 1967.
64. Penneys, N.S., Nayar, J.K., Bernstein, H., and Knight, J.W., Chronic pruritic eruption in patients with acquired immunodeficiency syndrome associated with increased antibody titers to mosquito salivary gland antigens, *J. Am. Acad. Dermatol.*, 21, 421, 1989.
65. Smith, K.J., Skelton, H.G., III, Vogel, P., Yeager, J., Baxter, D., and Wagner, K.F., Exaggerated insect bite reactions in patients positive for HIV, *J. Am. Acad. Dermatol.*, 29, 269, 1993.
66. Heng, M.C., Allen, S.G., Kim, A., and Lieberman, J., Alpha-1 antitrypsin deficiency in a patient with widespread prurigo nodularis, *Australas J. Dermatol.*, 32, 151, 1991.
67. Shibasaki, M., Sumazaki, R., and Takita, H., Hypersensitive reactions to mosquito bites in congenital agammaglobulinemia, *Ann. Allergy,* 56, 81, 1986.
68. Weed, R.I., Exaggerated delayed hypersensitivity to mosquito bites in chronic lymphocytic leukemia, *Blood*, 26(3), 257, 1965.
69. Tokura, Y., Ishihara, S., Tagawa, S., Seo, N., Ohshima, K., and Takigawa, M., Hypersensitivity to mosquito bites as the primary clinical manifestation of a juvenile type of Epstein Barr virus associated natural killer cell leukemia/lymphoma, *J. Am. Acad. Dermatol.*, 45, 569, 2001.

70. Reunala, T., Brummer-Korvenkontio, H., Lapalainen, P., Rasanen, L., and Palosuo, Y., Immunology and treatment of mosquito bites, *Clin. Exp. Allergy*, 20, 19, 1990.
71. Simons, F.E.R. and Peng, Z.P., Skeeter syndrome, *J. Allergy Clin. Immunol.*, 104, 705, 1999.
72. Howard, R. and Frieden, I., Papular urticaria in children, *Pediatr. Dermatol.*, 13, 246, 1996.
73. Gaig, P., Garcia-Ortega, P., Enrique, E., Benet, A., Bartolome, B., and Palacios, R., Serum sickness like syndrome due to mosquito bite, *J. Invest. Allergol. Clin. Immunol.*, 9, 190, 1999.
74. Gluck, J.C. and Pacin, M.P., Asthma from mosquito bites: a case report, *Ann. Allergy*, 56, 492, 1986.
75. McCormack, D.R., Salata, K.F., Hershey, J.N., Carpenter, G.B., and Engler, R.J., Mosquito bite anaphylaxis: immunotherapy with whole body extracts, *Ann. Allergy Asthma Immunol.*, 74, 39, 1995.
76. Galindo, P.A., Gomez, E., Borja, J., Feo, F., Garcia, R., Lombardero, M., and Barber, D., Mosquito bite hypersensitivity, *Allergol. Immunopathol.*, 26, 251, 1998.
77. Hassoun, S., Drouet, M., and Sabbah, A., Anaphylaxis caused by a mosquito: 2 case reports. *Allerg. Immunol.* (Paris), 31, 285, 1999.
78. Diven, D.G., Newton, R.C., and Ramsey, K.M., Heightened cutaneous reactions to mosquito bites in patients with acquired immunodeficiency syndrome receiving zidovudine, *Arch. Intern. Med.*, 148, 2296, 1988.
79. Davis, M.D.P., Perniciaro, C., Dahl, P.R., Randle, H.W., McEvoy, M.T., and Leiferman, K.M., Exaggerated arthropod-bites lesions in patients with chronic lymphocytic leukemia: a clinical, histopathologic and immunopathologic study of eight patients, *J. Am. Acad. Dermatol.*, 39, 27, 1998.
80. Tokura, Y., Tamura, Y., Takigawa, M., Koide, M., Satoh, T., Sakamoto, T., and Horiguchi, D., Severe hypersensitivity to mosquito bites associated with natural killer cell lymphocytosis, *Arch. Dermatol.*, 126, 362, 1990.
81. Hudson, B.W., Feingold, B.F., and Kartman, L., Allergy to flea bites. I. Experimental induction of flea-bite sensitivity in guinea pigs, *Exp. Parasitol.*, 9, 18, 1960.
82. Allen, J.R., Some Properties of Oral Secretion of Mosquitoes, doctoral thesis, Queen's University, Kingston, Ontario, Canada, 1964.
83. Penneys, N.S., Nayar, J.K., Bernstein, H., Knight, J.W., and Leonardi, C., Mosquito salivary gland antigens identified by circulating human antibodies, *Arch. Dermatol.*, 125, 219, 1989.
84. Brummer-Korvenkontio, H., Lappalainen, P., Reunala, T., and Palosuo T., Clinical aspects of allergic disease. Detection of mosquito saliva-specific IgE and IgG4 antibodies by immunoblotting. *J. Allergy Clin. Immunol.*, 93, 551, 1994.
85. Peng, Z. and Simons, F.E.R., Comparison of proteins, IgE and IgG binding antigens, and skin reactivity in commercial and laboratory-made mosquito extracts, *Ann. Allergy Asthma Immunol.*, 77, 371, 1996.
86. Peng, Z., Xu, W., James, A.A., Lam H, Sun, D., Cheng, L., and Simons, F.E., Expression, purification, characterization and clinical relevance of rAed a 1-a 68-kDa recombinant mosquito *Aedes aegypti* salivary allergen. *Int. Immunol.*, 13, 1445, 2001.
87. Reunala, T., Brummer-Korvenkontio, H., Palosuo, K., Miyanij, M., and Ruiz-Maldonado, R., Frequent occurrence of IgE and IgG4 antibodies against saliva of *Aedes communis* and *Aedes aegypti* mosquitoes in children, *Int. Arch. Allergy Immunol.*, 104, 366, 1994.
88. Brummer-Korvenkontio, H., Palosuo, T., Francois, G., and Reunala, T., Characterization of *Aedes communis, Aedes aegypti* and *Anopheles stephensi* mosquito saliva antigens by immunoblotting, *Int. Arch. Allergy Immunol.*, 112, 169, 1997.
89. Peng, Z. and Simons, F.E.R., Cross-reactivity of skin and serum specific IgE responses and allergen analysis for three mosquito species with worldwide distribution, *J. Allergy Clin. Immunol.*, 100, 192, 1997.
90. Docena, G.H., Benitez, P., Campos, R.E., Macia, A., Fernandez, R., and Fossati, C.A., Detection of allergens in *Aedes albifasciatus* mosquito (Diptera: Culicidae) extracts by immunological methods, *J. Invest. Allergol. Clin. Immunol.*, 9, 165, 1999.
91. Jeon, S.-H., Park, J.W., and Lee, B.H., Characterization of human IgE and mouse IgG1 responses to allergens in three mosquito species by immunoblotting and ELISA, *Int. Arch. Allergy Immunol.*, 126, 206, 2001.
92. Malafronte, Rdos, Calvo, E., James, A., and Marinotti, O., The major salivary gland antigens of Culex quinquefasciatus are D7-related proteins, *Insect. Biochem. Mol. Biol.*, 33, 63, 2003.
93. Racioppi, J., and Spielman, A., Secretory proteins from the salivary glands of adult Aedes aegypti mosquitoes, *Insect. Biochem.*, 17, 503, 1987.

94. Peng, Z., Lam, H., Xu, W., Cheng, L., Chen, Y.L., and Simons, F.E.R, Characterization and clinical relevance of two recombinant mosquito *Aedes aegypti* salivary allergens, rAed a 1 and rAed a 2, *J. Allergy Clin. Immunol.*, 101, S1, 32, 1998.
95. Xu, W., Peng, Z., and Simonns, F.E.R., Isolation of a cDNA encoding a 30 KD binding protein of mosquito *Aedes aegypti* saliva, *J. Allergy Clin. Immunol.*, 101, S203, 1998.
96. Wang, H., Mao, X., Simons, F.E.R., and Peng Z., Induction of IgE responses using a recombinant mosquito salivary allergen rAed a 2 without adjuvant in mice, *Int. Arch. Allergy Immunol.*, 120, 135, 1999.
97. Chen, Y.L., Simons, F.E.R., and Peng, Z., A mouse model of mosquito allergy for study of antigen-specific IgE and IgG subclass responses, lymphocyte proliferation and IL-4 and IFN-γ production, *Int. Arch. Allergy. Immunol.*, 116, 269, 1998.
98. Ohtsuka, E., Kawai, S., Ichikawa, T., Nojima, H., Kitagawa, K., Shirai, Y., and Kamimura, K., Roles of mast cells and histamine in mosquito bite induced allergic itch associated responses in mice, *Jpn. J. Pharmacol.*, 86, 97, 2001.
99. Peng, Z., Yang, M., and Simons, F.E.R., Immunologic mechanisms in mosquito allergy: correlation of skin reactions with specific IgE and IgG antibodies and lymphocyte proliferation response to mosquito antigens, *Ann. Allergy Asthma. Immunol.*, 77, 238, 1996.
100. Ohtaki, N. and Oka, K., A quantitative study of specific immunoglobulins to mosquito salivary gland antigen in hypersensitive and common types of mosquito bite reaction, *J. Dermatol.*, 21, 639, 1994.
101. Mathews, G.V., Sidjanski, S., and Vanderberg, J.P., Inhibition of mosquito salivary gland apyrase activity by antibodies produced in mice immunized by bites of *Anopheles stephensi* mosquitoes, *Am. J. Trop. Med. Hyg.*, 55, 417, 1996.
102. Reunala, T., Brummer-Korvenkontio, H., Rasanen, L., Francois, G., and Palosuo, T., Passive transfer of cutaneous mosquito-bite hypersensitivity by IgE anti-saliva antibodies, *J. Allergy Clin. Immunol.*, 94, 902, 1994.
103. Oka, K., Correlation of *Aedes albopictus* bite reaction with IgE antibody assay and lymphocyte transformation test to mosquito salivary antigens, *J. Dermatol.*, 16, 341, 1989.
104. Allen, J.R., Passive transfer between experimental animals of hypersensitivity to *Aedes aegypti* bites, *Exp. Parasitol.*, 19, 132, 1966.
105. Reunala, T., Brummer-Korvenkontio, H., and Palosuo, T., Are we really allergic to mosquito bites? *Ann. Med.*, 26, 301, 1994.
106. Frew, A.J. and Kay, A.B., Eosinophils and T-lymphocytes in late-phase allergic reactions, *J. Allergy Clin. Immunol.*, 85, 533, 1990.
107. Owhashi, M., Harada, M., Suguri, S., Ohmae, H., and Ishii, A., The role of saliva of *Anopheles stephensi* in inflammatory response: identification of a high molecular weight neutrophil chemotactic factor, *Parasitol. Res.*, 87, 376, 2001.
108. Agarwal, M.K., Chaudhry, S., Jhamb, S., Gaur, S.N., Chauhan, U.P., and Agarwal, H.C., Etiologic significance of mosquito (*Anopheles stephensi*) in respiratory allergy in India, *Ann. Allergy*, 67, 598, 1991.
109. Palosuo, T., Brummer-Korvenkontio, H., Lappalainen, P., Rasanen, L., Makinen-Kiljunen, S., and Reunala, L., Humoral and cell mediated immune response to mosquito antigens in man, *Clin. Exp. Allergy*, 20, 4s, 1990.
110. Fadok, V.A. and Greiner, E.C., Equine insect hypersensitivity: skin test and biopsy results correlated with clinical data, *Equine Vet. J.*, 22, 236, 1990.
111. Kurotaki, T., Narayama, K., Oyamada, T., Yoshikawa, H, and Yoshikawa, T., Immunopathological study on equine insect hypersensitivity ("kasen") in Japan, *J. Comp. Pathol.*, 110, 145, 1994.
112. Foster, A.P., Lees, P., and Cunningham, F.M., Platelet activating factor mimics antigen induced cutaneous inflammatory responses in sweet itch horses, *Vet. Immunol. Immunopathol.*, 44, 115, 1995.
113. Marti, E., Urwyler, A., Neuenschwander, M., Eicher, R., Meier, D., de Weck, A.L., Gerber, H., Lasary, S., and Dahinden, C.A., Sulfidoleukotriene generation from peripheral blood leukocytes of horses affected with insect bite dermal hypersensitivity, *Vet. Immunol. Immunopathol.*, 71, 307, 1999.
114. Van der Haegen, A., Griot-Wenk, M., Velle, M., Busato, A., and von Tscharner, C., Immunoglobulin-E bearing cells in skin biopsies of horses with insect bite hypersensitivity, *Equine Vet. J.*, 33, 699, 2001.
115. Wilson, A.D., Harwood, L.J., Bjornsdottir, S., Mari, E., and Day, M.J., Detection of IgG and IgE serum antibodies to *Culicoides* salivary gland antigens in horses with insect dermal hypersensitivity (sweet itch), *Equine Vet. J.*, 33, 707, 2001.

116. McKelvie, J., Foster, A.P., Cunningham, F.M., and Hamblin, S.A., Characterization of lymphocyte subpopulations in the skin and circulation of horses with sweet itch. (*Culicoides* hypersensitivity), *Equine Vet. J.*, 31, 466, 1999.
117. Benarafa, C., Collins, M.E., Hamblin, A.S., and Cunningham, F.M., Role of the chemokine eotaxin in the pathogenesis of equine sweet itch, *Vet. Rec.*, 151, 691, 2002.
118. Yeruham, I., Braverman, Y., and Orgad, U., Field observations in Israel on hypersensitivity in cattle, sheep and donkeys caused by *Culicoides, Aust. Vet. J.,* 70, 348, 1993.
119. Simons, F.E.R. and Peng, Z., Mosquito allergy: recombinant mosquito salivary antigens for new diagnostic tests, *Int. Arch. Allergy Immunol.*, 124, 403, 2001.
120. Peng, Z. and Simons, F.E.R., A prospective study of naturally acquired sensitization and subsequent desensitization to mosquito bites and concurrent antibody responses, *J. Allergy Clin. Immunol.*, 101, 284, 1998.
121. Sousa, C.A.. Fleas, flea allergy, and flea control: a review. *Dermatol. Online J.*, 3, 7, 1997.
122. Beck, W. and Clark, H.H., Differential diagnosis of medically relevant flea species and their significance in dermatology, *Hautarzt,* 48, 714, 1997.
123. Benjamini, E., Feingold, B.F., and Kartman, L., Antigenic property of the oral secretion of fleas, *Nature*, 188, 959, 1960.
124. Lee, S.E., Johnstone, I.P., Lee, R.P., and Opdebeeck, J.P., Putative salivary allergens of the cat flea, *Ctenocephalides felis felis, Vet. Immunol. Immunopathol.,* 69, 229, 1999.
125. McKeon, S.E. and Opdebeeck, J.P., IgG and IgE antibodies against antigens of the cat flea, *Ctenocephalides felis felis* in sera of allergic and non-allergic dogs, *Int. J. Parasitol.,* 24, 259, 1994.
126. Greene, W.K., Carnegie, R.L., Shaw, S.E., Thompson, R.C., and Penhale, W.J., Characterization of allergens of the cat flea, *Ctenocephalides felis:* detection and frequency of IgE antibodies in canine sera, *Parasite Immunol.,* 15, 69, 1993.
127. Von Ruedorffer, U., Fisch, R., Peel, J., Roosje, P., Griot-Wenk, M., and Welle, M., Flea bite hypersensitivity: new aspects on the involvement of mast cells, *Vet. J.*, 165, 149, 2003.
128. Croce, J., Hypersensitivity to flea bites, in *Adv. Allergy Appl. Immunol.*, Oehling, A., Glazer, Y., Mathov, E., and Arbesman, C., Eds., Pergamon Press, Oxford, 1980, 449.
129. De Almeida, F.A. and Croce, J., Estudo da hipersensibilidade dos doentes com prurigo de Hebra a picada de pulga, *Med. Cutan. Ibero Lat. Am.*, 18, 132, 1990.
130. Rohr, A.S., Marshall, N.A., and Saxon, A., Successful immunotherapy for *Triatoma protracta*-induced anaphylaxis, *J. Allergy Clin. Immunol.*, 73, 369, 1984.
131. Stevens, W.J., van den Abbeele, J., and Bridts, C.H., Anaphylactic reaction after bites by *Glossina morsitans* (tsetse fly) in a laboratory worker, *J. Allergy Clin. Immunol.*, 98, 700, 1996.
132. Hemmer, W., Focke, M., Vieluf, D., Berg-Drewniok, B., Gotz, M., and Jarisch, R., Anaphylaxis induced by horsefly bites: identification of a 69 kd IgE-binding salivary gland protein from *Chrysops* spp. (Diptera Tabanidae) by Western blot analysis, *J. Allergy Clin. Immunol.*, 101, 134, 1998.
133. Lavaud, F., Bouchet, F., Mertes, P.M., and Kochman, S., Allergy to the bites of blood sucking insects: clinical manifestations, *Allerg. Immunol.* (Paris), 31, 311, 1999.
134. Wikel, S.K., Host immunity to ticks, *Annu. Rev. Entomol.,* 41, 1, 1996.
135. Ghosh, K.N. and Mukhopadhyay, J., The effect of anti-sandfly saliva antibodies on *Phlebotomus argentipes* and *Leishmania donovani, Int. J. Parasitol.*, 28, 275, 1998.
136. Belkaid, Y., Valenzuela, J.G., Kamhawi, S., Rowton, E, Sacks, D.L., and Ribeiro, J.M., Delayed type hypersensitivity to *Phlebotomus papatasi* sand fly bite: an adaptive response induced by the fly? *Proc. Natl. Acad. Sci. U.S.A.*, 97, 6704, 2000.
137. Soares, M.B., Titus, R.G., Shoemaker, C.B., David J.R., and Bozza, M., The vasoactive peptide maxadilan from sand fly saliva inhibits TNF-$\alpha$ and induced IL-6 by mouse macrophages through interaction with the pituitary adenylate cyclase-activating polypeptide (PACAP) receptor, *J. Immunol.*, 160, 1811, 1998.
138. Wikel, S.K., Ramachandra, R.N., and Bergman, D.K., Tick induced modulation of the host immune response, *Int. J. Parasitol.,* 24, 59, 1994.
139. Belkaid, Y., Kamhawi, S., Modi, G., Valenzuela, J., Noben-Trauth, N., Rowton, E., Ribeiro, J., and Sacks, D.L., Development of a natural model of cutaneous leishmaniasis: powerful effects of vector saliva and saliva preexposure on the long-term outcome of *Leishmania major* infection in the mouse ear dermis, *J. Exp. Med.*, 188, 1941, 1998.

140. Kalvachova, P., Hribalova, V., Kodym, P., and Volf, P., Modulation of murine lymphocyte responsiveness by the saliva of *Rhodnius prolixus* (Hemiptera: Reduviidae), *J. Med. Entomol.,* 36, 341, 1999.
141. Marshall, N., Liebhaber, Z., Dyer, A., and Saxon, A., The prevalence of allergic sensitization to *Triatoma protracta* (Heteroptera: Reduviidae) in a Southern California, USA, community, *J. Med. Entomol.,* 23, 117, 1986.
142. Paddock, C.D., McKerrow, J.H., Hansell, E., Foreman, K.W., Hsieh, I., and Marshall, N., Identification, cloning and recombinant expression of procalin, a major triatomine allergen, *J. Immunol.*, 167, 2694, 2001.
143. De Lello, E. and Boulard, C., Rabbit antibody responses to experimental infestation with *Dermatobia hominis, Med. Vet. Entomol.*, 4, 303, 1990.
144. De Lello, E. and Peracoli, M.T., Cell-mediated and humoral immune responses in immunized and/or *Dermatobia hominis* infested rabbits, *Vet. Parasitol.,* 47, 129, 1993.
145. Ockenhouse, C.F., Samlaska, C.P., Benson, P.M., Roberts, L.W., Eliasson, A., and Malane, S., *Cutaneous myasis* caused by the African tumbu fly (Cordylobia Anthropophaga), *Arch. Dermatol.*, 126, 199, 1990.
146. Grogan, T.M., Payne, C.M., Payne, T.B., Spier, C., Cromey, D.W., Rangel, C., and Richter, L., Cutaneous myasis: immunohistologic and ultrastructural morphometric features of a human botfly lesion, *Am. J. Dermatopathol.*, 9, 232, 1987.
147. Arlian, L.G., Vyszenski-Moher, D.L., Ahmed, S.G., and Estes, S.A., Cross-antigenicity between the scabies mite, *Sarcoptes scabiei,* and the house dust mite, *Dermatophagoides pteronyssinus, J. Invest. Dermatol.*, 96, 349, 1991.
148. Falk, E.S., Dale, S., Bolle, R., and Haneberg, B., Antigens common to scabies and house dust mites, *Allergy*, 36, 233, 1981.
149. Harumal, P., Morgan, M., Walton, S.F., Holt, D., Rode, J., Arlian, L.G., Currie, B.J., and Kemp, D.J., Identification of a homologue of a house dust mite allergen in a cDNA library from *Sarcoptes scabiei* var. hominis and evaluation of its vaccine potential in a rabbit/*S. scabiei* var. canis model, *Am. J. Trop. Med. Hyg.,* 68, 54, 2003.
150. Falk, E.S., Serum IgE before and after treatment for scabies, *Allergy*, 36, 167, 1981.
151. Dahl, M.V., The immunology of scabies, *Ann. Allergy,* 51, 560, 1983.
152. Frentz, G., Veien, N.K., and Eriksen, K., Immunofluorescence studies in scabies, *J. Cutaneous Pathol.*, 4, 191, 1977.
153. Hancock, B.M. and Ward, M., Serum immunoglobulin in scabies, *J. Invest. Dermatol.*, 63, 482, 1974.
154. Schindo, K., Kono, T., Kitajima, J., and Hamada, T., Crusted scabies in acquire selective IgA deficiency, *Acta Derm. Venereol.,* 71, 250, 1991.
155. Arlian, L.G., Morgan, M.S., Vyszenski-Moher, D.L., and Stemmer, B.L., *Sarcoptes scabiei*: the circulating antibody response and induced immunity to scabies, *Exp. Parasitol.*, 78, 37, 1994.
156. Arlian, L.G. and Morgan, M.S., Serum antibody to *Sarcoptes scabiei* and house dust mite prior to during infestation with *S. scabiei, Vet. Parasitol.*, 90, 315, 2000.
157. Van Neste, D. and Salmon, J., Immune complexes in scabies, *Dermatologica*, 160, 131, 1980.
158. Konishi, N., Suzuki, K., Tokura, Y., Hashimoto, T., and Takigawa, M., Bullous eruption associated with scabies: evidence for scabietic induction of true bullous pemphigoid, *Acta Derm. Venereol.*, 80, 281, 2000.
159. Mellanby, K., *Scabies,* 2nd ed., E.W. Classey, London, 1972.
160. Dick, G., Burgdorf, W., and Gentry, W., Norwegian scabies in Bloom's syndrome, *Arch. Dermatol.*, 115, 212, 1979.
161. Clayton, R. and Farrow, S., Norwegian scabies following topical steroid therapy, *Postgrad. Med. J.*, 51, 657, 1975.
162. Ting, H.C. and Wang, F., Scabies and systemic lupus erythematous, *Int. J. Dermatol.,* 22, 473, 1983.
163. Donabedian, H. and Khazan, U., Norwegian scabies in a patient with AIDS, *Clin. Infect. Dis.*, 14, 162, 1992.
164. Barnes, L., McCallister, R.E., and Lucky, A.W., Crusted (Norwegian) scabies. Occurrence in a child undergoing a bone marrow transplant, *Arch. Dermatol.*, 123, 95, 1987.
165. Cabrera, R., Agar, A., and Dahl, M. V., The immunology of scabies, *Semin. Dermatol.,* 12, 15, 1993.
166. Liu, H.N., Sheu, W.J., and Chu, T.L., Scabietic nodules: a dermatopathologic and immunofluorescent study, *J. Cutaneous Pathol.*, 19, 124, 1992.

167. Hashimoto, K., Fujiwara, K., Punwaney, J., DiGregorio, F., Bostrom, P., El-Hoshy, K., Aronson, P., and Schoenfeld, R.J., Post-scabietic nodules: a lymphohistiocytic reaction rich in indeterminate cells, *J. Dermatol.*, 27, 181, 2000.
168. Cabrera, R.A., Agar, A., Wegmann, M., Zapata, S., and Sepulveda, C., Lymphoproliferative response of patients with vulgar scabies and crusted scabies, *Proc. 9th International Congress of Immunology*, 1995, 129.

# 36 Tumors of Skin-Homing Lymphocytes

*Rein Willemze*

## CONTENTS



## I. INTRODUCTION

Previous chapters have highlighted the many cell types that play an active role within the skin immune system. Tumors of immunocompetent cells therefore include an enormous variety of benign and malignant neoplasms originating from lymphocytes, Langerhans and related skin dendritic cells, endothelial cells, epithelial cells, and so on (Table 36.1). The skin immune system plays a crucial role in the development and progression of these tumors by the local production of tumor growth-promoting factors, and in some tumors by providing an effective antitumor response. The importance of an effective host immune response is illustrated by the increased incidence and the more aggressive clinical behavior of epithelial tumors and cutaneous malignant

0-8493-1959-5/05/$0.00+$1.50

**TABLE 36.1**
**Malignant Tumors of Skin Immunocompetent Cells**

| |
|---|
| Skin-homing lymphocytes |
| Cutaneous T-cell lymphoma |
| Cutaneous B-cell lymphoma[a] |
| Langerhans cells/dendritic cells/monocytes/macrophages |
| Langerhans cell histiocytosis |
| Non-Langerhans cell histiocytosis |
| Acute/chronic (myelo)monocytic leukemia[b] |
| Keratinocytes |
| Basal cell carcinoma |
| Squamous cell carcinoma |
| Endothelial cells |
| Angiosarcoma |
| Kaposi's sarcoma |
| Mast cell |
| Mast cell leukemia |
| Malignant mastocytosis |

[a] B lymphocytes are only found in the skin after antigenic challenge.
[b] May present in the skin before peripheral blood and/or bone marrow involvement are detectable (aleukemic leukemia cutis).

lymphomas in immunocompromised patients. The effect of immunosuppression on the development of epithelial tumors has already been discussed in Chapter 22. In this chapter, we focus on the group of cutaneous lymphomas.

## II. CUTANEOUS LYMPHOMAS: TUMORS OF SKIN-HOMING LYMPHOCYTES

Recent progress in our understanding of the mechanisms involved in the recirculation and tissue-specific homing of lymphocytes has resulted in the concept that malignant lymphomas arising in different tissues should be considered clonal proliferations of distinct populations of tissue-related lymphocytes.[1] In this concept, primary cutaneous lymphomas are thus derived from a subset of lymphocytes endowed with the capacity to infiltrate specifically into the skin (skin-homing lymphocytes), whereas lymphomas arising at other sites (e.g., lymph nodes, mucosa-associated tissue) are derived from a subset of lymphocytes with different homing characteristics.[2] Studies demonstrating that the cutaneous lymphocyte antigen (CLA), a skin-homing receptor expressed by T cells in normal and inflamed human skin[3,4], is also expressed by most primary cutaneous T-cell lymphomas (CTCL),[3,5] but not by extracutaneous T-cell lymphomas[5] are consistent with this view. This concept also explains why morphologically identical lymphomas arising at different sites may differ from one another not only in the expression of adhesion molecules mediating this tissue-specific homing, but also in the presence of specific translocations, the expression of oncogenes and viral antigens, and, most important, in clinical behavior and prognosis.[1] These new insights also indicate that primary cutaneous lymphomas should be considered as a separate group, and that differentiation between primary lymphomas and systemic lymphomas involving the skin secondarily (secondary cutaneous lymphomas) is essential. Recent clinicopathologic studies on selected groups of primary cutaneous lymphomas resulted in the delineation of new well-defined types of cutaneous T- and B-cell lymphomas, and formed the basis for a separate classification for this group of disorders.[1]

In this chapter, three major groups of primary cutaneous lymphomas are discussed: first, the group of classical CTCL, including mycosis fungoides (MF) and Sézary's syndrome (SS); second, the group of primary cutaneous CD30$^+$ T-cell lymphoproliferative disorders, which includes the primary cutaneous CD30$^+$ large T-cell lymphoma and lymphomatoid papulosis (LyP); and, third, the group of primary cutaneous B-cell lymphoma (CBCL). Characteristic clinical, histological, immunophenotypical, and genetic features are presented, and immunological mechanisms operative in tumor development and progression are emphasized.

## III. MYCOSIS FUNGOIDES AND SÉZARY'S SYNDROME

### A. Clinical Features

MF is the most common subtype within the group of CTCL. Characteristically, MF evolves through three clinical stages: the eczematous or patch stage, the plaque stage, and the tumor stage. Patients may have patch stage disease for years or even decades, before more infiltrated plaques develop. In only a proportion of patients, skin tumors develop and dissemination to lymph nodes and/or visceral organs is observed. In most patients, MF runs an indolent clinical course.[6,7]

SS is defined historically by the triad of a pruritic erythroderma, generalized lymphadenopathy, and the presence of malignant clonal T cells (Sézary cells) in skin, lymph nodes, and peripheral blood.[8] Alopecia, onychodystrophy, and palmoplantar hyperkeratosis are common findings. Patients with SS have a much poorer prognosis than patients with MF.[1,8]

### B. Histology and Immunophenotype

Histologically, the plaque stage of MF is characterized by the presence of medium-sized to large atypical lymphoid cells with indented (cerebriform) nuclei, which generally infiltrate into the epidermis and may form small intraepidermal aggregates (Pautrier microabscesses). In the early stages of the disease, the percentage of tumor cells is low, and based on the results of T-cell receptor gene rearrangement studies, probably does not exceed 1 to 3% of the total number of infiltrating cells.[9] In these early stages, there is an extensive inflammatory infiltrate of both CD4$^+$ and CD8$^+$ T cells, Langerhans/dendritic cells, and macrophages.[10,11] With progression to more infiltrated plaques and tumors, the dermal infiltrates become more diffuse; they contain an increasing number of tumor cells, including blast cells; and demonstrate a steady decrease in the proportion of inflammatory cells. In addition, the tendency of the neoplastic T cells to infiltrate into the epidermis may become lost. The histological features of SS are roughly similar to those of MF. However, the cellular infiltrates in SS are more often monotonous, containing a higher proportion of neoplastic T cells, and epidermotropism may be absent.

Characteristically, the neoplastic T cells in MF and SS have the phenotype of activated skin-homing memory T cells (CD3$^+$, CD4$^+$, CD8$^-$, CD45RO$^+$, CLA$^+$).[12] In the more advanced stages of MF, the neoplastic T cells may exhibit an aberrant phenotype with variable loss of one or more T-cell antigens.[10]

### C. Immunopathogenesis and Tumor Progression

The etiology and pathogenetic mechanisms involved in the development and stepwise progression of MF are largely unknown. Genetic, environmental, and immunologic factors all must be considered.

#### 1. Genetic Factors

Lymphomagenesis is considered a multifactorial process, in which a stepwise accumulation of genetic abnormalities may result in clonal proliferation, malignant transformation, and ultimately progressive and widely disseminated disease. Although the successive clinical steps in tumor progression in MF were described more than a century ago, the molecular events underlying these different steps in tumor progression are still poorly understood. Many genetic abnormalities involving oncogenes, tumor-suppressor genes, cell cycle-regulating genes, and DNA repair genes have been reported in patients with MF, but a consistent pattern has not emerged.[13–19] Many of these genetic alterations, including those in p53, p15, and p16 genes, have been reported in the advanced, but not in the early stages of MF suggesting that they play a role in tumor progression rather than in the early development of these lymphomas.[18,19]

## 2. Environmental Factors

Persistent antigenic stimulation has been demonstrated to play a crucial role in the development of various malignant lymphomas, including gastric mucosa-associated lymphoid tissue (MALT) lymphomas (*Helicobacter pylori* infection), CBCL (*Borrelia burgdorferi* infection), and enteropathy-type T-cell lymphoma (celiac disease). Patients with MF and SS generally have nondiagnostic skin lesions for several years before a definite diagnosis of MF or SS is made.[20] Whether these so-called premycotic eruptions represent an inflammatory dermatosis that harbors an increased risk to eventuate into genuine CTCL or whether they should be regarded as a host response to few tumor cells that cannot yet be recognized by routine histology is as yet unknown. Based on these clinical observations, also in MF persistent antigenic stimulation has been proposed as an initial event, but the nature of the antigen(s) involved is unknown. Large case-controlled studies do not support a relationship between industrial or environmental exposure and the development of MF.[21] Whereas the etiological role of human T-cell leukemia virus 1 in adult T-cell lymphoma/leukemia and of Epstein–Barr virus in nasal natural killer (NK)/T-cell lymphoma has been firmly established, conclusive evidence for a primary etiologic role of these viruses in MF is lacking.[22] Studies suggesting that chronic stimulation by bacterial superantigens or *Chlamydia* species play an important role in the development of MF need further confirmation.[23,24]

## 3. Immunological Factors

The affinity of the neoplastic T cells for the epidermis in the early stages of MF/SS is one of the most characteristic features of this group of diseases. Interactions between the different cell types in this compartment, either by direct cell–cell contact or by the production of soluble factors, are considered to play a critical role in the pathogenesis and progression of these CTCL.[25] The recruitment and/or retention of the neoplastic T cells in the epidermis is probably mediated by ICAM-1, expressed on the keratinocyte surface, and its ligand LFA-1, present on both benign and malignant T cells, but other adhesion molecules might be involved as well.[2,26] In addition, the chemokine interferon-inducible protein 10 (IP-10; CXCL10), which is highly expressed by the epidermal keratinocytes in the early stages of MF, has been implicated in the preferential infiltration of T cells expressing CXCR3, the receptor for CXCL10, into the epidermis.[27,28] Local production of interferon-gamma (IFN-γ) by activated T cells is considered responsible for the induction of both ICAM-1 and CXCL10 on keratinocytes. IL-2, IL-7, and IL-15 all have been implicated in the promotion of viability and proliferation of the neoplastic T cells, but their exact role remains to be defined.[29–31]

Recent studies suggest that the neoplastic T cells in SS and tumor stage MF are derived from $CD4^+$ T-cells with a Th2 cytokine profile (production of IL-4, IL-5, and IL-10). In accordance with this concept, a shift from a predominant type 1 cytokine profile in early MF plaques (relatively few neoplastic T cells; abundant inflammatory infiltrate) to a predominant type 2 cytokine profile in MF tumors (predominance of neoplastic T cells; relatively few inflammatory cells) has been suggested.[32–34] These observations offer an explanation for the clinical and histological changes observed during progression of these CTCL. The transition from epidermotropic to non-epidermotropic disease may be explained by the steady decrease in the proportion of IFN-γ producing $CD8^+$

T cells, resulting in decreased ICAM-1 expression by keratinocytes. Increased levels of Th2 cytokines may impair the Th1 cell-mediated antitumor response and contribute to the immunosuppression in patients with advanced MF and SS.

## 4. Antitumor Response

The protracted clinical course in most patients with MF, the beneficial effects of immunomodulating agents such as retinoids and interferons, and the disease progression observed in patients treated with such immunosuppressive agents as cyclosporine suggest the presence of an effective antitumor immune response in these lymphomas. Recent studies suggest that CD8+ cytotoxic T cells (CTL) play a crucial role in this antitumor response.[11,35] *In vitro* studies demonstrated that the malignant cells in MF display tumor-specific antigens that can be recognized by autologous CD8+ CTL.[36,37] An influx of CD8+ CTL was noted in MF tumors showing regression upon intralesional administration of IL-12.[38] Finally, a relationship between high percentages of CD8+ CTL in the dermal infiltrates and a better survival has been described.[11,35] These CD8+ T cells exert their antitumor effect both by a direct cytotoxic effect and by the production of cytokines, particularly IFN-γ. They can mediate tumor cell lysis by exocytosis of cytotoxic granules containing perforin, granzymes, and T-cell-restricted intracellular antigen (TIA-1), and by expression of Fas ligand (FasL), which interacts with Fas (CD95; APO-1) on the neoplastic T cells.[35] Both pathways ultimately lead to activation of caspase 3 and tumor cell death.

IFN-γ produced by these CD8+ CTL plays an important role in the Th1-mediated antitumor response by augmenting T-cell- and NK-cell-mediated killing and increasing phagocytosis by macrophages. Moreover, IFN-γ increases the sensitivity of the tumor cells to the immune response by inducing the expression of Fas, co-stimulatory molecules, and HLA class I molecules by these cells. Finally, IFN-γ is responsible for the induction of CXCR3-targeting chemokines, such as CXCL10 (IP-10), CXCL9 (Mig), and CXCL11 (IP-9; I-TACK), which play a critical role in the accumulation of activated T cells and NK cells at tumor sites.[39] Recent *in situ* hybridization studies showed high expression of CXCL10 and CXCL9 mRNA in MF plaques, whereas expression in MF tumors was generally absent.[28]

## 5. Evasion of Antitumor Immune Response

Neoplastic cells can develop several mechanisms to escape from an efficient immune response. These include evasive strategies to avoid immune recognition, the production of immunosuppressive cytokines, such as IL-10, unresponsiveness to growth inhibitory factors such as transforming growth factor-beta (TGF-β), and resistance to apoptosis.

In B-cell lymphomas loss of HLA class I and II molecules and of co-stimulatory molecules have been associated with disseminated disease and poor survival.[40,41] However, such mechanisms have not been described in MF or SS.

There is accumulating evidence that loss of Fas expression or function by the neoplastic T cells is an important mechanism, by which tumor cells can escape from an effective antitumor response.[42–45] Loss of Fas expression has been noted particularly in advanced stages of CTCL.[43] However, recent studies described a splice variant resulting in a dysfunctional Fas protein in skin biopsies of both early and advanced CTCL suggesting that impairment of Fas-induced apoptosis may be an early event in the pathogenesis of MF.[44] Mutations in the Fas gene are, however, infrequently found.[45] Elimination of tumor-specific CD8+ T cells expressing the Fas receptor by neoplastic T cells expressing high levels of Fas ligand has been suggested as another mechanism by which the neoplastic T cells escape from the antitumor response.[46] Gene expression studies using cDNA microarrays in MF biopsies revealed upregulation of multiple genes involved in tumor necrosis factor (TNF) signaling and having antiapoptopic activity.[47]

### 6. Therapeutic Implications

These new insights in the pathogenesis of these CTCL also have therapeutic implications. The concept that these classical CTCL represent a proliferation of malignant Th2 cells that can be controlled effectively for a long period of time by tumor-infiltrating Th1 cells offers a rationale for treating these lymphomas with immunomodulating agents with the capacity to augment the Th1-mediated antitumor response and vaccination strategies with peptides or peptide-loaded dendritic cells.[48–50] These immunomodulating agents include retinoids, IFN-α, IFN-γ, and IL-12, which is the most potent inducer of IFN-γ.[48,49] It is expected that these immunomodulatory therapies will become increasingly important in the treatment of these CTCL. Other new therapies such as immunotoxins (e.g., $DAB_{389}$IL-2) and monoclonal antibodies (e.g., anti-CD52) exert their beneficial effect most likely by inducing apoptosis of the neoplastic T cells. $DAB_{389}$IL-2 (Denileukin Diftitox) is a fusion protein, in which diphtheria toxin is linked to IL-2.[48,49] It binds to the high-affinity IL-2 receptor expressed by the neoplastic T cells in MF, which results in inhibition of protein synthesis and cell death, and clinically in overall and complete response rates of approximately 30 and 10%, respectively. Alemtuzumab (Campath-1H), a humanized $IgG_1$ monoclonal antibody against CD52, which is expressed on most malignant B cells and T cells, has recently been introduced for the treatment of patients with advanced MF and SS.[51]

## IV. PRIMARY CUTANEOUS CD30$^+$ LYMPHOPROLIFERATIVE DISORDERS

### A. Clinicopathologic Features

Primary cutaneous CD30$^+$ lymphoproliferative disorders represent the second most common group of CTCL, accounting for approximately 30% of CTCL.[1] This group includes primary cutaneous CD30$^+$ large T-cell lymphoma, lymphomatoid papulosis (LyP), and borderline cases. The term *borderline case* refers to a case, in which there is a discrepancy between the clinical features and the histologic appearance.[52] These include cases with the clinical presentation of a CD30$^+$ large T-cell lymphoma, but with histologic features suggestive of LyP, and vice versa. It follows that differentiation between primary cutaneous CD30$^+$ large T-cell lymphoma and LyP cannot only be based on histologic criteria. The clinical appearance and course are used as decisive criteria for the definite diagnosis and choice of treatment. The overlapping clinical, histological, and immunophenotypical features have resulted in the view that CD30$^+$ cutaneous large T-cell lymphomas and LyP are parts of a spectrum of primary cutaneous CD30$^+$ T-cell lymphoproliferative disorders.[52]

### 1. Primary Cutaneous CD30$^+$ (anaplastic) Large T-Cell Lymphoma

Clinically, most patients present with solitary or localized nodules or tumors, and sometimes papules, and often show ulceration. The skin lesions may show partial or complete spontaneous regression, as in LyP. These lymphomas frequently relapse in the skin. Extracutaneous dissemination occurs in approximately 10% of the patients, and mainly involves the regional lymph nodes. The prognosis is usually favorable with a 10-year disease-related survival exceeding 90%[52]

Histologically, these lymphomas generally show dense non-epidermotropic infiltrates with large clusters of CD30$^+$ tumor cells with round, oval, or irregularly shaped nuclei, one or several prominent often eosinophilic nucleoli, and abundant cytoplasm.[53] Inflammatory cells, mainly small lymphocytes, are generally found at the periphery of these clusters.

The tumor cells have the phenotype of activated, skin-homing helper T cells (CD30$^+$, CD4$^+$, CLA$^+$), with variable loss of CD2, CD3, and CD5 antigens.[53] CD30 must be expressed by the majority (>75%) of neoplastic cells.[1] Expression of cytotoxic proteins (granzyme B, TIA-1, perforin) is noted in approximately 70% of the cases.[54] Unlike systemic CD30$^+$ lymphomas, most primary cutaneous CD30+ large T-cell lymphomas express the CLA, but do not express EMA and ALK (anaplastic lymphoma kinase), indicative of the 2;5 chromosomal translocation, which is predominantly found in systemic CD30+ anaplastic large cell lymphomas in children.[52,55] Unlike Hodgkin and Reed-Sternberg cells in Hodgkin's disease, staining for CD15 is generally negative.

### 2. Lymphomatoid Papulosis

LyP is defined as a chronic, recurrent, self-healing papulonecrotic or papulonodular skin disease with the histologic features of a malignant lymphoma.[56] Clinically, LyP is characterized by the presence of papules and small nodules that may develop central hemorrhage, necrosis, and crusting, and subsequently disappear spontaneously within 3 to 8 weeks. In approximately 20% of patients, LyP may be preceded, associated with, or followed by another type of malignant lymphoma, almost invariably MF, Hodgkin's disease, or a CD30+ large cell lymphoma.[57]

Histologically, most cases of LyP contain large CD30+ tumor cells, similar to those observed in the CD30+ large cell lymphoma, that are surrounded by an extensive inflammatory infiltrate of neutrophils, sometimes eosinophils, histiocytes, and small lymphocytes (LyP, type A).[58,59] Some cases of LyP show epidermotropic infiltrates that are predominantly composed of atypical cerebriform mononuclear cells with the phenotype of activated, but CD30− helper T cells, similar to those observed in MF (LyP type B).[58]

Finally, in approximately 10% of patients the skin lesions may demonstrate a monotonous population or large clusters of large CD30+ T cells with relatively few admixed inflammatory cells, a histologic appearance typically found in primary cutaneous CD30+ large T-cell lymphomas (LyP, type C).[52] In such cases the definite diagnosis depends on the clinical appearance and course of the disease.

## B. Immunopathogenesis and Tumor Progression

The mechanisms involved in the development of these primary cutaneous CD30+ lymphoproliferative disorders are unknown. In view of the concept that the development of a malignant lymphoma is a multistep phenomenon, LyP might be considered a first step in tumor development. In most patients this initial step, which involves activation and (clonal) expansion of (CD30+) T cells, is controlled effectively by the host immune response, resulting in spontaneous regression of the skin lesions. Further progression occurs only when the tumor cells acquire a growth advantage either by additional chromosomal alterations or when the host immune response becomes deficient. In this concept the development of a primary cutaneous CD30+ large T-cell lymphoma not regressing spontaneously might be considered a second step in lymphomagenesis.

The initiating event in the development of these conditions is unknown. No causative agent has been identified thus far. Since viral antigens may strongly induce CD30 expression in both T cells and B cells, a viral etiology has been suggested. However, studies for an etiological role of HTLV-1, EBV, and other herpes viruses, including herpes simplex virus type 1 and type 2 and human herpesvirus-6, 7, and 8 have been consistently negative.[60–63] Spontaneous remission of skin lesions is one of the most characteristic features of these CD30+ lymphomas, occurring by definition in all patients with LyP and in approximately 25% of primary cutaneous CD30+ large T-cell lymphomas.[52] The mechanisms involved in the spontaneous disappearance of skin lesions, or in tumor progression, as observed in some patients, have not yet been identified. Histological and immunohistochemical studies suggested that a cell-mediated immune response plays an important role in the spontaneous regression of skin lesions in LyP.[64] Interactions between CD30 and its ligand (CD30L) may contribute to apoptosis of the neoplastic T cells and the subsequent regression of the skin lesions, but the exact mechanism is as yet unknown.[65] Unresponsiveness to the growth inhibitory effects of TGF-β by point mutations and deletions in the TGF-β type I and II receptors,[66,67] as well as high levels of bcl-2 expression by the CD30+ tumor cells[68] have been suggested as possible mechanisms in tumor progression. Recent studies demonstrated amplification and overexpression of JUNB, one of the principal components of the AP-1 transcription factor complex, in skin biopsies of primary cutaneous CD30+ large T-cell lymphomas as well as MF and SS.[69] The functional significance of JUNB overexpression remains, however, to be determined. Other studies using cDNA microarrays demonstrated differential gene expression profiles between T-cell lines derived from clinically indolent and aggressive stages of a cutaneous CD30+ large T-cell lymphomas.[70] The cell line derived from advanced stage disease showed higher expression of genes involved in cell proliferation, cell survival, and drug resistance, whereas the cell line obtained from the indolent stage of disease showed higher expression of genes involved in cell cycle inhibition, cell adhesion, apoptosis, and DNA repair. Similar studies on fresh skin biopsy samples of patients with a different clinical behavior and outcome may provide essential information to understand the pathogenesis of these conditions and to define novel targets for diagnosis and treatment.

## V. PRIMARY CUTANEOUS B-CELL LYMPHOMA

B lymphocytes are not found in normal skin, and therefore are not considered a normal constituent of the skin immune system.[71] This may have contributed to the traditional view that malignant B-cell lymphomas in the skin should always be considered as secondary cutaneous involvement of a systemic B-cell lymphoma.[72] The introduction of immunohistochemistry in diagnostic pathology in the late 1970s had a major effect on the diagnosis and classification of B-cell proliferations in the skin. Accepting the presence of monotypic immunoglobulin (Ig) light chain expression as the gold standard for the diagnosis of a malignant B-cell lymphoma, not only facilitated differentiation between malignant B-cell lymphomas and reactive B-cell proliferations (pseudolymphoma, cutaneous lymphoid hyperplasia, lymphadenosis benigna cutis), but also led to the recognition that malignant B-cell lymphomas can present in the skin without concurrent extracutaneous disease (primary cutaneous B-cell lymphoma). These primary CBCL appeared to have a much better prognosis than B-cell lymphomas involving the skin secondarily. In European studies these CBCL constitute approximately 20% of all primary cutaneous lymphomas, whereas a recent report suggest a frequency of only 5 to 10% in the United States.[1,73]

In recent years, several distinct types of CBCL have been described. In the EORTC classification for primary cutaneous lymphomas, primary cutaneous marginal zone B-cell lymphomas (previously termed primary cutaneous immunocytomas) and the group of primary cutaneous follicle center cell lymphomas are recognized as indolent types of CBCL, whereas primary cutaneous large B-cell lymphomas presenting on the leg are included as a separate group with an intermediate prognosis.[1]

### A. Clinicopathologic Features

#### 1. Primary Cutaneous Marginal Zone B-Cell Lymphoma (MZL)

Clinically, primary cutaneous MZL may present with a solitary nodule or tumor, or not infrequently with multifocal nodular skin lesions.[74–76] Association with *Borrelia burgdorferi* infection has been reported particularly in European studies, but seems quite rare in the United States.[77–80] Cutaneous relapses are common, but dissemination to extracutaneous sites is exceedingly rare. The prognosis is excellent.

Histologically, these lymphomas are characterized by the presence of small to medium-sized neoplastic B cells with round or cleaved nuclei, and in most cases monotypic plasma cells particularly at the periphery of the infiltrates. Reactive germinal centers are typically present. The neoplastic B cells express monotypic sIg, CD79a, CD20 (plasma cells negative), bcl-2, but not bcl-6 and CD10.[81,82]

#### 2. Primary Cutaneous Follicle Center Cell Lymphoma (PCFCCL)

PCFCCL has been introduced as an encompassing term for CBCL consisting of cells with the morphological features of follicle center cells (small and large centrocytes or cleaved cells; centroblasts or large noncleaved cells). Characteristically, these patients present with nodules or tumors confined to a rather circumscribed skin area, preferentially on the trunk or on the scalp.[83–85] The nodules or tumors are often surrounded by and preceded by papular lesions and/or annular erythemas. These PCFCCL are slowly progressive and extracutaneous dissemination is rare. They have an excellent prognosis with an estimated 5-year-survival of more than 95%.[1,86]

Histologically, early and small lesions often show diffuse infiltrates with a predominance of small B cells, few centroblasts, and many admixed T cells. However, most skin lesions, in particular rapidly growing tumors, show diffuse infiltrates of large centrocytes and/or centroblasts.[1,84,85] In the WHO classification such cases are classified as diffuse large B-cell lymphoma.[87] A follicular growth pattern, characteristic of follicular lymphomas in lymph nodes, is rarely observed. Characteristically, the neoplastic B cells have a $CD20^{+}$, $CD79a^{+}$, bcl-$6^{+}$, $CD10^{-/+}$, bcl-$2^{-/+}$ phenotype.[81,82]

### 3. Primary Cutaneous Large B-cell Lymphoma of the Leg

This group includes generally elderly patients presenting with one or several tumors on the legs. Initially, these cases were considered a subgroup of PCFCCL with a more unfavorable prognosis.[83] In the EORTC classification they were included as a separate subgroup, which is a subject of ongoing controversy.[1]

As compared to the PCFCCL with a large cell morphology localized on the head or trunk these lymphomas are more refractory to radiotherapy, more often disseminate to extracutaneous sites, and have a worse prognosis (5-year-survival: approximately 50%).[88,89]

Histologically, these lymphomas also display the histology of a diffuse large B-cell lymphoma.[88–89] There is often a considerable admixture with immunoblasts, whereas admixed inflammatory cells are few. These lymphomas almost without exception have a bcl-$6^{+}$, bcl-$2^{+}$, $CD10^{-}$ phenotype.[82]

## B. Immunopathogenesis and Tumor Progression

Although normal human skin does not contain B lymphocytes, several antigenic stimuli are known to result in a reactive B-cell response. These reactions are designated variously as cutaneous lymphoid hyperplasia, lymphadenosis benigna cutis, or pseudo B-cell lymphoma, and may be caused by insect bites, in particular tick bites transmitting a *B. burgdorferi* infection, acupuncture, antigen injections, and tattoo pigments.[90] Interestingly, *B. burgdorferi* infection[76–79,91] and tattoo pigment[92,93] have also been implicated in the development of primary CBCL, in particular some marginal zone B-cell lymphomas and follicle center cell lymphomas. There is accumulating evidence to suggest that these low-grade malignant CBCL and cutaneous lymphoid hyperplasia represent a spectrum of cutaneous B-cell lymphoproliferative disorders with a stepwise progression from a reactive to a neoplastic state.[90,93] This also explains why it can be so difficult to differentiate early stages of these low-grade CBCL from cutaneous lymphoid hyperplasias. Apart from clinical and histological similarities, and the shared association with *B. burgdorferi* infection and tattoo pigments, clonal Ig gene rearrangements have been demonstrated not only in primary CBCL, but also in a proportion of pseudo-B-cell lymphomas, as defined by immunohistochemical criteria.[93–95]

These *B. burgdorferi*-associated CBCL resemble in many ways gastric MALT lymphomas that develop in association with *Helicobacter pylori* infection, including resolution of the skin lymphoma after antibiotic therapy.[78,79] However, the different translocations associated with the subsequent steps of evolution of the gastric MALT lymphomas are not or are rarely found in these primary CBCL.[75]

The genetic abnormalities involved in the development of primary CBCL are largely unknown. The t(14;18) interchromosomal translocation, which is normally found in follicular lymphomas in lymph nodes, and which results in the overexpression of the bcl-2 protein, is rarely found in primary cutaneous follicle center cell lymphomas.[96–98] It is not found in the group of primary cutaneous large B-cell lymphomas on the leg, although strong bcl-2 expression is common in this group.[97] Recent studies reported inactivation of p15 and p16 tumor suppressor genes, most frequently as a result of promotor hypermethylation, in 8 (23%) and 15 (43%) of 35 CBCL, respectively.[99] Comparative genomic hybridization (CGH) analysis showed chromosomal imbalances in 40 to 60% of CBCL.[100,101] Gains in 18q and 7p and loss of 6q were most commonly found. In one of these studies chromosomal imbalances were found in only 3 of 9 PCFCCL, compared to 11 of 13 (85%) of primary cutaneous large B-cell lymphomas on the leg, which further supports that these latter cases should be considered as a separate group.[101]

## VI. CONCLUSION

It is now well accepted that the development of a malignant lymphoma is a multistep process, in which accumulating genetic alterations and an increasingly failing host response may result in progressive and finally metastatic and fatal disease. The three groups of diseases presented herein illustrate that this concept also holds true for the group of primary cutaneous lymphomas. The molecular mechanisms that provide the neoplastic cells with a growth advantage are now beginning to be unraveled; however, consistent genetic abnormalities have not been detected thus far. It is important to note that interchromosomal translocations found in some nodal lymphomas, such as the t(2;5) in CD30$^+$ anaplastic large cell lymphomas and the t(14;18) in follicular lymphomas, are not found in their primary cutaneous counterparts, which underscores the view that these morphologically identical lymphomas arising at different sites derive from different T- and B-cell populations.[1] It is expected that in the next few years gene and protein expression profiling will not only contribute to the elucidation of the molecular pathways involved in the development of the different types of primary cutaneous lymphomas, but will also provide new molecular targets for diagnosis and therapeutic intervention.

## REFERENCES


1. Willemze, R. et al., EORTC classification for primary cutaneous lymphomas. A proposal from the Cutaneous Lymphoma Study Group of the European Organization for Research and Treatment of Cancer (EORTC). *Blood*, 90, 354, 1997.
2. Drillenburg, P. and Pals, S.T., Cell adhesion receptors in lymphoma dissemination. *Blood,* 95, 1900, 2000.
3. Picker, L.J. et al., A unique phenotype of skin-associated lymphocytes in human. Preferential expression of the HECA-452 epitope by benign and malignant T-cells at cutaneous sites. *Am. J. Pathol.*, 136, 1053, 1990.
4. Bos, J.D. et al., Skin-homing T-lymphocytes: detection of cutaneous lymphocyte associated antigen (CLA) by HECA-452 in normal human skin. *Arch. Dermatol. Res.*, 285, 179, 1993.
5. Noorduyn, L.A. et al., Differential expression of the HECA-452 antigen (cutaneous lymphocyte antigen, CLA) in cutaneous and noncutaneous T-cell lymphomas. *Histopathology*, 21, 59, 1992.
6. van Doorn, R. et al., Mycosis fungoides: disease evolution and prognosis of 309 Dutch patients. *Arch. Dermatol.,* 136, 504, 2000.
7. Kim, Y.H. et al., Long-term outcome of 525 patients with mycosis fungoides and Sézary syndrome. *J. Am. Acad. Dermatol.*, 139, 857, 2003.
8. Wieselthier, J.S. and Koh, H.K., Sézary syndrome: diagnosis, prognosis, and critical review of treatment options. *J. Am. Acad. Dermatol.*, 22, 381, 1990.
9. Wood, G.S. et al., Detection of clonal T-cell receptor gene rearrangements in early mycosis fungoides/Sézary syndrome by polymerase chain reaction and denaturing gradient gel electrophoresis (PCR/DGGE). *J. Invest. Dermatol.*, 103, 34, 1994.
10. Preesman, A.H. et al., Immunophenotyping on simultaneously occurring plaques and tumors in mycosis fungoides and Sézary syndrome. *Br. J. Dermatol.*, 129, 660, 1993.
11. Hoppe, R.T. et al., CD8-positive tumor-infiltrating lymphocytes influence the long-term survival of patients with mycosis fungoides. *J. Am. Acad. Dermatol.*, 32, 448, 1995.

12. Rook, A.H. and Heald, P., The immunopathogenesis of cutaneous T-cell lymphoma. *Hematol. Oncol. Clin. North Am.*, 9, 997, 1995.
13. Thangavelu, M. et al., Recurring structural chromosome abnormalities in peripheral blood lymphocytes of patients with mycosis fungoides/Sezary syndrome. *Blood,* 89, 3371, 1997.
14. Karenko, L. et al., Chromosomal abnormalities in cutaneous T-cell lymphoma and in its premalignant conditions as detected by G-banding and interphase cytogenetic methods. *J. Invest. Dermatol.,* 108, 22, 1997.
15. Karenko, L. et al., Notable losses at specific regions of chromosomes 10q and 13q in the Sezary syndrome detected by comparative genomic hybridization. *J. Invest. Dermatol.,* 112, 392, 1999.
16. Scarisbrick, J.J. et al., Loss of heterozygosity on 10q and microsatellite instability in advanced stages of primary cutaneous T-cell lymphoma and possible association with homozygous deletion of PTEN. *Blood,* 95, 2937, 2000.
17. Navas, I.C. et al., p16(INK4a) gene alterations are frequent in lesions of mycosis fungoides. *Am. J. Pathol.,* 156, 1565, 2000.
18. Whittaker, S., Molecular genetics of cutaneous lymphomas. *Ann. N.Y. Acad. Sci.*, 941, 39, 2001.
19. Li, G. et al., Overexpression of p53 protein in cutaneous T-cell lymphoma: relationship to large cell transformation and disease progression. *J. Invest. Dermatol.,* 110, 767, 1998.
20. Lambert, W. C., Premycotic eruptions. *Dermatol Clin.*, 3, 629, 1985.
21. Weinstock, M.A., Epidemiology of mycosis fungoides. *Semin. Dermatol.,* 13, 154, 1994.
22. Li, G. et al., Failure to detect human T-lymphotropic virus type I (HTLV-I) proviral DNA in cell lines and tissues from patients with cutaneous T-cell lymphoma. *J. Invest. Dermatol.,* 107, 308, 1996.
23. Jackow, C.M. et al., Association of erythrodermic cutaneous T-cell lymphoma, superantigen-positive *Staphylococcus aureus*, and oligoclonal T-cell receptor V beta gene expansion. *Blood*, 89, 32, 1997.
24. Abrams, J.T., Balin, B.J., and Vonderheid, E.C., Association between Sezary T cell-activating factor, *Chlamydia pneumoniae* and cutaneous T-cell lymphoma. *Ann. N.Y. Acad. Sci.,* 941, 69, 2001.
25. Hansen, E.R., Immunoregulatory events in skin of patients with cutaneous T-cell lymphoma. *Arch. Dermatol.,* 132, 554, 1996.
26. Nickoloff, B.J. et al., Markedly diminished epidermal keratinocyte expression of intracellular adhesion molecule-1 (ICAM-1) in Sézary syndrome. *J. Am. Med. Assoc.,* 261, 2217, 1989.
27. Sarris, A. et al., Cytokine loops involving interferon-gamma and IP-10, a cytokine chemotactic for $CD4^+$ lymphocytes: an explanation for the epidermotropism of cutaneous T-cell lymphoma? *Am. Soc. Haematol.,* 86, 651, 1995.
28. Tensen, C.P. et al., Epidermal Interferon-$\gamma$ inducible protein-10 (IP-10) and monokine induced by $\gamma$-interferon (Mig) but not IL-8 mRNA expression is associated with epidermotropism in cutaneous T-cell lymphomas. *J. Invest. Dermatol.,* 111, 222, 1998.
29. Moller, P. et al., Interleukin-7, biology and implications for dermatology. *Exp Dermatol.,* 5, 129, 1996.
30. Dobbeling, U. et al., Interleukin-15 is an autocrine/paracrine viability factor for cutaneous T-cell lymphoma cells. *Blood,* 92, 252, 1998.
31. Qin, J.Z. et al., Interleukin-7 and interleukin-15 regulate the expression of the bcl-2 and c-myb genes in cutaneous T-cell lymphoma cells. *Blood,* 98, 2778, 2001.
32. Saed, G. et al., Mycosis fungoides exhibits a Th1-type cell-mediated cytokine profile, whereas Sézary syndrome expresses a Th2-type profile. *J. Invest. Dermatol.,* 103, 29, 1994.
33. Vowels, B.R. et al., Th2 cytokine mRNA expression in skin in cutaneous T-cell lymphoma. *J. Invest. Dermatol.,* 103, 669, 1994.
34. Asadullah, K. et al., Progression of mycosis fungoides is associated with increasing cutaneous expression of interleukin-10 mRNA. *J. Invest. Dermatol.,* 107, 833, 1996.
35. Vermeer, M.H. et al., $CD8^+$ T-cells in cutaneous T-cell lymphoma: expression of cytotoxic proteins, FAS ligand and killing inhibitory receptors and relationship with clinical behaviour. *J. Clin. Oncol.,* 19, 4322, 2001.
36. Berger, C.L. et al., Tumor-specific peptides in cutaneous T-cell lymphoma: association with class I major histocompatibility complex and possible derivation from the clonotypic T-cell receptor. *Int. J. Cancer,* 76, 304, 1998.
37. Bagot, M. et al., Isolation of tumor specific cytotoxic $CD4^+$ and $CD4^+$ $CD8dim^+$ T-cell clones infiltrating a cutaneous T-cell lymphoma. *Blood,* 11, 4331, 1998.

38. Rook, A.R. et al., Interleukin-12 therapy of cutaneous T-cell lymphoma induces lesion regression and cytotoxic T-cell responses. *Blood,* 94, 902, 1999.
39. Luster, A.D. and Leder, P., IP-10, a C-X-C chemokine, elicits a potent thymus-dependent anti-tumor response *in vivo*. *J. Exp. Med.,* 178, 1057, 1993.
40. Slymen, D.J. et al., Immunobiologic factors predictive of clinical outcome in diffuse large cell lymphoma. *J. Clin. Oncol.,* 8, 986, 1990.
41. Horst, E. et al., Adhesion molecules in the prognosis of diffuse large cell lymphoma: expression of a lymphocyte homing receptor (CD44), LFA-1 (CD11a/CD18) and ICAM-1 (CD54). *Leukemia*, 4, 595, 1990.
42. Zoi-Toli, O. et al., Expression of Fas and Fasl in primary cutaneous T-cell lymphomas: association between lack of Fas expression and aggressive types of CTCL. *Br. J. Dermatol.,* 143, 313, 2000.
43. Dereure, O. et al., Decreased expression of Fas (APO-1/CD95) on peripheral blood $CD4^+$ T-lymphocytes in cutaneous T-cell lymphomas. *Br. J. Dermatol.,* 143, 1205, 2000.
44. van Doorn, R. et al., A novel splice variant of the Fas gene in patients with cutaneous T-cell lymphoma. *Cancer Res.*, 62, 5389, 2002.
45. Dereure, O. et al., Infrequent Fas mutations but no Bax or p53 mutations in early mycosis fungoides: a possible mechanism for the accumulation of malignant T-lymphocytes in the skin. *J. Invest. Dermatol.*, 118, 949, 2002.
46. Ni, X. et al., Fas ligand expression by neoplastic T lymphocytes mediates elimination of $CD8^+$ cytotoxic T lymphocytes in mycosis fungoides: a potential mechanism of tumor immune escape? *Clin. Cancer Res.*, 7, 2682, 2001.
47. Tracey, L. et al., Mycosis fungoides show concurrent deregulation of multiple genes involved in the TNF signaling pathway: an expression profile study. *Blood*, 102, 1042, 2003.
48. Duvic, M. and Cather, J.C., Emerging new therapies for cutaneous T-cell lymphoma. *Dermatol. Clin.*, 18, 147, 2000.
49. Muche, J.M., Gellrich, S., and Sterry, W., Treatment of cutaneous T-cell lymphoma. *Semin. Cutaneous Med. Surg.*, 19, 142, 2000.
50. Maier, T. et al., Vaccination of cutaneous T-cell lymphoma patients using intranodal injection of autologous tumor lysate pulsed dendritic cells. *Blood,* 102, 2338, 2003.
51. Lundin, J. et al., Phase II study of alemtuzumab anti-CD52 monoclonal antibody (Campath-1H) in patients with advanced mycosis fungoides/Sezary's syndrome. *Blood,* 101, 4267, 2003.
52. Bekkenk, M. et al., Primary and secondary cutaneous CD30-positive lymphoproliferative disorders: long term follow-up data of 219 patients and guidelines for diagnosis and treatment. A report from the Dutch Cutaneous Lymphoma Group. *Blood*, 95, 3653, 2000.
53. Beljaards, R.C. et al., Primary cutaneous CD30-positive large cell lymphomas: definition of a new type of cutaneous lymphoma with a favorable prognosis. An European multicenter study on 47 cases. *Cancer*, 71, 2097, 1993.
54. Kummer, J.A. et al., Most primary cutaneous CD30-positive lymphoproliferative disorders have a CD4-positive cytotoxic T-cell phenotype. *J. Invest. Dermatol.,* 109, 636, 1997.
55. DeCouteau, J.F. et al., The t(2;5) chromosomal translocation is not a common feature of primary cutaneous $CD30^+$ lymphoproliferative disorders: comparison with anaplastic large cell lymphoma of nodal origin. *Blood*, 87, 3437, 1996.
56. McCaulay, W.L., Lymphomatoid papulosis, a self healing eruption, clinically benign, histologically malignant. *Arch. Dermatol.,* 97, 23, 1968.
57. Beljaards, R.C. and Willemze, R., The prognosis of patients with lymphomatoid papulosis associated with other types of malignancies. *Br. J. Dermatol.,* 126, 596, 1992.
58. Willemze, R. et al., The clinical and histologic spectrum of lymphomatoid papulosis. *Br. J. Dermatol.,* 107, 131, 1982.
59. Kaudewitz, P. et al., Atypical cells in lymphomatoid papulosis express the Hodgkin cell associated antigen Ki-1. *J. Invest. Dermatol.,* 86, 350, 1986.
60. Lange Wantzin, G., Thomsen, K., and Nissen, N.L., Occurrence pf human T-cell lymphotropic virus (type I) antibodies in cutaneous T-cell lymphoma. *J. Am. Acad. Dermatol.,* 15, 598, 1986.
61. Brice, S.L. et al., Examination of cutaneous T-cell lymphoma for human herpesviruses by using the polymerase chain reaction. *J. Cutaneous Pathol.,* 20, 304, 1993.

62. Kadin, M.E., Vonderheid, E.C., and Weiss, L.M., Absence of Epstein-Barr viral RNA in lymphomatoid papulosis. *J. Pathol.,* 170, 145, 1993.
63. Kempf, W. et al., Lymphomatoid papulosis and human herpesviruses-PCR-based evaluation for the presence of human herpesvirus 6, 7 and 8 related herpesviruses. *J. Cutaneous Pathol.,* 28, 29, 2001.
64. Agnarsson, B.A. and Kadin, M.E., Host response in lymphomatoid papulosis. *Hum. Pathol.,* 20, 747, 1989.
65. Mori, M. et al., CD30-CD30L interaction in primary cutaneous $CD30^+$ T-cell lymphomas: a clue to the pathophysiology of clinical regression. *Blood,* 94, 3077, 1999.
66. Knaus, P. et al., A dominant inhibitory mutant of the type II transforming growth factor-beta receptor in the malignant progression of a cutaneous T-cell lymphoma. *Mol. Cell. Biol.,* 16, 3480, 1996.
67. Schieman, W.P. et al., A deletion in the gene for transforming growth factor beta type I receptor abolishes growth regulation by transforming growth factor beta in cutaneous T-cell lymphoma. *Blood,* 94, 2854, 1999.
68. Paulli, M. et al., Cutaneous $CD30^+$ lymphoproliferative disorders: expression of bcl-2 and proteins of the tumor necrosis factor receptor superfamily. *Hum. Pathol.,* 29, 1223, 1998.
69. Mao, X. et al., Amplification and overexpression of JUNB is associated with primary cutaneous T-cell lymphomas. *Blood,* 101, 1513, 2003.
70. Li, S. et al., Comparative genome-scale analysis of gene expression profiles in T-cell lymphoma cells during malignant progression using a complementary DNA microarray. *Am. J. Pathol.,* 158, 1231, 2001.
71. Bos, J. et al., The skin immune system (SIS): distribution and immunophenotype of lymphocyte subpopulations in normal human skin. *J. Invest. Dermatol.,* 88, 569, 1987.
72. Evans, H., Winkelmann, R., and Banks, P., Differential diagnosis of malignant and benign cutaneous infiltrates. *Cancer,* 44, 699, 1979.
73. Zackheim, H.S. et al., Relative frequency of various forms of primary cutaneous lymphomas. *J. Am. Acad. Dermatol.,* 43, 793, 2000.
74. Cerroni, L. et al., Primary cutaneous marginal zone B-cell lymphoma: a recently described entity of low-grade malignant cutaneous B-cell lymphoma. *Am. J. Surg. Pathol.,* 21, 1307, 1997.
75. Li, C. et al., Primary cutaneous marginal zone B-cell lymphoma. A molecular and clinicopathologic study of 24 cases. *Am. J. Surg. Pathol.,* 27, 1061, 2003.
76. Cerroni, L. et al., Infection by *Borrelia burgdorferi* and cutaneous B-cell lymphoma. *J. Cutaneous Pathol.,* 24, 457, 1997.
77. Goodlad, J.R. et al., Primary cutaneous B-cell lymphoma and *Borrelia burgdorferi* infection in patients from the Highlands of Scotland. *Am. J. Surg. Pathol.,* 24, 1279, 2000.
78. Kutting, B., Borrelia burgdorferi-associated primary cutaneous B-cell lymphoma: complete clearing of skin lesions after antibiotic pulse therapy or intralesional injection of interferon alfa-2a. *J. Am. Acad. Dermatol.,* 36, 311, 1997.
79. Roggero, E. et al., Eradication of *Borrelia burgdorferi* infection in primary marginal zone B-cell lymphoma of the skin. *Hum. Pathol.,* 31, 263, 2000.
80. Wood, G.S. et al., Absence of *Borrelia burgdorferi* DNA in cutaneous B-cell lymphomas from the United States. *J. Cutaneous Pathol.,* 28, 502, 2001.
81. de Leval, L. et al., Cutaneous B-cell lymphomas of follicular and marginal zone types: use of Bcl-6, CD10, Bcl-2, and CD21 in differential diagnosis and classification. *Am. J. Surg. Pathol.,* 25, 732, 2001.
82. Hoefnagel, J.J. et al., Bcl-2, bcl-6 and CD10 expression in cutaneous B-cell lymphoma: further support for a follicle center cell origin and differential diagnostic significance. *Br. J. Dermatol.,* 149, 1183, 2003.
83. Willemze, R. et al., Primary cutaneous large cell lymphomas of follicular center cell origin. *J. Am. Acad. Dermatol.,* 16, 518, 1987.
84. Berti, E. et al., Reticulohistiocytoma of the dorsum. *J. Am. Acad. Dermatol.,* 19, 259, 1988.
85. Santucci, M., Pimpinelli, N., and Arganini, L., Primary cutaneous B-cell lymphoma: a unique type of low-grade lymphoma: clinicopathologic and immunologic study of 83 cases. *Cancer,* 67, 2311, 1991.
86. Rijlaarsdam, J.U. et al., Treatment of primary cutaneous B-cell lymphomas of follicular center cell origin. A clinical follow-up study of 55 patients treated with radiotherapy or polychemotherapy. *J. Clin. Oncol.,* 14, 549, 1996.

87. Jaffe, E.S. et al., *World Health Organisation Classification of Tumours of Haematopoietic and Lymphoid Tissues,* IARC Press, Lyon, France, 2001.
88. Vermeer, M.H. et al., Primary cutaneous large B-cell lymphomas of the legs. A distinct type of cutaneous B-cell lymphoma with an intermediate prognosis. *Arch. Dermatol.,* 132, 1304, 1996.
89. Grange, F. et al., Prognostic factors in primary cutaneous large B-cell lymphomas: a European multicenter study of 145 cases. *J. Clin. Oncol.,* 19, 3602, 2001.
90. Rijlaarsdam, J.U. and Willemze, R., Cutaneous pseudolymphomas: classification and differential diagnosis. *Semin. Dermatol.,* 13, 187, 1994.
91. Garbe, C. et al., *Borrelia burgdorferi* associated cutaneous B cell lymphoma: clinical and immunohistochemical characterization of four cases. *J. Am. Acad. Dermatol.,* 24, 584, 1991.
92. Sangueza, O.P. et al., Evolution of B-cell lymphoma from pseudolymphoma. *Am. J. Dermatopathol.,* 14, 408, 1992.
93. Gilliam, A.C. and Wood, G.S., Cutaneous lymphoid hyperplasias. *Semin. Cutaneous Med. Surg.,* 19, 133, 2000.
94. Rijlaarsdam, J.U. et al., Demonstration of clonal immunoglobulin gene rearrangements in cutaneous B-cell lymphomas and pseudo-B-cell lymphomas: differential diagnostic and pathogenetic aspects. *J. Invest. Dermatol.,* 99, 749, 1992.
95. Hammer, E. et al., Immunophenotypic and genotypic analysis in cutaneous lymphoid hyperplasias. *J. Am. Acad. Dermatol.,* 28, 426, 1993.
96. Cerroni, L. et al., bcl-2 protein expression and correlation with the interchromosomal 14;18 translocation in cutaneous lymphomas and pseudolymphomas. *J. Invest. Dermatol.,* 102, 231, 1994.
97. Geelen, F.A.M.J. et al., Bcl-2 protein expression in primary cutaneous large B-cell lymphoma is site-dependent. *J. Clin. Oncol.,* 16, 2080, 1998.
98. Child, F.J. et al., Absence of the t(14;18) chromosomal translocation in primary cutaneous B-cell lymphoma. *Br. J. Dermatol.,* 144, 735, 2001.
99. Child, F.J. et al., Inactivation of tumor suppressor genes p15(INK4b) and p16(INK4a) in primary cutaneous B cell lymphoma. *J. Invest. Dermatol.,* 118, 941, 2002.
100. Mao, X. et al., Comparative genomic hybridization analysis of primary cutaneous B-cell lymphomas: identification of common genomic alterations in disease pathogenesis. *Genes Chromosomes Cancer,* 35, 144, 2002.
101. Hallermann, C. et al., Chromosomal aberration patterns differ in subtypes of primary cutaneous B-cell lymphomas. *J. Invest. Dermatol.,* 122, 1495, 2004.

# Part VI

## Immunotherapy in Dermatology

# 37 Immunomodulatory Drugs

*Lionel Fry*

## CONTENTS



0-8493-1959-5/05/$0.00+$1.50

## I. INTRODUCTION

Until recently, drugs affecting the immune system have all been immunosuppressive and, thus, as a group were referred to as immunosuppressive drugs. However, pharmacological agents that stimulate the immune system are now being developed and the term *immunomodulatory* has been coined. This latter term is also preferred by the pharmaceutical industry even when it is known that a product is immunosuppressive as that term has negative connotations.

The history of immunosuppressive drugs is linked to that of organ transplantation. It was in the early 1950s that Billingham, Krohn, and Medawar showed that adrenocorticosteroids were able to prolong skin graft survival. Thus, it can be claimed that corticosteroids were the first immunosuppressive drugs, and are still probably the most widely used for this purpose. In the later 1950s, Schwartz and Dameshek demonstrated that 6 mercaptopurine could suppress immunoreactivity and prolong survival of skin grafts in animals. Azathioprine, a derivative of 6 mercaptopurine, is still widely used. However, the drug that revolutionized organ transplantation was cyclosporine, which was discovered and used for human transplantation in the 1970s.

Apart from their value in transplantation, immunosuppressive drugs are also of value in immunologically mediated disorders. Two of the most common disorders presenting in dermatological clinics are eczema and psoriasis and they are both mediated via immune mechanisms. Thus, not surprisingly, immunosuppressive drugs have proved to be highly effective in the treatment of these diseases.

In this chapter, the currently used immunosuppressive drugs are reviewed. Immunosuppressive drugs are also used for autoimmune bullous and the connective tissue disorders, although these conditions are more rarely seen than eczema and psoriasis. In fact, now that bacterial infections are no longer a major problem in dermatology, a large proportion of the medical conditions are immunologically mediated. Thus, it is important to have some knowledge of how immunosuppressive agents work and the problems that may ensue.

Not discussed in this chapter are drugs used in immune-mediated skin disorders but whose mechanism of action has not been clearly defined even though it is possible they have some immunomodulating effects. These drugs would include retinoids, vitamin D analogues, and thalidomide. In addition, dapsone and sulfonamides, which are effective in the bullous disorders of dermatitis herpetiformis and linear IgA diseases, are not reviewed. Although, these latter disorders have immunological mechanisms as part of their pathogenesis, dapsone and sulfonamides appear to act on the end stage of the disease process by interfering with neutrophil migration and activation. The recently developed monoclonal antibodies, cytokines, and immunoglobulin treatments are not discussed in this chapter but elsewhere in this book under the term *biologicals*.

## II. ADRENOCORTICOSTEROIDS

Adrenocortical steroids are classified into those whose main effects are on salt retention and potassium excretion (mineralocortical steroids) and those whose action is involved with hepatic glycogen deposition (glucocorticosteroids). It is the second group that is anti-inflammatory and immunomodulating, and this dual action is beneficial in immune-mediated disorders, which often have an anti-inflammatory component.

Glucocorticosteroids (GCS) have many actions on the immune system and the net result tends to be one of immunosuppression. Nearly all nucleated cells have cytosolic GCS receptors.[1] Once the steroid binds to the receptor, there is a conformational change in GCS receptor complex, which moves to the nucleus. The GCS receptor now binds to segments of DNA cell glucocorticoid-responsive elements. As a result, certain parts of the genome are affected, leading to increased or decreased transcription. Depending on the cell and cell processes involved, there may be increased or decreased protein production (e.g., interleukins in lymphocytes). Because the GCS receptors are ubiquitous, it is expected that corticosteroids will affect most cells in the body and this accounts for the many beneficial effects of these substances, but also the many side effects. One of the many actions of GCS complexes is to increase IkB expression thereby curtailing activation of NF-κB, which results in increased apoptosis of activated cells.[2] In addition, downregulation of NF-κB leads to a decrease of the pro-inflammatory cytokines: interferon-gamma (IFN-γ), granulocyte-macrophage colony-stimulating factor (GM-CSF), interleukin-1 (IL-1), IL-2, IL-3, IL-6, IL-8, IL-12, and tumor necrosis factor-alpha (TNF-α). The downregulation of IL-2 will lead to decreased T-cell proliferation.

Although GCS are usually considered immunosuppressive, there is a suggestion that in the physiological response to stress, they may upregulate the humoral component of the immune response, e.g., antibody production, but decreasing the cellular component of the immune response.[3] The mechanism underlying this switch is unclear, but it has been suggested that there may be change from a Th1 to Th2 response. However, GCS suppress atopic eczema, which is thought to be mediated by Th2 cells, so in this situation there is suppression of Th2 cells.

## A. Effect of Glucocorticosteroids on Cells

### 1. Macrophages and Monocytes

These cells produce inflammatory mediators, prostaglandins, and leukotrienes from arachidonic acid. This process is inhibited by GCS, which induces a protein (Cipocortin) that inhibits the enzyme phospholipase A2, which is necessary for the production of prostaglandins and leukotrienes. GCS will also inhibit the production of the cytokines IL-1, IL-6, and TNF-α by macrophages and monocytes and, thus, impair the immune response.

GCS also inhibit the expression of Fc receptors and release of pro-inflammatory mediators such as collagenase, elastase, and plaminogen activator.[4]

### 2. Lymphocytes

GCS inhibit the production of a large number of cytokines but, principally, IL-1, IL-2, IL-3, IL-6, TNF-α, GM-CSF, and IFN-γ. These cytokines are concerned with a Th1 response rather than a Th2 but it is well known that GCS are highly effective in atopic disorders, and thus other actions of the GCS are likely to be operative in the beneficial effect in atopic diseases. It has been suggested that the effect of GCS on IL-2 production is not a direct one, but it is due to the inhibition of IL-1 by macrophages and the specialized antigen-presenting cells.

### 3. Endothelial Cells

T-cell immune-mediated responses in the skin are dependent on T-cell trafficking. GCS downregulates the expression of endothelial leukocyte-adhesion molecule-1 (ELAM-1) and intracellular adhesion molecule-1 (ICAM-1), both of which are necessary for lymphocytes to move out of the capillaries and travel through the skin. GCS also inhibit cytokine production by the endothelial cells.

### 4. Fibroblasts

GCS will suppress fibroblast proliferation and growth factor-induced DNA synthesis. This inhibition of fibroblast activity will in the long term lead to inhibition of connective tissue formation and thinning of the skin. GCS will also downregulate cytokine production and the production of prostaglandins and leukotrienes by fibroblasts.

### 5. Neutrophils and Eosinophils

The response of these cells to chemotactic factors, release of enzymes, and phagocytosis is not affected by GCS.[5] However, recruitment of these cells into the skin will be affected by the downregulation of the receptors for leukocyte trafficking and, thus, tissue damage caused by these cells will be decreased.

### 6. B Cells and Plasma Cells

There is very little effect of GCS on antibody production unless they are taken for a long time.

### 7. Effects on Circulating Cell Numbers

GCS decrease the number of circulating lymphocytes, eosinophils, basophils, and monocytes but induce an increase in neutrophils. These effects are partly due to decreased production by the bone marrow of eosinophils, basophils, and monocytes but the decrease in lymphocytes is mainly due to sequestration of the lymphocytes in the reticloendothelial system. The neutrophilia is partly due to increased production by the bone marrow and, also, due to decreased margination of neutrophils along the vessel walls.[1] All these changes will lead to a decrease in the immune response.

## B. Indications for Glucocorticosteroids

In dermatology, GCS may be used topically, intralesionally, or orally.

### 1. Topical

The most widely used drugs in dermatology are topical corticosteroids. It should be remembered that the corticosteroids activity varies considerably between the weak and most potent topical GCS available. The strength of the GCS to be used depends on the nature of the condition, the anatomical site, and the likely duration of treatment. Side effects are directly proportional to the duration of use and strength of the GCS.

The two most common inflammatory skin disorders are eczema and psoriasis, and in both the pathogenic processes are due to immunological mechanisms, which are suppressed by GCS. Both eczema and psoriasis will respond to topical GCS, providing the strength is appropriate. Other skin disorders in which GCS have a therapeutic role are lichen planus, discoid lupus erythematosus, and possibly alopecia areata and vitiligo.

### 2. Intralesional GCS

This route of administration is highly effective for keloids, where the pathology is mainly dermal and is not influenced by topical GCS. Intralesional GCS may be helpful in hypertrophic lichen planus and lichen simplex. The lesions are so thick that the topically applied preparation will not reach the lower parts of the skin to have a therapeutic effect.

Intralesional GCS are also indicated in patchy alopecia areata but not in alopecia totalis or universalis. The route of administration is also helpful in granuloma annulare and acne cysts.

### 3. Systemic Glucocorticosteroids

With the advent of more specific immunosuppressive drugs and monoclonal antibody treatment, the indications are less than they were previously. GCS are still the initiating treatment of choice for pemphigus, pemphigoid, and herpes gestationis. The mechanism of action that GCS have in these bullous disorders is still uncertain. They may eventually decrease antibody production but they also seem to have a direct effect on the local pathology.

Systemic GCS are also used in the collagenoses, systemic lupus erythematosus and dermatomyositis, vasculitis, eosinophilic faciitis, and relapsing polychondritis. Short courses of systemic GCS are also indicated for acute flares of widespread atopic and pompholyx eczema and acute contact eczema. The duration of treatment is often only 1 to 2 weeks for these flares. Oral GCS are also effective in acute polymorphic light eruption and pyoderma gangrenosum.

## C. Side Effects

### 1. Topical Use

The side effects on the skin are due to the breakdown of collagen and inhibition of the fibroblasts so that new collagen is not formed. As already mentioned, the side effects from topical steroids are proportional to the strength of steroid times duration of use. In addition, the anatomical site is important as the thinner the skin, the more likely that the side effects will occur. Clinically, the side effects are manifested as striae, erythema, telangiectasia, purpura, and ecchymoses. Reversal of these side effects following withdrawal of topical GCS is very slow and may take years.

It has been estimated that less than 2% of the topically applied GCS is absorbed into the circulation and, thus, systemic side effects are uncommon. However, if large areas of the skin are involved in the disease and potent GCS are used, then suppression of the pituitary–adrenal axis may occur and on rare occasions if the treatment is continued for long periods cushingoid features may be produced.

### 2. Intralesional Use

If too great a quantity of proprietary GCS preparations for intralesional use is injected into one site, e.g., 0.5 ml or more of the standard preparations, then atrophy of the dermis may occur, which clinically presents as depressions in the skin. Thus, 0.1 ml of the standard preparation should be used per injection site. Erythema and telangiectasia may also be seen.

### 3. Systemic GCS

There are numerous side effects associated with the use of systemic GCS but may well only be seen with long-term use. In addition, the higher the dose, the more likely the side effects. The clinical side effects can be divided into the various systems and/or organs.

**Musculoskeletal:** Osteoporosis with fractures particularly of the vertebra, myopathy and avascular necrosis particularly of the head of the femur

**Cardiovascular:** Hypertension; fluid retention

**Ophthalmic:** Glaucoma and cataracts

**Gastrointestinal:** Peptic ulceration and pancreatitis

**Endocrine and Metabolic:** Diabetes mellitus, truncal obesity, buffalo hump, fatty liver, acne, hirsuitism, suppression of growth in children, menstrual irregularities, negative balance of potassium, nitrogen and calcium, sodium retention, and secondary adrenal insufficiency

**Neuropsychiatric:** Confusional state, alteration in mood, benign intracranial hypertension

**Dermatological:** Thinning of the skin, ecchymosis, purpura, striae, facial redness, and telangiectasia

**Immunity/Infections:** Increased susceptibility to infections

## III. METHOTREXATE

Methotrexate (MTX) belongs to the antimetabolite group of drugs that were developed in the 1940s and 1950s for use in malignant neoplasms. MTX is a folic acid antagonist that was originally shown to be effective for leukemia and choriocarcinoma. It was first used in psoriasis in the 1960s when it was considered that psoriasis was due to a primary defect of mitosis in the keratinocytes leading to uncontrolled proliferation. It was subsequently shown that this was not the primary mechanism of action in psoriasis as it was shown that improvement in the histological features of psoriasis occurred prior to a fall in the mitotic index of the keratinocytes.[6]

MTX is an inhibitor of the dihydrofolate reductase and the folate-dependent enzymes of *de novo* purine and thymidylate synthesis. Thus, MTX will inhibit DNA synthesis by cells and is likely to have a greater effect on rapidly dividing cells. In normal individuals, MTX will affect the bone marrow and gastrointestinal epithelium and is likely to be effective in diseases associated with rapidly dividing cells. However, MTX will also suppress inflammatory immune disorders, as these are associated with proliferation of T lymphocytes, which will be inhibited or reduced by MTX. It is possible that MTX may have a dual action in psoriasis, affecting both the lymphocytes and the keratinocytes; although studies suggest that the main effect is via the immune system because, although the mitotic index is similar in the intestinal epithelial cells and keratinocytes of the psoriatic epidermis, the response of the proliferating cells at the two sites is different.[7] This suggests that the proliferation of the keratinocytes is under the control of the cytokines released by the activated T cells in psoriasis, whereas in the intestine it is the inherent nature of the epithelial cells, which is necessary to maintain the integrity of the epithelium.

### A. Indications

MTx is most commonly used for severe psoriasis, which is not controlled by topical measures or ultraviolet (UV) light regimens. It is also used in autoimmune disorders as a steroid-sparing drug, particularly in pemphigus. The mechanism of action in the latter may be on the T and B cells inhibiting antibody production.

### B. Dosage and Monitoring

Prior to commencing MTX it is essential that a full blood count, liver function tests, and renal functions tests be performed, and if they are not normal, MTX should not be given. MTX is excreted via the kidneys and if renal function is impaired there is an increased risk of hepatotoxicity and bone marrow suppression.

It is important to note that in dermatological conditions MTX is given weekly and not daily. It was shown more than 30 years ago that, if the same dose of MTX was given by infusion over a 24-h period compared to a single injection, the continuous exposure of the tissues to the drug was far more likely to induce tissue damage. However, the effect of MTX on proliferating cells when given weekly was sufficient to produce a clinical response.

A test dose of 5 mg (2.5 mg in elderly people) of MTX should be given and a full blood count and liver function test performed after 6 days; if these are satisfactory, the next weekly test dose may be given. The dose may be gradually increased until a satisfactory clinical response is achieved. The dose should not exceed 30 mg weekly. There is evidence that the hepatoxicity of MTX is dose related and, thus, the lower the dose, the less likely there is to be liver damage.

Patients established on a regular dose of MTX should be seen every 3 months and a full blood count and liver function tests performed.

## C. Side Effects

**Subjective:** Lethargy and nausea may occur in the first 24 to 48 h after taking MTX. These symptoms are often dose related and decreasing the dose may abolish the symptoms. If these side effects are severe, it may be necessary to discontinue treatment.

**Hepatotoxity:** MTX is hepatotoxic and this appears to be dose related. Transient rise of liver enzymes may occur 2 to 3 days after taking MTX but these elevated levels have usually returned to normal within a week. The long-term effects of continuous MTX treatment are of most concern, as fibrosis or even cirrhosis may occur. Liver function tests must be carried out before treatment and then at regular intervals. If liver function tests are persistently elevated, then referral to a hepatologist and liver biopsy is necessary. However, it has been shown that fibrosis may occur with normal routine liver function tests. Thus, the question of routine liver biopsies arises. It was previously suggested that liver biopsies should be performed before starting MTX for psoriasis and then performed yearly. These guidelines suggesting this frequency of liver biopsy are now thought to be overcautious. Rheumatology guidelines for the use of MTX in rheumatoid arthritis do not consider liver biopsies necessary.[8] Monitoring patients by measuring serum type III procollagen aminopeptide before and during treatment has been advocated as an alternative to liver biopsy.[9,10]

**Atherosclerosis:** Long-term MTX has been shown to raise the level of homocysteine in patients with rheumatoid arthritis.[11] Increased levels of homocysteine may promote atherosclerosis and thrombosis. In a study of patients with rheumatoid arthritis treated with MTX, there was an increase in cardiovascular co-morbidity, which was attributed to the raised level of homocysteine due to MTX.[12] This effect of MTX can be countered by giving patients folic acid and should be routine for those with psoriasis receiving long-term MTX.

**Bone Marrow Suppression:** This is a potential hazard, and regular monitoring with a full blood count is required while patients take MTX. As with all drugs that may affect DNA, there is a risk of malignant change in bone marrow cells leading to leukemia and lymphoma with long-term treatment; although this is more likely to occur in patients who are given high doses of MTX for malignant disease.

**Pregnancy:** Methotrexate is contraindicated in pregnancy, as it is mutagenic. It has been suggested that MTX may also affect oogenesis and spermatogenesis. However, studies on semen in patients with psoriasis treated with MTX have not shown any abnormalities.[13]

# IV. CALCINEURIN INHIBITORS

Currently there are three calcineurin inhibitors used for dermatological disorders. They are cyclosporine, tacrolimus, and pimecrolimus. They are immunosuppressive drugs and their main site of action is on activated T lymphocytes.

These drugs bind to immunophilins in the cytoplasm: cyclosporine to cyclophilin, tacrolimus and pimecrolimus to FK506-binding proteins, the FKBP-12 (macrophilin 12).[14] Once the drugs are bound to the immunophilins, they form a complex that binds to calcineurin, inhibiting calcium-stimulated dephosphorylation of the cytosolic component of the nuclear factor of activated T cells (NFAT).[15] Normally, when the cytoplasmic component of NFAT is dephosphorylated, it translocates to the nucleus, where it complexes with nuclear components required for complete T-cell activation, including transactivation of IL-2 and lymphokine genes. Calcineurin enzymatic activity is inhibited following physical interaction with the drug/immunophilins complex. This results in the blockade of NFAT dephosphorylation; thus, the cytoplasmic component of NFAT does not enter the nucleus, gene transcription is not activated, and the T cell fails to respond to antigenic stimulation.

The calcineurin inhibitors not only decrease the production of Th1 cytokines (IL-2 and IFN-$\gamma$) but also the Th 2 cytokines (IL-4, IL-5, and IL-10).

## A. Cyclosporine

Cyclosporine (CyA) is a neutral lipophilic cyclic polypeptide and was isolated from the fungus *Tolypocladium inflatum* in 1972. Then, 4 years later Borel and colleagues[16] reported the immunosuppressive action of CyA and its apparent selective action on T-cell-dependent immune response. CyA revolutionized transplantation by improving survival of the donor organ to an extent that had not been possible with previous available immunosuppressive drugs.

### 1. Indications

The primary indication for CyA is psoriasis. Since it was suggested that psoriasis was a T-cell-mediated disorder,[17] it was logical to use CyA. CyA is indicated when the psoriasis is either extensive or incapacitating (e.g., involvement of the palms and soles) and is nonresponsive to topical measures and UV light regimens. CyA is also effective in severe atopic eczema, and it has been used in both children and adults. It is also effective in pyoderma gangrenosum and lichen planus; although it is only indicated if other measures are not successful.

### 2. Dosage

The initial dose of CyA for dermatological conditions should be 3 mg/kg/day. The dose may be titrated up or down depending on the clinical response and side effects but it should not exceed 5 mg/kg/day.

### 3. Side Effects

These two main side effects are nephrotoxicity and hypertension. It is important that patients be monitored on a regular basis, i.e., every 2 to 3 months, to check the renal function and blood pressure. Both these side effects are dose and duration related, but as with most biological responses to drugs, there is considerable patient variability in the degree of toxicity and the time when it becomes manifest. In a cohort of patients with psoriasis followed up for a period of 5 years, 50% had evidence of nephrotoxicity and, at 10 years, all patients showed this effect.[18]

Because CyA is a potent immunosuppressive drug, there are risks to patients from this effect. The greatest concern is of the risk of developing malignancy. It is well known that, in patients who have undergone organ transplantation and received long-term immunosuppressive medication, there is an increased incidence of malignancy, particularly lymphoma and skin malignancies. It has recently been shown that in patients with psoriasis treated with CyA for as long as 5 years, there is an increased incidence of nonmelanoma skin cancers.[19] This increase was greater in patients who had preceding photochemotherapy and had taken other immunosuppressive drugs.

## B. Tacrolimus

Tacrolimus was isolated from *Streptomyces tsukubaensis* in 1984. It is a macrolide with immunosuppressive properties 10 to 100 times greater than CyA *in vitro*. Its mechanism of action has been described above and it is classified as a calcineurin inhibitor.

The toxicity of tacrolimus is greater than CyA and, although its use in transplantation can be justified, it is considered to be too toxic for dermatological conditions such as psoriasis and eczema. The main toxic effects are: nephrotoxicity, gastrointestinal problems, hypertension, hyperkalemia, hyperglycemia, and diabetes. The last is considered to be due to a negative effect on the pancreatic islet beta cells. As with other immunosuppressive drugs, there is an increased risk of malignant neoplasms and opportunistic infections.

Unlike CyA, topical tacrolimus is absorbed into the skin and has been shown to have a beneficial effect on atopic eczema but not psoriasis. This may be due to the different properties of the stratum corneum in psoriasis.

It is accepted that activated T cells are an essential feature of atopic eczema and, therefore, tacrolimus would be expected to be effective in atopic eczema. However, it has been claimed that topical tacrolimus also has an inhibitory effect on dendritic cells, which are also increased and activated in atopic eczema.[20] Whether this is a primary effect on dendritic cells or whether it is secondary to the downregulation of cytokine production by the T cells is also a possibility.

Topical tacrolimus has been shown to be effective in the treatment of atopic eczema when compared to placebo.[21,22] Two strengths of topical tacrolimus are available: the 0.03% ointment and the 0.1% ointment. Both strengths produce a significant improvement in eczema, but the stronger preparation is more effective.[21] The efficacy of tacrolimus has been shown to be greater than 1% hydrocortisone acetate (a weak topical corticosteroids)[23] and approximately the same as 0.1% hydrocortisone butyrate, a moderate strength topical.[24]

The most commonly seen side effect of topical tacrolimus is a transient burning or itching sensation at the site of application, but this usually stops after a few days despite treatment being continued. Other side effects include flu-like symptoms, skin erythema, and headache. Studies on blood levels of tacrolimus in patients with 5 to 60% of the body affected by atopic eczema did not show any significant absorption. With the weaker concentration of topical tacrolimus (0.03% ointment) only 1.6% of patients, and in the stronger concentration (0.1% ointment) 11.3% of patients, showed a concentration of 1 ng/ml or greater. The highest value recorded was 2.8 ng/ml in the 0.1% ointment. These figures were taken to be minimal and not likely to cause any toxicity.[25]

As a result of the trials on topical tacrolimus, it has been suggested that this preparation is suitable for treatment of atopic eczema on the face and intertrigenous areas, sites where potent topical steroids should not be used because of the risk of dermal atrophy. This side effect is not seen with topical tacrolimus and is considered appropriate for these sites.[23–25] However, what these latter authors do not discuss is the possibility of skin neoplasms from the long-term use of topical immunosuppressive drugs, such as tacrolimus. It is known that long-term treatment with systemic immunosuppressive agents will increase the risk of skin malignancies. If the concentration of the topically applied agent (tacrolimus) in the skin is the same as that from oral intake, then the risk of malignancy in the skin may be similar. As yet, there are no published figures comparing the concentration of tacrolimus in the skin when given orally or used topically in therapeutic doses. Development of skin cancers is not usually seen for many years after initiation and prolonged use of immunosuppressive drugs. However, what is not known is whether these malignancies only develop with long-term and continuous use or whether a short period of exposure to these drugs might be able to induce a malignant clone of cells, which only manifests as a clinical malignant lesion years later. If the latter situation is biologically feasible, then the risk of developing malignant neoplasms with topical immunosuppressive drugs becomes more likely.

Although topical tacrolimus is so far licensed only for the treatment of atopic eczema, there are reports of it being beneficial in vitiligo, alopecia areata, and oral lichen planus. These are uncontrolled studies and controlled studies are needed to evaluate the use of topical tacrolimus in the above conditions. Providing it is absorbed into the skin, it should prove effective in T-cell-mediated disorders.

## C. Pimecrolimus

Pimecrolimus (SDZ ASM 981) has been developed as a topical immunosuppressive drug as cyclosporine is not absorbed into the skin. Pimecrolimus inhibits the production of both Th1 and Th2 cytokines and has also been reported to inhibit mediator release from human dermal mast cells and peripheral blood eosinophils.[26]

Pimecrolimus 1% cream has been shown to be effective in atopic dermatitis compared to vehicle alone in children[27–29] and adults.[30] However, it was less effective than the potent topical steroid betamethasone-17-valerate.[30] The most common side effect with topical pimecrolimus is a burning sensation at the site of initial application, which was transitory in nature. The symptoms disappeared with subsequent applications. No serious side effects have been reported and blood levels have been found to be low and considered not to be hazardous.[27]

The indications for topical pimcrolimus are the same as for topical tacrolimus. As yet, there has been no study comparing these two preparations to see which is more effective. The potential long-term risk for skin malignancies applies to pimecrolimus because of its immunosuppressive action.

Pimecrolimus has also recently been used orally in a placebo-controlled trial in psoriasis.[31] It was found to be highly effective when given for 4 weeks. The drug was well tolerated and there were no serious side effects reported. However, only long-term studies will determine the safety profile of the drug. Whether there are any specific toxicity effects as with tacrolimus and cyclosporine will emerge with time, but the side effects of long-term immunosuppression will certainly exist.

## V. AZATHIOPRINE

6-Mercaptopurine (6-MP) was developed as an antileukemic drug in the 1940s by Ellion and Hitchings (for which they were awarded the Noble prize). It was subsequently shown that 6-MP has immunosuppressive properties.[32] A 6-MP derivative — 6-(I-methyl-4-nitro-5-imidazolyl) thiopurine — named azathioprine was the most widely used immunosuppressive drug until 1979 when cyclosporine was introduced for transplantation. Azathioprine is cleaved to 6-MP by red blood cell gluthathione. 6-MP is then converted into a series of mercaptopurine-containing nucleotides, among them thioguanylic acid, which interferes with DNA synthesis and polyadenylate-containing RNA. Thioguanylic acid leads to thioguanosine triphosphate and its derivative, which can be incorporated into nucleic acid and produce chromosome breaks.[33] By interfering with DNA synthesis and mitosis, azathioprine will affect the proliferation of both T and B lymphocytes. However, thiopurines seem to be selective in blocking immune responses; the primary rather than the secondary response is more susceptible.[34]

### A. Indications

In dermatology, azathioprine has been used mainly in autoimmune bullous disorders, in an attempt to lower the dose of corticosteroids required to control the eruption. It is often used routinely in pemphigus and pemphigoid in combination with corticosteroids. It has also been used in cicatricial pemphigoid and adult linear IgA disease, but its benefit in these disorders is less clear-cut and most of the reports are anecdotal rather than controlled studies. Prior to cyclosporine, azathioprine was used in psoriasis and eczema, particularly photosensitive eczema in adults (so-called actinic reticuloids). The clinical response to cyclosporine is superior in these latter two disorders compared to azathioprine, and thus azathioprine is now very rarely used for eczema and psoriasis.

### B. Dosage

The dose of azathioprine in pemphigus and pemphigoid is 1 to 2 mg/kg/day. In pemphigus, in particular, treatment with azathioprine must be considered long term, and it is not uncommon to try and reduce the dose or even stop corticosteroids while continuing with azathioprine. It is important to measure the serum thiopurine methyl fransterase level before commencing treatment. If this enzyme is low, it will result in an increased incidence of side effects due to azathioprine.

### C. Side Effects

The main side effect of azathioprine is bone marrow suppression; neutropenia is the most common side effect. The toxic effect on bone marrow may be delayed, and if the white count falls to 3000 then the drug should be discontinued. Thus, regular blood counts are necessary during treatment particularly at the beginning of therapy.

Hepatotoxicity has also been described with azathioprine, and therefore regular liver function tests should also be preformed.

Patients receiving azathioprine particularly with corticosteroids are immunosuppressed and, therefore, more susceptible to infections. In long-term use, as with most form of immunosuppression, there is an increased risk of malignancies, particularly skin cancers and lymphomas.

## VI. CYCLOPHOSPHAMIDE

Cyclophosphamide is an alkylating agent and belongs to the group of drugs known as nitrogen mustards. The drug has the ability to interfere with mitosis in rapidly dividing cells.[35] Its site of action is on the S phase (DNA synthesis) of the cell cycle, and the cells are subsequently blocked in G2. Cyclophosphamide blocks both humoral and cellular immunological responses[36] and has a significant effect on antibody production.[37]

Although the primary action of cyclophosphamide is inhibition of DNA synthesis, it has a cytotoxic action, which may result in death. This cytotoxicity is due to metabolites of cyclophosphamide, phospharamide, and acrolein.

### A. Indications

Cyclophosphamide is mainly used in combination with other drugs as an anticancer drug, particularly in lymphomas. In dermatology, it has been used after plasmaphoresis in pemphigus to decrease subsequent antibody formation. It can be used with steroids in autoimmune disorders such as pemphigus, cicatricial pemphigoid, and systemic lupus erythematosus.

### B. Dosage

As an immunosuppressive agent, the dose is 2 to 3 mg/kg/day. Higher doses have been used in transplantation and in the treatment of cancer.

### C. Side Effects

Bone marrow suppression is the most common side effect with the principal effect on precursors of polymorphonuclear cells, although red blood cell and platelet precursors may also be affected. Nausea and vomiting are not uncommon and mucosal ulceration of the GI tract may occur. The drug has a relatively high potential for inducing sterility, mutations, and cancers; it is also teratogenic. Hemorrhagic cystitis is a well-recognized complication. Its use in children and pregnancy should be avoided.

## VII. MYCOPHENOLATE MOFETIL

Mycophenolate mofetil (MMF) is a prodrug that is hydrolyzed to the active drug mycophenolic acid (MPA). MPA acid was introduced as an anticancer drug in the early 1970s and was first used for psoriasis in 1975.[38] The drug was shown to be effective, but its use for psoriasis was not pursued because of its gastrointestinal side effects. MMF, an ester of MPA, was synthesized, introduced as an immunosuppressive in the early 1990s,[39] and was found to have fewer gastrointestinal side effects than MPA.

MPA is a selective, uncompetitive, and reversible inhibitor of monophosphate dehydrogenase, an important enzyme in the *de novo* pathway of guanine nucleotide synthesis. B and T cells are highly dependent on this pathway for cell proliferation, while other cell types can use salvage pathways. MPA, therefore, selectively inhibits lymphocyte proliferation and function, including antibody formation, cellular adhesion, and migration.

### A. Indications

MMF is used primarily in transplantation to stop rejection. In dermatology, it has been used with good effect in psoriasis, atopic eczema, and pemphigus. It should be effective in T-cell-mediated disorders and those autoimmune diseases where the antibodies are pathogenic. However, in psoriasis it does not appear to be as effective as cyclosporine.[40] MMF may have a place in the treatment of patients with psoriasis who cannot tolerate methotrexate or cyclosporine or who have significant hepatotoxicity from methotrexate and nephrotoxicity from cyclosporine.

### B. Dosage

The initial dose of MMF is 1 G bd and this may be increased to 1.5 G bd if the clinical response is not satisfactory.

### C. Side Effects

The two main side effects are gastrointestinal (diarrhea, nausea, and vomiting) and hematological (suppression of the bone marrow with leukopenia common). There is also an increased risk of infections, especially cytomegalovirus. As with the immunosuppressive drugs, the long-term risk of malignancy exists.

## VIII. IMIQUIMOD

Imiquimod and resiquimod (R-848) belong to the imidazoquinoline amine family, which has been termed immune response modifiers (IRM). They are reported to have antiviral and antitumor activity.

Imiquimod has been shown to act via the TLR-7 receptor (Toll-like receptor 7),[41] which is part of the innate immune system. Once bound to the receptor, signaling via IkB and NF-κB results in induction of gene transcription in the nucleus for IFN-α, TNF-α, and IL-12. The cells, which express TLR-7 and respond to IRM, are dendritic cells, macrophages, and monocytes.[42] The production of these cytokines activates natural killer cells of the innate immune system and induces production of IFN-γ, which upregulates acquired cell-mediated immunity.

In a study on peripheral blood mononuclear cells, imiquimod was also shown to induce the cytokines IL-1, IL-6, IL-8, and IL-10.[43] It has no effect on the T-cell growth factors IL-2 or IL-4.

Thus, the IRM imidazoquinoline amines affect both the innate and acquired immunity systems and it is these actions that are used for the treatment of both viral diseases and neoplasms.

### A. Indications

#### 1. Viral Infections

Imiquimod has been licensed for the treatment of anogenital warts and is an effective treatment for these lesions. Imiquimod has also been used for viral warts elsewhere with varied results. The failure with imiquimod to treat viral warts successfully appears to be due to the inability of the drug to penetrate thick keratotic surfaces. Attempts to improve these results have led to the use of occlusion and salicylic acid in combination with imiquimod.[44]

The IRM drug resiquimod has been shown to reduce genital recurrences in herpes simplex infection in guinea pigs.[45] If this result can be repeated for humans, it would be helpful in the management of patients with this disorder.

There are also reports that imiquimod is helpful in treating molluscum contagiosum in both immunocompetent subjects[46] and in HIV-infected persons.[47]

### 2. Malignancies

Imiquimod has been shown to have antitumor properties in animal studies. In humans, it has been claimed in phase II trials carried out by the drug company that markets imiquimod that there was an 87% complete response rate in superficial basal cell carcinomas and this was histologically proven.[48]

It has been claimed that in basal cell carcinomas there is downregulation of ICAM-1, IL-10, FasL, and BCL-2. This downregulation has been termed an "escape mechanism," which does not allow T cells to function and clear the lesion. Imiquimod, by upregulating cytokine production, counteracts the escape mechanisms and allows the immune system to eradicate the tumor.[49]

Imiquimod has been used for the treatment of actinic keratoses with success rates higher than 80% claimed.[50,51] One of the disadvantages of imiquimod in the treatment of actinic keratoses is the length of time that treatment has to be used. In the study by Stockfleth et al.,[51] treatment was three times a week for 12 weeks, while in the study by Salasche et al.[50] imiquimod was applied three times a week for 4 weeks and then another treatment period for 4 weeks, if the actinic keratoses has not cleared in the first course. In fact, total clearance was achieved in 46% of patients after one 4-week treatment period and in 82% after the second period.

Reports are now appearing of the use of imiquimod in a variety of other premalignant and malignant conditions including lentigo maligna,[52] extra mammary Paget's disease,[53] and mycosis fungoides.[54]

Imiquimod has been used in HIV immunosuppressed patients to treat HPV warts, molluscum contagiosum, bowenoid papulosis, and cervical neoplasia.

## B. Side Effects

The mechanism of action of imiquimod depends on cytokine production, which generates an inflammatory reaction and subsequent clearance of the lesion. Clinically, there is erythema of the lesion and surrounding skin and, subsequently, edema and induration and, finally, erosions, crusting, and ulceration of the lesions. All patients will experience some side effects. These side effects may appear as early as the second week of treatment peaking at 6 weeks. The side effects settle promptly when treatment is discontinued.

## C. Future Role of Imiquimod

The role of imiquimod in viral, dysplastic, and neoplastic conditions has yet to be determined. One of the problems is the length of time required to successfully treat lesions like actinic keratoses and superficial basal cell carcinomas. In addition, long-term data on the recurrence rates following treatment of these conditions are necessary before advising imiquimod as opposed to the standard treatments for actinic keratoses and superficial basal cell carcinomas.

# IX. CONCLUSION

The drugs discussed in this chapter are all immunosuppressive except imiquimod, which could be claimed to be an immunostimulator. Many of the common skin diseases seen in dermatological clinics, e.g., eczema, psoriasis, and lichen planus, are immunologically mediated and, thus, immunosuppressive drugs will have a beneficial effect. However, the immune mechanisms in these disorders may not represent the primary abnormality so that when these drugs are discontinued the diseases usually relapse. It is well known and accepted that the state of immunosuppression may lead to other disorders, e.g., infections and malignancies. Even the newer treatments with monoclonal antibodies directed against certain cytokines or their receptors are not specific enough for psoriasis and eczema. They are also effective in many other immunologically mediated disorders such as rheumatoid arthritis and Crohn's disease.

Thus, the answer to eczema and psoriasis is not going to be immunosuppression but more specific therapies that will not interfere with the immune system or any other vital functions, which may have a deleterious effect. These newer treatments will depend on a greater understanding of the pathogenetic mechanisms involved in these common disorders.

Immunostimulation by drug treatment is a newer concept and shows promise for the treatment of viral diseases and malignancy. Newer and more effective drugs than imiquimod may well play a role in the future management of viral and malignant disorders.

## REFERENCES


1. Claman, N.N., Corticosteroids as immunomodulators. *Ann. N.Y. Acad. Sci.,* 685, 288, 1993.
2. Auphan, N., Didarato, J.A., Caridad, R., Helmberg, A., and Karin, M., Immunosuppression by glucosteroids inhibition of NF-kB, activity through induction of IkB synthesis. *Science,* 270, 286, 1995.
3. Elenkov, I.J. and Chrousos, G.P., Stress hormones, Th1/Th2 patterns pro/anti inflammatory cytokines and susceptibility to disease. *Trends Endocrinol. Metab.*, 10, 359, 1999.
4. Werb, Z., Biochemical actions of glucosteroids on macrophages in culture: specific inhibitions of elastase, collagenase, and plasminogen activator secretions. *J. Exp. Med.,* 147, 1695, 1978.
5. Schleimer, R.P., Glucocorticosteroids; their mechanism of action and use in allergic diseases, in *Allergy, Principles and Practice,* 3rd ed., Middleton, E., Reed, C.E., and Ellis, E.F., Eds., C.V. Mosby, St. Louis, MO, 1992, 739.
6. Fry, L., The nature of psoriasis. *Br. J. Dermatol.,* 80, 833, 1968.
7. Fry, L. and McMinn, R.M.H., Action of methotrexate on the skin and intestinal mucosa. *Arch. Dermatol.*, 93, 726, 1966.
8. Kremer, J., Alarcom, G., Lightfoot, R. et al., Methotrexate for rheumatoid arthritis: suggested guidelines for measuring liver toxicity. *Arthritis Rheum.,* 37, 316, 1994.
9. Zachariae, H., Heinkendorff, L., and Sogaard, H., The value of amino-terminal propeptide of type III procollagen in routine screening for methotrexate-induced liver fibrosis: a ten-year follow-up. *Br. J. Dermatol.,* 143, 100, 2001.
10. Boffa, M.J., Smith, A., and Chalmers, R.J.G., Serum type III procollagen aminopeptide for assessing liver damage in methotrexate treated patients. *Br. J. Dermatol.,* 135, 538, 1996.
11. Haagsma, C.J., Bloom, H.J., Riel, P.L.C.M. van et al., Influence of sulfasalazine methotrexate and the combination of both on plasma homocysteine concentration in patients with rheumatoid arthritis. *Ann. Rheum. Dis.*, 58; 79. 1999.
12. Andeure, R.B.M., van den Borne, B.E.E.M., Breedveld, F.C., and Dijkmans, B.A.C., Methotrexate effects in patients with rheumatoid arthritis with cardiovascular co-morbidity. *Lancet,* 355, 1616, 2000.
13. Zachariae, H., Methotrexate, in *Textbook of Psoriasis*, Van de Kerkhof, P., Ed., Blackwell Science, Oxford, 196–232, 2003.
14. Grassberger, M., Baumruker, T., Enz, A. et al., SDZASM 981, for the treatment of skin diseases, *in vitro* pharmacology. *Br. J. Dermatol.,* 141, 264, 1999.
15. Schreiber, S.L. and Crabtree, G.R., The mechanism of action of cyclosporin A and FK 506. *Immunol. Today,* 13, 136, 1992.
16. Borel, J.F., Feurer, C., Gubler, H.U., and Stahelin, H., Biological effect of cyclosporin A: a new antilymphocytic agent. *Agents Action,* 6, 468, 1976.
17. Valdimarsson, H., Baker, B.S., Jonsdottir, I., and Fry, L., Psoriasis: a disease of abnormal keratinocytes proliferation induced by lymphocytes. *Immunol. Today,* 13, 136, 1986.
18. Powles, A.V., Hardman, C.M., Porter, V.M. et al., Renal function after 10 years treatment with cyclosporin for psoriasis. *Br. J Dermatol.,* 138, 443, 1998.
19. Paul, C.G., Ho, V.C., McGowan, C. et al., Risk of malignancies in psoriasis patients treated with cyclosporin: a 5-year cohort study. *J. Invest. Dermatol.,* 120, 211, 2003.
20. Wollenberg, A., Sharma, S., Von Bubnoff, D. et al., Topical Tacrolimus (FK506) leads to profound phenotypic and functional alterations of epidermal antigen-presenting dendritic cells in atopic eczema. *J. Allergy Clin. Immunol.,* 107; 519, 2001.

21. Hanifin, J.M., Ling, M.R., Langley, R. et al., Tacrolimus ointment for the treatment of atopic dermatitis in adult patients. Part 1, efficacy. *J. Am. Acad. Dermatol.*, 44, 28, 2001.
22. Paller, A.P., Eichenfield, L.F., Leung, D.Y.M. et al., A 12-week study of tacrolimus ointment for the treatment of atopic dermatitis in pediatric patients. *J. Am. Acad. Dermatol.,* 44, 547, 2001.
23. Reitamo, S., Van Leent, E.J.M., Ho, V. et al., Efficacy and safety of tacrolimus ointment compared with that of hydrocortisone acetate ointment in children with atopic dermatitis. *J. Allergy Clin. Immunol.,* 109, 539, 2002.
24. Reitamo, S., Rustin, M., Ruzicka, T. et al., Efficacy and safety of tacrolimus ointment compared with that of hydrocortisone butyrate ointment in adult patients with atopic dermatitis. *J. Allergy Clin. Immunol.,* 109, 547, 2002.
25. Soter, N.A., Fleischler, A.B., Webster, G.F. et al., Tacrolimus ointment for the treatment of atopic dermatitis in adult patients: Part II, safety. *J. Am. Acad. Dermatol.*, 44, S39, 2001.
26. Zuberbier, T., Chang, S.U., Grunow, K. et al., The ascomycin macrolactam primecrolimus (Elidel, SDZ ASM 981) is a potent-inhibitor of mediator release from human dermal mast cells and peripheral blood basophils. *J. Allergy Clin. Immunol.,* 108, 275, 2001.
27. Harper, J., Green, A., Scott, E. et al., First experience of topical SDZ ASM 981 in children with atopic dermatitis. *Br. J. Dermatol.,* 144, 178, 2001.
28. Kapp, A., Papp, K., Bingham, A. et al., Long-term management of atopic dermatitis in infants with topical pimecrolimus, a non-steroid anti-inflammatory drug. *J. Allergy Clin. Immunol.*, 110, 277, 2002.
29. Eichenfield, L.F., Lucky, A.W., Boguniewicz, M. et al., Safety and efficacy of pimecrolimus (ASM 981) cream in the treatment of mild to moderate atopic dermatitis in children and adolescents. *Am. J. Acad. Dermatol.,* 46, 504, 2002.
30. Luger, T., Van Leent, E.J.M., Graeber, M. et al., SDZ ASM 981: an emerging safe and effective treatment for atopic dermatitis. *Br. J. Dermatol.,* 144, 788, 2001.
31. Rappersberger, K., Kormat, M., Ebelin, M.E. et al., Pimecrolimus identifies a common genomic anti-inflammatory profile, is clinically highly effective in psoriasis and is well-tolerated. *J. Invest. Dermatol.,* 119, 876, 2002.
32. Schwartz, R. and Damashek, W., Drug induced immunological tolerance. *Nature,* 183, 1682, 1959.
33. Marino, I.R. and Doyle, H.R., Conventional immunosuppressive drugs, in *Immunosuppressive Drugs,* Thomas, A.W. and Starzl, T.E., Eds., Edward Arnold, London, 1994, chap. 1.
34. Schwartz, R.S., Eisner, A., and Dameshek, W., The effect of 6-mercaptopurine on primary and secondary immune responses. *J. Clin. Invest.,* 38, 1394, 1959.
35. Calabresi, P. and Chabner, B.A., Chemotherapy of neoplastic diseases, in *The Pharmacological Basis of Therapeutics*, Gilman, A.G., Rall, T.W., Nies, A.S., and Taylor, P., Eds., Pergamon Press, New York, 1990, chap. 52.
36. Turk, J.L., Studies on the mechanism of action of methotrexate and cyclophosphamide on contact sensitivity in the guinea pig. *Int. Arch. Allergy,* 24, 191, 1964.
37. Stender, H.S., Ringleb, D., Strauch, D., and Winter, H., Die Beeinflussung der Antikorpebildung durch Zytostatika und Rontgenbestrahlung. *Strahlen Ther.,* 43, 392, 1959.
38. Jones, E.L., Eppinette, W.W., Hackney, V.C. et al., Treatment of psoriasis with oral mycophenolic acid. *J. Invest. Dermatol.,* 65, 537, 1975.
39. Allison, A.C. and Eugui, E.M., Immunosuppressive and other effects of mycophenolic acid and an ester prodrug, mycophenolate mofetil. *Immunol. Rev.*, 136, 5, 1993.
40. Davison, S.C., Morris-Jones, R., Powles, A.V., and Fry, L., Change of treatment from cyclosporin to mycophenolate mofetil in severe psoriasis. *Br. J. Dermatol.,* 143, 405, 2000.
41. Hemmi, H.T., Kaisho, O., Takeuchi, S. et al., Small anti-viral compounds activate immune cells via TLR7 MyD88-dependent signalling pathways. *Nat. Immunol.*, 3, 196, 2002.
42. Ito, T., Amakawa, R., Kaisho, T. et al., Interferon alpha and interleukin-12 are induced differentially by T cell-like receptor 7 ligands in human blood dendritic cell types. *J. Exp. Med.,* 195, 1507, 2002.
43. Gibson, S.J., Imbertson, L.M., Wagner, T.L. et al., Cellular requirements for cytokine production in response to the immunomodulators Imiquimod and S 27609. *J. Interferon Cytokine Res.,* 15, 337, 1995.
44. Tucker, S.B., Ali, A., and Ransdell, B.L., Plantar wart treatment with combination Imiquimod and salicylic acid. *J. Drugs Dermatol.,* 2, 70, 2003.

45. Bernstein, D.I., Harrison, C.J., Tomai, M.A., and Miller, L., Daily or weekly therapy with resiquimod (R-484) reduces genital recurrences in herpes simplex virus–infected guinea pigs during and after treatment. *J. Infect. Dis.,* 183, 844, 2001.
46. Edward, L., Imiquimod in clinical practice. *J. Am. Acad. Dermatol*., 43, 12–17, 2000.
47. Conant, M., Immunomodulatory therapy in the management of viral infections in patients with HIV infection. *J. Am. Acad. Dermatol.,* 43, 527, 2000.
48. Cornelson, R.L., Pivotal data and experience of imiquimod in superficial basal cell carcinoma, presented at Satellite Symposium, British Association Dermatology Meeting. Brighton, 2003 (abstr.).
49. Miller, R.L., Updated mode of action of immune response modifiers, presented at Satellite Symposium, British Association of Dermatology Meeting. Brighton, 2003 (abstr.).
50. Salasche, S.J., Levine, N., and Morrison, L., Cycle therapy of actinic keratoses of the face and scalp with 5% imiquimod cream: an open trial. *J. Am. Acad. Dermatol.,* 47, 571, 2002.
51. Stockfleth, E., Meyer, T., Benninghoff, B. et al., A randomised, double blind vehicle controlled stuffy to assess 5% Imiquimod cream for the treatment of multiple actinic keratoses. *Arch. Dermatol.,* 138, 1498, 2002.
52. Chapman, M.S., Spencer, M.K., and Brennick, J.B., Histological resolution of melanoma *in situ* (lentigo maligna) with 5% imiquimod cream. *Arch. Dermatol*., 139, 943, 2003.
53. Qian, Z., Zeitoun, N.C., Shieh, S. et al., Successful treatment of extra mammary Paget's disease with Imiquimod. *J. Drugs Dermatol.,* 2, 73, 2003.
54. Dummer, R., Unosevic, M., Kempt, W. et al., Imiquimod induces complete clearance of a PUVA resistant plaque in mycosis fungoides. *Dermatology,* 207, 2003.

# 38 Therapeutic Manipulation of the Complement System in Dermatology

*Syed Shafi Asghar*

## CONTENTS



0-8493-1959-5/05/$0.00+$1.50

# I. INTRODUCTION

The complement (C) system is one of the most powerful immunological effectors involved in the body's defenses. This system has briefly been described by Asghar and co-workers in Chapter 14 of this volume and has been reviewed in detail elsewhere.[1–3] In normal individuals this system remains dormant except for a very low level continuous activation of alternative pathway. In a wide variety of diseases, however, such as infectious, immune complex, and autoimmune diseases and some immunodeficiency diseases (e.g., factor H and factor I deficiencies) there is extensive activation of plasma C. In some diseases C is activated for a long or indefinite time, while in others for a short time; in some it is activated systemically, in others locally; in some the whole cascade is activated, in others only few components are activated. In some diseases the classical, lectin, or alternative pathway is activated; in others more than one pathway is activated. In many diseases the otherwise advantageous biological activities of C fragments become detrimental, resulting in tissue injury and disease.

It is believed that the inhibition of early steps of C in classical-, lectin-, or alternative-pathway-mediated diseases by C inhibitors will suppress the disease process. From this point of view, some laboratories are engaged in the development of low-molecular-weight synthetic inhibitors whereas others are developing high-molecular-weight natural human C inhibitors and their recombinant forms for therapeutic purposes.

# II. LOW-MOLECULAR-WEIGHT INHIBITORS

An extensive review of the earlier literature on low-molecular-weight C inhibitors has been presented by Asghar.[4] Several compounds have been shown to inhibit C *in vitro* and *in vivo* and some of them have been shown to suppress complement-mediated diseases in several experimental models. After the appearance of the above review, some additional low-molecular-weight inhibitors of C have been developed. They include sulfated and acetylated low-molecular-weight heparin (heptasulfated hexasaccharide; Hep-NAc),[5] a natural product of fungal origin, namely, terpenoid 6,7-diformyl-3′,4′,4a′,5′,6′, 7′,8′,8a′-octahydro-4,6′,7′-trihydroxy-25′,5′,8a′-tetramethylspirol (1′(2′H)-naphthalene-2(3H)-benzofuran) referred to as K-76 and its monocarboxylate sodium salt K76COONa,[6] several A/C/D-ring analogues of K 76COONa,[7] a derivative of earlier described serine protease inhibitor compound FUT 175,[4] namely, 6-amidino-2-naphthyl-4-((4,5-di-hydro-1H-imidazole-2-yl) amino)-benzoate (FUT 187)[8] and a natural pentacyclic triterpene known as boswellic acid.[9] Recently, a highly selective peptidomimetic low-molecular-weight (m.w. 520.5) inhibitor (C1s-INH-248)[10] derived from thrombin inhibitor D-Phe-Pro-Arg has been developed (under patent) that inhibits C1r and C1s but not MASP-1 and other serine esterases such as Xa and XIIa. This compound was active *in vivo* as seen by its ability to inhibit ischemia and reperfusion injury that requires C. A C3-binding 13-amino acid residue cyclic compound, complastatin, inhibited C3 activation in primates[11] and prolonged survival of *ex vivo* perfused xenograft,[12] suggesting that this compound inhibits C *in vivo* and may have potential for various clinical applications.

Attempts have been made to produce C5a-receptor antagonists.[13] These attempts have largely been unsuccessful because of the associated agonistic activity in the newly developed molecules. Some of the C5a-receptor antagonists were peptides. Short peptides had the disadvantage of short half-life *in vivo*. Cyclic peptides may have a longer half-life but at least one of them, L-156,602, a 19-membered cyclic hexapeptide, had associated agonistic activity; others need thorough testing. Two synthetic compounds, RPR-121154 (phenylguanidine) and L-584,020 (a substituted 4,6-diaminoquinoline) were found to possess strong C5a-receptor antagonistic activity without associated agonistic activity. They also inhibit interleukin-8 (IL-8) binding to its receptor. This additional activity calls into question the specificity of antagonism but may perhaps be an added advantage in suppressing inflammation. Konteatis et al.[14] have produced a hexapeptide NMePhe-Lys-Pro-dCha-Trp-dArg-COOH (NMePhe = *N*-methylphenylalanine, Cha = cyclohexylalanine), namely,

C089 that inhibited C5a-induced degranulation of neutrophils and G protein activation and was free of the agonist activity in the assay systems used. Recently, several low-molecular-weight peptidic and cyclic C5a-receptor antagonists were synthesized, the most potent of which was a hexapeptide-derived compound AcPh [Orn-Pro-D-cyclohexylalanine-Trp-Arg], also referred to as AcF(OPdChaWR).[15] This compound inhibited C *in vivo* as seen by its ability to suppress antigen-induced monoarticular arthritis,[16] immune-complex-mediated dermal inflammation,[17] and ischemia/reperfusion injury[18] in rat models. It is hoped that C089 and AcF(OPdChaWR) will inhibit all the diverse activities of C5a, which is excessively generated in several inflammatory diseases such as systemic lupus erythematosus (SLE)[19] and psoriasis.[20,21]

Recently, two low-molecular-weight inhibitors of factor D, BCX-1470[22] and 3,4-dichloroisocoumarin,[23] were developed that inhibit this enzyme by binding to its active site. BCX-1470 also binds to C1s and inhibits the development of reverse passive Arthus reaction–induced edema in rat.[24] 3,4-Dichloroisocoumarin inhibits most serine proteases and many esterases. In view of the limited number of known inhibitors of factor D and lack of their specificity, development of specific, reversible, and relatively nontoxic inhibitors of this enzyme to suppress alternative-pathway-mediated disease processes remains a highly desirable task.

All these newly described C inhibitors inhibit C *in vitro* and *in vivo*. They, except C089, RPR-121154, and L-584,020, have been tested and shown to inhibit experimental models of C-mediated diseases. The possible use of some of the above-mentioned compounds in human skin diseases has to await further toxicity and pharmacokinetic studies.

Development of low-molecular-weight inhibitors of C for use in human diseases has been slow. This led to the development of high-molecular-weight C-inhibitory biomolecules some of which are already in clinical use. Because they are natural molecules, many of them are nontoxic and have minimal side effects, if any.

## III. HIGH-MOLECULAR-WEIGHT BIOMOLECULES THAT INHIBIT COMPLEMENT

### A. C1-Inhibitor (C1-INH)

The regulation of C at C1 stage is abrogated most prominently in the genetic deficiency of C1-INH, which leads to a disease known as hereditary angioneurotic edema (HANE). Asghar and coworkers (Chapter 14) have briefly described HANE. C1-inhibitor levels are decreased also in some severe inflammatory situations such as in patients with cancer undergoing immunotherapy with IL-2, sepsis, and burn. C1-INH has been tried and found to be beneficial in these situations.

#### 1. Treatment of HANE

C1-INH concentrates prepared from normal plasma have been in use for more than 30 years as replacement therapy for the treatment of HANE. C1-INH is used as a short-term preventive therapy of HANE; it is a life-saving drug in laryngeal edema.[4,25] Long-term preventive therapy is now largely based on the use of an attenuated androgen, danazol, that increases C1-INH levels in a few days and is effective in the prophylaxis of attack.[4,26] Serum C parameters improve during therapy. Patients with the inherited form of angioedema have a uniform good response to both these treatments. C1-INH and danazol are effective only in a minority of patients with the acquired deficiency of C1-INH. In these subjects C1-INH needs to be given in higher doses and prevention of attacks is obtained with antifibrinolytic agents (e.g., tranexamic acid).

As antifibrinolytic agents and attenuated hormones are not recommended for children because of their side effects, C1-INH therapy appears to be especially useful in the treatment of attacks of HANE in children.[27,28] In a recent study, acute attacks of six children were treated with a dose of 500 units of C1-INH concentrate. Progression of facial and laryngeal edema was halted in 30 to

60 min after infusion. Edema disappeared in 24 to 36 h. Necessity to repeat the dose to treat the progression of laryngeal edema arose on two occasions and the necessity for antifibrinolytic therapy arose in one patient.

Because surgery can precipitate attack of HANE, dental and other types of surgery can be safely performed after the C1-INH replacement therapy[29] or after prophylactic treatment with danazol.[30] C1-INH therapy is especially useful in pregnancy associated with attacks of angioedema.[31]

### 2. Treatment of Severe Inflammation

#### *a. Control of Toxicity Caused by Interleukin-2 Immunotherapy*

IL-2 treatment of advanced melanoma and renal carcinoma induces partial or complete remission.[32] Its use has been limited by its toxicity including a life-threatening vascular leakage syndrome characterized by hypotension, capillary leakage, and hydrodynamic changes similar to those seen in septic shock. During IL-2 therapy, two inflammatory systems, namely, C and contact system (factor XII, prekallikrein, low-molecular-weight kininogen, and factor XIa), are activated. Both are inhibited by C1-INH. As C activation during IL-2 therapy takes place via the classical pathway, the effect of administration of C1-INH to patients on hypotension, and C activation was studied in a pilot study with six patients with metastatic melanoma and renal cell carcinoma. The results showed that C1-INH administration during IL-2 treatment can prevent C activation as assessed by C3a levels but did not influence hypotension. They warrant further study to evaluate the ability of C1-INH to ameliorate IL-2-induced toxicity.

#### *b. Treatment of Sepsis*

C and contact systems are activated by microorganisms in septic shock.[33] C1-INH suppresses septic shock in a number of experimental models including in nonhuman primates.[34] This led to its trial in humans. High doses of C1-INH (2000 units followed by 100 units every 12 h) could safely be administered to patients with septic shock[35] and were found to inhibit C and contact systems in sepsis. C1-INH reduced hypotension and mortality. In another study on five cases with streptococcal shock, C1-INH (10,000 units) rapidly decreased the need for androgenic agents and caused a marked fluid shift from extravasal to intravasal space.[36] In a recent double-blind study,[37] 20 patients with severe sepsis or shock were treated with C1-INH and 20 with placebo. C1-INH was administered in 1-h infusion starting with 6000 IU followed by 3000 IU, 2000 IU, and 1000 IU at 12-h intervals. Multiple organ dysfunction and sepsis-related organ failure assessment scores were less pronounced in patients treated with C1-INH. C1-INH attenuated renal impairment. But the mortality rate was similar in C1-INH- and placebo-treated groups.

#### *c. Treatment of Burn*

Thermal injury is known to cause C activation and consumption of C1-INH.[38] Complement breakdown products such as C5a cause further injury in the host at distant sites such as lung. Efficacy of C1-INH in burn in humans has so far been tested only in one study;[39] treatment of 15 severely burned patients with C1-INH increased their long-term survival rate and improved clinical outcome.

## B. Mannose-Binding Lectin

As mannose-binding lectin (MBL) deficiency (see Chapter 14) contributes to the progression of infection in children and adults and is thought to be linked to the severity of disease in rheumatoid arthritis, cystic fibrosis, and systemic lupus erythematosus, the therapeutic potential of MBL in conditions associated with MBL deficiency is beginning to be explored.

Clinical-grade MBL, purified from pooled donor plasma, was first administered to an MBL-deficient 38-year-old adult male volunteer (Patient 1).[40] Patient 1 (MBL < 50 ng/ml; normal ~1.5 μg/ml) was defective in opsonization of *Saccharo myces cerevisiae*. He did not suffer from abnormal infections but had moderately severe psoriasis accompanied with chronic fatigue, headache, and irritable bowel symptoms. Patient 1 was initially given 60 μg MBL as an intravenous bolus dose. No change was noted in any of his clinical or laboratory parameters including C. Two days later, he received an infusion of 6 mg MBL. Concentrations of serum MBL increased to 800 ng/ml immediately after infusion but declined rapidly to ~400 ng/ml over the first 24 h. A half-life of 5 to 7 days was estimated. Opsonic activity normalized soon after infusion and remained normal until MBL concentrations reached 300 ng/ml. No MBL antibodies were seen when tested up to 4 weeks. All clinical and laboratory parameters including C components remained normal at all times.

Two years later MBL was administered to Patient 1 again, this time at a higher dose (18 mg as daily infusions of 6 mg on consecutive days). Soon after administration, serum MBL concentration increased to 1.35 μg/ml followed by a rapid decrease and subsequent slower decline with an estimated half-life of 6 days. No adverse effect was observed. CH50 and C3d levels remained normal. C-mediated opsonization of *S. cerevisiae* was normalized. Anti-MBL antibodies could not be detected after 1 year. This time another MBL-deficient patient, a 2-year-old girl (Patient 2), was also included in the study. Patient 2 (MBL < 10 ng/ml) had suffered from frequent infections from the age of 4 months. Her IgA level was in the lower normal range (0.37 mg/ml) for her age (0.2 to 1.44 mg/ml). Treatment with MBL (0.1 mg followed by 2 mg each day for 3 days; whole treatment repeated 10 days after the first infusion) resulted in normalization of C-mediated opsonization. No adverse effects were observed. Following these six MBL infusions, she remained healthy for more than 3 years. No significant abnormalities in C levels were observed before, during, or after infusions. No anti-MBL antibodies could be detected in the serum when tested up to 3 months after the last infusion.

Because MBL deficiency is associated with increased severity in autoimmune diseases, it is hoped that, in autoimmune dermatological diseases (e.g., SLE) associated with MBL deficiency, MBL will reduce the severity of the disease processes.

## C. Intravenous Immunoglobulin Preparation

Intravenous immunoglobulin (IvIg)[41] is prepared from pools of plasma of a large number of healthy donors. It contains 95% monomorphic IgG with the same proportion of subclasses as that present in normal serum. It also contains small amounts of IgA and IgM. There are substantial firm-to-firm and lot-to-lot differences in the number of donors, methods of preparation, use of additives, pH (4 to 6), cytomegalovirus neutralizing titers, and IgA levels.

Human IgG prepared from a single donor contains only traces (<1%) of dimers whereas that prepared from large pools (100,000 donations) contain up to 30 to 40% of the IgG dimers. These dimers are thought to be the complexes of idiotype (Id) IgG and anti-Id antibody. Because of the large number of donors, IvIg is expected to have a wide variety of antibodies directed against external antigens, self-antigens (natural autoantibodies), and self-antibodies (anti-idiotypic antibodies).

Beneficial effects of IvIg in different diseases may be mediated by its different properties[41] such as its antibody activity and its ability to (1) inhibit the release and activities of cytokines, (2) interact with idiotypes of autoantibodies, (3) block Fc-$\gamma$ receptors, (4) inhibit activation of T, B, and natural killer (NK) cells, (5) inhibit antibody production, and (6) inhibit the C system. In which disease which property is efficacious is not well defined. As IvIg is effective in most of the diseases in which C activation occurs in fluid phase or on tissues and cells, the ability of IvIg to inhibit C may be one of the most important properties of IvIg.

IvIg inhibits C activation at various stages. It appears to inhibit C activation at C1 stage[42] and at a stage of binding of C fragments, C3b and C4b, to target cells *in vitro* in a dose-dependent manner.[43] Serum from a patient treated with IvIg showed reduced C3b and C4b uptake (to baseline value) onto sensitized homologous erythrocytes. IvIg can perhaps inhibit C activation also at other sites of the cascade; this has yet to be explored. IvIg inhibits C *in vivo* in experimental models of complement-mediated diseases.[44]

IvIg has variously been used to treat a large array of immunological diseases.[41] It has well-established use as replacement therapy in primary immunodeficiencies for prevention of infections.

The efficacy of IvIg in many dermatological diseases has been tested either in individual patients or in small groups of patients.[45,46] Unfortunately, in none of the skin diseases have large-scale double-blind clinical trials been performed. However, several case reports on individual diseases and the results in small groups of patients do indicate that IvIg exerts beneficial effects and that many of these diseases are potential candidates for large-scale clinical trials.

### 1. Dermatomyositis

Dermatomyositis is the most thoroughly studied dermatological disease with regard to IvIg. In this disease membrane attack complex (MAC) formation is important in both muscle and skin inflammation. A placebo-controlled and several uncontrolled trials and case reports covering more than 100 patients show a high response rate.[47] The effects are long lasting in a minority of patients; the majority of patients require further treatment within weeks or months. This therapy has an immunosuppressive therapy–sparing effect. The response rate is higher in patients receiving adjunctive treatment.

### 2. Vasculitis

In a recent study, ten patients with vasculitis, in which other therapeutic means had failed, were treated with IvIg.[48] C is known to play a prominent role in vasculitis. One to six treatment courses of 400 mg/kg for 5 days were given on a monthly basis. In six patients beneficial clinical responses were seen. Levels of antimyeloperoxidase and antineutrophil cytoplasmic antibody decreased with clinical improvement in patients with Chug Straus vasculitis and Wagener's granulomatosis, respectively. In an earlier study,[49] treatment of 26 patients with active systemic vasculitis resulted in full remission in 13 patients and partial remission in 13. Clinical benefits were maintained for 12 months in 18 patients. Clinical benefits were associated with decrease in the levels of C-reactive protein and antinuclear cytoplasmic antibody. In another study with seven cases of systemic vasculitis (four with Wagner granuloma, two with microscopic polyarteritis, and one with rheumatoid vasculitis), all patients improved with high-dose IvIg treatment within 2 to 21 days.[50] The improvement was transient in one case. Relapse did not occur up to a mean of 12 months in four patients. Antinuclear cytoplasmic antibody levels first increased, probably due to its presence in IvIg preparation, and then decreased to a mean of 50% of pretreatment level and remained at this level. C-reactive protein levels, which were high in four cases, fell to normal. Radiologic pulmonary clearance occurred in two cases. The $(Fab')_2$ fragment of IvIg inhibited antinuclear cytoplasmic antibody *in vitro*.

Two Caucasian females with livedoid vasculitis were treated with IvIg.[51] Initially a dose of 0.4 g/kg for 5 days was given to patient 1 (30 years old). Infusions of a dose of 1 g/kg were repeated initially at 6-week and then at 8-week intervals. Active lesions healed within 4 weeks and there was relief of pain. The patient remained in remission at least for a year after six infusions. Patient 2 (46 years old) was first treated with 0.4 g/kg for 5 days. She became free of active lesions. A dose of 1 g/kg was then tried on monthly basis that resulted in a less dramatic improvement, and therefore subsequent doses were given at 0.4 g/kg daily for 5 days. The treatment was discontinued after 1 year. The patient was then successfully treated with cyclophosphamide.

### 3. Pemphigoid and Pemphigus

IvIg was tried in 11 patients (400 mg/kg for 5 days to 9 patients; 0.1 and 0.3 g/kg/day to 2 patients) with pemphigoid.[52] The response in 8 patients who received the high dose was good. Effect of prolonged treatment was not studied. Better results were obtained in another study[53] after prolonged treatment of 15 patients who were unresponsive to conventional therapy. IvIg was infused at a dose of 2 g/kg/cycle every 4 weeks until all previous lesions had healed and then after an increasing interval of 6, 8, 10, 12, 14, and 16 weeks. The end point of therapy was defined as the time at which the patient remained free of lesion. All the patients reached end point and achieved a sustained remission. IvIg also appears to be effective in oral pemphigoid.[54] When a group of seven patients with severe oral pemphigoid was treated with IvIg in the same way as described above[53] and a comparable control group of seven patients treated with conventional therapy, effective clinical response was observed after 4.5 months of treatment and a sustained clinical remission in all the seven patients after a mean treatment of 26.9 months. A significant reduction in the antibody titers was observed after 4 months of treatment, in both groups.

IvIg was tried in 15 patients with pemphigus.[55] The dose was 1 to 2 g/kg/cycle, each cycle divided in three equal doses given on 3 consecutive days. Each cycle was repeated every 3 to 4 weeks until effective clinical response was achieved. For maintenance therapy, the interval between the infusion cycles was increased to 6, 8, 10, 12, 14, and 16 weeks. The effective clinical response was achieved in 3.2 to 5.4 months and the maintenance period lasted 15 to 27 months. All patients reached end point when they remained free of lesion after two consecutive cycles. IvIg therapy had a corticosteroid-sparing effect. Similar observations were made in a previous study on a single patient and in 13 patients reviewed[56] who were resistant to conventional therapy. Following therapy, lowering of IgG antibodies was seen in all patients. Corticosteroid-sparing effect was seen. A dosage of 300 mg/kg for 5 days every 15 to 30 days was recommended. If large-scale double-blind studies confirm these findings, high-dose IvIg can be used as an alternative treatment in patients who are dependent on systemic corticosteroids or who develop side effects against corticosteroids.

### 4. Atopic Dermatitis

IvIg has been used to treat 32 patients with atopic dermatitis.[57] An improvement was observed in 61% patients. Of the responding patients, 48% of the adults responded and 90% of the children. Duration of response was longer in children. If the efficacy of IvIg in atopic dermatitis is confirmed by double-blind, controlled large-scale trials, it can perhaps be frequently used to treat cases, especially children, who do not respond to other treatments.

### 5. Pyoderma Gangrenosum

A patient with pyoderma gangrenosum,[58] who was previously unsuccessfully treated with prednisone, dapsone, cyclosporine, clobetasol propionate/triamcinolone cream, and methyl prednisone in various regimens, was treated with 0.4 g/kg/day of IvIg for 5 days while therapy with cyclosporine and prednisone continued. Improvement was seen within 2 weeks. Patient was then given a second course of 1 g/kg/day for 2 days. Pyoderma gangrenosum continued to improve, allowing gradual reduction of the cyclosporine and prednisone, and resolved completely. The disease did not recur at least until 8 months later. In another patient[59] with multiple ulcers on lower extremities in whom immunosuppressive therapy had to be discontinued because of side effects, IvIg (400 mg/kg for 5 days) caused arrest of the progression of ulcers and pain in 1 week and clinical improvement (improvement in one ulcer and healing in other) in the next 2 weeks. IvIg was given again at a dose of 1 g/kg for 2 consecutive days. There are also reports of lack of success in treatment of pyoderma gangrenosum with IvIg.

### 6. Epidermolysis Bullosa Acquisita

A patient with epidermolysis bullosa acquisita (EBA),[60] who was previously unsuccessfully treated with several therapeutic regimens of dapsone, cyclosporine and cyclophosphamide/dexamethasone, prednisone, azathioprine, and colchicine, was treated with 400 mg/kg IvIg for 5 days, repeated every 4 weeks. After three courses, there was a marked reduction in blistering. By the end of the study, nine therapy courses were administered, which resulted in continuous inhibition of blister formation and in enhanced healing of older lesions as well as in markedly decreased fragility. The titer of antibodies to collagen type VII was not affected, suggesting that beneficial effects could be due to inhibition of C activation at dermal–epidermal junction. Another patient with EBA[61] who had extensive infection of the lesion and a history of pulmonary tuberculosis was similarly treated with IvIg with satisfactory results.

### 7. Psoriasis and Psoriatic Arthritis

Three white women with psoriasis and psoriatic arthritis were treated with 2 g/kg IvIg on a monthly basis.[62] Patient 1 (40 years old) had severe psoriasis for 10 years and psoriatic arthritis for 5 years, Patient 2 (73 years old) had psoriasis and psoriatic arthritis for 3 years, and Patient 3 (31 years old) had severe psoriasis and psoriatic arthritis for 24 years. Following the first infusion, a fall in inflammatory markers and an improvement in joint symptoms were observed in all patients. In Patient 1 psoriasis was resolved after the third infusion, in patient 2 after the first infusion, and in Patient 3 it was hoped that psoriasis would be resolved after subsequent infusions.

### 8. Autoimmune Chronic Urticaria

Ten patients with severe chronic urticaria associated with histamine-releasing antibodies were tested for the efficacy of IvIg.[63] They were poorly responsive to conventional treatment. They received a dose of 0.4 kg/kg per day for 5 days. Clinical benefit subsequent to treatment was noted in nine patients; complete remission in three (3-year follow-up), temporary complete remission in two, and an improvement in symptoms in four. The decrease in urticarial activity in the majority of patients was associated with reduced weal-and-flare response to intradermal injection of autologous post-treatment serum compared with the pretreatment serum, indicating a decrease in histamine-releasing antibody following treatment.

It is obvious from the foregoing that double-blind clinical trials in a large number of patients with the above-mentioned diseases are needed to confirm the efficacy of IvIg.

## D. Factor I, Factor H, and C4-Binding Protein

The clinical effects and dysregulation of the C system caused by the deficiencies of Factor I, Factor H, and C4-binding protein (C4BP) have been described briefly by Asghar and co-workers in Chapter 14.

Factor I has been administered as substitution therapy in Factor I deficiency[64] in which C3 is fragmented to C3b and factor B is also consumed. Administration of 6.4 mg Factor I to one of the patients resulted in disappearance of almost all the C3b within 4 to 5 h. Native C3, C5, and classical pathway activities rose to normal or near normal levels over 4 days and remained normal for an additional week. Factor B levels were normalized within 24 h and fell over the next 5 days as were properdin, opsonic activity, and bactericidal activity. A recombinant form of Factor I has been produced[65] but has not been tried in Factor I deficiency.

Although a recombinant form of Factor H has been produced,[66] neither natural nor recombinant Factor H has been tried as substitution therapy in Factor H deficiency. A recombinant human Factor H (GPI-mini-Factor H)[67] consisting of only first to fourth short consensus repeats (SCRs). SCRs[68] are repeating domains of approximately 60 amino acids believed to be involved in protein–protein interaction; Factor H is made up of 20 SCRs. When cDNA of this GPI-mini-Factor H was transfected into a porcine endothelial cell line, the cells showed a high degree of expression. This expression blocked the lysis of transfected cells by human C. Thus, if transgenic pigs expressing GPI-mini-Factor H (and co-expressing other C-regulatory molecules) are produced, their organs may have a potential use in clinical xenotransplantation. C4BP has not yet been tried as replacement therapy in C4BP deficiency.

A recombinant human monomeric C4b-binding protein containing a GPI anchor (GPI-C4BP) has been engineered. When cDNA of this GPI-C4BP was transfected into a porcine endothelial cell line, the cells showed a high degree of expression. This expression blocked the lysis of porcine endothelial cells by human C.[69] These results showed that GPI-C4BP if expressed in vascular organs

**TABLE 38.1**
**Several Versions of Recombinant DAF, MCP, and CD59**

| Name | Characteristics | Ref. |
|---|---|---|
| | **Soluble** | |
| GPI-DAF or mDAF | GPI-bearing human (hu) DAF isolated from GPI-DAF-CHO cells[a] | 70 |
| sDAF | Soluble huDAF released from GPI-DAF-CHO cells, analogous to urine DAF | 70 |
| seDAF | A secretary form of huDAF lacking 28-COOH terminal residues required for attachment of GPI anchor | 70 |
| Ig $(DAF)_2$ | Fc part of rat IgG1 bearing rat DAF on each arm in place of Fab arm | 71 |
| Ig $(CD59)_2$ | Fc part of rat IgG1 bearing CD59 on each arm | 71 |
| Ig (DAF)(CD59) | Fc part of rat IgG1 bearing rat DAF on one arm and CD59 on the other | 71 |
| Ig-MPCS-DAF | Chimeras made up of Fc part of human Ig, metalloprotein cleavage sites, and three N-terminal SCRs of DAF | 72 |
| CD46-CD55 chimera (CAB-2) | Chimera composed of human MCP and DAF | 73, 74 |
| CD46CD(55-46) chimera | Encompassing four SCRs of MCP, SCR-1-2 of DAF, and SCR4 of MCP (and the STP, membrane and cytoplasmic tail of MCP) | 75 |
| CD46-C4BPα chimera | A recombinant soluble chimera consisting of CD46 and C4BPα | 75 |
| | **Cell Membrane Bound (transfected)** | |
| GPI-DAF-CHO | GPI-anchored huDAF expressed in CHO cells | 70 |
| GPI-MCP | GPI-bearing MCP expressed on CHO cells | 76 |
| TM-MCP | Transmembrane MCP expressed on CHO cells | 76 |
| GPI-(Delta-1-MCP) | Expressed on swine endothelial cells | 77 |
| CD59-TM | Transmembrane form of CD59 expressed on CD59-deficient melanoma cells (MeWo) | 78 |

[a] CHO cells = Chinese hamster ovary cells.

of transgenic pigs (especially in combination with other cell surface C-regulatory molecules) might have a potential therapeutic use in clinical xenotransplantation.

## E. Decay-Accelerating Factor (DAF), Membrane Cofactor Protein (MCP), and CD59

Recombinant forms of several versions of DAF, MCP, and CD59 have been produced. These are listed in Table 38.1.

Moran et al.[70] engineered and expressed human DAF (huDAF) in Chinese hamster ovary (CHO) cells. They extracted three types of huDAF from these cells. These were GPI-moiety-bearing membrane DAF (mDAF), soluble DAF (sDAF) that was analogous to DAF found in urine, and secretory form of DAF (seDAF) lacking 28-COOH terminal residues required for the attachment of GPI anchor (Table 38.1). mDAF was a more potent inhibitor of C on the cell surface than either sDAF or seDAF. In contrast, C activation in the fluid phase was inhibited by sDAF and seDAF but not by mDAF. seDAF inhibited classical and alternative pathway-mediated generation of C5a very efficiently. Harris et al.[71] produced three recombinant proteins, Ig $(DAF)_2$, Ig $(CD59)_2$, and Ig (DAF) (CD59), bearing Fc domain of rat IgG1, and rat C-regulatory molecules. All three fusion proteins inhibited C activation *in vitro* although less efficiently than C-regulatory protein lacking an Fc domain. Ig-$(DAF)_2$ had a much more extended half-life in circulation in rats than DAF. Harris et al.[72] also designed prodrugs Ig-MPCS-DAF and Ig-ACCS-DAF in which matrix metalloproteinases and aggrecanases cleavage sites, respectively, were incorporated between the human Fc domain and huDAF (three N-terminal SCRs). These fusion proteins had long half-lives *in vivo*, had little or no DAF activity probably due to steric constraints in binding to its large substrate, but was efficiently cleaved at inflammatory sites by metalloproteinases and aggrecanases to release active DAF to inhibit C and suppress inflammation. Recently, a recombinant CD46-CD55 chimera (CAB-2) has been constructed that inhibits C3/C5-convertases of classical and alternative pathways.[73,74] A soluble octameric CD46-C4BPα has also been constructed but its effects on C *in vitro* and *in vivo* have not been described.[75] A long chimera consisting of the four SCRs of MCP linked via a flexible hinge to a segment of DAF consisting of SCR1 and SCR2 and a segment of MCP consisting of SCR3, SCR4, STP, transmembrane, and cytoplasmic tail have been expressed on cell surfaces, but has not yet been studied for its possible use in any clinical situation.[75] Transmembrane and GPI-anchored forms of MCP have been expressed in CHO cells[76] (Table 38.1) and shown to protect these cells from C attack. Human MCP deleted of SCR-1 but bearing GPI-anchor GPI(Delta-1-MCP)[77] has been expressed on swine endothelial cells by transfection of cDNA. The expressed MCP protected the endothelial cells from C and was devoid of measles virus receptor activity, which resides in sCR1 of MCP. A transmembrane form of CD59 was expressed on a CD59-deficient melanoma cell line, MeWo.[78]

### 1. Inhibition of Inflammation

Some of the recombinant versions of C-regulatory proteins listed in Table 38.1 have been tested in animal models of human inflammatory conditions.

seDAF was able to inhibit reverse passive Arthus reaction (RPAR) in guinea pigs.[70] It significantly slowed the development of RPAR vasculitis and reduced its intensity in a dose-dependent manner as is apparent from the decrease in vascular permeability, neutrophil infiltration, and edema. The effective dose of seDAF was quite high, probably because of species specificity of DAF. A dose range of 75 to 150 μg/site caused 60 to 80% reduction in the intensity of the lesions.

Ig-$(DAF)_2$ was able to reduce the severity of the disease in a rat model of arthritis.[71] Thus, the human counterpart of this fusion protein is likely to have the potential for therapy of human inflammatory disorders. Ig-$(CD59)_2$ and Ig-(DAF)(CD59) were not tested for their anti-inflammatory effects perhaps because of the action of CD59 at late stage of C activation.

CD46-CD55 chimera (CAB-2) reduces tissue injury in pig to human xenotransplantation models,[73,74] indicating that it may prove to be effective in other inflammatory conditions as well.

### 2. Inhibition of Hyperacute Rejection Phase of Xenotransplantation

The serious shortage of human organs available for transplantation has generated a heightened interest in the use of animal organs for transplantation.[79] Transfected cells expressing human C-regulatory proteins have been found to be resistant to human C. These results and the ability to produce transgenic animals expressing human C-regulatory proteins in the endothelial and other cells of various organs have provided hope that the idea of xenotransplantation could perhaps one day be brought into practice. Here the discussion will be limited to the progress made in the production of pigs transgenic for human C-regulatory proteins; pig is viewed as the most suitable animal for this purpose.[80]

Transplantation of vascularized organs between discordant animals results in hyperacute rejection that is mediated by natural antibodies directed against antigens present on endothelial cells. Antibodies and C mediate hyperacute rejection via the classical pathway that results in severe endothelial cell injury. In some species combinations, the alternative pathway may mediate hyperacute rejection. Since membrane regulators of C are species specific, pig MCP, DAF, and CD59 present on the endothelium of pig organs can effectively inhibit pig C but not human C on pig endothelium. Thus, they cannot prevent hyperacute rejection of transplanted pig organs to a human host. The organs of the pigs that transgenically express human membrane regulators of C in endothelial cells may prove to be suitable for transplantation into humans.

Several laboratories have developed transgenic pigs expressing membrane complement regulatory proteins.[81–83] The cells and tissues of pigs transgenic for individual membrane C-regulatory proteins show significantly higher resistance to human C than those of nontransgenic pigs.[84–86] They are, however, not totally resistant. It is therefore desirable to produce pigs transgenic for not only single but multiple molecules, DAF, MCP, CD59 (and CR1), and to identify promoters that provide higher levels of expression of these molecules on endothelial cells. The organs of such transgenic pigs may have higher chances of finding their way from laboratory to the clinic for organ transplantation. Organs from transgenic swine expressing huDAF as well as huCD59 did not undergo hyperacute rejection when perfused with human or baboon plasma[86] or when transplanted to baboons.[87,88] Porcine endothelial cells obtained from pigs transgenic for huDAF when transfected with huCD59 and huCD46 became more resistant to hyperacute rejection than unmodified pig endothelial cells or endothelial cells transgenic for hDAF.[89]

Elimination of xenoantigens such as Gal-α-1,3-gal with simultaneous transgenic expression of multiple C-regulatory molecules may even be a better approach to achieve clinical xenotransplantation. Transgenic expression of α-1,2-fucosyltransferase (H-transferase) that reduces xenoantigen expression or eliminating α-1,3-galactosytransferase expression that synthesizes pig xenoantigen carbohydrate epitope gal-α-1,3-gal, with simultaneous transgenic expression of multiple C-regulatory molecules on endothelial cells may also prove to be a very effective approach. Transgenic pigs expressing H-transferase and CD59 have been produced.[90] Co-expression of the two molecules increased their resistance to hyperacute rejection in comparison to the expression of a single molecule.

Production of transgenic pigs expressing DAF, MCP, and CD59 (and CR1 and H-transferase) is awaited to find out whether such transgenic expression completely overcomes the barrier of hyperacute rejection and whether the time has come to go ahead with attempts to overcome other aspects of xenograft rejection such as acute vascular rejection.

If the problems associated at present with xenotransplantation are solved, the question arises whether patients requiring skin grafts will ever like to have pigskin on their bodies? Perhaps in very invalidating conditions when there is no alternative and the graft is required for the treatment of large and deep skin wounds such as third degree burns in the covered areas of the body, pigskin transplantation may be acceptable to the patient.

### 3. Purging of Tumor

C-activating monoclonal antibodies directed against tumor-specific antigens have been tried for immunotherapy of tumors but without success. The reasons for poor results could have been manifold. Some tumor cells may be expressing a low density of tumor-specific antigen; C attack on these may not be robust enough to be able to kill them. Monoclonal antibodies to tumor-specific antigens may not be able to penetrate effectively in solid tumors and may not be able to react with all tumor cells. Tumor-specific antigens and the C activation products (e.g., C3b, C4b, C5b-C9) that would have fixed on tumor cells as a result of antibody attack may be shed or internalized. Soluble C inhibitors may also prevent C activation on tumor cells and prevent their C-mediated killing. More importantly, expression of membrane regulators of C activation is deregulated in cancer; some tumor cells show weaker than normal expression of one or more regulators and others show strong overexpression of other regulators.[91] The overall result is the increased resistance to attack by C. CD59 is heterogeneously expressed in melanomas and represents the main restriction factor of C-mediated lysis of melanoma cells.[92] The major problem in immunotherapy of human tumors by means of C is the need to get tumor cells specifically attacked by antibodies to tumor-specific antigens and at the same time to inhibit C-regulatory membrane proteins specifically on C-attacked tumor cells without inhibiting these regulators present on normal cells. Attempts are being made to initiate C activation on tumor cells and at the same time to overcome the effect of overexpression of C-regulatory proteins. Monoclonal antibodies to tumor-specific antigen conjugated with CoVF have been shown to lyse tumor cells in the presence of C more effectively than unconjugated antibodies.[93,94] Biphasic monoclonal antibody constructs against tumor-specific antigen and DAF or tumor-specific antigen and CD59 increase killing of tumor cells.[95] A combination of both constructs was more effective. A recombinant bispecific antibody directed against a tumor-associated antigen G250 and CD59 was effective in lysing tumor cells in the presence of C.[96] Junnikkala et al.[97] developed a procedure to induce development of MAC and at the same time inhibit CD59 on human melanoma cells *in vitro*. A monoclonal antibody (R 24), directed against a tumor-specific antigen GD3-ganglioside present on G361 melanoma cells, was linked to biotinylated anti-CD59 through avidin as linker. Biotinylated anti-CD59 lost its ability to activate C but retained its CD59-neutralizing activity. The R24-anti-CD59 conjugate did not cause nonspecific lysis of surrounding erythrocytes and endothelial cells but neutralized CD59 on tumor cells. As a result, the tumor cells were effectively killed by the conjugate and C while the bystander cells remained viable. These results suggest that in the future it might become possible to purge cancer cells from the body by targeting an extensive C attack against tumor-associated antigens and at the same time inhibiting membrane regulators specifically on melanoma or other cancer cells.

The above approach can perhaps be modified in the light of some new observations. A synthetic peptide, C9H, corresponding to a region of C9 has been shown to bind specifically to CD59 and inhibit it.[98] It interferes with the C9 binding to CD59 and with insertion of C9 into the membrane and exhibits species specificity. This peptide may replace biotinylated anti-CD59 in the above-mentioned model of selective killing of melanoma cells.[97] Similarly, since the $\alpha$ chain of C8 and the b-domain of C9 bind to CD59, they may replace biotinylated anti-CD59 in the above-mentioned model.[97]

Another approach to kill tumor cells would be to reduce the expression of C-regulatory molecules specifically on tumor cells by pharmaceutical means and simultaneously attack tumor cells with monoclonal antibody and C. However, to date very little knowledge has been gained about the effective reagents that can specifically downregulate the expression of C-regulatory molecules in a given cell. Levamisole is known to downregulate CD59 in human colorectal adenocarcinoma cell lines.[99] Mevalonate prevents statin-induced upregulation of DAF in endothelial cells,[100] but it is not known whether it can normalize the overexpression of DAF or any other C-regulatory molecule in any tumor cell.

An ideal tool for killing tumor cells would be a biphasic monoclonal antibody construct in which Fc is linked with one arm to antibody directed against tumor-specific antigen without any steric constraint and the other arm fused to anti-DAF through an inflexible hinge region in which anti-DAF remains inactive due to steric constraints in binding to its large substrate. Anti-DAF should, however, become active due to removal of steric constraints as soon as the other arm reacts with the tumor-specific antigen. Such a construct will not react with any normal cell, will react with only tumor-specific antigen-bearing tumor cells, and will activate C specifically on them. It will selectively kill tumor cells. Other identical constructs except having anti-MCP and anti-CD59 should also be produced and the cocktail of all the three is likely to purge cancer cells from the body. This idea looks far-fetched but is theoretically sound and the technology for generating such constructs already exists.[71,72,95–97]

## F. Complement Receptor-1 (CR1)

The observation that a soluble form of CR1 (sCR1) found in body fluids[101] was a regulator of fluid-phase C activation led to the idea that sCR1 may be used to inhibit C in C-mediated diseases. This in turn led to the development of several versions of recombinant forms of human CR1, which are listed in Table 38.2.

Full-length CR1 and its derivatives[102–105] (Table 38.2) were able to bind to C3b and C4b, serve as cofactor for the enzyme Factor I for cleavage of C3b and C4b, and inhibit classical and alternative pathways at very low concentrations. However, CR1 lacking SCR 1-7[106,107] and its Sle x derivative

**TABLE 38.2**
**Several Versions of Recombinant Soluble and Membrane-Bound CR1**

| Name | Characteristics | Ref. |
|---|---|---|
| | **1. Soluble CR1 (sCR1)** | |
| sCR1 | Lacks transmembrane and cytoplastic domains | 102 |
| $s(CR1)_2$-$F(ab')_2$ | Lacks transmembrane and cytoplastic domains | 103 |
| sCR1-BA chimera | sCR1 fused to albumin-binding terminus of protein G | 104 |
| sCR1-slex[a] | sCR1 decorated with slex | 105 |
| sCR1 (des LHR[b]-A) | Lacks seven N-terminal short consensus repeats SCR1-7 | 106 |
| sCR1 (des LHR-A)-slex | sCR1 packing LHR-A and decorated with slex | 107 |
| | **2. Membrane-Bound CR1** | |
| GPI-mini-CR1 | Glycosyl-phosphatidyl-inositol (GPI) moiety of DAF linked to SCR 8-11 of CR1 expressed on a swine endothelial cell line | 108 |

[a] slex: N-linked oligosaccharide moiety (Neu 5 Ac α2-3 Gal 1-4(Fuc α1-3) GlcNAc-) referred to as sialyl Lewis x.

[b] LHR: long homologous repeat; 28 of the 30 SCR3 of CR1 are organized into four LHRs (A, B, C, and D) each of which is composed of seven SCRs.

[c] SCR: short consensus repeat;[68] repeating domains of approximately 60 amino acids believed to be involved in protein–protein interaction. Extracellular domain of CR1 is made up of 30 SCRs.

*Source:* Adapted from Asghar, S.S. and Pasch, M.C., *Frontiers Biosci.* 5, 63–81, 2000.

also lacked C4b-binding site and were only effective in inhibiting the alternative pathway. sCR1 chimeras had longer half-life. sCR1-slex[105] and sCR1(des LHR-A)-slex[107] were decorated with slex so that CR1 parts of these preparations inhibit C and carbohydrate moiety slex inhibits selectin-mediated interactions of neutrophils and lymphocytes with endothelium and their migration. These two properties in one molecule control inflammation efficiently.[105,107] GPI-mini-CR1 was able to inhibit human C-mediated lysis of the cells on which it was expressed by 50 to 70%.

Because sCR1 is not species specific, human sCR1 was active in animals and could be used in several experimental models of C-mediated human diseases. It gave promising results in experimental models of many C-mediated nondermatological diseases including ischemia/reperfusion damage, alveolitis, allergic encephalomyelitis, adult respiratory distress syndrome (ARDS), myocardial infarction, hyperacute graft rejection, and glomerulonephritis. It also suppressed acute arthritis induced by blocking of CD59.[109] It was also effective in dermatological models described below.

### 1. Treatment of Thermal Trauma

C is activated in burn injury.[38,39] In an experimental model of thermal injury[110] in which 25 to 30% of the body surface area of rat was subjected to thermal trauma, sCR1 reduced short-term (4 h) dermal and pulmonary vascular permeability and hemorrhage by about 45%. Thus, sCR1 inhibits local dermal injury as well as C5a-mediated distal injury in the lung, in this model of ARDS. The protective effect was related to reduced neutrophil content. sCR1 has not yet been tried in the treatment of thermal injury in humans but it is hoped that sCR1 or any of its more effective recombinant versions alone or in combination with C1-INH[39] will prove to be useful in the treatment of burn patients.

### 2. Inhibition of Immune-Complex-Induced Inflammation

sCR1 has been shown to inhibit immune-complex- and C-mediated inflammation in reverse passive Arthus reaction in rats.[110] Administration of sCR1 at dermal sites reduced the intensity of reverse passive Arthus reaction vasculitis in a dose-dependent manner as apparent from a decrease in vascular permeability, neutrophil infiltration, and edema. It also caused a decrease in C3 and C5-C9 (C9 neoantigen) deposition. A dose of 0.3 μg/site or higher was required to inhibit reverse passive Arthus reaction. This concentration is much lower than the effective concentration of seDAF needed to inhibit reverse passive Arthus reaction in guinea pigs.[70]

### 3. Inhibition of Hyperacute Rejection Phase of Xenotransplantation

Full-length sCR1 has been shown to inhibit hyperacute rejection and prolong survival of a porcine xenograft perfused with human blood.[112,113] sCR1 (des LHR-A), which selectively inhibits the alternative pathway, protects rabbit organs from damage by human C.[108] Swine endothelial cells moderately expressing GPI-mini-CR1 (Table 38.2) were appreciably resistant to human C,[108] indicating that organs transgenic for GPI-mini-CR1 (together with other C-regulatory proteins and H-transferase) may prove to be useful in clinical transplantation. It is hoped that the skin of pigs transgenic for multiple membrane regulators of C including sCR1 (and H-transferase) may be resistant to hyperacute rejection (also see above).

All these results of dermatological and nondermatological experimental models taken together suggest that sCR1 can limit C-mediated tissue damage in experimental animals. As sCR1 is not antigenic and is safe for therapeutic purposes, this molecule may prove to be highly useful in many C-mediated human diseases including dermatological ones. The U.S. Food and Drug Administration has approved sCR1 as an orphan drug for the treatment of ARDS and for infants undergoing cardiac surgery.[115]

### G. Antibody to Fifth Component of Complement

A monoclonal antibody (h 5G1.1) binds to C5 and prevents its cleavage during the activation of the C cascade.[116] It allows opsonization of pathogens by C3b for their phagocytosis but does not allow C5a and MAC formation. A recombinant humanized single-chain Fv portion of this antibody has recently been tried in patients undergoing cardiopulmonary bypass in which C activation and systemic inflammatory response occur. It was safe and well tolerated. There was dose-dependent (0.2 to 2.0 mg/kg) inhibition of C activation and C5b-9 formation. C5 inhibition caused inhibition of leukocyte activation and attenuation of postoperative myocardial injury. Thus, this single-chain Fv is also likely to be efficacious in many C-mediated skin diseases such as dermatomyositis in which MAC attack is important in muscle and skin inflammation and SLE in which C deposits including C5b-9 occur in skin. It is especially interesting to investigate its effect on the development of psoriatic lesions in which excessive amounts of C5a and C5b-9 are generated in the lesion and C5b-9 complex is found in circulation.[15,16]

## IV. MOLECULES THAT CAN ALTER THE EXPRESSION OF CELL-SURFACE REGULATORS OF THE COMPLEMENT

Expression of cell-surface C-regulatory proteins is downregulated in several human diseases,[117,118] including dermatological ones.[117] Expression of MCP and DAF is downregulated in the endothelium of lesional and nonlesional skin of patients with systemic sclerosis,[119] in the endothelium of lesional skin of patients with morphea,[120] and in whole lesional epidermis in patients with vitiligo.[121] These abnormalities are thought to be the part of the mechanisms of pathogenesis of these diseases. Compounds that can upregulate MCP, DAF, and/or CD59 on endothelial cells, melanocytes, and other epidermal cells may prove to be useful in suppressing disease activities in systemic sclerosis, morphea, and vitiligo. Compounds that can upregulate these molecules on cells of other organs on which C-regulatory molecules are downregulated in some nondermatological clinical conditions may also prove to be of high therapeutic value. From this point of view studies have begun to design and develop such molecules. Recently, three statins, atrovastatin, simvastatin, and mevastatin, have been shown to upregulate the expression of DAF on normal human umbilical vein and aortic endothelial cells at the protein and mRNA levels.[100] The increase in expression resulted in reduction of complement-mediated lysis of antibody-coated endothelial cells. The concentrations of statins necessary to upregulate DAF were almost in the same range that is achieved in plasma during statin treatment. This property of statins is believed to reduce the morbidity and mortality associated with athrosclerosis and may perhaps also reduce the morbidity and mortality in systemic sclerosis. This needs to be tested. The effect of statins on the expression of DAF and other C-regulatory molecules on other skin and body cells also needs to be tested. A geranylgeranyl transferase inhibitor GGTI-286 significantly increased endothelial surface DAF.[100] Doxorunicin[122] increases resistance of human SK-MEL-170 melanoma cells against human C but it is not known whether it can upregulate C-regulatory molecules on melanocytes. 5-Azacytidine[123] upregulates CD59 on CD59-negative Burkitt lymphoma cell line but it is not known whether it can upregulate CD59 on any epidermal or dermal cell. *N*-(Chloroetyl)-*N*′-cyclohexyl)-*N*-nitrosourea[124] induces the expression of clusterin and DAF mRNAs in tumor cells, but it is not known whether it can increase the resistance of epidermal and dermal cells to C attack *in vitro* and *in vivo*. Some cytokines (tumor necrosis factor-$\alpha$ and interferon-$\gamma$)[125] and growth factors (basic fibroblast growth factor and vascular endothelial growth factor)[126] upregulate C-regulatory molecules on endothelial cells. Intestinal trefoil factor induces DAF expression intestinal epithelial cells[127] and transforming growth factor-beta isoforms upregulate the expression of CD46 and CD59 on human keratinocytes,[128] but their possible therapeutic use seems to be unlikely because of their effects on a large array of biochemical reactions in the body. In short, expression of C-regulatory molecules on epidermal cells has been tested in few diseases and on dermal cells in none of the skin diseases and low-molecular-weight compounds that can alter the expression of C-regulatory molecules in epidermal and dermal cells are yet to be developed.

## V. CONCLUSION

Although several low-molecular-weight inhibitors of C have been shown to suppress experimental models of C-mediated dermatological and nondermatological diseases,[4] strenuous efforts to develop them for human use have not been made. A very limited number of them are used in some clinical conditions but they have not yet been tried in C-mediated human diseases. Slow development of low-molecular-weight inhibitors has turned attention toward high-molecular-weight natural inhibitors of C, some of which are already in clinical use and have promise of application in other diseases. Among those with possible wide clinical application in the future are C1-INH, IvIg, and sCR1. They do not cause susceptibility to infection and are nontoxic and non-immunogenic. They deserve to be tested in many C-mediated dermatological diseases in which they have not yet been tested. In addition, recombinant membrane inhibitors of C may find their way into the clinic to inhibit C. Some cell-surface human C regulators expressed in organs of transgenic pigs may prove to be useful in xenotransplantation of organs including skin. Strategies are beginning to be developed to induce C attack and at the same time inhibit membrane C-regulatory molecules specifically on cancer cells without affecting normal cells. This type of approach, although in its infancy, may eventually provide means of purging cancer cells from the body.

From the foregoing it is apparent that pharmacological manipulation of C for controlling C-mediated dermatological diseases is a fertile field. Many advances are likely to be made in near future.

## REFERENCES

1. Liszewski, M.K., Farries, T.C., Lublin, D.M., Rooney, I.A. and Atkinson, J.P., Control of the complement system. *Adv. Immunol.* 61, 201, 1996.
2. Morgan, B.P., The complement system: an overview. *Methods Mol. Biol.* 150, 1, 2000.

3. Holmskov, U., Thiel, S., and Jensenius, J.C., Collectins and ficolins: humoral lectins of the innate immune defense. *Annu. Rev. Immunol.* 21, 647, 2003.
4. Asghar, S.S., Pharmacological manipulation of the complement system. *Pharm. Rev.* 36, 223, 1984.
5. Weiler, J.M., Edens, R.E., Linhardt, R.J., and Kapelanski, D.P., Heparin and modified heparin inhibit complement activation *in vivo*. *J. Immunol.* 148, 3210, 1992.
6. Miyagawa, S., Shirakura, R., Matsumiya, G., Kitagwa, S., and Fukushima, N., Effect of anti-complementary agent K-76COOH and FUT 175 on discordant xenograft survival. *Transpl. Proc.* 24, 483, 1992.
7. Kaufman, T.S., Srivastava, R.P., and Sindlelar, R.D., Design, synthesis and evaluation of A/C/D- ring and analogues of the fungal metabolite K-76 as potential complement inhibitors. *J. Med. Chem.* 38, 1437, 1995.
8. Nakayama, T., Taira, S., Ikeda, M., Ashizawa, H., Oda, M., Arakawa, K., and Fujii, S., Synthesis and structure-activity study of protease inhibitors. V. Chemical modification of 6-amidino-2-naphthyl 4-guanidinobenzoate. *Chem. Pharm. Bull.* 41, 117, 1993.
9. Kapil, A. and Moza, N., Anticomplementary activity of boswellic acid(s) — an inhibitor of C3-convertase of the classical complement pathway. *Int. J. Immunopharmacol.* 14, 1139, 1992.
10. Buerke, M., Schwertz, H., Seitz, W., Mayer, J., and Darius, H., Novel small molecule inhibitor of C1s exerts cardioprotective effects in ischemia-reperfusion injury in rabbits. *J. Immunol.* 167, 5375, 2001.
11. Sahu, A., Soulika, A.M., Morikis, D., Spruce, L., Moore, W.T., and Lambris, J.D., Binding kinetics, structure activity relationship and biotransformation of complement inhibitor complastatin. *J. Immunol.* 165, 2491, 2000.
12. Fiane, A.E., Mollnes, T.E., Videm, V., Hovig, T., Hogasen, K., Mellbye, O.J., Sruce, L., Moore, W.T., Sahu, A., and Lambris, J.D. Prolongation of *ex vivo*-perfused pig xenograft survival by the complement inhibitor complastatin. *Transpl. Proc.* 31, 934, 1999.
13. Pellas, T.C. and Wennogle, L.P., C5a receptor antagonists. *Curr. Pharm. Design* 5, 737, 1999.
14. Konteatis, Z.D., Siciliano, S.J., Riper, G.V., Molineaux, C.J., Pandya, S., Fischer, P., Rosen, H., Mumfort, R.A., and Springer, M.S., Development of C5a receptor antagonists. Differential loss of functional responses. *J. Immunol.* 153, 4200, 1994.
15. Finch, A.M., Wong, A.K., Paczkowski, N.J., Wadi, S.K., Craik, D.K., Fairlie, D.P., and Taylor, S.M., Low-molecular-weight peptidic and cyclic antagonists of the receptor for the complement factor C5a. *J. Med. Chem.* 42, 1965, 1999.
16. Woodruff, T.M., Strachan, A.J., Dryburgh, N., Shiels, I.A., Reid, R.C., Fairlie, D.P., and Taylor, S.M., Anti-arthritic activity of an orally active C5a receptor antagonist against antigen-induced monarticular arthritis in the rat. *Arthritis Rheum.* 46, 2476, 2002.
17. Strachan, A.J., Shiels, I.A., Reid, R.C., Fairlie, D.P., and Taylor S.M., Inhibition of immune complex mediated dermal inflammation in rats following either oral or topical administration of a small molecule C5a receptor antagonist. *Br. J. Pharmacol.* 134, 1778, 2001.
18. Arumugam, T.V., Shiels, I.A., Strachan, A.J., Abbenante, G., Fairlie, D.P., and Taylor, S.M., A small molecule C5a receptor antagonist protects kidneys from ischemia/reperfusion injury in rats. *Kidney Int.* 63, 134, 2003.
19. Hopkins, P., Belmont, H.M., Buyon, J., Phillips, M., Weissmann, G., and Abramson, S.B., Increased levels of plasma anaphylatoxins in systemic lupus erythematosus predict flares of the disease and may elicit vascular injury in lupus cerebritis. *Arthritis Rheum.* 31, 632, 1988.
20. Takematsu, H. and Tagami, H., Quantification of chemotactic peptides (C5a anaphylatoxin and IL-8) in psoriatic lesional skin. *Arch. Dermatol.* 129, 74, 1993.
21. Bergh, K., Iverson, O.J., and Lysvand, H., Surprisingly high levels of anaphylatoxin C5a des Arg are extractable from psoriatic scales. *Arch. Dermatol. Res.* 285, 131, 1993.
22. Kalpatrick, J.M., Development of small molecule inhibitors of factor D, paper presented at New Therapeutic Targets Based on Control of Complement System, June 9–11, 1997.
23. Cole, L.B., Kilpatrick, J.M., Chu, N., and Babu, Y.S., Structure of 3,4-dichloroisocoumarin-inhibited factor D. *Acta Crystallogr. D. Biol. Crystallogr.* 54, 511, 1998.
24. Szalai, A.J., Digerness, S.B., Agarwal, A., Kearney, J.F., Bucy, R.P., Niwas, S., Kilpatrick, J.M., Babu, Y.S., and Volankis, J.E., The Arthus reaction in rodents: species specific recruitment of complement. *J. Immunol.* 164, 463, 2000.

25. Bork, K. and Barnstedt, S.E., Treatment of 193 episodes of laryngeal edema with C1-inhibitor concentrate in patients with hereditary angioedema. *Arch. Intern. Med.* 161, 714, 2001.
26. Robinson, L.C. and Hart, L.L., Danazol in hereditary angioedema. *Ann. Pharmacother.* 26, 1251, 1992.
27. Farkas, H., Harmat, G., Fust, G., Varga, L., and Visy, B., Clinical management of hereditary angio-oedema in children. *Pediatr. Allergy Immunol.* 13, 153, 2002.
28. Abinum, M., Hereditary angioedema in children. *Lancet* 353, 2242, 1999.
29. Alvarez, J.M., Successful use of C1-esterase inhibitor protein in a patient with hereditary angioneurotic edema requiring coronary artery bypass surgery. *J. Thoracic Cardiovasc. Surg.* 119, 168, 2000.
30. Farkas, H., Gyeney, L., Gidofalvy, E., Fust, G., and Varga L., The efficacy of short-term danazol prophylaxis in hereditary angioedema patients undergoing maxillofacial and dental procedures. *J. Oral Maxillofac. Surg.* 57, 404, 1999.
31. Hsieh, F.H. and Sheffer, A.L., Episodic swelling in a pregnant woman from Bangladesh: evaluation and management of angioedema in pregnancy. *Allergy Asthma Proc.* 23, 157, 2002.
32. Hack, C.E., Ogilia, A.C., Eisele, B., Jansen, P.M., Wagstaff, J., and Thijs, L.G., Initial studies on administration of C1-esterase inhibitor to patients with septic shock or with a vascular leakage syndrome, induced by interleukin-2 therapy. *Prog. Clin. Biol. Res.* 388, 335, 1994.
33. Kaplan, A.P., Joseph, K., Shibayama, Y., Reddigari, S., Ghebrehiwet, B., and Silverberg, M., The intrinsic coagulation/kinin-forming cascade: assembly in plasma and cell surfaces in inflammation. *Adv. Immunol.* 66, 225, 1977.
34. Jansen, P.M., Eisele, B., De Jong, I., Chang, A., Delvos, U., Taylor, F.B., and Hack, C.E., Effect of C1-esterase inhibitor on inflammatory and physiologic response patterns in primates suffering from lethal septic shock. *J. Immunol.* 160, 475, 1998.
35. Hack, C.E., Voerman, H.J., Eisele, B., Keinecke, H.O., Nuijens, J.H., Evenberg, A.J., Ogilivie, A., Strack van Schijndel, R.J., Delvos, U., and Thijs, L.G., C1-esterase inhibitor substitution in sepsis. *Lancet* 339, 378, 1992.
36. Walger, P.S., Fronhoffs, S., Steuer, K., and Vetter, H., The effect of C1-esterase inhibitor in five patients with streptococcal toxic syndrome. *Ann. Haematol.* 74 (Suppl.), A160, 1997.
37. Caliezi, C., Zeeleder, S., Redondo, M., Regli, B., Rothen, H.-U., Zurcher-Zenklusen, R., Rieben, R., Devay, J., Hack, C.E., Lammle, B., and Wuillemin, W.A., C1-inhibitor in patients with severe sepsis and septic shock: beneficial effect on renal dysfunction. *Crit. Care Med.* 30, 1722, 2002.
38. Kowel-Vern, A., Walenga, J.M., Sharp-Pucci, M., Hoppenstaedt, D., and Gameli, R.L., Postburn edema and related changes in interleukin-2, leukocytes, platelet activation, endothelin-1, and C1-esterase inhibitor. *J. Burn Care Rehabil.* 18, 99, 1997.
39. Jostkleigrewe, F., Brandt, K.A., and Janssen, A.C., C1-esterase inhibitor (C1-INH) as adjuvant therapy for septic shock following severe thermal trauma. *Ann. Haematol.* 74 (Suppl.), A159, 1997.
40. Valdimarsson, H., Stefansson, M., Vikingsdottir, T., Arason, G.T., Koch, C., Thiel, S., and Jensenius, J.C., Reconstitution of opsonizing activity by infusion of mannan-binding lectin (MBL) to MBL-deficient humans. *Scand. J. Immunol.* 48, 116, 1998.
41. Rauova, L., Rovenski, J., and Schoenfield, Y., Immunomodulation of autoimmune diseases by high-dose intravenous gammaglobulin. *Springer Semin. Immunopathol.* 23, 447, 2001.
42. Qi, M. and Schifferli, J. A., Inhibition of complement activation by intravenous immunoglobulins. *Arthritis Rheum.* 38, 146, 1995.
43. Basta, M., Fries, L.F., and Frank, M.M., High doses of intravenous Ig inhibit *in vitro* uptake of C4 fragments onto sensitized erythrocytes. *Blood* 77, 376, 1991.
44. Basta, M., Modulation of complement-mediated immune damage by intravenous immunoglobulin. *Clin. Exp. Immunol.* 104(Suppl. 1), 21, 1996.
45. Jolles, S., Hughes, J., and Wittekar, S., Dermatological uses of high-dose intravenous immunoglobulin. *Arch. Dermatol.* 134, 80, 1998.
46. Glied, M. and Rico, M.J., Treatment of autoimmune blistering diseases. *Dermatol. Clin.* 17, 431, 1999.
47. Dalakas, M.C., Controlled studies with high-dose intravenous immunoglobulin in the treatment of dermatomyositis, inclusion body myositis and polymyositis. *Neurology* 51(Suppl. 5), S37, 1998.
48. Levy, Y., Sherer, Y., George, J., Langevitz, P., Ahmad, A., Bar-Dayan, Y., Fabbrizzi, F., Terryberry, J., Peter, J., and Schoenfeld, Y., Serological and clinical responses to treatment of systemic vasculitis and associated disease with intravenous immunoglobulin. *Intern. Arch. Allergy Immunol.* 119, 231, 1999.

49. Jayne, D.R. and Lockwood, C.M., Pooled intravenous immunoglobulin in the management of systemic vasculitis. *Adv. Exp. Med. Biol.* 336, 469, 1993.
50. Jayne, D.R., Davies, M.J., Fox, C.J., Black, C.M., and Lockwood, C.M., Treatment of systemic vasculitis with pooled intravenous immunoglobulin. *Lancet* 337, 1137, 1991.
51. Ravat, F.E., Evans, A.V., and Russell-Jones, R., Response of livedoid vasculitis to intravenous immunoglobulin. *Br. J. Dermatol.* 147, 166, 2002.
52. Godard, W., Roujeau, J.C., Guillot, B., Andre, C., and Rifle, G., Bullous pemphigoid and intravenous gammaglobulin. *Ann. Intern. Med.* 103, 964, 1985.
53. Ahmed, A.R., Intravenous immunoglobulin therapy for patients with bullous pemphigoid unresponsive to conventional immunosuppressive treatment. *J. Am. Acad. Dermatol.* 45, 625, 2001.
54. Sami, N., Bhol, K.C., and Ahmed, A.R., Treatment of oral pemphigoid with intravenous immunoglobulin as monotherapy. Long-term follow-up: influence of treatment on antibody titers to human a6 integrin. *Clin. Exp. Immunol.* 129, 533, 2002.
55. Sami, N., Qureshi, A., Ruocco, E., and Ahmed, A.R., Corticosteroid-sparing effect of intravenous immunoglobulin therapy in patients with *Pemphigus vulgaris. Arch. Dermatol.* 138, 1158, 2002.
56. Colona, L., Cianchini, G., Frezzolini, A., De Pita, O., Di Lella, G., and Puddu, P., Intravenous immunoglobulin for pemphigus vulgaris: adjuvant or first choice therapy? *Br. J. Dermatol.* 38, 1102, 1998.
57. Jolles, S., A review of high-dose intravenous immunoglobulin treatment for atopic dermatitis. *Clin. Exp. Dermatol.* 27, 3, 2002.
58. Gupta, A.K., Shear, N.H., and Sauder, D.N., Efficacy of human intravenous immune globulin in pyoderma gangrenosum. *J. Am. Acad. Dermatol.* 32, 140, 1995.
59. Hagman, J.H., Carozzo, A.M., Campione, E., Romanelli, P., and Chimenti, S., The use of high dose immunoglobulin in the treatment of pyoderma gangrenosum. *J. Dermatol. Treat.* 12, 19, 2001.
60. Mohr, C., Sunderkotter, C., Hilderbrand, A., Biel, K., Rutter, A., Rutter, G.H., Leuger, T.A., and Kolde, G., Successful treatment of epidermolysis bullosa acquisita using intravenous immunoglobulins. *Br. J. Dermatol.* 132, 824, 1995.
61. Gourgiotou, K., Exadaktylou, D., Aroni, K., Rallis, E., Nicolaidou, E., Paraskevakou, H., and Katsambas, A.D., Epidermolysis bullosa acquisita: treatment with intravenous immunoglobulins. *J. Eur. Acad. Dermatol. Venereol.* 16, 77, 2002.
62. Gurmin, V., Mediwake, R., Fernando, M., Whittaker, S., Rustin, M.H.A., and Beynon, H.L.C., Psoriasis: response to high-dose intravenous immunoglobulin in three patients. *Br. J. Dermatol.* 147, 554, 2002.
63. O'Donnell, B.F., Barr, R.M., Kobza Black, A., Francis, D.M., Kermani, F., Niimi, N., Barlow, R.J., Winkelmann, R.K., and Greaves, M.W., Intravenous immunoglobulin in autoimmune chronic urticaria. *Br. J. Dermatol.* 138, 101, 1998.
64. Ziegler, J.B., Alper, C.A., Rosen, R.S., Lachmann, P.J., and Sherington, L., Restoration by purified C3b inactivator of complement mediated function *in vivo* in a patient with C3b inactivator deficiency. *J. Clin. Invest.* 55, 668, 1975.
65. Ullman, C.G., Chamberlin, D., Ansari, A., Emery, V.C., Haris, P.I., Sim, R.B., and Perkins, S.J., Human complement factor I: its expression by insect cells and its biochemical and structural characterization. *Mol. Immunol.* 35, 503, 1998.
66. Sharma, A.K. and Pangburn, M.K., Biologically active recombinant factor H: synthesis and secretion by baculovirus system. *Gene* 143, 301, 1994.
67. Yoshitatsu, M., Miyagawa, S., Mikata, S., Matsunami, K., Yamada, M., Koresawa, Y., Sawa, Y., Ohtake, S., Matsuda, H., and Shirakura, R., Expression of PI-anchored Mini-Factor H on porcine endothelial cells: potential use in xenotransplantation. *Transpl. Proc.* 31, 2812, 1999.
68. Janatova, J., Reids, K.B.M., and Willis, A.C., Disulphide bonds are localized within short consensus repeat units of complement regulatory protein: C4 binding protein. *Biochemistry* 28, 4754, 1989.
69. Mikata, S., Miyagawa, S., Iwata, K., Nagasawa, S., Hatanaka, M., Matsumoto, M., Kamiika, W., Matsuda, H., Shirakura, R., and Seya, T., Regulation of complement-mediated swine endothelial cell lysis by a surface-bound form of a human C4b binding protein. *Transplantation* 65, 363, 1998.
70. Moran, P., Beasley, H., Gorrell, A., Martin, E., Gribling, P., Fuchs, H., Gillet, N., Burton, L.E., and Caras, I.W., Human recombinant soluble decay accelerating factor inhibits complement activation *in vitro* and *in vivo. J. Immunol.* 149, 1736, 1992.

71. Harris, C.L., Williams, A.S., Linton, S.M., and Morgan, B.P., Coupling complement regulators to immunoglobulin domains generates effective anti-complement reagents with extended half-life *in vivo*. *Clin. Exp. Immunol.* 129, 198, 2002.
72. Harris, C.L., Fraser, D.A., and Morgan, B.P., Tailoring anti-complement therapeutics. *Biochem. Soc. Trans.* 30, 1019, 2002.
73. Salerno, C.T., Kulick, D.M., Yeh, C.G., Guzman-Paz, M., Higgins, P.J., Benson, B.A., Park, S.J., Shumway, S.J., Bolman, R.M., III, and Dalmasso, A.P., A soluble chimeric inhibitor of C3 and C5 convertases, complement activation blocker-2, prolongs graft survival in pig-to-rhesus monkey heart transplantation. *Xenotransplantation* 9, 125, 2002.
74. Kroshus, T.J., Salerno, C.T., Yeh, C.G., Higgins, P.J., Bolman, R.M., III, and Dalmasso, A.P., A recombinant soluble chimeric complement inhibitor composed of human CD46 and CD55 reduces acute cardiac tissue injury in models of pig-to-human heart transplantation. *Transplantation* 69, 2282, 2000.
75. Christiansen, D., De Sousa, E.R., Loveland, B., Kyriakou, P., Lanteri, M., Wild, F.T., and Gerlier, D., A CD46CD(55-46) chimeric receptor, eight short consensus repeats long, acts as an inhibitor of both CD46 (MCP)- and CD150 (SLAM)-mediated cell-cell fusion induced by CD46-using measles virus. *J. Gen. Virol.* 83, 1147, 2002.
76. Lubin, D.M. and Coyne, K.E., Phospholipid anchored and transmembrane versions of either decay-accelerating factor or membrane cofactor protein show equal efficiency in protection from complement mediated cell damage. *J. Exp. Med.* 174, 35, 1991.
77. Begum, N.A., Murakami, Y., Mikata, S., Matsumoto, M., Hatanaka, M., Nagasawa, S., Kinoshita, T., and Seya, T., Molecular remodeling of human CD46 for xenotransplantation: designing a potent complement regulator without measles virus receptor activity. *Immunology* 100, 131, 2000.
78. De Nardo, C., Fonsatti, E., Sigalotti, L., Calabro, L., Colizzi, F., Cortini, E., Coral, S., Altomonte, M., and Maio, M., Recombinant transmembrane CD59 (CD59-TM) confers complement resistance to GPI-protein defective melanoma cells. *J. Cell Physiol.* 190, 200, 2002.
79. Platt, J.L., A perspective on xenograft rejection and accommodation. *Immunol. Rev.* 141, 127, 1994.
80. Sachs, D.H., The pig as a potential xenograft donor. *Vet. Immunol. Immunopathol.* 43, 185, 1994.
81. Lavitrano, M., Bacci, M.L., Forni, M., Lazzereschi, D., Di Stefano, C., Fioretti, D., Giancotti, P., Marfe, G., Pucci, L., Renzi, L., Wang, H., Stoppacciaro, A., Stass, G., Sargiacomo, M., Sinibaldi, P., Turchi, V., Giovannoni, R., Della Casa, G., Seren, E., and Rossi, G., Efficient production by sperm-mediated gene transfer of human decay accelerating factor (hDAF) transgenic pigs for xenotransplantation. *Proc. Natl. Acad. Sci. U.S.A.*, 99, 14230, 2002.
82. Zhou, C.Y., McInnes, E., Parsons, N., Langford, G., Lancaster, R., Richards, A., Pino-Chavez, G., Dos Santo Cruz, G., Copeman, L., Carrington, C., and Thompson, S., Production and characterization of a pig line transgenic for human membrane cofactor protein. *Xenotransplantation* 9, 183, 2002.
83. Niemann, H., Verhoeyen, E., Wonigeit, K., Lorenz, R., Hecker, J., Schwinzer, R., Hauser, H., Hues, W.A., Halter, R., Lemme, E., Herrmann, D., Winkler, M., Wirth, D., and Paul, D., Cytomegalovirus early promotor induced expression of hCD59 in porcine organ provides protection against hyperacute rejection. *Transplantation* 72, 1898, 2001.
84. Kadner, A., Chen, R.H., Fariver, R.S., Santerre, D., and Adams, D.H., Transplantation of MCP cardiac xenografts into baboon recipients. *Transpl. Proc.* 33, 770, 2001.
85. Diamond, L.E., Quinn, C.M., Martin, M.J., Lawson, J., Platt, J.L., and Logan, J.S., A human CD46 transgenic pig model system for the study of discordant xenotransplantation. *Transplantation* 71, 132, 2001.
86. Yeatman, M., Dagget, C.W., Lau, C.L., Byrne, G.W., Logan, J.S., Platt, J.L., and Davis, R.D., Human complement regulatory proteins protect swine lungs from xenogeneic injury. *Ann Thorac. Surg.* 67, 769, 1999.
87. Byrne, G.W., Mc Curry, K.R., Martin, M.J., McClellan, S.M., Platt, J.L., and Logan, J.S., Transgenic pigs expressing human CD59 and decay accelerating factor produce an intrinsic barrier to complement mediated damage. *Transplantation* 63, 149, 1997.
88. Yeatman, M., Dagget, C.W., Parker, W., Byrne, G.W., Logan, J.S., Platt, J.L., and Davis, R.D., Complement mediated pulmonary xenograft injury: studies in swine-to-primate orthrotropic single lung transplant model. *Transplantation* 65, 1084, 1998.

89. Chen, S., Chen, G., Cai, C.C., Wang, X.M., Guo, H., Shen, S.Q., Wang, H., Wu, Y., Li, G.X., Huang, J., Li, W.X., Wei, Q.X., and Sun, F.Z., A study of human transgene in xenotransplantation. *Transpl. Proc.* 33, 3851, 2001.
90. Costa, C., Zhao, L., Burton, W.V., Rosas, C., Bondiolo, K.R., Williams, B.L., Hoagland, T.A., Dalmasso. A.P., and Fodor, W.L., Transgenic pigs designated to express CD59 and H-transferase to avoid humoral xenograft rejection. *Xenotransplantation* 9, 45, 2002.
91. Durrant, L.G. and Spendlove, I., Immunization against tumor cell surface complement regulatory proteins. *Curr. Opin. Invest. Drugs* 2, 859, 2001.
92. Carol, S., Fonsatti, E., Sigalotti, L., De Nardo, C., Visintin, A., Nardi, G., Colizzi, F., Colombo, M.P., Romano, G., Altomonte, M., and Mio, M., Overexpression of protectin (CD59) downregulates the susceptibility of human melanoma cells to homologous complement. *J. Cell Physiol.* 185, 317, 2000.
93. Fu, Q. and Gowda, D.C., Carbohydrate directed conjugation of cobra venom factor to antibody by selective derivatization of the terminal galactose residues. *Bioconjug. Chem.* 12, 271, 2001.
94. Juhl, H., Petrella, E.C., Cheung, N.K., Bredehorst, R., and Vogel, C.-W., Additive cytotoxicity of different monoclonal antibody-cobra venom factor conjugates for human neuroblastoma cells. *Immunobiology* 197, 444, 1997.
95. Harris, C.L., Kan, K.S., Stevenson, G.T., and Morgan, B.P., Tumor cell killing using chemically engineered antibody constructs specific for tumor cells and the complement inhibitor CD59. *Clin. Exp. Immunol.* 107, 364, 1997.
96. Block, V.T., Daha, M.R., Tijsma, O., Harris, C.L., Morgan, B.P., Fleuren, G.J., and Gorter, A., A bispecific monoclonal antibody directed against both the membrane bound complement regulators CD59 and CD55 and the renal tumor associated antigen 250 enhances C3 deposition and tumor cell lysis by complement. *J. Immunol.* 160, 3437, 1998.
97. Junnikala, S., Hakulinen, J., and Meri, S., Targeted neutralization of complement membrane attack complex inhibitor CD59 on the surface of human melanoma cell. *J. Immunol.* 24, 611, 1994.
98. Tomlinson, S., Whitlow, M.B., and Nussenzweig V.A., Synthetic peptide from complement protein C9 binds to CD59 and enhances lysis of human erythrocytes by C5b-9. *J. Immunol.* 152, 1927, 1994.
99. Bjorge, L. and Matre, R., Down-regulation of CD59 (protectin) expression on human colorectal adenocarcinoma cell lines by levamisole. *Scand. J. Immunol.* 42, 512, 1995.
100. Mason, J.C., Ahmad, Z., Mankoff, R., Lidington, E.A., Ahmad, S., Bhatia, V., Kinderlerer, A., Randi, A.M., and Haskard, D.O., Statin-induced expression of decay accelerating factor protects vascular endothelium against complement-mediated injury. *Circ. Res.* 91, 696, 2002.
101. Yoon, S. and Fearon, D.T., Characterization of a soluble form of the C3b/C4b receptor (CR1) in human plasma. *J. Immunol.* 134, 3332, 1985.
102. Weisman, H.F., Bartow, T., Leppo, M.K., Marsh, H.C., Jr., Carson, G.R., Concino, M.F., Boyle, M.P., Roux, K.H., Weisfeltdt, M.L., and Fearon, D.T., Soluble human complement receptor type 1: *in vivo* inhibitor of complement suppressing post-ischemic myocardial inflammation and necrosis. *Science* 249, 146, 1990.
103. Kalli, K.R., Hsu, P.H., Bartow, T.J., Ahearn, J.M., Matsumoto, A.K., Klickstein, L.B., and Fearon, D.T., Mapping of the C3b-binding site of CR1 and construction of a (CR1)2-F(ab′)2 chimeric complement inhibitor. *J. Exp. Med.* 174, 1451, 1991.
104. Makrides, S.C., Nygren, P.-A., Andrews, B., Ford, P.J., Evans, K.S., Hayman, E.G., Adari, H., Levin, J., Uhlen, M., and Toth, C.A., Extended *in vivo* half life of human soluble complement receptor type-1 fused to a serum albumin-binding receptor. *J. Pharmacol. Exp. Ther.* 277, 534, 1996.
105. Mulligan, M.S., Warner, R.L., Rittershaus, C.W., Thomas, L.J., Ryan, U.S., Foreman, K.E., Crouch, L.D., Till, G.O., and Ward, P.A., Endothelial targeting and enhanced anti-inflammatory effects of complement inhibitors possessing Lewis x moieties. *J. Immunol.* 162, 4952, 1999.
106. Scesney, S.M., Makrides, S.C., Gosselin, M.L., Ford, P.J., Andrews, B.M., Hayman, E.G., and Marsh, H.C., Jr., A soluble deletion mutation of the human complement receptor type 1, which lacks the C4b binding site, is a selective inhibitor of the alternative pathway. *Eur. J. Immunol.* 26, 1729, 1996.
107. Rittershaus, C.W., Thomas, L.J., Mitter, D.P., Picard, M.D., Geoghegan-Barek, K.M., Scesney, S.M., Henry, L.D., Sen, A.C., Bertino, A.M., Hanning, G., Adari, H., Mealey, R.A., Gosselin, M.L., Conto, M., Hayman, E.G., Levin, J.L., Reinhold, V.N., and Marsh, H.C., Jr., Recombinant glycoproteins that inhibit complement activation and also bind the selectin adhesion molecules. *J. Biol. Chem.* 274, 11237, 1999.

108. Mikata, S., Miyagawa, M., Yoshitatsu, M., Ikawa, M., Okabe. M., Matsuda, H., and Shirakura, R., Prevention of hyperacute rejection by phosphatidylinositol-anchored mini-complement receptor type 1. *Transpl. Immunol.* 6, 107, 1998.
109. Mizuno, M., Nishikaawa, K., Morgan, B.P., and Matsuo, S., Comparison of the suppressive effects of soluble CR1 and C5a receptor antagonist in acute arthritis induced in rats by blocking of CD59. *Clin. Exp. Immunol.* 119, 368, 2000.
110. Mulligan, M.S., Yeh, C.G., Rudolph, A.R., and Ward, P.A., Protective effects of soluble CR1 in complement and neutrophil-mediated injury. *J. Immunol.* 148, 1479, 1992.
111. Yeh, G.C., Marsh, H.C., Jr., Carson, G.R., Berman, L., Concino, M.F., Scesney, S.M., Kuestner, R.E., Skibbens, R., Donahue, K.A., and Ip, S.H., Recombinant soluble human complement receptor type 1 inhibits inflammation in the reverse passive Arthus reaction in rats. *J. Immunol.* 146, 250, 1991.
112. Pruitt, S.K., Kirk, A.D., Bollinger, R.R., Marsh, H.C., Collins, B.H., Levin, J.L, Mault, J.R., Heinle, J.S., Ibrahim, S., Rudolph, A.R., Baldwin, W.M., and Sanfilippo, F., The effect of soluble complement receptor type 1 on hyperacute rejection of porcine xenografts. *Transplantation* 57, 363, 1994.
113. Levine, J.L., Marsh, H.C., Jr., and Rudolph, A.R., sCR1, a novel complement inhibitor: development of potential applications for treating hyperacute rejection of transplanted organ, in *Principles of Drug Development in Transplantation and Autoimmunity,* Lieberman, R. and Mukherjee, A., Eds., R.G. Landes, Austin, TX, 1996, 695.
114. Gralinski, M.R., Wiater, B.C., Assenmacher, A.N., and Lucchesi, B.R., Selective inhibition of the alternative complement pathway by sCR1 (des LHR-A) protects the rabbit isolated heart from human complement mediated damage. *Immunopharmacology* 34, 79, 1996.
115. Rioux, P., TP-10 (AVANT Immunotherapeutics). *Curr. Opin. Invest. Drugs* 2, 364, 2001.
116. Fitch, J.C., Rollins, S., Matis, L., Alford, B., Aranki, S., Collard, C.D., Dewar, M., Elefteriades, J., Hines, R., Kopf, G., Kraker, P., Li, L., O'Hara, R., Rinder, C., Rinder, H., Shaw, R., Smith, B., Stahl, G., and Shernan, S.K., Pharmacology and biological efficiency of a recombinant, humanized, single chain antibody C5 complement inhibitor in patients undergoing coronary artery bypass graft surgery with cardiopulmonary bypass. *Circulation* 100, 2499, 1999.
117. Asghar, S.S., Membrane regulators of complement activation and their aberrant expression in disease. *Lab. Invest.* 72, 254, 1995.
118. Singhrao, S.K., Neal, J.W., Rushmere, N.K., Morgan, B.P., and Gasque, P., Spontaneous classical pathway activation and deficiency of membrane regulators render human neurons susceptible to complement lysis. *Am. J. Pathol.* 157, 905, 2000.
119. Venneker, G.T., van den Hoogen, F.H., Boerbooms, A.M., Bos, J.D., and Asghar, S.S., Aberrant expression of membrane cofactor protein and decay-accelerating factor in the endothelium of patients with systemic sclerosis. A possible mechanism of vascular damage. *Lab. Invest.* 70, 830, 1994.
120. Venneker, G.T., Das, P.K., Naafs, B., Tigges, A.J., Bos, J.D., and Asghar, S.S., Morphea lesions are associated with aberrant expression of membrane cofactor protein and decay accelerating factor in vascular endothelium. *Br. J. Dermatol.* 131, 237, 1994.
121. van den Wijngaard, R.M.J.G.J., Asghar, S.S., Pijnenborg, A.C.L.M., Tigges, A.J., Westerhof, W., and Das, P.K., Aberrant expression of complement regulatory proteins, membrane cofactor protein and decay accelerating factor, in the involved epidermis of patients with vitiligo. *Br. J. Dermatol.* 146, 80, 2002.
122. Panneerselvam, M., Bredehorst, R., and Vogel, C.W., Resistance of human melanoma cells against the cytotoxic and complement-enhancing activities of doxorubicin. *Cancer Res.* 47, 4601, 1987.
123. Kuraya, M., Minarovits, J., Okada, H., and Klein, E., HRF20/CD59 complement regulatory protein expression is phenotype-dependent and inducible by the hypomethylating agent 5-azacytidine on Burkitt's lymphoma cell lines. *Immunol. Lett.* 37, 35, 1993.
124. Kumar, S., Vinci, J.M., Pytel, B.A., and Baglioni, C., Expression of messenger RNAs for complement inhibitors in human tissues and tumors. *Cancer Res.* 53, 348, 1993.
125. Mason, J.C., Yarwood, H., Sugars, K., Morgan, B.P., Davies, K.A., and Haskard, D.O., Induction of decay accelerating factor by cytokines or the membrane attack complex protects endothelial cells against complement deposition. *Blood* 94, 1673, 1999.
126. Mason, J.C., Lidington, E.A., Ahmad, S.R., and Haskard, D.O., BFGF and VEGF synergistically enhance endothelial cytoprotection via decay-accelerating factor induction. *Am. J. Physiol. Cell Physiol.* 282, C578, 2002.

127. Andoh, A., Kinoshita, K., Rosenberg, I., and Podolsky, D.K., Intestinal trefoil factor induces decay accelerating factor expression and enhances the protective activities against complement activation in intestinal epithelial cells. *J. Immunol.* 167, 3887, 2001.
128. Pasch, M.C., Bos, J.D., Daha, M.R., and Asghar, S.S., Transforming growth factor-β isoforms regulate the surface expression of membrane cofactor protein (CD46) and CD59 on human keratinocytes. *Eur. J. Immunol.* 29, 100, 1999.

# 39 Immunological Strategies to Fight Skin Cancer

*Dirk Schadendorf, Annette Paschen, and Stefan Eichmüller*

## CONTENTS



## I. INTRODUCTION

Epithelial skin cancers such as squamous cell and basal cell carcinomas can usually be treated easily by performing surgery and local application of therapeutic ointments such as 5-FU, imiquimod, etc., as well as by using photosensitizers combined with ultraviolet (UV) or radiation (reviewed in Reference 1). Cutaneous malignant melanoma and cutaneous lymphomas are much harder to treat successfully, as this can only be achieved in the early clinical stages. In the advanced stages,

0-8493-1959-5/05/$0.00+$1.50

particularly in the case of melanoma, there is currently no cure available.[2,3] Because the effectiveness of surgery, chemotherapy, and radiotherapy as treatment for these diseases is so limited, an extensive search for alternative therapy strategies has been launched, and this has stimulated the search for molecular structures that are detected by the immune system. This chapter reviews the recent progress made in the identification and characterization of human tumor antigens detected by T cells and antibodies in cutaneous lymphoma and melanoma, and the therapeutic strategies emerging from these findings are briefly outlined.

## II. IDENTIFICATION AND CHARACTERIZATION OF TUMOR ANTIGENS IN SKIN CANCERS

The prerequisite of specific immunotherapies is the knowledge of specific targets. Once these are available, two different therapeutic strategies can be applied:

1. *Induction of a cellular immune response.* Cytotoxic T cells (CTLs) can recognize peptide epitopes derived from tumor antigens presented by histocompatability leukocyte antigen (HLA) molecules on the tumor cells and specifically lyse the identified target cell. Defined peptides from tumor-specific antigens can be applied as synthetic peptide, naked DNA, or loaded onto dendritic cells to activate the cellular immune response.
2. *Application of tumor-specific, therapeutic antibodies.* Membrane-bound antigens can serve as targets for therapeutic antibodies, which may be coupled to toxins or radioactive substances.

The requirements of tumor antigens used for both strategies differ in some respect. In both cases, the expression of the target protein has to be tumor specific, at least from an immunological point of view. There is, for example, a large group of genes expressed only in tumor cells and healthy testis, probably due to strong demethylation in both tissues.[4] As testis is immune privileged with a low level or even lack of HLA molecules, CTLs specific for epitopes derived from these gene products will only detect tumor cells. These proteins have been called cancer germline genes or cancer-testis antigens (CTA),[5,6] although others avoid the designation *antigens*, as in testis these proteins do not function as antigens. MAGE-A1, A2, and A3 were the first antigens of this group, identified by tumor-specific CTLs from a melanoma patient.[7] Meanwhile, a large number CTAs have been published,[6] including 15 genes of the MAGE-A group.

Antibody-mediated immunotherapy is a still young field, with the first successful examples of therapeutic antibodies.[8,9] The subcellular localization is essential in case of antibody-based strategies, as only membrane-bound antigens exposed to the cell surface can function as targets. This is irrelevant in the case of CTL-based immune therapies; instead, an HLA-dependent epitope derived from the tumor antigen is needed. A large number of such epitopes have meanwhile been identified for different tumor antigens, most of them were originally isolated from malignant melanomas.[10] As the various peptides from one tumor antigen presented by different HLA molecules differ substantially, a bundle of immunogenic epitopes must be identified for each tumor antigen and peptides for therapy must be selected depending on the HLA type of the patient.

The question arises, how tumor antigens can be identified and how we can select the most promising ones as targets for therapy. A classification of tumor antigens should provide orientation in this respect.

### A. Classification

A first rough classification of tumor antigens refers to their expression pattern: Antigens, which are expressed on tumor cells, but not on normal cells are called *tumor-specific antigens* (TSAs), whereas the term *tumor-associated antigens* (TAAs) delineates all kinds of tumor antigens including

**TABLE 39.1**
**Classification of Tumor-Associated Antigens for Malignant Melanoma**

| | | Relevance for Malignant Melanoma Proven by: | | |
|---|---|---|---|---|
| **Type of Antigen** | **Examples** | **Expression Analysis** | **Specific CTLs** | **Clinical Usage** |
| Proto-oncogenes | *Ras* (mutated) | 48, 14 | 47, 175 | 47 |
| Cancer testis antigens (CTA) | MAGE genes | 176, 177, 57, 58 | Many published reviews: 16, 10 | 178, 179 |
| Differentiation antigens | Tyrosinase, Melan-A | 19, 20 | e.g., 10, 180 | 178, 110 |
| Oncofetal antigens | CEA | Not expressed in melanoma, 181 | 22, 24* | 182* |
| Mutations, alternative splicing | CAMEL, cTAGE-5a | 26, 28 | 26 | None |

* This work is not on melanoma.

those proteins detected in tumors and also in normal cells. This distinction reflects the important issue of expression specificity. Notably, many tumor antigens, which are already successfully used in the clinics, are overexpressed only on the protein level (e.g., Her2/neu), or are expressed during oncogenesis or at immune-privileged sites (e.g., CTA, see above). These tumor antigens are still tumor specific from an immunological point of view and are thus also often termed TSA.

Alternatively, tumor antigens are classified on the basis of their function and source. A number of categories have been suggested (see, e.g., Reference 11); the most important are outlined in the following. Table 39.1 gives examples and references for clinical use in respect to skin cancers, especially malignant melanoma.

1. Oncogenes genes like *Ras* or *Her2/neu*.[12] Oncogenes are derived from normal genes, which are then called proto-oncogenes.[13] Various mutational mechanisms can lead to this transformation: Point mutations can alter the function of the protein (e.g., Ras); translocations can result in fusion proteins with new functions (BCR-ABL); gene amplification or overexpression of the gene product due to increased transcriptional activity can lead to increased amount of the protein (e.g., growth factors like bFGF). Due to the mutation the oncogene is a tumor-specific protein. A number of oncogenes have been described in melanoma.[14]
2. Mutated antigens, not involved in tumorigenesis, like the β-catenin in malignant melanoma.[15] Mutations may also be the reason for the existence of antibodies in cancer patients' sera against proteins belonging to self-proteins: Tolerance must not be broken, because the mutated region is non-self, but the antibodies against this mutated protein may also cross-react with the wild-type protein.
3. CTA are expressed only within tumor cells and testis tissue (see above). Almost all CTA have been described to be expressed in melanoma,[10,16] but recently some have also been described for cutaneous T-cell lymphoma CTCL.[17,18] CTA can be detected in most types of tumors, although to different frequencies and preferences.[6]
4. A number of differentiation antigens have been described for malignant melanoma, e.g., tyrosinase, tyrosinase-related peptide 1 (TYRP-1) and 2 (TYRP-2), and Melan-A/MART-1.[19,20] These genes are specific for melanocytes, and can also be found in the malignant derivative.
5. Products of oncogenic viruses, like papillomavirus E6 and E7 proteins.[21]
6. Oncofetal antigens like CEA (carcinoembryogenic antigen) or AFP (alpha-fetoprotein).[22–24]
7. Another source for tumor antigens might be an atypical protein translation: A growing number of tumor antigens are described as products from alternative open reading frames,

cryptic start sites, alternative splicing, and even the reverse strand.[25–28] It remains to be elucidated whether these proteins are possibly not recognized as self-proteins by the immune system and thus be advantageous for therapeutic purposes.

Several of the examples mentioned have meanwhile been applied during clinical trials (see Table 39.1) and it became apparent that successful targets do not have to be expressed in a strictly tumor-specific fashion, although side effects have to be analyzed and monitored very carefully. For example, vitiligo was an expected side effect, when melanocytic differentiation antigens were used for immunotherapy of malignant melanoma, as the induced immune response should also recognize normal melanocytes.[29]

## B. Screening for Tumor Antigens

Different approaches have been employed for the identification of tumor antigens (Figure 39.1). Two of these use the help of the tumor patient's immune system by utilizing either the cellular (CTL approach) or the humoral response (SEREX approach). Besides this, differential gene expression analysis has been applied,[30] which may become more important in the future due to the invention of chip technology.

Interestingly, a number of TAA have been shown to be recognized only by antibodies from patients' sera and not control sera, despite their expression in control tissues (see, e.g., References 31 through 34). Recently, this serological specificity could be confirmed for a number of TAA by analyzing many sera from patients with colon carcinoma and healthy controls.[33] A serological

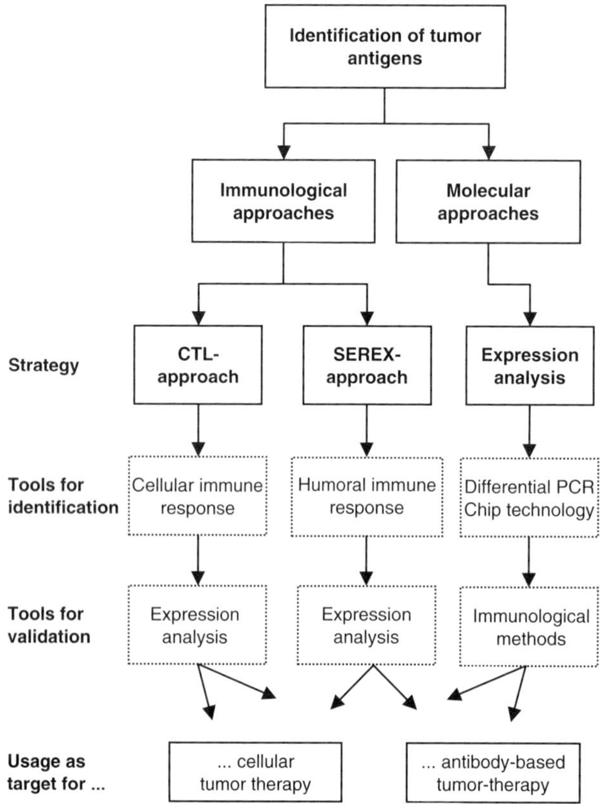


**FIGURE 39.1** Flowchart of different possible approaches for the identification, validation, and usage of tumor antigens.

specificity despite an unspecific expression pattern of the target protein might be explained by an overexpression of the protein in tumor tissue, by the danger context or by generation of antibodies against a mutated protein of the tumor, which cross-react with the wild-type protein as has been shown for p53.[35] In any case, the measurement of specific antibodies in the serum of tumor patients might be useful as diagnostic or prognostic factor.[33,36]

The CTL approach was the first to be used with the classical study by van der Bruggen and colleagues[7] to identify MAGE-1 as the first tumor-associated antigen. In the meantime, there are a number of variations, but all need CTLs for validation of the targets. The invention of the SEREX method[37] has unraveled a very large number of TAAs. Whether an antigen is identified by cellular or humoral approaches does not necessarily determine the later use in immunological therapy (CTL vs. antibodies): For example, NY-ESO-1 was originally discovered by SEREX, but subsequently CTL epitopes have been defined and active CTLs against these epitopes were observed.[38]

### 1. Screening by CTLs

The first tumor antigens identified by immunological methods were MAGE-1, 2, and 3 published in a hallmark paper by van der Bruggen and colleagues 15 years ago.[7] These authors used tumor-specific CTLs for the identification of tumor antigens. This approach has since been used in a multitude of studies and has led to a large number of identified T-cell epitopes (reviewed in Reference 10).

A necessary step for antigen screening by CTLs is the establishment of a CTL cell line. This can be done by isolating an already generated CTL from a tumor patient using autologous tumor cells as outlined in Figure 39.2. Briefly, lymphocytes are restimulated weekly with irradiated tumor cells leading to amplification of tumor-specific CTLs, which are cloned by dilution. The corresponding epitopes can then be identified by the biochemical or the genetic approach.[16]

The genetic approach utilizes cDNA libraries, which are transfected into target cells and then searched by the CTL clone. This technique most likely discovers the whole gene, or at least a large part of it.

The biochemical approach aims at the isolation of the presented peptides of the tumor cells. These peptides are separated and subsequently loaded onto target cells to be eventually recognized by the CTL clone. By this method, the actual epitope is directly identified, but it is difficult to find the corresponding gene from starting from a known, 9- to 10-amino-acid-long peptide. The biochemical approach has been performed to identify natural epitopes using a CTCL cell line (MyLa) and CTLs from three different patients, but the authors failed to identify any immunogenic epitope.[39] On the other hand, in melanoma several reports describe the identification of T-cell epitopes using this strategy (see, e.g., Reference 40).

### 2. Screening by Antibodies

A different approach is the serological screening of recombinantly expressed cDNA clones derived from tumor mRNA (SEREX), which was established by Sahin et al.[37] following the observation of serological responses to tumor antigens made long before.[41] SEREX uses the humoral response of the patient's immune system to identify tumor-associated or tumor-specific proteins and has been used by a number of research groups leading to a large number of antigens (reviewed by Chen[42]). Many of these are associated with cancer, but not expressed in a tumor-specific fashion when analyzed on the mRNA level by reverse-transcription polymerase chain reaction (RT-PCR). A public library established at the Ludwig Institute for Cancer Research described in August 2003 about 2160 SEREX-defined clones belonging to 1156 genes as defined by HUGO (Human Genome Organization; a list of regularly updated resources in the Internet is given in Table 39.2).

The SEREX protocol is outlined in Figure 39.3. Briefly, a cDNA phage library is made from tumor mRNA and expressed in *Escherichia coli* leading to plaques by phage-dependent lyses of

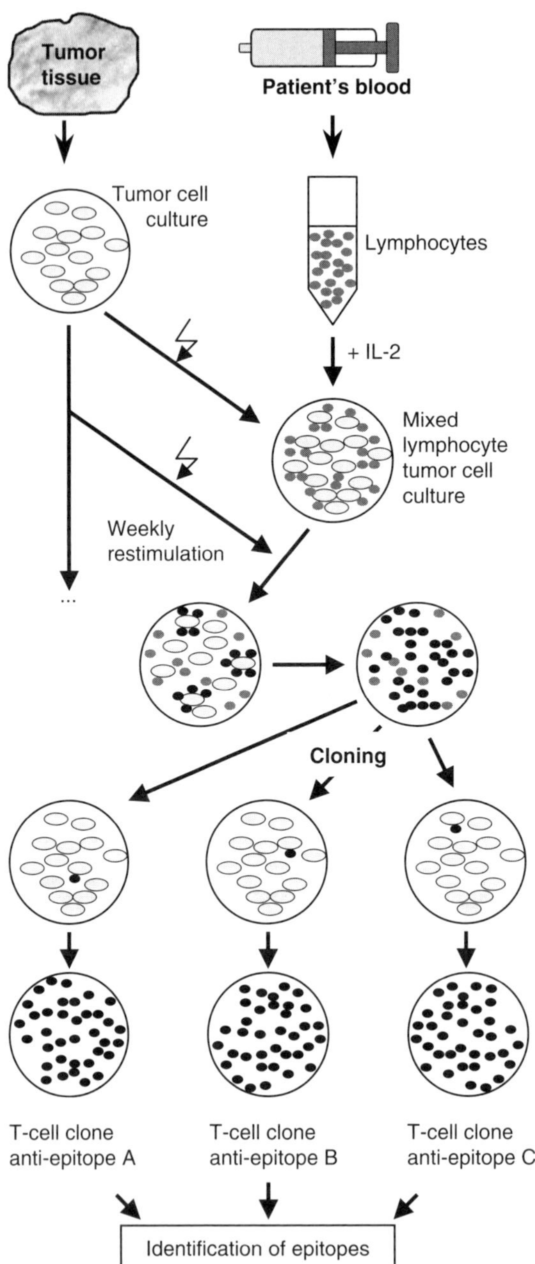


**FIGURE 39.2** Generation of peptide-specific T-cell lines. Lymphocytes are isolated from peripheral blood, supplemented with IL-2, and stimulated with irradiated tumor cells weekly. By diluting the cells a peptide-specific T-cell clone is established. By this method, CD-4 T-cell clones or CTLs may be established. (Adapted from Eichmüller, S., *Onkologie*, 25, 448, 2002. With permission.)

the bacteria. During phage protein translation in *E. coli*, recombinant tumor proteins are also expressed, which are then blotted to a nitrocellulose membrane and tested for recognition by preabsorbed tumor patients' sera. The cDNA insert of the positive phage is sequenced, and subsequent RT-PCR using insert-specific primers evaluates the expression of the identified TAA in human tissues in order to proof for tumor specificity.

**TABLE 39.2**
**Actualized Resources in the Internet**

| Title | Address | Description |
|---|---|---|
| Cancer Immunome Database | http://www2.licr.org/CancerImmunomeDB/ | Tumor-associated antigens identified by SEREX |
| Cancer Genome Anatomy Project | http://cgap.nci.nih.gov/ | Gene expression profiling |
| Peptide Database by Cancer Immunity | http://www.cancerimmunity.org/peptidedatabase/Tcellepitopes.htm | CTL epitope database |
| SYFPEITHI | http://syfpeithi.bmi-heidelberg.com/ | CTL epitope database and epitope predictions |
| BIMAS | http://www-bimas.dcrt.nih.gov/molbio/hla_bind/index.html | CTL epitope predictions |
| NetChop | http://www.cbs.dtu.dk/services/NetChop/ | Prediction of proteasomal cleavage |
| PAPROC | http://www.paproc.de/ | Prediction of proteasomal cleavage |
| NCI | http://www.nci.nih.gov/search/clinicaltrials/ | Clinical trials on melanoma |
| NCBI | http://www.ncbi.nlm.nih.gov/ | Many databases, e.g., Online Mendelian Inheritance in Man |

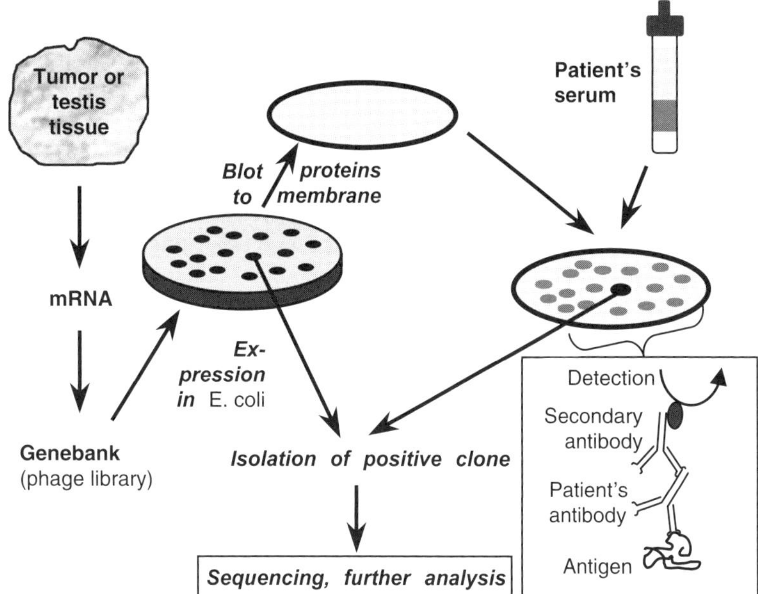


**FIGURE 39.3** The SEREX approach for identifying tumor antigens. For details see text. (Adapted from Eichmüller, S., *Onkologie*, 25, 448, 2002. With permission.)

## C. Humoral and Cellular Targets in Melanoma

Malignant melanoma was one of the first tumors used for identifying tumor antigens. Melanoma is addressed as very immunogenic, but this might also be due to the longer experimental familiarity with this tumor.[43]

### 1. Identification of Melanoma Antigens and Corresponding Epitopes

Tumor antigens for melanoma have been identified by all the methods described above: Tumor-specific CTLs have been used in many attempts (e.g., MAGE-A1),[7] subtractive methods led to

LAGE-1,[30] and the SEREX approach confirmed the immunogenicity of MAGE-A1[37] and MAGE-A4a.[44] Comprehensive lists of tumor antigens for malignant melanoma can be found in Reference 10.

We have recently investigated the humoral response against tumor antigens in patients with melanoma immunized with autologous, gene-modified tumor cells.[45] Interestingly, we found an induction of antibodies against a variety of antigens in these patients during the course of treatment. This response was rather individual, suggesting a diverse repertoire of antigens in different tumors and/or a discrete immunological reaction in different patients.

A promising attempt for immunotherapy activates the cellular tumor defense by antigen-specific CTLs preferentially done by using a vaccine with peptide-loaded dendritic cells (DCs; see below).[46] For this approach the actual HLA-dependent epitope has to be identified, irrespective of the method used to identify the tumor antigen (genetic CTL approach, differential expression screening, or SEREX).

Starting from a known tumor antigen, an HLA-dependent epitope is predicted, e.g., by computer programs referring to binding strength and proteasomal cleavage (for programs, see Table 39.2). The predicted peptides are synthesized and loaded onto DCs. Autologous CTLs are generated with the help of these peptide-loaded antigen-presenting cells and are confirmed to kill peptide-loaded target cells. Finally, the significance of the epitope has to be established by several tests: (1) blocking of killing the target cells by an anti-HLA antibody, (2) killing of target cells transfected with a plasmid encoding the antigen without external loading of peptides, (3) prevention of target cell-detection in case of the wrong HLA type, and (4) establishing of killing such target cells by transfecting them with a plasmid encoding the suitable HLA molecule. The whole strategy has been called reverse immunology.

## 2. Known Melanoma Antigens

The long-lasting experience with malignant melanoma may also account for the fact that tumor antigens of almost all classes have been identified for this type of tumor. Moreover, many tumor antigens were first described for melanoma.

A number of proto-oncogenes, which become oncogenic through mutations, have been described for melanoma, e.g., Ras,[14,47,48] CDK4,[49] and β-catenin.[15] Specific CTLs have been described to be generated in patients with melanoma against these oncogenes, but hot-spot mutations, which might be used as shared targets, have been described only in melanoma: for example, N-RAS codon 61 is mutated in 28% of patients with melanoma.[50] Omholt et al.[50] found three different amino acid replacements of codon 61 (Gln) by Lys (48% if the mutations), Arg (43%), or His (4.5%). Thus, in case of this hot-spot mutation one variant would cover 13% of patients with melanoma and two variants might be detected in one quarter of the patients.

As a result of the individuality of most mutated antigens, this class of targets has not been used in clinical trials, so far. An increasing number of publications during recent years could show a specific immune response against epitopes derived from the mutated region of tumor antigens via $CD8^+$,[51,52] or $CD4^+$ T cells.[53,54] The epitope may also derive from an intronic region in case of alternative splicing of the antigen, as has been shown for gp100.[55]

Most CTA were originally described in malignant melanoma. Prominent examples are the MAGE-A gene family,[7,56–58] GAGE,[20,59] or the LAGE-1/NY-ESO-1 group.[26,30,60,61] At present, 20 groups or individual genes are attributed to CTA.[6] As especially MAGE-A genes have been investigated for more than a decade, the listing of known T-cell epitopes is very long.[10]

Melanoma is derived from its normal cellular counterpart, the melanocyte, and shares with this lineage its differentiation genes. Proteins of quite a number of these genes have been proved to be usable as antigens for a cellular immune defense against the tumor. Most of these differentiation antigens belong to proteins involved in melanogenesis:[62] tyrosinase is the rate-limiting enzyme in melanin biosynthesis, tyrosinase-related protein-1 (TYRP-1/gp75) stabilizes tyrosinase, TYRP-2/DCT is a DOPAchrome tautomerase, and gp100/pmel17 is involved in melanin polymerization.

**TABLE 39.3**
**Tumor Antigens of CTCL Putatively Suitable for Therapy**

| Name | Type of Antigen | Identification | Expression | Ref. |
|---|---|---|---|---|
| SCP-1 | CTA | SEREX | 6% of CTCL tissues<br>Testis | 32 |
| cTAGE-1 | CTA | SEREX | 35% of CTCL tissues<br>Testis | 32 |
| GBP-5ta | Unknown | SEREX | 47% of CTCL tissues<br>Protein not in controls | 34 |
| SC5 | Transmembrane receptor | Monoclonal antibody | CTCL cells and minority of PBLs | 70 |
| LAGE-1<br>NY-ESO-1<br>GAGE-3-7<br>MAGE-A9 | Known CTA or tumor antigens | Identified in other tumors | 15% to 35% of CTCL tissues and testis | 18 |

It has been known since 1983 that melanoma differentiation antigens (TYRP-1) can be detected by IgG antibodies from the patient.[63] Moreover, numerous HLA class I- and class II-dependent epitopes have been identified from all melanoma differentiation antigens.[10]

Melan-A/MART-1, another antigenic melanomosomal protein, is recognized in patients with melanoma. Interestingly, it has been shown that T cells specific for the 27-35 epitope of Melan-A/MART-1 respond to a variety of epitopes including bacterial and viral.[64] Epitope mimicry may be an important factor for the possible strength of an induced immune response against a given tumor antigen.

A comprehensive overview on T-cell epitopes is available online at the Web site of "Cancer Immunity" (for address, see Table 39.2).

## D. Humoral and Cellular Targets in Cutaneous T-Cell Lymphoma

Cutaneous lymphomas (CLs) summarize a variety of malignant tumors originating from T or B lymphocytes with primary manifestation in the skin. They can be subspecified into CTCL or cutaneous B-cell lymphoma (CBCL) depending on the lymphocyte lineage involved (cutaneous T-/B-cell lymphoma). After gastrointestinal lymphoma, CLs are the second most frequent extranodal non-Hodgkin lymphomas (NHL; 25% of all NHL) and have an incidence of 0.5 to 1/100,000.[65] A detailed description of CL is given in Chapter 36.

The clonality of the malignant cells has been shown for CTCL of different stages by determining a clonal T-cell receptor rearrangement.[66] This opens the possibility to search for unique expression profiles of the tumor cells. Clinical observations correlating CD8$^+$ T-cells within CD4$^+$ CTCL tumor lesions with good prognosis[67] and the demonstration of CTCL-specific CD8$^+$ infiltrates[68] indicated a possible tumor defense by the patient's immune system. Recently, the induction of immune defense by tumor-loaded DC could be shown for CTCL.[69] Thus, immunological therapies such as vaccination with peptides or peptide-loaded DC[46] could be a promising new concept for CL, but tumor-specific antigens need to be identified. Putatively suitable tumor antigens in CTCL for therapy are listed in Table 39.3.

### 1. Tumor Antigens Identified by Antibodies

Nikolova et al.[70] have used a monoclonal antibody generated against a natural killer cell line and isolated a new CTCL tumor antigen. They identified SC5, a 96-kDa transmembrane receptor, which is expressed on tumor cells and a minority of peripheral blood lymphocytes. SC5 is one of the rare examples, where interaction with the tumor antigen provokes a physiological effect associated with tumor growth: ligation of SC5 inhibits anti-CD3-induced proliferation.[70]

Our group has recently performed two different SEREX approaches to determine CL-associated tumor antigens. First, a cDNA phage library made from mRNA from a healthy testis was screened with sera from patients with CTCL. The rationale behind this approach is to directly look for CTA relevant for CTCL. This attempt led to 15 TAAs, 2 of which were CTA, while 13 were also expressed in a variety of control tissues.[32] One showed high homology to SCP-1, which has also been identified by others using SEREX and which is expressed in a variety of tumors.[71] Unfortunately, SCP-1 was expressed in only one tumor specimen ($n$ = 20). The second was a new CTA named cTAGE-132, which could be detected in 35% of CTCL specimen ($n$ = 20) and also in several other types of tumors including colorectal, ovarian, mamma, and head and neck squamous cell carcinomas, and malignant melanoma. Interestingly, cTAGE-1 is a member of a larger gene family comprising both tumor-specific and widely expressed genes.[28] cTAGE-5 is another, especially promising target for CTCL and other types of tumors.[28]

In a second attempt we generated a phage library from tumor mRNA using several CTCL and CBCL specimen. This screening led to an additional nine TAAs, one of which is presumably tumor specific on protein level and has been named GBP-5ta.[34] GBP-5 has high homology to the well-characterized guanylate-binding proteins, which belong to the GTPase superfamily including Ras.[72]

### 2. Antigens Known from Other Tumors

A variety of tumor antigens are known from different types of tumors, in particular from malignant melanoma, and for many of those proven CTL epitopes have already been published.[10] Thus, it is tempting to check possible expression of these tumor antigens in CLs. We have performed RT-PCR using specific primers for a variety of individual tumor antigens or groups of antigens, mostly belonging to the CTA comprising MAGE-A genes, MAGE-B genes, GAGE genes, SCP-1, LAGE-1, NY-ESO-1, and the RAGE family.[18] Interestingly, we found only selected tumor antigens expressed in relevant numbers of CTCL tissues, namely, LAGE-1 (55% splicing variant A and/or B) and the GAGE-3-7 group (35%), as well as NY-ESO-1 and the MAGE-A group, although to a lower degree. Moreover, we could show that several of these tumor antigens were detected by patients' antibodies, when expressed as recombinant proteins: cTAGE-1 (34% patients seropositive; $n$ = 29), MAGE-A9 (22%; $n$ = 18), and truncated GAGE (16%; $n$ = 19). In contrast, MAGE-A1, A3, and A6 recognition was observed only to a lower frequency (6 to 11%) and no serum could detect recombinant LAGE-1a.[18]

### 3. The Idiotype as Target

The T-cell receptor (TCR) has been suggested as an antigen for CTCL,[73] which could function as a specific target like the idiotype immunoglobulins do for B-cell lymphoma-specific T cells. In both cases treatment regimens face the disadvantage that the antigen/TCR would have to be identified for each patient individually. Currently, sequencing of the variable chain of the TCR can easily be done and has been suggested to be performed during diagnostic procedures;[66] thus, the sequence of the TCR would be available to search for epitopes in CTCL clones.

The existence of CTLs against epitopes derived from the CDR3 region of the TCR has been proved by Berger and co-workers.[74] In a very recent publication Winter et al.[75] showed that epitopes derived from the beta chain of the TCR can be targeted by patients' CTLs. Further experiments will have to prove whether the individual TCR as unique identifier of the malignant cells is a valuable target in the clinical setting, especially as failures in attempting to identify such targets have also been published.[39]

## E. Targets in Other Skin Cancers

Melanoma rather dominates research on epithelial malignancies. This explains why all other types of skin cancers are summarized as nonmelanoma skin cancers (NMSC). This heterogeneous group is mainly composed of basal cell carcinoma (BCC) and squamous cell carcinoma (SCC), together accounting for more than 95% of all NMSC. While these types of cancer are more frequent than prostate carcinoma in men and also outnumber breast cancer in women, the mortality is conversely low.[76] NMSC grow slowly and rarely metastasize, which makes them easier to manage clinically, especially as surgery achieves a very high cure rate when the histopathological margins are tumor-free.[77]

A number of treatment modalities are available for NMSC: Simple excision, Mohs micrographic surgery, curettage and electrodesiccation, cryosurgery, and irradiation therapy. However, the areas in which NMSC often arise are cosmetically "important" for the patient, leading to disfigurement in the classical therapies, especially in case of multiple tumors.[78] Thus, although the classical treatment regimens are very effective, they may not always be applicable, as they are associated with pain and scarring and may be cosmetically deforming under certain circumstances.

Notably, numerous prerequisites for the application of immune therapies are fulfilled by NMSC.[78] The tumor is growing slowly, spontaneous regression can be observed, and some specific targets have been detected, e.g., p53,[79] Her2/neu,[80,81] and Ep-CAM.[82]

In contrast to malignant melanoma (and probably also CTCL), NMSC is often associated with viral infections, especially several subtypes of human papilloma viruses (HPV).[83–85] This is opening the possibility for true nonself proteins being used as targets for immunotherapy, although the applicability has still to be proved.

## III. STRATEGIES TO FIGHT SKIN CANCER

The identification of tumor antigens and their epitopes provided the basis for the experimental development of specific cancer immunotherapies, from which a large number have already been translated into clinical application. The continuously growing knowledge available on the mechanisms essentially contributing to the induction of a potent, long-term T-cell activation and on the molecular characteristics of tumors and their interaction with the hosts' immune system is still directly transferred into intense preclinical investigations. The whole of these treatment approaches can be subdivided into active and passive immunization strategies. Active immunotherapy (vaccination) encompasses strategies to deliver tumor antigens or their epitopes to the cancer patient's immune system, which should induce an *in vivo* mobilization of antigen-specific effector lymphocytes against the tumor. In contrast, passive immunization delineates the transfer of *ex vivo* generated or expanded effectors (T cells or antibodies) for tumor cell destruction into the patient. In the following, strategies that have already been applied to skin cancer and especially malignant melanoma are discussed.

### A. Specific Immune Responses against Malignant Melanoma

Strategies to achieve specific immune responses against melanoma have been extensively investigated in preclinical models. The great majority of these experimental studies have been performed in the transplantable B16 melanoma system. Comparable to the human situation, this tumor, as well as its syngeneic mouse recipient, expresses melanoma-differentiation antigens (MDA, e.g., gp100, TRP1, TRP2, tyrosinase). Therefore, immunotherapies targeting these antigens have to deal with the problem of T cell tolerance toward self-antigens. These tolerance mechanisms lead to a deletion and/or anergy of high-avidity self-reactive T cells, indicating that the residual T-cell repertoire responding to immunotherapy might be of low avidity. But several studies in the B16 melanoma model repeatedly demonstrated that by proper immunotherapeutic activation these T cells can be mobilized to mediate effective prophylactic and therapeutic tumor immunity.[86–88] Although conclusions drawn from treatment of transplantable animal tumors cannot be translated directly into the human situation, where tumors develop spontaneously, this model resembles, at least to a certain degree, the barriers of immune responses toward human MDA, which have to be overcome by immunotherapy.

Indeed, spontaneously *in vivo* sensitized T cells recognizing MDA have repeatedly been isolated from tumors and from the peripheral blood of patients with melanoma indicating that tolerance toward these antigens is also not absolute in humans.[89–93] Especially reactive T cells against the MelanA/MART-1 antigen can be frequently observed in patients with HLA-A2-positive melanoma. The immunodominance of T-cell responses against the HLA-A2-restricted MelanA/MART-127-35 epitope can at least partially be attributed to the exceptionally high frequency of T-cell precursors even detectable in healthy individuals. Whereas in normal donors these T-cell precursors are naive, a high percentage of MelanA/MART-127-35-specific T cells from patients with melanoma detectable in the peripheral blood compartment, lymph nodes, and tumors exhibits an antigen-experienced phenotype.[94–96]

Treatment of patients with melanoma with vaccines targeting MDA has been demonstrated to enhance preexisting spontaneous T-cell responses and to be capable of inducing primary antigen-specific T-cell immunity, which was associated with clinical responses at least in some individuals (see next sections). As these antigens are expressed in a lineage-specific pattern, immunity toward them potentially bears the risk of inducing autoimmunity. Indeed, vitiligo has been demonstrated to occur spontaneously in patients with melanoma but can also be vaccine induced,[97,98] but this risk seems to be acceptable as long as the normal tissue is not essential for life.

In contrast, autoimmunity should be no problem for immunotherapies targeting the group of CTA. Spontaneous T-cell responses against the antigens can also be observed in patients with melanoma.[7,99] Especially for the NY-ESO-1 antigens, spontaneous humoral and cellular immune responses occur in a high percentage of patients with melanoma.[60,100] Antigens belonging to the category of MDA or CTA are the most frequently used targets for T-cell-based immunotherapy of melanoma.

## B. Requirements for T-Cell-Based Immunotherapies

The first generations of clinically applied vaccines exclusively focused on the activation of tumor antigen-specific cytotoxic $CD8^+$ T lymphocytes (CTL), which are still defined to be the most essential mediators of destructive antitumor immunity. But during the last years it has been demonstrated that *in vivo* induction of a potent, long-lasting cytotoxic immune response requires the interaction of at least three cellular players: DC, antigen-specific $CD4^+$ T helper (Th) lymphocytes, and antigen-specific CTL. Basic immunological findings led to the following actual concept of antigen-specific T-cell immunity against tumors: To become properly activated and to differentiate into cytotoxic effectors, naive CTL simultaneously have to receive the antigen signal (peptide–HLA complex) in combination with certain co-stimulatory signals. Consequently, tumors, which usually do not express co-stimulatory molecules, cannot induce initial T-cell activation; in contrast, antigen stimulation in the absence of co-stimulation contributes to T-cell tolerance. Antigen and co-stimulatory signals can only be properly provided by activated professional antigen-presenting cells (APC), especially DC. To become inductors of antigen-specific immune responses, immature DC have to sample and process the tumor antigen and in addition have to receive a maturation signal. This signal can be delivered by the interaction of the CD40 surface molecule on DC with the CD40 ligand (CD40L) expressed on activated $CD4^+$ T helper cells.[101,102] The Th cell itself becomes activated by specifically recognizing its antigenic peptide presented on HLA class II molecules by DC. Recent data indicate that antigen-specific Th not only contribute to primary CTL sensitization and proliferation via DC activation and cytokine secretion (e.g., interleukin-2, or IL-2), but also play an essential role in the generation of specific $CD8^+$ T cell memory by the interaction of CD40L with CD40 being transiently expressed on activated $CD8^+$ T cells.[103,104]

Based on this model, the ideal T-cell-based vaccines should target both the antigen-specific $CD4^+$ and the $CD8^+$ T-cell subset. Therefore, research laboratories dedicate their efforts to the improvement of clinically applied therapies as well as to the development of new T-cell-based immunotherapies. As described in the following the great majority of these strategies belong to the category of active immunotherapies (see above).

## C. Peptide and Protein Vaccines

To date, peptide vaccination has been the most frequently applied antigen-specific treatment regimen for patients with melanoma. The first vaccine generations consisted of synthetic peptide epitopes recognized by CD8+ T cells, which are the simplest and easiest to produce. In several clinical studies, patients with melanoma received peptide vaccines consisting of a single epitope from one tumor antigen or of a mixture of synthetic peptides derived from several antigen targets. In general, peptides were given in combination with adjuvants to increase vaccine-induced T-cell response.[105,106] The analysis of T-cell responses in patients with metastatic melanoma receiving the Melan-A/MART-127-35 peptide either with or without incomplete Freund's adjuvants (IFA) allowed detection of vaccine-specific T-cell responses only when peptide plus adjuvant was administered.[105] In addition to IFA, recombinant cytokines were included in many peptide vaccination trials to strengthen the adjuvant effect. Rosenberg et al.[107] observed a twofold increase in clinical responses toward a gp100 peptide (+ IFA) vaccine when patients additionally received high doses of IL-2. Because of its ability to mobilize immature DC and to contribute to their maturation, granulocyte-macrophage colony-stimulating factor (GM-CSF) has been included as a cytokine adjuvant in several peptide immunization regimens.[108–110] However, a recent phase I study by Scheibenbogen et al.[111] with patients with high-risk melanoma, clinically free of disease, questions the influence of GM-CSF on the T-cell-stimulatory capacity of a tyrosinase peptide vaccine. Tyrosinase-specific T-cell responses could be detected in patients receiving the peptide alone (three of nine patients) as frequently as in patients receiving the peptide plus GM-CSF (four of nine patients). Accordingly, clinical responses could be observed in 7 of 25 patients with metastatic melanoma receiving an HLA-A1-restricted MAGE-3 peptide vaccine without any adjuvant, with three patients exhibiting complete responses.[112] The detailed analysis of CTL responses in one of the patients with tumor regression demonstrated the existence of a monoclonal low-level CTL response against MAGE-3 after vaccination. This indicates (1) that even those effectors that are more difficult to detect might initiate tumor rejection and (2) that evaluation of the frequency of specific T-cell responses in patients before and after vaccination has to be carried out very carefully and probably requires a combined application of different highly sensitive technologies (e.g., limiting dilution, tetramer staining, enzyme-linked immunospot).[113] Indeed, some encouraging results have been obtained by peptide vaccination, but overall clinical responses were observed only in 10 to 30% of the treated patients, raising the question of vaccine efficacy.

Although CTL peptide epitopes have been identified to be target structures of *in vivo* sensitized T cells, their natural immunogenicity is often very low, which might lead to an ineffective T-cell stimulation during immunotherapy. It has been demonstrated that peptide immunogenicity can be improved either by increasing the binding affinity of the peptide to its HLA restriction element or by strengthening the interaction of the peptide–HLA complex with the TCR. An altered variant of the Melan-A/MART-127-35 peptide ligand (Melan-A/MART-127-35/27L) exhibits increased immunogenicity, presumably through a more efficient interaction of the peptide–HLA complex with the TCR. Increased binding affinity has been demonstrated for the Melan-A/MART-126-35/27L and the gp100209-217/210M epitope,[114,115] the latter being already applied in different clinical trials.[107]

With respect to the essential role of antigen-specific CD4+ T cells in the process of induction and maintenance of an antigen-specific cytotoxic immunity it was postulated that the efficacy of peptide immunotherapy might be improved by including synthetic peptide sequences recognized by Th cells into the vaccine. Until recently, the knowledge about HLA class II-restricted epitopes from tumor antigens was very limited. To overcome this deficit foreign helper epitopes (e.g., tetanus helper epitope)[116,117] or proteins (e.g., KLH, or keyhole limpet hemocyanin)[111] were included in the vaccine as a source for Th stimulation. As a result of the great efforts directed toward the identification of tumor-antigen-specific HLA class II epitopes, it can be expected that this information will soon be translated into the design of new clinical trials.[118,119]

In contrast to synthetic peptide epitopes, protein vaccines have the advantage of a broad application. The administration of entire antigens obviates the need to define epitopes for each patient's HLA genotype, as multiple HLAclass I and class II epitopes can be processed from the protein *in vivo*. So far patients with metastatic melanoma have only been immunized with recombinant MAGE-3 protein, in most cases in combination with the SBAS-2 adjuvant.[120] Tumor responses to vaccination could be observed only in the minority of patients. But $CD4^+$ T-cell clones recognizing an HLA-DR1 restricted MAGE-3 epitope could be isolated from one selected patient, who exhibited partial responses upon vaccination.[121]

## D. Naked DNA Vaccines

Naked DNA vaccines simply consist of eukaryotic expression plasmids encoding the tumor antigen or its epitopes. The plasmid DNA, isolated from bacteria, contains immunostimulatory, unmethylated CpG motifs, which at least in mouse studies have been demonstrated to have an adjuvant effect by activating certain players of the immune system, including dendritic cells.[122] After administration the DNA is most probably taken up by nonprofessional APC, which then produce the antigen that has to be taken up, sampled, and cross-presented by DC.[123]

Recently, the results of two clinical studies of naked DNA immunization of patients with melanoma were published. In one study, plasmid DNA-encoding native gp100 was administered either intradermally or intramuscularly to the patients. No anti-gp100 was detectable in any of the 13 analyzed recipients, which might at least partially be attributed to the low immunogenicity of the native gp100 sequence (see next section).[124] In the second study, patients received repeated infusions of a DNA vaccine, encoding multiple HLA-A2-restricted epitopes of the tyrosinase antigen, into a lymph node. T-cell responses toward a tyrosinase epitope could be detected in 11 of 26 patients by tetramer analysis.[125] As the available information on clinically applied DNA vaccines is very limited, further clinical trials must be performed to estimate the capacity of DNA vaccines to induce antigen-specific T-cell responses in patients with tumor.

## E. Recombinant Viral Vaccines

Different viruses have already been employed in clinical trials as recombinant vector systems for tumor antigens, including adenovirus,[126] vaccinia virus,[127] fowlpox virus,[128] and canarypox virus.[129]

As a result of the relative ease of genetically modifying and amplifying fowlpox virus, which is replication-defective in mammalian cells, the Rosenberg's group[128] recently vaccinated patients with melanoma with recombinant fowlpox virus encoding different forms of the gp100 tumor antigen. Only one of seven patients receiving a virus encoding the native gp100 sequence exhibited T-cell responses toward the antigen. However, gp100-specifc immunity was detectable in the majority of patients immunized with a fowlpox virus encoding either the anchor-modified gp100209-217/210M epitope variant (see section on peptide and protein vaccines) or the full-length gp100 with anchor-modified epitope sequences. Induction of antigen-specific T-cell responses has also been reported for patients immunized with a vaccinia virus encoding co-stimulatory molecules and HLA-A2-restricted epitopes derived from the gp100, Melan-A/MART-1, and tyrosinase antigens.[127]

When employing viral vectors for vaccination, it has to be taken into account that in some cases preexisting neutralizing antibodies and T-cell responses toward viral antigens might reduce the strength of T-cell responses to the tumor antigen, limiting the repeated administration of the same recombinant vector to the patient. To overcome this, different viral vectors that do not share antigenic structures except for the tumor antigen might be used for immunization. Alternatively, sequential applications of naked DNA and viral vaccines encoding the same antigen might be useful. In preclinical studies it has been demonstrated that these so-called prime and boost regimens induce a tremendous increase in the frequency of tumor antigen-specific T cells.[130]

An alternative to viral systems might be the use of bacterial vector systems.[131] Several studies in the B16 melanoma mouse model performed by Reisfeld's group[132] impressively demonstrated the capability of *Salmonella* to efficiently deliver eukaryotic expression plasmids to the infected host, thereby inducing immune responses toward plasmid-encoded MDA.

## F. DC Vaccines

In spite of the promising results reported for early clinical trials, DC vaccination is still in an early stage of development. The understanding of the biology of DC has increased dramatically and, as a consequence, the techniques for generating DC cells have improved steadily. However, it will take some time to test all the newly developed techniques and possibilities in various clinical trials in a clinical setting. Nevertheless, sufficient evidence has been provided to show that DC do have the capacity to induce and expand immune responses against cancer cells. In the rest of this chapter the key variables involved are explicated and the clinical achievements briefly summarized. For a more extensive review see Schuler et al.[133]

In is now clear that the maturation status of DC has a decisive influence on the success of DC vaccination and its reproducibility. Immature DC induce predominantly regulatory T cells and tolerance,[134,135] whereas mature DC induce Th1 responses. There is still no general agreement among researchers on the best source for obtaining DC precursors (monocytes, $CD34^+$ precursors, Langerhans cells, or bone marrow). Furthermore, it has become increasingly clear that human blood contains several subsets of DC,[136] but only since it just recently became possible to use magnetic cell sorting to separate the cells has it been possible to identify and characterize these DC subsets and to compare the DC vaccines produced in accordance with various DC generation protocols at different disease stages. At present DC derived from $CD14^+$ monocytes, which are first exposed to GM-CSF and IL-4 and subsequently to IL-1$\beta$, tumor necrosis factor-alpha (TNF-$\alpha$), IL-6, and prostaglandin $E_2$ ($PGE_2$) are used widely.[137] DC matured with this cocktail were shown to have some migrating capacity mediated by the induction of CCR7 surface expression,[138,139] but they exhibited only weak bioactive IL-12 secretion[140] and some capacity to induce Th1 responses.

There is still no commonly accepted knowledge on the number of DC needed for effective vaccination and no general agreement on the best route of administration. Immunization over the subcutaneous route is the easiest and has been shown to induce CTL responses,[118] although only a small number of mature DC migrate to the lymph nodes.[133] There has still been no adequate systematic exploration of the optimal loading of DC with antigens. Peptides of various lengths, recombinant proteins, RNA, as well as lysates of necrotic or apoptotic cells or exosomes have been investigated for loading, but no comparative data are available. The same applies to data on dosage and optimal frequency of vaccination.

The results of more that 50 clinical trials using DC have proved that DC vaccination is safe and occasionally leads to impressive clinical regression. Almost all of these trials are clinical phase I and II studies testing safety and feasibility but not analyzing efficacy. A single injection of 2 to 4 million mature monocyte-derived DC in healthy volunteers proved to be sufficient to induce a strong Th1 response,[141] and these findings could be reproduced in various clinical trials with patients suffering from advanced cancers including melanoma (reviewed in Reference 133). Several reports described an association between clinical responses and detected T-cell responses, but there is still some controversy on this subject. These results must be viewed with some caution because most of these studies are quite small and include only a very selected patient cohort. Whether these encouraging results translate into greater success in treating patients with cancer cannot be determined until the results of clinical phase III trials testing the efficacy of this novel treatment have been analyzed. Possibly, these studies will reveal that only certain subsets of patients, for example, patients with melanoma with a high risk of recurrence (stage III or stage IV with no evidence of disease) or with a limited tumor burden (AJCC, M1a)[142] would be the ideal patient population for vaccination treatment. Recent advances in the understanding of the biology of DC, first results showing that DC vaccination combined with cytokine treatment[143,144] or that other immunomodulatory measures improve treatment efficacy, along with improvements made in standardized DC generation will be incorporated in the designs of new clinical phase II and III studies. These studies in turn will provide more direct and revealing comparisons of the vaccination approaches in question and ultimately make it possible to decide whether DC vaccination has a future as a new standard in cancer treatment.

## G. Adoptive T-Cell Transfer

In addition to the different approaches of active immunotherapy, passive T-cell-based treatments have received new interest. Therefore, autologous cytotoxic T cells are expanded *in vitro,* which are then adoptively transferred into the patient to mediate tumor cell destruction. The therapeutic capacity of T cells infused into patients with advanced metastatic melanoma was recently demonstrated by Dudley et al.[145] In this study HLA-A2$^+$ patients, after a nonmyeloablative conditioning regimen, received *in vitro* expanded TIL (tumor-infiltrating lymphocytes), exhibiting cytolytic activity toward autologous tumor cells or allogenic HLA-A2$^+$ melanoma cell lines. Most TIL cultures, although consisting of heterogeneous populations of CD8$^+$ and CD4$^+$ T cells, exhibited specificity toward the MART-1/MelanA and/or gp100 antigens. T cells were applied with high doses of IL-2 and induced tumor regressions in 8 of 13 patients. Massive clonal expansion of adoptively transferred T cells was detectable in the peripheral blood of two selected patients, probably due to the disturbance of T-cell homeostasis after lymphodepletion.

In a second phase I study of Yee et al.[146] patients with HLA-A2$^+$ melanoma were treated with *in vitro* expanded autologous CD8$^+$ T cell clones from the peripheral blood exhibiting a defined specificity for either the MART-1/MelanA or the gp100 antigen. It was demonstrated that these T cells persisted *in vivo* in response to low systemic doses of IL-2 and preferentially migrated to the tumor site. In eight of ten patients this treatment led to minor, mixed, or stable responses. Immunohistochemical analysis of antigen expression in biopsies obtained pre- and post-treatment from some patients demonstrated that loss of antigen expression might have prevented a more extensive tumor mass destruction. Although results obtained in this study clearly demonstrate the destructive activity of T-cell clones against autologous tumor mass and that immunity toward MDA can restrict tumor growth, it also indicates limitations of immunotherapies due to immune escape mechanisms by the tumor.

## H. Obstacles of T-Cell-Based Immunotherapy

Application of T-cell-based immunotherapies so far has produced some encouraging clinical responses but only in the minority of patients. Therefore, one task of future studies will be the identification of (1) mechanisms mediating successful immunotherapy in a small subset of patients and (2) mechanisms preventing successful immunotherapy in the majority of patients.

One obstacle to the induction of a potent therapeutic CTL immunity might be the administration of ineffective vaccines. Although in many patients with melanoma T-cell responses against tumor antigens have been induced by vaccinations, these responses were only weak and transient. Vaccines must be potent enough to break antigen-specific T-cell tolerance and to mobilize also low-affinity T cells, which can only be achieved when antigen loading and activation of professional APC during vaccination occurs efficiently.

Another barrier preventing effective destruction of tumors by CTL is the genetic instability of the malignant cells, which allows the outgrowth of a heterogeneous tumor cell population. Therefore, antigen-specific cytotoxic T cells activated by the vaccine might be able to kill only some cells expressing the antigen but variants having lost antigen expression will continuously grow out.[147,146] This might to a certain extent be prevented by the application of vaccines consisting of a mixture of antigens or by targeting antigens that are essential for maintenance of the malignant phenotype.

The genetic instability of tumors has also been demonstrated to lead to mutations in the cellular antigen-processing and presentation machinery preventing antigenic peptide presentation to T lymphocytes.[148,149] Reduced surface presentation of HLA class I molecules and even total loss of expression, the last mainly originating from mutations in the β2-microglobulin gene encoding the light chain of HLA class I molecules, can frequently be observed for melanoma.[150,151]

Another mechanism that might enable the tumor to escape the destructive mechanisms of adaptive immunity has recently been described by Andreola et al.[152] Melanoma cells were demonstrated to secrete microvesicles containing FasL. Ligation of FasL to its receptor Fas induces programmed cell death. Since Fas is expressed on most cells of the immune system, including T cells, secretion of the vesicles might be a strategy to induce T-cell death.

## I. Antibody-Based Immunotherapies

Immunological therapies using antibodies are especially attractive, as they do not need to be patient specific, if shared antigens are used as targets. The main difficulty of this therapy is the selection of good targets, which need to be overexpressed in the tumor, membrane bound, accessible from the outside of the cell by an antibody, and — as all shared targets — should be expressed in a high percentage of tumor cells and in tumors of many patients. The generated antibody should possess a high immunogenicity, a long half-life, and the ability to recruit immune effector functions.[9]

The usage of antibodies as a clinical device has been classified as passive or active antibody therapy, referring to whether or not the immune system of the patient has to react against the therapeutic antibody (active/indirect) or the antibody mediates the therapeutic effect directly (passive).

The aim of active/indirect antibody therapy is to resemble the target by an antibody (called Ab2), which is then detected by newly generated anti-idiotype antibodies from the patient (Ab3).[153] Ab2 is generated against the idiotype of a target-specific antibody (Ab1) and should thus mimic the natural target. The rationale of using Ab2 instead of the natural target is to overcome tolerance against the weakly immunogenic self-antigens presented on the tumor cell. Ab3, which is generated as an immunological response within the patient, will detect not only the idiotype of Ab2, but also the natural target on the tumor cell, which is mimicked by Ab2. Active antibody therapy harks back to an idea published in the early 1970s.[154] A theory on this issue called the "network of the immune system" has been elaborated on by Jerne.[155] The therapeutic effect mediated by Ab3 might act through antibody-dependent cell-mediated cytotoxicity (ADCC) or complement activation (CDC) or other yet unknown mechanisms.

Since the introduction of the "network of the immune system," a number of targets have been selected to be used for indirect antibody therapy and several studies have also been performed for malignant melanoma.[156] Especially ganglioside-mimicking Ab2 antibodies have been used. In a recently published clinical study safety and an immunological response in terms of specific Ab3 could be shown, but no objective clinical responses were observed.[157] In spite of the long tradition on indirect antibody therapy, to date no phase III/IV studies have been performed for malignant melanoma.[156]

Direct (passive) antibody immune therapy aims at mediating the therapeutic effect through an antibody specific for the target on the tumor cell. This antibody is comparable to Ab3 in the indirect antibody therapy concept with the important difference that the therapeutic antibody is artificially generated and thus amenable for further modifications. These include generation of bispecific antibodies[158] and coupling to toxins[159] or to radioisotopes like yttrium (90Y) or iodine (131I).[160,161]

In spite of the name passive, direct antibody therapy needs a very active immune system in several variants applied today. First, all kinds of antibody therapies can induce ADCC and/or CDC, which can, for example, be induced strongly by murine antibodies.[162] Second, bispecific antibodies, which are directed against membrane-bound targets on the tumor cell and components of T cells like the CD3 molecule, act through the close localization of tumor and T cell.[158] And even in case of the toxin-coupled antibodies part macrophages are responsible for the eradication of killed cells and antigen-presenting cells may mediate a cytotoxic bystander effect.

Radioimmunotherapy or toxin-coupled antibodies have been generated against a variety of targets (e.g., CD20, CD22, CD52, CD80, CD30, and HLA-DR) and are at present applied in various clinical studies.[159,160,161,163–166] Much new hope in the field of antibody therapy has been brought by antibodies against CD20 (Rituximab) and Her2/Neu (Trastuzumab). Rituximab has also been applied for a dermatological malignancy: CBCL has been treated by the chimeric CD20 antibody both systemically[167] and intralesionally[168] with objective clinical responses. The murine monoclonal antibody has been humanized (human IgG1 (κ) heavy and light chain) and exerts its effect on the binding of CD20-mediating cell cycle arrest and apoptosis. In addition, the human Fc part of the antibody is recognized by the immune system and induces CDC, phagocytosis by mononuclear cells, and activation of natural killer cells.[167]

Specific antibody therapy in malignant melanoma has been performed using gangliosides as targets. Initial phase I/II trials have used a murine monoclonal antibody (3F8) against glycosphingolipid GD2 and reported clinical responses comprising ADCC and CDC.[169] Also, intralesional injection of the human monoclonal anti-GD2 antibody L72-mediated CDC.[170] A therapeutic murine antibody directed against GD3 (R24) produced clinical response rates no greater than 10%, which was even worsened by various strategies applied to improve the effectiveness of the clinical application of R24.[156]

Another mouse/human chimeric antibody against GD2 (ch14.18) has been fused to lymphotoxin-α and applied to the B16 mouse melanoma model by Schrama and colleagues.[171] In contrast to the control group, which obtained the lymphotoxin alone, the application of ch14.18-lymphotoxin-α resulted clearance of tumor and prevention of lung metastasis depending on dose and time of application (latest successful treatment 1 week after tumor inoculation). Extensive investigations were performed to delineate the mechanisms involved in the antitumor effect of the fusion-antibody treatment unraveling a number of immunological mediators: First, a T-cell response was evident even against other tumor antigens than GD2, as proved by a Trp-2-derived epitope (Trp-2180-188). Second, the induction of a peripheral lympoid-like tissue in the tumor mass due to the antibody application was observed containing naive T cells. If antibody-lymphotoxin-dependent lymphoid neogenesis would be confirmed for humans, this may provide the possibility of priming T cells in the periphery close to the tumor in a microenvironment with predominance of tumor antigens and a reduction in time between priming and expansion.

Recently, an antimelanoma single-chain Fv antibody fused to the toxin gelonin has been reported.[172] Because of the small size of the antibody part and the short half-life in the circulation, Rosenblum and colleagues hope that the immunogenicity of their construct is low, as this would allow a prolonged application of the fusion toxin. In other therapeutic antibodies fused to toxins, duration of therapy had often been hampered by side effects resulting from the immunogenicity of the construct.

Antibodies are used not only for mediating therapy by guiding effector cells or toxins to the malignant cell, but also for mediating adjuvant effects through interacting with immunoregulatory components. Recently, an antibody directed against cytotoxic T-lymphocyte-associated antigen 4 (CTLA-4) has been used in parallel with a vaccination with HLA-dependent peptides in 14 patients.[173] The anti-CTLA-4 antibody has been made responsible for the induction of three objective clinical responses (two complete, one partial) and two mixed responses, as the application of the same peptides in a former study did not result in any clinical responses. In parallel, the antibody-induced grade III/IV autoimmune reactions in 43% of the patients, which could be cured by discontinuation of the treatment cycles and supportive care.[173] This report underlines the notion that successful immunotherapy against self-proteins represented on the malignant cells will often be associated with autoimmune responses.

## IV. CONCLUSION

Antigen-specific immunotherapy of patients with tumor follows different strategies; even clinical trials targeting the same tumor antigen by the same vaccine (synthetic peptide epitope) are extremely heterogeneous, e.g., with respect to vaccine formulation, vaccine dose, and route of vaccine application. Therefore, results obtained by these studies have to be compared with caution, especially when different technologies have been applied to characterize spontaneous and vaccine-induced T-cell responses, e.g., tetramer staining, intracellular interferon-$\gamma$ staining, or ELISPOT analysis. Consequently, multicenter clinical trials will be needed to obtain reliable results on the efficacy of different immunotherapies.

To define precisely the requirements necessary to induce a therapeutic potent and durable immunity against the tumor, preclinical studies in animal model systems more related to the human situation will be needed. So far, experimental studies have been performed in a prophylactic setting in which the animals have to be protected against a lethal challenge with tumor cells. To leave these artificial systems and come closer to tumorgenesis in humans, these analyses should be performed in recently developed model systems where tumors occur that are genetically driven "spontaneously."[174] Nevertheless, encouraging results from animal studies obtained in a prophylactic setting might provide the rationale to think about immunizations to prevent formation of tumors. Under these conditions highly effective antigen-specific immune responses might be easier to achieve as immune suppression by the tumor does not occur, although a precise selection of target antigens would be required to prevent severe side effects.

## REFERENCES


1. Fleming, I.D. et al. Principles of management of basal and squamous cell carcinoma of the skin, *Cancer*, 75, 699, 1995.
2. Schadendorf, D., Is there a standard for the palliative treatment of melanoma? *Onkologie*, 25, 74, 2002.
3. Eigentler, T.K. et al., Palliative therapy of disseminated malignant melanoma: a systematic review of 41 randomised clinical trials, *Lancet Oncol*, 4, 748, 2003.
4. De Smet, C. et al., The activation of human gene MAGE-1 in tumor cells is correlated with genome-wide demethylation, *PNAS*, 93, 7149, 1996.
5. Old, L.J., Cancer/Testis (CT) antigens — a new link between gametogenesis and cancer, *Cancer Immun.*, 1, 1, 2001.
6. Scanlan, M.J. et al., Cancer/testis antigens: an expanding family of targets for cancer immunotherapy, *Immunol. Rev.*, 188, 22, 2002.
7. van der Bruggen, P. et al., A gene encoding an antigen recognized by cytolytic T lymphocytes on a human melanoma, *Science*, 254, 1643, 1991.
8. Hartmann, F., Renner, C., and Pfreundschuh, M., Tumor Immunotherapy with bispecific antibodies, *Onkologie*, 19, 114, 1996.
9. White, C.A., Weaver, R.L., and Grillo-Lopez, A.J., Antibody-targeted immunotherapy for treatment of malignancy, *Annu. Rev. Med.*, 52, 125, 2001.
10. Renkvist, N. et al., A listing of human tumor antigens recognized by T cells, *Cancer Immunol. Immunother.*, 50, 3, 2001.
11. Sahin, U., Türeci, Ö., and Pfreundschuh, M., Serological identification of human tumor antigens, *Curr. Opin. Immunol.*, 9, 709, 1997.
12. Bos, J.L., Ras oncogenes in human cancer: a review, *Cancer Res.*, 49, 4682, 1989.
13. Varmus, H.E., Viruses, genes, and cancer. I. The discovery of cellular oncogenes and their role in neoplasia, *Cancer*, 55, 2324, 1985.
14. Polsky, D. and Cordon-Cardo, C., Oncogenes in melanoma, *Oncogene*, 22, 3087, 2003.
15. Robbins, P.F. et al., A mutated beta-catenin gene encodes a melanoma-specific antigen recognized by tumor infiltrating lymphocytes, *J. Exp. Med.*, 183, 1185, 1996.

16. Castelli, C. et al., T-cell recognition of melanoma-associated antigens, *J. Cell Physiol.*, 182, 323, 2000.
17. Häffner, A.C. et al., Expression of cancer/testis antigens in cutaneous T cell lymphomas, *Int. J. Cancer*, 97, 668, 2002.
18. Eichmüller, S. et al., Tumor-specific antigens in cutaneous T-cell lymphoma: expression and sero-reactivity, *Int. J. Cancer*, 104, 482, 2003.
19. Coulie, P.G. et al., Genes coding for tumor antigens recognized by human cytolytic T lymphocytes, *J. Immunother.*, 14, 104, 1993.
20. Dalerba, P. et al., High homogeneity of MAGE, BAGE, GAGE, tyrosinase and Melan-A/MART-1 gene expression in clusters of multiple simultaneous metastases of human melanoma: implications for protocol design of therapeutic antigen-specific vaccination strategies, *Int. J. Cancer*, 77, 200, 1998.
21. Fehrmann, F. and Laimins, L.A., Human papillomaviruses: targeting differentiating epithelial cells for malignant transformation, *Oncogene*, 22, 5201, 2003.
22. Tsang, K.Y. et al., Generation of human cytotoxic T cells specific for human carcinoembryonic antigen epitopes from patients immunized with recombinant vaccinia-CEA vaccine, *J. Natl. Cancer Inst.*, 87, 982, 1995.
23. Lamerz, R., AFP isoforms and their clinical significance (overview), *Anticancer Res.*, 17, 2927, 1997.
24. Nagorsen, D. et al., Natural T-cell response against MHC class I epitopes of epithelial cell adhesion molecule, her-2/neu, and carcinoembryonic antigen in patients with colorectal cancer, *Cancer Res.*, 60, 4850, 2000.
25. Wreschner, D.H. et al., Human epithelial tumor antigen cDNA sequences. Differential splicing may generate multiple protein forms, *Eur. J. Biochem.*, 189, 463, 1990.
26. Aarnoudse, C.A. et al., Interleukin-2-induced, melanoma-specific T cells recognize CAMEL, an unexpected translation product of LAGE-1, *Int. J. Cancer*, 82, 442, 1999.
27. van den Eynde, B.J. et al., A new antigen recognized by cytolytic T lymphocytes on a human kidney tumor results from reverse strand transcription, *J. Exp. Med.*, 190, 1793, 1999.
28. Usener, D. et al., cTAGE: a cutaneous T-cell lymphoma associated antigen family with tumor-specific splicing, *J. Invest. Dermatol.*, 121, 198, 2003.
29. Jäger, E., Jäger, D., and Knuth, A., Peptide Vaccination in Clinical Oncology, *Onkologie*, 23, 410, 2000.
30. Lethé, B. et al., LAGE-1, a new gene with tumor specificity, *Int. J. Cancer*, 76, 903, 1998.
31. Scanlan, M.J. et al., Antigens recognized by autologous antibody in patients with renal-cell carcinoma, *Int. J. Cancer*, 83, 456, 1999.
32. Eichmüller, S. et al., Serological detection of cutaneous T-cell lymphoma-associated antigens, *PNAS*, 98, 629, 2001.
33. Scanlan, M.J. et al., Cancer-related serological recognition of human colon cancer: identification of potential diagnostic and immunotherapeutic targets, *Cancer Res.*, 62, 4041, 2002.
34. Hartmann, T.B. et al., SEREX identification of new tumour-associated antigens in cutaneous T-cell lymphoma, *Br. J. Dermatol.*, 150, 252, 2004.
35. Labrecque, S. et al., Analysis of the anti-p53 antibody response in cancer patients, *Cancer Res.*, 53, 3468, 1993.
36. Eichmüller, S., Towards defining specific antigens for cutaneous lymphomas, *Onkologie*, 25, 448, 2002.
37. Sahin, U. et al., Human neoplasms elicit multiple specific immune responses in the autologous host, *PNAS*, 92, 11810, 1995.
38. Jäger, E. et al., Induction of primary NY-ESO-1 immunity: $CD8^+$ T lymphocyte and antibody responses in peptide-vaccinated patients with NY-ESO-$1^+$ cancers, *PNAS*, 97, 12198, 2000.
39. Linnemann, T. et al., Identification of epitopes for CTCL-specific cytotoxic T lymphocytes, *Adv. Exp. Med. Biol.*, 451, 231, 1998.
40. Falk, K. et al., Identification of naturally processed viral nonapeptides allows their quantification in infected cells and suggests an allele-specific T cell epitope forecast, *J. Exp. Med.*, 174, 425, 1991.
41. Pfreundschuh, M. et al., Serological analysis of cell surface antigens of malignant human brain tumors, *PNAS*, 75, 5122, 1978.
42. Chen, Y.T., Cancer vaccine: identification of human tumor antigens by SEREX, *Cancer J. Sci. Am.*, 6(Suppl. 3), S208, 2000.
43. Houghton, A.N., Gold, J.S., and Blachere, N.E., Immunity against cancer: lessons learned from melanoma, *Curr. Opin. Immunol.*, 13, 134, 2001.

44. Chen, Y.T. et al., Identification of multiple cancer/testis antigens by allogeneic antibody screening of a melanoma cell line library, *PNAS*, 95, 6919, 1998.
45. Ehlken, H., Schadendorf, D., and Eichmüller, S., Humoral immune response against melanoma antigens induced by vaccination with cytokine gene-modified autologous tumor cells, *Int. J. Cancer*, 108, 307, 2004.
46. Rosenberg, S.A., Progress in human tumour immunology and immunotherapy, *Nature*, 411, 380, 2001.
47. Hunger, R.E. et al., Successful induction of immune responses against mutant ras in melanoma patients using intradermal injection of peptides and GM-CSF as adjuvant, *Exp. Dermatol.*, 10, 161, 2001.
48. Gorden, A. et al., Analysis of BRAF and N-RAS mutations in metastatic melanoma tissues, *Cancer Res.*, 63, 3955, 2003.
49. Wölfel, T. et al., A p16INK4a-insensitive CDK4 mutant targeted by cytolytic T lymphocytes in a human melanoma, *Science*, 269, 1281, 1995.
50. Omholt, K. et al., Screening of N-ras codon 61 mutations in paired primary and metastatic cutaneous melanomas: mutations occur early and persist throughout tumor progression, *Clin. Cancer Res.*, 8, 3468, 2002.
51. Bergmann-Leitner, E.S. et al., Identification of a human $CD8^+$ T lymphocyte neo-epitope created by a ras codon 12 mutation which is restricted by the HLA-A2 allele, *Cell Immunol.*, 187, 103, 1998.
52. Zorn, E. and Hercend, T., A natural cytotoxic T cell response in a spontaneously regressing human melanoma targets a neoantigen resulting from a somatic point mutation, *Eur. J. Immunol.*, 29, 592, 1999.
53. Robbins, P.F. et al., Multiple HLA class II-restricted melanocyte differentiation antigens are recognized by tumor-infiltrating lymphocytes from a patient with melanoma, *J. Immunol.*, 169, 6036, 2002.
54. Novellino, L. et al., Identification of a mutated receptor-like protein tyrosine phosphatase kappa as a novel, class II HLA-restricted melanoma antigen, *J. Immunol.*, 170, 6363, 2003.
55. Robbins, P.F. et al., The intronic region of an incompletely spliced gp100 gene transcript encodes an epitope recognized by melanoma-reactive tumor-infiltrating lymphocytes, *J. Immunol.*, 159, 303, 1997.
56. De Plaen, E. et al., Structure, chromosomal localization, and expression of 12 genes of the MAGE family, *Immunogenetics*, 40, 360, 1994.
57. Gibbs, P. et al., MAGE-12 and MAGE-6 are frequently expressed in malignant melanoma, *Melanoma Res.*, 10, 259, 2000.
58. Eichmüller, S. et al., mRNA expression of tumor-associated antigens in melanoma tissues and cell lines, *Exp. Dermatol.*, 11, 292, 2002.
59. van den Eynde, B.J. and Boon, T., Tumor antigens recognized by T lymphocytes, *Int. J. Clin. Lab. Res.*, 27, 81, 1997.
60. Jäger, E. et al., Simultaneous humoral and cellular immune response against cancer-testis antigen NY-ESO-1: definition of human histocompatibility leukocyte antigen (HLA)-A2-binding peptide epitopes, *J. Exp. Med.*, 187, 265, 1998.
61. Rimoldi, D. et al., Efficient simultaneous presentation of NY-ESO-1/LAGE-1 primary and nonprimary open reading frame-derived CTL epitopes in melanoma, *J. Immunol.*, 165, 7253, 2000.
62. Thomson, T.M. et al., Differentiation antigens of melanocytes and melanoma: analysis of melanosome and cell surface markers of human pigmented cells with monoclonal antibodies, *J. Invest. Dermatol.*, 90, 459, 1988.
63. Mattes, M.J. et al., A pigmentation-associated, differentiation antigen of human melanoma defined by a precipitating antibody in human serum, *Int. J. Cancer*, 32, 717, 1983.
64. Loftus, D.J. et al., Identification of epitope mimics recognized by CTL reactive to the melanoma/melanocyte-derived peptide MART-1(27-35), *J. Exp. Med.*, 184, 647, 1996.
65. Willemze, R. et al., EORTC classification for primary cutaneous lymphomas: a proposal from the Cutaneous Lymphoma Study Group of the European Organization for Research and Treatment of Cancer, *Blood*, 90, 354, 1997.
66. Dippel, E. et al., Clonal T-cell receptor gamma-chain gene rearrangement by PCR-based GeneScan analysis in advanced cutaneous T-cell lymphoma: a critical evaluation, *J. Pathol.*, 188, 146, 1999.
67. Hoppe, R.T. et al., CD8-positive tumor-infiltrating lymphocytes influence the long-term survival of patients with mycosis fungoides, *J. Am. Acad. Dermatol.*, 32, 448, 1995.
68. Berger, C.L. et al., The immune response to class I-associated tumor-specific cutaneous T-cell lymphoma antigens, *J. Invest. Dermatol.*, 107, 392, 1996.

69. Berger, C.L. et al., Induction of human tumor-loaded dendritic cells, *Int. J. Cancer*, 91, 438, 2001.
70. Nikolova, M. et al., Increased expression of a novel early activation surface membrane receptor in cutaneous T cell lymphoma cells, *J. Invest. Dermatol.*, 116, 731, 2001.
71. Türeci, Ö. et al., Identification of a meiosis-specific protein as a member of the class of cancer testis antigens, *PNAS*, 95, 5211, 1998.
72. Fellenberg, F. et al., GBP-5 splicing variants: new guanylate-binding proteins with tumor-specific expression and antigenicity, *J. Invest. Dermatol.,* 122, 1510, 2004.
73. Berger, C.L. et al., Tumor-specific peptides in cutaneous T-cell lymphoma: association with class I major histocompatibility complex and possible derivation from the clonotypic T-cell receptor, *Int. J. Cancer*, 76, 304, 1998.
74. Berger, C.L. et al., The clonotypic T cell receptor is a source of tumor-associated antigens in cutaneous T cell lymphoma, *Ann. N.Y. Acad. Sci.*, 941, 106, 2001.
75. Winter, D. et al., Definition of TCR Epitopes for CTL-mediated attack of cutaneous T cell lymphoma, *J. Immunol.*, 171, 2714, 2003.
76. Marcil, I. and Stern, R.S., Risk of developing a subsequent nonmelanoma skin cancer in patients with a history of nonmelanoma skin cancer: a critical review of the literature and meta-analysis, *Arch. Dermatol.*, 136, 1524, 2000.
77. Goldman, G.D., Squamous cell cancer: a practical approach, *Semin. Cutaneous Med. Surg.*, 17, 80, 1998.
78. Urosevic, M. and Dummer, R., Immunotherapy for nonmelanoma skin cancer: does it have a future? *Cancer*, 94, 477, 2002.
79. Black, A.P. and Ogg, G.S., The role of p53 in the immunobiology of cutaneous squamous cell carcinoma, *Clin. Exp. Immunol.*, 132, 379, 2003.
80. Liu, B. et al., The expression of c-erbB-1 and c-erbB-2 oncogenes in basal cell carcinoma and squamous cell carcinoma of skin, *Chin. Med. Sci. J.*, 11, 106, 1996.
81. Ahmed, N.U., Ueda, M., and Ichihashi, M., Increased level of c-erbB-2/neu/HER-2 protein in cutaneous squamous cell carcinoma, *Br. J. Dermatol.*, 136, 908, 1997.
82. Piyathilake, C.J. et al., The expression of Ep-CAM (17-1A) in squamous cell cancers of the lung, *Hum. Pathol.*, 31, 482, 2000.
83. Jackson, S. et al., Reduced apoptotic levels in squamous but not basal cell carcinomas correlates with detection of cutaneous human papillomavirus, *Br. J. Cancer*, 87, 319, 2002.
84. Feltkamp, M.C. et al., Seroreactivity to epidermodysplasia verruciformis-related human papillomavirus types is associated with nonmelanoma skin cancer, *Cancer Res.*, 63, 2695, 2003.
85. Forslund, O. et al., A broad spectrum of human papillomavirus types is present in the skin of Australian patients with non-melanoma skin cancers and solar keratosis, *Br. J. Dermatol.*, 149, 64, 2003.
86. Schreurs, M.W. et al., Dendritic cells break tolerance and induce protective immunity against a melanocyte differentiation antigen in an autologous melanoma model, *Cancer Res.*, 60, 6995, 2000.
87. Sutmuller, R.P. et al., Synergism of cytotoxic T lymphocyte-associated antigen 4 blockade and depletion of CD25(+) regulatory T cells in antitumor therapy reveals alternative pathways for suppression of autoreactive cytotoxic T lymphocyte responses, *J. Exp. Med.*, 194, 823, 2001.
88. Davila, E., Kennedy, R., and Celis, E., Generation of antitumor immunity by cytotoxic T lymphocyte epitope peptide vaccination, CpG-oligodeoxynucleotide adjuvant, and CTLA-4 blockade, *Cancer Res.*, 63, 3281, 2003.
89. Kawakami, Y. et al., Cloning of the gene coding for a shared human melanoma antigen recognized by autologous T cells infiltrating into tumor, *PNAS*, 91, 3515, 1994.
90. Kawakami, Y. et al., Identification of a human melanoma antigen recognized by tumor-infiltrating lymphocytes associated with *in vivo* tumor rejection, *PNAS*, 91, 6458, 1994.
91. Lupetti, R. et al., Translation of a retained intron in tyrosinase-related protein (TRP) 2 mRNA generates a new cytotoxic T lymphocyte (CTL)-defined and shared human melanoma antigen not expressed in normal cells of the melanocytic lineage, *J. Exp. Med.*, 188, 1005, 1998.
92. Castelli, C. et al., Novel HLA-Cw8-restricted T cell epitopes derived from tyrosinase-related protein-2 and gp100 melanoma antigens, *J. Immunol.*, 162, 1739, 1999.
93. Khong, H.T. and Rosenberg, S.A., Pre-existing immunity to tyrosinase-related protein (TRP)-2, a new TRP-2 isoform, and the NY-ESO-1 melanoma antigen in a patient with a dramatic response to immunotherapy, *J. Immunol.*, 168, 951, 2002.

94. Romero, P. et al., *Ex vivo* staining of metastatic lymph nodes by class I major histocompatibility complex tetramers reveals high numbers of antigen-experienced tumor-specific cytolytic T lymphocytes, *J. Exp. Med.*, 188, 1641, 1998.
95. Anichini, A. et al., An expanded peripheral T cell population to a cytotoxic T lymphocyte (CTL)-defined, melanocyte-specific antigen in metastatic melanoma patients impacts on generation of peptide-specific CTLs but does not overcome tumor escape from immune surveillance in metastatic lesions, *J. Exp. Med.*, 190, 651, 1999.
96. Pittet, M.J. et al., High frequencies of naive Melan-A/MART-1-specific CD8(+) T cells in a large proportion of human histocompatibility leukocyte antigen (HLA)-A2 individuals, *J. Exp. Med.*, 190, 705, 1999.
97. Ogg, G.S. et al., High frequency of skin-homing melanocyte-specific cytotoxic T lymphocytes in autoimmune vitiligo, *J. Exp. Med.*, 188, 1203, 1998.
98. Yee, C. et al., Melanocyte destruction after antigen-specific immunotherapy of melanoma: Direct evidence of T cell- mediated vitiligo, *J. Exp. Med.*, 192, 1637, 2000.
99. van den Eynde, B. et al., A new family of genes coding for an antigen recognized by autologous cytolytic T lymphocytes on a human melanoma, *J. Exp. Med.*, 182, 689, 1995.
100. Valmori, D. et al., Naturally occurring human lymphocyte antigen-A2 restricted $CD8^+$ T-cell response to the cancer testis antigen NY-ESO-1 in melanoma patients, *Cancer Res.*, 60, 4499, 2000.
101. Ridge, J.P., Di Rosa, F., and Matzinger, P., A conditioned dendritic cell can be a temporal bridge between a $CD4^+$ T-helper and a T-killer cell, *Nature*, 393, 474, 1998.
102. Schoenberger, S.P. et al., T-cell help for cytotoxic T lymphocytes is mediated by CD40-CD40L interactions, *Nature*, 393, 480, 1998.
103. Bourgeois, C., Rocha, B., and Tanchot, C., A role for CD40 expression on $CD8^+$ T cells in the generation of $CD8^+$ T cell memory, *Science*, 297, 2060, 2002.
104. Janssen, E.M. et al., $CD4^+$ T cells are required for secondary expansion and memory in $CD8^+$ T lymphocytes, *Nature*, 421, 852, 2003.
105. Cormier, J.N. et al., Enhancement of cellular immunity in melanoma patients immunized with a peptide from MART-1/Melan A [see comments], *Cancer J. Sci. Am.*, 3, 37, 1997.
106. Wang, F. et al., Phase I trial of a MART-1 peptide vaccine with incomplete Freund's adjuvant for resected high-risk melanoma, *Clin. Cancer Res.*, 5, 2756, 1999.
107. Rosenberg, S.A. et al., Immunologic and therapeutic evaluation of a synthetic peptide vaccine for the treatment of patients with metastatic melanoma, *Nat. Med.*, 4, 321, 1998.
108. Jäger, E. et al., Granulocyte-macrophage-colony-stimulating factor enhances immune responses to melanoma-associated peptides *in vivo*, *Int. J. Cancer*, 67, 54, 1996.
109. Jäger, E. et al., Monitoring CD8 T cell responses to NY-ESO-1: correlation of humoral and cellular immune responses, *PNAS*, 97, 4760, 2000.
110. Scheibenbogen, C. et al., Phase 2 trial of vaccination with tyrosinase peptides and granulocyte-macrophage colony-stimulating factor in patients with metastatic melanoma, *J. Immunother.*, 23, 275, 2000.
111. Scheibenbogen, C. et al., Effects of granulocyte-macrophage colony-stimulating factor and foreign helper protein as immunologic adjuvants on the T-cell response to vaccination with tyrosinase peptides, *Int. J. Cancer*, 104, 188, 2003.
112. Marchand, M. et al., Tumor regressions observed in patients with metastatic melanoma treated with an antigenic peptide encoded by gene MAGE-3 and presented by HLA-A1, *Int. J. Cancer*, 80, 219, 1999.
113. Coulie, P.G. et al., A monoclonal cytolytic T-lymphocyte response observed in a melanoma patient vaccinated with a tumor-specific antigenic peptide encoded by gene MAGE-3, *PNAS*, 98, 10290, 2001.
114. Parkhurst, M.R. et al., Improved induction of melanoma-reactive CTL with peptides from the melanoma antigen gp100 modified at HLA-A*0201-binding residues, *J Immunol*, 157, 2539, 1996.
115. Valmori, D. et al., Enhanced generation of specific tumor-reactive CTL *in vitro* by selected Melan-A/MART-1 immunodominant peptide analogues, *J. Immunol.*, 160, 1750, 1998.
116. Slingluff, C.L., Jr. et al., Phase I trial of a melanoma vaccine with gp100(280-288) peptide and tetanus helper peptide in adjuvant: immunologic and clinical outcomes, *Clin. Cancer Res.*, 7, 3012, 2001.
117. Yamshchikov, G.V. et al., Evaluation of peptide vaccine immunogenicity in draining lymph nodes and peripheral blood of melanoma patients, *Int. J. Cancer*, 92, 703, 2001.

118. Schuler-Thurner, B. et al., Rapid induction of tumor-specific type 1 T helper cells in metastatic melanoma patients by vaccination with mature, cryopreserved, peptide-loaded monocyte-derived dendritic cells [erratum in *J. Exp. Med.*. 197(3):395, 2003], *J. Exp. Med.*, 195, 1279, 2002.
119. Phan, G.Q. et al., Immunization of patients with metastatic melanoma using both class I- and class II-restricted peptides from melanoma-associated antigens, *J. Immunother.*, 26, 349, 2003.
120. Marchand, M. et al., Immunisation of metastatic cancer patients with MAGE-3 protein combined with adjuvant SBAS-2: a clinical report, *Eur. J. Cancer*, 39, 70, 2003.
121. Zhang, Y. et al., A MAGE-3 peptide presented by HLA-DR1 to $CD4^+$ T cells that were isolated from a melanoma patient vaccinated with a MAGE-3 protein, *J. Immunol.*, 171, 219, 2003.
122. Akira, S., Takeda, K., and Kaisho, T., Toll-like receptors: critical proteins linking innate and acquired immunity, *Nat. Immunol.*, 2, 675, 2001.
123. Gurunathan, S., Klinman, D.M., and Seder, R.A., DNA vaccines: immunology, application, and optimization, *Annu. Rev. Immunol.*, 18, 927, 2000.
124. Rosenberg, S.A. et al., Inability to immunize patients with metastatic melanoma using plasmid DNA encoding the gp100 melanoma-melanocyte antigen, *Hum. Gene Ther.*, 14, 709, 2003.
125. Tagawa, S.T. et al., Phase I study of intranodal delivery of a plasmid DNA vaccine for patients with stage IV melanoma, *Cancer*, 98, 144, 2003.
126. Rosenberg, S.A. et al., Immunizing patients with metastatic melanoma using recombinant adenoviruses encoding MART-1 or gp100 melanoma antigens, *J. Natl. Cancer Inst.*, 90, 1894, 1998.
127. Oertli, D. et al., Rapid induction of specific cytotoxic T lymphocytes against melanoma-associated antigens by a recombinant vaccinia virus vector expressing multiple immunodominant epitopes and costimulatory molecules *in vivo*, *Hum. Gene Ther.*, 13, 569, 2002.
128. Rosenberg, S.A. et al., Recombinant fowlpox viruses encoding the anchor-modified gp100 melanoma antigen can generate antitumor immune responses in patients with metastatic melanoma, *Clin. Cancer Res.*, 9, 2973, 2003.
129. Coulie, P.G. and Bruggen, P., T-cell responses of vaccinated cancer patients, *Curr. Opin. Immunol.*, 15, 131, 2003.
130. Ramshaw, I.A. and Ramsay, A.J., The prime-boost strategy: exciting prospects for improved vaccination, *Immunol. Today*, 21, 163, 2000.
131. Paschen, A., Bacteria as vectors for gene therapy of cancer, in *Gene Therapy: Therapeutic Mechanisms and Strategies*, 2nd ed., Paschen, A., Schadendorf, D., and Weiss, S., Eds., Marcel Dekker, New York, 2004, 199.
132. Xiang, R. et al., An autologous oral DNA vaccine protects against murine melanoma, *PNAS*, 97, 5492, 2000.
133. Schuler, G., Schuler-Thurner, B., and Steinman, R.M., The use of dendritic cells in cancer immunotherapy, *Curr Opin Immunol*, 15, 138, 2003.
134. Jonuleit, H. et al., A comparison of two types of dendritic cell as adjuvants for the induction of melanoma-specific T-cell responses in humans following intranodal injection, *Int. J. Cancer*, 93, 243, 2001.
135. Dhodapkar, M.V. and Steinman, R.M., Antigen-bearing immature dendritic cells induce peptide-specific CD8(+) regulatory T cells *in vivo* in humans, *Blood*, 100, 174, 2002.
136. Shortman, K. and Liu, Y.J., Mouse and human dendritic cell subtypes, *Nat. Rev. Immunol.*, 2, 151, 2002.
137. Jonuleit, H. et al., Pro-inflammatory cytokines and prostaglandins induce maturation of potent immunostimulatory dendritic cells under fetal calf serum-free conditions, *Eur. J. Immunol.*, 27, 3135, 1997.
138. Luft, T. et al., Functionally distinct dendritic cell (DC) populations induced by physiologic stimuli: prostaglandin E(2) regulates the migratory capacity of specific DC subsets, *Blood*, 100, 1362, 2002.
139. Scandella, E. et al., Prostaglandin E2 is a key factor for CCR7 surface expression and migration of monocyte-derived dendritic cells, *Blood*, 100, 1354, 2002.
140. Kalinski, P. et al., Prostaglandin E(2) is a selective inducer of interleukin-12 p40 (IL-12p40) production and an inhibitor of bioactive IL-12p70 heterodimer, *Blood*, 97, 3466, 2001.
141. Dhodapkar, M.V. et al., Mature dendritic cells boost functionally superior CD8(+) T-cell in humans without foreign helper epitopes, *J. Clin. Invest.*, 105, R9, 2000.
142. Balch, C.M. et al., Final version of the American Joint Committee on Cancer staging system for cutaneous melanoma, *J. Clin. Oncol.*, 19, 3635, 2001.
143. Shimizu, K. et al., Systemic administration of interleukin 2 enhances the therapeutic efficacy of dendritic cell-based tumor vaccines, *PNAS*, 96, 2268, 1999.

144. Eggert, A.O. et al., Specific peptide-mediated immunity against established melanoma tumors with dendritic cells requires IL-2 and fetal calf serum-free cell culture, *Eur. J. Immunol.*, 32, 122, 2002.
145. Dudley, M.E. et al., Cancer regression and autoimmunity in patients after clonal repopulation with antitumor lymphocytes, *Science*, 298, 850, 2002.
146. Yee, C. et al., Adoptive T cell therapy using antigen-specific $CD8^+$ T cell clones for the treatment of patients with metastatic melanoma: *in vivo* persistence, migration, and antitumor effect of transferred T cells, *PNAS*, 99, 16168, 2002.
147. de Vries, T.J. et al., Heterogeneous expression of immunotherapy candidate proteins gp100, MART-1, and tyrosinase in human melanoma cell lines and in human melanocytic lesions, *Cancer Res.*, 57, 3223, 1997.
148. Ruiz-Cabello, F. et al., Impaired surface antigen presentation in tumors: implications for T cell-based immunotherapy, *Semin. Cancer Biol.*, 12, 15, 2002.
149. Seliger, B. et al., HLA class I antigen abnormalities and immune escape by malignant cells, *Semin. Cancer Biol.*, 12, 3, 2002.
150. Hicklin, D.J. et al., beta2-Microglobulin mutations, HLA class I antigen loss, and tumor progression in melanoma, *J. Clin. Invest.*, 101, 2720, 1998.
151. Paschen, A. et al., Complete loss of HLA class I antigen expression on melanoma cells: a result of successive mutational events, *Int. J. Cancer*, 103, 759, 2003.
152. Andreola, G. et al., Induction of lymphocyte apoptosis by tumor cell secretion of FasL-bearing microvesicles, *J. Exp. Med.*, 195, 1303, 2002.
153. Green, M.C., Murray, J.L., and Hortobagyi, G.N., Monoclonal antibody therapy for solid tumors, *Cancer Treat. Rev.*, 26, 269, 2000.
154. Binz, H., Ramseier, H., and Lindenmann, J., Anti-alloantibodies: a *de novo* product, *J. Immunol.*, 111, 1108, 1973.
155. Jerne, N., Towards a network theory of the immune system, *Ann. Immunol.* (Paris), 125, 373, 1974.
156. Altomonte, M. and Maio, M., European approach to antibody-based immunotherapy of melanoma, *Semin. Oncol.*, 29, 471, 2002.
157. Alfonso, M. et al., An anti-idiotype vaccine elicits a specific response to *N*-glycolyl sialic acid residues of glycoconjugates in melanoma patients, *J. Immunol.*, 168, 2523, 2002.
158. Segal, D.M., Weiner, G.J., and Weiner, L.M., Bispecific antibodies in cancer therapy, *Curr. Opin. Immunol.*, 11, 558, 1999.
159. Frankel, A.E. et al., Immunotoxin therapy of hematologic malignancies, *Semin. Oncol.*, 30, 545, 2003.
160. Emmanouilides, C., Radioimmunotherapy for non-Hodgkin's lymphoma, *Semin. Oncol.*, 30, 531, 2003.
161. Siegel, A.B. et al., CD22-directed monoclonal antibody therapy for lymphoma, *Semin. Oncol.*, 30, 457, 2003.
162. Gorter, A. and Meri, S., Immune evasion of tumor cells using membrane-bound complement regulatory proteins, *Immunol. Today*, 20, 576, 1999.
163. Blum, K.A. and Bartlett, N.L., Antibodies for the treatment of diffuse large cell lymphoma, *Semin. Oncol.*, 30, 448, 2003.
164. Dechant, M., Bruenke, J., and Valerius, T., HLA class II antibodies in the treatment of hematologic malignancies, *Semin. Oncol.*, 30, 465, 2003.
165. Lin, T.S., Lucas, M.S., and Byrd, J.C., Rituximab in B-cell chronic lymphocytic leukemia, *Semin. Oncol.*, 30, 483, 2003.
166. Moreton, P. and Hillmen, P., Alemtuzumab therapy in B-cell lymphoproliferative disorders, *Semin. Oncol.*, 30, 493, 2003.
167. Heinzerling, L.M. et al., Reduction of tumor burden and stabilization of disease by systemic therapy with anti-CD20 antibody (rituximab) in patients with primary cutaneous B-cell lymphoma, *Cancer*, 89, 1835, 2000.
168. Heinzerling, L. et al., Intralesional therapy with anti-CD20 monoclonal antibody rituximab in primary cutaneous B-cell lymphoma, *Arch. Dermatol.*, 136, 374, 2000.
169. Cheung, N.K. et al., Ganglioside GD2 specific monoclonal antibody 3F8: A phase I study in patients with neuroblastoma and malignant melanoma, *J. Clin. Oncol.*, 5, 1430, 1987.
170. Irie, R.F. and Morton, D.L., Regression of cutaneous metastatic melanoma by intralesional injection with human monoclonal antibody to ganglioside GD2, *PNAS*, 83, 8694, 1986.

171. Schrama, D. et al., Targeting of lymphotoxin-alpha to the tumor elicits an efficient immune response associated with induction of peripheral lymphoid-like tissue, *Immunity*, 14, 111, 2001.
172. Rosenblum, M.G. et al., Design, expression, purification, and characterization, *in vitro* and *in vivo*, of an antimelanoma single-chain Fv antibody fused to the toxin gelonin, *Cancer Res.*, 63, 3995, 2003.
173. Phan, G.Q. et al., Cancer regression and autoimmunity induced by cytotoxic T lymphocyte-associated antigen 4 blockade in patients with metastatic melanoma, *PNAS*, 100, 8372, 2003.
174. Chin, L., The genetics of malignant melanoma: lessons from mouse and man, *Nat. Rev. Cancer*, 3, 559, 2003.
175. Linard, B. et al., A ras-mutated peptide targeted by CTL infiltrating a human melanoma lesion, *J. Immunol.*, 168, 4802, 2002.
176. Brasseur, F. et al., Expression of MAGE genes in primary and metastatic cutaneous melanoma, *Int. J. Cancer*, 63, 375, 1995.
177. Basarab, T. et al., Melanoma antigen-encoding gene expression in melanocytic naevi and cutaneous malignant melanomas, *Br. J. Dermatol.*, 140, 106, 1999.
178. Mackensen, A. et al., Phase I study in melanoma patients of a vaccine with peptide-pulsed dendritic cells generated *in vitro* from CD34(+) hematopoietic progenitor cells, *Int. J. Cancer*, 86, 385, 2000.
179. Gajewski, T.F. et al., Immunization of HLA-A2+ melanoma patients with MAGE-3 or MelanA peptide-pulsed autologous peripheral blood mononuclear cells plus recombinant human interleukin 12, *Clin. Cancer Res.*, 7, 895s, 2001.
180. Romero, P. et al., Antigenicity and immunogenicity of Melan-A/MART-1 derived peptides as targets for tumor reactive CTL in human melanoma, *Immunol. Rev.*, 188, 81, 2002.
181. Ravindranath, M.H. et al., Does human melanoma express carcinoembryonic antigen? *Anticancer Res.*, 20, 3083, 2000.
182. Horig, H. et al., Phase I clinical trial of a recombinant canarypoxvirus (ALVAC) vaccine expressing human carcinoembryonic antigen and the B7.1 co-stimulatory molecule, *Cancer Immunol. Immunother.*, 49, 504, 2000.

# 40 Photo(chemo)therapeutic Modulation of the Skin Immune System

*Menno A. de Rie and Jan D. Bos*

## CONTENTS



## I. INTRODUCTION: PRINCIPLES OF ULTRAVIOLET-MEDIATED IMMUNOSUPPRESSION

The skin is almost daily exposed to visible light and ultraviolet radiation (UVR) from different sources. The sun is the most important source of UV radiation, and it is therefore not surprising

0-8493-1959-5/05/$0.00+$1.50

**TABLE 40.1**
**Major UVR-Mediated Effect on Constituents of the SIS**

| Target | Result |
|---|---|
| **Chromophores** | |
| DNA | Dimer formation/reduction of DNA synthesis |
| *trans*-Urocanic acid | *cis*-Urocanic acid formation |
| **Cell membranes** | Nuclear factor-kappa B activation |
| | Increased apoptosis (esp. in T cells) |
| | Increased membrane permeability |
| | Generation of reactive oxygen species |
| **Keratinocytes** | |
| IL-1 | Increased production |
| IL-1Receptor I | Decreased expression |
| IL-1Receptor II | Increased expression |
| TNF-α | Increased production |
| IL-10 | Increased production |
| GM-CSF/IL-3 | Increased production |
| α-MSH | Increased synthesis |
| Prostaglandins (esp. $PGE_2$) | Increased production |
| Adhesion molecules | Decreased expression |
| **T-Lymphocytes** | |
| Number of circulating cells | Decreased |
| Helper/suppressor ratio | Decreased |
| Viability | Decreased |
| Apoptosis | Increased |
| **Langerhans Cells** | |
| Number | Decreased |
| Function | Decreased |
| Adhesion molecules | Decreased expression |
| **Mast Cells** | |
| Histamine release | Dose dependent |
| **Macrophages** ($CD1a^-$, $CD11b^+$) | Influx in the epidermis |
| Adhesion molecules | Decreased expression |
| **Monocytes** | |
| Adhesion molecules | Decreased expression |
| **Endothelial Cells** | Uncertain |
| **Fibroblasts** | Increased matrix metalloproteinasen (MMP)-1 expression |

that ancient Egyptian and Indian healers knew about the treatment of vitiligo by using extracts of plants (*Ammi majus*) and subsequent exposure to sunlight.[1] Modern phototherapy started about a century ago when Finsen observed the beneficial effect of UVR on lupus vulgaris.[2]

We now know that UVR has major local and systemic immunosuppressive effects. Ample evidence has been presented that UVR induces skin cancers by formation of pyrimidine dimers and subsequent DNA changes[3–7] combined with induction of immunosuppression.[8–12] Although most of the initial studies were performed in mice, little doubt exists that a causal relation between UVR and immunosuppression is also true for humans.[13–15]

Modulation of the skin immune system (SIS) by UVR or combinations of UVR with psoralens is the basis of phototherapy of various T-cell-mediated dermatoses, among which psoriasis and atopic dermatitis are the most important. Since the physiology of skin photoimmunology is discussed in great detail elsewhere in this book, only the major findings related to photo(chemo)therapeutic modulation of the SIS are discussed here (Table 40.1).

## A. Chromophores

To exert its effect on the skin, UVR must be absorbed by certain molecules (chromophores). Changes within these molecules will eventually lead to metabolic and cellular modifications and finally sometimes to visible alterations of the skin. The absorption spectra of these chromophores are different and therefore the basic mechanisms of various types of phototherapy using UVA (315–400 nm) including UVA-1 (340–400 nm) and UVA-2 (315–340 nm), UVB (290–315 nm), and visible light (400–760 nm) differ also. The major chromophores with immunological importance are DNA, *trans*-urocanic acid (UCA), and cell membranes.

DNA is an important chromophore.[16] Absorption by DNA of UVB leads to the formation of pyrimidine dimers and immunosuppression.[17] Most of these pyrimidine dimers are cyclobutane dimers, while C-C (6-4) photoproducts constitute only a minority of the total UVR-induced DNA damage. Pyrimidine dimers can give rise to tumors.[5]

Despite the quantitative predominance of these pyrimidine dimers, the pyrimidine (6-4) pyrimidone photoproduct may prove to be of greater biological significance.[18]

The consequence of DNA photoproduct formation is that cell cycle progression is inhibited and growth arrest for cell-fate decision is induced. This leads to reduction of DNA synthesis and alteration of cell-cycle control mechanisms.

Next to these DNA changes, the tumor suppressor gene product p53 is upregulated by UVB exposure (see Chapter 21, Physiology and Pathology of Skin Photoimmunology). Since p53 is involved in the control of the cell cycle, upregulation of this tumor suppressor gene may be responsible for the reversal of the shortened cell cycle in keratinocytes of the psoriatic epidermis.[19]

*trans*-UCA is formed after deamination of histidine and is found in high concentrations in the epidermis. On UVR, *trans*-UCA is photoisomerized to *cis*-UCA and can subsequently be found in the serum and urine.[20] *cis*-UCA has immunosuppressive effects via modulation of keratinocytes and skin Langerhans cells, or systemically on lymphocytes, monocytes, circulating dendritic cells, or natural killer cells.[21,22] We demonstrated that formation of *cis*-UCA in the skin takes places over a broad spectrum of UVA and UVB up to at least 363 nm.[23]

The role of unsaturated lipids within cell membranes, which — upon UVR — lead to immunosuppression, is uncertain. Activation of nuclear factor-kappa B at the cell membrane after UVR and the UVR-induced generation of reactive oxygen species within cell membranes may play a role in this perspective (see Chapter 12, Free Radicals).[24,25] Evidence has also been put forward that UVR, especially UVA-1 (340–400 nm) radiation, leads to immediate apoptosis and increased membrane permeability.[26]

## B. Cellular Targets of Ultraviolet Radiation

### 1. Keratinocytes

From cytokine studies in keratinocytes, we know that UVR stimulates the production of at least two important pro-inflammatory cytokines: interleukin-1 (IL-1)[27,28] and tumor necrosis factor-α (TNF-α).[29,30] IL-1a and TNF-α suppress Langerhans cells and thereby induce immunosuppression.[30,31] Evidence has been produced indicating that UVB-irradiated Langerhans cells are unable to present antigen to Th1 cells in particular.[32] Whether the IL-1 immunomodulation effects can be blocked by the IL-1 inhibitor, which is produced by UVB-irradiated keratinocytes, is not known.[33] UVB radiation increases the type II IL-1 receptor (IL-1R II) expression, which leads to increased IL-1 binding but has no functional consequences. On the other hand, IL-1R I expression is decreased by UVR and consequently limits excessive UV-induced IL-1 responses.[34]

In addition to the two pro-inflammatory cytokines IL-1 and TNF-α, IL-6, IL-8, IL-10, IL-12, IL-15, granulocyte-macrophage colony-stimulating factor (GM-CSF), and prostaglandins are produced by UV-irradiated keratinocytes. IL-10 is released by irradiated mouse keratinocytes and has immunosuppressive effects by interfering with Langerhans cell antigen presentation.[35,36] However, in contrast to their murine counterparts, some controversy exists whether human keratinocytes are also able to produce IL-10.[37] The immunosuppressive effects in mice of the hematopoietic factor GM-CSF and the lymphopoietic factor IL-3 have not yet been demonstrated in humans.[38]

Increased expression of the adhesion molecule intercellular adhesion molecule-1 (ICAM-1), which is a predominant sign in inflammatory dermatoses, is inhibited by UVR.[39,40]

*In vitro* exposure of human keratinocytes to UVA/B radiation increases the synthesis of propiomelanocorticotropin-derived peptides including $\alpha$-melanocyte-stimulating hormone ($\alpha$-MSH). $\alpha$-MSH has anti-inflammatory and immunosuppressive effects that result from its capacity to inhibit cell-mediated immune responses.[41]

Radiation of keratinocytes also induces the production of prostaglandins.[42] Prostaglandin $E_2$ ($PGE_2$) is an especially potent immunosuppressant that inhibits the expression of co-stimulatory molecules on the surface of antigen-presenting cells and thereby prevents the activation of T cells.[43]

### 2. T Cells

Erythemogenic doses of UVB decrease the number of circulating T cells.[44] Both natural sunlight and UVA affect T-cell subsets, resulting in an increase in T-cell suppressor cell activity.[14,15] Both solar-simulated UV irradiation and UVB preferentially induce the recruitment of memory $CD4^+$ T cells.[45,46]

Different studies have shown that human peripheral blood T cells are highly susceptible to UV-induced apoptosis compared to other cell populations.[47,48] The apoptosis mechanisms induced by UVB, PUVA, and UVA-1 are different. PUVA and UVB induced late apoptosis, which requires *de novo* protein synthesis, while UVA-1 induces both early apoptosis (protein synthesis independent) and late apoptosis.[49,50]

Different investigators have now demonstrated that therapeutic UVB doses suppress the T helper I axis, as defined by IL-12, interferon-gamma (IFN-), and IL-8.[51,52] This view is supported by the finding that UVB irradiation favors the development of type II helper T cells *in vivo* and induces the appearance of IL-$4^+$ neutrophils, which also increases T helper II responses.[53,54]

### 3. Monocytes/Macrophages and Langerhans Cells

UVR can lead to induction of T-suppressor cells as the end result of influx in the dermis of macrophages (CD1a$^-$, CD11b$^+$).[55] In addition, this type of macrophage is able to stimulate the production of IL-10 in the epidermis.[56]

*In vivo* UVR decreases the density of Langerhans cells in the skin, and also affects the antigen presentation by these cells.[57,58] In addition, UVB radiation has been found to suppress adhesion molecule expression by both epidermal Langerhans cells and monocytes/macrophages.[59] UVR-induced changes of Langerhans cells can thus suppress the *in vivo* SIS.

### 4. Mast Cells

Erythemogenic doses of UVB affect membranes of mast cells and stimulate direct degranulation and release of histamines.[60] Low doses of UVB, however, suppress histamine release and prevent the UV-induced vasodilation.[61]

### 5. Fibroblasts

*In vitro* studies with human dermal fibroblasts have shown that both UVB and UVA radiation lead to increased matrix metalloproteinasen (MMP)-1 expression. Induction of MMP-1 is considered to be the key factor in the UVA-1-induced softening and disappearance of sclerotic skin.[62]

The net result of UVR on the SIS is immunosuppression as demonstrated *in vivo* by suppression of contact allergy, delayed-type hypersensitivity, and immunosurveillance against UV-induced nonmelanoma skin carcinoma. It is believed that this concept of immunosuppression is the basis of modern phototherapy. In this chapter, various forms of photo(chemo)therapy, in relation to specific dermatoses, are further discussed.

## II. ULTRAVIOLET B THERAPY

UV therapy utilizing a carbon arc lamp was introduced at the beginning of this century for psoriasis.[2] Later, medium-pressure mercury arc lamps and finally fluorescent UV lamps were developed for UVB therapy. UVB (290–315 nm) is now widely used in psoriasis, atopic dermatitis, pruritus, pityriasis lichenoides acuta, and chronic and eosinophilic pustular folliculitis. Other less well established indications are chronic hand eczema, parapsoriasis, mycosis fungoides, chronic urticaria, polymorphous light eruption, solar urticaria, and lichen ruber planus.[63] The therapeutic effects of UVB are thought to be accomplished via interactions with the chromophore DNA and related biochemical events. Together, this leads to immunosuppression in the skin itself and components of the immune system, in general, that interact with the SIS (see also Section I of this chapter and Chapter 21, Physiology and Pathology of Skin Photoimmunology).[64,65] The actual mechanistic pathways of UVB phototherapy, however, in most skin diseases are not known in detail.

### A. Psoriasis

In patients suffering from moderate to severe psoriasis, UVB plus coal tar has the best therapeutic index with a minimal risk of inducing skin cancer.[66] Daily in-patient treatment with UVB and crude coal tar leads to remission in at least 80% of patients.[67] However, because of economic, practical, and cosmetic reasons, UVB therapy alone is used more frequently in patients with psoriasis.

Wavelengths shorter than 295 nm are mostly absorbed by the upper epidermis and have no therapeutic effect in psoriasis. Wavelengths around 313 nm have optimal efficacy in treatment of psoriasis.[68] UVB directly inhibits DNA synthesis and mitosis in the hyperproliferating epidermal cells that are characteristic of psoriasis. This decrease in DNA, RNA, and subsequent protein synthesis and upregulation of the tumor suppressor gene product p53, is followed by a temporary return to normal cell kinetics of the psoriatic keratinocyte.[19,69] Other mechanisms that contribute to the beneficial effects of UVB therapy are (1) alterations in the level of prostaglandins and leukotrienes that mediate the inflammatory state in psoriatic skin,[70] (2) effects on the vitamin D metabolism,[71] and (3) immunosuppression. The mechanisms of immunosuppression have been described in Section I of this chapter. Several lines of evidence indicate that psoriasis is not only a T-cell-mediated disease but that T-cell inhibition is of therapeutic value.[72] Since T cells are highly susceptible to UVB irradiation,[47,48] it is not surprising that psoriasis, which is characterized by intraepidermal and perivascular T-cell infiltrates of the papillary dermis, can be effectively cleared with penetrating, e.g., long-wavelength UVB.

#### 1. Combination Therapies

UVB therapy can be combined with emollients (to enhance UVB penetration), anthralin, tar, and calcipotriol.[73] The mechanism by which anthralin clears psoriasis is not well understood and the effect of UVB irradiation is merely additive. Crude coal tar is the distillation product of coal tar and contains more than 10,000 compounds. Most of these compounds have not been identified. Crude coal tar has a negative effect on DNA synthesis.[74] Although crude coal tar contains carcinogenic polyaromatic hydrocarbons, no clear data on the carcinogenicity of UVB–coal tar combination therapy have been reported. Calcipotriol is the most recent, well-established topical antipsoriatic drug.[75] This vitamin $D_3$ analogue not only affects keratinocytes but also inhibits T-cell activation and subsequent IL-2, IL-6, and IFN-$\gamma$ production.[76] Indeed, UVB has a synergistic effect on topical calcipotriol therapy and this combination therapy is now considered by many dermatologists as first-choice treatment in patients with moderate to severe psoriasis.[77] However, this synergistic effect is limited if optimal narrowband UVB doses are used.[78] Recently, data have been presented indicating that calcipotriol ointment should be introduced with caution in patients already receiving UVB phototherapy, because of the risk of photosensitivity.[79] Because the vehicle of calcipotriol cream and ointment have a UVB-blocking effect, they should not be applied immediately before irradiation.[80]

Combinations of UVB phototherapy with corticosteroids, UVA, PUVA, methotrexate, retinoids, cyclosporine, or fish-oil show no additional effect compared to UVB phototherapy alone.[63] Moreover, because of increased risk of carcinogenicity, combination with immunosuppressive treatments is undesirable.

### 2. Narrowband Ultraviolet B Phototherapy

Because UVB wavelengths situated near 313 nm showed the most beneficial effects, Van Weelden together with Philips developed a lamp excluding shorter erythemogenic UVB wavelenths.[81] Current published data support the view that the TL-01 lamp is more effective and has no greater long-term risk than broadband UVB.[82–84] Narrowband UVB phototherapy (311 nm) using the Philips TL-01 lamp is now routinely used to treat psoriasis, atopic dermatitis, and photodermatoses.[85–87]

Narrowband UVB studies in mice suggested that exposure to TL-01 irradiation not only resulted in local immunosuppression but also had systemic effects.[88] However, randomized within-subject comparison in patients with psoriasis treated with narrowband UVB has shown that if UVB therapy has any systemic effect capable of improving psoriasis, this effect is small.[89] These authors therefore concluded that narrowband UVB phototherapy works for chronic plaque psoriasis through local effects.[89] Indeed, we have previously shown that even therapeutic but low-dose narrowband UVB did not affect systemic T-cell activation.[90]

## B. Atopic Dermatitis

Atopic dermatitis (AD) is part of the atopic syndrome, which has a genetic background. It is one of the most common skin diseases and it can invalidate patients by the occurrence of chronic relapsing episodes of itching that can be provoked by environmental factors including exposure to allergens and bacterial infection of the skin.[91] Patients suffering from AD show immune dysfunction: elevated T-cell activation, hyperstimulation of Langerhans cells, defective cell-mediated immunity, and IgE overproduction.[92] The mainstay of treatment is aimed at immunosuppression by topical application of corticosteroids and new emerging topical therapies like tacrolimus and pimecrolimus. Phototherapy is especially helpful in patients unresponsive to topical treatment.[93] Broadband UVB, broadband UVA, narrowband UVB, UVA-1, and photochemotherapy with psoralen and UVA can be useful adjuncts in treatment of atopic dermatitis.

UVB exerts its action in AD by immunosuppression mediated via (1) inhibition of Langerhans cell function and reduction in number of the antigen-presenting cells, (2) inhibition of degranulation of histamine, (3) direct phototoxic effect on T cells present in the dermoepidermal junction and modulation of cytokine production by keratinocytes (see Section I of this chapter). Interestingly, UVB is also effective at reducing *Staphylococcus aureus* colonization.[94] Addition of UVA to UVB was found to be more effective than UVB alone in treatment of AD.[95,96] Principles of UVA phototherapy, high-dose UVA1 (340–400 nm), and PUVA photochemotherapy are discussed in Sections III and IV of this chapter.

## C. Pruritus and Other Dermatological Disorders

Pruritus can be the result of a variety of diseases, and therefore different mechanisms of action can be involved. Nevertheless, most patients suffering from pruritus can improve by UVB phototherapy. In general, UVA phototherapy is not effective in pruritus especially not in patients suffering from pruritus caused by chronic renal failure.[97] UVB phototherapy is effective in uremic pruritus[98] and in patients suffering from primary biliary cirrhosis,[99] although the mechanisms of actions are not well understood. Since UVB treatment of one body half led to bilateral improvement, a systemic effect of UVB has been postulated.[98]

UVB irradiation induces local and systemic immunosuppressive effects and has proved to be effective in treatment of cell-mediated (type IV) nickel contact dermatitis.[100] In addition, it was found that UVB reduced the increased number of Langerhans cells in patients suffering from both allergic and irritant dermatitis of the hands.[101]

Because of the potential long-term side effects of PUVA and the effectiveness of UVB, narrowband UVB is becoming the first-choice treatment in vitiligo and mycosis fungoides, after several decades of PUVA hegemony. Details of photo(chemo)therapy are discussed in Section IV.

Pityriasis rosea is an idiopathic self-limiting disease and therefore phototherapy is almost never indicated. However, UVB phototherapy is sometimes given to relief pruritus.[102]

Pityriasis lichenoides et varioliformis acuta, pityriasis lichenoides chronica, and eosinophilic pustular folliculitis in HIV-infected persons can be treated with UVB.[63] Since the pathogenesis of these disorders is at present not well understood, it is hard to explain the mechanism of action of UVB in these diseases other than immunosuppression. Although UVB phototherapy may itself aggravate symptoms in photosensitive dermatoses (e.g., polymorphous light eruption and solar urticaria), repeated UVB exposure may relieve symptoms eventually.[103] This is accomplished by acanthosis of the epidermis, stimulation of melanogenesis, inhibition of degranulation of mast cells, and modulation of cytokine production by keratinocytes.

## III. ULTRAVIOLET A THERAPY

Since sunlight leads to improvement of a majority of patients suffering from a chronic state of AD, UVB (see Section II), UVA, and combinations of UVA and UVB have been employed as a therapeutic modality. Jekler and Larkö[104] showed that monotherapy using conventional broad-band UVA radiation equipment was effective in treatment of AD patients and superior to UVB treatment.[96,104] This has led to the development of high dose UVA-1 (340–400 nm; 130 J/cm$^2$) radiation equipment for monotherapy in patients with AD.[105–107] Kowalzick[108] showed that the effect of UVA-1 therapy is dose dependent. At this moment, UVA-1 treatment is not exclusively used in patients with AD. Experience with treatment in patients suffering from lupus erythematosus[109,110] and urticaria pigmentosa[107] is limited but very promising. Recent studies have shown that both low- (<20 J/cm$^2$) and medium-dose (20-50 J/cm$^2$) UVA-1 can be effective for treatment of sclerotic plaques in patients with localized scleroderma.[111,112]

The risks of high-dose UVA-1 radiation treatment of the skin of patients with AD have not been established yet. From studies on conventional UVA radiation, i.e., indoor tanning machines, it is known that UVA itself can also induce skin cancers, although UVB is three to four orders of magnitude more potent in inducing skin malignancies.[113] There is no question that high-dose UVA can produce tumors in experimental animals.[113] In addition, chronic UVA radiation of the skin leads to photoaging, which is histologically characterized by dermal aggregates of degraded elastic fibers.[114]

Experience with UVA-1 treatment is limited. The value of this new modality in comparison to conventional photochemotherapy (see Section IV) and other effective systemic treatments with immunosuppressive drugs (i.e., cyclosporine A) needs more widespread investigations.

## IV. PHOTOCHEMOTHERAPY

### A. Principles of PUVA Therapy

PUVA is a combination therapy of psoralen and long-wave UV radiation (UVA: 320–400). Psoralens may be applied topically or can be used orally. PUVA is used to treat a number of diseases among

**TABLE 40.2**
**PUVA-Responsive Diseases**

| Therapy | Prevention |
|---|---|
| Psoriasis | Polymorphous light eruption |
| Palmoplantar pustulosis | *Hydroa vacciniforme* |
| Lichen ruber planus | *Solar urticaria* |
| Pityriasis rubra pilaris | Chronic actinic dermatitis |
| Pityriasis lichenoides | Persistent light reaction |
| CTCL (Mycosis fungoides stages I + II) | |
| Actinic reticuloid | Actinic reticuloid |
| Lymphomatoid papulosis | |
| Vitiligo | |
| Graft-vs.-host disease (cutaneous) | |
| Atopic dermatitis | |
| Granuloma annulare | |
| Urticaria pigmentosa | |

*Source:* Adapted from Hönigsmann et al.[115]

which psoriasis, AD, vitiligo, and cutaneous T-cell lymphoma are well-established indications (Table 40.2).[115]

The most widely used psoralens are psoralen, 8-MOP (8-methoxypsoralen), TMP (4,5′,8-trimethylpsoralen), and 5-MOP (5-methoxypsoralen). For the treatment of psoriasis, 8-MOP is most frequently used; TMP is often used for vitiligo. 5-MOP is now used experimentally in treatment of psoriasis and seems to be less erythemogenic than 8-MOP; moreover, it does not induce intolerance reactions. Psoralens intercalate between DNA base pairs and, after absorption of photons in the UVA range, induce bifunctional adducts with interstrand cross-links of the double helix. The net result of this interaction with DNA of epidermal cells is suppression of DNA synthesis and subsequent inhibition of cell proliferation.[115] However, since PUVA is also effective in nonproliferating diseases, e.g., vitiligo, other mechanisms of action may be involved. Indeed, psoralens have been shown to undergo photoaddition reactions with other cellular components, thus leading to altered protein processing via enhanced major histocompatibility complex (MHC) class I synthesis, and transcription factor induction.[116] In addition to the direct antiproliferative effect on keratinocytes, several other effects of photoactivated psoralens on the immune system have been demonstrated (Table 40.3).[117–125]

**TABLE 40.3**
**Effect of Photoactivated Psoralens on the SIS**

Direct photoinactivation of T cells[117]
Specific T-suppressor cell induction[118]
Impairment of IL-2 production by T cells[119]
Inhibition of epidermal growth factor activity[120]
Inhibition of chemotactic activity of polymorphonuclear neutrophils to anaphylatoxin C5a[121]
Inhibition of antigen recognition via negative effects on the number and function of Langerhans cells (decreased ATPase activity and MHC class II expression)[122]
Systemic immunosuppression[123,124]
Apoptosis[125]

Marks and Fox[125] have suggested that treatment of cells with PUVA could lead to apoptosis together with expression of new oligopeptides in surface MHC molecules. This process may be responsible for a higher level of antigenicity of these cells. This hypothesis is valid not only for PUVA, but also for understanding the mechanism of extracorporeal photopheresis.

Details of psoralen photochemistry, pharmacokinetics, and psoralen photosensitization have been reviewed elsewhere.[115]

## B. PUVA for Psoriasis

Histologically, a psoriasis skin lesion is characterized by hyperproliferation of keratinocytes together with reduced differentiation. Another histological hallmark of psoriasis is the perivascular inflammation and infiltration of the epidermis with mononuclear cells.[126] The mononuclear cell infiltrate is mainly composed of activated T lymphocytes as described in detail in Chapter 32, Psoriasis.[127,128] Polymorphonuclear neutrophils also migrate toward the epidermis and characteristic microabcesses are formed in the upper portion of the epidermis. Photochemotherapy inhibits the hyperproliferation of epidermal cells and also has local and systemic immunosuppressive effects via negative effects on T cells and inhibition of migration of polymorphonuclear neutrophils (see above). It is therefore not surprising that photochemotherapy is very effective in treatment of psoriasis. Large-scale clinical trials have demonstrated its effectiveness in inducing and maintaining remissions of psoriasis, as was recently confirmed in two controlled studies comparing narrowband UVB and photochemotherapy [129,130]

Together with the introduction of photochemotherapy in 1974, a discussion started regarding the carcinogenic potential of PUVA. It is now well established that PUVA using oral psoralen derivates is associated with long-term risks.[131] To reduce possible side effects such as risk of carcinogenesis and intolerance, PUVA therapy with bath-water delivery of TMP and 8-MOP was developed.[132,133] In addition, psoralen-delivery systems were developed for treatment of localized psoriasis.[134] The actual risk of development of skin malignancies after topical and bath-PUVA has not yet been established.

The relation between carcinogenesis and PUVA is well recognized. UVA itself induces pyrimidine dimers in human skin. Psoralens form unstable complexes in the DNA molecule and subsequent UVA exposure causes DNA cross-links. Together with local immunosuppression and inhibition of immune surveillance, photochemotherapy increases the risk of nonmelanoma skin cancer. The risk of nonmelanoma skin cancer in patients with psoriasis treated with systemic PUVA is not simply dose related. Several risk factors have been identified: skin type, geographic location, arsenic exposure, ionizing radiation therapy, and a history of skin cancer.[131,135–137] Based on data from the literature, guidelines of care for photochemotherapy have been presented by British and American dermatologists.[138,139]

To increase the effectiveness of photochemotherapy and to reduce the cumulative PUVA dose, combination therapies have been developed. Calcipotriol in combination with PUVA (= D-PUVA) may be considered a real contribution to the management of psoriasis.[140] Combination with other topical antipsoriasis therapies (corticosteroids, tar preparations) has no significant beneficial effect, although combination of PUVA with anthralin may be worthwhile.[115] Combination with immunosuppressive therapies, including methotrexate and cyclosporine A, is not recommended because of synergistic carcinogenic potential. Re-PUVA, i.e., oral retinoids (0.5 to 1 mg/kg bodyweight) combined with photochemotherapy accelerates clearing of the lesions, thus reducing the number of treatments by 30% and reduction of the cumulative PUVA dose by 50%.[141] The mechanism of the synergistic action of retinoids and PUVA is unknown. The long-term toxicity of this combination therapy has not been established. The acute adverse events of retinoids (dry skin, chapping of the lips, diffuse hair loss) and potential teratogenic effects of retinoids are obviously more important than the long-term effects.

## C. PUVA beyond Psoriasis

As discussed in Section II.B of this chapter, PUVA acts not only by way of inhibition of hyperproliferation or epidermal cells but also via suppression of local and systemic immunity. Diseases that are thought to have a pathogenesis that involves a disturbance of immune function are therefore also treated with PUVA. Among these diseases are atopic dermatitis, mycosis fungoides, and vitiligo. The spectrum of PUVA-responsive diseases was reviewed by Honig et al.[142]

### 1. Atopic Dermatitis

Oral psoralen photochemotherapy is an effective treatment for both adults and children with severe AD.[143–145] The immunopathogenesis of AD has been discussed in Section II.B of this chapter. It is generally believed that PUVA acts in AD by suppression of immune responses and modulation of function and distribution of lymphocytes (see Section IV.A). Although AD is more difficult to treat than psoriasis, the guidelines for treatment are essentially the same. In children, PUVA is not easily recommended because of potential risks such as increased skin aging and carcinogenicity.[137]

### 2. Vitiligo

In ancient cultures, vitiligo was treated with topical photosensitizing extracts of plants, e.g., *Ammi majus*. Based on these observations, oral photochemotherapy was developed and has now been found an effective therapeutic modality for vitiligo.[1]

PUVA stimulates the proliferation of melanocytes, which leads to repopulation of the epidermis. In addition, PUVA induces hypertrophy of melanocytes and stimulation of tyrosinase activity. Modulation of the SIS may also be beneficial in vitiligo, which is frequently associated with autoimmune disorders and is sometimes also regarded as an autoimmune disease. Indeed, not only induction of local immunosuppression by corticosteroids, but also immunosuppression, mediated by systemic and local PUVA, acts beneficially in vitiligo.[115] PUVA therapy in combination with epidermal grafting can be used for areas of vitiligo that are unresponsive to PUVA therapy alone.[146]

A meta-analysis of the literature performed by Njoo et al. demonstrated that oral PUVA, narrowband UVB and broad-band UVB are not statistically different in terms of success rate.[147] In addition, a retrospective analysis has confirmed these data.[148] Because of the potential long-term side effects of PUVA, UVB especially narrowband UVB is becoming the first choice treatment of vitiligo, after several decades of PUVA hegemony.

### 3. Mycosis Fungoides

Mycosis fungoides (MF) is an epidermotropic form of cutaneous T-cell lymphoma in which a malignant clone of helper T cells invades the skin. Since the initial report in 1976 by Gilchrest,[149] successful treatment has been reported by several investigators.[142] Patients with stage I and II MF respond best to PUVA compared to other topical therapies.[150] Although PUVA may also affect cytokine production in MF, the beneficial effect appears to be mainly due to the direct cytotoxic effect on the epidermotropic T-cell infiltrate.[151] In addition, PUVA also mediates the downregulation of the expression of "homing receptors" (HECA) of epidermotropic malignant T cells.[152]

Similar to vitiligo, narrowband UVB is now successfully used to treat mycosis fungoides.[153] A retrospective study in patients with early MF demonstrated that both modalities are equally effective and therefore narrowband UVB is preferred to PUVA.[154]

### 4. Miscellaneous

Photochemotherapy is applied in different dermatological conditions as reviewed by Honig et al.[142] and De Rie et al.[155] Recently, we have shown that topical psoralen plus UVA is also effective in patients suffering from necrobiosis lipoidica.[156]

## V. EXTRACORPOREAL PHOTOPHERESIS

Extracorporeal photopheresis (ECP) using UVA irradiation of leukocyte-enriched blood in the presence of psoralens (e.g., 8-MOP) was originally introduced by Edelson[157] as a therapeutic regimen for cutaneous T-cell lymphoma. ECP is now also used for the treatment of other T-cell-mediated diseases such as systemic sclerosis, pemphigus vulgaris, psoriasis arthritis, rheumatoid arthritis, systemic lupus erythematosus, and AIDS-related complex.[158] Although case reports have claimed otherwise, a randomized controlled study was unable to demonstrate that ECP is effective in patients with systemic sclerosis.[159]

The principle of treatment of ECP is similar to PUVA therapy; the difference lies in the UVA exposure of the lymphocytes concentrated in the leukapheresed blood fraction in ECP. Psoralens can be administered orally or directly to the leukocyte/plasma concentrate in the treatment bag of the ECP apparatus before irradiation with UVA.[160]

Although the mechanism of action of ECP is not fully understood, photodamage and modulation of the immune system have been reported. The principle of PUVA therapy is formation of photo-adducts that inhibit cell replication, photodamage, apoptosis, and modulation of the immune system (see Section IV.A). These principles are also true for ECP. In addition, evidence has been presented indicating that ECP modifies cytokine release by lymphocytes,[161] suppresses immunity,[162] and induces apoptosis in lymphocytes.[163] These observations have led to the hypothesis that reinfusion of ECP-treated lymphocytes induces autovaccination against the pathogenic T-cell clones. Details of the therapeutic procedure have been described elsewhere.[158]

## VI. PHOTODYNAMIC THERAPY

In photodynamic therapy (PDT), a photosensitizer, for example, porphyrins, is administered and following its uptake by the target tissue illuminated by a specific light source, preferably laser.[164] This leads to selective tissue destruction, without damage of surrounding tissue. PDT was first used for tumor ablation but is now also used in dermatological conditions like psoriasis, actinic keratosis, basal cell carcinoma, and condylomata acuminata.

The mechanism of PDT-induced tissue damage is not fully understood but involves the generation of reactive oxygen intermediates, followed by cell lysis and an inflammatory response.[165,166] A number of nonspecific mediators of inflammation such as histamine, serotonin, proteases, eicosanoids, and TNF-$\alpha$ have been documented.[167] More specific immunosuppressive effects of PDT have been demonstrated in a murine contact hypersensitivity model.[168] It has been demonstrated that PDT *in vitro* inhibits cutaneous mast cells in rats[169] and activation (CD25 expression) of human peripheral blood T cells.[170]

The selectivity of PDT can be further enhanced by using macromolecular carrier systems: immunoconjugates of photosensitizers with specific monoclonal antibodies can be employed for tissue-specific targeting and destruction. Since experience with PDT is almost exclusively limited to treatment of malignancies, little is known about the effect on the SIS in health and benign inflammatory diseases.

## VII. CONCLUSION

Since Finsen noticed the beneficial effects of artificial UVR on lupus vulgaris, phototherapy has developed from nonselective broadband irradiation to tailor-made narrowband applications of electromagnetic radiation, which includes not only the UV spectrum but also visible light. Moreover, not only has the differentiation in irradiation sources grown but also the number of diseases that are found to be responsive to phototherapy has expanded. Consequently, the pathomechanisms of some of these diseases are now better understood and it can be anticipated that further therapeutic improvements are to be expected. Immunosuppression and inhibition of cell division used to be the main principles of phototherapy. We now know from basic photoimmunology studies that other mechanisms, for example, increase of matrix metalloproteinases expression, are key factors in localized scleroderma and possibly other connective diseases as well. On the other hand, optimizing existing phototherapies (combination therapies, dosing, choice of wavelength) will still be needed to reduce long-term side effects such as photoaging and carcinogenesis. Therefore, further studies on both clinical and basic photoimmunology will be needed to reach these goals.

## REFERENCES

1. Fitzpatrick, T.B. and Pathak, M.A., Research and development of oral psoralen and longwave radiation photochemotherapy 2000 B.C.–1982 A.D., *Monogr. Natl. Cancer Inst.*, 66, 3, 1984.
2. Roelandts, R., The history of phototherapy: something new under the sun? *J. Am Acad. Dermatol.*, 46, 926, 2002.
3. Tan, E.M. and Stoughton, R.B., Ultraviolet light-induced damage to deoxyribonucleic acid in human skin, *J. Invest. Dermatol.*, 52, 537, 1969.
4. Tan, E.M., Freeman, R.G., and Stoughton, R.B., Action spectrum of ultraviolet light-induced damage to nuclear DNA *in vivo*, *J. Invest. Dermatol.*, 55, 439, 1970.
5. Hart, R.W., Setlow, R.B., and Woodhead, A.D., Evidence that pyrimidine dimers in DNA can give rise to tumors, *Proc. Natl. Acad. Sci. U.S.A.*, 74, 5574, 1977.
6. Sutherland, B.M., Harber, L.C., and Kochevar, I.E., Pyrimidine dimer formation and repair in human skin, *Cancer Res.*, 40, 3181, 1980.
7. Brash, D.E. and Haseltine, W.A., UV-induced mutation hotspots occur at DNA damage hotspots, *Nature* (London), 298, 189, 1982.
8. Burnet, F.M., Immunological surveillance in neoplasia, *Transpl. Rev.*, 7, 3, 1971.
9. Urbach, F., in *The Biologic Effects of Ultraviolet Radiation*, Urbach, F., Ed., Pergamon Press, Oxford, 1978, 635.
10. Kripke, M.L., Immunological mechanisms in UV radiation carcinogenesis, *Adv. Cancer Res.*, 34, 69, 1981.
11. Kripke, M.L., Immunobiology of UV-radiation-induced skin cancer, in *Photoimmunology,* Parrish, J.A., Kripke, M.L., and Morison, W.L., Eds., Plenum Press, New York, 1983, 154.
12. Friedmann, P.S., Effects of ultraviolet radiation on immune response of skin, *Photobiochem. Photobiophys. Suppl. Proc.,* 463, 1987.
13. Morison, W.L. et al., *In vivo* effects of UVB on lymphocyte function, *Br. J. Dermatol.*, 101, 513, 1979.
14. Hersey, P. et al., Alteration of T-cell subsets and induction of suppressor T-cell activity in normal subjects after exposure to sunlight, *J. Immunol.*, 131, 171, 1983.
15. Hersey, P. et al., Immunological effects of solarium exposure, *Lancet*, 1, 545, 1983.
16. Hruza, L.L. and Pentland, A.P., Mechanisms of UV-induced inflammation, *J. Invest. Dermatol.*, 100, 35S, 1993.
17. Kripke, M.L. et al., Pyrimidine dimers in DNA initiate systemic immunosuppression in UV-irradiated mice, *Proc. Natl. Acad. Sci. U.S.A.*, 89, 7516, 1992.
18. Petit Frere, C. et al., Inhibition of RNA and DNA synthesis in UV-irradiated normal human fibroblasts is correlated with pyrimidine (6-4) pyrimidone photoproduct formation, *Mutat. Res.*, 87, 354, 1996.
19. Liu, M. and Pellingo, J.C., UV-B/A irradiation of mouse keratinocytes results in p53-mediated WAF1/CIP expression, *Oncogene,* 10, 1955, 1995.
20. Kammeyer, A. et al., Retention of increased cis-urocanic acid levels in human body upon UV-B exposure, *Photochem. Photobiol.*, 59, 27S, 1994.
21. Noonan, F.P. and De Fabo, E.C., Immunosuppression by ultraviolet B radiation: initiation by urocanic acid, *Immunol. Today,* 13, 250, 1992.
22. Norval, M, Gibbs, N.K., and Gilmour, J., The role of urocanic acid in UV-induced immunosuppression: recent advances (1992–1994), *Photochem. Photobiol.*, 62, 209, 1995.
23. Kammeyer, A. et al., Photoisomerization spectrum of urocanic acid in human skin and *in vitro*: effects of simulated solar and artificial ultraviolet radiation, *Br. J. Dermatol.*, 132, 884, 1995.
24. Devary, Y. et al., NF-kappa B activation by ultraviolet light on dependent on a nuclear signal, *Science*, 261, 1442, 1993.

25. Picardo, M. et al., Squalene peroxides may contribute to ultraviolet light-induced immunological effects, *Photodermatol. Photoimmunol. Photomed.*, 8, 105, 1991.
26. Godar, D.E. and Lucas, A.D., Spectral dependence of UV-induced immediate and delayed apoptosis: the role of membrane and DNA damage, *Photochem. Photobiol.*, 62, 108, 1995.
27. Gahring, L. et al., The effect of ultraviolet radiation on production of epidermal cell thymocyte-activating factor/interleukin 1 *in vivo* and *in vitro*, *Proc. Natl. Acad. Sci. U.S.A.*, 81, 1198, 1984.
28. Kupper, T.S. et al., Interleukin 1 gene expression in cultured human keratinocytes is augmented by ultraviolet irradiation, *J. Clin. Invest.*, 80, 430, 1987.
29. Köck, A., Schwarz, T., and Kirnbauer, R., Human keratinocytes are a source for tumor necrosis factor alpha: Evidence for synthesis and release upon stimulation with endotoxin or ultraviolet light, *J. Exp. Med.*, 172, 1609, 1990.
30. Yoshikawa, T., Kurimoto, I., and Streilein, J.W., Tumor necrosis factor-alpha mediates ultraviolet light B-enhanced expression of contact hypersensitivity, *Immunology*, 76, 262, 1992.
31. Daynes, R.A. et al., Alpha-melanocyte stimulating hormone exhibits target cell selectivity in its capacity to affect interleukin-1-inducible responses *in vivo* and *in vitro*, *J. Immunol.*, 139, 103, 1987.
32. Simon, J.C. et al., Low dose ultraviolet B-irradiated Langerhans cells preferentially activate $CD4^+$ cells of the T helper 2 subset, *J. Immunol.*, 145, 2087, 1990.
33. Schwartz, T. et al., UV-irradiated epidermal cells produce a specific inhibitor of interleukin 1 activity, *J. Immunol.*, 138, 1457, 1987.
34. Grewe, M. et al., Interleukin-1 receptors type I and type II are differentially regulated in human keratinocytes by ultraviolet B radiation, *J. Invest. Dermatol.*, 107, 865, 1996.
35. Rivas, J.M. and Ullrich, S.E., Systemic suppression of delayed-type hypersensitivity by supernatants from UV-irradiated keratinocytes, an essential role for keratinocyte-derived IL-10, *J. Immunol.*, 149, 3865, 1992.
36. Enk, A.H. et al., Inhibition of Langerhans cell antigen-presenting function by IL-10, *J. Immunol.*, 151, 2390, 1993.
37. Teunissen, M.B.M. et al., Inability of human keratinocytes to synthesize interleukin-10, *J. Invest. Dermatol.*, 102, 632, 1994.
38. Gallo, R.L. et al., Regulation of GM-CSF and IL-3 production from the murine keratinocyte cell line Pam 212 following exposure to ultraviolet radiation, *J. Invest. Dermatol.*, 97, 203, 1991.
39. Roza, L., Stege, H., and Krutmann, J., Role of UV-induced DNA damage in phototherapy, in *The Fundamental Bases of Phototherapy,* Hönigsmann, H., Jori, G., and Young, A.R., Eds., OEMS spa, Milan, 1996, 145.
40. Stege, H. et al., Enzyme plus light therapy to repair DNA damage in ultraviolet-B-irradiated human skin, *Proc. Natl. Acad. Sci. U.S.A.*, 97, 1790, 2000.
41. Luger, T.A. and Schwarz, T., Effects of UV light on cytokines and neuroendocrine hormones, in *Photoimmunology,* Krutmann, J. and Elmets, C.A., Eds., Blackwell Science, Oxford, 1995, 55.
42. Grewe, M. et al., Analysis of the mechanism of ultraviolet B radiation induced prostaglandin E2 synthesis by human epidermoid carcinoma cells, *J. Invest. Dermatol.*, 101, 528, 1993.
43. Grewe, M. et al., Involvement of direct and indirect mechanisms in ultraviolet B radiation (UVBR)-induced inhibition of ICAM-1 expression in human antigen presenting cells, *J. Invest. Dermatol.*, 106, 933, 1996.
44. Morison, W.L. et al., *In vivo* effects of UVB on lymphocyte function, *Br. J. Dermatol.*, 101, 513, 1979.
45. Di Nuzzo, S. et al., Solar-simulated ultraviolet irradiation induces selective influx of $CD4^+$ T lymphocytes in normal human skin, *Photochem. Photobiol.*, 64, 988, 1996.
46. Di Nuzzo, S. et al., UVB radiation preferentially induces recruitment of memory $CD4^+$ T cells in normal human skin: long-term effect after a single exposure. *J. Invest. Dermatol.*, 110, 978, 1998.
47. Teunissen, M.B.M. et al., Effect of low-dose ultraviolet-B radiation on the function of human T lymphocytes *in vitro*, *Clin. Exp. Immunol.*, 94, 208, 1993.
48. Krueger, J.G. et al., Successful ultraviolet B treatment of psoriasis is accompanied by a reversal of keratinocytes pathology and by selective depletion of intraepidermal T cells, *J. Exp. Med.*, 182, 2057, 1995.
49. Godar, D.E., Preprogrammed and programmed cell death mechanisms of apoptosis: UV-induced immediate and delayed apoptosis, *Photochem. Photobiol.*, 63, 825, 1996.

50. Godar, D.E., UVA 1 radiation mediates singlet-oxygen and speroxide-anion production which trigger two different final apoptotic pathways: the S and P site of mitochondria, *J. Invest. Dermatol.*, 112, 3, 1999.
51. Walters, I.B. et al., Narrowband (312-nm) UV-B suppresses interferon and interleukin (IL) 12 and increases IL-4 transcripts, *Arch. Dermatol.*, 139, 155, 2003.
52. Piskin, G. et al., Dermal T cell contribution to the changes in interferon (IFN)- and interleukin (IL)-4 expression in psoriatic skin after narrow band-ultraviolet b therapy: *in vitro* and *in situ* findings, *Br. J. Dermatol.*, 147, 1069, 2002.
53. Teunissen, M.B.M. et al., Ultraviolet B radiation induces a transient appearance of IL-$4^+$ neutrophils, which support the development of Th2 responses, *J. Immunol.*, 168, 3732, 2002.
54. Di Nuzzo, S. et al., UVB Irradiation of normal human skin favors the development of type-2 T-cells *in vivo* and in primary dermal cell cultures, *Photochem. Photobiol.*, 76, 301, 2002.
55. Cooper, K.D. et al., UV exposure reduces immunization rates and promotes tolerance to epicutaneous antigens in humans: relationship to dose, CD1aDR$^+$ epidermal macrophage induction, and Langerhans cell depletion, *Proc. Natl. Acad. Sci. U.S.A.*, 89, 8497, 1992.
56. Kang, K. et al., CD11b$^+$ macrophages that infiltrate human epidermis after *in vivo* ultraviolet exposure potently produce IL-10 and represent the major secretory source of epidermal IL-10 protein, *J. Immunol.*, 153, 5256, 1994.
57. Aberer, W. et al., Ultraviolet light depletes surface markers of Langerhans cells, *J. Invest. Dermatol.*, 76, 202, 1981.
58. Granstein, R.D., in *Dermatology in General Medicine*, 5th ed., Freedberg, I.M. et al., Eds., McGraw-Hill, New York, 1999, 1562.
59. Simon, J.C. et al., Ultraviolet B irradiated antigen presenting cells display altered accessory signaling for T cell activation: relevance to immune responses initiated in the skin, *J. Invest. Dermatol.*, 98, 66S, 1992.
60. Gendimenico, G.J. and Kochevar, I.E., Degranulation of mast cells and inhibition of the response to secretory agents by phototoxic compounds and ultraviolet radiation, *Toxicol. Appl. Pharmacol.*, 76, 374, 1984.
61. Danno, K., Toda, K., and Horio, J., Ultraviolet-B radiation suppresses mast cell degranulation induced by compound 48/80, *J. Invest. Dermatol.*, 87, 775, 1986.
62. Wlascheck, M. et al., UVA-induced autocrine stimulation of fibroblasts derived collegenase/MMP-1 by interrelated loops of interleukin-1 and interleukin-6, *Photochem. Photobiol.*, 59, 550, 1994.
63. Coopman, S.A. and Stern, R.S., in *Clinical Photomedicine*, Lim, H.W. and Soter, N.A., Eds., Marcel Dekker, New York, 1993, chap. 18.
64. Morison, W.L., Effects of ultraviolet radiation on the immune system in humans, *Photochem. Photobiol.*, 50, 515, 1989.
65. Goettsch, W. et al., UV-B and the immune system, *Thymus*, 21, 93, 1993.
66. Stern, R.S., Zierler, S., and Parrish, J.A., Skin carcinoma in patients with psoriasis treated with topical tar and artificial ultraviolet radiation, *Lancet*, 1, 732, 1980.
67. Stern, R.S. et al., Effect of continued ultraviolet B phototherapy on the duration of remission of psoriasis: a randomized study, *J. Am. Acad. Dermatol.*, 15, 546, 1986.
68. Fisher, T., UV-light treatment of psoriasis, *Acta. Derm. Venereol.* (Stockholm), 56, 473, 1976.
69. Epstein, J.H., Fukuyama, K., and Fye, K., Effects of ultraviolet radiation on the mitotic cycle and DNA, RNA and protein synthesis in mammalian epidermis *in vivo*, *Photochem. Photobiol.*, 12, 57, 1970.
70. Katayama, H. and Hori, Y., The influence of ultraviolet B irradiation on the excretion of the main urinary metabolic metabolite of prostaglandin F1 alpha and F2 alpha in psoriatic and normal subjects, *Acta. Derm. Venereol.* (Stockholm), 64, 1, 1984.
71. Staberg, B. et al., Is the effect of phototherapy in psoriasis partly due to an impact on vitamin D metabolism? *Acta. Derm. Venereol.* (Stockholm), 68, 436, 1988.
72. Bos, J.D. and De Rie, M.A., The pathogenesis of psoriasis: immunological facts and speculations, *Immunol. Today*, 20, 40, 1999.
73. Greaves, M.W. and Weinstein, G.D., Treatment of psoriasis, *N. Engl. J. Med.*, 332, 581, 1995.
74. Farber, E.M., Abel, E.A., and Charuworn, A., Recent advances in the treatment of psoriasis, *J. Am. Acad. Dermatol.*, 8, 311, 1983.

75. Ashcroft, D.M. et al., Systematic review of comparative efficacy and tolerability of calcipotriol in treating chronic plaque psoriasis, *Br. Med. J.*, 320, 963, 2000.
76. Berth-Jones, J. and Hutchinson P.E., Vitamin D analogues and psoriasis, *Br. J. Dermatol.*, 127, 71, 1992.
77. Kerscher, M. et al., Combination phototherapy of psoriasis with calcipotriol and narrow-band UVB, *Lancet*, 342, 923, 1993.
78. Brands, S. et al., No additional effect of calcipotriol ointment on low-dose narrow-band UVB phototherapy in psoriasis, *J. Am. Acad. Dermatol.*, 41, 991, 1999.
79. McKenna, K.E. and Stern, R.S., Photosensitivity associated with combined UV-B and calcipotriene therapy, *Arch. Dermatol.*, 131, 1305, 1995.
80. De Rie, M.A. et al., Calcipotriol ointment and cream or their vehicles applied immediately before irradiation inhibit ultraviolet B-induced erythema, *Br. J. Dermatol.*, 142, 1160, 2000.
81. Van Weelden, H. et al., Comparison of narrow-band UV-B phototherapy and PUVA photochemotherapy in the treatment of psoriasis, *Acta. Derm. Venereol.* (Stockholm), 70, 212, 1990.
82. Ferguson, J., The use of narrowband UV-B (tube lamp) in the management of skin disease, *Arch. Dermatol.*, 135, 589, 1999.
83. British Photodermatology Group, An appraisal of narrowband (TL-01) UVB phototherapy. British Photodermatology Group Workshop Report (April 1996), *Br. J. Dermatol.*, 137, 327, 1997.
84. Walters, I.B. et al., Suberythemogenic narrow-band UVB is markedly more effective than conventional UVB in treatment of psoriasis vulgaris, *J. Am Acad. Dermatol.*, 40, 893, 1999.
85. Green, C. et al., 311 nm UVB phototherapy — an effective treatment for psoriasis, *Br. J. Dermatol.*, 119, 691, 1988.
86. Collins, P. and Ferguson, J., Narrow-band UVB (TL-01) phototherapy: an effective preventative treatment for the photodermatoses, *Br. J. Dermatol.*, 132, 956, 1995.
87. Reynolds, N.J. et al., Narrow-band ultraviolet B and broad-band ultraviolet A phototherapy in adult atopic eczema: a randomised controlled trial, *Lancet*, 357, 2012, 2001.
88. El-Ghorr, A.A. et al., The effect of chronic low-dose UVB radiation on Langerhans cells, sunburn cells, urocanic acid isomers, contact hypersensitivity and serum immunoglobulins in mice, *Photochem. Photobiol.*, 62, 326, 1995.
89. Dawe, R.S. et al., UV-B phototherapy clears psoriasis through local effects, *Arch. Dermatol.*, 138, 1071, 2002.
90. De Rie, M.A., Out, T.A., and Bos, J.D., Low-dose narrow-band UVB phototherapy combined with topical therapy is effective in psoriasis and does not inhibit systemic T-cell activation, *Dermatology*, 196, 412, 1998.
91. Leung, D.Y.M. and Bieber, T., Atopic dermatitis, *Lancet*, 361, 151, 2003.
92. Leung, D.Y.M. and Soter, N.A., Cellular and immunologic mechanisms in atopic dermatitis, *J. Am. Acad. Dermatol*, 44, S1, 2001.
93. Rudikoff, D. and Lebwohl, M., Atopic dermatitis, *Lancet*, 351, 1715, 1998.
94. Faergemann, J. and Larkö, O., The effect of UV-light on human skin microorganisms, *Acta. Derm. Venereol.* (Stockholm), 67, 69, 1987.
95. Midelfart, K., Stenvold, S.-E., and Volden, G., Combined UVB and UVA phototherapy of atopic eczema, *Dermatologica*, 171, 95, 1985.
96. Jekler, J. and Larkö, O., Combined UVA-UVB versus UVB phototherapy for atopic dermatitis: a paired-comparison study, *J. Am. Acad. Dermatol.*, 22, 49, 1990.
97. Krutmann, J., in *Dermatology in General Medicine*, 5th ed., Freedberg, I.M. et al., Eds., McGraw-Hill, New York, 1999, 2870.
98. Gilchrest, B.A. et al., Ultraviolet phototherapy of uremic pruritus: long-term results and possible mechanisms of action, *Ann. Intern. Med.*, 91, 17, 1979.
99. Cerio, R. et al., A combination of phototherapy and cholestyramine for the relief of pruritus in primary biliary cirrhosis, *Br. J. Dermatol.*, 117, 265, 1987.
100. Sjovall, P. and Christensen, O.B., Local and systemic effect of ultraviolet irradiation (UVA and UVB) on human allergic contact dermatitis, *Acta. Derm. Venereol.* (Stockholm), 66, 290, 1986.
101. Rosén, K. et al., Langerhans cells in chronic eczematous dermatitis of the palms treated with PUVA and UVB, *Acta. Derm. Venereol.* (Stockholm), 69, 200, 1989.
102. Arndt, K.A. et al., Treatment of pityriasis rosea with UV radiation, *Arch. Dermatol.*, 119, 381, 1983.

103. Harber, L.C. and Bickers, D.R., *Photosensitivity Diseases. Principles of Diagnosis and Treatment*, 2nd ed., B.C. Decker, Toronto, 1989.
104. Jekler, J. and Larkö, O., Phototherapy for atopic dermatitis with ultraviolet A (UVA), low-dose UVB and combined UVA and UVB: two paired-comparison studies, *Photodermatol. Photoimmunol. Photomed.*, 8, 151, 1991.
105. Krutmann, J. et al., High-dose UVA1 therapy in the treatment of patients with atopic dermatitis, *J. Am. Acad. Dermatol.*, 26, 225, 1992.
106. Krutmann, J. et al., High-dose UVA-1 therapy for atopic dermatitis: results of a multicenter trial, *J. Am. Acad. Dermatol.*, 38, 589, 1998.
107. Krutmann, J., Ultraviolet A1 radiation-induced immunomodulation: high-dose UVA1 therapy in atopic dermatitis, in *Photoimmunology*, Krutmann, J. and Elmets, C.A., Eds., Blackwell Science, Oxford, 1995, 246.
108. Kowalzick, L. et al., Low dose versus medium dose UV-A1 treatment in severe atopic eczema, *Acta. Derm. Venereol.* (Stockholm), 75, 43, 1995.
109. McGrath, H., Jr., Ultraviolet-A1 irradiation decreases clinical disease activity and autoantibodies in patients with systemic lupus erythematosus, *Clin. Exp. Rheum.*, 12, 129, 1994.
110. Sönnichsen, N. et al., UV-A-1-Therapie bei subakut-kutanem Lupus erythematodes, *Hautartzt,* 44, 723, 1993.
111. Kerscher, M. et al., Low-dose UVA1 phototherapy for treatment of localized scleroderma, *J. Am. Acad. Dermatol.*, 38, 21, 1998.
112. De Rie, M.A. et al., Evaluation of medium-dose UVA-1 phototherapy in localized scleroderma with the cutometer and fast Fourier transform method, *Dermatology*, 207, 298, 2003.
113. Spencer, J.M., Indoor tanning: risks, benefits, and future trends, *J. Am. Acad. Dermatol.*, 33, 288, 1995.
114. Fisher, G.J. et al., Mechanisms of photoaging and chronological skin aging, *Arch. Dermatol.*, 138, 1462, 2002.
115. Hönigsmann, H. et al., in *Dermatology in General Medicine*, 5th ed., Freedberg, I.M. et al., Eds., McGraw-Hill, New York, 1999, 2880.
116. Schmitt, I.M., Chimenti, S., and Gasparro, F.P., Psoralen-protein photochemistry — a forgotten field, *J. Photochem. Photobiol.*, 227, 101, 1995.
117. Ullrich, S.E., Photoinactivation of T-cell function with psoralen and UVA radiation suppresses the induction of experimental murine graft-versus-host disease across major histocompatibility barriers, *J. Invest. Dermatol.*, 96, 303, 1991.
118. Edelson, R.L., Photopheresis: present and future aspects, *J. Photochem. Photobiol.*, 10, 165, 1991.
119. Okamoto, H., Alteration of lymphocyte functions by 8-methoxypsoralen and long-wave ultraviolet radiation. II. The effect of *in vivo* PUVA on IL-2 production, *J. Invest. Dermatol.*, 89, 24, 1987.
120. Mermelstein, F.H., Abidi, T.F., and Laskin, J.D., Inhibition of epidermal growth factor receptor tyrosine kinase activity in A 431 human epidermoid cells following psoralen/ultraviolet light treatment, *Mol. Pharmacol.*, 36, 848, 1989.
121. Esaki, K. and Mizuno, N., Effect of psoralen + ultraviolet-A on the chemotactic activity of polymorphonuclear neutrophils towards anaphylatoxin C5a des Arg, *Photochem. Photobiol.*, 55, 783, 1992.
122. Moss. C., Friedmann, P.S., and Shuster, S., How does PUVA inhibit delayed cutaneous hypersensitivity? *Br. J. Dermatol.*, 107, 511, 1982.
123. Morison, W.L. et al., Transient impairment of peripheral lymphocyte function during PUVA therapy, *Br. J. Dermatol.*, 101, 391, 1979.
124. Friedmann, P.S. and Rogers, S., Photochemotherapy of psoriasis: DNA damage in blood lymphocytes, *J. Invest. Dermatol.*, 74, 440, 1980.
125. Marks, D.I. and Fox, R.M., Mechanism of photochemotherapy-induced apoptotic cell death in lymphoid cells, *Biochem. Cell. Biol.*, 69, 754, 1991.
126. Bos, J.D. and De Rie, M.A., The pathogenesis of psoriasis: immunological facts and speculations. *Immunol. Today*, 20, 40, 1999.
127. Bos, J.D., The pathomechanisms of psoriasis, the skin immune system, and cyclosporin, *Br. J. Dermatol.*, 118, 141, 1988.
128. De Rie, M.A. et al., Expression of the T-cell activation antigens CD27 and CD28 in normal and psoriatic skin, *Clin. Exp. Dermatol.*, 21, 104, 1996.

129. Tanew, A. et al., Narrowband UV-B phototherapy vs photochemotherapy in the treatment of chronic plaque-type psoriasis, *Arch Dermatol.*, 135, 519, 1999.
130. Markham, T., Rogers, S., and Collins, P., Narrowband UV-B (TL-01) phototherapy vs. oral 8-methoxypsoralen psoralen-UV-A for the treatment of chronic plaque psoriasis, *Arch. Dermatol.,* 139, 325, 2003.
131. Stern, R.S. and the PUVA follow up study, The risk of melanoma in association with long-term exposure in PUVA, *J. Am. Acad. Dermatol.*, 44, 755, 2001.
132. Hannuksela, M. and Karvonen, J., Trioxsalen bath plus UVA is effective and safe in the treatment of psoriasis, *Br. J. Dermatol.*, 99, 703, 1978.
133. Lowe, N.J. et al., PUVA therapy for psoriasis: comparison of oral and bath-water delivery of 8-methoxypsoralen, *J. Am. Acad. Dermatol.*, 3, 406, 1980.
134. De Rie, M.A. et al., A new psoralen containing gel for topical PUVA therapy: development and treatment results of patients with palmoplantar and plaque-type psoriasis, and hyperkeratotic eczema, *Br. J. Dermatol.*, 132, 964, 1995.
135. Studniberg, H.M. and Weller, P., PUVA, UVB, psoriasis, and nonmelanoma skin cancer, *J. Am. Acad. Dermatol.*, 29, 1013, 1993.
136. Stern, R.S. et al., The persistent risk of genital tumors among men treated with psoralen plus ultraviolet (PUVA) for psoriasis, *J. Am. Acad. Dermatol.*, 47, 33, 2002.
137. Stern, R.S., Actinic degeneration and pigmentary change in association with psoralen and UVA treatment: a 20-year prospective study, *J. Am. Acad. Dermatol.*, 48, 61, 2003.
138. British Photodermatology Group, British Photodermatology Group Guidelines for PUVA, *Br. J. Dermatol.*, 130, 246, 1994.
139. Drake, L.A. et al., Guidelines of care for phototherapy and photochemotherapy, *J. Am. Acad. Dermatol.*, 31, 645, 1994.
140. Frappaz, A. and Thivolet, J., Calcipotriol in combination with PUVA: a randomized double blind placebo study in severe psoriasis, *Eur. J. Dermatol.*, 3, 351, 1993.
141. Wolff, K. and Hönigsmann, H., Clinical aspects of photochemotherapy, *Pharmacol. Ther.*, 12, 381, 1981.
142. Honig, B., Morison, W.L., and Karp, D., Photochemotherapy beyond psoriasis, *J. Am. Acad. Dermatol.*, 31, 775, 1994.
143. Morison, W.L., Parrish, J.A., and Fitzpatrick, T.B., Oral psoralen photochemotherapy of atopic eczema, *Br. J. Dermatol.*, 98, 25, 1978.
144. Atherton, D.J. et al., The role of psoralen photochemotherapy (PUVA) in the treatment of severe atopic eczema in adolescents, *Br. J. Dermatol.*, 118, 791, 1988.
145. Sheehan, M.P. et al., Oral psoralen photochemotherapy in severe childhood atopic eczema: an update, *Br. J. Dermatol.*, 129, 431, 1993.
146. Skouge, J.W. et al., Autografting and PUVA, *J. Dermatol. Surg. Oncol.*, 18, 357, 1992.
147. Njoo, D. and Westerhof, W., Vitiligo. Pathogenesis and treatment, *Am. J. Clin. Dermatol.*, 2, 167, 2001.
148. Scherschun, L., Kim, J.J. and Lim, H.W., Narrow-band ultraviolet B is a useful and well-tolerated treatment for vitiligo, *J. Am. Acad. Dermatol.*, 44, 999, 2001.
149. Gilchrest, B.A. et al., Oral methoxsalen photochemotherapy of mycosis fungoides, *Cancer*, 38, 683, 1976.
150. Herrmann, J.J. et al., Treatment of mycosis fungoides with photochemotherapy (PUVA): long-term follow-up, *J. Am. Acad. Dermatol.*, 33, 234, 1995.
151. Hansen, E.R. et al., Epidermal interleukin 1a functional activity and interleukin 8 immunoreactivity are increased in patients with cutaneous T-cell lymphoma, *J. Invest. Dermatol.*, 97, 818, 1991.
152. Picker, L.J. et al., A unique phenotype of skin-associated lymphocytes in humans, *Am. J. Pathol.*, 136, 1053, 1990.
153. Hofer, A. et al., Narrowband (311-nm) UV-B therapy for small plaque parapsoriasis and early-stage mycosis fungoides, *Arch. Dermatol.*, 135, 1377, 1999.
154. Diederen, P.V.M.M. et al., Narrowband UVB and psoralen-UVA in the treatment of early-stage mycosis fungoides: a retrospective study, *J. Am. Acad. Dermatol.*, 48, 215, 2003.
155. De Rie, M.A. and Bos, J.D., Photochemotherapy for systemic and localized scleroderma, *J. Am. Acad. Dermatol.*, 43, 725, 2000.

156. De Rie, M.A. et al., Treatment of necrobiosis lipoidica with topical psoralen plus ultraviolet A., *Br. J. Dermatol.*, 147, 743, 2002.
157. Edelson, R.L. et al., Treatment of cutaneous T-cell lymphoma by extracorporeal photochemotherapy, *N. Engl. J. Med.*, 316, 297, 1987.
158. Knobler, R. and Heald, P., Extracorporeal photochemotherapy, in *Dermatological Phototherapy and Photodiagnostic Methods*, Krutmann, J. et al., Eds., Springer, Berlin, 2001, 248.
159. Enomoto, D.N.H. et al., Treatment of patients with systemic sclerosis with extracorporeal photochemotherapy (photopheresis), *J. Am. Acad. Dermatol.*, 41, 915, 1999.
160. Knobler, R.M. et al., Parenteral administration of 8-methoxypsoralen in photopheresis, *J. Am. Acad. Dermatol.*, 28, 580, 1993.
161. Vowels, B.R. et al., Extracorporeal photochemotherapy induces the production of tumor necrosis factor alpha by monocytes: implications for the treatment of cutaneous T-cell lymphoma and systemic sclerosis, *J. Invest. Dermatol.*, 98, 686, 1992.
162. Perez, M.I., Effects of UV light, in *Mechanisms of Regulation of Immunity*, Granstein. R., Ed., Karger, Basel, 1997, 121.
163. Enomoto, D.N.H. et al., Extracorporeal photochemotherapy (photopheresis) induces apoptosis in lymphocytes: a possible mechanism of action of PUVA therapy, *Photochem. Photobiol.*, 65, 177, 1997.
164. Kalka, K., Merk, H., and Mukhtar, H., Photodynamic therapy in dermatology, *J. Am. Acad. Dermatol.*, 42, 389, 2000.
165. Athar, M. et al., A novel mechanism for the generation of superoxide anions in hematoporphyrin derivative-mediated cutaneous photosensitization: activation of xanthine oxidase pathway, *J. Clin. Invest.*, 83, 1137, 1989.
166. Zhou, C., New trends in photobiology: mechanisms of tumor necrosis induced by photodynamic therapy, *J. Photochem. Photobiol.* B., 3, 299, 1989.
167. Mukhtar, H. et al., Photoimmunology of photodynamic therapy, in *Photoimmunology*, Krutmann, J. and Elmets, C.A., Eds., Blackwell Science, Oxford, 1995, 257.
168. Elmets, C.A. and Bowen, K.D., Immunological suppression in mice treated with hematoporphyrin derivative photoradiation, *Cancer Res.*, 46, 1608, 1986.
169. Yen, A., Gigli, I., and Barrett, K.E., Dual effects of protoporphyrin and longwave ultraviolet light on histamine release from rat peritoneal and cutaneous mast cells, *J. Immunol.*, 144, 4327, 1990.
170. Barrett, K.E. et al., Inhibition of human peripheral blood lymphocyte function by protoporphyrin and longwave ultraviolet light, *J. Immunol.*, 153, 3286, 1994.

# 41 Biologicals for the Treatment of Immune-Mediated Skin Disease

*Menno A. de Rie and Jan D. Bos*

## CONTENTS



0-8493-1959-5/05/$0.00+$1.50

# I. INTRODUCTION

Biologicals are engineered proteins that are used to modify immune reactions. Antibodies, fusion proteins, and recombinant cytokines are examples of these biologicals. Biologicals, which are sometimes also called "biological response modifiers," are designed to modify defined (patho)physiological pathways that regulate pivotal immunological processes such as lymphocyte activation, interactions with antigen-presenting cells (APC) and endothelial cells (adhesion and migration), and production and action of cytokines and chemokines.

In dermatology, biologicals have been used to treat inflammatory skin diseases such as psoriasis, atopic dermatitis, and cutaneous T cell lymphoma (CTCL). Biologicals are especially interesting as they may have remittive effects, inducing long-term remissions. In addition, they may have a favorable side-effect profile. Treatment with conventional drugs (systemic steroids, acitretine, methotrexate, cyclosporine) or photochemotherapy may have severe short- or long-term side effects. The increased understanding of the immunopathology of inflammatory skin diseases such as psoriasis and atopic dermatitis, together with the development of biotechnology has led to the rapid development of these engineered proteins, not only in dermatology, but also in rheumatology, gastroenterology, and transplantation medicine.

## A. Nomenclature

Although the generic names of the biologicals may be confusing, a strict nomenclature has been applied. Generic names of chimeric monoclonals end with "-ximab," humanized monoclonals end with "-zumab," and human monoclonal antibodies (Mab) end with "-umab." Receptor–antibody fusion proteins end with "-cept."

Table 41.1 lists biologicals that are approved for dermatologic indications or are at present under investigation for treatment of dermatologic conditions. Biologicals can be divided in three main groups: Mab, fusion proteins, and cytokines.

## B. Monoclonal Antibodies

Mab used to be from murine origin. Monoclonal antibody therapies were in the 1990s handicapped by their adverse events related to their murine origin. Patients that were treated with these allogeneic proteins induced immune responses with development of neutralizing antibodies, allergic reactions, and the cytokine-release syndrome.[1] This has now changed with the possibility to produce fully humanized Mab. Nowadays, Mab in therapeutic trials are chimeric (fused segments of mouse and human antibodies), humanized (individual amino acids in a human backbone replaced with specific sequences derived from murine Mab), or human sequence (generated in genetically engineered mice).[2,3]

## C. Fusion Proteins

Fusion proteins are typically composed of a fusion of two protein parts: a human cellular receptor or a specific toxin and an immunoglobulin. The ligand-binding domains of human cellular receptors or the toxin bind directly to the specific target. This part is coupled to another protein, in most cases the CH2/CH3 constant region domain of human IgG, thus improving the stability of the fusion protein or facilitating the binding to an Fc-receptor expressed by an immunological effector cell by inducing antibody-dependent cell-mediated cytotoxicity (for example, a natural killer cell). Fusion proteins are also potential immunogenic proteins because of reasons mentioned above. The best-known example of the first kind is $DAB_{389}$IL-2 fusion protein in which the receptor-binding domain of diphtheria toxin is replaced by human interleukin-2 (IL-2) but where the membrane-translocating and cytotoxic domains have been retained.[4] Etanercept is an example of the second

**TABLE 41.1**
**Overview of Biologicals Used in Dermatology**

| Binding Characteristics | Generic Name | Brand Name/Synonym | Protein Characteristics | Mode of Action |
|---|---|---|---|---|
| | | **Monoclonal Antibodies** | | |
| Anti-CD2 | Siplizumab (Medi-507) | | Humanized Mab | Binds to CD2; induces T-cell depletion |
| Anti-CD3 | Muromab-CD3 (OKT3) | Orthoclone-OKT3 | Murine Mab | Binds to CD3; induces T-cell depletion and anergy |
| | Visilizumab (HuM291) | Nuvion | Humanized Mab | Binds to CD3; induces T-cell anergy and apoptosis |
| Anti-CD4 | OKTcdr4a | IMUCLONE | Humanized Mab | Binds to CD4; induces CD4 downmodulation? |
| Anti-CD11a | Efalizumab (hu1124) | Xanelim Raptiva | Humanized Mab | Binds to α subunit of LFA-1; blocks CD11a–ICAM-1 interaction |
| Anti-CD20 | Rituximab | Mabthera | Chimeric Mab | Binds to CD20 (pan B-cell antigen) |
| Anti-CD25 | Daclizumab anti-TAC | Zenapax | Humanized Mab | Binds to α subunit of IL-2R; inhibition of T-cell proliferation |
| | basiliximab | Simulect | Chimeric Mab | |
| Anti-CD40L | IDEC-131 | | Humanized Mab | Binds to CD40L |
| Anti-CD80 (B7-1) | IDEC-114 | | Humanized Mab | Blocks CD28 (T-cells) – CD80 (APC) interaction |
| Anti-E-selectin | CDP850 | | Humanized Mab | Blocks CLA (T cells)–E-selectin (endothelial cells) interaction |
| Anti-IL-8 | ABX-IL-8 | | Fully human Mab | Binds IL-8; inhibits leukocyte chemotaxis and T-cell proliferations |
| Anti-TNF-α | Infliximab | Remicade | Chimeric Mab | Binds TNF-α and mediates lysis of TNF-α⁺ cells |
| | Adalimumab | Humira | Human recombinant IgG1 | Binds TNF-α |
| Anti-IFN-γ | HuZAF SMART anti-IFN-γ | | Humanized Mab | Neutralizes IFN-γ |
| | | **Fusion Proteins** | | |
| Anti-TNF-α | Etanercept | Enbrel | Extracellular domain of human TNF-αR-Fc part human IgG1 | Binds TNF-α |
| Anti-TNF-α and | Onercept | | Fusion protein | Binds TNF-α and |
| Anti-CD2 and natural killer cells (Fc- receptor) | Alefacept | Amevive | First extracellular domain of human LFA-3–Fc part human IgG1 | Inhibits LFA-3 (APC)–CD2 (T cell) interaction; induces T-cell apoptosis (via natural killer cells) |
| Anti-CD25 | Denileukin difitox ($DAB_{389}$IL-2) | ONTAK | Cytokine (IL-2)-toxin fusion protein | Binds to high-affinity IL-2R (CD25) and releases diphtheria toxin |
| Anti-CD80 (B7-1) and anti-CD86 (B7-2) | CTLA4-Ig (BMS 188667) | | CTLA4–human IgG fusion protein | Inhibits CD28 (T cells) CD80 (APC) interaction |

**TABLE 41.1 (Continued)**
**Overview of Biologicals Used in Dermatology**

| Binding Characteristics | Generic Name | Brand Name/Synonym | Protein Characteristics | Mode of Action |
|---|---|---|---|---|
| | | **Recombinant Cytokines and Interferons** | | |
| IL-4 | rhu-IL-4 | | Recombinant human Th2 cytokine | Immune deviation from Th1 to Th2 |
| IL-10 | rhu-IL-10 | Tenovil | Recombinant human Th2 cytokine | Immune deviation from Th1 to Th2 |
| IL-11 | Oprelvekin rhu-IL-11 | Neumega | Recombinant human Th2 cytokine | Immune deviation from Th1 to Th2 |
| IL-12 | rhu-IL-12 | | Recombinant human cytokine | Activates Th1 cells; enhances IFN-γ production |
| GM-CSF | Sargramostine | Leukine | | Immune adjuvans |
| IFN-α | IFN-α 2a or 2b | Roferon-A Intron-A | Recombinant cytokine | Immune adjuvans |
| IFN-γ | IFN- 1b | | | Immune adjuvans |
| | | **Other** | | |
| Soluble IL-4 R | Altrakincept | | | Binds IL-4 |
| IL-18 binding protein | r-hIL-18BP | | Recombinant human IL-18-binding protein | Binds IL-18 |
| Antiangiogenic peptide | Æ-941 | | Shark cartilage molecular fraction (<500 kDa) | Blocks VEGF |

*Abbreviations:* APC: antigen-presenting cell; Fc: constant region; GM-CSF: granulocyte-macrophage colony-stimulating factor; IFN: interferon; IgG: immunoglobulin G; IL: interleukin; L: ligand; Mab: monoclonal antibody; R: receptor; Th: T helper cell; VEGF: vascular endothelial growth factor.

*Nomenclature:* *-umab* indicates human Mab, *-zumab* indicates humanized Mab, *-ximab* indicates chimeric Mab, and *–cept* indicates receptor-antibody fusion protein.

type of fusion proteins and uses the extracellular domain of the tumor necrosis factor-alpha (TNF-α) receptor that is linked to the Fc portion of the human IgG1 immunoglobulin.[5]

### D. Recombinant Cytokines and Interferons

In addition, not only humanized Mab but also human cytokines can be made. One of the first cytokines used for psoriasis treatment is IL-10, which acts by deviation of the T helper 1-type immune response toward a T helper 2-type response.[6] These recombinant human proteins are molecules that are identical to normal human proteins and function by interacting with normal cellular receptors.

Interferons (especially IFN-α) have been widely used for treatment of viral diseases (not discussed in this chapter) and have recently been employed in other conditions such as atopic dermatitis and CTCL (see Section IV Clinical Uses).

## II. MECHANISM OF ACTION

The main goal of biologic therapy is to prevent pathologic effector immune responses in skin tissue. Biologicals have been developed to affect one or more of the different steps of a cutaneous immune response. These steps are (1) Langerhans cell maturation and T-cell activation, (2) T-cell receptor

(TCR) stimulation, (3) T-cell activation by co-stimulation (second, or accessory, signals), (4) T-cell differentiation and proliferation by regulatory cytokines, (5) T-cell adhesion and migration, and (6) effector actions of T cells in skin tissue. This subject has recently been reviewed extensively.[7] In addition, Mab directed against other (cellular) targets are also employed. For example, anti-B-cell Mab, originally used in hemato-oncology, are now successfully used to treat cutaneous B-cell lymphomas and autoimmune (bulleous) diseases. The therapeutic aspects of the biologicals are further discussed in Section IV of this chapter.

### A. Langerhans Cell Maturation and T-Cell Activation

A cutaneous immune response may be initiated by Langerhans cells. After antigen uptake and processing these APC migrate to skin-draining lymph nodes, where naive T cells (CD45RO-negative) are activated and differentiated into memory T cells (CD45RO-positive). The lymphocyte function-associated antigen-1 (LFA-1) (CD11a)/ICAM binding is the initial interaction of T cells with Langerhans cells. This binding can be prevented by the humanized anti-CD11a monoclonal antibody efalizumab.[8] LFA-1 is also an important adhesion molecule in T-cell trafficking and T-cell adhesion to keratinocytes (step 5). It is therefore not surprising that anti-CD11a antibodies are effective immunosuppressive biologicals.

### B. T-Cell Receptor Stimulation

Antibodies to various protein subunits of the TCR complex are used for therapeutic immune modulation. Initially, murine anti-CD3 but today humanized anti-CD3 Mab are used in transplantation medicine, psoriasis, and refractory graft-vs.-host disease patients.

### C. T-Cell Activation by Co-Stimulation

TCR stimulation by antigen is not sufficient for T-cell activation; accessory signals (co-stimulation) are required. These signals are delivered by physical contact between cell surface molecules present on Langerhans cells and T cells. Examples of these molecules are CD80 (B7-1) and CD86 (B7-2; expressed by Langerhans cells), and the T-cell molecules CD28 and CTLA4. T-cell co-stimulation can be reduced or blocked by Mab to CD80 and CD86, as well as by the fusion protein CTLA4Ig. The B7/CD28 co-stimulatory pathway can be inhibited by the primatized anti-B7-1 Mab IDEC-114.

### D. T-Cell Differentiation and Proliferation by Regulatory Cytokines

Activated T cells may be differentiated into type 1 effectors (which synthesize IFN-$\gamma$) or type 2 effectors (IL-4) in lymph nodes. By administration of IL-4 or IL-10, T cells may be directed toward a type 2 effector cell, while IL-12 stimulates type 1 T-cell growth and IFN-$\gamma$ production. This principle ("immune deviation") has been used successfully to manipulate psoriasis, which is thought to be a type 1 disease, toward type 2 T-cell differentiation.

Proliferation of T cells after activation is mainly due to stimulation of the $\alpha$ protein subunit of the IL-2R (CD25). Daclizumab, a humanized anti-CD25 and the chimeric monoclonal antibody basiliximab have shown efficacy, not only in renal allograft rejection, but also in psoriasis patients. The fusion protein denileukin difitox ($DAB_{389}$ IL-2) is also specific for CD25. After binding to CD25 and receptor-mediated endocytosis, an enzymatic fragment of the diphtheria toxin is released that inhibits protein synthesis, eventually leading to T-cell apoptosis.

### E. T-Cell Adhesion and Migration

Differentiated and CLA (cutaneous lymphocyte antigen)-positive T cells return to the skin via the bloodstream. Via adhesion molecules (E-selectin and P-selectin) expressed by postcapillary venules and integrins such as LFA-1, T cells bind to endothelial cells. Next, T cells migrate in the dermis and become effector cells. A humanized antibody to E-selectin (CDP850) has been developed and was tested in patients with psoriasis, but was not effective. Integrin blockade and consequent clinical efficacy has been accomplished in patients with psoriasis with the anti-CD11a monoclonal antibody efalizumab (see above). Antisense oligonucleotides to the counterpart of LFA-1, ICAM-1, are under investigation.

### F. Effector Actions of T Cells in Skin Tissue

Once effector T cells have entered the dermis or epidermis, they can recognize antigen and subsequently start releasing cytokines, such as IFN-γ and TNF-α. These cytokines then trigger various inflammatory pathways that affect proliferation and differentiation of endothelial cells, keratinocytes, mast cells, etc. (reviewed by Krueger).[7] Different strategies have now been developed to block some of these effector cytokines (especially IFN-γ and TNF-α) and chemokines (IL-8). TNF blockade was first demonstrated to be effective in rheumatoid arthritis. Nowadays, different types of TNF antagonists exist (see Table 41.1). Numerous studies have been published showing efficacy in rheumatologic, gastrointestinal, and dermatologic conditions. Especially, Mab against TNF-α (infliximab: a chimeric Mab) and a fusion protein called etanercept (a TNF-receptor–Ig fusion protein) has demonstrated promising effects.

A fully human anti-IL-8 Mab (ABX-IL-8) has been tested in psoriasis. IL-8, which is a chemokine and a chemoattractant for neutrophils, was indeed partly neutralized by ABX-IL-8, demonstrating the validity of this concept.

## III. ADVERSE EVENTS

Potentially, all biologicals including fully human Mab are immunogenic because of variation in constant region amino acid sequences (allovariation) or glycosylation differences produced by cultured cell lines that are used to produce the products.[3] Thus, immediate IgE-mediated or T-cell-mediated delayed hypersensitivity reactions can occur and neutralizing antibodies may be produced. In addition, several T-cell-binding biologicals can induce a first-dose reaction, which consists of flu-like symptoms due to release of cytokines such as TNF-α, IFN-γ, and IL-6. Anyone administering biologicals should be aware of these side effects and be prepared to treat anaphylactic reactions that may be life-threatening.

Administration of these proteins may lead to the formation of neutralizing antibodies, thus reducing the efficacy of the biological. This has been demonstrated clearly in patients with Crohn's disease treated repeatedly with the chimeric Mab infliximab.[9] Injection-site reactions and rashes are seen with many biologicals. These reactions may be mechanistic or due to hypersensitivity.

Since most biologicals affect the immune system, an increased risk of lymphoma development and immunosuppressive side effects can be expected. Not only myelosuppression and decreases of circulating immunocompetent cells (T cells) can be seen, but also opportunistic infections have been reported, especially after treatment with TNF-blocking biologicals. In addition, treatment with TNF-blocking agents has been associated with development of autoantibodies, nonmelanoma skin cancer, development or exacerbation of multiple sclerosis, drug-induced lupus erythematodes-like diseases, or vasculitis (see Anticytokines subsection of Section IV).

Biologicals, as with all drugs, may lead to different and unpredictable side effects. At this moment the long-term safety of T-cell-depleting and immunosuppressive biologicals has not been established. Long-term safety studies will be needed to establish the safety of these biologicals. Because it is not rare that patients suffering from skin diseases have been treated with other (mutagenic) therapies (psoriasis patients and photo(chemo)therapy, special attention for possible long-term side effects is needed.

## IV. CLINICAL USES

Biologicals can be applied for any skin disease that is immune mediated. However, to date most biologicals have been tested and registered in patients suffering from plaque-type psoriasis and psoriatic arthritis. In theory, many antipsoriatic biologicals may also be beneficial in other T-cell-mediated diseases such as atopic dermatitis, CTCL, alopecia areata, lichen ruber planus, etc., but have not been studied in randomized controlled trials, so far. In this section an overview of biologicals now under investigation or already established is presented, focused on psoriasis. As this field is rapidly changing, the reader is encouraged to check recent literature for updates.

### A. Psoriasis

#### 1. T-Cell-Targeted Therapies

##### *a. Anti-CD2*

Siplizumab (Medi-507) is a humanized monoclonal antibody to a conformational epitope of CD2, which is also expressed by natural killer cells. Treatment with siplizumab leads to depletion of activated T cells and blocking of co-stimulatory signals between APC and T cells by inhibiting CD2-LFA-3 interaction.[10] Siplizumab has been shown to be effective in a small number of patients with approximately 50% of patients achieving 75% or more improvement of psoriasis.[11] The drug can be administered subcutaneously and intravenously. Early phase 1 and 2 studies have just been completed.

##### *b. Anti-CD3*

OKT3 was one of the first murine Mab used in transplantation patients and later on also in patients with psoriasis.[12] Recently, the humanized anti-CD3 Mab visilizumab (HuM291) was developed. Visilizumab leads to apoptosis and consequently T-cell depletion.[13] In addition, visilizumab partly activates the TCR complex via binding to the epsilon subunit of CD3. This results in T-cell anergy.[14] Visilizumab has been shown to be effective in clearing of cutaneous lesions in graft-vs.-host disease.[15] An initial study with visilizumab in psoriasis has been initiated.

##### *c. Anti-CD4*

Anti-CD4 Mab interfere with the APC–CD4$^+$ T-cell interaction. Treatment with anti-CD4 antibodies can be effective as was demonstrated in 1992.[16] More recent studies have reported reductions in psoriasis area and severity in patients with high-dose humanized anti-CD4 Mab (OKTcdr4a; two courses of 750 mg).[17,18] There was no complete CD4$^+$ T-cell depletion and measurement of CD4 saturation showed that sustained saturation was not needed to obtain a clinical response. Side effects were mild and included fever and headache during infusion.

##### *d. Anti-CD25*

Binding of IL-2 to the $\alpha$ subunit of the IL-2-receptor (CD25) is pivotal in T-cell activation and proliferation. Prevention of binding of IL-2 to CD25 thus inhibits T-cell proliferation. Recently, a humanized Mab to CD25, termed daclizumab, has been developed. A vehicle-controlled study with daclizumab demonstrated that this therapy may be effective in patients with severe psoriasis — psoriasis area and severity index (PASI) > 36.[19] The overall antipsoriatic effect was moderate (30% PASI reduction). Complete blockade of CD25 was needed; when dosing was reduced variable receptor saturation was found, which correlated with exacerbation of psoriasis. Another and older chimeric anti-CD25 Mab, termed basiliximab, which is also used in transplantation medicine, has been given together with cyclosporine to patients with (pustular) psoriasis.[20–22] It has been suggested that monotherapy with anti-CD25 Mab is less effective in stable plaque-type psoriasis.[23] The value of anti-CD25 therapy may be limited to combination therapy in patients with flaring pustular psoriasis.

### e. *Denileukin diftitox*

Anti-CD25-targeted therapy has also been tried with fusion proteins of which $DAB_{389}$IL-2 (synonym: denileukin diftitox) is the best example.[4,24] Clinical efficacy was first demonstrated by Gottlieb et al.[4] in a placebo-controlled trial in 41 patients. Denileukin diftitox doses of 5, 10, and 15 μg/kg/day administered for 3 consecutive days every week for 4 weeks resulted in a PASI reduction of ≥50% in 44% of the patients, but also in serious adverse events in three patients (hypersensitivity reactions with hypotension). Recently, an alternative regimen was investigated and showed that doses of 5 μg/kg/day of denileukin diftitox resulted in PASI reductions of 50% or more in 7 of 15 patients.[25] However, again serious adverse developed, such as vascular leak syndrome. Thus, it seems that at higher doses (≥5 μg/kg/day), denileukin diftitox is too problematic for routine use in patients with psoriasis.

## 2. Co-Stimulatory Molecules (accessory cell signals)

### a. *Alefacept*

Recently, the fusion protein alefacept (LFA-3TIP, Amevive®) was developed (reviewed by Krueger).[26] LFA-3TIP is a protein comprising the first LFA-3 extracellular domain ("tip") fused to the hinge, CH2 and CH3 regions of a human IgG1. LFA-3TIP binds to CD2, thus leading to inhibition of proliferation of human T cells *in vitro*.[27] Efficacy was first demonstrated in a placebo-controlled phase II trial in 229 patients with chronic plaque psoriasis.[28] The mechanism of action of alefacept is not completely understood. The therapeutic activity of alefacept is partly explained by the blockade of co-stimulation between CD2 on T cells and LFA-3 on APC. Since the expression of CD2 is increased on activated, proliferating memory-effector $CD45RO^+$ T cells in psoriatic lesions, these pathogenic T cells are affected by alefacept to a greater extent as compared to other non-activated T cells.[29] In addition, treatment with alefacept results in a depletion of circulating memory ($CD4^+CD45RO^+$) T cells. It has been suggested that apoptosis of these T cells is mediated by natural killer cells that bind alefacept by their Fc receptors, resulting in a release of cytotoxic granules.[30]

Although alefacept affects memory T cells, no signs of opportunistic infections have been reported. Studies have demonstrated that alefacept not only marginally affects naive T cells but in addition does not affect antibody responses to novel and recall antigens.[31] The increased expression of CD2 on memory-effector $CD45RO^+$ provides a specific marker for pathogenic T cells that are targeted by alefacept. Clinical responses in patients with chronic plaque psoriasis correlate with alefacept-induced decreases in circulating blood lymphocyte counts, thus supporting the hypothesized mechanism of action of this fusion protein.[32]

Several randomized, placebo-controlled phase III trials with alefacept in more than 1300 patients suffering from chronic plaque-type psoriasis have been completed by different study groups.[33–35] In patients receiving two 12-weeks intravenous courses of 15 mg alefacept, 40 and 71%, achieved a 50% or greater and a 75% or greater PASI reduction, respectively. The median duration of the remission was 7 months. No serious side effects or signs of increased risk of infection were reported.

In a pilot study in 11 patients suffering from psoriatic arthritis, alefacept was found to have a positive effect on arthritis as well; 6 of 11 patients (56%) fulfilled the disease activity score (DAS) response criteria. Of the 11 patients, 9 (82%) fulfilled the DAS response criteria at any point during study. Serial synovial tissue biopsies showed a significant reduction in $CD4^+$ and $CD8^+$ T cells and $CD68^+$ macrophages.[36]

### b. *CTLA4-Ig (BMS 188667) and Anti-CD80*

CTLA4-Ig is a chimeric fusion protein that combines the extracellular domain of CTLA4 (cytotoxic T-lymphocyte-associated antigen 4, = CD28) with an IgG heavy-chain and binds with high affinity to both CD80 (B7-1) and CD86 (B7-2) expressed on activated APC.[37,38] Binding of CTLA4-Ig to its ligands inhibits T-cell co-stimulation. In an open-label dose-finding trial, intravenously administered CTLA4-Ig resulted in >50% improvement of psoriasis in 9 of 11 patients with long-lasting remission (mean 147 days).[37] CTLA4-Ig was well tolerated by most patients. According to the authors, the efficacy of CTLA4-Ig is similar to both cyclosporine and photochemotherapy. CTLA4-Ig will be further developed for transplantation medicine and rheumatoid arthritis only.

Anti-CD80 (IDEC 114) is a humanized monoclonal antibody directed against CD80 (B7-1), which is expressed primarily on activated APC and thereby inhibits the T-cell (CD28)–CD80 interaction. In addition, without binding of CD28 through CD80, T cells may become anergized and irresponsive to stimuli.[39] Efficacy of IDEC-114 was first demonstrated in a phase I trial with a single-dose regimen (0.05 to 15 mg/kg).[40] In a phase I/II trial 35 patients received four biweekly infusions at various doses. Of the patients, 40% achieved at least 50% PASI reduction.[41] Patients showed continued improvement with maximal effect 12 weeks after treatment. No serious adverse events were seen. A phase II trial with single-dose treatment has recently been published confirming the efficacy of anti-CD80 treatment.[42]

### 3. Adhesion Molecules

#### a. *Efalizumab*

Efalizumab is a humanized Mab directed against the CD11a component (α subunit) of LFA-1 (reviewed by Leonardi).[8] In phase I studies pharmacokinetics and pharmacodynamics of single and multiple doses of efalizumab were established.[43] A placebo-controlled trial in 75 patients with psoriasis using 0.3 mg/kg efalizumab given intravenously, weekly for 8 weeks, demonstrated its efficacy.[44] About 48% of patients achieved 50% clinical improvement in psoriasis and 25% reached >75% improvement. Efalizumab was well tolerated. In this clinical study the mechanism of action of efalizumab was further elucidated; it was demonstrated that efalizumab blocks T-cell trafficking into the skin.[44] In addition, it was found that at therapeutic doses efalizumab not only blocks binding of LFA-1 to ICAM-1, but also downregulates surface expression of CD11a by about 90%.[45]

The efficacy of efalizumab has been confirmed by randomized, placebo-controlled phase III studies of 12 weekly subcutaneous doses of efalizumab in more than 1000 patients. The majority of patients relapsed within 12 weeks of completing therapy. No significant infectious complications that might suggest an immunosuppressive effect due to treatment with efalizumab have as yet been reported.[46–48]

#### b. *Anti-E-Selectin and Anti-CLA Monoclonal Antibodies*

T cells need to bind first with their membrane adhesion molecules CD11a and CLA to their ligands ICAM-1 and E-selectin, respectively, expressed on activated endothelial cells, in order to leave the circulation and enter the dermis. Efalizumab is able to inhibit the CD11a–ICAM-1 interaction (see above). Although an anti-CLA Mab has become available, clinical studies have not yet been presented. A humanized Mab directed against E-selectin has been tested in a double-blind, placebo-controlled trial in 13 patients but was found ineffective.[49] The inability of an anti-E-selectin antibody to improve psoriasis, despite high skin and blood levels, suggests that this adhesion pathway is not pivotal in the pathogenesis of psoriasis.

#### c. *Antisense Oligonucleotides to ICAM-1*

Animal studies with antisense oligonucleotides to ICAM-1 have demonstrated their positive effect in lung transplantation and contact hypersensitivity. Human studies in inflammatory conditions such as psoriasis have not been presented yet.

### 4. Cytokine-Targeted Therapies

#### a. *Cytokine Switching/Immune Deviation*

*Interkeukin-4 (IL-4).* A pilot study with IL-4 showed that this Th2 cytokine can be successfully used in patients suffering from plaque-type psoriasis.[50] In a dose-escalating study (0.05, 0.1, 0.2, 0.3, 0.5 rhu IL-4/kg) in 20 patients with plaque-type psoriasis, PASI 50 was reached in 19 of 20 patients and PASI 68 in 15 of 20 patients. Only one relapse was seen 6 weeks after treatment. Mild adverse events (fever, headache, and edema of hands; 2 of 20) were reported.[51]

*IL-10.* IL-10 is an important Th2 cytokine capable of downregulation of the ongoing Th1 immune response in psoriasis.[52] Early phase I/II trials with subcutaneous injections of recombinant IL-10 three times a week showed a mean PASI reduction of 55%.[53–55] In a controlled study ($n$ = 30) rhu IL-10 was found not to be effective, although a shift toward Th2-type cytokine production could be demonstrated.[56]

*IL-11.* Recombinant human IL-11 (oprelvekin) is an FDA-approved therapy for the treatment of thrombocytopenia. In early studies with subcutaneously injected IL-11, it was found that IL-11 may act to induce immune deviation in Th1-type diseases such as psoriasis.[57] In a phase I trial, 7 of 12 patients demonstrated a significant reduction of their psoriasis.[58]

#### b. Anticytokines

*Anti-IL-8.* The human high-affinity anti-IL-8 monoclonal ABX-IL-8 blocks leukocyte chemotaxis and T-cell proliferation via binding and deactivation of free IL-8 in the skin. Phase I and II trials with anti-IL-8 have been conducted. Treatment with 3 and 6 mg/kg every 3 weeks showed a PASI reduction of >50% in 33 and 17% of the patients, respectively.[59,60] The drug was well tolerated.

*Infliximab.* Infliximab is a chimeric monoclonal IgG antibody that binds TNF-α and mediates lysis of TNF-α-expressing cells (reviewed by Gottlieb).[61] Infliximab is FDA approved for the treatment of Crohn's disease and rheumatoid arthritis. TNF-α is a central cytokine that drives the immune response toward aberrant proliferation and differentiation of keratinocytes in psoriasis.[62] Indeed, treatment with infliximab of a patient suffering from both Crohn's disease and psoriasis led to dramatic decreases of clinical activity.[63] Subsequently, a small randomized, controlled study in 33 patients demonstrated a greater than 80% response rate with minimal adverse effects after three intravenous treatments with 5 or 10 mg infliximab/kg.[64] The efficacy of treatment with infliximab has been demonstrated by two controlled studies.[65,66] Clearance of methotrexate-resistant skin lesions has also been demonstrated in six patients suffering from psoriatic arthritis.[67]

*Etanercept.* Etanercept is a fusion protein that is composed of the TNF-α type II receptor and the Fc part of a human IgG antibody (reviewed by Goffe).[68] Etanercept, which is also FDA approved for rheumatoid arthritis and Crohn's disease, binds soluble TNF-α and forms a complex similar to infliximab but less stable than infliximab.[69] In addition, etanercept is FDA approved for psoriatic arthritis. In a phase II trial of etanercept (25 mg twice weekly, 12 weeks) in 60 patients with psoriatic arthritis a median PASI improvement of 46% was achieved. More than 75% PASI improvement was seen in 26% of patients; 73% of these etanercept-treated patients met the American College of Rheumatology criteria for improvement (ACR 20). No serious side effects were reported.[70] In a phase III trial these results have been confirmed, although in this multicenter study concomitant therapy was permitted.[71]

*Side effects of anti-TNF-α-directed therapies.* Of great concern are the reports of tuberculosis infection reactivation in patients treated with TNF-blocking agents.[72] Etanercept has recently been associated with drug-induced subacute cutaneous lupus erythematodes (15% of patients develop anti-double-stranded-DNA antibodies), drug-induced systemic lupus erythematosus, and rapid onset of cutaneous squamous cell carcinoma.[73,74]

*Anti-IFN-γ.* A humanized IgG1 Mab against IFN-γ (HuZAF) has been developed but so far no results of these phase I trials have been published.

### B. Atopic Dermatitis

Atopic dermatitis is characterized by immunologic abnormalities. A major immunological abnormality is the skewing of Th0 toward Th2 lymphocytes upon antigenic challenge and consequent increased IgE production, reduced IFN-γ, and increased IL-4 and IL-5 production (see Chapter 30, Atopic Dermatitis).

### 1. Interferon-γ

Several clinical studies have focused on the therapeutic effects of IFN-γ. In 1993 Hanifin et al.[75] demonstrated that recombinant IFN-γ given by daily subcutaneous injection over a 12-week period was safe, well accepted, and effective in reducing inflammation, clinical symptoms, and eosinophilia in severe atopic dermatitis. In a clinical and immunohistochemical study it was demonstrated that a higher dosage ($1.5 \times 10E6$ IU/m$^2$) was more effective for the maintenance of clinical improvement than a lower dosage ($0.5 \times 10E6$ IU/m$^2$).[76]

### 2. Anti-IL-4 and Anti-IL-5 Therapy

To date, no trials have been conducted with anti-IL-4-directed therapies in patients with atopic dermatitis. However, promising results with soluble IL-4 receptor (altrakincept) and anti-IL-5 Mab (mepolizumab) treatment in patients with atopic asthma have been published.[77] It can therefore be anticipated that these biologicals will also be investigated in patients with atopic dermatitis.

### 3. Anti-IgE Therapy

Humanized Mab against IgE (rhuMAb-E25) block the interaction of free IgE with mast cells and basophiles, and has in placebo-controlled studies shown a clinical effect in patients with allergic rhinitis and moderate to severe asthma.[78,79] So far, there are no published results concerning anti-IgE antibodies treatment in atopic dermatitis.

## C. Cutaneous T-Cell Lymphoma

In recent years several new therapies for cutaneous lymphomas have been described. CTCL is a condition of unregulated proliferation of T cells with Th2 characteristics. Thus, not only are new antiproliferative therapies being developed, but also immune stimulators (IFN) and Th1-stimulating biologicals such as IL-12. Although some promising results have been achieved, most of these new treatments with Mab, fusion proteins, cytokines, and IFN can still be considered as experimental. Conclusions regarding which patient will benefit most from these new therapies are unknown because of the lack of controlled clinical trials.

### 1. Anti-CD20 Therapy

Rituximab, a chimeric Mab directed against the pan B-cell antigen CD20, has a high therapeutic value in refractory/relapsed low-grade or follicular B-cell non-Hodgkin's lymphoma. Recent studies indicate that monotherapy and combination therapy with rituximab, administered intralesionally or intravenously, is effective in treatment of cutaneous B-cell lymphomas.[80–82]

### 2. Anti-CD25-Directed Therapies

The anti-CD25 Mab daclizumab binds to the α subunit of the IL-2 receptor, which is present on activated and malignant T cells only. Monotherapy in patients with CTCL was not found to be effective.[83] Further with studies with radioactive-labeled anti-CD25 Mab are ongoing.

The fusion protein denileukin difitox ($DAB_{389}$IL-2) has not only been employed in patients with psoriasis (see above) but also in a phase III study in 71 patients suffering from mycosis fungoides.[84] As the response rate was only 30%, with 10% reaching complete remission, and most patients suffering from severe adverse events (vascular leak syndrome), this treatment is only indicated when standard therapies fail, although recently complete and durable responses have been described.[85]

TABLE 41.2
**Summary of Skin Diseases Treated with Anti-TNF Agents**

| Infliximab | Etanercept |
|---|---|
| **Psoriasis (plaque-type and arthritis)*** | |
| Psoriasis pustulosa | Scleroderma |
| Pyoderma gangrenosum | Cicatricial pemphigoid |
| Graft-vs.-host disease | Common variable immunodeficiency |
| Synovitis, acne, pustulosis, hyperostosis, and osteitis (SAPHO) syndrome | Langerhans cell histiocytosis |
| Subcorneal pustular dermatosis (Sneddon–Wilkinson disease) | |
| Toxic epidermal necrolysis | |
| Hidradenitis suppurativa | |
| Cutaneous manifestations of Crohn's disease (pyostomatitis vegetans) | |
| Sarcoidosis | |
| Behçet's disease | |

* Randomized controlled studies have been published (see text).

### 3. Interferon-α

Monotherapy with IFN-α has been registered for treatment of CTCL for many years. Recent studies with high-dose IFN-α (3 to 6 × 10E6 IU/3 times per week) indicate that higher response rate (62%) can be achieved in patients suffering from plaque-stage mycosis fungoides and 43% of patients with tumor-stage mycosis fungoides.[86]

### 4. Interleukin-12

Phase I and II studies with IL-12 showed some effectivity in patients suffering from mycosis fungoides, while intralesional treatment showed complete disappearance.[87] Further studies are needed to establish the value of this treatment.

## D. Miscellaneous

### 1. Anti-TNF-Blocking Agents in Nonpsoriatic Skin Diseases

It is clear from the central role of TNF-α in inflammation that TNF-α-blocking agents should be effective in nonpsoriatic skin diseases. Indeed, many studies have recently been published showing beneficial responses in various inflammatory skin conditions.[88] A summary of inflammatory conditions treated with the fusion protein etanercept and the anti-TNF-α Mab infliximab is listed in Table 41.2. Unfortunately, no randomized controlled trials with these agents in relation to these diseases have been published.

### 2. Anti-CD20 Therapy

Targeting of pemphigus-specific $CD20^+$ memory B cells with rituximab, as demonstrated by different investigators, seems to be a promising therapy in patients with resistant pemphigus vulgaris.[89,90] It can be anticipated that treatment with anti-CD20 antibodies is not only effective in pemphigus vulgaris but also in other autoantibody-related (blistering) skin disorders.

# V. CONCLUSION

Although the value of the biologicals, as discussed in this chapter, has not yet been established, it is clear that they have elucidated the pathogenesis of several skin diseases. This is strikingly true in psoriasis where 10 years ago nobody would have suspected that TNF could be so pivotal in the pathogenesis, as treatment with TNF-blocking agents has now clearly demonstrated. In addition, development of these biologicals for common skin diseases such as psoriasis will give us sufficient experience to safely use these new drugs in other less common, but difficult-to-treat conditions such as scleroderma and hidradenitis suppurativa.

Most biologicals are now being developed for treatment of psoriasis. Since long-term experience with these drugs is lacking, physicians should be careful especially as most patients suffering from moderate to severe psoriasis have been treated previously with mutagenic modalities. In addition, some biologicals interfere with essential steps in our innate immunity as was demonstrated with infliximab and the development of opportunistic infections. Because some biologicals (anti-IL-18- and anti-IL-23-directed therapies) affect similar pathways, great caution is indicated. Although some new biologicals employed in patients with psoriasis show not only suppressive but also remittive effects (alefacept, efalizumab), this does not mean that established suppressive systemic therapies (methotrexate, cyclosporine, and retinoids) should be forgotten. Only recently the first randomized controlled trial in patients with psoriasis treated with methotrexate and cyclosporine A was published.[91] A careful evaluation of the new and costly biological therapies in relation to these standard therapies is needed before these new drugs can be used in daily practice.

## REFERENCES


1. Breedveld, F.C., Therapeutic monoclonal antibodies, *Lancet*, 355, 735, 2002.
2. Bruggemann, M. and Neuberger, M.S., Strategies for expressing human antibody repertoires in transgenic mice, *Immunol. Today*, 17, 391, 1996.
3. Isaacs, J.D., From bench to bedside: discovering rules for antibody design, and improving serotherapy with monoclonal antibodies, *Rheumatology*, 40, 724, 2001.
4. Gottlieb, S.L. et al., Response of psoriasis to a lymphocyte-selective toxin (DAB389IL-2) suggests a primary immune, but not keratinocyte, pathogenic basis, *Nat. Med.*, 1, 442, 1995.
5. Mease, P.J., Tumour necrosis factor (TNF) in psoriatic arthritis: pathophysiology and treatment with TNF inhibitors, *Ann. Rheum. Dis.*, 61, 298, 2002.
6. Seifert, M. et al., The antipsoriatic activity of IL-10 is rather caused by effects on peripheral blood cells than by a direct effect on human keratinocytes, *Arch. Dermatol. Res.*, 292, 164, 2000.
7. Krueger, J.G., The immunologic basis for the treatment of psoriasis with new biologic agents, *J. Am. Acad. Dermatol.*, 46, 1, 2002.
8. Leonardi, C.L., Efalizumab: an overview, *J. Am. Acad. Dermatol.*, 49, S98, 2003.
9. Baert, F. et al., Influence of immunogenicity on the long-term efficacy of infliximab in Crohn's disease, *N. Engl. J. Med.*, 348, 601, 2003.
10. Branco, L. et al., Selective depletion of antigen-specific activated T cells by a humanized MAB to CD2 (MEDI-507) is mediated by NK cells, *Transplantation*, 68, 1588, 1999.
11. Langley, R. et al., Phase I results of intravenous MEDI-507, an anti-T-cell-monoclonal antibody, for the treatment of psoriasis, *J. Invest. Dermatol.*, 117, 817, 2001.
12. Weinshenker, B.G. et al., Remission of psoriatic lesions with muromab-CD3 (Orthoclone OKT3) treatment, *J. Am. Acad. Dermatol.*, 6, 1132, 1989.
13. Yu, X.Z. et al., Anti-CD2 epsilon F(ab′)2 prevents graft-versus-host disease by selectively depleting T cells activated by recipient alloantigens, *J. Immunol.*, 166, 5835, 2001.
14. Chau, L.A. et al., HuM291 (Nuvion), a humanized Fc receptor-nonbinding antibody against CD3, anergizes peripheral blood T cells as partial agonist of the T cell receptor, *Transplantation*, 15, 941, 2001.
15. Carpenter, P.A. et al., A humanized non-FcR-binding anti-CD3 antibody, visilizumab, for treatment of steroid-refractory acute graft-versus-host disease, *Blood*, 99, 2712, 2002.
16. Morel, P. et al., Anti-CD4 monoclonal antibody therapy in severe psoriasis, *J. Autoimmun.*, 5, 465, 1992.
17. Bachelez, H. et al., Treatment of recalcitrant plaque psoriasis with a humanized non-depleting antibody to CD4, *J. Autoimmun.*, 11, 53, 1998.

18. Gottlieb, A.B. et al., Anti-CD4 monoclonal antibody treatment of moderate to severe psoriasis vulgaris: results of a pilot, multicentre, multiple-dose, placebo-controlled study, *J. Am. Acad. Dermatol.*, 43, 595, 2002.
19. Krueger, J.G. et al., Successful *in vivo* blockade of CD25 (high-affinity interleukin 2 receptor) on T cells by administration of humanized anti-TAC antibody to patients with psoriasis, *J. Am. Acad. Dermatol.*, 43, 448, 2002.
20. Owen, C.M. and Harrison, P.V., Successful treatment of severe psoriasis with basiliximab, an interleukin-2 receptor monoclonal antibody, *Clin. Exp. Dermatol.*, 25, 195, 2002.
21. Mrowietz, U., Zhu, K., and Christophers, E., Treatment of severe psoriasis with anti-CD25 monoclonal antibodies, *Arch. Dermatol.*, 136, 675, 2000.
22. Salim, A., Emerson, R.M., and Dalziel, K.L., Successful treatment of severe generalized pustular psoriasis with basiliximab (interleukin-2 receptor blocker), *Br. J. Dermatol.*, 143, 1121, 2000.
23. Kirby, B. and Griffiths, C.E.M., Novel immune-based therapies for psoriasis, *Br. J. Dermatol.*, 146, 546, 2002.
24. Bagel, J. et al., Administration of DAB389IL-2 to patients with recalcitrant psoriasis: a double-blind, phase II multicenter trial, *J. Am. Acad. Dermatol.*, 38, 938, 1998.
25. Martin, A. et al., A multicenter dose-escalation trial with denileukin difitox (ONTAK, $DAB_{389}$IL-2) in patients with severe psoriasis, *J. Am. Acad. Dermatol.*, 45, 871, 2001.
26. Krueger, G.G. and Callis, K.P., Development and use of alefacept to treat psoriasis, *J. Am. Acad. Dermatol.*, 49, S87, 2003.
27. Majeau, G.R. et al., Mechanism of Lymphocyte Function-Associated molecule 3-Ig fusion proteins inhibition of T cell responses, *J. Immunol.*, 152, 2753, 1994.
28. Ellis, C.N. and Krueger, G.G. for the Alefacept Clinical Study Group, Treatment of chronic plaque psoriasis by selective targeting of memory effector T lymphocytes, *N. Engl. J. Med.*, 292, 519, 2001.
29. Robbert, C. and Kupper, T.S., Inflammatory skin diseases, T cells, and immune surveillance, *N. Engl. J. Med.*, 341, 1817, 1999.
30. Da Silva, A.J. et al., Alefacept, an immunomodulatory recombinant LFA-3/IgG1 fusion protein, induces CD16 signaling and CD2/CD16-dependent apoptosis of $CD2^+$ cells, *J. Immunol.*, 168, 4462, 2002.
31. Gottlieb, A.B. et al., Impact of a 12-week course of alefacept therapy on primary and secondary responses in psoriasis patients, *J. Eur. Acad. Dermatol. Venereol.*, 15(Suppl. 2), 242, 2001.
32. Ortonne, J.P., Lebwohl, M., and Griffiths C., Alefacept-induced decreases in circulating blood lymphocyte counts correlate with clinical response in patients with chronic plaque psoriasis, *Eur. J. Dermatol.*, 13, 117, 2003.
33. Krueger, G.G. et al., A randomised, double-blind, placebo-controlled phase III study evaluating efficacy and tolerability of 2 courses of alefacept in patients with chronic plaque psoriasis, *J. Am. Acad. Dermatol.*, 47, 821, 2002.
34. Krueger, G.G. and Ellis C.N., Alefacept therapy produces remission for patients with chronic plaque psoriasis, *Br. J. Dermatol.*, 148, 784, 2003.
35. Lowe, N.J. et al., Repeat courses of intravenous alefacept in patients with chronic plaque psoriasis provide consistent safety and efficacy, *Int. J. Dermatol.*, 42, 224, 2003.
36. Kraan, M.C. et al., Alefacept treatment in psoriatic arthritis, *Arthritis Rheum.*, 46, 2776, 2002.
37. Abrams, J.R. et al., CTLA4Ig-mediated blockade of T-cell costimulation in patients with psoriasis vulgaris, *J. Clin. Invest.*, 103, 1243, 1999.
38. Abrams, J.R. et al., Blockade of T lymphocyte costimulation with cytotoxic T lymphocyte-associated antigen 4-immunoglobulin (CTLA4Ig) reverses the cellular pathology of psoriatic plaques, including the activation of keratinocytes, dendritic cells, and endothelial cells, *J. Exp. Med.*, 192, 681, 2000.
39. Mitra, R.S. et al., Psoriatic skin-derived dendritic cell function is inhibited by exogenous IL-10: differential modulation of B7-1 (CD80) and B7-2 (CD86) expression, *J. Immunol.*, 154, 2668, 1995.
40. Gottlieb, A.B. et al., Results of a single-dose, dose-escalating trial of an anti-B7 monoclonal antibody (IDEC-114) in patients with psoriasis, *J. Invest. Dermatol.*, 114, 840, 2000.
41. Gottlieb, A.B. et al., Results of a multiple-dose, multiple schedule trial of anti-CD80 monoclonal antibody (IDEC-114) in patients with psoriasis, poster presented at the annual meeting of the American Academy of Dermatology, Washington, D.C., March 2, 2001.

42. Gottlieb, A.B. et al., Clinical and histologic response to single-dose treatment of moderate to severe psoriasis with an anti-CD80 monoclonal antibody, *J. Am. Acad. Dermatol.*, 47, 692, 2002.
43. Gottlieb, A.B. et al., Effects of administration of a single dose of a humanized monoclonal antibody to CD11a on the immunobiology and clinical activity of psoriasis, *J. Am. Acad. Dermatol.*, 42, 428, 2000.
44. Papp, K. et al., The treatment of moderate to severe psoriasis with a new anti-CD11a monoclonal antibody, *J. Am. Acad. Dermatol.*, 45, 665, 2000.
45. Gottlieb, A.B. et al., Psoriasis as a model for T-cell-mediated disease: immunobiologic and clinical effects of treatment with multiple doses of efalizumab, an anti-CD11a antibody, *Arch. Dermatol.*, 138, 591, 2002.
46. Leonardi, C.L. et al., Efalizumab (anti-CD11a): results of a 12 week trial of subcutaneous administration in patients with moderate to severe plaque psoriasis, poster presented at the annual meeting of the American Academy of Dermatology, Washington, D.C., March 2, 2001.
47. Gottlieb, A.B. et al., Clinical and histologic effects of subcutaneously administered anti-CD11a (hu1124) in patients with psoriasis, *J. Invest. Dermatol.*, 114, 840, 2000.
48. Gottlieb, A.B. et al., Subcutaneously administered efalizumab (Anti-CD11a) improves signs and symptoms of moderate to severe plaque psoriasis, *J. Cutaneous Med. Surg.*, April 30, 2003.
49. Bhushan, M. et al., Anti-E-selectin is ineffective in the treatment of psoriasis: a randomised trial, *Br. J. Dermatol.*, 146, 824, 2002.
50. Ghoreschi, K. et al., Interleukin-4 induced immune deviation as therapy for psoriasis, *J. Invest. Dermatol.*, 117, 465, 2001.
51. Ghoreschi, K. et al., Interleukin-4 therapy of psoriasis induces Th2 responses and improves human autoimmune disease, *Nat. Med.*, 9, 40, 2003.
52. Asadullah, K. et al., IL-10 is a key cytokine in psoriasis: proof of principle by IL-10 therapy: a new therapeutic approach, *J. Clin. Invest.*, 101, 783, 1998.
53. Reich, K. et al., Treatment of psoriasis with interleukin-10, *J. Invest. Dermatol.*, 111, 1235, 1998.
54. Asadullah, K. et al., Interleukin 10 treatment of psoriasis: clinical results in a phase II trial, *Arch. Dermatol.*, 135, 187, 1999.
55. Asadullah, K. et al., Clinical and immunological effects of IL-10 therapy in psoriasis, *Br. J. Dermatol.*, 141, 989, 1999.
56. Kimball, A.B. et al., Clinical and immunological assessment of patients with psoriasis in a randomised, double-blind, placebo-controlled trial using recombinant human interleukin 10, *Arch. Dermatol.*, 138, 1341, 2002.
57. Vial, T. and Descotes, J., Immune-mediated side effects of cytokines in humans, *Toxicology*, 105, 31, 1995.
58. Trepicchio, W.L. et al., Interleukin-11 therapy selectively downregulates type I cytokine proinflammatory pathways in psoriasis lesions, *J. Clin. Invest.*, 104, 1527, 1999.
59. Lohner, M.E. et al., Clinical trials of a fully human anti-IL-8 antibody for the treatment of psoriasis, *Br. J. Dermatol.*, 141, 989, 1999.
60. Krueger, G.C. et al., Clinical trial results: a fully human anti-IL-8 antibody in patients with moderate to severe psoriasis, poster presented at the annual meeting of the American Academy of Dermatology, Washington, D.C., March 2, 2001.
61. Gottlieb, A.B., Infliximab for psoriasis, *J. Am. Acad. Dermatol.*, 49, S112, 2003.
62. Ettehadi, P. et al., Elevated tumour necrosis factor-alpha (TNF-alpha) biological activity in psoriatic skin lesions, *Clin. Exp. Immunol.*, 96, 146, 1994.
63. Oh, C.J., Das, K.M., and Gottlieb, A.B., Treatment with anti-tumor necrosis factor alpha (TNF-alpha) monoclonal antibody dramatically decreases the clinical activity of psoriasis lesions, *J. Am. Acad. Dermatol.*, 42, 829, 2000.
64. Chaudhari, U. et al., Efficacy and safety of infliximab monotherapy for plaque-type psoriasis: a randomised trial, *Lancet*, 357, 1842, 2001.
65. Schopf, R.E., Aust, H., and Knop, J., Treatment of psoriasis with the chimeric monoclonal antibody against tumor necrosis factor $\alpha$, infliximab, *J. Am. Acad. Dermatol.*, 46, 886, 2002.
66. Gottlieb, A.B. et al., Infliximab monotherapy provides rapid and sustained benefit for plaque-type psoriasis, *J. Am. Acad. Dermatol.*, 48, 829, 2003.

67. Ogilvie, A.L. et al., Treatment of psoriatic arthritis with antitumour necrosis factor-alpha antibody clears skin lesions of psoriasis resistant to treatment with methotrexate, *Br. J. Dermatol.*, 144, 587, 2001.
68. Goffe, B. and Cather, J.C., Etanercept: an overview, *J. Am. Acad. Dermatol.*, 49, S105, 2003.
69. Scallon, B.J. et al., New comparisons of two types of TNFα antagonists approved for rheumatoid arthritis, *Arthritis Rheum.*, 43, S226, 2000.
70. Mease, P.J. et al., Etanercept in the treatment of psoriatic arthritis and psoriasis: a randomised trial, *Lancet*, 356, 385, 2000.
71. Mease, P.J. et al., Improvement in disease activity in patients with psoriatic arthritis receiving etanercept (Enbrel): results of a phase 3 multicenter clinical trial, *Arthritis Rheum.*, 44, S90, 2001.
72. Keane, J. et al., Tuberculosis associated with infliximab, a tumor necrosis factor alpha-neutralizing agent, *N. Engl. J. Med.*, 345, 1098, 2001.
73. Shakoor, N. et al., Drug-induced systemic lupus erythematosus associated with etanercept therapy, *Lancet*, 359, 579, 2002.
74. Smith, K.J. and Skelton, H.G., Rapid onset of cutaneous squamous cell carcinoma in patients with rheumatoid arthritis after starting tumor necrosis factor alpha receptor IgG1-Fc fusion complex therapy, *J. Am. Acad. Dermatol.*, 45, 953, 2001.
75. Hanifin, J.M. et al., Recombinant interferon gamma therapy for atopic dermatitis, *J. Am. Acad. Dermatol.*, 28, 189, 1993.
76. Jang, I.G. et al., Clinical improvement and immunohistochemical findings in severe atopic dermatitis treated with interferon gamma, *J. Am. Acad. Dermatol.*, 42, 1033, 2003.
77. Borish, L.C. et al., Efficacy of soluble IL-4 receptor for the treatment of adults with asthma, *J. Allergy Clin. Immunol.*, 107, 963, 2001.
78. Casale, T.B. et al., Use of an anti-IgE humanized monoclonal antibody in ragweed-induced allergic rhinitis, *J. Allergy Clin. Immunol.*, 100, 110, 1997.
79. Milgrom, H. et al., Treatment of allergic asthma with monoclonal anti-IgE antibody. Rhum-ab-E25 study group, *N. Engl. J. Med.*, 341, 1966, 1999.
80. Heinzerling, L.M. et al., Reduction of tumor burden and stabilization of disease by systemic therapy with anti-CD20 antibody (rituximab) in patients with primary cutaneous B-cell lymphoma, *Cancer*, 89, 1835, 2000.
81. Paul, T. et al., Intralesional rituximab for cutaneous B-cell lymphoma, *Br. J. Dermatol.*, 144, 1239, 2001.
82. Fierro, M.T. et al., Systemic therapy with cyclophosphamide and anti-CD20 antibody (rituximab) in relapsed primary cutaneous B-cell lymphoma: a report of 7 cases, *J. Am. Acad. Dermatol.*, 49, 281, 2003.
83. Waldmann, T.A., T-cell receptors for cytokines: targets for immunotherapy of leukemia/lymphoma, *Ann. Oncol.*, 11, 101, 2000.
84. Olsen, E. et al., Pivotal phase III trial of two dose levels of denileukin diftitox for the treatment of cutaneous T-cell lymphoma, *J. Clin. Oncol.*, 19, 376, 2001.
85. Carretero-Margolis, C.D. and Fivenson, D.P., A complete and durable response to denileukin difitox in a patient with mycosis fungoides, *J. Am. Acad. Dermatol.*, 48, 275, 2003.
86. Jumbou, O. et al., Long-term follow-up in 51 patients with mycosis fungoides and Sézary's syndrome treated with interferon-alfa, *Br. J. Dermatol.*, 140, 427, 1999.
87. Rook, A.H. et al., Interleukin-12 therapy in cutaneous T-cell lymphoma induces lesion regression and cytotoxic T-cell responses, *Blood*, 94, 902, 1999.
88. Williams, J.D.L. and Griffiths, C.E.M., Cytokine blocking agents in dermatology, *Clin. Dermatol.*, 27, 585, 2002.
89. Cooper, H.L. et al., Treatment of resistant pemphigus vulgaris with an anti-CD20 monoclonal antibody (rituximab), *Clin. Exp. Dermatol.*, 28, 366, 2003.
90. Herrmann, G., Engert, A., and Hunzelmann, N., Treatment of pemphigus vulgaris with anti-CD20 monoclonal antibody (rituximab), *Br. J. Dermatol.*, 148, 602, 2003.
91. Heydendael, V.M.R. et al., Methotrexate versus cyclosporine in moderate-to-severe chronic plaque psoriasis, *N. Engl. J. Med.*, 349, 658, 2003.

# Index

## NUMBERS



## A

## B

## C

## D



## E

## F

## G



## H

## I

## J



## K

## L

## M

## N



## O

## P

## R

## S

## T

## U

## V



## W



## X



## Z